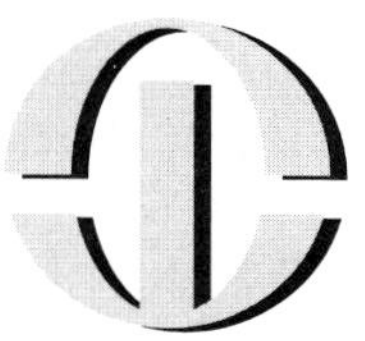

RUSH University

Review of SURGERY

Daniel J. Deziel, M.D.
Professor of Surgery, Rush Medical College of Rush University;
Senior Attending Surgeon, Department of General Surgery
Rush-Presbyterian-St. Luke's Medical Center, Chicago, Illinois

Thomas R. Witt, M.D.
Associate Professor of Surgery, Rush Medical College of Rush University;
Associate Attending Surgeon, Department of General Surgery
Rush-Presbyterian-St. Luke's Medical Center, Chicago, Illinois

Steven D. Bines, M.D.
Associate Professor of Surgery, Rush Medical College of Rush University;
Associate Attending Surgeon, Department of General Surgery
Rush-Presbyterian-St. Luke's Medical Center, Chicago, Illinois

Theodore J. Saclarides, M.D.
Professor of Surgery, Rush Medical College of Rush University;
Head, Section of Colon & Rectal Surgery;
Senior Attending Surgeon, Department of General Surgery
Rush-Presbyterian-St. Luke's Medical Center, Chicago, Illinois

Edgar D. Staren, M.D., Ph.D.
Professor of Surgery, Chairman, Department of Surgery; Medical Director
Medical College of Ohio, Toledo, Ohio

José M. Velasco, M.D.
Professor of Surgery, Rush Medical College of Rush University;
Senior Attending Surgeon, Department of General Surgery
Rush-Presbyterian-St. Luke's Medical Center, Chicago, Illinois;
Chairman, Department of Surgery
Rush North Shore Medical Center, Skokie, Illinois

Keith W. Millikan, M.D.
Associate Professor of Surgery, Rush Medical College of Rush University;
Associate Attending Surgeon and Director, Undergraduate Surgical Education
Department of General Surgery
Rush-Presbyterian-St. Luke's Medical Center, Chicago, Illinois

Richard A. Prinz, M.D.
Helen Shedd Keith Professor, Rush Medical College of Rush University;
Chairman, Department of General Surgery
Rush-Presbyterian-St. Luke's Medical Center, Chicago, Illinois

Steven G. Economou, M.D.
Professor of Surgery, Rush Medical College of Rush University;
Chairman Emeritus, Department of General Surgery
Rush-Presbyterian-St. Luke's Medical Center, Chicago, Illinois

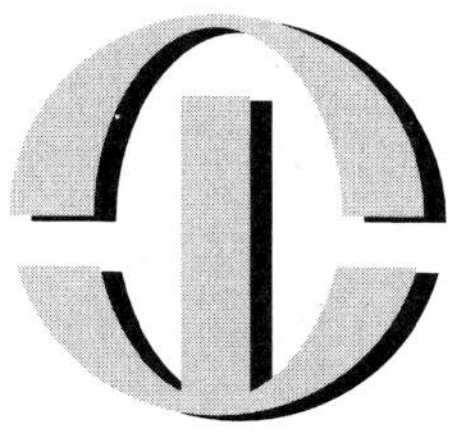

RUSH University

Review of SURGERY

Third Edition

W.B. SAUNDERS COMPANY
An Imprint of Elsevier Science
Philadelphia London New York St. Louis Sydney Toronto

W.B. SAUNDERS COMPANY
An Imprint of Elsevier Science

The Curtis Center
Independence Square West
Philadelphia, Pennsylvania 19106

Library of Congress Cataloging-in-Publication Data

Rush University review of surgery / Daniel J. Deziel — [et al.]. — 3rd ed.
p. cm.
Includes bibliographical references.
ISBN 0-7216-7581-6
1. Surgery Examinations, questions, etc. I. Deziel, Daniel J. II. Rush University. III. Title: Review of surgery.
[DNLM: 1. Surgery Examination Questions. WO 18.2 R953 2000]
RD31.R85 2000
617′.0076—dc21
DNLM/DLC 99-23140

RUSH UNIVERSITY REVIEW OF SURGERY, THIRD EDITION ISBN 0–7216–7581–6

Printed in the United States of America.

Last digit is the print number: 9 8 7 6 5

All of us are keenly aware of the many persons in our lives—parents, wives and children, teachers and mentors, residents and students, and surely others—who, at different times and in varying ways, have so critically molded our lives and influenced our careers. We are honored to dedicate this book to them.

Contributing Editors

Joseph J. Amato, M.D.
Professor of Cardiovascular/Thoracic Surgery, Rush Medical College of Rush University; Senior Attending Surgeon and Head, Section of Pediatric Cardiovascular Surgery, Rush-Presbyterian-St. Luke's Medical Center, Chicago, Illinois

Katherine F. Baker, M.D.
Assistant Professor of Radiation Oncology, Rush Medical College of Rush University; Assistant Attending Radiation Oncologist, Department of Radiation Oncology, Rush-Presbyterian-St. Luke's Medical Center, Chicago, Illinois

Kathryn D. Bass, M.D.
Assistant Professor of Pediatric Surgery and Pediatrics, Rush Medical College of Rush University; Assistant Attending Surgeon and Head, Section of Pediatric Surgery, Department of General Surgery, Rush-Presbyterian-St. Luke's Medical Center, Chicago, Illinois

Sami Bittar, M.D.
Associate Professor of Plastic and Reconstructive Surgery, Rush Medical College of Rush University; Associate Attending Surgeon, Department of Plastic & Reconstructive Surgery, Rush-Presbyterian-St. Luke's Medical Center, Chicago, Illinois

Gregory Bormes, M.D.
Fellow in Plastic and Reconstructive Surgery, Department of Plastic & Reconstructive Surgery, Rush-Presbyterian-St. Luke's Medical Center, Chicago, Illinois

Marc I. Brand, M.D.
Assistant Professor of Surgery, Rush Medical College of Rush University; Assistant Attending Surgeon, Department of General Surgery, Section of Colon and Rectal Surgery, Rush-Presbyterian-St. Luke's Medical Center, Chicago, Illinois

Donald P. Braun, Ph.D.
Administrative Director of the Cancer Center, Professor, Department of Surgery, Medical College of Ohio, Toledo, Ohio

Charles A. Bush-Joseph, M.D.
Associate Professor of Orthopaedic Surgery, Rush Medical College of Rush University; Associate Attending, Department of Orthopaedic Surgery, Rush-Presbyterian-St. Luke's Medical Center, Chicago, Illinois

Richard W. Byrne, M.D.
Assistant Professor of Neurosurgery, Rush Medical College of Rush University; Assistant Attending, Department of Neurosurgery, Rush-Presbyterian-St. Luke's Medical Center and Cook County Hospital, Chicago, Illinois

Chester Cheng, M.D.
Fellow in Plastic and Reconstructive Surgery, Department of Plastic and Reconstructive Surgery, Rush-Presbyterian-St. Luke's Medical Center, Chicago, Illinois

Melody A. Cobleigh, M.D.
Associate Professor of Medicine, Rush Medical College of Rush University; Director, Comprehensive Breast Center, Rush Cancer Institute, Rush-Presbyterian-St. Luke's Medical Center, Chicago, Illinois

James A. Colombo, M.D.
Assistant Professor of Anesthesiology, Rush Medical College of Rush University; Assistant Attending, Department of Anesthesiology and Director, Division of Critical Care, Rush-Presbyterian-St. Luke's Medical Center, Chicago, Illinois

Christopher L. Coogan, M.D.
Assistant Professor of Urology, Rush Medical College of Rush University; Assistant Attending Surgeon, Department of Urology, Rush-Presbyterian-St. Luke's Medical Center, Chicago, Illinois

Shawn M. Davies, M.D.
Instructor of Obstetrics and Gynecology, Rush Medical College of Rush University; Adjunct Attending, Department of Obstetrics and Gynecology, Rush-Presbyterian-St. Luke's Medical Center, Chicago, Illinois

Gordon H. Derman, M.D.
Assistant Professor of Plastic and Reconstructive Surgery, Rush Medical College of Rush University; Assistant Attending, Department of Plastic and Reconstructive Surgery, Rush-Presbyterian-St. Luke's Medical Center, Chicago, Illinois

Utpal Desai, M.D.
Instructor of Cardiovascular/Thoracic Surgery, Rush Medical College of Rush University; Fellow in Cardiovascular and Thoracic Surgery, Rush-Presbyterian-St. Luke's Medical Center, Chicago, Illinois

Philip Donahue, M.D.
Lecturer, Rush Medical College of Rush University; Professor of Surgery, University of Illinois at Chicago; Chairman, Division of General Surgery, Cook County Hospital; Senior Attending Surgeon, Department of General Surgery, Rush-Presbyterian-St. Luke's Medical Center, Chicago, Illinois

Alexander Doolas, M.D.
Steven G. Economou, M.D. Professor of Surgery, Rush Medical College of Rush University; Senior Attending Surgeon and Associate Chairman, Department of General Surgery, Rush-Presbyterian-St. Luke's Medical Center, Chicago, Illinois

William I. Douglas, M.D.
Assistant Professor of Cardiovascular/Thoracic Surgery, Rush Medical College of Rush University; Assistant Attending Surgeon, Department of Cardiovascular/Thoracic Surgery; Section of Pediatric Cardiovascular Surgery, Rush-Presbyterian-St. Luke's Medical Center, Chicago, Illinois

Kambiz Dowlat, M.D.
Associate Professor of Surgery, Rush Medical College of Rush University; Associate Attending Surgeon, Department of General Surgery, Rush-Presbyterian-St. Luke's Medical Center, Chicago, Illinois

S. Reneé Edwards, M.D.
Assistant Professor of Gynecology, Rush Medical College of Rush University; Assistant Attending Surgeon, Department of Obstetrics and Gynecology; Head, Section of Urogynecology and Reconstructive Pelvic Surgery, Rush-Presbyterian-St. Luke's Medical Center, Chicago, Illinois

L. Penfield Faber, M.D.
Professor of Cardiovascular/Thoracic Surgery, Rush Medical College of Rush University; Senior Attending Surgeon, Department of Cardiovascular Thoracic Surgery; Director, Section of General Thoracic Surgery, Rush-Presbyterian-St. Luke's Medical Center, Chicago, Illinois

Scott Fisher, M.D.
Chief Resident, Department of General Surgery, Rush-Presbyterian-St. Luke's Medical Center, Chicago, Illinois

Darius S. Francescatti, M.D.
Assistant Professor of Surgery, Rush Medical College of Rush University; Assistant Attending Surgeon, Department of General Surgery, Rush-Presbyterian-St. Luke's Medical Center, Chicago, Illinois

Maija G. Freimanis, M.D.
Associate Professor of Radiology, Rush Medical College of Rush University; Associate Attending Radiologist and Director, Section of Ultrasound, Department of Diagnostic Radiology, Rush-Presbyterian-St. Luke's Medical Center, Chicago, Illinois

Michael Friedman, M.D.
Professor of Otolaryngology and Bronchoesophagology, Rush Medical College of Rush University; Attending Surgeon, Department of Otolaryngology and Bronchoesophagology; Chairman, Section of Head and Neck Surgery, Rush-Presbyterian-St. Luke's Medical Center, Chicago, Illinois

Constantine V. Godellas, M.D.
Assistant Professor of Surgery, Rush Medical College of Rush University; Assistant Attending Surgeon, Department of General Surgery, Rush-Presbyterian-St. Luke's Medical Center; Attending Surgeon, Cook County Hospital, Chicago, Illinois

Stephen P. Haggerty, M.D.
Chief Resident, Department of General Surgery, Rush-Presbyterian-St. Luke's Medical Center, Chicago, Illinois

Marella L. Hanumadass, M.D.
Assistant Professor of Surgery, University of Illinois College of Medicine; Chairman, Division of Burn Surgery; Director, Sumner L. Koch Burn Center, Cook County Hospital, Chicago, Illinois

Tina J. Hieken, M.D.
Assistant Professor of Surgery, Rush Medical College of Rush University; Assistant Attending Surgeon, Department of General Surgery, Rush-Presbyterian-St. Luke's Medical Center, Chicago, Illinois; Attending Surgeon, Rush North Shore Medical Center, Skokie, Illinois

Timothy James, M.D.
Fellow in Cardiovascular/Thoracic Surgery, Department of Cardiovascular/Thoracic Surgery, Rush-Presbyterian-St. Luke's Medical Center, Chicago, Illinois

Richard R. Keen, M.D.
Assistant Professor of Surgery, Rush Medical College of Rush University; Assistant Attending Surgeon, Department of Cardiovascular Thoracic Surgery, Rush-Presbyterian-St. Luke's Medical Center, Chicago, Illinois; Senior Attending Surgeon, Division of Vascular Surgery, Cook County Hospital, Chicago, Illinois

Barbara D. Loris, M.D.
Instructor, Rush Medical College of Rush University; Adjunct Attending Surgeon, Department of General Surgery, Rush-Presbyterian-St. Luke's Medical Center, Chicago, Illinois

James A. Madura II, M.D.
Assistant Professor of Surgery, Rush Medical College of Rush University; Assistant Attending Surgeon, Department of General Surgery, Rush-Presbyterian-St. Luke's Medical Center; Attending Surgeon, Cook County Hospital, Chicago, Illinois

Ahmed Mahmoud, M.D.
Instructor in Cardiovascular/Thoracic Surgery, Rush Medical College of Rush University; Adjunct Attending Surgeon, Department of Cardiovascular/Thoracic Surgery, Rush-Presbyterian-St. Luke's Medical Center, Chicago, Illinois

Robert J. March, M.D.
Assistant Professor of Cardiovascular/Thoracic Surgery, Rush Medical College of Rush University; Assistant Attending Surgeon in the Department of Cardiovascular/Thoracic Surgery; Director of Cardiovascular Research, Rush-Presbyterian-St. Luke's Medical Center, Chicago, Illinois

Walter A. McCarthy, III, M.D.
Associate Professor of Cardiovascular/Thoracic Surgery, Rush Medical College of Rush University; Chief, Section of Vascular Surgery, Department of Cardiovascular/Thoracic Surgery, Rush-Presbyterian St. Luke's Medical Center; Chairman, Division of Vascular Surgery, Department of Surgery, Cook County Hospital, Chicago, Illinois

Lawrence P. McChesney, M.D.
Associate Professor, Chief, Division of Transplantation Surgery, Department of Surgery, Medical College of Ohio, Toledo, Ohio

Bruce McLeod, M.D.
Professor of Medicine and Pathology, Rush Medical College of Rush University; Director of Blood Bank, Rush-Presbyterian-St. Luke's Medical Center, Chicago, Illinois

Janet Deselich Millikan, M.S., R.D., L.D.
Formerly, Nutrition Support Team, Department of Food and Nutrition Services, Rush-Presbyterian-St. Luke's Medical Center, Chicago, Illinois

Deepak Mital, M.B.B.S., M.S., F.R.C.S. (Edin.)
Assistant Professor of Surgery, Rush Medical College of Rush University; Adjunct Attending Surgeon, Department of General Surgery, Section of Transplantation Surgery, Rush-Presbyterian-St. Luke's Medical Center, Chicago, Illinois; Director, Transplant Fellowship Program; Attending Surgeon, Department of General Surgery, Division of Vascular Surgery, Cook County Hospital, Chicago, Illinois

Douglas Norman, M.D.
Assistant Professor of Cardiovascular/Thoracic Surgery, Rush Medical College of Rush University, Chicago, Illinois; Attending Surgeon, Section of Cardiovascular/Thoracic Surgery, Department of Surgery, Rush North Shore Medical Center, Skokie, Illinois

William Piccione Jr., M.D.
Associate Professor of Cardiovascular/Thoracic Surgery, Rush Medical College of Rush University; Associate Attending Surgeon, Department of Cardiovascular/Thoracic Surgery, Rush-Presbyterian-St. Luke's Medical Center, Chicago, Illinois

David B. Rubin, M.D.
Associate Professor of Medicine and Radiation Oncology, Rush Medical College of Rush University; Associate Attending Physician, Department of Internal Medicine, Section of Pulmonary and Critical Care; Assistant Attending, Radiation Oncology, Department of Radiation Oncology, Section of Radiation Biology, Rush-Presbyterian-St. Luke's Medical Center, Chicago, Illinois

Michael S. Sabel, M.D.
Junior Faculty Associate, Division of Surgical Oncology, Roswell Park Cancer Institute, Buffalo, New York

Howard N. Sankary, M.D.
Associate Professor of Surgery, Rush Medical College of Rush University; Associate Attending Surgeon, Department of General Surgery, Section of Transplantation, Rush-Presbyterian-St. Luke's Medical Center, Chicago, Illinois

Jonathan C. Silverstein, M.D., M.S.
Assistant Professor of Surgery, Division of General Surgery, University of Illinois at Chicago; Assistant Professor of Information Sciences, School of Biomedical and Health Information Sciences, University of Illinois at Chicago, Chicago, Illinois

Jonathan Somers, M.D.
Assistant Professor of Cardiovascular/Thoracic Surgery, Rush Medical College of Rush University; Attending Surgeon, Department of Cardiovascular/Thoracic Surgery, Rush-Presbyterian-St. Luke's Medical Center, Chicago, Illinois; Director of Cardiovascular and Thoracic Surgery, Rush North Shore Medical Center, Skokie, Illinois

Anil K. Srivastava, M.D.
Senior Burn Fellow, Burn Surgery, Sumner L. Koch Burn Center, Cook County Hospital, Chicago, Illinois

Nelson H. Stringer, Jr., M.D.
Assistant Professor of Surgery, Rush Medical College of Rush University; Assistant Attending Surgeon, Department of Obstetrics and Gynecology, Rush-Presbyterian-St. Luke's Medical Center, Chicago, Illinois

Michael Sullivan, M.D.
Instructor in Vascular Surgery, Rush Medical College of Rush University; Adjunct Attending Surgeon, Department of Cardiovascular/Thoracic Surgery, Rush-Presbyterian-St. Luke's Medical Center, Chicago, Illinois

Kenneth J. Tuman, M.D.
The Max S. Sadove M.D. Professor of Anesthesiology, Rush Medical College of Rush University; Vice-Chairman, Department of Anesthesiology, Rush-Presbyterian-St. Luke's Medical Center, Chicago, Illinois

Leonard Valentino, M.D.
Associate Professor of Medicine, Pediatrics, and Immunology/Microbiology, Rush Medical College of Rush University; Associate Attending in Medicine, Pediatrics and Immunology/Microbiology, Rush-Presbyterian-St. Luke's Medical Center, Chicago, Illinois

T. K. Venkatesan, M.D.
Fellow, Department of Otolaryngology and Bronchoesophagology, Rush-Presbyterian-St. Luke's Medical Center, Chicago, Illinois

James W. Williams, M.D.
Professor of Surgery, Rush Medical College of Rush University; Senior Attending Surgeon, Department of General Surgery, Section of Transplantation, Rush-Presbyterian-St. Luke's Medical Center, Chicago, Illinois

Edward S. Yastrow, M.D.
Associate Professor of Anesthesiology, Rush Medical College of Rush University; Attending Anesthesiologist, Department of Anesthesiology, Rush North Shore Medical Center, Skokie, Illinois

Preface

The first two editions of *Rush Review of Surgery* were favorably received. They provided their targeted audiences—residents in training, young surgeons preparing for General Surgery Boards, those already certified or preparing for recertification, and those simply wishing to remain abreast of current surgical knowledge—an encompassing yet concise and self-contained review of surgery and its subspecialties in a format that stimulates self-examination. At the same time they encouraged further reading of more comprehensive texts and current periodical literature.

Since publication of the Second Edition, surgical information has increased appreciably, and new subjects about which surgeons should be knowledgeable have expanded dramatically. This has led to heightened expectations for the Third Edition, to which we have responded appropriately. The entire book was examined minutely to ensure that it continues to contain the fullest information in the field of general surgery. With respect to the subspecialties, we have focused on fundamental information that a general surgeon might wish to know or be required to know by accreditation boards. Thus this edition can serve residents in general surgery and in most of the subspecialties. Subspecialty residents reading the *Rush Review* before sitting for their board examination can expect an exposition of subjects in general surgery that should satisfy most of their needs. In similar fashion, a general surgeon can feel confident of a rich storehouse of information on general surgery and exposure to the fundamentals of the surgical subspecialties.

This comprehensive offering was developed by extensively rewriting many chapters and bringing the remaining ones to a current state. We believe that these numerous additions and revisions were necessary, not only because of the dictates of newer and more precise information but also because of the practical expectation that those who already have access to the first and second editions can combine them with the third edition for an even fuller compendium of ready surgical information.

In addition, an important decision with this edition was to achieve an even greater emphasis on basic science. This is in keeping with the increased sophistication of care of patients and with the need for surgeons to be well versed in the fundamental scientific components of clinical practice. From the practical standpoint, it is logical to expect that accrediting bodies will rightfully have higher expectations in this respect as well.

Finally, whereas in the previous edition we relied mostly on several popular surgical textbooks, in this edition we set no restrictions on the reference base of suggested reading. Just as the wealth of surgical knowledge of which one must be aware came to us from many and varied sources and because the keen minds of our readers no doubt expect the most current views—even competing ones—it was prudent for us to include any information we believed valuable and pertinent and from whatever source.

As a consequence of these changes, we expect that the Third Edition will enable the reader to gain a breadth of knowledge in general surgery and closely associated subspecialty subjects in a manner that can be readily translated to clinical use as well as provide a deeper understanding of the fundamentals of surgical diseases and practices.

The Editors

Acknowledgments

The Third Edition of *Rush Review of Surgery* was written in a whirlwind of separate and then converging activity by the editors, augmented by a sizeable supportive team of talented contributors. An integral part of all this was a huge flow of manuscripts, revised drafts and new writing, resulting in penultimate copies that were then refined and assembled into the final chapters. This daunting project was made logistically possible and infinitely easier for us by the unmatched skill and dedication of our secretaries, Linda Wahrer, Jan Nunnally, Kathy Martin, Eileen Pehanich, Joan Cummings, Delores Miller, Eulonda Lacey and Cindy Adams. We express our sincere gratitude to them for this marvelous effort. We wish to also thank Berta Steiner for her significant editorial contributions.

Finally, we are especially indebted to our editor, Lisette Bralow, whose steady and unerring guidance was critical to the completion of this edition of *Rush Review of Surgery*.

How To Use This Text

A reader's approach to any book may vary from rapid scanning for basic concepts to meticulous outlining, note-taking, and underlining for detail. In an effort to satisfy these needs, this book includes an appropriate mixture of detail (found primarily in the Questions) and conceptual information (found primarily in the Comments).

The questions are organized principally in an organ-system manner. None of the questions is intentionally "tricky"; many, however, require the careful attention to detail that should characterize all students of surgery. To allow readers the opportunity to answer the question on their own and yet enable them to check their response without the ponderous flipping back and forth of pages, the correct answer is spatially separated from the question by the interposed Comment. For readers who wish to go to the basic source material before answering the question, such material is referenced immediately after the question. Although a number of popular textbooks serve as sources for further reading, many additional references (e.g., more specialized monographs and review articles) are cited in this Third Edition as supplemental sources of information. All of the sources used in a given chapter are listed at the end of the chapter and are referred to by number, as appropriate, after each question. Because sufficient factual information is provided in the Comments section to answer each question, the referenced materials do not include specific page numbers but are offered as sources of general reading on the topic at hand, so overall conceptual knowledge can be enhanced.

The Comments are offered to provide amplification and elucidation of the facts brought out in the Question and to provide a conceptual framework within which to view the factual data. Of necessity, several Comments have the latitude of editorial license and reflect individual and pooled clinical experiences that amplify the cited references. As there are many areas of controversy in surgery, the reader may disagree with some of the more judgmental statements made in the Comments. We trust, however, that our editorial and consultant review of the Comments has successfully resulted in the avoidance of factual errors.

We hope that readers will find this book an enjoyable means by which not only to test their knowledge of the art and science of surgery but to expand it as well.

NOTICE

Medicine is an ever-changing field. Standard safety precautions must be followed, but as new research and clinical experience broaden our knowledge, changes in treatment and drug therapy become necessary or appropriate. Readers are advised to check the product information currently provided by the manufacturer of each drug to be administered to verify the recommended dose, the method and duration of administration, and contraindications. It is the responsibility of the treating physician relying on experience and knowledge of the patient to determine dosages and the best treatment for the patient. Neither the Publisher nor the editors assume any responsibility for any injury and/or damage to persons or property.

THE PUBLISHER

Contents

CHAPTER 1

Cell Biology

1. Match the cellular structures named below with the appropriate structure labeled on the figure.

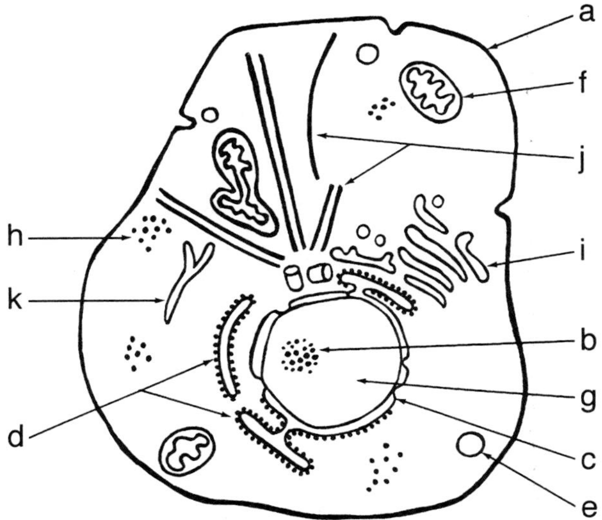

A. Nuclear envelope.
B. Lysosome.
C. Mitochondria.
D. Nucleus.
E. Golgi complex.
F. Smooth endoplasmic reticulum.
G. Ribosome.
H. Nucleolus.
I. Plasma membrane.
J. Rough endoplasmic reticulum.
K. Cytoskeleton: microtubules and filaments.

Ref.: 1, 2, 3, 4

2. Match the descriptions of cellular structures with the appropriate structure labeled on the figure in Question 1.

Description

A. Lipid bilayer that surrounds cell.
B. May have attached ribosomes; involved in protein synthesis.
C. Membrane-bound collection of catabolic enzymes.
D. Involved in transport and assembly of glycoproteins and lysosomal synthesis.
E. Synthesizes ATP, which is a major cellular storage form of energy.
F. Involved in energy-generating reactions, including oxidation of fatty acids and oxidative phosphorylation.
G. Double membrane sheath whose pores regulate passage of materials to and from the nucleus.
H. Depot of RNA and protein that will be assembled into preribosomal subunits.

Ref.: 1, 2, 3, 4

COMMENTS: The **plasma membrane** is made up of a **lipid bilayer** (a) in which proteins are floating. The lipid bilayer surrounds the cell and comprises approximately 20% of the cell's weight. The **nucleus** (g) of the cell is composed of a surrounding double-membrane **nuclear envelope** (c) (which approximates at points called pores and regulates the passage of materials in and out of the nucleus), a **nucleolus** (b) (which is divided into a fibrillar and granular zone and acts as a depot of RNA and protein that is being assembled into preribosomal subunits), chromatin, and a structural network known as the matrix. **Lysosomes** (e) are membrane-bound intracellular organelles that contain two or more acid hydrolases and are engaged in the catabolism of intra- and extracellular substrates. **Mitochondria** (f), intracellular organelles bounded by two membranes, are involved in storage of energy as ATP by oxidative phosphorylation. The **Golgi complex** (i) is a system of membranes that work in cooperation with the endoplasmic reticulum for transport and assembly of glycoproteins. The Golgi complex is also involved in the synthesis of lysosomes. The **endoplasmic reticulum** is found in a *smooth* form (k) (without attached ribosomes) and a *rough* form (d) (with attached ribosomes). Rough endoplasmic reticulum is the site for synthesis of membrane-associated proteins or secreted proteins, whereas smooth endoplasmic reticulum is the site for a variety of synthetic reactions and chemical modifications, including steroid production. Cytoplasmic proteins are synthesized on free **ribosomes** (h). The **cytoskeleton** (j) is a network of fiber systems made up of microtubules and filaments that may be involved in various cellular activities ranging from movement to transport.

ANSWER:
Question 1: A-c; B-e; C-f; D-g; E-i; F-k; G-h; H-b; I-a; J-d; K-j
Question 2: A-a; B-d; C-e; D-i; E-f; F-f; G-c; H-b

3. With regard to plasma membranes, which of the following statements is/are correct?

A. Plasma membranes are composed of a single layer of lipid and protein.
B. Approximately 60% of the plasma membrane is composed of carbohydrate.
C. The major lipids in the membrane are phospholipids, glycolipids, and cholesterol.
D. The ability of proteins to move around in the plasma membrane depends primarily on the amount of cholesterol in the membrane.
E. Plasma membrane lipids have a high degree of polarity.

Ref.: 1, 2, 3

COMMENTS: Plasma membranes are a common feature of all cells. They are composed of a lipid bilayer in which proteins are essentially floating. Carbohydrate is a minor component (approximately 1–10%), whereas approximately 60% is protein and 40% is lipid. The major lipids in the plasma membrane are the phospholipids, glycolipids, and cholesterol. Specific examples of the most common phospholipids include phosphatidylcholine and phosphatidylethanolamine. The more cholesterol in the membrane, the greater is the membrane fluidity and therefore the easier it is for intramembrane proteins to move and interact. Plasma membrane lipids are quite polar, containing both hydrophilic and hydrophobic components. The hydrophilic portions of the lipid generally orient in a direction perpendicular to the membrane plane and point toward either the cytoplasm or the extracellular space; the hydrophobic lipid chains are sandwiched between the hydrophilic portions.

ANSWER: C, D, E

4. Which of the following statements regarding plasma membrane proteins is/are correct?

A. Transmembrane proteins traverse the entire lipid bilayer.
B. Membrane proteins are always attached by a covalent bond to a membrane lipid.
C. The transmembrane protein within the membrane plane is in an α-helical configuration.
D. Membrane proteins within the membrane plane are free to move in a fluid mosaic.
E. The outer surface of the cell generally has a positive charge.

Ref.: 5

COMMENTS: Membrane proteins can be divided into a few basic types. **Transmembrane** proteins extend across the lipid bilayer one or more times; this group includes receptor molecules linked to intracellular enzymes, transport molecules, and ion conductance channels. Some proteins are **covalently** attached to the lipid bilayer by a direct covalent link to a lipid or, less commonly, indirectly through an oligosaccharide link to a lipid. Some proteins are associated with the plasma membrane by **noncovalent** interactions with transmembrane proteins; proteins linking the cytoskeleton to membrane junctions are examples of this type. The proteins that pass through the membrane are generally in an α-helical configuration. The proteins and lipids within the plane of the membrane are not covalently bound but are free to move in a fluid mosaic. Although some complex polysaccharides are noncovalently associated with the membrane, glycolipids and glycoproteins generally have covalently linked carbohydrate chains that are oriented toward the extracellular space. On glycoproteins, sialic acid residues comprise the terminal residue on the oligosaccharide chain. Sialic acid residues help maintain a negative charge on the outer cell surface and may be involved in maintaining cell independence and inhibiting cell contact.

ANSWER: A, C, D

5. Which of the following statements about the electrical properties of cell membranes is/are correct?

A. Ions flow through hydrophilic channels formed by specific transmembrane proteins.
B. The ability to store electrical charge (capacitance) is required for maintenance of a resting membrane potential.
C. The ionic gradients necessary for a resting potential are maintained by active ionic pumps.
D. Large numbers of sodium ions rush in during the initial phase of a nerve action potential.

Ref.: 4, 5

COMMENTS: The lipid component of the plasma membrane provides the capability of storing electrical charge (capacitance), and the protein component provides the capability of resisting electrical charge (resistance). Specific transmembrane proteins provide hydrophilic paths for the ions (primarily Na^+, K^+, Ca^{2+}, and Cl^-) involved in electrical signaling. The amino acid sequence in specific regions of these proteins determines the selectivity for specific ions. The establishment and maintenance of a resting cell membrane potential require the separation of charge maintained by membrane capacitance, selective permeability of the plasma membrane, concentration gradients (intracellular versus extracellular) of the permeant ions, and impermeant intracellular anions. The ionic concentration gradients are generally maintained by active pumping by the sodium (Na^+/K^+-ATPase) or Ca^{2+} pumps. Action potentials are regenerative (self-sustaining) transient depolarizations caused by activation of voltage-sensitive sodium and potassium channels. Only a small volume of sodium ions is necessary to initiate an action potential; in fact, the amount of sodium ions that flow into a typical nerve cell during an action potential would change the intracellular Na^+ concentration by only a few parts per million.

ANSWER: A, B, C

6. With regard to cell surface antigens, which of the following statements is/are true?

A. Cell surface antigens are generally glycoproteins or glycolipids.
B. ABO blood group antigens and histocompatibility antigens are two common examples of cell surface antigens.
C. ABO antigens are glycoproteins.
D. HLA antigens have an extracellular hydrophobic region and an intracellular hydrophilic region.

Ref.: 1, 2, 3

COMMENTS: Cell surface antigens are generally glycoproteins or glycolipids that are anchored to either a protein or a lipid. Common examples include the ABO blood group antigens and the histocompatibility antigens. Antigens of the ABO system are glycolipids whose oligosaccharide portions are responsible for the antigenic properties. The structures of the blood group oligosaccharides occur commonly in nature and lead to the stimulation needed to produce anti-A or anti-B antibodies after a few months of life. HLA antigens are two-chain glycoproteins that are anchored into the cell membrane at the carboxy terminal. These antigens contain an extracellular hydrophilic region, a transmembrane hydrophobic region, and an intracellular hydrophilic region. It is thought that this transmembrane structure may allow extracellular signals to be transmitted to the interior of the cell.

ANSWER: A, B

7. Which of the following statements regarding "second messenger" systems is/are correct?

A. Inositol triphosphate (IP_3) inhibits intracellular calcium release.
B. Adenylate cyclase stimulates conversion of cyclic adenosine monophosphate (cAMP) to ATP.
C. Diacylglycerol (DAG) and calcium lead to the activation of protein kinase C.
D. cAMP mediates its second messenger effect by regulating the activation of protein kinase C.
E. Thyroid stimulating hormone (TSH) release is mediated by conversion of IP_3 to membrane phospholipid.
F. The receptors (e.g., muscarinic acetylcholine receptors) that increase intracellular cAMP activate adenylate cyclase directly.

Ref.: 1, 2, 3, 4

COMMENTS: The interaction of ligands with cell surface receptors results in activation of so-called second messenger systems. Well described examples of second messengers include IP_3, DAG, calcium, and cAMP. Stimulation of the cell surface receptor leads to increased calcium concentration in the cytoplasm by either causing a membrane permeability change that increases calcium influx from outside the cell or allowing intracellular organelle calcium release. In the latter system, receptor stimulation activates the enzyme phospholipase C, which converts membrane phospholipids (i.e., phosphoinositols) to IP_3 and DAG. IP_3 mediates release of calcium from intracellular reservoirs, such as the endoplasmic reticulum, sarcoplasmic reticulum in muscle, and mitochondria. • DAG works in concert with calcium to activate protein kinase. • Cell surface receptor activation stimulates the enzyme adenylate cyclase, which breaks down ATP to cAMP with release of pyrophosphate. cAMP regulates the activation of protein kinases, which in turn stimulate a variety of metabolic pathways by activation of many other enzymes via phosphorylation. Examples of cAMP-dependent hormones include adrenocorticotrophic hormone (ACTH) and TSH. Receptors that increase cAMP are coupled to adenylate cyclase through intermediary guanosine triphosphate (GTP)-binding proteins (G-proteins). The interaction with G-proteins may be a site of normal regulation (permissive actions of hormones) or toxin action (pertussis toxin).

ANSWER: C, D

8. Which of the following statements regarding mechanisms of cell transport is/are correct?

A. Simple diffusion is generally greater with more hydrophilic substances.
B. Facilitated diffusion requires a carrier for transport and does not require ATP.
C. Facilitated diffusion requires ATP.
D. The sodium/potassium pump is an example of active transport down a concentration gradient and therefore does not require ATP hydrolysis.

Ref.: 1

COMMENTS: There are two basic types of **cell transport**: **diffusion** and **active transport**. The driving force of diffusion is simply a concentration gradient; therefore it does not require energy in the form of ATP. • *Simple* diffusion is generally greater with more hydrophobic substances, whereas hydrophilic substances penetrate less easily, and larger molecules are limited by pores of specific size. Oxygen, carbon dioxide, and urea pass easily through the membrane by diffusion. • *Facilitated* (carrier-mediated) diffusion requires a carrier for transport. In addition, unlike simple diffusion, which is not saturable, facilitated diffusion is limited by the number of carrier proteins. • **Active transport** requires ATP for energy. The sodium/potassium pump, in which a higher potassium concentration and lower sodium concentration are maintained on the inside of the cell relative to that in the extracellular space, is an example of active transport. In this case, both sodium and potassium are pumped against concentration gradients, an effect accomplished as a result of energy released by ATP hydrolysis.

ANSWER: B

9. Match the major types of cell junction on the left with the characteristic(s) on the right.

A. Gap junctions	a. Cell adhesion point
B. Desmosomes	b. Linked by transmembrane linkers
C. Tight junctions	c. Most common type of cell junction
	d. Help maintain cells in a polar state
	e. Involved in intercellular communication
	f. Point of true cell fusion

Ref.: 1, 2, 3

COMMENTS: There are three major types of cell junction: gap junctions, desmosomes, and tight junctions. **Gap** junctions are the most common type and function primarily for intercellular communication but also for cellular adhesion. The connection between cells maintained by the gap junction is not particularly stable; it depends on a variety of complexes on each cell but not on connecting proteins (hence the term "gap"). Gap junctions serve as a pathway of permeability between cells for many different molecules up to weights of 1000 daltons. **Desmosomes** function as cellular adhesion points but do not provide a pathway of communication. They are linked by filaments that function as transmembrane linkers, but desmosomes are not points of true cell fusion. **Tight junctions**, in contrast, are true points of cell fusion and are impermeable barriers. They prevent leakage of molecules across the epithelium in either direction. They also limit the movement of membrane proteins within the lipid bilayer of the plasma membrane and therefore maintain cells in a differentiated polar state.

ANSWER:
A-a,c,e; B-a,b; C-d,f

10. Which of the following statements regarding the endoplasmic reticulum is/are correct?

A. The rough endoplasmic reticulum is characterized by a ribosomal coating.
B. Rough endoplasmic reticulum is the site of lipid synthesis.
C. Smooth endoplasmic reticulum mediates synthetic reactions and chemical modifications of protein synthesis.
D. Endoplasmic reticulum may be differentiated from plasma membrane by its higher protein/lipid ratio and having less cholesterol.
E. There are three general shapes of endoplasmic reticulum: lamellar, vesicular, and tubular.

Ref.: 1, 2, 3

COMMENTS: Endoplasmic reticulum is part of a network that includes mitochondria, lysosomes, microbodies, the Golgi complex, and the nuclear envelope. This network forms an intracellular circulatory system that allows vital substrates to reach the cell interior for transportation and assembly. There are **two types** of endoplasmic reticulum: *rough* endoplasmic reticulum, which is coated with ribosomes and functions as the site for synthesis of membrane and secreted proteins, and *smooth* endoplasmic reticulum, which is the site for synthetic reactions and chemical modifications of protein synthesis. As such, cells that produce a lot of protein have a lot of rough endoplasmic reticulum, whereas cells that make a lot of steroids (e.g., those in the adrenal cortex) generally have a lot of smooth endoplasmic reticulum. • Endoplasmic reticulum is found in **three general forms**: *lamellar*, which is made up of collections of flattened membrane sacs and is the most common; *vesicular*, which is particularly common with smooth endoplasmic reticulum; and *tubular*, which also is mainly a form of smooth endoplasmic reticulum. • Endoplasmic reticulum may be differentiated from plasma membrane in that it has a higher protein/lipid ratio and a lower concentration of cholesterol. Both of these properties give it more structural stability. The endoplasmic reticulum, however, is thinner than the plasma membrane.

ANSWER: A, C, D, E

11. Which of the following statement(s) concerning microbodies is/are correct?

A. Peroxisomes contain catalases and oxidases.
B. The membrane in the microbody is essentially impermeable.
C. The enzymes in microbodies are a specialized group of hydroxylation enzymes.
D. Microbodies use molecular oxygen to oxidize substrate with generation of hydrogen peroxide.
E. Microbodies degrade hydrogen peroxide to water and oxygen.

Ref.: 1, 2, 3

COMMENTS: Microbodies may be distinguished from other cell organelles by the fact that they contain catalase. There are two microbody classes: the **peroxisome**, which is found in both plants and animals and contains catalases and oxidase, and the **glyoxisome**, which is found mainly in plants and contains part or all of the enzymes of the glyoxylate cycle. Like the endoplasmic reticulum, the microbody membrane is thinner than that of the plasma membrane. The membrane of microbodies is freely permeable to a number of substances that are natural substrates of the enzymes within. These substances include amino acids, hydroxy acids, and uric acid. In general, the enzymes in microbodies are a specialized group of oxidation enzymes that act on a fairly limited number of substrates in a degradative manner. Microbodies protect cells from high oxygen toxicity and function to compartmentalize purine/pyrimidine catabolism as well as amino acid destruction. They use molecular oxygen to oxidize a given substrate with the generation of hydrogen peroxide. They then degrade the hydrogen peroxide to water and oxygen to protect the cell from the toxic effect of hydrogen peroxide.

ANSWER: A, D, E

12. With regard to phagocytosis, which of the following statements is/are correct?

A. Phagocytosis may be defined as engulfment of particulate matter, whereas pinocytosis is the engulfment of soluble materials.
B. Increased hydrophilicity of a foreign particle, in comparison to the phagocyte, increases phagocytosis.
C. An opsonin increases phagocytosis by binding with the foreign particle and exposing the hydrophobic tail portion of the antibody.
D. The particle is engulfed by the phagocyte to form a phagosome.
E. Phagocytosis is not temperature-dependent, whereas pinocytosis is.

Ref.: 1, 2, 3

COMMENTS: Phagocytosis is accomplished by several cells in the body, including macrophages and polymorphonuclear leukocytes. **Endocytosis** is, generally, cellular engulfment of *foreign* particles. **Phagocytosis** specifically refers to the engulfment of *particulate* material; **pinocytosis** is the engulfment of *soluble* materials. Increased hydrophobicity of a foreign particle or increased hydrophilicity of the phagocyte increases phagocytosis. **Opsonins** are antibody molecules that increase phagocytosis as a result of combining the hydrophilic antigen-binding portion of the antibody with a foreign particle, thereby exposing the hydrophobic tail of the antibody. Once a particle is engulfed by a phagocyte, it forms a **phagosome**, which then combines with a **lysosome** to form a **phagolysosome**. Phagocytosis is temperature-dependent in that it does not occur below a critical temperature threshold. Because pinocytosis involves the uptake of already soluble molecules, it is not affected by this critical temperature threshold.

ANSWER: A, C, D

13. Which of the following is/are true regarding lysosomes?

A. Lysosomes generally contain only oxidative enzymes.
B. Heterolysosomes are involved in the endocytosis of extracellular material.
C. Primary lysosomes are those formed by fusion of a phagosome and are referred to as phagolysosomes.
D. Acid phosphatase is a marker enzyme for lysosomes.

Ref.: 1, 2, 3

COMMENTS: A lysosome is a membrane-bound cellular structure that contains two or more acid hydrolases. Heterolysosomes are involved in the endocytosis and digestion of extracellular material, whereas autolysosomes are involved in digestion of the cell's own intracellular material. A primary lysosome is formed by the cell before digestive activity. Combining a primary lysosome with a phagosome creates a secondary lysosome, or phagolysosome. Lysosomal enzymes are hydrolases that are resistant to autolysis; acid phosphatase is the principal marker enzyme for lysosomes.

ANSWER: B, D

14. Which of the following is/are true regarding lysosomes?

A. Lysosomal membranes have a high proportion of lipids in a micellular configuration.
B. It is suggested that steroids may work by facilitating the breakdown of lysosomal membranes with release of contained enzymes.
C. Cathepsins are a form of oxidative enzyme found in lysosomes.
D. Lysosomes are produced in the Golgi complex.

Ref.: 1, 2, 3

COMMENTS: One of the distinguishing characteristics of lysosomal membranes is their ability to fuse with other cell membranes. Lysosomal membranes have a high proportion of lipids in a micellular configuration, primarily because of the presence of the phospholipid lysolecithin. This increased micellular configuration in the membrane facilitates membrane fusion of lysosomes with phagosomes for digestion and with the plasma membrane for secretion. Steroids are thought to work partially by stabilizing lysosomal membranes, thereby inhibiting membrane fusion and enzyme release. Cathepsins are a type of acid hydrolase found in lysosomes. Lysosomes may engage in some autophagocytosis, which is thought to be responsible for cell turnover, cell remodeling, and tissue changes. Lysosomes are formed in the Golgi complex by the packaging of enzymes formed in the rough endoplasmic reticulum.

ANSWER: A, D

15. Which of the following is/are true regarding the Golgi complex?

A. The Golgi complex is a system of round membrane sacs scattered throughout the cytoplasm.
B. The Golgi complex is oriented so a forming face is close to the endoplasmic reticulum, whereas a mature face points toward the cell surface.
C. The Golgi complex is responsible for assembly of carbohydrate-rich macromolecules.
D. The Golgi complex is involved in the breakdown of integral membrane proteins and lysosomes.

Ref.: 1, 2, 3

COMMENTS: The Golgi complex is a highly pleomorphic system of membrane sacs arranged in a stacked form. It is surrounded by vesicles and tubules, with an orientation such that the forming face is close to the endoplasmic reticulum, and the mature face points toward the cell surface, where secretory materials may be exported. The Golgi complex contains a variety of enzymes, including glycosyltransferase, which is its best marking enzyme. The Golgi complex is responsible for the assembly of carbohydrate-rich macromolecules. It is partially responsible for the synthesis of integral membrane glycoproteins and the synthesis of lysosomes.

ANSWER: B, C

16. Which of the following statements regarding mitochondria is/are true?

A. Mitochondria have two discontinuous spaces: the intermembrane space and the matrix.
B. The matrix contains soluble enzymes of the tricarboxylic acid cycle.
C. There is an inverse relation between the number of mitochondria and the metabolic demands on a cell.
D. Ribosomes are rarely found in association with the mitochondrial matrix.
E. The lamellar form of cristae is common in steroid-producing cells.

Ref.: 1, 2, 3

COMMENTS: Mitochondria are organelles bounded by two membranes separated by a space called the **intermembrane space**. Although the membranes appear separate, they are in fact continuous. The highly invaginated inner membrane, or **crista**, projects into the innermost space of the organelle, referred to as the **matrix**. The matrix contains soluble enzymes of the tricarboxylic acid cycle. Although the matrix appears smooth, it may also contain ribosomes and filaments of DNA. There are two forms of mitochondrial cristae: the lamellar form, which is relatively stacked and the most common, and the tubular form, which is common in steroid-producing cells. The inner membranes contain all the enzymes necessary for electron transport, from reduced coenzymes to molecular oxygen, as well as the coupled process of phosphorylation. There appears to be a direct relation between the number of mitochondria per cell and the metabolic demands on the cell.

ANSWER: A, B

17. Which of the following statements regarding oxidative phosphorylation and mitochondria is/are true?

A. Metabolic products from glycolytic reactions outside mitochondria enter the mitochondria and are acted on by matrix enzymes of the tricarboxylic acid (TCA) cycle.
B. Oxyreductase enzymes sequester electrons and then load onto electron carriers reduced nicotinamide adenine dinucleotide phosphate (NADPH) and flavine adenine dinucleotide phosphate (FADPH).
C. Electrons flow through a system of membranes, thereby releasing energy, which is captured by phosphorylation of ADP to ATP.
D. Twelve ATP molecules are generated per mole of oxygen consumed.

Ref.: 1, 2, 3

COMMENTS: Metabolic products from outside the mitochondria in reactions of glycolysis enter the mitochondria and are acted on by enzymes of the TCA cycle located in the matrix. Oxyreductase enzymes sequester electrons from these substrates and then load onto electron carriers. The electrons flow through three membrane systems, the energy being released and stored by the phosphorylation of ADP to ATP. This electron flow is coupled to phosphorylation in such a way that three ATP molecules are generated for each mole of oxygen consumed. In the mitochondria of muscle cells, the process of aerobic glycolysis breaks down glycogen to carbon dioxide and water, releasing the energy necessary for conversion of ADP to ATP.

ANSWER: A, C

18. Which of the following statements about cellular motility and contractility is/are correct?

A. Actin is found only in muscle cells.
B. The interactions between actin and myosin that underlie the contraction of skeletal muscle require Ca^{2+} but not ATP.
C. The proteins kinesin and dynein are required for directional transport of cellular components along the microtubules.
D. Microtubules are involved in the movement of cilia and flagella.
E. The spindle apparatus is formed by cytoskeletal microtubules.

Ref.: 4, 5

COMMENTS: **Actin** is found in many cell types in addition to muscle cells. Actin microfilaments form a cortical layer underneath the plasma membrane of most cells in addition to forming the stress fibers of fibroblasts and the cytoskeleton of microvilli of intestinal epithelial cells. The cycle of interaction between the heads of **myosin** (''thick filaments'') and actin (''thin filaments'') in skeletal muscle requires hydrolysis of ATP to separate the myosin from the actin filament at the end of the power stroke. Calcium and troponin C (an actin-associated protein) are required to expose the binding site for myosin on the actin filament. • Cilia and flagella contain a column of doublet microtubules in a ''9 + 2'' arrangement (nine doublets in a circle surrounding two central doublets). Movement is accomplished by the doublets sliding along each other, mediated by *dynein*, an associated protein and requiring the hydrolysis of ATP. • Microtubules form part of the cytoskeletal network and arise from the microtubule organizing center (sometimes called the *centrosome*). The microtubule organizing center is found near the nucleus and contains a pair of *centrioles*. Movement of cellular components such as vacuoles along the microtubules requires ATP and the involvement of either of two associated proteins: *kinesin* for movement away from the microtubule organizing center and *dynein* for movement toward it. Microtubules are in a constant dynamic equilibrium between assembly from subunits and disassembly. Assembly of the mitotic spindle involves (1) replication and splitting of the microtubule organizing center into the two spindle poles and (2) reorganization of the cytoskeletal microtubules to form the spindle apparatus.

ANSWER: C, D, E

19. Match the intermediate filament with the appropriate cell type or location.

A. Nuclear lamins	a. Epithelial cells and epidermal derivatives such as hair and nails
B. Vimentin	b. Neurons
C. Keratin	c. Fibroblasts and other cells of mesenchymal origin
D. Glial fibrillary acidic protein	d. Nuclear lamina of all cells
E. Neurofilaments	e. Astrocyte glial cells

Ref.: 4, 5

COMMENTS: Intermediate filaments are a group of related molecules that form stable mechanical components of the cytoskeleton. Nuclear lamins are also intermediate filaments, but they form the nuclear lamina on the inner surface of the nuclear envelope. One or more specific intermediate filaments are characteristic of certain cell types. Immunocytochemical identification of intermediate filament proteins is used to determine the cell type origin of some tumors. **Desmin** is an important intermediate filament protein found in smooth muscle cells and in the mechanical junctions (**desmosomes**) that link epithelial cells. **Vimentin** is an intermediate filament characteristic of fibroblasts and other mesenchymal cells. **Keratin** is characteristic of epithelial cells and of epidermal derivatives such as hair and nails. **Glial protein**, or glial fibrillary acidic protein, is found in all glial cells (e.g., astrocytes). **Neurofilaments** are characteristic of neuronal tissue (e.g., neurons).

ANSWER: A-d; B-c; C-a; D-e; E-b

20. Match the following structure concerning cell–cell and cell–matrix interactions with the appropriate statement or statements.

A. Fibrous proteins	a. Example of an adhesion molecule that sticks to itself on other cells
B. Neural cell adhesion molecule	b. Structural or adhesive proteins of the extracellular matrix
C. Laminin	c. Specific membrane receptor proteins that interact with extracellular matrix proteins on other cells
D. Integrins	d. Extracellular matrix protein secreted by epithelial cells

Ref.: 4, 5

COMMENTS: The **extracellular matrix**, a meshwork of various macromolecules, is particularly prominent in connective tissue, where it is secreted by fibroblasts. The two components of the extracellular matrix are the **matrix** (*glycosaminoglycans*, linked to proteins to form *proteoglycans*) and **fibrous** proteins, which can be primarily structural (e.g., *collagen* and *elastin*) or primarily adhesive (e.g., *fibronectin* and *laminin*). Some adhesive molecules are found on cell membranes and bind not to distinct receptor molecules but to identical molecules on the membranes of adjacent cells. Thus cells with the same cell adhesion molecules stick to each other, to the exclusion of other cell types. The best known example of this class is the *neural cell adhesion molecule* (N-CAM). Several extracellular matrix proteins are involved in providing a substrate for cell adhesion. Examples include fibronectin, which is secreted by fibroblasts in connective tissue; *tenascin*, which is secreted by glial cells; and laminin, which is secreted by epithelial cells. Cells interacting with these substrates have specific membrane receptor proteins, generically called *integrins*.

ANSWER: A-b; B-a; C-d; D-c

21. Which of the following statements regarding the nuclear envelope is/are correct?

A. The nuclear envelope is a double-membrane sheath that joins at several areas called tight junctions.
B. The space between the two nuclear envelope membranes is called the perinuclear space.

C. Pore complexes are made up of a cylindrical structure called the annulus and a central granule.
D. The nuclear envelope is impermeable to inorganic ions and small organic molecules.
E. The nucleus moves throughout the cell because of its free-floating nature.

Ref.: 1, 2, 3

COMMENTS: The nuclear envelope, which surrounds the nucleus, is made up of two membranes that are essentially parallel except in areas where they join as a pore complex. The space between the membranes is referred to as the **perinuclear space**. The outer membrane of the nuclear envelope occasionally has attached ribosomes and may be continuous with the endoplasmic reticulum. The nuclear side of the inner membrane is a fibrous layer of electron dense material and is referred to as the **nuclear lamina**. The nuclear lamina is thought to function as an organizing frame for the nuclear envelope and as a site of attachment for chromosomes. The **pore complexes** are composed of a cylindrical structure called the **annulus**, which forms the rim of the pore, and an inner **central granule**. A large number of pore complexes is associated with heavy traffic between the nucleus and the cytoplasm. There are fewer pore complexes in slowly metabolizing or nonproliferating cells than in highly proliferating cells. The nuclear envelope is highly permeable to inorganic ions and small organic molecules and may permit passage of materials up to the molecular weight of proteins needed inside the nucleus for nucleic acid replication and transcription. The nucleus does not appear to be free-floating in the cell; it may be held in position by a web of filaments from the surface throughout the cell interior.

ANSWER: B, C

22. Which of the following regarding the nucleus is/are true?

A. The nucleus is made up of a nuclear envelope, a nucleolus, chromatin, and a structural network called the matrix.
B. The matrix is thought to be involved in replication, transcription, and posttranscriptional processing and transport.
C. The matrix functions as a depot for RNA and protein being assembled into preribosomal subunits.
D. The nucleolus contains a fibrillar zone in which ribosomes are condensed with RNA.

Ref.: 1, 2, 3

COMMENTS: The nuclear region is divided into a **nuclear envelope**, a **nucleolus**, **chromatin**, and a structural network called the **matrix**. The **matrix** is proposed to be involved in replication, transcription, and posttranscriptional processing and transport. The **nucleolus** functions as a depot for RNA and protein being assembled into preribosomal subunits. The nucleolus is divided into a fibrillar zone and a granular zone. The fibrillar zone has sites where ribosomal RNA is transcribed, and the granular zone has sites where ribosomes and proteins are condensed with the ribosomal RNA.

ANSWER: A, B

23. Which of the following statements about chromosomes is/are correct?

A. The nucleus contains all of the cellular DNA.
B. Chromosomes contain a single strand of DNA.
C. Interactions between DNA and proteins stabilize chromosome structure.
D. Interactions between DNA and proteins expose specific genes and control their expression.
E. During mitosis, the spindle apparatus attaches to the chromosome at a region called the centromere.

Ref.: 4, 5

COMMENTS: Chromosomes are formed by the combination of double-stranded helical **DNA** with histones and other proteins. The interactions between DNA and proteins stabilize the chromosomal structure. Most cellular DNA is located in the **nucleus**, although a small portion is found in the mitochondria. Each chromosomal double helix contains approximately 10^8 basepairs. There are several levels of organizational restructuring: progression from the DNA and histones forming chromatin to the complex folded structure of the chromosome. To express a gene, that portion of the chromosome must be unfolded and unwrapped, exposing the DNA double helix. Gene expression is regulated by the binding of nonchromosomal proteins (*transcription factors*) to specific regions of the DNA (*enhancer elements* and *promoter elements*). Several distinct regions of chromosomes are identifiable: *origins of replication* (sites of initiation of DNA synthesis), the *centromere* (site of spindle attachment during mitosis), and *telomeres* (specialized end structures that maintain the length of the chromosome through replication cycles).

ANSWER: C, D, E

24. Which of the following statements regarding the nucleolus is/are true?

A. The nucleolus is the functional site for the generation of DNA.
B. The nucleolus is limited by a double-membrane sheath.
C. The fibrillar component of the nucleolus is involved in associating genes for ribosomal RNA.
D. The nucleolus is characterized by a granular component, which is a site for RNA transcription and protein synthesis.

Ref.: 1, 2, 3

COMMENTS: The primary function of the nucleolus is generation of ribosomes. It is functionally and structurally associated with the nuclear envelope and the lamina. The nucleolus has no limiting membrane. The nucleolus is made up of a fibrillar component and a granular component. The fibrillar center of the nucleolus functions to associate nucleolar organizing regions, which are genes for ribosomal RNA. The dense fibrillar component is involved in the transcription of ribosomal RNA genes and the assembly of preribosomal subunits. The granular component is involved in the processing and maturation of preribosomes.

ANSWER: C

25. Match each of the following phases of mitosis on the left with the appropriate characteristics on the right.

A. Prophase
B. Anaphase
C. Metaphase
D. Telophase

a. Centromeres migrate toward opposite poles
b. Centromeres align at the equatorial plate
c. Shortening of chromosomes followed by disappearance of the nucleolus and nuclear envelope
d. Lengthening of chromosomes with re-formation of the nucleolus and nuclear envelope
e. Formation of the spindle apparatus
f. Replication of centrioles

Ref.: 1, 2, 3

COMMENTS: Mitosis is a progressive cell change characterized by several phases, which leads to two identical daughter cells. **Prophase**, the first phase, includes shortening of the chromosomes, followed by disappearance of both the nucleolus and the nuclear envelope and formation of the spindle apparatus. Centrioles replicate, and the two centrioles move to opposite ends. At this stage the shortened chromosomes are referred to as chromatids and are held together by a centromere; the chromatids are identical chromosomes temporarily joined by the centromere. **Metaphase** occurs with movement of the chromosomes toward the center, so the centromeres align on a plane called the *equatorial plate*. The centromeres then attach to spindle fibers from the spindle apparatus. At the same time, the centromeres of each chromatid duplicate. **Anaphase**, the next portion of mitosis, is marked by migration of the chromatids to opposite poles. When separated, the chromatids are referred to as chromosomes. **Telophase** occurs shortly thereafter and involves decondensation of the chromosomes with simultaneous nucleolar and nuclear envelope re-formation.

ANSWER: A-c,e,f; B-a; C-b; D-d

26. Match the cell phase in the left column with the appropriate activity in the right column.

A. S
B. G_1
C. G_2
D. M

a. DNA replication
b. RNA and protein synthesis
c. Characterized by four subphases that lead to two identical daughter cells

Ref.: 1, 2, 3

COMMENTS: The cell cycle is composed of a long **interphase** and the comparatively short **mitosis** phase. Interphase is initiated by a G_1 phase followed by an *S* phase (during which DNA synthesis occurs and two sister chromosomes are generated) and then by a G_2 quiescent phase. RNA and protein synthesis occurs during both the G_1 and G_2 phases. Mitosis (characterized by a prophase, metaphase, anaphase, and telophase, during which two identical daughter cells are generated) then occurs, and the cycle is repeated.

ANSWER: A-a; B-b; C-b; D-c

27. Regarding protein synthesis, which of the following statements is/are true?

A. Transcription takes place in the nucleus.
B. Messenger RNA moves from the nucleus to the cytoplasm and attaches to free ribosomes in the cytoplasm.
C. Introns initiate protein synthesis by attaching the ribosome to the rough endoplasmic reticulum.
D. The enzyme RNA polymerase catalyzes the transcription of messenger RNA from DNA.
E. Free ribosomes are involved in the synthesis of proteins that insert into the endoplasmic reticulum.

Ref.: 1, 2, 3, 4

COMMENTS: The sequence of nucleotides in DNA determines the amino acid sequence of the protein. Protein synthesis involves (1) *transcription* of messenger RNA from the gene that codes for the protein, (2) *translation* of the messenger RNA into a protein, and (3) *posttranslational processing* of the protein, in which there may be enzymatic cleavage or glycosylation of the protein. *Transcription* takes place in the nucleus, whereas translation and posttranslational processing occur in the rough endoplasmic reticulum, Golgi complex, or free ribosomes in the cytoplasm. Transcription of messenger RNA from DNA occurs by assembly of complementary basepairs on the DNA template one nucleotide at a time. This step is catalyzed by the enzyme RNA polymerase. Eukaryotic genes are interrupted by noncoding regions called *introns*. Introns are removed from the RNA transcript by *splicing*. The resulting messenger RNA is moved to the cytoplasm, in which it binds to ribosomes to begin *translation*. Ribosomes are composed of proteins and ribosomal RNA. Ribosomal RNA is transcribed in the *nucleolus*. There it is combined with ribosomal proteins to form ribosomal subunits. These ribosomal subunits are transported to the cytoplasm, where they are assembled into two populations of ribosomes: *free ribosomes*, which are engaged in the synthesis of proteins that remain in the cytoplasm, and *membrane-bound ribosomes*, which become attached to the *rough endoplasmic reticulum* and are involved in the synthesis of proteins that are inserted into the endoplasmic reticulum. The initial step of protein synthesis is attachment of the messenger RNA to a ribosome that is preloaded with a *transfer RNA* that recognizes the start codon (three bases) AUG and thus sets the reading frame for the translation. Subsequent binding of aminoacyl-transfer RNA to the ribosomes that match the three nucleotide codons that specify each amino acid results in peptide synthesis as the ribosome moves along the messenger RNA molecule. The first portion of the protein that is synthesized is an amino terminal leader called the *signal peptide*. At this stage the ribosome becomes attached to the rough endoplasmic reticulum through interactions between the signal peptide, a cytoplasmic signal recognition peptide (SRP), and an SRP receptor protein in the rough endoplasmic reticulum. As translation continues, the signal peptide is inserted into the rough endoplasmic reticulum membrane by another transmembrane protein and later cleaved as the peptide elongates.

ANSWER: A, B, D

REFERENCES

1. Thorpe NO: *Cell Biology*. John Wiley, New York, 1984.
2. Carroll M: *Organelles*. Guilford Press, New York, 1989.
3. Karp G: *Cell Biology*. McGraw-Hill, New York, 1984.
4. Darnell J, Lodish H, Baltimore D: *Molecular Cell Biology*. Scientific American Books, New York, 1990.
5. Alberts B, Bray D, Lewis J, et al: *Molecular Biology of the Cell*. Garland Publishing, New York, 1989.

CHAPTER 2

Fluids and Electrolytes

1. With regard to total body water, which of the following statements is/are true?

   A. Approximately 50–70% of total body weight is water.
   B. In general, the percentage of total body weight that is water is higher in males than in females.
   C. Lean individuals have a greater proportion of water (relative to body weight) than do obese individuals.
   D. The percentage of total body weight that is water increases with age.
   E. Body water is divided into extracellular (i.e., intravascular and interstitial) and intracellular functional compartments.

Ref.: 1, 2

COMMENTS: Management of fluid and electrolyte balance depends on an understanding of the size and composition of various body fluid compartments, usually expressed as a percentage of body weight. About 50–75% of body weight is water. It varies according to sex, age, and lean body mass; 60% of body weight in males and 50% of body weight in females is water (± 15%). This difference relates in part to the fact that fat contains little water, and lean individuals have a greater proportion of body water than do fat individuals of the same weight. Because females have more subcutaneous fat in relation to lean mass than do males, they have less body water. Total body water decreases with age as a result of decreasing lean muscle mass. Infants have an unusually high ratio of total body water to body weight: up to 75–80%. By 1 year of age, however, the percentage of body water approaches that of the adult. • Body water is divided into three functional compartments: the *intracellular* fluid compartment (40% of body weight), the *interstitial* (extravascular) fluid compartment (15% of body weight), and the *intravascular* (plasma) fluid compartment (5% of body weight). Together, the interstitial and intravascular compartments constitute the *extracellular* fluid compartment.

ANSWER: A, B, C, E

2. With regard to the distribution and composition of the body fluid compartments, which of the following statements is/are correct?

   A. Most intracellular water is in skeletal muscle.
   B. The major intracellular cation is sodium.
   C. The major intracellular anions are proteins and phosphates.
   D. The major extracellular cation is sodium.
   E. The major extracellular anions are chloride and bicarbonate.

Ref.: 1, 2

COMMENTS: The intracellular fluid compartment (comprising 40% of total body weight) is contained mostly within skeletal muscle. The principal intracellular cations are potassium and magnesium, whereas the principal anions are proteins and phosphates. In the extracellular fluid compartment (20% of total body weight), subdivided into the interstitial compartment (extravascular) and the intravascular compartment (plasma), the principal cation is sodium, and the principal anions are chloride and bicarbonate. The interstitial compartment has a rapidly equilibrating functional component and a slowly equilibrating, relatively nonfunctional component, i.e., fluid within connective tissue and that contained in cerebrospinal (CSF) and joint fluids. The water in the CSF and joint spaces is called transcellular water. The nonfunctional component represents only one-half of body weight. Intravascular fluid (plasma) has a higher concentration of nondiffusible organic proteins than do interstitial fluids. These plasma proteins act as multivalent anions. As a result, the concentration of *inorganic* anions is lower, but the total concentration of cations is higher, in intravascular fluid than in interstitial fluid. This relation is explained by the **Gibbs-Donnan** equilibrium equation (the product of the concentrations of any pair of diffusible cations and anions on one side of a semipermeable membrane equals the product of the same pair on the other side).

ANSWER: A, C, D, E

3. With regard to the chemical composition and osmolarity of the body fluids, which of the following statements is/are true?

   A. From a physiologic standpoint, the numbers of millimoles, milliequivalents, and milliosmoles are interchangeable.
   B. The osmolality of body fluids is between 290 and 310 mOsm.
   C. The effective osmotic pressure of a body compartment is determined by the presence of nondiffusible proteins.
   D. Because water diffuses freely between compartments, the effective osmotic pressures within the various fluid compartments are considered to be equal.

Ref.: 1, 2

COMMENTS: From a physiologic and a chemical standpoint, the terms milliosmoles, milliequivalents, and millimoles are not interchangeable. Millimoles (mM) refer to the number of particles per unit volume. Millequivalents (mEq) refer to the number of electrical charges per unit volume. Milliosmoles (mOsm) refer to the number of osmotic active particles per unit volume. In solution, the number of milliequivalents of cations present is balanced by the same number of milliequivalents of anions (a balance that the body maintains in a steady state). In each body compartment, the concentration of osmotically active particles is 290–310 mOsm. Although total osmotic pressure represents the sum of osmotically active particles in a fluid compartment, the effective osmotic pressure depends on osmotically active particles that do not freely pass between the semipermeable membranes of the body. Nonpermeable proteins in plasma are responsible for the effective osmotic pressure between the plasma and interstitial fluid compartment (the colloid osmotic pressure). The effective osmotic pressure between extracellular fluid (ECF) and intracellular fluid (ICF) compartments is contributed to mainly by sodium, the major extracellular cation, which does not freely cross the cell membrane. Because water moves freely between compartments, the effective oncotic pressures within the various body fluid compartments are considered to be equal. An increase in the effective oncotic pressure of the ECF compartment, as would result from an increase in sodium concentration, would cause movement of water from the intracellular space to the extracellular space until the osmotic pressures equalize. Conversely, loss of sodium (hyponatremia) from the extracellular space would result in a movement of water into the intracellular space. Thus, the ICF contributes to correcting the concentration and composition changes in the ECF. Isotonic extracellular volume losses (volume loss without change in concentration) generally do not cause transfer of water from the intracellular space so long as the osmolarity remains unchanged. Isotonic volume losses result in ECF volume changes.

ANSWER: B, C, D

4. With regard to volume status changes of the extracellular fluid compartment, which of the following statements is/are true?

A. Hyponatremia is diagnostic of extracellular fluid volume excess.
B. Hypernatremia is diagnostic of extracellular fluid volume depletion.
C. Tissue signs of acute volume loss appear early after acute volume loss.
D. Extracellular volume excess is usually iatrogenic.

Ref.: 1, 2

COMMENTS: The concentration of serum sodium is not necessarily related to the volume status of the extracellular fluid. Volume deficit or excess can exist with high, low, or normal serum sodium concentrations. **Volume deficit** is the most common volume disorder encountered during surgery; loss of isotonic fluid (fluid having the same composition as extracellular fluid) is the most common cause (examples: hemorrhage, vomiting, diarrhea, fistulas, third spacing). With acute volume loss, central nervous system (CNS) symptoms (sleepiness and apathy progressing to coma) and cardiovascular signs (orthostasis, hypotension, tachycardia, coolness in the extremities) appear first, along with a decreasing urine output. Tissue signs such as decreased turgor, softness of the tongue with longitudinal wrinkling, and atonicity of muscles usually do not appear during the first 24 hours. In response to hypovolemia, the body temperature may be decreased slightly (varying with the environmental temperature); it is therefore important to monitor the body temperature of hypovolemic patients. Signs and symptoms of sepsis may be depressed in the volume-depleted patient. The abdominal pain, fever, and leukocytosis associated with peritonitis may be absent until the extracellular fluid volume is restored. **Volume overload** generally is either iatrogenic or the result of renal insufficiency or heart failure. Both plasma and interstitial fluid spaces are involved. The signs are those of circulatory overload and include distended veins, bounding pulse, functional murmurs, edema, and basilar rales. These signs may be present in young, healthy patients, but these patients can compensate for moderate to severe volume excess without developing overt failure or pulmonary edema. In elderly patients, however, congestive heart failure with pulmonary edema may develop quite rapidly.

ANSWER: D

5. With regard to prerenal versus renal azotemia, which of the following statements is/are true?

A. Urine osmolality is higher in prerenal oliguria.
B. The BUN/creatinine ratio is higher with prerenal azotemia.
C. The urine/plasma urea ratio is higher in prerenal azotemia.
D. Renal failure index (RFI) is calculated as the urine sodium divided by the urine/plasma creatinine ratio.

Ref.: 1, 2

COMMENTS: Volume loss can cause renal hypoperfusion and oliguria (prerenal azotemia). It is important to distinguish this type of oliguria from that caused by intrinsic renal disease, renal azotemia. In the patient with healthy kidneys, the BUN rises disproportionately to the creatinine and the kidney preserves its ability to concentrate urine and preserve sodium. When comparing the urine of patients with prerenal azotemia to the urine of patients with renal oliguria, the urine osmolality is generally higher (>500 mOsm vs. <350 mOsm), the sodium concentration is lower (<20 mEq/L vs. >40 mEq/L), the BUN/serum creatinine ratio is higher (>15 vs. <10), the urine/plasma urea ratio is higher (>8 vs. <3), the urine/plasma creatinine ratio is higher (>40 vs. <20), the renal failure index (RFI) (urine sodium divided by the urine/plasma creatinine ratio) is lower (<1 vs. >1.5), and the fractional excretion of sodium (FE-sodium = urine/plasma sodium ratio divided by the urine/plasma creatinine ratio $\times$ 100) is lower (<1 vs. >1.5). Loss of concentrating ability in the elderly may compromise the usefulness of some of these tests in older patients with hypovolemia. The RFI and the FE-sodium are the most accurate tests.

ANSWER: A, B, C, D

6. With regard to derangement of the serum sodium concentration, which of the following statements is/are true?

A. Changes in serum sodium concentration usually produce changes in the status of the extracellular fluid volume.
B. The chloride ion is the main determinant of the osmolarity of the extracellular fluid space.
C. Extracellular hyponatremia leads to depletion of intracellular water.

D. Dry, sticky mucous membranes are characteristic of hypernatremia.

***Ref.*:** 1, 2

COMMENTS: Whereas extracellular volume may change without a change in serum sodium concentration (as occurs after isotonic volume losses), changes in serum sodium concentration usually produce changes in extracellular fluid volume. This is because the serum sodium concentration is the main determinant of the **osmolarity** of the extracellular fluid space. Alterations in its concentration produce concomitant shifts in water volume. Signs and symptoms of hyper- and hyponatremia generally are not present until the changes are severe or if the change in sodium concentration occurs rapidly. **Hyponatremia** is caused by excessive intake of hypotonic fluids or salt losses in excess of water loss. With hyponatremia, decreased extracellular osmolarity causes a shift of water *into* the intracellular compartment. When this occurs, CNS symptoms caused by increased intracranial pressure develop, and tissue signs of excess water are noted. The CNS symptoms include muscle twitching, hyperactive tendon reflexes, and, when severe, convulsions and hypertension (caused by the increased intracranial pressure). Tissue signs include salivation, lacrimation, watery diarrhea, and "fingerprinting" of the skin. When hyponatremia develops rapidly, signs and symptoms may appear at sodium concentrations of less than 130 mEq/L. Chronic hyponatremia develops slowly, and patients may develop sodium levels as low as 120 mEq/L before becoming symptomatic. Severe hyponatremia may be associated with the onset of irreversible oliguric renal failure. Patients with a closed head injury are sensitive to even mild hyponatremia owing to increased intracellular water, which exacerbates the increased intracranial pressure associated with the head injury. In symptomatic patients, the administration of hypertonic (3%) solutions of sodium salt may be indicated to correct the acute problem. In less severe cases, free water restriction and judicious infusion of normal saline usually are sufficient. **Hypernatremia** is the result of excessive free water loss or salt intake. The signs and symptoms associated with hypernatremia include such CNS signs as restlessness, weakness, delirium, and maniacal behavior. The tissue signs are characteristic and include dryness and stickiness of mucous membranes, decreased salivation and tear production, and redness and swelling of the tongue. The body temperature is usually elevated, occasionally to a lethal level. The treatment consists of water replacement.

ANSWER: A, D

7. With regard to mixed volume and concentration abnormalities, match the clinical situation in the left column with the appropriate clinical condition in the right column:

A. Excess sweating; no fluid intake volume deficit
B. Prolonged evaporative loss; saline volume deficit, solution replacement
C. Renal failure; hypotonic fluid volume excess, replacement
D. Isotonic volume loss; hypotonic volume excess, fluid replacement

a. Extracellular volume deficit, hypernatremia
b. Extracellular volume deficit, hyponatremia
c. Extracellular volume excess, hypernatremia
d. Extracellular volume excess, hyponatremia

***Ref.*:** 1, 2

COMMENTS: Extracellular fluid deficit combined with hyponatremia is one of the most commonly seen mixed volume and concentration abnormalities, occurring in patients who drink large volumes of water to replace gastrointestinal losses (such as patients who replace diarrheal loss with tap water) or in postoperative patients who receive prolonged hypotonic saline infusions. **Extracellular volume deficit combined with hypernatremia** can occur when hypotonic fluid is lost, as during excessive sweating, in the absence of fluid intake. When hypotonic fluid losses (such as losses resulting from sweating or excessive insensible evaporative loss during long operative procedures) are treated by replacement with saline-containing solutions only, **extracellular fluid volume excess combined with hypernatremia** may result. **Extracellular volume excess combined with hyponatremia** can result from the excessive infusion of water or hypotonic saline solutions into a patient with oliguric renal failure. Normal kidneys can minimize these mixed abnormalities, but patients in oliguric or anuric renal failure are particularly prone to their development. The signs and symptoms of mixed volume and concentration abnormalities tend to be additive, and opposing signs often nullify one another. Good clinical judgment and a thorough review of a patient's underlying disease and fluid replacement history are essential for making the diagnosis.

ANSWER: A-a; B-c; C-d; D-b

8. With regard to the acid-base buffering system of the extracellular fluid, which of the following statements is/are true?

A. The bicarbonate-carbonic acid system is the primary extracellular buffering system.
B. The base bicarbonate/carbonic acid ratio determines the extracellular fluid pH.
C. The functions of the extracellular buffering system are expressed in the Henderson-Hasselbalch equation.
D. A bicarbonate/carbonic acid ratio of 20:1 is associated with a normal pH (7.4).

***Ref.*:** 1, 2

9. The Henderson-Hasselbalch equation is properly expressed by which equation?

A. $pK = pH + \log BHCO_3/H_2CO_3$
B. $pK = pH + \log H_2CO_3/BHCO_3$
C. $pH = pK + \log H_2CO_3/BHCO_3$
D. $pH = pK + \log BHCO_3/H_2CO_3$

***Ref.*:** 1, 2

COMMENTS: Assessment of complex acid-base disorders requires an understanding of the given clinical situation and of acid-base physiology. Important intracellular buffers include proteins and phosphates, whereas the bicarbonate-carbonic acid system is the primary extracellular buffering system. In extracellular fluids, acids (inorganic acids such as hydrochloric, sulfuric, or phosphoric acids, and organic acids such as lactic, pyruvic, and keto acids) combine with sodium bicarbonate to form the sodium salt of the acid and carbonic acid. Carbonic acid then dissociates into water and carbon dioxide. In equation form, this interaction is as follows:

$$\underset{\text{HCl}}{\text{(acid)}} + \underset{\text{NaHCO}_3}{\text{(base)}} \leftrightarrow \underset{\text{NaCl}}{\text{(acid anion)}} + H_2CO_3 \leftrightarrow H_2O + CO_2$$

The CO_2 is excreted by the lungs (this occurs quickly, and respiratory compensation for excess CO_2 production is rapid); the acid anion (chloride in the case of hydrochloric acid) is excreted by the kidney (this occurs slowly and hence metabolic compensation is slow) with hydrogen or ammonium ions. Extracellular fluid pH is determined mainly by the ratio of the base bicarbonate to the amount of carbonic acid in the blood. The function of this buffer system is expressed in the Henderson-Hasselbalch equation, in which bicarbonate is the numerator (affected mainly by metabolic/renal events) and carbonic acid is the denominator (affected mainly by respiratory events). At a body pH of 7.4, this ratio is 20:1. So long as this ratio is kept at 20:1, the pH remains 7.4 regardless of the absolute values. The relation between the buffering reactions of bicarbonate and carbonic acid and their respective positions in the Henderson-Hasselbalch equation are important for understanding acid-base physiology; this point cannot be overemphasized. As an example, *addition of an acid* (such as the lactic acid that accumulates during periods of hypoperfusion) shifts the bicarbonate/carbonic acid equation to the right [H lactate + $NaHCO_3$ (consumed) Na lactate + H_2CO_3 (increased) $\leftrightarrow$ H_2O + CO_2], consuming bicarbonate (which lowers the numerator) and increasing the concentration of carbonic acid (which increases the denominator). As a result, the 20:1 ratio decreases, and pH falls. Increased ventilation then occurs, eliminating the excess CO_2 and thereby decreasing the concentration of carbonic acid, restoring the 20:1 ratio and bringing the pH back to 7.4. This is an example of the changes in pH associated with metabolic acidosis. In this setting, the ability of the lungs to eliminate excess CO_2 rapidly provides rapid compensation for the pH disturbance. Slower compensation is provided by the kidney, in which excretion of excess acid occurs in exchange for bicarbonate.

ANSWER:
Question 8: A, B, C, D
Question 9: D

10. Match the acute metabolic condition in the left column with the changes in the HCO_3/H_2CO_3 ratio in the right column.

A. Respiratory acidosis — a. HCO_3 decrease
B. Respiratory alkalosis — b. HCO_3 increase
C. Metabolic acidosis — c. H_2CO_3 decrease
D. Metabolic alkalosis — d. H_2CO_3 increase

Ref.: 1, 2

11. With regard to respiratory acid-base abnormalities, which of the following statements is/are true?

A. Respiratory acidosis is caused by decreased alveolar ventilation.
B. Respiratory alkalosis is caused by increased alveolar ventilation.
C. Hyperkalemia is a frequent complication of respiratory alkalosis.
D. Potassium restriction is an important adjunct in the treatment of respiratory alkalosis.

Ref.: 1, 2

COMMENTS: There are four types of acid-base disturbances: respiratory acidosis, respiratory alkalosis, metabolic acidosis, and metabolic alkalosis. **Respiratory acidosis** is a result of CO_2 retention secondary to decreased alveolar ventilation; it leads to increased carbonic acid production, which in turn increases the denominator of the Henderson-Hasselbalch ratio. This lowers the 20:1 ratio, and the pH falls. Acute forms of this problem in previously healthy individuals can be corrected by restoring alveolar ventilation to normal values, such as by reversing CNS depression, removing mechanical airway obstruction, or increasing the rate of mechanical ventilation. Compensation for chronic forms of decreased alveolar ventilation occurs in the kidney, in which increased resorption of bicarbonate occurs. This resorbed bicarbonate raises the numerator, thus restoring the 20:1 ratio and raising the pH to a normal value. In this compensated form, the plasma bicarbonate level is *higher* than in the normal noncompensated state. **Respiratory alkalosis** is caused by excessive loss of CO_2 secondary to increased alveolar ventilation. It is characterized by a fall in arterial CO_2 pressure (PCO_2) and a rise in pH. Carbonic acid production falls, lowering the denominator of the Henderson-Hasselbalch ratio; and the 20:1 ratio increases, leading to increased pH. Renal compensation occurs when acid is *resorbed* in exchange for increased bicarbonate excretion. This renal excretion of bicarbonate lowers the numerator, restores the 20:1 ratio, and brings the pH back down to 7.4. In the acute phase of respiratory alkalosis, pH is elevated, PCO_2 falls, and the bicarbonate level may be normal. In the compensated phase, pH normalizes, and the bicarbonate concentration falls and is *lower* than normal. Of central importance when dealing with alkalosis is the avoidance of hypokalemia. Potassium is in competition with hydrogen ions for resorption of sodium bicarbonate at the level of the renal tubule. With alkalosis (where there is a relative lack of hydrogen ions) preferential excretion of potassium in exchange for sodium occurs at the level of the distal convoluted tubule. Also, hypokalemia itself may contribute to alkalosis, because in hypokalemic states hydrogen ion rather than potassium is, by necessity, excreted for sodium resorption. An additional factor in the development of hypokalemia in alkalotic states is the exchange of extracellular potassium for intracellular hydrogen ions (these changes are more pronounced for metabolic alkalosis than they are for respiratory alkalosis). It becomes clear that part of the treatment for alkalosis, whether it be respiratory, metabolic, or a combination of the two, is adequate potassium replacement. Adjusting the ventilatory rate and volume and adding deadspace to the ventilation circuit are methods used to avoid respiratory alkalosis. Adding 5% CO_2 to inspired air is poorly tolerated and not used.

ANSWER:
Question 10: A-d; B-c; C-a; D-b
Question 11: A, B

12. True or False: Respiratory alkalosis has few, if any, effects other than causing an alteration of the blood pH.

Ref.: 1, 2

COMMENTS: Respiratory alkalosis can be associated with severe cardiovascular and cerebral complications. Cardiac arrhythmia and arrest are possible complications of the hypokalemia associated with respiratory alkalosis. This is particularly true in patients who are digitalized or who have unrecognized preexisting hypokalemia. Cardiac arrhythmias are further exacerbated by the effect alkalosis has on ionized calcium. Acute alkalosis causes a fall in the level of ionized calcium. Sudden onset of severe respiratory alkalosis can cause cerebral vasoconstriction leading to cerebral ischemia and acidosis, which can be particularly serious in patients who have obstructed arterial blood flow to the brain or during performance of a carotid endarterectomy. Complicating this effect is the fact that respiratory alkalosis causes a shift of the oxygen dissociation curve to the left, which limits the ability of hemoglobin to give up oxygen to the tissues.

ANSWER: False

13. With regard to metabolic acidosis, which of the following statements is/are true?

A. Metabolic acidosis results from the loss of bicarbonate or a gain of fixed acids.
B. The most common cause of acid excess is prolonged nasogastric suction.
C. The acute compensation for metabolic acidosis is primarily renal.
D. Restoration of blood pressure with vasopressors corrects the metabolic acidosis associated with circulatory failure.

Ref.: 1, 2

COMMENTS: Metabolic acidosis has several causes. It results from retention or gain of fixed acids (through diabetic acidosis, lactic acidosis) or the loss of bicarbonate (through diarrhea, small bowel fistula, renal tubular dysfunction). Increased acid consumes bicarbonate, thereby lowering the numerator of the Henderson-Hasselbalch ratio and lowering the pH. Bicarbonate loss causes the same change. Initial compensation is respiratory (hyperventilation), which lowers carbonic acid concentration, decreasing the denominator and restoring the 20:1 ratio. Renal compensation is slower and occurs through the same means as the renal compensation for respiratory acidosis, that is, excretion of acid salts and retention of bicarbonate. This compensation depends on normal renal function. When kidney damage interferes with the ability to excrete acid and resorb bicarbonate, metabolic acidosis may rapidly progress to profound levels. The most common cause of metabolic acidosis in surgical patients is circulatory failure with accumulation of lactic acid. It results from tissue hypoxia and anaerobic metabolism. Resuscitation with vasopressors or infusion of bicarbonate does not correct the underlying problem. Volume replacement with a balanced electrolyte solution or blood (or both) results in restoration of the circulation, hepatic clearance of lactate, consumption of the formed bicarbonate, and clearance of carbonic acid by the lung. The excessive use of bicarbonate for resuscitation of patients can lead to severe metabolic alkalosis, which, in association with other possible sequelae such as hypothermia and low levels of 2,3-diphosphoglycerate in banked blood, shifts the oxygen hemoglobin distribution curve farther to the left, compromising oxygen delivery. Acidosis resulting from circulatory arrest is well tolerated if the patient is well ventilated and has not previously been acidotic. The use of excessive bicarbonate in such situations may induce a hypernatremic, hyperosmotic state. It is therefore recommended that the initial dose of bicarbonate not exceed 50 ml of a 7.5% solution and that administration of additional doses be based on results of serial blood gas analysis.

ANSWER: A

14. With regard to the anion gap, which questions is/are true?

A. Gap anions include sulfate, phosphate, and lactate.
B. Loss of bicarbonate or gain of chloride causes a widened anion gap.
C. Shock and renal failure are associated with a normal anion gap.
D. The anion gap equals the sum of serum chloride plus serum bicarbonate levels subtracted from the serum sodium concentration.

Ref.: 1, 2

COMMENTS: A useful tool for assessing patients with acid-base disorders is the anion gap, which is calculated from the sum of serum chloride plus bicarbonate levels subtracted from the serum sodium concentration. Normal anion gap values range between 10 and 15 mEq/L. The unmeasured anions that account for the anion gap are sulfate, phosphate, lactate, and other organic anions. Acidosis caused by loss of bicarbonate or gain of chloride is associated with a normal anion gap. Acidosis due to increased production of organic acids (e.g., lactic acid in patients with hypovolemic shock) or retention of acids (e.g., phosphoric acid retention in renal failure) causes the gap to increase. Causes of metabolic acidosis that are associated with a normal anion gap include diarrhea and fistulas, proximal and distal renal tubular acidosis, and exogenous administration of hydrogen ion. Causes of metabolic acidosis that are associated with an elevated anion gap include hypovolemic shock, diabetes, starvation, alcohol intoxication, and uremia. The most common cause of metabolic acidosis in surgical patients associated with an increased anion gap is circulatory failure (which leads to accumulation of lactic acid). Diabetes and starvation lead to an increase in keto acids, and uremia is associated with retention of sulfuric and phosphoric acids.

ANSWER: A, D

15. With regard to metabolic alkalosis, which of the following statements is/are true?

A. Metabolic alkalosis is a result of loss of fixed acid or gain of bicarbonate.
B. Compensation is mainly renal.
C. A common cause is prolonged nasogastric suctioning.
D. Hydrochloric acid infusion to correct this disturbance is no longer used because of the high incidence of arrhythmias.

Ref.: 1, 2

16. A 70-kg man with pyloric obstruction resulting from ulcer disease is admitted to the hospital for resuscitation after 1 week of persistent vomiting. What acid-base disturbance is expected to be seen?

A. Hypokalemic hyperchloremic metabolic acidosis.
B. Hyperkalemic hypochloremic metabolic alkalosis.
C. Hyperkalemic hyperchloremic metabolic acidosis.
D. Hypokalemic hypochloremic metabolic alkalosis.

Ref.: 1, 2

17. The same patient is found to have a serum chloride level of 80 mEq/L (normal is 103 mEq/L). What is his chloride deficit?

A. 23.
B. 183.
C. 640.
D. 322.

Ref.: 1, 2

COMMENTS: Metabolic alkalosis results from the loss of fixed acids (as with prolonged nasogastric suction of an obstructed stomach) or from the gain of bicarbonate (as occurs when renal tubular damage prevents its normal excretion). Loss of acid or gain of bicarbonate leads to a relative increase in the numerator of the Henderson-Hasselbalch equation, an increase in the 20:1 ratio, and a rise in pH. Compensation is mainly renal and occurs through the same mechanisms discussed for respiratory alkalosis (see Question 11). Again, with alkalosis, avoidance of hypokalemia is important. Occasionally, there is a component of respiratory compensation that leads to hypercarbia. • A common problem seen in patients with persistent emesis in the presence of an obstructive pylorus is hypokalemic, hypochloremic metabolic alkalosis. To compensate for the alkalosis associated with the loss of chloride and hydrogen ion-rich fluid from the stomach, there is an increase in bicarbonate excretion in the urine. The bicarbonate usually is excreted as the sodium salt; but in an attempt to conserve intravascular volume, aldosterone-mediated sodium absorption occurs accompanied by potassium and hydrogen excretion, compounding the alkalosis and leading to a paradoxical aciduria. The principles of management of this derangement include resuscitation with isotonic saline solutions and aggressive replacement of lost potassium. • Severe metabolic alkalosis (such as that caused by renal or liver failure) may respond to infusions of dilute hydrochloride formulated by the addition of 150 ml of a 0.1 N hydrochloride solution in 1 liter of normal saline or 5% dextrose. When formulated with the use of normal saline, the additional chloride in the saline must be taken into account. Such a solution (with 5% dextrose) yields 300 mEq of hydrogen and chloride ions and is infused over a 6- to 24-hour period, with measurement of the pH, PCO_2, and electrolytes every 4–6 hours. To determine the volume of solution that should be infused, the **chloride deficit** can be calculated using the plasma chloride concentration and the presumed volume in which the chloride is dispersed (a volume equal to 20% of body weight). For a 70-kg man with a serum chloride level of 80 mEq/L (normal being 103 mEq), the deficit would be 20% of body weight × (normal chloride level − observed plasma chloride level), which equals $(0.2 \times 70) \times (103 - 80) = 322$ mEq.

ANSWER:
Question 15: A, B, C
Question 16: D
Question 17: D

18. With regard to respiratory acidosis and alkalosis, which of the following statements is/are true?

A. Respiratory acidosis is associated with an increased denominator of the Henderson-Hasselbalch ratio that is due to CO_2 retention, resulting in a ratio of less than 20:1.
B. Respiratory alkalosis is associated with a decreased denominator that is due to loss of CO_2, resulting in a ratio of more than 20:1.
C. Compensation for respiratory acidosis is primarily renal.
D. Compensation for respiratory alkalosis is primarily pulmonary.

Ref.: 1, 2

COMMENTS: As previously discussed, respiratory causes of acid-base imbalance relate to changes in CO_2, which correspond to changes in carbonic acid. The carbonic acid concentration is represented in the denominator of the Henderson-Hasselbalch ratio. **Respiratory alkalosis**, caused by CO_2 retention, increases the denominator resulting in a ratio of less than 20:1, with an associated fall in pH. **Respiratory alkalosis**, caused by excessive loss of CO_2, lowers the denominator, with an increase in the 20:1 ratio and a resultant rise in pH. In both settings, for patients with normal underlying pulmonary function acute defects can usually be corrected by improving ventilation and avoiding hyperventilation. Compensation for chronic respiratory acid-base disturbances is primarily renal.

ANSWER: A, B, C

19. With regard to metabolic acidosis and alkalosis, which of the following statements is/are true?

A. Metabolic acidosis results from retention of fixed acid or a loss of bicarbonate, which causes a fall in the numerator of the Henderson-Hasselbalch ratio, leading to a ratio of less than 20:1.
B. Metabolic alkalosis results from loss of fixed acid or gain of bicarbonate, causing an increase in the numerator of the Henderson-Hasselbalch ratio and leading to a ratio greater than 20:1.
C. With metabolic acidosis or alkalosis, rapid compensation is brought about by pulmonary mechanisms.
D. With metabolic acidosis or alkalosis, slow compensation occurs via renal mechanisms.

Ref.: 1, 2

COMMENTS: The major effects of metabolic acid-base derangements are exerted on the numerator of the Henderson-Hasselbalch ratio. **Metabolic acidosis** due to retention of fixed acid or loss of bicarbonate causes a fall in the numerator relative to the denominator, a ratio of less than 20:1, and a fall in pH. **Metabolic alkalosis** results from a loss of fixed acid or a gain of bicarbonate, which causes a relative increase in the numerator and produces a ratio of more than 20:1 with an associated rise in pH. Rapid compensation for metabolic acid-base disturbances is provided via pulmonary mechanisms. Increased ventilation compensates for metabolic acidosis; and decreased ventilation compensates for metabolic alkalosis. In both instances, slow compensation is via renal mechanisms, as for respiratory acidosis and respiratory alkalosis.

ANSWER: A, B, C, D

20. With regard to potassium, which of the following statements is/are true?

A. Normal dietary intake of potassium is 50–100 mEq daily.
B. In patients with normal renal function, most ingested potassium is excreted in the urine.
C. More than 90% of potassium in the body is located in the extracellular compartment.
D. Dangerous hyperkalemia (> 6 mEq/L) is rarely encountered if renal function is normal.

Ref.: 1, 2

21. With regard to hyperkalemia, which of the following statements is/are true?

A. Potassium levels up to 8 mEq/L are well tolerated.
B. The most significant complications of hyperkalemia are gastrointestinal.
C. Cation-exchange resins produce the most rapid decrease in serum potassium levels.
D. The definitive treatment of hyperkalemia in patients with compromised renal function is dialysis.

Ref.: 1, 2

COMMENTS: The average daily dietary intake of potassium is 50–100 mEq. In patients with normal renal function and normal serum potassium levels, most ingested potassium is excreted in the urine. More than 90% of the body's potassium is within the intracellular compartment at a concentration of 150 mEq/L. Although the total extracellular potassium concentration is only 50–70 mEq (4.5 mEq/L), this concentration is critical for cardiac and neuromuscular function. Significant quantities of intracellular potassium are released in response to severe injury, surgical stress, acidosis, and a catabolic state; however, dangerous hyperkalemia (> 6 mEq/L) is rarely encountered if renal function is normal. The signs of hyperkalemia are generally limited to cardiovascular and gastrointestinal (GI) symptoms. GI symptoms include nausea, vomiting, intermittent intestinal colic, and diarrhea. Cardiovascular symptoms are electrocardiographic and include high-peaked T waves, a widened QRS complex, and depressed ST segments. These may be seen with potassium concentrations of more than 6 mEq/L. At higher levels of potassium concentration, the T wave may disappear, heart block follows, and diastolic cardiac arrest may ultimately develop. The treatment of hyperkalemia consists of withholding exogenous potassium, correcting the underlying cause, and instituting measures to reduce levels of serum potassium. Sudden, rapid rises can be treated with the infusion of sodium lactate, calcium gluconate, and dextrose-insulin solutions (1 unit/5 gm glucose). Sodium lactate raises the pH and shifts potassium intracellularly; the calcium gluconate counteracts the myocardial effects of hyperkalemia; and the insulin stimulates uptake of dextrose by the cell with concurrent intracellular uptake of potassium. **Exogenous** insulin (used in the ratio described earlier) is clearly indicated in patients who are hyperglycemic. **Endogenous** insulin production may be sufficient in patients with normal glucose metabolism. Selection of the appropriate glucose solution (either 10% or 50%) and the decision of whether to use exogenous insulin is directed toward the avoidance of hyper- or hypoglycemia. Treatment of slow, chronic increases in serum potassium levels can be controlled by the use of cation-exchange resins, such as sodium polystyrene sulfonate (Kayexalate).

ANSWER:
Question 20: A, B, D
Question 21: D

22. With regard to hypokalemia, which of the following statements is/are true?

A. Potassium is in competition with hydrogen ion for renal tubular excretion in exchange for sodium resorption.
B. Tubular excretion of potassium may be increased when large quantities of sodium are available for resorption.
C. Flattening of the T waves and suppression of the ST segments are characteristic electrocardiographic (ECG) changes associated with hypokalemia.
D. Intravenous administration of potassium should never exceed 40–60 mEq/hr.

Ref.: 1, 2

COMMENTS: Surgical patients exhibit hypokalemia more frequently than hyperkalemia. This is the result of excessive renal excretion, prolonged administration of potassium-free parenteral fluids, parenteral hyperalimentation with inadequate potassium replacement, and loss of GI secretions. Some acid-base disturbances, including respiratory and metabolic alkalosis, result in excess excretion. Potassium is in competition with hydrogen ion for renal tubular excretion in exchange for sodium. With alkalosis the potassium ion is preferentially excreted in an attempt to preserve the hydrogen ion. Another setting leading to increased tubular excretion of potassium exists when there is a large quantity of sodium available for resorption from the renal tubule; potassium is exchanged for sodium, and the serum potassium levels fall. The loss of GI fluids can be a significant cause of potassium depletion. This problem is compounded if potassium-free fluids are used for replacement. Signs of potassium deficit are related to failure of contractility of skeletal, smooth, and cardiac muscle. Such signs include paralytic ileus and diminishing or absent tendon reflexes or weakness that may progress to flaccid paralysis. Sensitivity to digitalis and ECG signs of low voltage, such as flattening of the T waves and suppression of ST segments, are characteristic. The best treatment for hypokalemia is prevention. GI losses should be treated by replacement with fluids containing potassium in quantities sufficient to replace the daily obligatory loss (20 mEq/day) as well as the additional loss related to the volume of GI drainage. As general guidelines, no more than 40–60 mEq of potassium should be added to each liter of intravenous fluid; the rate of administration should never exceed 40–60 mEq/hr; the ECG should be monitored during infusion; and potassium administration to the oliguric patient should be withheld during the first 24 hours after severe surgical stress or trauma.

ANSWER: A, B, C, D

23. With regard to calcium metabolism, which of the following statements is/are true?

A. The normal daily intake of calcium is 1–3 gm.
B. Most dietary calcium is excreted in the urine.
C. Nonionized calcium is the portion of serum calcium responsible for neuromuscular stability.
D. Unless there is prolonged immobilization, routine administration of calcium to the surgical patient is not needed in the absence of specific indications.

Ref.: 1, 2

COMMENTS: The body contains approximately 1000–1200 gm of calcium. Most of it is in the bone in the form of calcium carbonate and calcium phosphate. Normal daily intake of calcium is 1–3 gm, most of which is excreted via the GI tract; 200 mg or less is excreted in the urine. Approximately half of the normal serum calcium level (9–11 mg/ml) is nonionized and bound to plasma protein. An additional 5% of nonionized calcium is bound to other substances in the plasma. The remaining 45% is ionized and is the portion responsible for neuromuscular stability. It is therefore important to determine the plasma protein level when assessing serum calcium levels. A drop of 1 gm of protein results in a 0.8 mg/dl decrease in measured total serum calcium. Conversely, total serum calcium *increases* by 0.8 mg/dl for every 1 gm/dl increment of serum albumin above a normal value of 4 gm/dl. The ratio of ionized to nonionized calcium is affected by the pH; acidosis increases and alkalosis decreases the ionized fraction. Routine administration of calcium to the surgical patient is not needed unless there is a specific indication. An exception is the skeletal loss of calcium, which results in hypocalcemia in patients subjected to prolonged immobilization.

ANSWER: A, D

24. With regard to hypocalcemia, which of the following statements is/are true?

A. The symptoms do not develop until serum levels fall below 6 mg/dl.
B. Typical ECG changes include prolongation of the QT interval.
C. Neuromuscular symptoms can occur in patients with normal serum calcium levels.
D. For patients receiving rapid transfusions of blood, calcium should be administered at a dose of 0.2 gm for each 500 ml of blood transfused.

Ref.: 1, 2

COMMENTS: The signs and symptoms of hypocalcemia generally are seen at serum levels of less than 8 mg/dl. The symptoms include numbness and tingling of the circumoral area and in the tips of the fingers and toes. The signs include hyperactive deep tendon reflexes, positive Chvostek's sign, muscle and abdominal cramps, tetany with carpal pedal spasm, convulsions, and prolongation of the QT interval on the ECG. Symptoms may appear with a normal serum calcium level in patients with severe alkalosis as the result of a decrease in the ionized fraction of the total serum calcium. Conversely, hypocalcemia without signs or symptoms may be present in patients with hypoproteinemia and a normal ionized fraction. Common causes of hypocalcemia include acute pancreatitis, necrotizing fasciitis, renal failure, GI fistula, and hypoparathyroidism. (It can transiently develop in patients who have a parathyroid adenoma removed because of atrophy of the remaining glands.) Acute symptoms can be relieved by intravenous administration of calcium gluconate or calcium chloride. Patients requiring prolonged replacement can be treated with oral calcium lactate given with or without vitamin D. At present it is believed that most patients receiving slow, elective blood transfusions do not require calcium supplementation. Citrate binding of ionized calcium is compensated for by mobilization of body stores. An exception is the patient receiving blood rapidly (500 ml over 10 minutes); in this setting, calcium should be replaced at a dose of 0.2 gm per 500 ml of blood transfused. The total calcium dose should not exceed 3 gm unless obvious signs and symptoms of hypocalcemia are present. Under ideal circumstances, calcium replacement should be monitored by measuring the concentration of ionized calcium.

ANSWER: B, C, D

25. With regard to hypercalcemia, which of the following statements is/are true?

A. The symptoms are of GI, renal, musculoskeletal, and central nervous system (CNS) origin.
B. The major causes of hypercalcemia are hyperparathyroidism and cancer with bony metastases.
C. Metastatic prostate cancer is the most common cause of hypercalcemia associated with metastases.
D. Intravenous mithramycin is the treatment of choice for rapid reduction of acute hypercalcemia.

Ref.: 1, 2

COMMENTS: The symptoms of hypercalcemia arise from the GI, renal, musculoskeletal, and central nervous systems. Early symptoms include fatigability, lassitude, weakness, anorexia, nausea, and vomiting. CNS symptoms can progress to stupor and coma. Other symptoms may include headaches and the "three P's": **pain**, **polydipsia**, and **polyuria**. The critical serum calcium level for hypercalcemia is 16–20 mg/ml. Prompt treatment must be instituted at this level; otherwise the symptoms may progress to death. • The two major causes of hypercalcemia are hyperparathyroidism and cancer with bony metastases. Metastatic breast cancer in patients receiving estrogen therapy is the most common cause of hypercalcemia associated with metastases. In many patients there is an associated volume deficit due to vomiting and polyuria. Rapid volume replacement with saline quickly lowers the calcium level by dilution and by increasing renal excretion of calcium (saline diuresis). Renal clearance of calcium can be increased by giving furosemide. Oral or intravenous phosphates are useful for reducing hypercalcemia by inhibiting bone resorption and forming calcium phosphate complexes that are deposited in the soft tissues. Intravenous phosphorus, however, has been associated with acute development of hypocalcemia, hypotension, and renal failure. For this reason, it should be given slowly over 8–12 hours once daily for no more than 2–3 days. Intravenous sodium sulfate is effective but no more so than is saline diuresis. Corticosteroids decrease resorption of calcium from bone and reduce intestinal absorption; thus they are useful for treating patients with sarcoidosis, myeloma, lymphoma, or leukemia who have hypercalcemia. Their effects, however, may not be apparent for 1–2 weeks. • Mithramycin lowers serum calcium in 24–48 hours by direct action on the bones. A single dose may maintain a normal serum calcium level for up to several weeks. • Calcitonin can produce a moderate decrease in serum sodium, but the effect is lost with repeated administration. • Acute hypercalcemic crisis in hyperparathyroidism is treated by immediate corrective operation after the patient is stabilized to the point at which anesthesia can be safely administered.

ANSWER: A, B

26. With regard to magnesium, which of the following statements is/are true?

A. The distribution of nonosseous magnesium is similar to that of potassium.
B. Obligate renal loss is 15–20 mEq/day.
C. Magnesium depletion is characterized by depression of the neuromuscular and central nervous systems.
D. The treatment of choice for magnesium deficiency is the oral administration of magnesium phosphate.

Ref.: 1, 2

COMMENTS: The total body content of magnesium is 2000 mEq, half of which is in bone. Of the remaining magnesium, most is intracellular (a distribution similar to potassium). Plasma levels range between 1.5 and 2.5 mEq/L. Normal dietary intake is 240 mg/day, most of which is excreted in the feces. The kidneys excrete some magnesium and effectively conserve magnesium in the presence of deficiency, excreting less than 1 mEq/day if necessary. Hypomagnesemia is characterized by neuromuscular and central nervous system (CNS) hyperactivity—signs and symptoms similar to those of calcium deficiency. Deficiency is known to occur with starvation, malabsorption, protracted loss of GI fluid, and prolonged parenteral therapy without proper magnesium supplementation. When there is an accompanying calcium deficiency, the latter cannot be successfully treated until the hypomagnesemia is corrected. Magnesium deficiency is treated by parenteral administration of magnesium sulfate or magnesium chloride. In a patient with normal renal function, up to 2 mEq magnesium per kilogram body weight can be given on a daily basis. When large doses of magnesium are given, vital signs and the ECG should be monitored for signs of magnesium toxicity, which can lead to cardiac arrest (increased PR interval, widening QRS, elevated T waves). Magnesium toxicity is treated by infusion of calcium chloride or calcium gluconate. In fact, these substances should be on hand when magnesium is administered intravenously to severely depleted patients. In depleted states, the extracellular concentration can be rapidly restored, but therapy must be continued for 1–2 weeks to replenish the intracellular component. To avoid the development of magnesium deficiency, patients on hyperalimentation should receive 12–24 mEq magnesium daily. Finally, magnesium should not be given to oliguric patients unless magnesium depletion has been demonstrated. Oral supplementation (magnesium oxide 800 mg/day) or intramuscular injection (magnesium sulfate—very painful) are alternative routes for replacement but are not preferred.

ANSWER: A, B

27. With regard to hypermagnesemia, which statements is/are true?

A. It is most commonly seen in patients with severe renal insufficiency.
B. It occasionally occurs in patients with severe alkalosis.
C. The acute symptoms can be controlled by intravenous administration of calcium chloride or calcium gluconate.
D. Persistent symptoms may be an indication for dialysis.

Ref.: 1, 2

COMMENTS: Symptomatic hypermagnesemia is most commonly seen in patients with severe renal insufficiency. The serum magnesium levels tend to *parallel* changes in *potassium* concentration in these cases. The use of magnesium-containing antacids and laxatives can produce symptomatic hypermagnesemia in patients with impaired renal function, and so these drugs should be avoided. Other causes of symptomatic hypermagnesemia include burns, massive trauma, surgical stress, severe extracellular volume deficit, and severe acidosis. The signs and symptoms include lethargy, weakness, and progressive loss of deep tendon reflexes. The ECG changes resemble those seen with hyperkalemia. In extreme cases, somnolence leading to coma and muscular paralysis may occur. Treatment is aimed at correcting any existing acidosis, restoring depleted extracellular volume deficit, and withholding exogenous magnesium. Acute symptoms can be temporarily controlled by the infusion of 5–10 mEq calcium chloride or calcium gluconate. If elevated levels of magnesium or the symptoms persist, peritoneal dialysis or hemodialysis may be required.

ANSWER: A, C, D

28. Regarding water exchange: Please match the item in the left column with the appropriate choice in the right column. Each item in the right column is used only once.

A. Average stool loss	a. 250 ml
B. Average insensible loss	b. 2000–2500 ml
C. Average urine volume	c. 800–1500 ml
D. Daily water consumption	d. 600 ml
E. Percent of daily insensible loss: skin	e. 25%
F. Percent of daily insensible loss: lung	f. 75%

Ref.: 1, 2

COMMENTS: The average individual has an intake of 2000–2500 ml of water per day: 1500 ml is ingested orally and the remainder through solid food. Daily losses include 250 ml in the stool, 800–1500 ml in urine, and approximately 600 ml as insensible loss. To excrete the products of normal daily catabolism, an individual must produce at least 500–800 ml of urine. In normal individuals 75% of insensible loss is through the skin and 25% through the lungs. Insensible loss from the skin is by loss of water vapor through the skin and not the evaporation of water secreted by sweat glands. In febrile patients insensible skin loss may increase to 250 ml per day for each degree of fever. Losses from sweating can be as high as 4 L/hr. In a patient with a tracheostomy who is ventilated with unhumidified air, insensible loss from the lung may increase to 1500 ml per day.

ANSWER: A-a; B-d; C-c; D-b; E-f; F-e

29. With regard to gain and loss of sodium, which of the following statements is/are true?

A. The intake of sodium normally is 50–90 mEq/day.
B. Normal kidneys can reduce sodium loss to less than 1 mEq/day.
C. Sweat represents a hypertonic loss of fluids and sodium.
D. Gastrointestinal losses are usually isotonic or slightly hypotonic.

Ref.: 1, 2

30. Match items in the left column with the *best* choice from the right column. Items in the right column may be used more than once.

A. Stomach secretions	a. High in potassium
B. Saliva	b. High in bicarbonate
C. Pancreatic secretions	c. Hypotonic
D. Sweat	d. Isotonic
E. Duodenal secretions	e. Low sodium, high chloride
F. Ileal secretions	
G. Colonic secretions	

Ref.: 1, 2

COMMENTS: Normal daily salt intake varies from between 50 and 90 mEq sodium chloride; normal kidneys maintain balance and excrete excess salt as it is encountered. Under conditions of reduced intake or increased extrarenal loss, the kidney can reduce sodium excretion to less than 1 mEq/day. Conversely, in patients with nonfunctioning kidneys, sodium loss may be as high as 200 mEq/L of urine. • Knowing the approximate composition of the various body fluids is extremely important. When fluid disorders result from this loss, successful resuscitation depends on proper selection of replacement solutions. This selection is determined by the type of fluid lost in a given clinical situation. • Sweat represents a hypotonic loss of fluids. The average sodium concentration is 15–60 mEq/L. Insensible loss from skin and lungs is pure water. Note that *insensible* skin loss is not the same as water lost from sweat glands. • Although the various gastrointestinal (GI) secretions vary in composition (the more obvious differences are highlighted in Question 30), GI losses are usually isotonic or slightly hypotonic. Pancreatic fluids and bile have high bicarbonate concentrations; stomach, small intestine, and biliary fluids have relatively high chloride concentrations. Duodenal, ileal, pancreatic, and biliary fluids contain levels of sodium that approximate those seen in the plasma. Saliva is relatively high in potassium, a fact important to remember for managing a patient with a salivary fistula.

ANSWER:
Question 29: A, B, D
Question 30: A-e; B-a; C-b; D-c; E-d; F-d; G-d

31. Match the solution in the left column with its appropriate composition in the right column.

A. 0.9% saline	a. 130 mEq sodium, 109 mEq chloride, 28 mEq lactate
B. Lactated Ringer's solution	b. 154 mEq sodium, 154 mEq chloride
C. M/6 Sodium lactate	c. 167 mEq sodium, 167 mEq lactate
D. 3% Sodium chloride	d. 513 mEq sodium, 513 mEq chloride
E. D_5 .45% sodium chloride	e. 77 mEq sodium, 77 mEq chloride

Ref.: 1, 2

COMMENTS: For delivering fluid and electrolyte therapy, the choice of fluids depends on the patient's volume status and the type of fluid and electrolyte abnormality present. Lactated Ringer's solution is an excellent isotonic salt solution for replacing isotonic GI losses and preexisting volume deficits when a patient has normal or near-normal electrolyte levels. Isotonic sodium (0.9% saline) is ideal for the initial correction of depleted extracellular fluid volume associated with hyponatremia, hypochloremia, and metabolic alkalosis. The high chloride concentration may exceed the capacity of the kidney to excrete it and has the potential to cause a dilutional acidosis (remember that chloride is an acid anion that reduces bicarbonate concentrations in relation to carbonic acid content). M/6 Sodium lactate is an alternative fluid for hyponatremic, hypochloremic states associated with moderate metabolic acidosis. Molar sodium lactate or 3% sodium chloride may be useful for rapidly correcting symptomatic hyponatremic states. The choice of lactate or chloride depends on the accompanying acid-base disorder (chloride for alkalosis and lactate for acidosis).

ANSWER: A-b; B-a; C-c; D-d; E-e

32. A 30-year-old 70-kg woman has symptomatic hyponatremia. Her serum sodium level is 120 mEq/L (normal is 140 mEq/L). Her sodium deficit is calculated to be:

A. 500 mEq/L.
B. 600 mEq/L.
C. 700 mEq/L.
D. 800 mEq/L.

Ref.: 1

COMMENTS: Correction of concentration changes depends in part on whether the patient is symptomatic. If symptomatic hypernatremia or hyponatremia is present, attention is focused on prompt correction of the concentration abnormality to the point that symptoms are relieved. Then attention is shifted to correction of the associated volume abnormality. The sodium deficiency in this patient is estimated by multiplying the sodium deficit (normal sodium concentration minus observed sodium concentration) by total body water in liters (60% of body weight in males and 50% of body weight in females). For the patient in question, the calculation is as follows: total body water = 70 kg × 0.5 = 35 liters. Sodium deficit = (140 − 120 mEq/L) × 35 liters = 700 mEq sodium chloride. Initially, half the calculated amount of sodium is infused by means of 3% sodium chloride. The infusion is given slowly. Rapid infusion can be associated with symptomatic hypovolemia. Rapid correction of hyponatremia can be associated with irreversible CNS injury (central pontine and extrapontine myelinolysis). Once symptoms are alleviated, the patient should be reassessed before additional infusion of sodium salt is begun. In cases of profound hyponatremia a correction of no more than 12 mEq/L/24 hr should be achieved. If the original problem was associated with a volume deficit, the remainder of the resuscitation can be accomplished with isotonic fluids (sodium chloride in the presence of alkalosis; M/6 sodium lactate in the presence of acidosis). Care must be taken when hyponatremia associated with volume excess is treated. In this setting, after symptoms are alleviated with a small volume of hypertonic saline, water restriction is the treatment of choice. Infusion of hypertonic saline in this setting (hyponatremia with volume excess) has the potential to further expand extracellular intravascular volume and is contraindicated in patients with severely compromised cardiac reserve. In such a case, peritoneal dialysis or hemodialysis may be preferred for removing excess water.

ANSWER: C

33. True or False: Using 5% dextrose in water for rapid correction of severe symptomatic hypernatremia associated with volume deficit may result in convulsions and coma.

Ref.: 1, 2

COMMENTS: The rapid correction of symptomatic hypernatremia associated with volume deficit can be achieved by slow, cautious infusion of 5% dextrose in water. However, this treatment can cause a rapid reduction in extracellular osmolarity. If this occurs too rapidly, it may cause convulsions and coma. It may therefore be safer to correct the hypernatremia and the volume deficit with half-strength sodium chloride or half-strength lactated Ringer's solution. In the absence of significant volume deficit, hypervolemia may result with the injudicious infusion of water. When treating symptomatic hypernatremia, frequent clinical observation and determination of serum sodium concentrations are mandatory.

ANSWER: True

34. With regard to distributional shifts during an operation, which of the following statements is/are true?

A. Distributional shifts include edema, fluid in the bowel wall and lumen, and fluid in the peritoneal cavity.
B. The surface area of the peritoneum is not great enough to account for significant third space loss.
C. Sequestered extracellular fluid is predominantly isotonic.
D. The formula for replacing intraoperative fluid loss follows strict guidelines based on body weight and serum sodium concentration.
E. Third-space volume losses include evaporative loss from the open wound.

Ref.: 1, 2

35. With regard to intraoperative management of fluids, which of the following statements is/are true?

A. In a healthy person, up to 500 ml of blood loss may be well tolerated without the need for blood replacement.
B. During an operation, the functional extracellular fluid volume relates directly to the volume lost to suction.
C. Functional extracellular fluid losses should be replaced with plasma.
D. Administration of albumin plays an important role in the replacement of functional extracellular fluid volume loss.

Ref.: 1, 2

COMMENTS: The functional extracellular fluid volume decreases during major abdominal operations largely as the result of sequestration of fluid into the operative site as a consequence of (1) extensive dissection, (2) fluid collection within the lumen and wall of the small bowel, and (3) accumulations of fluid in the peritoneal cavity. The surface area of the peritoneum is 1.8 m^2. When irritated, it can account for the functional loss of several liters of fluid that is not readily apparent. It is generally agreed that this lost volume should be replaced during the course of an operation with isotonic saline solution as a "mimic" for sequestered extracellular fluid. Although there is no set formula for intraoperative fluid therapy, useful guidelines for replacement include the following: (1) Blood is replaced as it is lost, regardless of additional fluid therapy. (2) Lost extracellular fluid should be replaced during the operative procedure; delay of replacement until after the operation is complicated by adrenal and hypophyseal compensatory mechanisms that respond to operative trauma during the immediate postoperative period. (3) Approximately 0.5–1.0 liter of fluid per hour is needed during the course of an operation, but only to a *maximum* of 2–3 liters during a 4-hour procedure, unless there are measurable losses. It is now believed that the addition of albumin to blood and extracellular fluid replacement intraoperatively is not indicated and may be potentially harmful. Maintenance of cardiac and pulmonary function by replacing blood with blood products and extracellular fluid with "mimic" solutions can be obtained without the addition of albumin. In general, it is believed that blood should be replaced as it is lost. However, it is usually unnecessary to replace blood loss of less than 500 ml. Operative blood loss is usually underestimated by the operative surgeon by a factor of 15–40% less than when isotopically measured, a factor that may contribute to the detection of anemia during the immediate postoperative period. There is an understandable hesitancy to perform transfusions unless absolutely necessary. In cases involving rapid loss of large volumes of blood, there is not much room for debate. In more controlled situations, careful clinical judgment is needed.

ANSWER:
Question 34: A, C
Question 35: A

36. With regard to postoperative fluid management, which of the following statements is/are true?

A. Insensible loss is approximately 600 ml/day.
B. Insensible loss may increase to 1500 ml/day.
C. About 800–1000 ml of fluid is needed to excrete the catabolic end-products of metabolism.
D. Lost urine should be replaced milliliter for milliliter.
E. Lost gastrointestinal fluids should be replaced milliliter for milliliter.
F. In a healthy individual, potassium administration should be approximately 40 mEq/day to replace renal losses and 20 mEq for each liter of gastrointestinal loss.

Ref.: 1, 2

COMMENTS: Administration of fluids to the postoperative patient begins with an assessment of the patient's volume status and a check for concentration or compositional disorders. Familiarity with the usual routes of fluid loss is of central importance, a point that cannot be repeated too often. All measured and insensible losses should be treated by replacement with appropriate fluids. In patients with normal renal function, the amount of potassium given is 40 mEq daily for replacement of renal excretion. An additional 20 mEq should be given for each liter of gastrointestinal loss. Insensible water loss is usually constant in the range of 600 ml/day; it can be increased to 1500 ml/day by hypermetabolism, hyperventilation, or fever. Insensible loss is replaced with 5% dextrose in water. Insensible loss may be offset by an insensible gain of water from excessive catabolism in postoperative patients who require prolonged intravenous fluid therapy. Approximately 800–1000 ml of fluid per day is needed to excrete the catabolic end-products of metabolism. Because the kidneys are able to conserve sodium in a healthy individual, this can be replaced with 5% dextrose in water. A small amount of salt is usually added, however, to relieve the kidneys of the stress of sodium resorption. If there is a question regarding urinary sodium loss, measurement of urinary sodium helps determine the type of fluid that can best be used. Urine volume should not be replaced milliliter for milliliter, because a high output may represent diuresis of fluids given during operation or the diuresis that takes place to eliminate excessive fluid administration. Sensible or measurable losses such as those from the gastrointestinal tract are usually isotonic and therefore should be treated by replacement in equal volumes with isotonic salt solutions. The type of salt solution selected depends on the determination of serum sodium, potassium, and chloride levels. In general, replacement fluids are administered at a steady rate over 18–24 hours as losses are incurred.

ANSWER: A, B, C, E, F

37. With regard to volume excess in the postoperative patient, which of the following statements is/are true?

A. This situation can be produced by the overadministration of isotonic salt in excess of volume loss.
B. Acute overexpansion of the extracellular fluid space is usually well tolerated in healthy individuals.

C. Avoidance of volume excess requires daily monitoring of intake and output and determinations of serum sodium concentrations to guide accurate fluid administration.
D. The earliest sign of volume excess is peripheral edema.

Ref.: 1, 2

COMMENTS: The earliest sign of volume excess during the postoperative period is **weight gain**. Normally during this period the patient is in a catabolic state and is expected to *lose weight* (¼ to ½ pound per day). Circulatory and pulmonary signs of overload appear late and usually represent a massive overload. Peripheral edema does not necessarily indicate volume excess. In a patient with edema but without additional evidence of volume overload, other causes of peripheral edema should be considered. The commonest cause of volume excess in a surgical patient is administration of isotonic salt solutions in excess of volume loss. In a healthy individual this overload is usually well tolerated; but if excess administration of fluid continues for several days the ability of the kidneys to secrete sodium may be exceeded, and hypernatremia may result.

ANSWER: A, B, C

38. With regard to postoperative hyponatremia, which of the following statements is/are true?

A. It may easily occur when water is used to replace sodium-containing fluids or when the water given exceeds the water lost.
B. In patients with head injury, hyponatremia despite adequate salt administration is usually caused by occult renal dysfunction.
C. In oliguric patients, cellular catabolism with resultant metabolic acidosis increases cellular release of water and can contribute to hyponatremia.
D. Bacterial sepsis may be a cause of hyponatremia.
E. Hyperglycemia may be a cause of hyponatremia.

Ref.: 1, 2

39. A postoperative patient has a serum sodium concentration of 125 mEq/L and a blood glucose level of 500 mg/dl (normal is 100 mg/dl). What would his serum sodium concentration be (assuming normal renal function and appropriate intraoperative fluid therapy) if his blood glucose level were normal?

A. 120 mEq/L.
B. 122 mEq/L.
C. 137 mEq/L.
D. 142 mEq/L.

Ref.: 1, 2

COMMENTS: Abnormalities of sodium concentration during the postoperative period usually do not occur if the functional extracellular fluid volume has been adequately replaced during operation. This is because the kidneys retain the ability to excrete moderate excesses of water and solute administered during the early postoperative period. Hyponatremia does occur when water is given to replace lost sodium-containing fluids or when the water given consistently exceeds water lost. • In patients with head injury, hyponatremia may develop despite adequate salt administration because of excessive secretion of antidiuretic hormone with resultant increased water retention. • Patients with preexisting renal disease and loss of concentrating ability may elaborate urine with a high salt concentration. This salt-wasting phenomenon is commonly encountered in elderly patients. Often is is not anticipated because the blood urea nitrogen and creatinine levels are within normal limits. When there is doubt, determination of urine sodium concentration can help clarify the diagnosis. • Oliguria reduces the daily water requirement and can lead to hyponatremia if not anticipated. • Cellular catabolism in the patient without adequate caloric intake can lead to the gain of significant quantities of water released from the tissues. • Systemic bacterial sepsis is often accompanied by a drop in serum sodium concentration, possibly due to interstitial or intracellular sequestration. It is treated by withholding free water, restoring extracellular fluid volume, and treating the source of sepsis. • Hyperglycemia may produce a depressed serum sodium level by exerting an osmotic force in the extracellular compartment whereby serum sodium levels become diluted. As a general rule, each 100 mg/dl rise in the blood glucose level above normal is equivalent to a 1.6–3.0 mEq/L fall in the apparent serum sodium concentration. As an example, the patient with a blood glucose level of 500 mg/dl has a blood glucose level of 400 mg/dl above normal. This is equivalent to a 12 mEq/L change in the serum sodium level. If, for example, this patient has a measured sodium concentration of 125 mEq/L, he would have in reality a 137 mEq/L concentration of sodium if the excess extracellular water were eliminated.

ANSWER:
Question 38: A, C, D, E
Question 39: C

40. With regard to postoperative hypernatremia, which of the following statements is/are true?

A. Hypernatremia may indicate a deficit of total body water.
B. It may be caused by a high protein intake.
C. Replacement of lost water with isotonic salt solutions can produce hypernatremia.
D. A common cause is excessive extrarenal water loss.

Ref.: 1, 2

COMMENTS: Hypernatremia can easily be produced when renal function is normal. In surgical patients hypernatremia most commonly arises from excessive or unexpected water loss, although it may result from the replacement of lost water with salt-containing solutions. Excessive extrarenal water loss is most often associated with loss of water from excessive sweating and failure to humidify the air used to ventilate patients with a tracheostomy. Another cause of water loss is the presence of granulating surfaces, and this loss may be significant in burn patients. Increased renal water loss results from hypoxic damage to the distal tubules and collecting ducts or from CNS injury causing diabetes insipidus (loss of antidiuretic hormone). High protein intake produces an osmotic load of urea, which necessitates secretion of large volumes of water. This can be avoided by allowing an intake of 7 ml of water per gram of dietary protein. Finally, isotonic salt solutions can produce hypernatremia if they are used to replace pure water loss.

ANSWER: A, B, C, D

41. With regard to high-output renal failure, which of the following statements is/are true?

A. The condition is characterized by uremia without a period of oliguria and a daily urine output of more than 1000–1500 ml/day.
B. Management requires serial measurement of blood urea nitrogen (BUN), serum electrolytes, and daily fluid outputs.
C. Replacement fluid should be administered with sodium chloride to avoid alkalosis.
D. Daily maintenance doses of potassium are given intravenously, because hyperkalemia is unlikely to develop as a result of the high urine output.

Ref.: 1, 2

COMMENTS: High-output renal failure is characterized by uremia that occurs without a period of oliguria and is accompanied by a daily urine output of more than 1000–1500 ml/day. It is managed by monitoring serial measurements of BUN and serum electrolytes, replacing fluids on the basis of these measurements, and accurately measuring the daily fluid output. Because of the kidneys' impaired ability to handle catabolic by-products, mild metabolic acidosis occurs. Therefore, sodium-containing fluids should be administered as lactate (not chloride) to control this metabolic derangement. Severe acidosis may develop if gastrointestinal or renal losses of sodium are replaced as sodium chloride. Despite the high urine output, potassium salt should not be administered unless a precise dose is calculated on the basis of a measured deficit. As little as 20 mEq of potassium given intravenously may produce cardiac side effects. If this happens, hemodialysis may be required. This type of renal dysfunction can occur in patients who experience one or more episodes of hypotension. If the urine output continues after these episodes, normal renal function may be mistakenly assumed. For this reason, administration of potassium during the first 24 hours postoperatively should be withheld unless a potassium deficit definitely exists.

ANSWER: A, B

REFERENCES

1. Sabiston DC Jr: *Textbook of Surgery*, 15th ed. WB Saunders, Philadelphia, 1997.
2. Schwartz SI, Shires GT, Spencer FC: *Principles of Surgery*, 7th ed. McGraw-Hill, New York, 1999.

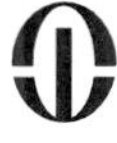

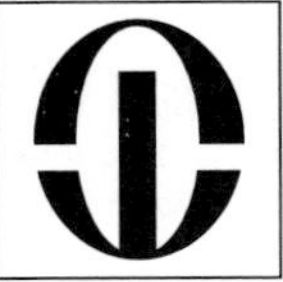

CHAPTER 3

Endocrine and Metabolic Response to Injury

1. Which of the following is the most important stimulus for triggering the endocrine response after injury?

A. Afferent nerve stimuli from the injured area.
B. Hypovolemia.
C. Tissue acidosis.
D. Local wound factors.
E. Temperature changes.

Ref.: 1, 2

COMMENTS: The response to injury involves an integrated series of endocrine and metabolic changes designed to maintain homeostasis; a variety of stimuli are involved in triggering these responses. Of these, one of the earliest and most important stimuli is the signal carried by the afferent sensory nerves from the injured area. This signal directly stimulates release of *adrenocorticotropic hormone* (ACTH) (which begins the adrenocortical response to injury) and elaboration of arginine vasopressin (AVP; formerly called *antidiuretic hormone*, or ADH). ACTH is synthesized and stored in the chromophobe cells of the anterior pituitary. Its release is stimulated by corticotropin-releasing factor (CRF) from the paraventricular nucleus of the hypothalamus. CRF release is induced by the neurogenic inputs (afferent nerve stimuli) generated by injury. This hormonal response can be ablated experimentally by division of the peripheral nerves to the injured area, and it may be diminished clinically in patients with spinal anesthesia. It is for this reason that paraplegic patients show a diminished corticosteroid response to injuries below the level of cord transection. Perception of injury need not be conscious. Individuals under general anesthesia are able to respond to stimuli present during injury.

ANSWER: A

2. In addition to decreased effective circulatory volume, which of the following can stimulate the reflexes associated with injury?

A. Oxygen, carbon dioxide, and hydrogen ion concentration.
B. Emotional arousal.
C. Hypoglycemia.
D. Alteration in body temperature.
E. Local response to wounds.

Ref.: 1, 2

COMMENTS: Although nearly all injuries are associated with loss of effective circulatory volume, which initiates the events previously discussed, there are stimuli other than hypovolemia and pain that are capable of initiating many of the reflexes associated with injury. Hypoxemia, hypercarbia, and acidosis are events sensed by chemoreceptors located in the carotid and aortic bodies. Activation of these receptors stimulates the hypothalamus and sympathetic nervous system and inhibits the parasympathetic nervous system. There is a resultant tachycardia and increased cardiac contractility. The respiratory rate increases, and ACTH and AVP release is stimulated. Hypoxemia potentiates the response to hypovolemia, and hyperventilation often accompanies these events. The perception or threat of possible injury, acting via the limbic system, affects the hypothalamus and stimulates secretion of injury-related hormones such as AVP, ACTH, cortisol, catecholamines, and aldosterone. Hypoglycemia acting via central and autonomic pathways stimulates the release of these same injury-related hormones. The inflammatory cells that accumulate and become activated in the environment around wounds can exert systemic effects that can stimulate a neurohormonal response such as those described above. Exotoxin (from gram-positive bacteria) and endotoxin (from gram-negative bacteria) can activate such substances as interleukin-1 and tissue necrosis factor and can stimulate the release of ACTH.

ANSWER: A, B, C, D, E

3. Please match the items in the left column with the appropriate items in the right column B.

Area	***Activity***
A. Posterior hypothalamic area	a. Controls ACTH and sympathetic activity
B. Paraventricular nucleus	b. Controls arginine vasopressin (AVP), oxytocin, and ACTH
C. Ventromedial nucleus	c. Controls growth hormone and ACTH
D. Arcuate nucleus	d. Controls gonadotropic releasing hormones
E. Supraoptic nucleus	e. Controls AVP and oxytocin
F. Superchiasmic nucleus	f. Controls circadian rhythms of ACTH and gonadotropins

Ref.: 1, 2

COMMENTS: The afferent impulses stimulated by injury act via input into various hypothalamic nuclei (refer to Question 3). The response to injury is variable and depends on the type of injury, its duration, and its severity. It is not an all-or-none phenomenon, and physiologic potentiation is common. An example of this potentiation is baroreceptor responsiveness to hypovolemia. Hypovolemia increases baroreceptor responsiveness, which initiates catecholamine release. Catecholamines, in turn, increase baroreceptor responsiveness.

ANSWER: A-a; B-b; C-c; D-d; E-e, F-f

4. True or False: The "fight or flight" response described by W. B. Cannon is a sympathetic event mediated by catecholamines.

Ref.: 1, 2

COMMENTS: The "fight or flight" response to danger or pain is an event mediated primarily by the sympathetic nervous system and catecholamines. It includes sweating, tremor, tachycardia, dry mouth, and pallor. This is in contrast to the vasovagal response mediated by the parasympathetic nervous system, which includes bradycardia and increased salivation.

ANSWER: True

5. With regard to the mediators of the response to injury, which of the following statements is/are true?

A. Steroid hormones interact only with cell surface receptors.
B. Peptide and amine hormones originally bind to cytosolic receptors in target cells.
C. The action of steroid hormones is faster and of shorter duration than the action of peptide hormones.
D. Peptide hormones act primarily via the second messenger system.
E. Cyclic adenosine monophosphate (cAMP) and calcium are the second messengers.

Ref.: 1, 2

COMMENTS: See Question 6.

6. True or False: G-proteins bind steroid hormones to the nuclear envelope.

Ref.: 1, 2

COMMENTS: Steroid hormones bind to cytosolic receptors. The receptor–steroid complex passes to the nucleus, where it binds to the nonhistone protein of nuclear chromatin, whereby it modulates the transcription of specific messenger RNA and ultimately the synthesis of effector proteins. This is why there is a 1- to 2-hour delay in the onset of action for most steroid hormones. Peptide hormones, in contrast, bind to cell surface receptors coupled to guanine nucleotide-binding proteins (G-proteins), causing alteration in the intracellular concentration of either cAMP or calcium, the so-called second messengers. Their onset of action is faster and of shorter duration than for steroid hormones; the second messengers activate or inactivate existing regulatory proteins and enzymes rather than initiate the synthesis of new proteins. G-proteins coupled to adenylate cyclase increase cAMP. G-proteins coupled to phospholipase C produce either diacylglycerol (DAG) or inositol triphosphate (IP_3). DAG activates protein kinase C, which in turn opens membrane calcium channels. IP_3 acts on the endoplasmic reticulum to release intracellular calcium. The free calcium binds to calmodulin, a calcium-binding protein that activates phosphorylase kinase, the final step in activating the target enzyme. The actions of cAMP and Ca^{2+} in the coupling of receptor activation with hormonal action is known as stimulus-response coupling.

ANSWER:
Question 5: D, E
Question 6: False

7. With regard to catecholamines, which of the following statements is/are true?

A. Catecholamine levels increase immediately after injury.
B. Catecholamine levels peak 24–48 hours after injury.
C. Epinephrine generally reflects the activity of the sympathetic nervous system.
D. Norepinephrine generally reflects the activity of the adrenal medulla.

Ref.: 1, 2

COMMENTS: Catecholamines include norepinephrine and epinephrine. Norepinephrine is released from sympathetic postganglionic neurons. Epinephrine is secreted by the adrenal medulla as a hormone acting at local and distant sites. The effects of catecholamines differ according to target cell receptor types. Plasma catecholamine levels after injury are correlated most closely with the volume of blood lost. There is a considerable psychological component that affects these levels, depending on the mechanisms of injury. Levels rise immediately and peak within 24–48 hours. In general, changes in norepinephrine reflect changes in the activity of the sympathetic nervous system, whereas changes in epinephrine reflect the activity of the adrenal medulla. Their actions, mediated by α- and β-adrenergic receptors, are primarily metabolic and hemodynamic. Epinephrine plays a major role in stress-induced hyperglycemia by increasing glucose production in the liver and decreasing glucose uptake in the periphery. Epinephrine and norepinephrine cause increased secretion of glucagon (from pancreatic alpha islet cells) and decreased secretion of insulin (from pancreatic beta islet cells). Hemodynamic effects include α_1-mediated vasoconstriction, β_2-mediated arterial vasodilatation, and β_1 receptor-mediated increases in heart rate, conductivity, and contractility. The effects are dose-dependent: Those of low-dose epinephrine are primarily β_1- and β_2-mediated, whereas those of high-dose epinephrine are primarily α_1-mediated.

ANSWER: A, B

8. Which of the following substances is/are elevated during the acute response to injury?

A. Glucagon.
B. Glucocorticoids.
C. Catecholamines.
D. Insulin.
E. Thyroid-stimulating hormone (TSH).

Ref.: 1, 2

COMMENTS: After injury, pain and hypovolemia are the primary stimuli that produce the subsequent neurohormonal events aimed at restoring hemodynamic stability and providing readily available energy substrates. Direct stimulation of the hypothalamic-pituitary axis results in prompt increases in circulating ACTH, cortisol, AVP, and growth hormone. Hypothalamic signals also result in sympathetic autonomic nerve stimulation that leads to the release of epinephrine and norepinephrine from the adrenal medulla and the sympathetic nerve endings themselves. • The catecholamines modulate glucagon (from pancreatic alpha islet cells) and insulin (from pancreatic beta islet cells) secretion via α- and β-adrenergic receptor stimulation (not related to the "alpha" and "beta" designation for islet cells). α-Adrenergic receptors mediate inhibition, whereas β-adrenergic receptors mediate stimulation of glucagon and insulin secretion. The alpha islet cell (the source of glucagon) is relatively rich in β-adrenergic (stimulatory) receptors; therefore the predominant response to adrenergic stimulation is glucagon secretion. The beta islet cell (the source of insulin) is relatively rich in α-adrenergic (inhibitory) receptors, and its response to adrenergic stimulation is inhibition of insulin secretion. This is one reason why the hyperglycemia observed with acute injury does not elicit a reflex insulin response. Elevated TSH levels are not thought to play an important role in the acute response to injury.

ANSWER: A, B, C

9. True or False: The neuroendocrine changes initiated by a loss of blood volume are proportional to the magnitude of the volume loss.

Ref.: 1, 2

COMMENTS: The neuroendocrine and cardiovascular changes in response to volume loss are proportional to the magnitude of the loss. Maximal response, however, is achieved when the volume is decreased by 30–40%.

ANSWER: True

10. True or False: The *rate* of change in volume loss is not an important parameter determining the neuroendocrine response to hypovolemia.

Ref.: 1, 2

COMMENTS: For small hemorrhages (10–20%) of blood volume, the neuroendocrine response is independent of the rate of hemorrhage. However, for larger volume losses (−20%), the rate of hemorrhage does affect response. Rapid losses are not as well tolerated as slow losses.

ANSWER: False

11. Hypothalamically mediated responses to hemorrhagic shock include production of which of the following substances?

A. ACTH.
B. AVP (arginine vasopressin, ADH).
C. Somatostatin.
D. Growth hormone.
E. Aldosterone.

Ref.: 1, 2

COMMENTS: When acute blood loss occurs, the decrease in the effective circulating volume activates high-pressure baroreceptors (in the aorta, carotid arteries, and renal arteries) and low-pressure stretch receptors (in the left atrium), which set into motion a series of compensatory responses. The pressure and stretch receptors exert a tonic inhibitory effect on the neuroendocrine system. Volume loss causes release or inactivation of this effect, initiating the compensatory cascade. Receptor activity exerts its effect via direct hypothalamic stimulation resulting in increases in ACTH, AVP, and growth hormone levels. AVP is synthesized in the hypothalamus and stored in the neurohypophysis. In addition to changes in the effective circulating volume, an increase in plasma osmolality is a major stimulus for its release. Other stimulators of ACTH activity are pain, catecholamines, angiotensin II, and cortisol. Its actions are *osmoregulatory* (via resorption of solute free water from the distal convoluted tubules and collecting ducts), *vasoactive* (via peripheral vasoconstriction, especially in the splanchnic bed), and *metabolic* (stimulating hepatic glycogenolysis and gluconeogenesis). Growth hormone is synthesized and released from acidophilic cells of the adenohypophysis. Decreased effective circulating volume causes its release after injury. It has many metabolic actions that lead to an increase in plasma glucose. One of the most important responses to hypovolemia is the release of aldosterone. Aldosterone is synthesized in the adrenal zona glomerulosa. It is released in response to a number of stimuli. The two important stimuli for its release after injury are ACTH and angiotensin II. ACTH stimulation is a calcium/cAMP-dependent event that is short-lived. Angiotensin II stimulation is a calcium-dependent, cAMP-independent event and is most important during injury. Generation of angiotensin II is the result of activation of the renin-angiotensin system by stimulation of the juxtaglomerular cells as a result of decreased renal arterial perfusion. ACTH is elevated as a result of hypothalamic stimulation in hypovolemic shock. Aldosterone increases Na^+ and Cl^- resorption in the early distal convoluted tubule and promotes Na^+ resorption and K^+ excretion in the late distal convoluted tubule and collecting ducts. Water follows the sodium, and the net effect is an increase in intravascular volume.

ANSWER: A, B, D, E

12. True or False: There are many stimuli associated with injury and many areas where input can be registered, but the afferent (output) arm of the injury response is under local tissue control.

Ref.: 1, 2

COMMENTS: There are several arms to the efferent limb of the neuroendocrine response to injury. The endocrine response includes hormones under hypothalamic-pituitary control (cortisol, thyroxine, growth hormone, AVP) and hormones under autonomic control (catecholamines, insulin, glucagon). Local tissue response includes release of cytokines such as the interleukins, tissue necrosis factor, and eicosanoids. Vascular endothelium can respond by releasing endothelial cell mediators including nitric oxide, endothelins, and prostaglandins.

ANSWER: False

13. Match the hormones in the left-hand column with their site of production in the right-hand column.

A. Growth hormone	a. Chromophobe cells anterior pituitary
B. Cortisol	b. Adrenal zona fasciculata
C. ACTH	c. Acidophilic cells anterior pituitary
D. Follicle-stimulating hormone/luteinizing hormone (FSH/LH)	d. Supraoptic and paraventricular nuclei
E. AVP	e. Basophilic cells anterior pituitary

14. Which of the following statements is/are true?

A. The cumulative effect of cortisol is "insulin like."
B. Peripheral conversion of thyroxine (T_4) to triiodothyronine (T_3) increases with injury.
C. Somatostatin potentiates growth hormone release.
D. Primary function of growth hormone is to promote protein synthesis.

Ref.: 1, 2

COMMENTS: The chromophobe cells of the anterior pituitary synthesize and store ACTH. It is stored as a large molecule, propiomelanocortin (POMC). This large molecule also contains γ- and β-lipotropin, α-melanocyte-stimulating hormone (αMSH), and β-endorphins. ACTH is responsible for stimulating the release of cortisol from the adrenal zona fasciculata. Cortisol's primary role is to maintain euglycemia during stress and injury. It has widespread effects on metabolism and the utilization of glucose, amino acids, and fatty acids. In the liver, cortisol stimulates gluconeogenic activity. In skeletal muscle it inhibits insulin-mediated glucose uptake. Cortisol inhibits amino acid uptake and stimulates amino acid release. In adipose tissue, cortisol stimulates lypolysis and decreases glucose uptake. Cortisol also exerts immunologic and inflammatory effects. It causes demargination of white blood cells and suppresses leukocyte synthesis of the cytokines associated with inflammation. Cortisol inhibits phospholipase A_2, limiting the production of prostaglandins and leukotrienes. • Peripheral conversion of T_4 to T_3 is impaired following injury, burns, and surgery, leading to reduced circulating concentrations of both free and total T_3. This is a cortisol-mediated event and decreases the metabolic impact thyroid hormone plays during injury. • Growth hormone is synthesized, stored, and released from acidophylic cells of the anterior pituitary. It exerts a direct action as growth hormone and secondarily due to release of insulin-like growth factors 1 and 2 (IGF-1 and IGF-2), formerly called somatomedins. Secretion of growth hormone is stimulated by a variety of factors including α-adrenergic stimulation, thyroxine, AVP, ACTH, αMSH, glucagon, and testosterone. Its release is suppressed by somatostatin, β-adrenergic stimulation, cortisol, hyperglycemia, and increased plasma fatty acid concentration. The primary action of growth hormone during stress is to promote protein synthesis (IGF-1-mediated) and enhance breakdown of lipid and carbohydrates. Plasma concentrations of growth hormone increase following injury, hemorrhage, and operative stress.

ANSWER:
Question 13: A-c; B-b; C-a; D-e; E-d.
Question 14: D

15. Which of the following is/are true?

A. Suppression of gonadotropic hormones is the cause of posttraumatic amenorrhea.
B. Prolactin inhibits T cell function.
C. Exogenous opioids act via a single receptor.
D. Head injury can cause both diabetes insipidus and syndrome of inappropriate secretion of ADH (SIADH).

Ref.: 1, 2

COMMENTS: Follicle-stimulating hormone (FSH) and luteinizing hormone (LH) are synthesized and stored by the basophilic cells of the anterior pituitary. Their secretion is suppressed after injury, which is responsible for the menstrual dysfunction and decreased libido observed after injury. • Prolactin is synthesized and released by acidophilic cells of the anterior pituitary. It acts metabolically to produce increased nitrogen retention and increased lipid mobilization. It also has been shown to stimulate T cell function. The importance of prolactin action following injury is not well understood. • Endogenous opioids arise from precursors whose secretion increases during the response to injury. ACTH is secreted as a large protein complex that includes β-endorphin activity. Endogenous opioids act on several receptors and exert multiple effects, as none shows complete specificity for a single receptor type. The endogenous opioids exert an analgesic effect and have cardiovascular, metabolic, and immunologic actions. β-Endorphin is hypotensive. The enkephalins are associated with hypertension. β-Endorphin is associated with hyperglycemia. Some opioid peptides have the ability to suppress immunologic function. Their precise actions in response to hemorrhage and sepsis are still under investigation. • Arginine vasopressin (AVP; formerly called antidiuretic hormone, or ADH) arises from the supraoptic and paraventricular nuclei of the anterior hypothalamus and is stored in the posterior pituitary. Primary stimulus for its secretion is increased plasma osmolality. Its release is enhanced by β-adrenergic and angiotensin II stimulation. Its actions are classified as osmoregulatory, vasoactive, and metabolic. It mediates resorption of solute-free water in the distal tubules and collecting ducts. It mediates peripheral vasoconstriction particularly in the splanchnic bed. It stimulates hepatic glycogenolysis and gluconeogenesis. Head injury can be associated with inappropriately high secretion (known as syndrome of inappropriate ADH secretion, SIADH) and can, conversely, also cause lack of its secretion, leading to diabetes insipidus (resulting from damage to the supraoptic hypophyseal system).

ANSWER: A, D

16. Metabolic effects of the neuroendocrine response to injury include which of the following events?

A. Gluconeogenesis.
B. Glycogen synthesis.
C. Lipolysis.
D. Proteolysis.
E. Hypoglycemia.

Ref.: 1, 2

COMMENTS: Glucose is the primary fuel for vital organs, such as the heart, peripheral nerves, renal medulla, red blood cells, and leukocytes. For the human organism to survive serious injury, a ready supply of glucose must be made available; this condition constitutes a critical effect of the many neurohormonal changes observed after injury. The supply of hepatic glucose stored as glycogen is rapidly depleted, and so glucose must be obtained from other sources. Gluconeogenesis occurs through the use of alanine and other amino acids generated from breakdown of skeletal muscle (proteolysis), glycerol derived from the breakdown of triglycerides in body fat (lipolysis), or lactate and pyruvate formed as a result of anaerobic glycolysis of glucose. In addition, glucose entry into cells is impaired by the action of catecholamines and cortisol and by the decrease in serum insulin; this impairment produces hyperglycemia rather than hypoglycemia.

ANSWER: A, C, D

17. Which of the following statements is/are true?

A. Insulin levels are elevated during the early phase of injury.

B. The postinjury elevation of insulin is mediated by epinephrine.
C. Serum glucose levels in the injured patient relate directly to insulin levels.
D. Serum insulin levels correlate well with the degree of injury.
E. The insulin/glucose level is a better predictor of survival than either level alone.

Ref.: 1, 2

COMMENTS: After injury there is initial suppression of insulin secretion mediated by catecholamines and sympathetic nervous system activity, followed by a period of normal or slightly increased secretion. Injury produces peripheral block of insulin action; therefore hyperglycemia can occur in the presence of a normal insulin level. The insulin/glucose ratio is a better predictor of survival than the insulin or glucose level alone.

ANSWER: E

18. Which of the following statements is/are true?

A. Insulin is the body's primary anabolic hormone.
B. Cortisol exerts its effect on insulin by direct action on the beta islet cells of the pancreas.
C. β-Endorphins contribute to stress-induced hyperglycemia by interfering with the peripheral action of insulin.
D. Insulin exerts its metabolic effects via carbohydrate, fatty acid, and amino acid metabolism.

Ref.: 1, 2

COMMENTS: Insulin is secreted by beta islet cells of the pancreas. Substrates that increase its secretion include glucose, amino acids, free fatty acids, and ketone bodies. Normally glucose is the most important stimulant. Sympathetic nervous cell stimulation and epinephrine secretion inhibit insulin secretion in the presence of hyperglycemia. Glucagon, somatostatin, β-endorphin, and interleukin-1 (IL-1) also inhibit insulin secretion via their effects on beta islet cells. Cortisol, estrogen, and progesterone enhance injury-related hyperglycemia by interfering with the peripheral action of insulin. Insulin is an anabolic hormone promoting storage of carbohydrates, proteins, and lipids. Carbohydrate effects include stimulation of glucose transfer into cells, stimulation of gluconeogenesis and glycolysis, and inhibition of hepatic gluconeogenesis. Insulin stimulates lipid synthesis and inhibits lipid degradation. Insulin promotes protein synthesis by increasing amino acid transfer into the liver and peripheral tissues and by inhibiting gluconeogenesis and amino acid oxidation.

ANSWER: A, D

19. Which of the following statements is/are true?

A. Major stimulants for secretion of glucagon include glucose, amino acids, and exercise.
B. Glucagon effects are inhibited by cortisol.
C. Glucagon plays a major role in the development of postinjury hyperglycemia.
D. Somatostatin potentiates glucagon effects.

Ref.: 1, 2

COMMENTS: Glucagon originates from the alpha islet cells of the pancreas. Its normal stimuli are glucose, amino acids, and exercise. Hypoglycemia causes its release, as does sympathetic nervous system α-adrenergic stimulation. Parasympathetic and β-adrenergic input inhibits its secretion. Glucagon stimulates glucogenolysis, gluconeogenesis, and ketogenesis in the liver. Its effects on hepatic carbohydrate metabolism are potentiated by cortisol. Although glucagon levels increase after injury, glucagon does not play an important part in postinjury hyperglycemia. Somatostatin is synthesized in delta islet cells and in central and peripheral neurons. It is an inhibitor of growth hormone, TSH, renin, insulin, and glucagon release.

ANSWER: A

20. Match the items in the left-hand column with the appropriate choice in the right-hand column. Items in the right column may be used more than once.

A. C-reactive protein	a. With copper, helps clear oxygen-free radicals
B. Ceruloplasmin	b. Protease inhibitor
C. α_1-Antitrypsin	c. Functions as an opsonin and complement activator
D. α_2-Macroglobulin	

Ref.: 1, 2

COMMENTS: See Question 21.

21. Which of the following items is/are true?

A. Both IL-1 and IL-2 act primarily as immunostimulants.
B. IL-2 is used to generate lymphokine-activated killer cells.
C. IL-6 is released from the anterior hypothalamus.
D. IL-6 is responsible primarily for splanchnic vasoconstriction.

Ref.: 1, 2

COMMENTS: Cells are capable of releasing a number of factors that participate in the response to injury, including cytokines, eicosanoids, and endothelial cell factors. Cytokines are primarily involved in cell-to-cell (paracrine) functions; however, some exert distant (hormonal) effects. Those that affect immune function are termed lymphokines and include primarily the interleukins, tissue necrosis factor (TNF), and the interferons. IL-1 activity is mediated by IL-1α and IL-1β and has a broad range of activities. IL-1 augments T cell proliferation. It induces fever by stimulating local release of prostaglandins in the anterior hypothalamus. Other centrally mediated effects include induction of anorexia, lessening pain perception (by increasing β-endorphin release), and increasing the basal metabolic rate and oxygen consumption. Together with IL-6, TNF, and interferon, IL-1 promotes synthesis of hepatic acute-phase proteins (ceruloplasmin, fibrinogen, haptoglobin, C-reactive protein, complement factors, α_1-antitrypsin and α_2-macroglobulin). IL-1 also promotes the breakdown of skeletal muscle into amino acids, some of which are oxidized and others are used by the liver for protein synthesis. The IL-1 effect on carbohydrate metabolism is a mild hyperglycemic response. IL-2 is the true lymphokine, acting mainly as an immunostimulant. Antigen stimulation of lymphocytes triggers its release. IL-2 is used to generate lymphokine-activated killer cells. IL-6 is a family of glycoproteins whose role is to enhance immune function and (with IL-1) to promote hepatic protein synthesis. Surgical stress, virus, bacterial products, and cytokines IL-1 and TNF cause its release by monocytes, fibroblasts, and endothelial cells.

ANSWER:
Question 20: A-c; B-a; C-b; D-b
Question 21: B

22. Which of the following statements is/are true?

A. TNF is also known as anabolin.
B. Interferon is released by macrophages.
C. TNF and interferon have similar effects.
D. TNF is active in dimer, trimer, and pentamer forms.

Ref.: 1, 2

COMMENTS: Tissue necrosis factor (TNF, cachectin) is produced as a pro-TNF molecule and undergoes proteolysis into dimer, trimer, and pentamer forms. Its production is stimulated by complement activation. Many cells can produce TNF, including monocytes, macrophages, Kupffer cells, mast cells, and endothelial cells. TNF acts with IL-1 to produce hypotension, tissue necrosis, and death. It causes prostaglandin E_2 (PGE_2) release and is cytotoxic for beta islet cells. TNF and IL-2 induce eicosanoids and platelet-activating factor. TNF may mediate the early phase, and IL-2 the late phase, of hypotension associated with sepsis. Interferon γ is a glycoprotein released by T lymphocytes. It activates macrophages to release IL-1 and TNF, increases monocyte IL-2 expression, and inhibits viral replication. It inhibits PGE_2 release, thereby reducing the immunosuppressive effects of PGE_2 secretion.

ANSWER: D

23. Which of the following is/are true?

A. Eicosanoids are known as the glycoprotein mediators of shock.
B. Eicosanoids are derived from arachidonic acid.
C. Eicosanoids are stored in hepatic Kupffer cells.
D. Eicosanoids include thromboxane and prostaglandins.

Ref.: 1, 2

COMMENTS: Eicosanoids, the lipid mediators of shock, are derived from arachidonic acid and are secreted by all enucleated cells except lymphocytes. Stimuli for their secretion include hypoxia, ischemia, injury, fibrinogens, endotoxin, norepinephrine, AVP, angiotensin II, bradykinin, serotonin, and histamine. The creation of eicosanoids begins with the action of the enzyme phosphorylase A on precursor fatty acids to form arachidonic acid. This enzyme is activated by epinephrine, angiotensin II, bradykinin, histamine, and thrombin; it is inhibited by lipocortin. Eicosanoids, which include prostaglandins, thromboxane, and leukotrienes, are created from arachidonic acid by the activity of cyclooxygenase, thromboxane synthetase, and lipoxygenase, respectively. The eicosanoids are not stored but are released de novo, and their effects depend on what stimulates their production and what cells produce them. Examples include vascular endothelial cell production of prostacyclin (PGI_2) by the action of prostacycline synthetase on arachidonic acid. This substance produces vasodilatation. Platelets use thromboxane synthetase to convert prostaglandin to thromboxane A_2 (TxA_2), a vasoconstrictor and platelet-aggregating stimulator. Leukotrienes include the slow-releasing substance of anaphylaxis; they produce capillary leakage, bronchospasm, and vasoconstriction. Prostaglandins are the major component of the inflammatory response: Eicosanoids have been proposed as the cause of adult respiratory distress syndrome (ARDS), pancreatitis, and some forms of renal failure. β-Kinin release is stimulated by hypoxia and ischemia. The kinins are vasodilators and produce capillary leakage, edema, pain, and bronchospasm.

ANSWER: B, D

24. True or false: Although the endothelium can elaborate a number of active substances, the endothelial mass is small, limiting its effect on the body's response to injury.

Ref.: 1, 2

COMMENTS: The endothelial cell mass is large, approximately 1.5 kg in weight and 400 square meters in surface area. The endothelium secretes substances whose primary action is vasomotor regulation and regulation of coagulation. Endothelium derived relaxing factor (EDRF) acts through the release of nitrous oxide (NO). NO production is dependent on L-arginine. The compound EDRF–NO is a potent vasodilator. Endothelins, which are produced in response to injury, counteract this vasodilatory effect. They are 21-amino-acid peptides and are 10 times more potent than angiotensin II. Endothelial cells also produce prostacyclin and PGE_2. These products promote vasodilatation and reduce platelet aggregation. Release of platelet-activating factor (PAF) from endothelial cells is stimulated by TNF, IL-1, AVP, and angiotensin II. PAF causes platelets to produce TxA_2 and increases endothelial cell permeability to albumin. PAF may mediate the hemodynamic and metabolic effects of endotoxin. Atrial natriuretic peptides (ANP) are released by atrial tissue in response to volume change. ANP is a potent inhibitor of aldosterone.

ANSWER: False

25. In which of the following situations is ACTH release not inhibited by high plasma cortisol levels?

A. Somatic pain.
B. Severe hypovolemia.
C. Sequential injury or operations.
D. Cushing's disease.
E. Endotoxic shock.

Ref.: 2

COMMENTS: The pituitary-adrenal axis is normally under control of a negative feedback mechanism, wherein increased cortisol levels inhibit further release of ACTH. This mechanism is operable in most situations of simple trauma, in which various stimuli lead to ACTH release. Important exceptions are severe hypovolemia and scenarios involving sequential traumatic events or sequential operations; in such settings, ACTH release is not cortisol-suppressible. The mechanism of this physiologic facilitation, termed *feed forward*, is not known. The secondary cortisol responses are often greater than the initial response (a phenomenon known as potentiation). Stimulation of ACTH persists until the intravascular volume has been replenished. Lack of ACTH suppression by cortisol is also seen in the nontraumatic condition of Cushing's disease as the result of ACTH production by a pituitary adenoma.

ANSWER: B, C, D

26. Chronic adrenal insufficiency is characterized by which of the following?

A. Hypothermia.
B. Hypertension.

C. Hyperkalemia.
D. Hyponatremia.
E. Hyperglycemia.

Ref.: 1, 2

COMMENTS: Adrenocortical response is a critical mechanism of survival in situations of shock, trauma, or sepsis. When endogenous corticosteroid production is impaired and exogenous replacement insufficient, profound cardiovascular collapse occurs. **Acute adrenal insufficiency** may result from bilateral adrenal hemorrhage (caused by severe sepsis or anticoagulation or occurring spontaneously), adrenalectomy, or, in particular, withdrawal of exogenous steroids that have been administered for a long time. **Chronic adrenal insufficiency** may result from autoimmune destruction of the adrenal glands or, less commonly, from tuberculous or fungal disease. The clinical manifestations of chronic adrenal insufficiency are those of combined mineralocorticoid and glucocorticoid deficiency. Characteristically, patients with chronic adrenal insufficiency have hyperpigmentation, weakness, weight loss, gastrointestinal symptoms, hyperkalemia, hyponatremia, and hypoglycemia. In injured patients with adrenal insufficiency, hyperkalemia, hyponatremia, and hypoglycemia predominate. The hyponatremia and hyperkalemia are a result of the loss of the sodium-retaining and kaliuretic properties of aldosterone. The hypoglycemia results from the loss of cortisol's effect on hepatic glucose production. Fever and hypotension are the most prominent features of acute adrenal insufficiency. Adrenal insufficiency must be recognized and promptly treated with exogenous supplementation; otherwise, affected patients may die as a result of any medically stressful situation, such as an operation, an injury, or an infection.

ANSWER: C, D

27. Death after severe injury often is the result of which of the following events?

A. Adrenal failure.
B. Respiratory failure.
C. Renal failure.
D. All of the above.

Ref.: 1, 2

COMMENTS: Death after injury does not result from adrenal exhaustion, except in patients with underlying insufficiency or those in whom acute adrenal failure develops during the course of their illness. Severe illness or injury is characterized by marked adrenocortical stimulation and release of cortisol under the control of ACTH. ACTH acts on the cells of the zona fasciculata via cAMP. Plasma levels of corticosteroids and their metabolites are elevated in these patients, and the normal circadian rhythm is lost. Levels remain elevated for up to 4 weeks after burns, 1 week after soft tissue injury, and a few days after hemorrhage. With pure hypovolemia, cortisol levels quickly return to normal when the patient becomes euvolemic. During recovery, plasma corticosteroid levels decline; a persistent elevation suggests ongoing injury or sepsis and is a bad prognostic sign. Death after critical illness often involves multisystem organ failure, particularly pulmonary and renal decompensation.

ANSWER: B, C

28. Which of the following processes is/are important in the restoration of blood volume after hypovolemia?

A. Transcapillary refill.
B. Increased interstitial osmolality.
C. Decreased interstitial osmolality.
D. Hepatic albumin synthesis.

Ref.: 1, 2

COMMENTS: Reduction of blood volume by 15–20% decreases capillary pressure and results in an initial shift of protein-free fluid from the interstitium back into the vascular compartments. This mechanism only partially compensates the volume loss, however, and is limited by the equilibrium established between intravascular oncotic pressure and interstitial fluid pressure. Further restoration of the intravascular volume depends on increases in plasma proteins, primarily albumin. This albumin comes from the interstitium itself but can be moved across capillary membranes into the vascular system only if the interstitial pressure (relative to the intravascular pressure) is adequate. Critical to increasing interstitial pressure to accomplish this is an increase in the extracellular interstitial osmolality that occurs after injury. This metabolic effect is the result of numerous hormonal influences, especially that of cortisol.

ANSWER: A, B

29. With regard to the renin-angiotensin system, which of the following statements is/are true?

A. Renin is an enzyme originating from the juxtaglomerular apparatus of the kidney.
B. Angiotensinogen is a potent vasoconstrictor synthesized in the liver.
C. Angiotensin I is converted to angiotensin II primarily in the kidney.
D. Angiotensin II stimulates aldosterone release from the adrenal cortex.
E. Aldosterone increases sodium resorption in the distal renal tubule.

Ref.: 2

30. Match each relation described in the left column to the appropriate physiologic effect in the right column.

A. Effect of decreased renal artery perfusion on renin release	a. Stimulates
B. Effect of vasopressin on renin release	b. Inhibits
C. Effect of angiotensin II on renin release	c. Neither
D. Effect of angiotensin II on ADH release	

Ref.: 1, 2

COMMENTS: The renin-angiotensin pathway is a physiologic mechanism critical for maintaining perfusion after hypovolemia. Renin is elaborated in an inactive form, prorenin, in the myoepithelial cells (juxtaglomerular cells) of afferent renal arterioles. It is converted to its active form in response to decreased perfusion pressure or to β-adrenergic stimulation of the juxtaglomerular body. It is also stimulated by decreased delivery of sodium chloride to the distal renal tubules as sensed by the macula densa. Renin acts on angiotensinogen (renin substrate), produced in the liver, to convert it to angiotensin I, which is an inactive intermediary peptide. In the lung, angiotensin-converting enzyme converts angiotensin I to the active angiotensin II. Angiotensin II is a potent vasoconstrictor, stimulates the heart rate and myocardial contractility, and increases vascular permeability. It stimulates the secretion and release of aldosterone from the adrenal cortex, which in turn increases sodium and water resorption from the renal tubules. Angiotensin II has other physiologic effects, including stimulating the release of vasopressin and ACTH from the pituitary. Metabolic activity includes stimulation of hepatic glycogenolysis and gluconeogenesis. By a negative feedback mechanism, angiotensin II inhibits the release of renin. Renin release is inhibited by vasopressin and potassium as well. Renin's normal circadian rhythm is lost after injury. Its release after injury can be suppressed by salt and water loading.

ANSWER:
Question 29: A, D, E
Question 30: A-a; B-b; C-b; D-a

31. With regard to protein loss after injury, which of the following statements is/are true?

A. It results from impaired protein synthesis.
B. It occurs primarily from skeletal muscle.
C. It occurs primarily from the site of injury.
D. It can be prevented by total parenteral nutrition.

Ref.: 1, 2

COMMENTS: Acute injury is associated with an obligatory nitrogen loss occurring primarily in the form of urinary nitrogen. Generalized catabolism of skeletal muscle is the primary cause of this protein loss; there is also impaired entry of amino acids into muscle cells as an effect of cortisol and other hormones. Protein may also be lost when there are large, open wounds, extensive areas of necrotic tissue, peritonitis, or ascites. Protein synthesis is not impaired after injury; in fact, it may be accelerated, but because of the marked increase in catabolism the net protein balance is negative.

ANSWER: B

32. Match the metabolic response in the left column with the appropriate clinical situation in the right column.

A. Hepatic glycogenolysis	a. Trauma
B. Hyperglycemia	b. Fasting
C. Protein catabolism in excess of energy needs	c. Both
D. Gluconeogenesis from glycerol	d. Neither
E. Fat is the main energy source	

Ref.: 1, 2

COMMENTS: Response to injury or fasting requires energy substrates. Normal circulating fuel sources in the form of glucose and plasma fats and triglycerides make up a small part of a person's total fuel composition and are not capable of providing the required calories. Stored sources of fuel include hepatic and muscle glycogen, protein, and fat. Hepatic glycogen stores are readily available but are limited and depleted within 24 hours. The largest potential calorie source is body fat, and following starvation or injury it is this source that becomes a main provider of energy through oxidation of fatty acids and generation of glycerol to be used in gluconeogenesis. A number of vital areas of the body, including the brain, renal medulla, red blood cells, leukocytes, and peripheral nerves are glycolytic tissues, meaning that they require a glucose source of energy for metabolism and are unable to utilize fatty acids. For this reason, a continuous supply of glucose must be available; when the limited glycogen stores are depleted, this availability is accomplished by gluconeogenesis and by recycling incompletely metabolized glucose. Primary sources of gluconeogenesis are (1) amino acids, derived from breakdown of muscle proteins, and (2) glycerol, derived from breakdown of triglycerides in adipose stores. These processes are fueled by the oxidation of fatty acids. With trauma, the hormonal milieu present results in catabolism of protein stores beyond that necessary for energy needs alone. With starvation, the body attempts to conserve proteins by adaptations that permit the use of fatty acids and ketones for fuel by nonglycolytic tissues and that promote gluconeogenesis. With prolonged fasting, ketone bodies such as acetoacetate and β-hydroxybutyrate can be used for brain metabolism in place of glucose. Lactate and pyruvate derived from incomplete utilization of glucose by glycolytic tissues can be regenerated into glucose through the use of energy provided by fatty acid oxidation; this process is known as the Cori cycle. The recycled glucose, in fact, becomes the main source of available glucose during late starvation. Another change observed during late starvation is a shift from the liver to the kidney as the primary source of gluconeogenesis; this occurs as alanine—the main source of gluconeogenesis from amino acids—is depleted in the liver. The human organism does not have the enzymes necessary to utilize free fatty acids directly for gluconeogenesis. The protein-conserving adaptations seen during late starvation do not occur with injury because of the hypermetabolic effects of cortisol, catecholamines, and other circulating hormones.

ANSWER: A-c; B-a; C-a; D-c; E-c

33. Match the statement in the left column with the appropriate response in the right column.

A. High urine output	a. Inappropriate ADH secretion
B. High urinary osmolarity	b. Diabetes insipidus
C. Hypernatremia	c. Both
D. Associated with head trauma	d. Neither

Ref.: 1, 2

COMMENTS: Afferent neural stimulation of the hypothalamus in response to injury or hypovolemia leads to release of antidiuretic hormone (ADH, or vasopressin) from the posterior pituitary gland. The physiologic action of ADH is to increase water resorption from the distal renal tubule and collecting ducts. A disturbance causing persistent release of ADH may produce a syndrome of inappropriate ADH (SIADH). The converse is diabetes insipidus, or absence of ADH secretion. Either of these conditions may be associated with head injury. With SIADH there is secretion of ADH in excess of that required for normal homeostasis. Consequently, there is *oliguria*, *urinary hyperosmolality*, and *dilutional hyponatremia*. Hyponatremia may occur in patients with normal ADH response if they are given excess hypotonic fluids. Diabetes insipidus, in contradistinction to SIADH, is a situation in which there is a failure of ADH secretion. It is characterized by the production of large volumes of *dilute urine*, with the urine osmolality lower than the plasma osmolality, which is abnormally high. If not recognized and treated appropriately, it leads to dehydration, hypernatremia, and hypotension. It is corrected by administering free water and exogenous vasopressin.

ANSWER: A-b; B-a; C-b; D-c

34. With regard to renal conservation of salt and water after injury, which of the following statements is/are true?

A. Normally, 25% of the cardiac output is directed to the kidneys.
B. Normally, 180 liters of plasma water are filtered per day.
C. Glomerular filtration can be increased by changes in pressure at the renal afferent arteriole.
D. Increased filtration fraction can maintain the glomerular filtration rate with renal perfusion pressure as low as 80 mm Hg.
E. Increased filtration fraction causes increased oncotic pressure of the blood perfusing the proximal tubule.

Ref.: 1, 2

COMMENTS: Volume loss causes a reflex increase in renal efferent arteriolar pressure, which allows maintenance of glomerular filtration rate by increasing filtration fraction. When the amount of plasma water removed at the glomerulus is increased, the oncotic pressure of the remaining blood passing out of the glomerulus to the proximal tubule is increased. This increased oncotic pressure of the capillary blood surrounding the proximal tubule causes a net transfer of water, sodium, chloride, and bicarbonate from the renal tubule into the blood. As a result, sodium, chloride, and fluid volume delivery to the loop of Henle are decreased. This, in turn, affects the normal osmotic gradient maintained in the renal medulla (this gradient depends on adequate delivery of Na^+ and Cl^- to the loop of Henle). This fall in the medullary oncotic gradient decreases the kidney's ability to concentrate urine and can lead to polyuric prerenal failure. Volume loss also leads to a shift of glomerular blood flow to the juxtamedullary nephrons, which possess much longer loops of Henle, thereby allowing increased resorption of sodium. This Na^+ resorption is dependent on the active resorption of chloride. If chloride delivery is decreased (as would occur with increased chloride resorption in the proximal tubule in response to increased filtration fraction), there is increased delivery of sodium to the distal tubules, which produces hypokalemia and alkalosis as sodium is resorbed and K^+ and H^+ are secreted; this process is augmented by the aldosterone secretion that accompanies injury. In summary, sodium retention, a hallmark of injury, results from increased secretion of corticosteroids and aldosterone, an increased glomerular filtration fraction with an attendant increase in proximal tubule resorption of sodium, and increased flow of blood to the juxtamedullary nephrons.

ANSWER: A, B, E

35. True or false: Injury and hypotension are characterized by an increase in water resorption.

Ref.: 1, 2

COMMENTS: Increased water resorption occurs after injury and is caused by several factors. One is sodium retention (discussed in the previous question), which is associated with the passive resorption of water. Another is the increased ADH secretion associated with injury. The increased levels last 3–5 days. Their return to normal is associated with a brisk diuresis of free water and resolution of edema, as is seen in surgical patients on the third to fifth postoperative day.

ANSWER: True

36. With regard to protein digestion and utilization, which of the following statements is/are true?

A. Approximately 40% of ingested protein is stored in nonfunctional energy reserves.
B. The stomach is unnecessary for protein digestion.
C. Amino acid absorption occurs primarily in the proximal ileum.
D. At least 10% of ingested protein is lost in the feces.

Ref.: 1, 2

COMMENTS: Nearly all protein in the body is functional. Although it represents a large potential source of energy, there is no nonfunctional storage analogous to the storage of triglycerides in fat globules. Protein digestion begins in the stomach, in which polypeptides are denatured and partially digested by the action of gastric acid and pepsin. The stomach, however, is not essential for protein digestion. Most enzymatic digestion of protein occurs in the duodenum as the result of pancreatic enzyme activity. More than 80% of protein absorption occurs in the first 100 cm of the jejunum. Absorption of ingested protein is nearly 100% complete. Almost all of the protein excreted in the feces is derived from bacteria, desquamated cells, and mucoproteins. Ultimately, all protein is absorbed as amino acids by an active carrier-mediated transport mechanism. Absorbed amino acids are necessary for daily protein synthesis to occur in a state of positive nitrogen balance. The normal nonstressed adult requires protein at 0.8–1.0 gm/kg/day to maintain this balance (the average diet provides 70–80 gm of protein per day). Daily synthesis is utilized to maintain skin and muscle mass, the structural proteins of the gut, plasma proteins, and enzymes; it also provides a circulating pool of amino acids. As the diagram indicates, little if any protein is used for daily energy requirements in the normal nonstressed adult, and nearly every molecule of protein has a specific function. An example of the disruption of this balance occurs during starvation, in which amino acids are shunted from muscle to liver to provide substrate for gluconeogenesis. When this occurs, urinary excretion of nitrogen (not protein) increases dramatically.

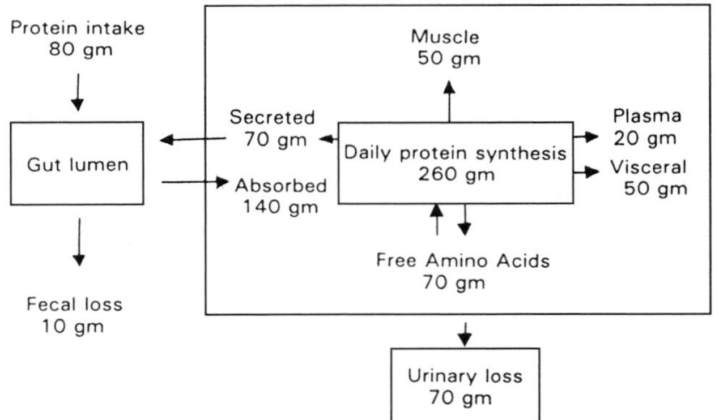

ANSWER: B

REFERENCES

1. Sabiston DC Jr: *Textbook of Surgery*, 15th ed. WB Saunders, Philadelphia, 1997.
2. Schwartz SI, Shires GT, Spencer FC: *Principles of Surgery*, 7th ed. McGraw-Hill, New York, 1999.

CHAPTER 4

Hemostasis and Transfusion

1. With regard to normal hemostasis and platelet function, which of the following statements is/are true?

   A. Vascular disruption is followed by vessel constriction mediated by vasoactive substances released by platelets.
   B. Platelet adhesion depends on the preformation of fibrin monomers.
   C. The endothelial surface supports platelet adhesion and thrombus formation.
   D. Heparin inhibits adenosine diphosphate (ADP)-stimulated platelet aggregation.
   E. A prolonged bleeding time may be due to thrombocytopenia, a qualitative platelet defect, or reduced amounts of von Willebrand factor.

Ref.: 1, 2, 3

COMMENTS: Blood fluidity is maintained by the action of inhibitors of blood coagulation, the nonthrombogenic vascular surface, and a high-flow (shear) rate preventing platelet adhesion. Three physiologic reactions mediate initial hemostasis following vascular injury: (1) vascular response to injury; (2) platelet adherence and aggregation; and (3) generation of thrombin. Injury exposes subendothelial components and induces vasoconstriction independent of platelet participation, resulting in decreased blood flow. Within seconds, platelets adhere to exposed subendothelial collagen by a mechanism dependent on the participation of von Willebrand factor. Adhesion stimulates release of platelet ADP, which initiates platelet aggregation. This requires calcium and magnesium and is not affected by heparin. The platelets then become densely packed, forming the primary hemostatic plug. Bleeding time measurements reflect the time it takes to form this plug. The bleeding time may be affected by platelet number and function, vascular integrity, and the amount and function of von Willebrand factor.

ANSWER: E

2. With regard to drug effects and platelet function, which of the following statements is/are true?

   A. Vasoconstricting agents such as epinephrine, prostaglandins G_2 and H_2 (PGG_2, PGH_2), and thromboxane A_2 cause lower levels of cyclic adenosine monophosphate (cAMP) and induce platelet aggregation.
   B. Vasodilators such as PGE_1, prostacyclin (PGI_2), theophylline, and dipyridamole elevate cAMP levels and block platelet aggregation.
   C. Aspirin and indomethacin interfere with platelet release of ADP and inhibit aggregation.
   D. Furosemide competitively inhibits PGG_2 and platelet aggregation.
   E. The effect of aspirin is reversible in 2–3 days.

Ref.: 1, 2, 3, 4

COMMENTS: Aspirin and indomethacin and most other nonsteroidal antiinflammatory drugs (NSAIDs) are inhibitors of prostaglandin synthesis. They block the formation of PGG_2 and PGH_2 from platelet arachidonic acid and, as a result, inhibit platelet aggregation. PGI_2, PGE_2, and thromboxane A_2 stimulate cAMP production, whereas dipyridamole and theophylline derivatives block its degradation. Aspirin inhibits thromboxane production, acetylates fibrinogen, interferes with fibrin formation, and makes fibrin susceptible to accelerated fibrinolysis. The effect of aspirin begins within 2 hours, is irreversible, and lasts the 7- to 9-day lifespan of affected platelets. The result clinically is increased bruising and bleeding and an increased risk of surgical bleeding. Platelet counts are normal, but there is a prolonged bleeding time. Furosemide competitively inhibits ADP-induced platelet aggregation and reduces the response of platelets to PGG_2. Furosemide can also cause thrombocytopenia. A wide variety of drugs inhibit platelet function.

ANSWER: A, B

3. With regard to blood coagulation, which of the following statements is/are true?

   A. The principal complex initiating blood coagulation is tissue factor–factor VIIa complex.
   B. Coagulation is initiated in the fluid phase of blood.
   C. Many cells including monocytes and fibroblasts express tissue factor.
   D. Factor Xa–Va complex converts prothrombin to thrombin in quantities sufficient to activate platelets.
   E. Antithrombin III is the main regulator of blood coagulation.

Ref.: 1, 2

COMMENTS: Coagulation is initiated on a phospholipid surface such as the monocyte or fibroblast membrane following expression of tissue factor (TF). Tissue factor binds factor VII, which is then activated by minor proteolysis through an autocatalytic mechanism or by the action of thrombin or other serine proteases. The TF–factor VIIa complex is a potent serine protease that activates factors X and IX. Factor Xa combines with factor Va at the phospholipid surface to convert prothrombin to thrombin. The amount of thrombin generated by this reaction is insufficient for formation of a stable fibrin clot. It is sufficient, however, to activate platelets, dissociate von Willebrand factor from factor VIII, activate factors V and VIII, and possibly activate factor XI. Factor IXa, formed by the action of the TF–factor VIIa complex, binds to activated platelets and associates with factor VIIIa, which then recruits circulating factor X to the platelet surface, converting it to factor Xa. Platelet-bound factor Xa and its cofactor factor Va generate sufficient quantities of thrombin to form a stable fibrin clot. The catalytic activity of TF–factor VIIa–factor Xa complex is regulated by tissue factor pathway inhibitor (RFPI). TFPI binds to factor Xa limiting the activity of the complex.

ANSWER: A, C, D

4. With regard to fibrinolysis, which of the following statements is/are true?

A. Plasmin is essential to fibrinolysis.
B. Plasminogen deficiency results in a clinical bleeding disorder.
C. Plasmin acts only on cross-linked fibrin polymers.
D. Ischemia is a potent activator of the fibrinolytic system.
E. There is no such thing as "physiologic" fibrinolysis.

Ref.: 1, 2, 3

COMMENTS: Plasminogen is converted to plasmin by a number of enzymes, including blood-borne activators and tissue activators such as thrombin, streptokinase, urokinase, and kallikrein. Ischemia is also a potent stimulator of the activation of the fibrinolytic system. Plasmin acts on fibrin, fibrinogen, factor V, and factor VIII. Physiologic fibrinolysis is the result of the natural affinity of plasminogen for fibrin. Plasminogen is incorporated into the clot, and fibrinolysis is locally controlled. Pathologic fibrinolysis occurs when plasminogen that is free in plasma is activated, resulting in proteolysis of fibrinogen, fibrin, and other coagulation factors. Unrestrained fibrinolysis can result in bleeding for several reasons: Small fibrin fragments are capable of interfering with normal platelet aggregation; large fibrin fragments join the clot instead of the normal monomers, producing an unstable clot; fibrin fragments interfere with thrombin cleavage of fibrinogen; and destruction of clotting factors other than fibrin result in a consumptive coagulopathy. Blood and platelets contain antifibrinolytic substances capable of plasminogen inhibition. Physiologic fibrinolysis plays an important role in tissue repair, cancer metastasis, ovulation, and embryo implantation. Disorders of fibrinolysis can result from excessive activity (bleeding) or insufficient activity (thrombosis).

ANSWER: A, D

5. With regard to the measurement of bleeding times, which of the following statements is/are true?

A. Spontaneous bleeding rarely occurs with platelet counts higher than 40,000/μl.
B. Platelet counts higher than 150,000/μl exclude the possibility of a primary hemostatic disorder.
C. Bleeding time is prolonged by a variety of drugs.
D. Platelet counts higher than 50,000/μl are usually associated with a normal bleeding time and adequate surgical hemostasis.
E. Normal bleeding time excludes von Willebrand disease as a potential factor affecting surgical hemostasis.

Ref.: 1, 3

COMMENTS: The bleeding time is a crude measure of platelet function, the number of platelets, or both. The normal value is 3–9 minutes and implies normal platelet function and counts of more than 50,000/μl. Bleeding time is prolonged in patients with normal platelet counts in whom qualitative abnormalities are present as a primary platelet disorder or one secondary to drugs, uremia, or liver disease or in those who have thrombasthenia or a variety of other platelet function defects. Patients with defective platelets or capillaries, those with von Willebrand disease, and those with a history of recent ingestion of aspirin, NSAIDs, antibiotics (penicillins and cephalosporins), and a wide variety of miscellaneous drugs also have prolonged bleeding times. False-negative (normal) bleeding times are frequently due to the technical difficulty of performing the test and its lack of sensitivity. For example, only 60% of patients with von Willebrand disease have a prolonged bleeding time. Other tests of platelet function include assessment of platelet aggregation in response to a variety of agonists and serotonin release.

ANSWER: A, C, D

6. Match each item in the left column with the appropriate item in the right column.

A. Prolonged in hemophilia and von Willebrand disease
B. Prolonged owing to factor VIII deficiency
C. Detects deficiencies of factors II, V, and X and fibrinogen
D. Detects deficiencies of factors II, V, X, VIII, IX, XI, and XII and fibrinogen
E. Preferred method for monitoring warfarin (Coumadin) anticoagulation
F. Prolonged by use of heparin

a. Prothrombin time (PT)
b. Partial thromboplastin time (PTT)
c. Both
d. Neither

Ref.: 1, 2

COMMENTS: The one-stage PT is used to measure the function of fibrinogen and factors II, V, X, and VII. The PTT reflects the function of fibrinogen and factors II, V, X, VIII, IX, XI, and XII. Fibrinogen and factors II, V, and X are common to both tests. Both tests require comparison with normal control values obtained daily in the laboratory. Even trace amounts of heparin, because of its antithrombin effect, prolong the PT, PTT, and thrombin time. At least 5 hours must elapse after the last dose of intravenous heparin before the PT can be reliably interpreted. The thrombin time is a measure of the ability to generate fibrin and is prolonged by deficiencies and abnormalities of fibrinogen, the presence of heparin or fibrinogen degradation products. Together, the thrombin time with the PT and PTT can distinguish deficiencies into the first stage or second stage of coagulation. A normal PT and thrombin time with an abnormal PTT in the absence of clinical bleeding suggests deficiencies of factor XII, high-molecular-weight kininogen, or prekallikrein or the presence of a lupus anticoagulant. The same laboratory values in a bleeding patient suggest deficiency of factor VIII, IX, or XI. A normal PTT and thrombin time with an abnormal PT suggests factor VII deficiency. A prolonged thrombin with abnormal PTT and PT suggests the presence of hepatocellular liver disease or a consumptive coagulopathy if the platelet count is decreased or an abnormality of fibrinogen if the platelet count is normal. Factor VIII is synthesized in endothelial cells of the liver and is therefore not affected by hepatocellular disease. A decrease in factor VIII can be used to differentiate consumptive coagulopathy (reduced levels of all factors) from hepatocellular liver disease (reduction in all factors except factor VIII). The PTT also is prolonged by heparin administration and can be used to monitor its efficacy. The INR calculated from the PT is the preferred method for controlling anticoagulation with warfarin (Coumadin). Vitamin K is necessary for the full function of factors II, VII, IX, and X, and therefore its deficiency is reflected by prolongation of both the PT and PTT.

ANSWER: A-b; B-a; C-c; D-b; E-a; F-c

7. True or false: Thrombin times aid in detecting qualitative abnormalities of fibrin, circulating anticoagulants, and inhibition of fibrin polymerization.

Ref.: 1, 2

COMMENTS: The thrombin time is a measurement of the clotting time of plasma. In the absence of heparin or the byproducts of fibrinolysis, fibrinogen abnormalities or deficiencies may be detected. Pathologic fibrinolysis causes a prolonged thrombin time as well as rapid whole blood clot dissolution. Whole blood clot lysis, which normally takes as long as 48 hours, may occur in as little as 2 hours in the presence of increased fibrinolysis. The presence of a paraprotein may cause false-positive results of the thrombin time and other tests based on whole blood clotting measurements.

ANSWER: True

8. With regard to evaluating bleeding in the surgical patient, which of the following statements is/are true?

   A. All surgical wounds, no matter how small, must be evaluated.
   B. The most common cause of surgical bleeding is incomplete mechanical hemostasis.
   C. ε-Aminocaproic acid is an excellent topical hemostatic agent.
   D. Isolated bleeding from the surgical wound implies poor local hemostasis.

Ref.: 1, 2, 4

COMMENTS: Bleeding from the surgical wound suggests ineffective local hemostasis, particularly if associated wounds (drain sites, tracheostomy wounds, intravenous infusion sites) are not bleeding. An exception is isolated bleeding from a resected prostatic bed, in which prostate-borne plasminogen activators can be activated by urokinase. Activation is inhibited to ε-aminocaproic acid. Blood transfusions can lead to bleeding via a number of mechanisms. Transfusion of more than one blood volume produces thrombocytopenia by dilution. Patients bleeding after a large number of blood transfusions should be considered thrombocytopenic and treated as such. Nonetheless, additional evaluation is indicated because an alternative explanation to transfusion-associated bleeding is a hemolytic transfusion reaction. In such an instance, disseminated intravascular coagulopathy (DIC) is caused by thromboplastic activity liberated from the stroma of lysed red blood cells. Extracorporeal circulation may induce hemostatic failure on the basis of thrombocytopenia, inadequate reversal of heparinization, or the overadministration of protamine. Septic surgical patients may bleed because of endotoxin-induced thrombocytopenia. Defibrination and bleeding may occur with meningococcemia, *Clostridium welchii* sepsis, or staphylococcal sepsis. Uncommonly, an operation on tissues rich in fibrinolytic activity, such as those of the pancreas, liver, or lungs, may lead to pathologic fibrinolysis and bleeding.

Table 4–1. Examples of DIC Syndromes

"Fast" DIC	"Slow" DIC
Amniotic fluid embolus	Acute promyelocytic leukemia
Abruptio placentae	Dead fetus syndrome
Septic abortion	Transfusion of activated prothrombin complex concentrates (APCC)
Septicemia	
Massive tissue injury	
Incompatible blood transfusion	Carcinomas
Purpura fulminans	Kasabach-Merritt syndrome
	Liver disease

ANSWER: A, B, D

9. With regard to the assessment of the patient who unexpectedly bleeds, which of the following statements is/are true?

   A. The most reliable way to detect patients at risk for bleeding is with a platelet count.
   B. Infants who do not bleed during circumcision have normal hemostatic function.
   C. An isolated episode of gastrointestinal bleeding is often associated with generalized hemostatic disorders.
   D. Menorrhagia is common in women with generalized hemostatic disorders.
   E. The presence of healthy parents and siblings does not exclude the possibility of a primary hemostatic disorder.

Ref.: 2, 3

COMMENTS: No single test for detecting the patient at risk for bleeding exists; the best protocol is a complete history and physical examination. Many normal individuals consider themselves to have a positive bleeding history. Aspirin is contained in a wide variety of over-the-counter medications; and as such its use is easily overlooked in the patient's medical history. • Circumcision typically involves significant trauma to tissues and activation of the tissue factor–factor VIIa pathway. Only 30% of affected males bleed following circumcision. • Only rarely do patients with a bleeding disorder undergo tooth extraction or tonsillectomy without encountering a bleeding problem; some patients with a severe bleeding disorder experience bleeding with tooth eruption. • Isolated gastrointestinal bleeding is unusual in patients with congenital bleeding disorders. Epistaxis is one of the most common symptoms of von Willebrand disease and platelet disorders. • Excessive menstrual flow (menorrhagia), but not intermenstrual bleeding, is common in patients with hemostatic disorders. • Because inherited bleeding defects may be autosomal dominant, autosomal recessive, or sex-linked recessive, an inquiry into the family history should account for grandparents, uncles, and cousins. • Because patients' assessment of severity is subjective, objective indicators should be sought, such as need for a prolonged hospital stay for minor surgery, transfusion, and anemia. A search for ecchymosis or petechiae, particularly near pressure points, is essential. • The lesions of hereditary hemorrhagic telangiectasia are found on the lips, underneath the fingernails, and around the anus. • Signs of liver disease suggest the presence of acquired deficiency of the prothrombin complex, not a predisposition to primary hemostatic disorders.

ANSWER: D, E

10. With regard to classic hemophilia, which of the following statements is/are true?

A. The incidence in the general population is 1:10,000.
B. A given patient's baseline factor VIII or IX level remains constant.
C. Muscle compartment bleeds are the most common orthopedic problem.
D. Factor VIII replacement therapy is required before any elective surgery.
E. Therapy with cryoprecipitated plasma is free of risk for hepatitis.

Ref.: 1, 2, 3

COMMENTS: Bleeding in hemophiliacs usually appears during early childhood; hemarthrosis is the most common problem. Epistaxis, hematuria, and intracranial bleeding may occur. Equinus contracture, Volkmann's contracture of the forearm, and flexion contracture of elbows or knees are sequelae of these bleeding episodes. Retroperitoneal or intramural intestinal bleeding may produce abdominal symptoms. The level of factor VIII in the plasma (which tends to remain stable throughout life) determines the tendency to bleed: spontaneous bleeding with severe disease, less than 1%; factor VIII or IX activity, 10%; bleeding with trauma in moderately severe disease, 1–5%; bleeding with major trauma or surgery with mild disease, 5–25%. A factor VIII or IX level of at least 30% must be achieved to control minor hemorrhage, 50% to control joint and muscle bleeding, and 80–100% to prepare patients for elective surgery. After elective surgery, levels of 25% should be maintained for at least 2 weeks. Transmission of hepatitis or human immunodeficiency virus (HIV), development of neutralizing antibodies, and qualitative platelet dysfunction are possible complications of factor replacement therapy.

ANSWER: A, B, D

11. A 12-year-old boy with known factor VIII deficiency has a painful, swollen, immobile right knee. You suspect a hemarthrosis; therapeutic options include which of the following?

A. Immediate aspiration and compression dressings to prevent cartilage necrosis.
B. Compression dressings and immobilization to prevent further bleeding.
C. Immediate aspiration after appropriate factor VIII replacement therapy.
D. Initial trial of factor VIII therapy, compression dressings, cold packs, and rest followed by active range-of-motion exercises.

Ref.: 1, 2

COMMENTS: Treatment of joint bleeding is aimed at preventing chronic synovitis and degenerative arthritis. Early, intensive factor VIII therapy is critical for limiting the extent of hemorrhage. Factor VIII replacement therapy is most effective when initiated prior to swelling of the joint capsule. Often replacement therapy is initiated prior to the onset of any objective physical findings, when the patient perceives only subtle signs of joint hemorrhage. Factor VIII therapy, joint rest, compression dressing (Ace wrap), and cold packs constitute the usual initial therapy. Aspiration is to be avoided. The goal of treatment of hemarthrosis is maintenance of range of motion. Active range of motion exercises should begin 24 hours after factor VIII therapy. Compression and cold packs should be continued for 3–5 days.

ANSWER: D

12. With regard to von Willebrand disease, which of the following statements is/are true?

A. It is more common than hemophilia.
B. It is best treated with cryoprecipitated plasma.
C. Factor VIII levels may vary over time in a given patient.
D. There is an associated platelet abnormality in 70% of patients.
E. Bleeding following elective surgery is rare.

Ref.: 1, 2

COMMENTS: Von Willebrand disease is the most common congenital bleeding disorder, affecting 1% of the population. The prevalence of patients with symptomatic bleeding is approximately 1:1000. Most patients have mild disease unless challenged by trauma or surgery. Von Willebrand disease is associated with a variable deficiency of both von Willebrand factor and factor VIII; a platelet defect is also present. The severity of coagulation abnormalities varies from patient to patient and from time to time for a given patient. In all but 1–2% of patients, bleeding manifestations are milder than those of classic hemophilia. In the same group of patients with type 3 von Willebrand disease, bleeding is more severe than in hemophilia. Bleeding is treated with desmopressin (DDAVP), which induces the release of von Willebrand factor from storage sites in endothelial cells and platelets. The effect of desmopressin is rapid, reaching maximal procoagulant effects in 1–2 hours. The effects dissipate quickly, necessitating repeated dosing at 12-hour intervals; when more than two or three doses of DDAVP are given, the effects diminish or are absent. Desmopressin is most effective for type 1 disease and is not effective for type 3 disease. Because of a risk of thrombocytopenia, DDAVP is specifically contraindicated for type 2B disease but may be effective for other forms of type 2 disease.

ANSWER: A, C, D

13. With regard to hereditary hemostatic disorders, which of the following statements is/are true?

A. Deficiencies of any of the four vitamin K-dependent factors (II, V, VII, X) may be treated with stored plasma.
B. Factor VII has the shortest intravascular half-life of any clotting factor.
C. Factor IX deficiency is clinically indistinguishable from factor VIII deficiency.
D. Factor V is known as a labile factor.
E. Factor XI deficiency is treated with plasma.

Ref.: 2, 4

COMMENTS: Factor V is not vitamin K-dependent. Factor VIII and IX deficiencies are clinically indistinguishable. Bleeding with factor IX deficiency (Christmas disease) is treated with recombinant factor IX concentrate. The use of prothrombin complex concentrate (PCC) may be complicated by thrombosis or disseminated intravascular coagulopathy (DIC). In older patients, administration of PCC should be accompanied by prophylactic administration of low-dose heparin. Deficiency of factor XI (Rosenthal syndrome) or factor V is treated with plasma. Because Factor V is labile and activity is lost with storage, fresh plasma is necessary. Deficiencies of factor VII, X (Stuart-Prower), or II are also treated with plasma. The duration and frequency of treatment with plasma-derived products is inversely proportional to the intravascular half-life.

ANSWER: B, C, D, E

14. True statements regarding acquired hypofibrinogenemia include which of the following?

A. Introduction of thromboplastic materials into the circulation is the most common cause of disseminated intravascular coagulation (DIC).
B. Release of excessive plasminogen activators causes pathologic fibrinolysis.
C. Primary fibrinolysis can be differentiated from DIC on the basis of the PT, PTT, and thrombin time.
D. The most important aspect of the treatment of DIC is adequate heparinization.

Ref.: 1, 2, 3

COMMENTS: DIC results from the introduction of thromboplastic materials into the circulation, leading to activation of the coagulation system with secondary "protective" fibrinolysis. Transfusion reactions, crush injuries, hemorrhagic perinatal complications, disseminated cancer, and bacterial sepsis have been implicated as causes. The release of excessive plasminogen-activating substances leads to primary pathologic fibrinolysis. Shock, hypoxia, sepsis, disseminated prostate cancer, cirrhosis, portal hypertension, and peritoneovenous shunts are possible causes. Differentiation between DIC and "protective" fibrinolysis on laboratory grounds alone is difficult, although thrombocytopenia is rarely seen with pure fibrinolysis. For both entities, treating the underlying medical or surgical problem is the most important single step. With DIC, maintenance of a patent microcirculation is important. Adequate fluid volumes and heparinization may be necessary. Active bleeding should be appropriately treated with factor replacement and does not accelerate DIC. Clotting factors can be replenished with fresh-frozen plasma. Heparin alone is rarely useful for treatment of acute DIC. Antithrombin III concentrates may be beneficial. Fibrinolytic inhibitors may be useful for DIC after appropriate heparinization. Giving heparin to patients with primary pathologic fibrinolysis can be dangerous, as is giving ε-aminocaproic acid to patients with secondary fibrinolysis. Correction of the underlying etiology is the most important component in the treatment of DIC.

ANSWER: A, B

15. With regard to polycythemia vera, which of the following statements is/are true?

A. Spontaneous thrombosis is a complication of polycythemia vera.
B. Spontaneous hemorrhage is a possible complication of polycythemia vera.
C. The reason for bleeding is a deficit of platelet function.
D. A hematocrit of less than 48% and a platelet count of less than 400,000/μl are desirable before an elective operation is performed on a patient with polycythemia vera.

Ref.: 2, 3

COMMENTS: Patients with untreated polycythemia vera are at high risk for postoperative bleeding or thrombosis. The complication rate is highest with uncontrolled erythrocytosis. Increased viscosity and platelet count along with a tendency toward stasis may explain the spontaneous thrombosis seen in patients with polycythemia vera. Patients most likely to bleed are those with platelet counts greater than 1.5 million/μl; it may be caused by a qualitative defect in platelet function. When possible, operation should be delayed until the hematocrit and platelet count can be medically reduced. Phlebotomy may help in acute situations. Complication rates as high as 46% have been reported among patients with polycythemia vera undergoing operation. Spontaneous hemorrhage, thrombosis, a combination of hemorrhage and thrombosis, and infection are the major complications.

ANSWER: A, B, C, D

16. With regard to anticoagulation, which of the following statements is/are true?

A. Warfarin (Coumadin) inhibits the activity of vitamin K-dependent factors (II, VII, IX, X).
B. Heparin impairs the effect of thrombin on fibrinogen.
C. Theoretically, 1.28 mg of protamine neutralizes 1 mg of heparin.
D. The effects of vitamin K reversal take 48 hours.
E. An international normalized ratio (INR) of more than 1.5 is considered safe for operation.

Ref.: 2

COMMENTS: With meticulous hemostatic technique, many operations can be performed on patients with an INR less than 1.5. Exceptions include operations on the eye or the prostate, neurosurgical procedures, or a blind needle aspiration. In these cases, an INR less than 1.2 is necessary. In patients who have recently undergone anticoagulant treatment with warfarin and who require emergency surgery, plasma may be given to reverse the warfarin effect immediately. Alternatively, vitamin K may be given orally or subcutaneously at least 6 hours preoperatively to reverse the effect of warfarin on vitamin K-dependent factors. An INR greater than 1.5 is a contraindication to intramuscular medications.

ANSWER: A, B, C, E

17. With regard to the storage of banked blood, which of the following statements is/are true?

A. Citrate phosphate dextrose (CPD) or CPD-adenine stored blood kept at 4°C is suitable for transfusion for up to 3 months.
B. Platelets in banked blood retain their function for only 3 days.
C. Factors II, VII, IX, and XI are stable in banked blood.
D. An increase in oxygen affinity occurs in stored blood as the result of a fall in 2,3-diphosphoglycerate (2,3-DPG) levels.

E. There is a significant rate of hemolysis in stored blood.

Ref.: 1, 2

COMMENTS: Whole blood properly collected and stored at 4°C is "good" for 21 days in CPD and 35 days in citrate-phosphate-dextrose-adenine (CPDA-1). The proportion of cells removed from the circulation within 24 hours of transfusion increases with the time the blood is in storage, reaching about 25–30% at 21 days in CPD (35 days in CPDA-1). These percentages define the shelf life of stored blood. However, any blood component stored in an "open" system (e.g., frozen blood) has a useful life of only 24 hours. The cells that survive the first 24 hours have a normal lifespan; cells can be detected for up to 120 days—the lifespan of the normal red blood cell. Red blood cell ATP and 2,3-DPG levels fall during storage. Factors II, VII, IX, and XI are stable in storage, whereas factors V and VIII are not, unless they are frozen immediately after the blood is drawn, as in fresh-frozen plasma. Lactic acid concentrations increase and pH falls during storage. Potassium and ammonia concentrations rise steadily during storage. The citrate used for preservation may reduce plasma-ionized calcium if large volumes are transfused. These metabolites are especially significant in pediatric patients and in patients with impaired liver or renal function (or both).

ANSWER: C, D

18. True or false: In a major crossmatch donor cells are compared with recipient serum, whereas in a minor crossmatch donor serum is compared with recipient cells.

Ref.: 2

COMMENTS: Because of the high degree of sensitivity of the indirect antiglobulin test performed on donor blood, virtually all unexpected antibodies are detected, and the minor crossmatch has been rendered unnecessary. Alloimmunization to "minor" antigens may occur after multiple transfusions. To detect alloimmunization, repeated recipient serum samples should be checked with the indirect antiglobulin test every 48–72 hours if multiple transfusions are given.

ANSWER: True

19. With regard to blood components, which of the following statements is/are true?

A. Frozen red blood cells maintain their ATP and 2,3-DPG levels.
B. Leukocyte- and platelet-poor red blood cells are prepared by removing plasma and the buffy coat.
C. Platelets should be transfused within 6 hours of donation.
D. Fresh-frozen plasma retains factor V and VII function.
E. Hydroxyethylstarch (HES) solution should not be used in place of plasma in hypovolemic patients.

Ref.: 2

COMMENTS: Fresh whole blood should be used within 24 hours of donation because its platelets remain useful for only the first 6 hours. Factors V and VIII remain active throughout the 24 hours. • Packed red blood cells reduce the danger of volume overload. Leukocyte- and platelet-poor red blood cells are used in patients with demonstrated hypersensitivity to white blood cells or platelets and in those who must be protected from HLA antigen sensitization, such as transplant recipients and chronic transfusion patients. The most effective method for reducing the leukocyte content is leukocyte filtration. • The recovery of platelets from a donor is less than 60% efficient. Platelet antibodies develop in 20% of patients after 10–20 platelet transfusions and can rise to close to 100% as the number of transfusions increases. • Fresh-frozen plasma is needed for factors V and VIII. • Volume expansion with fresh-frozen plasma is rarely indicated. HES, Ringer's lactate, or albumin is preferred for plasma expansion. HES volume should not exceed 1 liter per day to avoid bleeding complications.

ANSWER: A, B, D

20. With regard to hemolytic transfusion reactions, which of the following statements is/are true?

A. They are generally caused by ABO incompatibility.
B. Urticaria and pruritus are the most common symptoms.
C. Acidification of the urine prevents precipitation of hemoglobin.
D. Intravenous diphenhydramine (Benadryl) should be given immediately.
E. The laboratory findings include free hemoglobin concentrations higher than 5 mg/dl and serum haptoglobin concentrations of less than 50 mg/dl.

Ref.: 1, 2

COMMENTS: The most common cause of fatal hemolytic transfusion reaction is a clerical error that results in transfusion of the wrong ABO type of blood. Because the severity is proportional to the antigen dose, constant awareness, early recognition, and immediate intervention are important. Hemolytic transfusion reactions lead to the release of vasoactive amines through the activation of complement. This in turn leads to shock, renal ischemia, tubular necrosis, and renal failure proportional to the depth and duration of hypotension. Hemolytic reactions lead to red blood cell destruction, hemoglobinemia, and hemoglobinuria. Haptoglobin can bind 100 mg of hemoglobin per 100 ml of plasma; but when free hemoglobin concentration exceeds 25 mg/dl, it is excreted in the urine and can cause tubular necrosis. Red blood cell lipids initiate DIC in 8–30% of patients in whom a full unit of mismatched blood has been transfused. However, as little as 10 ml can produce serious hypotension and DIC. Typical signs and symptoms include chills, fever, lumbar and chest pain, pain at the infusion site, and hypotension. In anesthetized patients, diffuse bleeding and continued hypotension suggest the diagnosis. Laboratory criteria are hemoglobinuria with free hemoglobin concentrations higher than 5 mg/dl, serum haptoglobin concentrations of less than 50 mg/dl, and serologic confirmation of incompatibility. Because hemoglobin is a highly chromogenic molecule, small amounts (as little as 30 mg/dl) can be detected visually. The hemoglobin from as little as 5 ml of red blood cells makes the plasma pink and produces hemoglobinuria. Treatment includes stopping the transfusion, inserting a bladder catheter, and administering mannitol and bicarbonate to encourage excretion of an alkaline urine. This helps prevent precipitation of hemoglobin in the renal tubules. Should oliguria develop, appropriate fluid management and possibly dialysis are begun. The most important treatment is restoration of blood pressure and renal perfusion; vasopressors may be necessary. A sample of recipient blood is compared to pretransfusion samples to confirm incompatibility. Direct antiglobulin tests persist in being positive so long as incompatible red blood cells continue to circulate. The serum bilirubin level can be monitored to follow the increase in indirect bilirubin caused by hemolysis.

ANSWER: A, E

21. With regard to complications of transfusion, which of the following statements is/are true?

A. Febrile reactions are rare.
B. Gram-positive organisms are the most common contaminants of stored blood.
C. Even small amounts of intravenous air are poorly tolerated.
D. Transfusions lasting longer than 6 hours increase the risk of infection by contaminated blood.
E. Malaria, Chagas' disease, human T cell leukemia virus I (HTLV-I), acquired immunodeficiency syndrome (AIDS), and hepatitis can be transmitted by blood transfusions.

Ref.: 1, 4

COMMENTS: Febrile reactions are the most common reactions to red blood cell and platelet transfusions and occur once per 100 units given. Fever and chills are the usual symptoms. If mild, these symptoms respond to antipyretics; in severe cases they are treated with opiates. Urticarial reactions are the most common reaction to plasma transfusions. They usually respond to antihistamines. Anaphylactic reactions are rare and are treated with epinephrine and steroids. Although unusual, gram-negative organisms capable of surviving at 4°C are the most common cause of bacterial contamination of banked blood. Platelets, which are optimally stored at room temperature and are being used increasingly, are a more frequent source of sepsis. Air embolus has become rare since bottles have been replaced by collapsible plastic containers. Even small volumes of air have the potential to cause fatal complications and should be avoided whenever possible. Hepatitis viruses B and C (HBV and HCV), human immunodeficiency virus (HIV), HTLV I and II, malaria, Chagas' disease, and other infections can be transmitted by transfusion. Specific testing of donors is available for HBV, HCV, HIV, and HTLV; health, immigration, and travel history are used to exclude donors who might harbor malaria or Chagas' disease.

ANSWER: C, D, E

22. In cirrhotic patients who are actively bleeding, the coagulopathy of end-stage liver disease can be differentiated from DIC most readily by estimation of which of the following factors?

A. Factor II.
B. Factor V.
C. Factor VII.
D. Factor VIII:C
E. Factor X.

Ref.: 3

COMMENTS: Of all of the coagulation factors, only factor VIII:C is not produced by the hepatocyte. It is manufactured by reticuloendothelial cells, and levels are typically increased in the presence of cirrhosis. Reductions in factor VIII:C are observed in patients with DIC because it is consumed along with the other coagulation factors.

ANSWER: D

REFERENCES

1. Sabiston DC Jr: *Textbook of Surgery*, 15th ed. WB Saunders, Philadelphia, 1997.
2. Schwartz SI, Shires GT, Spencer FC: *Principles of Surgery*, 7th ed. McGraw-Hill, New York, 1999.
3. Colman RW, Hirsh J, Marder VJ, et al: *Hemostasis and Thrombosis, Basic Principles and Practice*. JB Lippincott, Philadelphia, 1994.
4. Rossi EC, Simon TL, Moss GS: *Principles of Transfusion Medicine*, 2nd ed. Williams & Wilkins, Baltimore, 1996.

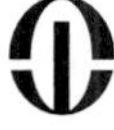

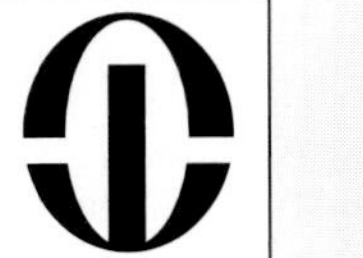

CHAPTER 5

Nutrition

1. In relation to body composition, which of the following is/are true?

   A. Fat stores cannot exceed 160,000 kcal in any individual.
   B. Carbohydrate reserves can be depleted quickly (24–48 hours) during simple starvation.
   C. Protein is the most efficiently stored nutrient, providing 9 kcal/gm.
   D. Carbohydrates, like fat, are stored in an anhydrous form, allowing a large energy potential.

Ref.: 1, 2

COMMENTS: Understanding the nutritional composition of the body is important for understanding metabolic changes that occur in different clinical situations. In a 70-kg man the lean body mass (LBM) is 75% of body weight with the other 25% of body weight composed of fat. Lean body mass is 40% body cell mass (skeletal muscle and viscera) and 35% extracellular mass (plasma proteins, extracellular fluids, and skeleton). Lean body mass contributes 13 kg of the body's protein stores and 30,000 kcal of the body's energy stores. Fat has energy stores that total 160,000 kcal in the average 70-kg man. Obese individuals can have higher (unlimited) stores of fat. Body composition can also be categorized as follows: 40% of body weight is organic material; 55% is total body water (32% intracellular and 23% extracellular); and 5% is minerals. Note that the amount of a substance in the body does not necessarily generate a proportional amount of energy. The largest body substrates, water and minerals, provide no energy. Protein and fat supply most of the body's energy. However, protein is an inefficient energy source in relation to its wet weight, providing 1–2 kcal/gm of weight. That is one-fourth the energy used for its synthesis. Carbohydrates are also stored in aqueous solution, providing only 1–2 kcal/gm of weight. Carbohydrates are the essential energy source during anaerobic glycolysis, and therefore their role as an energy substrate cannot be ignored. Fat is stored in an anhydrous state, allowing its large energy potential of 9 kcal/gm. Larger amounts of fat energy can be stored in the obese owing to this compact storage form. It should be noted that carbohydrate reserves can be depleted within 24–48 hours. Protein mobilization of 80–100 gm/day during starvation leads to LBM loss; thus when 7–10% of body weight is lost, organ and tissue function is compromised. The loss of 50–60% of body cell mass most likely leads to death.

ANSWER: B

2. Which of the following is/are true of hormonal regulation of blood glucose?

   A. Increased glucagon/insulin ratio allows mobilization of liver glycogen.
   B. Increased circulating insulin with glucose intake allows decreased glucagon secretion.
   C. Insulin allows tissues such as liver, muscle, and adipose tissue to release glucose.
   D. Glucagon stimulates the cAMP cycle to store glucose as glycogen to meet the body's future needs.

Ref.: 3, 4

COMMENTS: See Question 4.

3. Which two carbohydrates are monosaccharides?

   A. Glucose and fructose.
   B. Pectin and cellulose.
   C. Maltose and lactose.
   D. All of the above.
   E. None of the above.

Ref.: 3, 4

COMMENTS: See Question 4.

4. Which is/are true of carbohydrate metabolism?

   A. Dietary fiber is digested similarly to starch in that it can be readily digested into the small intestine and used as a source of energy.
   B. Digestion primarily occurs in the small intestine via pancreatic enzymes.
   C. To prevent stimulation of protein for use in gluconeogenesis during times of stress only 50 gm of glucose per day must be supplied exogenously.
   D. Glucagon secretion is increased with the intake of glucose, which allows uptake of glucose by the liver, muscle, and adipose tissue.

Ref.: 5

COMMENTS: Dietary carbohydrates (CHO) provide 4 kcal/gm and can be complex (polymeric) or simple (monomeric or dimeric). The major role of CHO in the body is to provide energy for body tissues to use for metabolic processes. Approximately 30–60% of calories consumed are in the form of CHO. Digestion of starches begins orally via salivary amylase. As the starches are passed from the stomach to the small intestine, pancreatic and intestinal enzymes (amylase and disaccharidases) reduce complex CHO to disaccharides (maltose, sucrose, lactose), which can then be hydrolyzed to primary derivatives of CHO, the monosaccharides or hexoses (glucose, fructose, galactose), via specific disaccharidases. Glucose is the preferred fuel in humans, with all metabolism beginning or ending with this hexose. The monosaccharides are absorbed into the intestinal mucosa and transported to the liver via the portal circulation. Their final fate is to be used to form pyruvate or glycogen or to be transported back to the blood for use by RBCs, brain, or formation of fat in adipose tissue. In a 70-kg man, the liver can store as much as 70 gm of glycogen (10% of the liver's wet weight), allowing a 12- to 24-hour nutritional reservoir during fasting. In the same 70-kg man, 120 gm (1–2%) of the wet weight of the muscle mass can be attributed to glycogen. Muscle glycogen has the role of maintaining fuel within that tissue. Release of muscle glycogen to the bloodstream, as seen with liver glycogen, cannot occur as muscle tissue lacks the necessary enzyme for release, glucose-6-phosphatase. Free glucose from muscle glycogen is not a significant contributor to plasma glucose; therefore liver glycogen is the glucose reserve used to maintain blood glucose levels as needed. Hormonal regulation of blood glucose levels in relation to carbohydrate intake is important as insulin secretion increases with intake of glucose, and glucagon secretion declines. This allows increased uptake of glucose by liver, muscle, and adipose tissue. Conversely, glucagon mobilizes liver glycogen via the cyclic adenosine monophosphate (cAMP) protein kinase system with decreases in blood glucose levels due to decreased intake. Glucose tolerance is determined by the rate at which mechanisms of glucose removal can operate. The protein-sparing effect of glucose intake is also important, as administration of 100 gm of glucose (or 1 mg/kg/min) can suppress nitrogen (amino acids, AA) use for gluconeogenesis. The major function of CHO is to provide energy for body tissues to perform their metabolic functions, and all major pathways of CHO metabolism start or end with glucose. The three major types of glucose metabolism are (1) glycolysis, a process by which all cells can oxidize glucose to pyruvate and lactate; (2) oxidation of acetyl coenzyme A (CoA) for use by the tricarboxylic acid (TCA) cycle where the acetyl CoA can come from CHO, fat, or protein; and (3) the hexose monophosphate shunt (pentose phosphate shunt) with the primary purpose of producing NADPH for its reducing power and allowing degradation of sugars other than hexoses. In addition to outside glucose sources, gluconeogenesis (formation of glucose from a large variety of non-CHO substrates including AAs, lactate, pyruvate, propionate, and glycerol) and glycogenolysis (formation of glucose from glycogen) allow glucose production endogenously when outside sources are not available. Endogenous glucose production allows maintenance of plasma glucose levels in the fasting state at a rate of approximately 2–3 mg/kg/min. Given the availability of endogenous glucose, excess infusion of parenteral glucose can lead to unwanted side effects, including (1) elevated blood glucose levels; (2) increased rate of fat synthesis leading to fatty liver; and (3) increased H_2O and CO_2 production, which can lead to respiratory compromise and possible H_2O overload. Glucose administration should be kept below 5 mg/kg/min to prevent these complications. Dietary fiber is a form of complex CHO, classified based on its structure; it is enzymatically digested and is not considered a source of nourishment. Fiber includes cellulose (insoluble) and noncellulose (soluble) forms (pectins, gums, mucilages, and hemicelluloses), which are broken down by bacterial flora of the gut and degraded primarily in the colon. Soluble fiber is thought to have numerous benefits, including (1) hypocholesterolemic effects; (2) production of short-chain fatty acids, which have trophic effects throughout the intestinal tract; (3) improvement of blood glucose levels due to decreasing the rate of glucose absorption; and (4) protection from bacterial translocation.

ANSWER:
Question 2: A, B
Question 3: A
Question 4: B

5. Which general statements is/are correct regarding amino acids?

A. Categorized as essential, nonessential, or conditionally essential depending on the body's ability to synthesize them.
B. Utilized for creating essential nitrogenous substances, growth, and maintenance.
C. Metabolized with the influence of endogenous mediators including glucagon and insulin.
D. Digested and absorbed completely in the stomach, allowing the small intestine to digest only fat and carbohydrates.

Ref.: 6

COMMENTS: See Question 6.

6. Which is/are true of the metabolism of proteins/amino acids?

A. Branched-chain amino acids (BCAAs) can be metabolized outside the liver by muscle.
B. The liver can biosynthesize nonessential amino acids important for maintaining the equilibrium of proteins in the body.
C. Cannot be oxidized for energy.
D. Regulate insulin production.

Ref.: 6

COMMENTS: Body proteins are made up of 20 different amino acids (AA) each of which has a different metabolic fate and different function in the body. AAs commonly have a central α-carbon atom with a carboxylic acid group, amino group, and hydrogen atom covalently bonded. The α-carbon atom is the site at which a side chain, different for each amino acid, is attached. Unlike carbohydrates and fat, protein (AAs) contain nitrogen. Three categories exist for AAs (Table 5–1): (1) essential amino acids: those AAs that cannot be synthesized by the body; (2) nonessential amino acids: those AAs that can be synthesized de novo in the body; and (3) conditionally essential amino acids: certain nonessential AAs that may be considered essential during stress or trauma in that an outside AA

Table 5–1. Common Body Amino Acids

Essential Amino Acids	Nonessential Amino Acids	Conditionally Essential Amino Acids
Isoleucine	Alanine	Cysteine
Leucine	Arginine	Histidine
Lysine	Aspartic acid	Tyrosine
Methionine	Asparagine	
Phenylalanine	Glutamic acid	
Threonine	Glutamine	
Tryptophan	Glycine	
Valine	Proline	
	Serine	

source is needed because use of that particular AA exceeds the body's capacity for synthesis. The **dietary** protein requirement for adults is 0.8 gm/kg/day; that is, approximately 20% of calories consumed should be in the form of protein. Overconsumption of protein is common in the Western diet, where dietary requirements are based only on the need for AAs not able to be synthesized by the body. Protein consumed is used as a source of AAs for: (1) creating essential nitrogenous substances; (2) growth; and (3) maintenance. Degradation and absorption of protein-derived AAs is efficient, with protein being recycled continuously. Protein digestion is a result of sequential hydrolysis of peptide bonds of the protein to form AAs and peptides; it begins in the stomach via pepsin and proceeds to the small intestine where pancreatic enzymes (trypsin, chymotrypsin, and carboxypolypeptidase) continue the process. All protein metabolism depends on numerous endogenous mediators, including endocrine hormones (insulin and glucagon), prostaglandins, cytokines, and lymphokines, with health status and intake determining which substance takes precedence. The resulting free AAs and small peptides of protein digestion are absorbed into the brush border of intestinal epithelial cells. Once in the portal system, free AAs distribute to the liver and muscles. Endogenous protein production is estimated at 70 gm/day with approximately 250 gm of protein mobilized daily within the body. Protein breakdown is thought to match protein input, with 60% of protein intake converted to urea, 25% used to form new AAs, and 15% used for new protein synthesis. Urine contains 90% of all nitrogen lost with small amounts lost via skin and stool. Cellular protein and AAs are thought to be in constant equilibrium in terms of degradation and synthesis. Continuous turnover of protein and AAs (amount of synthesis or degradation occurring over time) occurs at the following rates: 30% in muscle, 50% in the viscera, and 20% of plasma proteins without which daily protein requirements would be higher. In relation to proteins and AAs, the liver is the site for urea production, biosynthesis of nonessential AAs, and degradation of all AAs. Excess AAs can be oxidized for energy, stored as fat or glycogen, or excreted. Glutamate dehydrogenase is present in both the cytoplasm and mitochondria of the liver; it is the primary enzyme responsible for transamination of AAs to the end products α-ketoglutarate and ammonia. One special class of AAs are the branched-chain amino acids (BCAAs), which include leucine, isoleucine, and valine. The BCAAs are similar in terms of chemical structure, and degradation steps; and they are the only AAs metabolized outside the liver. BCAAs are extensively oxidized by muscle and adipose tissue and are a local source of energy for muscle, indicating their importance for patients with severe liver disease.

ANSWER:
Question 5: A, B, C
Question 6: A, B

7. Match the items in the two columns.

A. Cholesterol is primarily composed of this substance	a. Glycerides
B. The main forms of fat found in the body and diet	b. Phospholipids
C. Can be directly absorbed via portal blood, bypassing the lymphatic system	c. Sterols
	d. Medium-chain fatty acids
	e. All of the above

Ref.: 3, 7

COMMENTS: See Question 9.

8. Lipolysis is the breakdown of fat. Which of the following statements is/are true regarding this process?

A. Insulin stimulates fat breakdown.
B. Lipolysis results in the formation of glycerol.
C. Glucagon is a hormone that can stimulate lipolysis.
D. With increased lipolysis, ketones are formed and released into the circulation.

Ref.: 3, 7

COMMENTS: See Question 9.

9. Triglycerides are the storage form of fat. Which of these statements is/are true of triglycerides?

A. Most abundant form of fat found in foods.
B. Least efficient form of fat storage.
C. Primarily composed of cholesterol.
D. Essential fatty acids are a form of triglycerides.

Ref.: 3, 7

COMMENTS: Fat is considered the most calorie-dense macronutrient in the diet, providing 9 kcal/gm. The structure of fat is characterized by its relative lack of oxygen with longer oxidative processes necessary than the lesser calorie-yielding carbohydrates. Three main forms of fat are found in the body: (1) Glycerides, principally triglycerides or triglycerol (fatty acid and glycerol), are the fat storage form of fat and are the most abundant forms in food, comprising approximately 95–98% of ingested fat and tissues. Essential fatty acids (EFAs) are a form of triglyceride characterized by an unsaturated bond within the last seven carbons of the fatty acid chain at the methyl end. The EFAs (linoleic, linolenic, and arachidonic acids) cannot be synthesized by humans. (2) Phospholipids are ingested in small amounts and are mainly constituents of cell membranes and myelin sheaths. (3) Sterols are comprised primarily of cholesterol. The functions of each type of fat are as follows: Triglycerides are the most efficient form for storing calories. In adipose tissue they serve to protect organs, act as an insulator, and contribute to body shape. Cholesterol and phospholipids make up cell membranes and are substrates for other essential substances. Cholesterol is the substrate for the formation of bile acids (primary bile acids are cholate and chenodeoxycholate) and steroid hormones (aldosterone, progesterone, estrogen, androgens). Phospholipids are substrates for prostaglandins, leukotrienes, and thromboxanes. Dietary fat is digested in the small intestine where emulsification by bile salts greatly increases the surface area of fat globules, thereby allowing hydrolysis by lipases on the surface of fat. The end-products of triglyceride digestion are free fatty acid (FFA) and two monoglycerides. These end-products combine with bile salts to form micelles, which are then transported to brush borders of epithelial cells. Bile salts are released back to chyme when monoglycerides and FFAs make their way to the brush border. Cholesterol (esters) and phospholipids are hydrolyzed by pancreatic cholesterol ester hydrolase and phospholipase A_2, respectively; and bile salts once again form micelles to be delivered to the brush border. Once absorbed, the triglycerides, cholesterol esters, and phospholipids are formed and combined with small amounts of protein to form lipoproteins. Lipoproteins [very low density (VLDL), low density (LDL), high density (HDL)] act as transporters for various forms of fat to their ultimate destination (i.e., liver, adipose tissue). Note that only medium-chain fatty acids (MCFAs), which are made up of fewer than 12 carbons, can be directly absorbed via portal blood, bypassing the lymphatic system. Various hormonal and substrate factors influence rates of adipose tissue lipolysis. Utilization of fat energy relies on adipose cell lipase, which is regulated by epinephrine, norepinephrine, glucagon, and adrenocorticotrophic hormone (ACTH). Insulin inhibits the lipolysis. Lipolysis results in the formation of glycerol and eventually glucose or pyruvate in the liver. If fat breakdown exceeds carbohydrate degradation for energy, common in the diabetic patient or in the fasting state, fatty acids are converted to ketones (acetoacetate and β-hydroxybutyrate) and oxidation by the tricarboxylic acid cycle is decreased. The ketones are released into the circulation from the liver and converted back to acetyl CoA for use in the citric acid cycle in peripheral tissues. Heart, muscle, and the renal cortex prefer ketone acetoacetate to glucose, whereas in the brain and RBCs glucose is the preferred fuel.

ANSWER:
Question 7: A-c; B-e; C-d
Question 8: B, C, D
Question 9: A, D

10. Where in the cell does the tricarboxylic acid (TCA) cycle function?

A. Cytoplasm.
B. Mitochondria.
C. Golgi apparatus.
D. Sarcoplasm.

Ref.: 3, 4

COMMENTS: The major pathways of CHO metabolism begin or end with glucose, which is used as a source of energy at the cellular level. Glycolysis is the conversion of glucose to pyruvate in aerobic conditions and to lactate during anaerobic conditions; it occurs in the cytoplasm via a series of enzyme-catalyzed reactions. There are various subdivisions of carbohydrate metabolism to provide energy for cells, including glycolysis, the TCA cycle, electron transport and oxidative phosphorylation, gluconeogenesis, glycogenesis, the pentose phosphate shunt, glycogenolysis, and galactose and fructose metabolism. All cycles are linked in that they can accomplish the same thing under different metabolic conditions. The TCA cycle can ultimately utilize all three major substrates (fat, protein, carbohydrate) for energy. The Kreb's, or TCA, cycle is a complete system of oxidizing acetyl COA derived from fat, CHO, and protein to CO_2 in the mitochondria. Because oxidation of pyruvate, fatty acids, and glycolysis ends in the mitochondria, the energy capacity of most cells depends on the mitochondrial compartment. Acetic acid in the form of acetyl COA is converted via multiple steps, involving acids, coenzymes, and enzymes, to CO_2 and water. In addition, reducing equivalents are formed that are needed to generate ATP and energy in the electron transport system. Coenzymes reduced in the mitochondria (electron transport) drive the respiratory chain. The cycle allows utilization of glucose, fatty acids, and amino acids by conversion of each to acetyl CoA. Fatty acids cannot be converted to CHO owing to the irreversible reaction of pyruvate dehydrogenase. The TCA cycle also provides precursors necessary for the formation of various essential molecules, including nucleic acids and hemoglobin, synthesis of collagen, and activation of acetoacetate for use in extrahepatic tissues. The TCA cycle produces two-thirds of all ATP, with 12 ATPs per cycle.

ANSWER: B

11. A healthy 70-kg man with intact protein stores requires approximately how many grams of protein per day (gm/kg) in his oral diet to maintain adequate protein stores?

A. 0.8 gm/kg (56 gm/day).
B. 2.0 gm/kg (140 gm/day).
C. 3.8 gm/kg (266 gm/day).
D. 4.0 gm/kg (280 gm/day).

Ref.: 8, 9

COMMENTS: See Question 12.

12. When evaluating a patient's nutritional status, which would be an indicator of declining or poor nutritional status? Indicate all that are true.

A. One and a half weeks of poor or negligible oral intake without supplemental feedings and a serum albumin level of 2.1 gm/dl.
B. Nitrogen balance of −1.
C. Indirect calorimetry indicates the patient requires 1600 kcal/day, and the patient has been consuming 1600–1800 kcal/day.
D. Patient receiving tube feedings cannot meet the goal tube feeding rate of 1500 cc/day for 2 weeks, and problems with nausea and vomiting prevent oral intake.

Ref.: 8, 9

COMMENTS: Malnutrition in the hospitalized patient is common, with significant increases in morbidity and mortality in surgical or highly stressed patients. As many as 50% may have moderate malnutrition, causing a suboptimal response to surgery or medical therapies. Diagnosis of malnutrition is important early in the patient's care, as rapid depletion of the body's energy and protein stores can occur. Nutritional status can be determined via review of the patient's medical history, physical examination, anthropometrics, and laboratory data as they relate to ingestion, digestion, absorption, and excretion. There is no official formula for diagnosis of malnutrition, but surgical candidates and postoperative patients are highly susceptible to nutritional anomalies. **Medical history**: Evaluate how past and present medical problems and therapies can affect current nutritional status and have knowledge of each disease state as it relates to nutrition (i.e., medical problems including recent surgery, sepsis, chronic illness, gastrointestinal disorders, psychosocial problems, or abnormal diets). **Physical examination**: It can identify frank signs of malnutrition (i.e., marasmus or physical effects of specific vitamin or mineral deficiency). **Anthropometrics**: Height and weight help relate body size to nutritional needs. Drastic changes in weight within a short time (days) is an indication of fluid shifts and should be evaluated appropriately. Adjustments to weight expectations and macronutrient needs should be made for obese patients and those with amputations. Estimates of fat and muscle mass using the midarm circumference and triceps skinfold thickness are not widely used for assessment purposes in the hospitalized patient given issues with technique and time for data collection, but they have shown merit in patients followed long term. **Laboratory tests**: Visceral protein stores are commonly assessed when evaluating nutritional status. Various proteins can be evaluated: albumin (half-life of 18–21 days); transferrin (half-life of 8–10 days); thyroxine-binding prealbumin (half-life of 1–2 days), and retinol-binding protein (half-life of 10 hours). Albumin is the visceral protein universally used as an indicator of nutritional status and is typically the least expensive to obtain. Shorter half-life proteins are most useful in acute care settings. All can be affected by other variables unrelated to nutrient intake (i.e., surgery, fluid status), and these variables must be considered when evaluating protein status. The adequacy of protein supplied to maintain lean body mass is typically evaluated via the nitrogen balance, which is the state when protein intake (nitrogen in) and output of nitrogen are equal. Nitrogen output is monitored via 24-hour urine collections and the urinary urea nitrogen (UUN) levels. One gram of protein equals 6.25 gm of nitrogen; therefore the protein in (24-hour UUN + 4 for insensible losses) equals the nitrogen balance. A positive nitrogen balance is an indication of anabolism (goal of +2 to +4), and a negative nitrogen balance indicates catabolic or starvation state. Total lymphocyte count and delayed hypersensitivity testing to measure compromised immune function resulting from malnutrition can be affected by many nonnutritional factors. The validity of these tests as a measure of malnutrition is debated. The most common type of malnutrition seen in the hospitalized patient is protein-calorie malnutrition due to partial or total starvation. Seven days is the absolute maximum a patient should have severely limited nutritional intake. Therefore determination of the need for oral supplements or a more aggressive feeding regimen (parenteral or enteral nutrition) is important and requires knowledge of a patient's daily nutritional requirements. There are consequences for underfeeding (i.e., weight loss, nutrient deficiency) or overfeeding (i.e., hepatic lipogenesis, increased carbon dioxide production), indicating the importance of specific, individualized estimates of each patient's nutritional requirements. Many equations and formulas have been developed and studied to determine energy expenditure, including the most widely used Harris-Benedict equation for measuring basal energy expenditure (BEE). BEE is the energy required to fuel basic life functions in normal healthy individuals at rest in a neutral, thermal environment 10 hours or more after eating.

Male: 66 + 13.7 (wt) + 5 (ht) − 6.8 (age)
Female: 65 + 9.6 (wt) + 1.8 (ht) − 4.7 (age)

where wt is the weight in kilograms (pounds ÷ 2.2), ht is the height in centimeters, and age is recorded in years.

The BEE is typically adjusted for injury and activity factors, but overestimation of needs with these considerations do occur. The most accurate means to measure energy expenditure is via indirect calorimetry to measure resting energy expenditure (REE). REE is the energy needed for the specific action or thermogenic effect of food measured in the awake, resting individual receiving food. The REE equals oxygen consumed divided by carbon dioxide produced under these conditions. Indirect calorimetry is expensive and sometimes not possible; therefore indirect calorimetry is used to confirm the accuracy of the results obtained from equation estimates. Typically, calorie requirements of the hospitalized adult range from 25 to 35 kcal/kg. The recommended daily allowance (RDA) for protein is 0.8 gm/kg in healthy adults. An increased need for protein is seen with the catabolic response to injury with 1.2–1.5 gm protein per kilogram or higher necessary for protein synthesis in stressed patient populations (i.e., postsurgery or sepsis). Calculating nitrogen balance is the most common way to determine if protein needs are being met. Patients with severe injuries or burns typically require larger amounts of protein. Protein synthesis requires calories from sources other than protein to fuel production. A nonprotein calorie/nitrogen ratio of 150:1 or 100:1 is typically recommended. In patients with hepatic disease protein requirements are based on stress level. A patient with encephalopathic episodes requires use of BCAAs, as these amino acids do not require metabolism by the liver and can be converted to energy locally in the muscle. Patients with renal disease and in acute failure, without dialysis, are typically permitted only 0.4–0.6 gm/kg. Protein needs increase with dialysis, and the needs should be determined on an individual basis.

ANSWER:
Question 11: A
Question 12: A, B, D

13. Which is/are true of simple starvation?

A. It results in a respiratory quotient of 0.6–0.7, which is indicative of fat as a primary fuel source.
B. The Cori and alanine cycles provide carbon for gluconeogenesis in the liver.
C. Lipogenesis continues to allow future fat reserves.
D. Synthesis of glucose in the liver is closely linked to the synthesis of urea.

Ref.: 10, 11

COMMENTS: See Question 14.

14. Which tissues are obligatory glucose users?

A. Cardiac muscle.
B. RBCs.
C. Brain.
D. Skeletal muscle.

Ref.: 10, 11

COMMENTS: Simple starvation results when nutrient intake does not meet energy requirements. Energy expenditure characteristically decreases to help match energy intake. The metabolic responses that occur do so to preserve muscle mass. Initially, during early fasting, glycogen via glycogenolysis supplies glucose for obligatory glucose-using tissues (i.e., RBCs and brain). Lipogenesis is curtailed, as lactate, pyruvate, and AAs are not diverted to glucose production. The Cori cycle is then activated, which allows the glucose produced by gluconeogenesis in the liver to be converted back to lactate via glycolysis in the peripheral tissues. Skeletal muscle releases AAs via the alanine cycle, which provides carbon for gluconeogenesis in the liver. The Cori and alanine cycles are important, as tissues that use only glucose (brain, blood, renal medulla, bone marrow) are dependent on hepatic gluconeogenesis primarily from lactate, glycerol, and alanine during starvation. The alanine and Cori cycles supply glucose but do not provide carbon for net synthesis of glucose; they only replace the glucose that is used to produce lactate in peripheral tissues. Even as fuel in the gut is diminished, glucose is still mandatory. Glycerol and protein are important substrates for net glucose synthesis. Protein metabolism adapts to starvation, as follows: (1) synthesis of protein decreases, as energy sources to generate production are not available; (2) protein catabolism is reduced as other fuels become primary sources of energy for many tissues; (3) decreased ureagenesis and urinary nitrogen loss reflect protein sparing (initial starvation rates of urea nitrogen are more than 10 gm/day with a decline to less than 7 gm/day after weeks of starvation). To calculate protein losses, note that each gram of nitrogen lost in urine reflects 6.25 gm of protein lost. Alanine, glutamine, and glycine are released in large amounts to be used by the liver and kidney for net glucose formation. Glucose synthesis in the liver during simple starvation is linked to synthesis of urea because of the increased transamination. The adipose tissue during starvation is important because the insulin/glucagon ratio is decreased, which allows activation of lipolysis and suppression of lipogenesis. Levels of fatty acids are increased during starvation and are used as alternative fuels by many tissues that prefer fat as a fuel source (i.e., kidney, cardiac muscle, skeletal muscle). The liver uses fatty acids to meet energy needs for gluconeogenesis. The acetyl CoA generated by oxidation of fatty acids in the liver is converted to ketones. As ketones (acetoacetate and β-hydroxybutyrate) rise, they can cross the blood–brain barrier to supply fuel, though some glucose is still required. The use of fatty acids as a primary fuel source allows the sparing of body proteins for gluconeogenesis. This sparing effect is important for maintenance of immune functions and liver and respiratory muscle function. A respiratory quotient of 0.6–0.7 during simple starvation is reflective of fat being the body's primary fuel source during simple starvation.

ANSWER:
Question 13: A, B, D
Question 14: B, C

15. Hormonal changes that typically occur during stress include which of the following?

A. Increased cortisol.
B. Increased glucagon.
C. Increased catecholamines.
D. Increased insulin.

Ref.: 10, 11, 12, 13

COMMENTS: See Question 17.

16. Unsuppressible glucose production during stress can lead to which of the following problems?

A. Low rate of glycogen storage.
B. Low rate of lipolysis.
C. High rate of fat oxidation.
D. None of the above.

Ref.: 10, 11, 12, 13

COMMENTS: See Question 17.

17. Which of the following occurs during stress?

A. Hypoalbuminemia.
B. Decreased muscle mass.
C. Positive nitrogen balance.
D. Increased serum total protein.

Ref.: 10, 11, 12, 13

COMMENTS: Activation of stress hypermetabolism occurs following surgery, trauma, or sepsis to provide energy and substrates for tissue repair and to activate immune function and the inflammatory response. Initially (the ebb phase) a decline in oxygen consumption is seen along with poor circulation, fluid imbalance, and cellular shock lasting 24–36 hours. As the body adapts (flow phase), there is increased cellular activity and increased hormonal stimulation, which leads to an elevated metabolic rate, body temperature, and nitrogen loss. This phase can last days, weeks, or months. Nutrients are used during hypermetabolism in response to the stress hormonal and inflammatory mediator response to the injury. The earliest stages of response are characterized by increases in gluconeogenesis, resting energy expenditure, proteolysis, ureagenesis, and urinary nitrogen loss. Clinical signs include tachypnea, increased temperature, and tachycardia, with laboratory results showing increased leukocytosis, hyperlactatemia, azotemia, and hyperglycemia. Liver production of glucose during stress is increased secondary to gluconeogenesis and glycogenolysis (Cori cycle), which are stimulated by endocrine (hormonal) changes: increased cortisol, increased glucagon, increased catecholamines, and decreased insulin. Overall use of protein as an oxidative fuel source by liver is increased, and typically there is increased turnover of BCAAs. Hyperglycemia is characteristic during stress, with (1) increased glycogenolysis occurring initially to elevate blood glucose followed by (2) increased glucose production and (3) reduced peripheral utilization later in response to the stress. Gluconeogenesis in the liver continues despite hyperglycemia. Typically, neither glucose nor insulin infusion can control blood glucose levels (or gluconeogenesis) during times of extreme stress. Insuppressible glucose production leads to low rates of glycogen storage, lipolysis, and oxidation of fat. Continuous circulation of insulin secondary to high plasma glucose levels prevents extended use of the body's vast fat stores for energy. Increases in fatty acid oxidation does occur with hypermetabolism, resulting in decreased plasma linoleic and arachidonic acid levels, which can lead to essential fatty acid deficiency in 10 days if exogenous sources are not supplied. A respiratory quotient of 0.80–0.85 during hypermetabolism reflects oxidation of mixed fuel sources.

ANSWER:
Question 15: A, B, C
Question 16: A, B
Question 17: A, B

18. Which of the following is appropriate action when a patient experiences diarrhea with the initiation of tube feedings?

A. Stop tube feedings immediately to ensure that the patient does not become dehydrated.
B. Switch to a more concentrated formula to provide less free water to the patient.
C. Evaluate the patient's medications, if any, and determine if they contribute to the diarrhea.
D. Rule out *Clostridium difficile* colitis.
E. Slow the rate of feedings or consider antidiarrheal medications when *C. difficile* is ruled out as a cause of the diarrhea.

Ref.: 14, 15, 16

COMMENTS: Enteral nutrition is the provision of liquid formula diets by mouth or tube into some area of the gastrointestinal (GI) tract to maintain or improve nutritional status. The decision to use enteral nutrition is based on the premise that if the gut works—use it. Conditions contraindicating use of the GI tract include gastroparesis, intestinal obstruction, paralytic ileus, high-output enteric fistula, and short bowel syndrome. Once it has been established that the enteral route can be used and the patient cannot consume adequate nutrition by mouth, the next steps are to determine where in the GI tract to establish the feeding and which technique is required for tube placement. Nasogastric tubes are preferred for short-term feedings for less than 30 days. Gastrostomy can be temporary (Stamm) or permanent (Janeway). Endoscopic procedures are a viable alternative to surgery in some patients. Contraindications to endoscopically placed tubes include aspiration, gastroparesis, and head trauma. Jejunostomy tube placement is necessary for patients requiring enteric feedings. Techniques for jejunostomy placement include open laparotomy or radiologic, laparoscopic, or endoscopic placement. The patient's status, their ability to tolerate the procedure, the cost, and techniques available to the institution all influence selection of the tube feeding technique. Decisions regarding tube feeding rate, frequency, and amount depend on the patient and his or her condition, the tube feeding type, and the enteral feeding site. There are three methods for administering enteral feedings: (1) bolus or gravity: 250–500 ml of feeding administered quickly several times per day in patients with relatively normal digestion and absorption; (2) intermittent: also applied several times per day but given over at least 0.5 hour to allow gastic emptying similar to that seen with normal eating; and (3) continuous: requires a Kangaroo-type pump to administer feedings over 10–24 hours for patients who require consistent delivery of nutrients to prevent dumping. The formula is typically full strength, initiated at a slow rate (20–40 cc/hr), and advanced as tolerated to goal. A patient's goal rate is based on nutritional requirements for fluid, calories, and protein. A typical advancement schedule may include increasing the tube feeding rate by 20–30 cc every 6 hours, as tolerated, to goal, depending on the patient. Most complications associated with tube feedings can be prevented with proper monitoring. Complications can be metabolic (over- or underhydration), gastrointestinal (diarrhea, nausea, vomiting), or mechanical (wrong tube size, cracked tube). To prevent complications for gastrically fed patients, ensure that the patient is in a semiupright position for gastric feeds, confirm the tube position, and initiate feedings slowly with gastric residuals checked frequently (i.e., every 4–6 hours, with residuals of more than 150 ml rechecked and tube feedings or other contributing factors adjusted appropriately). All patients should be instructed about flushing to keep lines clear and to provide adequate hydration. Note that the typical tube feeding regimen requires additional water to ensure adequate hydration. Diarrhea has been estimated to occur in 2.3% of the enteral population and in 34–41% of critically ill patients. Diarrhea may be related to factors other than the tube feeding itself in the critically ill patient (e.g., hypoalbuminemia or medications). Diarrhea may be able to be controlled by: (1) medication, if not contraindicated, such as Lomotil, Imodium, or paregoric; (2) changing feedings to continuous; or (3) slowing the rate of tube feeding until tolerance is established. *Clostridium difficile* must be ruled out as a cause of the diarrhea prior to initiation of medication to control the problem. Concentrated tube feeding formulas (>1.5 kcal/cc of formula) may exacerbate or cause diarrhea. Careful monitoring of conditions surrounding the onset of diarrhea are important when evaluating the cause.

ANSWER: C, D, E

19. Which of the following statements is/are true? Categorically speaking, concentrated enteral formulas:

A. Do not contain fat sufficient to meet patients' nutritional requirements.
B. Contain less water than standard formulas.
C. Typically are used for regulation of bowel function.
D. Lower the volume required to meet patients' calorie needs compared to standard formulas.

Ref.: 17

COMMENTS: See Question 21.

20. Elemental tube feeding products contain hydrolyzed macronutrients. Which of the following statements is/are correct regarding these types of formulas?

A. Typically not palatable.
B. Typically used for patients with impaired digestion due to disease state or lengthy NPO status.
C. Typically not tolerated well in patients with partially functioning GI tracts.
D. Include Vivonex and Vital HN.

Ref.: 17

COMMENTS: See Question 21.

21. Fiber-containing formulas can help regulate bowel function. Which of these statements is/are true of formulas in this category?

A. Can eliminate diarrhea or constipation.
B. Include Sustacal and Peptamen.
C. Are not able to meet macronutrient requirements as efficiently as regular formulas due to the "bulk" of soy polysaccharides.
D. May contain soy polysaccharides as the fiber source.

Ref.: 5, 17

COMMENTS: Many formulas exist for use in the tube-fed patient. Whereas the hospital formulary dictates what is available for use in the hospital, any formula can be obtained for the tube-fed outpatient. Carbohydrate is usually provided from intact macronutrient sources, including maltodextrin, hydrolyzed cornstarch, corn syrup solids, and sucrose. Protein sources are casein, soy, whey, lactalbumin, or free amino acids. Fat content may be long-chain triglycerides derived from vegetable oil or medium-chain triglycerides from coconut or palm kernel oil. Appropriate selection is key to successful tube feeding. Six product categories exist for enteral formulas. **Standard**: a formula that mimics the American diet, with 50–60% of calories from CHO, 10–15% from protein, and 25–40% from fat. These formulas are isosmolar to blood (300 mOsmol/kg) and are used for patients with functioning GI tracts who have been NPO less than 7 days. Examples are Isocal and Osmolite. **Concentrated**: similar to standard products in terms of content to meet the patient's nutritional requirements, but the density per milliliter is greater than that of standard formulas because of the decreased water content. It is typically used for patients with fluid restrictions. Examples are Isocal HN and Two-Cal HN. **High nitrogen-protein** formulas contain more than 15% of calories supplied by nitrogen and protein. These formulas are used for patients with higher than normal protein needs (i.e., malnourished, catabolic, or elderly patients with increased protein requirements). Examples are Ensure, Osmolite HN, and Travasorb HN. **Elemental**: formulas advocated for patients who have been NPO more than 7 days or those with partially functioning GI tracts. They contain hydrolyzed macronutrients that require less digestion and are potentially better tolerated until the patient is able to transition back to intact nutrients. Generally, the formulas are low in fat or contain fewer long-chain triglycerides and are hyperosmolar (>450 mOsm/kg). Examples are Criticare HN, Vital HN, Vivonex TEN, Peptamen. **Fiber-containing or blenderized**: fiber supplied from added soy polysaccharides or natural food sources, respectively. Fiber formulas are intended to regulate bowel function by eliminating diarrhea and constipation. Examples are Jevity and Enrich (Ensure with fiber). Blenderized formulas can be distinguished from fiber formulas in that they are regular foods and therefore contain all components of nutrients naturally occurring in foods. Examples are Compleat and Vitaneed. **Specialty products**: These products are available for liver, renal, and pulmonary disease. Their composition varies depending on the disease state, but generally these products have high osmolality and are nutritionally inadequate. The benefit of such formulas remains controversial. Examples are for pulmonary disease, Pulmocare; for liver disease, Hepatic Aid; and for renal disease, AminAid. Some enteral products do contain lactose, which causes bloating, cramping, and diarrhea in some patients. Lactose-free products should be used if intolerance is expected or symptoms arise. Some patients have needs that cannot be met by available commercial products due to electrolyte imbalances or the need for varied macronutrient content. Enteral feeding modules can be used to create a patient-specific formula (*modular formula*). Carbohydrate modules include Sumacal and Polycose. Protein modules available include Promod and Propac. Fat sources are MCT oil and Microlipid. Vitamins and mineral products are available. Modular formulas are made by adding water to specific amounts of these products to best suit a patient's needs. Adding to the complexities of nutritional management of the tube-fed patient is the wide variety of enteral products available. Dietitians and nutrition support teams are typically responsible for determining the best formulas for a hospital formulary to carry based on current research and cost containment.

ANSWER:
Question 19: B, D
Question 20: A, B, D
Question 21: A, D

22. Which of the following is/are associated with enteral feedings (ENT) when compared to parenteral feedings (TPN)?

A. There is a decreased likelihood of bacterial translocation with ENT compared to TPN.
B. Increased risk of infection.
C. Reduced cost.
D. Preservation of gut integrity.

Ref.: 18, 19

COMMENTS: Although TPN is a valuable feeding technique, using the GI tract seems prudent. Research indicates that enteral nutrition is generally well tolerated and allows gut mucosal growth and development as well as maintenance of gut integrity. Moreover ENT costs less than TPN. Patients receiving enteral feedings tend to have fewer septic complications than those receiving TPN, most likely due to a reduction of bacterial translocation from the gut. Kudsk et al. showed that among severely injured patients only 14% of those fed enterally developed septic complications versus 52% of those on TPN. Bacterial translocation can be defined as the movement of microbes or their by-products across an intact intestinal barrier. Three factors known to predispose patients to bacterial translocation are (1) microscopic or structural harm to the gut directly (i.e., Crohn's disease or radiation therapy) or indirectly (i.e., burns or sepsis); (2) changes in gut (microbial) flora due to disuse with TPN or broad-spectrum antibiotic use; or (3) secretory immunoglobulin A (IgA), the immune system's primary enterocyte defense, is augmented in the nutritionally depleted or catabolic patient, and so the IgA cannot perform its primary role of coating the enterocyte to prevent attachment by pathogenic bacteria. Once gut permeability is increased (loss of GI tract integrity) owing to these factors, toxic substances or bacteria move (translocate) into the portal circulation or lymphatics. Moderate amounts may be acceptable (i.e., to upgrade the inflammatory response to injury), but large amounts can cause irreversible harm. Many former limitations to using enteral feedings have been discounted. Most importantly, the gut can be used immediately after trauma or surgery provided the patient is resuscitated initially. Traditionally, the early feeding approach was not considered possible during the early postoperative or posttrauma period, and TPN was typically administered. With respect to postoperative medications, it is suggested that the small intestine may be least affected by prescribed opiates, and enteral feed can be administered with close observation for intolerance. Initiation of tube feedings as early as postoperative day 1 have been successful. Some clinicians argue that postoperative ileus cannot be automatically assumed with lack of bowel sounds. Small bowel function may be intact despite a lack of colon activity postoperatively; therefore initiation of tube feedings seems appropriate early in the postoperative period. Of note when discussing bacterial translocation is the issue of multisystem organ failure (MOF), which is characterized by a rapid onset of malnutrition, high oxygen consumption, catabolic activity, and the development of infections as a response to shock, sepsis, tissue injury, and inflammation. One proposed mechanism for this type of septic morbidity is that the loss of integrity of the GI tract as a barrier may aggravate or cause MOF. At this point the cause of MOF (loss of gut integrity or otherwise) has yet to be established, but support for enteral feedings on the whole seems prudent when possible.

ANSWER: A, C, D

23. The anhydrous form of dextrose used in parenteral formulas contains how many calories per gram?

A. 3.4.
B. 4.0.
C. 7.0.
D. 9.0.

Ref.: 20

COMMENTS: See Question 25.

24. Which is true of peripheral venous nutrition (PVN) when compared to central venous nutrition (CVN)?

A. PVN is administered into small veins, typically in the arm, whereas CVN is administered into larger veins such as the superior vena cava.
B. PVN can be used for a long time (weeks or months), as it can usually meet patients' protein and calorie requirements adequately, as with CVN.
C. Due to rapid blood flow in peripheral veins, the PVN solution is rapidly diluted by blood, thereby allowing tolerance to the high osmolality of the solution.
D. Intravenous fat solutions are isotonic and can therefore be administered peripherally and centrally without concern for thrombosis.

Ref.: 20

COMMENTS: See Question 25.

25. How many calories are provided in one 500-cc bottle of 10% intravenous solution?

A. 150 kcal.
B. 550 kcal.
C. 800 kcal.
D. 1000 kcal.

Ref.: 20

COMMENTS: Parenteral nutrition (PN, TPN, hyperalimentation) is the provision of nutrients (CHO, protein, fat, vitamins and minerals, sterile water) via a hyperosmolar solution delivered into a central vein, typically the superior vena cava. All components must be individualized to the patient based on diagnosis, chronic disease state, fluid and electrolyte status, acid–base balance, and specific nutritional goals. The patient who cannot meet nutritional needs via the oral or enteral route requires TPN, with the basic goal of TPN being to meet nutritional needs of the patient and maintain or improve metabolic balance. Disease state indications for TPN include a nonfunctioning GI tract (i.e., short bowel syndrome, intractable vomiting, or diarrhea), the need for bowel rest (i.e., severe pancreatitis), and severe malnutrition where the patient is unable to eat for 5–7 days or more. Two types of solution exist: (1) traditional dextrose and amino acid solutions in which lipids are piggybacked into the solution; and (2) total nutrient admixture (TNA), where the solution contains all three macronutrients and is dispensed from a single container. An automated compounding device is needed for accurate mixing; and as will all TPN, mixing should be done under laminar airflow to control bacterial contamination. Various concentrations of macronutrients are available to develop a patient-specific, nutritional regimen that helps prevent overfeeding or underfeeding. The composition of TPN is limited by maximum concentrations of various amino acid (AA) and dextrose solutions that are physically achievable. Crystalline protein and synthetic AAs are the protein sources for TPN solutions with standard base solutions ranging from 8.5% to 10.0% AAs (0.5 liter of 8.5% solution would contain 42.5 gm protein). Hepatamine 8% is an AA solution sometimes used for patients with encephalopathy, as it contains an increased percentage of branched-chain amino acids. Commercially available dextrose solutions contain 5–70% glucose (50–700 gm/L). The final solution typically contains 15–35% dextrose. The monohydrate form of dextrose is used for TPN providing 3.4 kcal/gm upon oxidation. Dextrose can be provided peripherally (peripheral venous nutrition, or PVN) at concentrations of less than 10%, and should be administered only short term. Higher concentrations may promote thrombosis owing to low peripheral blood flow, thereby preventing the provision of adequate calories or protein (or both) via this method. Fat solutions are considered isotonic and can be administered peripherally or centrally without concern about thrombosis. Carbohydrates should be administered at a rate no greater than 5 mg/kg/min via TPN, which is the maximum oxidation rate of glucose. Fat solutions are available in 10% and 20% solutions, which provide 1.1 and 2.0 kcal/ml, respectively. Fats can be administered intermittently, continuously, or via TNA. Monitoring clearance via triglyceride levels is key to ensuring tolerance to lipid infusions. Patients should also be monitored for signs of chills, fevers, headaches, or back pain with initiation of fat to rule out intolerance. Fat should be administered at no more than 2.5 gm/kg/day. Lipid solutions should be administered cautiously to patients with respiratory distress syndrome, severe liver disease, or increased metabolic stress, as fat may exacerbate these conditions. Patients with hypertriglyceridemia (>250 mg/dl), lipid nephrosis, egg allergy, or acute pancreatitis associated with hyperlipidemia should not be given fat emulsions. Vitamins and minerals should be supplied to meet the recommended daily allowance (RDA). Vitamin K must be ordered separately based on coagulation status. Electrolytes are added to TPN to maintain or achieve electrolyte homeostasis with individual electrolyte needs depending on disease state, renal function, drug therapy, hepatic function, and nutritional status (Table 5–2). A problem sometimes seen in the malnourished patient with initiation of feedings is the refeeding syndrome, which is characterized by rapid depletion of potassium, phosphorus, and magnesium due to lean tissue synthesis and the shift of metabolism intracellularly with glucose administration. This problem can result in death if electrolytes are not carefully monitored. The increased need for various minerals and electrolytes seen with diarrhea, ostomies, fistulas, vomiting, and other GI losses can be met via TPN. Metabolic and nutritional factors should be evaluated for each patient receiving TPN. Metabolic monitoring can include serum or urine glucose levels (or both) several times daily and electrolytes daily until tolerance is established; other necessary laboratory tests include magnesium, phosphorus, calcium, bilirubin, SGOT, SGPT, alkaline phosphatase, BUN, and creatinine assays. Coagulation monitoring is done daily until the goal TPN reached, as are triglyceride levels to determine the patient's ability to clear lipids before and after lipid administration. Nutritional monitoring should include daily fluid balance evaluation, daily weight, the nitrogen balance as needed, and visceral protein status once per week. Institutional guidelines should be followed for monitoring TPN. A typical initiation plan may progress as follows: (1) check all laboratory values prior to starting TPN and all other related information; (2) initiate TPN at 1 liter at a final concentration needed to meet the patient's needs; (3) monitor tolerance to TPN initiation as outlined (i.e., laboratory tests); (4) increase to the goal TPN. Ongoing adjustments should be expected throughout the course of TPN administration. When calculating the specifics for ordering TPN, the following are taken into account: (1) all macronutrients and micronutrients are based on patients' individual needs; (2) fluid (water) is provided at a volume of 25–50 ml/kg depending on age, renal status, and so on; (3) dextrose solutions are available in 5–70% solutions, and amino acids are available in 3–10% solutions; (4) lipids come in 500 cc bottles with 10% solutions containing 550 kcal and 20% fat solutions containing 1000 kcal; minimal fat needs of 2–4% of the kilocalories as essential fatty acids can be met with weekly administration of lipids. The benefit of using perioperative nutrition remains controversial, with various studies showing conflicting results. It seems at this time that 7–10 days of perioperative nutrition for patients with severe malnutrition may help reduce the risk of postoperative complications and morbidity associated with malnutrition. Patients diagnosed with severe malnutrition (decreased visceral and somatic protein stores) and decreased oral intake prior to surgery who are not ready to undergo surgery, and for whom oral or enteral feedings are not an option, should be fed intravenously. When delay in feeding does not seem logical for those with a suspected postoperative need for TPN, administration should be considered.

Table 5–2. Suggested Initial Amounts of Electrolytes for TPN Solutions

Electrolytes	Usual Amount (mEq/L)	Amount/day (mEq)
Na^+ (sodium)	20–60	60+
Cl^- (chloride)	10–60	60+
K^+ (potassium)	20–50	60–120
Ca^{2+} (calcium)	2.5–10.0	10–20
Mg^+ (magnesium)	2.5–8.0	10–30
Acetate	36	80–120

ANSWER:
Question 23: A
Question 24: A, D
Question 25: B

26. Treatment of hyperglycemia in TPN patients may include:

A. Glucose control with long-lasting insulin.
B. Addition of regular insulin to the parenteral solution.
C. Use of sliding scale coverage with regular insulin.
D. None of the above.

Ref.: 21, 22

COMMENTS: See Question 28.

27. Refeeding syndrome is characterized by which of the following electrolyte abnormalities?

A. Hyponatremia, hypokalemia, hypercalcemia.
B. Hyperphosphatemia, hypokalemia, hypocalcemia.
C. Hypokalemia, hypomagnesemia, hypophosphatemia.
D. Hypocalcemia, hyponatremia, hypomagnesemia.

Ref.: 21, 22

COMMENTS: See Question 28.

28. Match the micronutrient on the left with the appropriate signs and symptoms of its clinical deficiency on the right.

A. Zinc	a. Night blindness; keratosis of the skin
B. Selenium	b. Glucose intolerance, peripheral neuropathy
C. Vitamin A	c. Alopecia, seborrheic dermatitis, neuritis
D. Chromium	d. Poor wound healing, impaired immunity
E. Biotin	e. Cardiomyopathy, weakness, hair loss

Ref.: 23, 24

COMMENTS: There are three areas of complication with use of TPN: (1) mechanical problems secondary to obtaining and continuing central venous access; (2) metabolic problems; and (3) catheter-related sepsis. **Mechanical**: Pneumothorax should not occur in more than 4% of patients with elective access. The incidence is usually higher in emergency situations and in nutritionally depleted patients. Artery injury, air embolism, brachial plexus injury, thoracic duct injury, lymphatic injury, catheter embolus, venous thrombosis, and poor catheter position, among others, are possible mechanically related problems. **Metabolic**: Standard use of vitamins and trace element solutions in TPN has eliminated the problem of deficiency states that were seen with extended use of TPN during the early stages of TPN usage. Excess glucose can (1) increase blood glucose levels and induce hyperosmolar nonketotic coma; (2) lead to dehydration; (3) lead to lipogenesis with subsequent hepatic abnormalities (i.e., fatty liver); and (4) increase CO_2 production, which may compromise respiratory function. Rebound hypoglycemia can occur with discontinuation of TPN; therefore weaning TPN to 50 ml/hr prior to complete discontinuation is important. Treatment for hyperglycemia in TPN patients is typically the addition of regular insulin (not long-acting insulin) to the parenteral solution with stringent monitoring of ACCU-CHECKS and serum blood glucose levels. Fat deficiency can occur if fat is not provided at least twice weekly to meet essential fatty acid requirements. Additional requirements for insulin in critically ill patients with large fluctuations in blood sugar levels benefit from combination of regular insulin in the TPN and sliding scale coverage, with regular insulin to control what the dosage in the TPN cannot. Clinical signs of essential fatty acid deficiency include dry skin, poor wound healing, and hair loss. Hepatic toxicity and benign transient liver function test abnormalities can occur. Gut atrophy and bacterial translocation can occur with gut disuse. Depletion of or excess vitamins and minerals can cause unwanted deficiencies or elevated levels of nutrients (i.e., hyper- or hypokalemia, hyper- or hypophosphatemia). Refeeding syndrome results when glucose is administered quickly to an individual with poor nutrient intake prior to TPN, the result being that glucose moves into the cells rapidly to be utilized and those nutrients required for metabolism of glucose rapidly follow to the intracellular spaces. Subsequent rapid serum depletion of magnesium, phosphorus, or potassium develops. Careful monitoring of the results of initial TPN administration is key. Immunologic impairment due to large doses or rapid lipid administration has been shown to occur. It is thought that once the lipoprotein lipase system becomes overloaded the reticuloendothelial system helps rid the body of excess amounts of lipids, causing neutrophils to become lipid-saturated, affecting their ability to function. Therefore careful monitoring of lipid levels is important. **Catheter-related sepsis**: One can expect to see the incidence of catheter-related sepsis at 2–5%; the rate of line sepsis is 20–30%. Important steps to help prevent line infections include appropriate skin preparation prior to an operative procedure; appropriate maintenance of the central line, frequent catheter changes, careful use of multiple-lumen catheters, and appropriate antibiotic and thrombolytic treatment if sepsis develops.

ANSWER:
Question 26: A, B, C
Question 27: C
Question 28: A-d; B-e; C-a; D-b; E-c

29. Which of the following can be associated with glutamine metabolism?

A. Glutamine's postsurgical uptake by the intestine is mediated by glucagon and glucocorticoids.
B. End-products of glutamine metabolism, ammonia, citrulline, and alanine are used for fuel by enterocytes.
C. Utilization of glutamine during stress occurs faster than the body's ability to synthesize it, which allows significant depletion of glutamine stores.
D. Stimulates protein degradation.

Ref.: 11, 25, 26

COMMENTS: Long-term use of TPN may lead to nutrient deficiencies not typically seen in patients with oral intake. A patient's nutrient status prior to TPN, available oral absorption, increased needs due to the disease state, and losses of vitamins and minerals through adherence to the delivery systems or renal or GI tract losses must be taken into consideration. Some common micronutrient deficiencies seen with the use of long-term TPN include (1) EFA: scaly dermatitis; (2) zinc: growth retardation, hypogonadism, poor healing, impaired immunity, night blindness; (3) copper: microcytic anemia, leukopenia, depigmentation, and osteopenia; (4) chromium: glucose intolerance, weight loss, peripheral neuropathy, ataxia, confusion; (5) molybdenum: confusional state due to toxic accumulation of sulfur-containing amino acid, cholestasis; (6) selenium: cardiomyopathy, proximal muscle pain, weakness, hair loss; (7) vitamin A: night blindness, xerophthalmia, testicular atrophy, skin keratosis; (8) vitamin D: osteomalacia, muscle weakness; (9) vitamin E: dystrophic changes of the retina and posterior column nuclei; (10) vitamin K: bleeding tendency; (11) biotin:

alopecia, seborrheic dermatitis, neuritis. Specific nutrients are being investigated as to their positive effects on enhancing the patient response to nutritional therapy. **Glutamine** is the most abundant amino acid in the plasma and skeletal muscle, comprising 50% of the body's free amino acid pool. Glutamine and alanine are the primary carriers of nitrogen from the skeletal muscle. In healthy individuals, glutamine is considered nonessential in that adipose tissue, lung, skeletal muscle, and sometimes liver can synthesize it. The glutamine "users" are kidney, liver, and small intestine. In the metabolically challenged patient, glutamine may be conditionally essential. Glutamine functions include the following: (1) carrier of nitrogen from organ to organ; (2) major fuel for small intestinal mucosa, lymphocytes, macrophages, fibroblasts, and endothelial and malignant cells; (3) provides nitrogen for nucleic acid of cells; (4) exerts trophic properties on intestinal mucosa; and (5) stimulates protein synthesis and inhibits protein degradation. Accelerated release and increased demand by tissues during critical illness result in large glutamine deficits. Intestinal glutamine metabolism after surgery is mediated by glucagon and glucocorticoid hormones. Sepsis and endotoxemia enchance gut mucosal barrier breakdown via impaired glutamine metabolism, which may lead to bacterial translocation. End-products of glutamine metabolism are ammonia, citrulline, and alanine, with the carbons produced from glutamine used for fuel by enterocytes. Intestinal mucosal atrophy and bacterial translocation in patients without oral intake are thought to be improved with the use of glutamine-containing TPN or tube feedings. Other improvements seen with the use of supplemental glutamine include (1) decreased loss of glutamine from skeletal muscle; (2) prevention of hepatic steatosis; (3) adequate immune function; and (4) regulation of pancreatic endocrine function via islet cell stimulation. Standard TPN solutions do not routinely contain glutamine at this time owing to issues with stability when in solution, but advances are being made that will allow ready availability of glutamine-containing TPN and tube feedings. **Arginine** is a nonessential amino acid produced by the body in the urea cycle. It is thought to stimulate hormonal secretory action, including increasing release of growth hormone and prolactin, glucagon and insulin, insulin growth factor, and catecholamines. Arginine may also improve T cell proliferation by its action on the thymus gland. Use of supplemental arginine has been advocated for the stressed patient to improve nitrogen balance, stimulate the immune system, and accelerate wound healing. Research continues in the area of supplemental arginine with some nutritional products already containing arginine. Immunomodulation and hypermetabolic response are thought to be improved by the use of **omega-3 fatty acids** (fish oil). A study by Daly et al. reported that tube feedings with omega-3 fatty acids, arginine, and RNA significantly improved subjects' nitrogen balance, infection rate, and wound complication rate compared to those on regular feedings. One criticism of the study was that the study group did not receive isonitrogenous feedings. Further research is needed. Evidence suggests that conventional nutritional support may not protect protein stores from depletion during stress. Administration of **growth factors** and other protein-synthesizing agents, such as anabolic steroids, are being studied to measure their ability to enhance protein accrual, improve immune function after surgery, improve wound healing, and enhance maintenance of the GI tract. Use of exogenous growth hormone has protein-sparing effects that seem to result from increased protein synthesis rather than decreased protein breakdown. Effects of growth hormone on fat and carbohydrate metabolism are less clearly understood, with long-term use resulting in intolerance and lipolysis. Studies continue in the area of growth factors and hormones.

ANSWER: A, B, C

REFERENCES

1. Van Way CW III: Basic nutrition, energy stores, and body composition. In: Van Way CW III (ed) *Handbook of Surgical Nutrition*. JB Lippincott, Philadelphia, 1992.
2. Shizgal HM: Body composition and nutritional support. *Surg Clin North Am* 61:727–741, 1981.
3. Jeejeebhoy KN: Nutrient metabolism. In: Kinney JN, Jeejeebhoy KN, Hill GL, et al (eds) *Nutrition and Metabolism in Patient Care*. WB Saunders, Philadelphia, 1988.
4. Harris RA: Carbohydrate metabolism. Major metabolic pathways and their control. In: Devlin TM (ed) *Textbook of Biochemistry with Clinical Correlations*. John Wiley, New York, 1986.
5. Compher C, Seto RW, Lew JI, et al: Dietary fiber and its clinical applications to enteral nutrition. In: Rombeau JL, Rolandelli RH (eds) *Clinical Nutrition: Enteral and Tube Feeding*, 3rd ed. WB Saunders, Philadelphia, 1997.
6. Matthews DE, Fong Y: Amino acid and protein metabolism. In: Rombeau JL, Caldwell MD (eds) *Clinical Nutrition: Parenteral Nutrition*, 2nd ed. WB Saunders, Philadelphia, 1993.
7. McGarry JD: Lipid metabolism. I. Utilization and storage of energy in lipid form. In: Devlin T (ed) *Textbook of Biochemistry with Clinical Correlations*. John Wiley, New York, 1986.
8. Jeejeebhoy KN, Detsky AS, Baker JP: Assessment of nutritional status. *J Parenter Enteral Nutr* 14(Suppl):1935–1965, 1990.
9. Daley BJ, Bistrian BR: Nutritional assessment. In: Zaloga G (ed) *Nutrition in Critical Care*. Mosby-Year Book, St. Louis, 1994.
10. Cerra FB: How nutrition intervention changes what getting sick means. *J Parenter Enteral Nutr* 14(Suppl):1966–1995, 1990.
11. Barton RG: Nutrition support in critical illness. *Nutr Clin Pract* 9:127–139, 1994.
12. Gefland RA, Matthews DE, Bier DM, Sherwin RS: Role of counterregulatory hormones in the catabolic response to stress. *J Clin Invest* 74:2238–2248, 1984.
13. VanWay CW III: Nutritional support in the injured patient. *Surg Clin North Am* 71:537–548, 1991.
14. ASPEN American Society for Parenteral and Enteral Nutrition Board of Directors: Guidelines for the use of parenteral and enteral nutrition in adult and pediatric patients. *J Parenter Enteral Nutr* 17(Suppl):5SA–26SA, 1993.
15. Kohn CL, Keithly JK: Techniques for evaluating and managing diarrhea in the tube-fed patient. *Nutr Clin Pract* 2:250–257, 1987.
16. Homann HH, Kemen M, Fuessenich MD, et al: Reduction in diarrhea incidence by soluble fiber in patients receiving total or supplemental enteral nutrition. *J Parenter Enteral Nutr* 18:486–490, 1994.
17. Bell SJ, Pasulka PS, Blackburn GL: Enteral formulas. In: Skipper A (ed) *Dietitian's Handbook of Enteral and Parenteral Nutrition*. Aspen Publishers, Rockville, MD, 1989.
18. Kudsk KS, Croce MA, Fabian TC, et al: Enteral vs. parenteral feeding: effects on septic morbidity after blunt and penetrating trauma. *Ann Surg* 215:503–513, 1992.
19. Moore EE, Moore FA: Immediate enteral nutrition following multisystem trauma: a decade perspective. *J Am Coll Nutr* 10:633–648, 1991.
20. Maillet JO: Calculating parenteral feedings: a programmed instruction. *J Am Diet Assoc* 11:1312–1323, 1984.
21. Giner M, Curtas S: Adverse metabolic consequences of nutritional support: macronutrients. *Surg Clin North Am* 66:1025–1047, 1986.
22. Solomon SM, Kirby DF: The refeeding syndrome: a review. *J Parenter Enteral Nutr* 14:90–97, 1990.
23. Hammond K: Physical assessment: a nuritional perspective. *Nurs Clin North Am* 32:779–790, 1997.
24. Howard L, Alger S, Michalek A, et al: Home parenteral nutrition in adults. In: Rombeau JL, Caldwell MD (eds) *Clinical Nutrition: Parenteral Nutrition*, 2nd ed. WB Saunders, Philadelphia, 1993.
25. O'Dwyer SO, Smith RJ, Hwang TL, et al: Maintenance of small bowel mucosa with glutamine enriched parenteral nutrition. *J Parenter Enteral Nutr* 13:579–585, 1989.
26. Van Der Hulst RRW, VanKrell DK, VonMeyenfeldt MF, et al: Glutamine and preservation of gut integrity. *Lancet* 341:1363–1365, 1993.

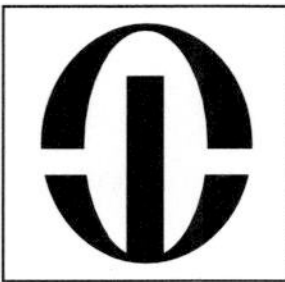

CHAPTER 6

Wound Healing

1. Arrange the following events in the healing of an uncomplicated wound into proper sequence.

   A. Proliferation
   B. Inflammation
   C. Maturation

Ref.: 1, 2, 3

COMMENTS: The process of wound healing is not a simple sequence of events but an array of simultaneously occurring metabolic and physiologic changes that are initiated at the time of injury and continue long after the process appears to have been completed. Wound repair events are conceptually defined as inflammation, epithelialization, granulation, fibroplasia, and contraction. The basic processes are similar for sutured wounds, which heal by primary intention, and wounds with tissue loss, which heal by secondary intention. In general, the process of wound healing is divided into three overlapping phases: inflammation, proliferation, and maturation. During **inflammation**, the capillary vessels become permeable to leukocytes and plasma proteins, which, within hours, fill the wound with an inflammatory exudate of neutrophils, monocytes, and protein. Meanwhile, the wound epithelializes by 48 hours as basal epithelial cells multiply and fill in the wound surface. On approximately the third day, fibroblasts appear in the wound in significant numbers, marking the beginning of the **proliferative** phase. The proliferative phase is sometimes referred to as the fibroplasia phase because it is then that the fibroblasts begin to multiply in number and release collagen and interstitial matrix. Meanwhile, endothelial cells begin to proliferate and form new vessels. Wound contraction, carried out by myofibroblasts, also occurs at this time. After approximately 3 weeks the fibroblasts and macrophages gradually disappear from the wound, and the relatively acellular collagen begins a continuous process of remodeling and **maturation**.

ANSWER: B, A, C

2. With regard to the inflammatory phase of wound healing, which of the following statements is/are correct?

   A. It begins 5–6 hours after the wound event.
   B. Bradykinin causes vasoconstriction, which inhibits neutrophil migration to the healing wound.
   C. The complement component C5a and platelet factor attract neutrophils to the wound.
   D. The presence of neutrophils in the wound is essential for normal wound healing.

Ref.: 1, 3, 4

COMMENTS: The inflammatory phase starts immediately after the wounding occurs. After the injury there is a transient period (about 10 minutes) of vasoconstriction followed by active vasodilatation. These events are mediated by substances released secondary to the local tissue injury. Vasoactive components such as histamine cause brief periods of vasodilatation and increased vascular permeability. The kinins (bradykinin and kallidin) are released by enzymatic action of kallikrein, which is formed after coagulation cascade activation. These components, in addition to those of the complement system, stimulate release of prostaglandins (particularly PGE and PGE_2), which work in concert to maintain more prolonged vessel permeability not only of the capillaries but of larger vessels as well. In addition, these substances, particularly the complement component C5a and platelet-derived factors such as platelet-derived growth factor (PDGF) act as chemotactic stimuli for neutrophils to enter the wound. Although neutrophils do phagocytize bacteria from a wound, results of studies involving clean wound healing show that healing can proceed normally without them. Monocytes, however, must be present for normal wound healing because, in addition to phagocytosis, they are required to trigger a normal fibroblast response.

ANSWER: C

3. Which of the following statements regarding wound inflammation is/are true?

   A. Platelets are responsible for the release of numerous, biologically active substances important for wound healing.
   B. Thrombin and fibrin fragments act as potent growth and chemoattractant factors.
   C. Monocytes differentiate into neutrophils by 24 hours after injury.
   D. In the healing wound, macrophages act primarily to clear tissue and bacterial debris.

Ref.: 1, 2

COMMENTS: Immediately after the creation of a wound, there is initially vasoconstriction, release of tissue thromboplastic factors, and activation of the coagulation and complement cascade. Trapped platelets degenerate, and several types of storage granules are released: (1) α-Granules contain growth factors such as PDGF, transforming growth factor-beta (TGF-β) and insulin-like growth factor-1 (IGF-1). The granules also contain several adhesive glycoproteins such as fibronectin, fibrinogen, thrombospondin, and von Willebrand factor. (2) Dense bodies release serotonin, which increases vascular permeability. This, in concert with the local release of kinins, complement components, and prostaglandins, reverses the initial vasoconstriction of the microcirculation. (3) Lysozomes release hydrolases and proteases. • Prothrombin converts to thrombin, which in turn converts fibrinogen to fibrin. This creates a stable clot that acts as a scaffolding for subsequent fibroblast in-growth. The clot also acts as an inducer of angiogenesis. Thrombin acts as a growth factor for endothelial cells and fibroblasts. Thrombin fragments stimulate monocytes and platelets. Fibrinogen acts as a chemoattractant for monocytes. • Neutrophils are the first cells to enter the wound and scavenge cellular debris and bacteria. Monocytes enter the wound later and differentiate into macrophages. They clean debris, but more importantly the monocytes release a number of growth factors that activate endothelial cells, fibroblasts, and epithelial cells, a sequence of events essential for the formation of granulation tissue.

ANSWER: A, B

4. Which of the following are constituents of the granulation tissue matrix?

A. Collagen.
B. Macrophages.
C. Fibroblasts.
D. Hyaluronic acid.

Ref.: 1, 2

COMMENTS: See Question 5.

5. Which statements regarding granulation is/are true?

A. Granulation tissue is primarily desiccated fibrin/platelet clot.
B. Fibroblasts involved in wound repair migrate into the wound from the systemic circulation after vasodilatation begins.
C. Most collagen in normal skin is type III.
D. Most collagen in healing wounds is type I.

Ref.: 1, 2

COMMENTS: Granulation starts with endothelial cell division and migration (angiogenesis) into the wound, creating a rich network of capillaries. At the same time, fibroblasts at the wound edge differentiate and migrate into the wound, moving along the previously deposited fibrin–fibrinonectin matrix. As fibroblasts proliferate, a process known as fibroplasia, they synthesize a new extracellular matrix. Both angiogenesis and fibroplasia are stimulated by platelet- and macrophage-derived growth factors. • The initial granulation tissue is composed, therefore, of collagen (secreted by fibroblasts), fibrinonectin, hyaluronic acid, macrophages, fibroblasts, and capillary endothelial cells. • Hyaluronic acid is a nonsulfated glycosaminoglycan (GAG). Glycosaminoglycans, along with adhesion glycoproteins such as fibronectin, laminin, and tenascin, create a scaffolding along which fibroblasts move and deposit collagen. Collagen types 1 and 3 are the major collagen types in the wound matrix. The major collagen type in normal skin extracellular matrix is type 1. Although there is relatively more type 3 collagen in the wound matrix, the predominant type of collagen there is type 1.

ANSWER:
Question 4: A, B, C, D
Question 5: D

6. With regard to epithelialization, which of the following statements is/are correct?

A. It produces a watertight seal of surgical incisions within 48 hours.
B. A reepithelialized wound develops hair follicles and sweat glands, like normal skin.
C. It is a process normally inhibited by surface contact with other epithelial cells.
D. Disruption of normal healing, such as in a chronic wound, may produce malignancy.

Ref.: 1, 2, 3

COMMENTS: Migration of epithelial cells is one of the earliest events in wound healing. Shortly after injury and during the inflammatory phase, basal epithelial cells begin to multiply and migrate across the defect, using fibrin strands as a support structure. • Meticulously coapted surgical incisions seal rather promptly and after 24 hours are protected from the external environment. Epithelialization of larger separations in wounds requires a long time. Early tensile strength is a result of blood vessel ingrowth, epithelialization, and protein aggregation. If the wound is not under excessive tension, this allows approximation until adequate collagen has been synthesized to provide significant structural strength. After covering the wound, the epithelial cells keratinize. The reepithelialized wound has no sweat glands or hair follicles, which distinguishes it from normal skin. • Control of the cellular process during wound epithelialization is not completely understood, but it appears to involve inhibition of surface contact with similar cells. Derangements in the control of this process can result in epidermoid malignancy. This has been observed particularly in wounds resulting from ionizing radiation or chemical injury, but it can occur in any wound when the healing process has been chronically disrupted, such as the development of squamous cell carcinoma in chronic burn wounds or osteomyelitis (Marjolin's ulcer).

ANSWER: C, D

7. Which statements regarding epithelialization is/are true?

A. Mitosis is the predominant event in the process of epithelialization.
B. Keratinocytes migrate over the top of the debris at the wound surface.
C. Keratinocytes move by an actin–myocin contractile system.
D. Epiboly refers to epithelial cell degranulation.
E. Like fibroblasts, keratinocytes lay down types 1 and 3 collagen to create a new basement membrane.

Ref.: 1, 2

COMMENTS: There are two major events in the process of epithelialization: migration and mitosis. Migration is the dominant process and is independent of mitosis. Keratinocytes responsible for epithelialization are derived from the basal layer of the epithelium in the skin, as well as the hair follicles and sweat glands present at the wound edge. The more superficial the wound, the more of these cells are present and the more rapid is the process of epithelialization. Epithelial cells lose their contact inhibition and begin to migrate. They are able to secrete collagenases and proteases, which facilitate movement under the debris of the wound surface. Migrating cells do not divide. Additional cells are recruited in the basal layer of the skin at the wound edge. Several growth factors stimulate keratinocyte migration and mitosis, including basic fibroblast growth factor (bFGF), PDGF, TGF-α, and epithelial growth factor (EGF). Epidermal cells contain a cytoskeleton and move by an actin–myocin contractile system. Epiboly is a process whereby keratinocytes at the leading edge of the migration pile up on top of one another and tumble forward over the top of the heap (like leap-frogging) to move forward. Keratinocytes lay down laminin and type 4 collagen to create a new basement membrane. When epithelial integrity is restored, the cells become columnar and start to divide. Keratin forms as the cells mature.

ANSWER: C

8. With regard to wound contraction, which of the following statements is/are true?

A. Wound dehydration is important to normal healing and contraction.
B. The amount of collagen content is directly proportional to the rate of wound contraction.
C. Myofibroblasts are modified fibroblasts that contact contractile protein similar to muscle.
D. Skin grafting tends to increase wound healing by facilitating contraction.
E. Older individuals generally have less contraction and deformity of facial wounds than children because they have more excess skin in this area.

Ref.: 1, 2

COMMENTS: Experimental evidence suggests that movement or contraction of wound edges occurs primarily as a result of the myofibroblast, which is a modified fibroblast with characteristics of both fibroblasts and smooth muscle cells. The hallmark of myofibroblasts is the expression of alpha-smooth muscle. This is the most prevalent formation of actin present in vascular smooth muscle cells. Wound dehydration is not responsible for contraction. Although collagen is a dynamic substance undergoing constant change during the healing process, contraction is not related to collagen content and is not inhibited by suppression of collagen synthesis or its cross-linking. Although the signals that initiate and terminate the contraction process have not been fully elucidated, wound contraction is a reproducible biologic phenomenon; it occurs in all wounds and does not always stop immediately with wound closure. Although some contraction still occurs, closure of an open wound by skin grafting or with a flap significantly reduces the amount of contraction. Young individuals tend to have less excess skin over their face and hands than do older individuals; as a consequence, the accompanying contraction of wounds in these areas, particularly in children, can produce significant distortion and permanent deformities.

ANSWER: C, E

9. Which statements regarding myofibroblasts is/are true?

A. A phenotypic characteristic shared by myofibroblasts and fibroblasts is the presence of gap junctions.
B. The fibronexus is an intracellular structure linking myofibroblast actin to the cell membrane.
C. Transmission of the force of contraction is via a paracrine event mediated by contractosomes.
D. Myofibroblasts are found in abundance in a number of fibroconnective tissue diseases.

Ref.: 1, 2

COMMENTS: Myofibroblasts are connected by *gap junctions*. These junctions are not found in normal fibroblasts. They also possess an entity called the fibronexus. The fibronexus crosses the cell membrane of the myofibroblasts, connecting intracellular microfilaments to extracellular *fibronectin*. One possible explanation of the mechanism of wound contraction is as follows: The force needed for contraction is generated by the actin bundles in the myofibroblasts. The force of this contraction is transmitted to the wound edge via the gap (cell–cell) junctions between myofibroblasts and the fibronexus (cell–matrix links) between myofibroblasts and the wound matrix fibronectin. • The myofibroblast is a classic feature of the contracting wound. It is also seen in several fibroconnective diseases, such as fibromatosis, hepatic cirrhosis, renal and pulmonary fibrosis, Dupuytren's contracture, and neoplasia-induced desmoplasia.

ANSWER: D

10. With regard to the proliferative phase of wound healing, which of the following statements is/are true?

A. The extracellular matrix is composed of both structural and adhesive proteins.
B. Fibronectin is a structural protein that inhibits fibroblast migration.
C. The fibroblast produces both an extracellular matrix and a hydrated polysaccharide gel.
D. The hydrated gel permits diffusion of nutrients to the cells.
E. Laminin is an adhesive protein that facilitates epithelial cell anchoring.

Ref.: 1, 3

COMMENTS: The proliferative, or fibroblastic, phase usually begins about the third to fourth day after injury. It is during this phase that fibrous collagen protein is produced. Mediators such as C5a, fibronectin (secreted by macrophages), FGF, and PDGF released during the inflammatory phase attract fibroblasts to the healing wound. Fibroblasts begin to proliferate and produce both an extracellular matrix and a hydrated polysaccharide gel into which the matrix is embedded. The matrix is composed of structural protein such as collagen and elastin and adhesive proteins such as fibronectin and laminin. The gel is composed of glycosaminoglycans (hyaluronic acid, chondroitin sulfate, keratin sulfate, and heparin sulfate) linked to proteoglycans. The gel permits diffusion of nutrients to the cells, and the structural proteins collagen and elastin act as a framework. The adhesive proteins are laminin, which facilitates epithelial cell anchoring, and fibronectin, which anchors the fibroblast, is chemotactic to macrophages, and facilitates phagocytosis. By virtue of its ability to bind the fibroblast and the matrix, fibronectin provides a sort of scaffold along which the fibroblasts can migrate.

ANSWER: A, C, D, E

11. The maturation phase of wound healing is characterized by which of the following?

A. An increase in net collagen deposition and a decrease in collagen degeneration.
B. An increase in hypertrophy and redness of the wound.
C. Steady increase in type III collagen.

D. Decreased hyaluronic acid and chondroitin sulfate compared to that during the proliferative phase.

Ref.: 1, 3, 5, 6

COMMENTS: In normally healing wounds the maturation phase starts approximately 3 weeks after the injury. By 6 weeks after injury, the rate of collagen deposition and degeneration are nearly balanced so the net collagen content remains the same but becomes progressively more organized in appearance. The red, raised scar of the proliferative phase starts to flatten, with a concomitant decrease in redness and itching. The amount of type III immature collagen, which is deposited during the proliferative phase, gradually decreases and is replaced by the more mature type I collagen. The ratio of type I to type III collagen, 8:1, is approximately equal to that normally found in skin that has not been injured. The intracellular matrix also changes to a more normal makeup. The large number of fibroblasts that dominated during the proliferative phase decrease, as do the substances produced by these cells, including the glycosaminoglycans, hyaluronic acid, and chondroitin sulfate.

ANSWER: D

12. Match each of the five major collagen types in the left column with its normal locations in the right column.

A. Collagen type I	a. Cornea
B. Collagen type II	b. Basement membrane
C. Collagen type III	c. Bones, skin, tendon
D. Collagen type IV	d. Cartilage
E. Collagen type V	e. Found in association with type I
	f. Found in association with type V

Ref.: 1, 2

COMMENTS: Up to 12 types of collagen have been found. The major collagen types are types I–V. Type I is the major structural collagen of bones, skin, and tendons. Type II is found primarily in cartilage. Type III is found in association with type I in bone, skin, and tendon. The ratio of type I to type III varies in different tissues, although type I predominates. Type IV is found in basement membranes in association with mucopolysaccharides in laminin, and type V is found in the cornea (in association with type III).

ANSWER: A-c; B-d; C-a,c,e,f; D-b; E-a

13. With regard to the role of collagen in wound healing, which of the following statements is/are correct?

A. Thermal shrinkage temperature and solubility in saline are correlated with the age of the collagen.
B. Net collagen content increases for up to 2 years after injury.
C. Tensile strength of the wound increases gradually for up to 2 years after injury.
D. Tensile strength is the force necessary to break the wound.

Ref.: 1, 2

COMMENTS: Collagen synthesis by fibroblasts begins as early as 10 hours after injury and increases rapidly, peaking by day 6 or 7 and then continuing more slowly until day 42. Collagen continues to mature and remodel for years. The solubility in saline and the thermal shrinkage temperature of collagen reflect the intra- and intermolecular cross links, which are directly proportional to collagen age. After 6 weeks there is no measurable increase in the net collagen content; however, synthesis and turnover is ongoing for life. Historical accounts of sailors with scurvy (and impaired collagen production) who developed reopening of previously healed wounds serve to further emphasize this fact. • Tensile strength correlates with total collagen content for approximately the first 3 weeks of wound healing. At 3 weeks the tensile strength of skin is 30% of normal. After this time, there is a much slower increase in the content of collagen until it plateaus at about 6 weeks. Nevertheless, tensile strength continues to increase as a result of intermolecular bonding of collagen and changes in the physical arrangement of collagen fibers. Although the most rapid increase in tensile strength is early during the first 6 weeks of healing, there is a slow gain for at least 2 years. The ultimate strength, however, never equals that of unwounded tissue, reaching a level only 80% of original skin strength. Tensile strength is measured as the strength per unit area of tissue. It may be differentiated from burst strength, which is the force required to break a wound and is independent of area. For example, in wounds of the face and back, the burst strengths are different because of the different thicknesses, although the tensile strengths may be similar.

ANSWER: A, C

14. Match the cell or protein involved in collagen synthesis in the left column with the appropriate activity in the right column.

A. Pro-α-chains	a. Formed by cleaning nonhelical portions of procollagen
B. Tropocollagen	b. Combine in a triple helix to form procollagen
C. Propyl hydroxylase	c. Cleaves nonhelical portions of procollagen
D. Procollagen peptidase	d. Site of collagen synthesis
E. Fibroblasts	e. Responsible for hydroxylation of proline

Ref.: 1, 2

COMMENTS: See Question 15.

15. Which of the following statements is/are true?

A. Lyceal hydroxylase is the rate-limiting enzyme responsible for α-chain polymerization.
B. Vitamin C deficiency causes decreased hydroxylation of proline.
C. Lyceal oxidase mediates lysl–lysine bond formation.
D. β-Aminopropionitrile inhibits lyceal oxidase.

Ref.: 1, 2

COMMENTS: Collagen is manufactured by the fibroblasts. The single-strand pro-α-chains are made intracellularly on ribosomes. They combine in a triple helix to form procollagen. The molecule has its nonhelical portion removed by procollagen peptidase, creating tropocollagen, a molecule that contains three α-peptide chains in a right-handed helix. It is then packed into secretory vesicles in the Golgi apparatus and secreted. In the extracellular space, enzymatic cleavage of the telopeptide end of the molecule occurs, allowing it to form intra- and intermolecular cross-links. While still in the cell before secretion, its proline molecules are hydroxylated by two dioxygenases called *lyceal hydroxylase* and *propyl hydroxylase*. One of them, propyl hydroxylase, is a rate-limiting enzyme in collagen synthesis. Its function depends on several cofactors, including iron, α-ketoglutarate, ascorbate, and oxygen. Without these cofactors there is insufficient hydroxylation, the α-chains cannot form a stable helix, and collagen cannot be exported out of the cell. Ascorbate deficiency (scurvy) and hypoxia affect collagen synthesis at this level. Collagen cross-linking occurs in the extracellular space. Lyceal oxygenase is an enzyme responsible for this. It mediates oxidation of lysine to form lysyl–lysine bonds. This cross-linking can be prevented by β-aminopropionitrile (BAPN), which inhibits lyceal oxidase, and *d*-penicillamine, which prevents cross-link formation by directly binding to collagen substrate.

ANSWER:
Question 14: A-b; B-a; C-e; D-c; E-d
Question 15: B, C, D

16. With regard to growth factors, which of the following statements is/are true?

A. Growth factors act in an endocrine manner.
B. Paracrine effects imply activation of complement.
C. Autocrine effects imply same-cell stimulation via cell surface receptors.
D. Intracrine effects imply same-cell stimulation via intracellular effects.

Ref.: 1, 2

COMMENTS: The term growth factor refers to any substance that stimulates growth. Growth factors act in a number of ways. They may be *paracrine*, that is, produced by one cell and acting on an adjacent target cell. They may be *autocrine*, secreted by a cell and then acting on cell surface receptors on the same cell. They may be *intracrine*, produced by a cell and staying active inside the cell. Hormones are released by cells that act on a distant target. • In general, growth factors are named according to their tissue of origin or their originally discovered action. Growth factors stimulate growth by interacting with specific membrane receptors. This process initiates a series of events that ultimately lead to the stimulation of cellular division. These intermediate events include a variety of second messenger systems mediated by agents such as inositol triphosphate, diacylglycerol, and cyclic adenosine monophosphate.

ANSWER: C, D

17. Which of the following statements is/are true?

A. Transforming growth factor-beta may have immunosuppressive effects.
B. Transforming growth factor-alpha binds to the same receptors as does transforming growth factor-beta.
C. Epidermal growth factor and keratinocyte growth factor stimulate epithelial growth and keratinization.
D. Urogastrone and epidermal growth factor have similar effects on gastric secretion.

Ref.: 1, 2, 3, 5, 6

COMMENTS: Transforming growth factor-beta (TGF-β) is produced by platelets, fibroblasts, endothelial cells, smooth muscle, keratinocytes, lymphocytes, and macrophages. It exerts an autocrine effect, thereby enhancing its own production. In the wound it is produced primarily by platelets, macrophages, and fibroblasts. It increases collagen synthesis by enhancing collagen and matrix component production by fibroblasts and inhibiting collagenase production. It also enhances angiogenesis and is chemotactic for fibroblasts, monocytes, and macrophages. It has been found to have a suppressive effect on a variety of immune activities. Increased production has been demonstrated in a variety of cancers and may explain some of the immunodeficiencies in individuals with these malignancies. Mammalian TGF-β exists in three isoforms. Isoform-1 is the most abundant. • Epithelialization is directly stimulated by at least two growth factors, epidermal growth factor (EGF), and keratinocyte growth factor (KGF). EGF is released by platelets, macrophages, and keratinocytes and acts in an autocrine fashion amplifying its own secretion. It stimulates epithelial cell migration and mitosis and is a mitogen for fibroblasts and endothelial cells. It also stimulates secretion of collagenase by fibroblasts. The end result is epithelial growth and keratinization. EGF is the same substance as urogastrone, a peptide in human urine that inhibits gastric secretion. TGF-α is closely related to EGF, acting via common receptors and having primarily the same function. TGF-α also has an angiogenic effect on endothelial cells. KGF is released by fibroblasts to stimulate keratinotype division and differentiation.

ANSWER: A, C, D

18. Which of the following statements is/are true?

A. Platelet-derived growth factor (PDGF) is released only by platelets.
B. PDGF is chemotactic for platelets.
C. Fibroblast growth factor (FGF) is produced by fibroblasts.
D. FGF is a potent angiogenesis factor.

Ref.: 1, 2, 3, 5, 6

COMMENTS: Platelet-derived growth factor is released by platelets at the site of vascular injury. It is also synthesized by macrophages, endothelial cells, and fibroblasts. It is chemotactic for fibroblasts, neutrophils, macrophages, and smooth muscle. It stimulates fibroblasts to synthesize noncollagenous extracellular matrix, such as glucoseaminoglycans, fibronectin, and hyaluronic acid. It also stimulates fibroblast secretion of collagenase and may stimulate contractions. • FGF is produced by endothelial cells and macrophages. There is an acidic and basic form whose actions are identical but whose strengths differ (basic FGF is 10 times stronger than acidic FGF). It is a potent angiogenesis factor, stimulating endothelial cells to divide and make new capillaries. It is chemotactic for keratinocytes and fibroblasts and may hasten wound contraction. It is stored in an inactive form in the basement membrane of the skin where it is released after injury.

ANSWER: D

19. With regard to angiogenesis, which of the following statements is/are correct?

A. Division of vascular smooth muscle cells is the key first step.
B. Hypoxia of macrophages stimulates angiogenesis.
C. Migration precedes breakdown of basement membrane and is followed by cell division to form new vessels.

D. Endothelial cells release proteases, which allow breakdown of basement membrane, followed by migration and division to form new vessels.
E. Fibroblast growth factor releases substances that stimulate fibroblasts, thereby inhibiting angiogenesis.

Ref.: 3, 7

COMMENTS: An important aspect of wound healing during the proliferative phase is angiogenesis, which is a process of vessel growth in a previously avascular area. The first step in angiogenesis is stimulation of endothelial cell proliferation. A stimulated endothelial cell must first break through the basal lamina and into the perivascular space. This process requires a protease enzyme. The endothelial cell subsequently migrates and divides. Vacuoles form in adjacent cells, which fuse to form capillary lumens. Capillaries sprout from larger vessels in response to further angiogenic stimulation by local factors. A variety of angiogenic factors can be isolated from diverse tissues. The factors most relevant to wound healing originate from leukocytes. Examples of angiogenesis factors include FGF, TGF-β, and TGF-α; the latter two stimulate endothelial cell proliferation in addition to angiogenesis. Many conditions probably regulate angiogenesis, but some of the best evidence indicates that the angiogenic process is regulated by a macrophage response to local oxygen tension. Hypoxia stimulates angiogenesis, whereas increasing the oxygen concentration in the tissues stops this activity.

ANSWER: B, D

20. With regard to the division of vascular endothelial cells, which of the following statements is/are correct?

A. It depends on activation by growth factor in S growth phase.
B. It depends on activation by growth factors in G_1 growth phase.
C. Both smooth muscle cells and endothelial cells depend on the same growth factors.
D. Fibroblast growth factor stimulates division of endothelial cells.
E. PDGF stimulates division of smooth muscle cells.

Ref.: 7

COMMENTS: See Question 21.

21. Angiogenesis is key in which one or more of the following?

A. Development of cartilage.
B. Maintaining chronic inflammatory states.
C. Ulcer healing.
D. Tumor growth.

Ref.: 7

COMMENTS: Normal vascular endothelial cells turn over physiologically at a low rate; however, under conditions that promote angiogenesis, endothelial cells are activated to divide. Such conditions include wound healing, tumor growth, revascularization following ischemia, chronic inflammation, and organogenesis. Angiogenesis, or formation of new blood vessels, occurs when endothelial cells sprout from existing vessels. First, the endothelial cells break down surrounding extracellular matrix with a variety of proteases. The cells then migrate and form tubes. Cell division is not required for these beginning steps of angiogenesis but is required for sustained blood vessel growth. • Whereas angiogenesis is key to maintaining chronic inflammatory states, ulcer healing, and tumor growth, cartilage contains *no* vessels; this fact led to the observation that antiangiogenesis growth factors exist in tissues. • Among the growth factors that stimulate endothelial cells to divide are FGF and macrophage-derived endothelial growth factor. Smooth muscle cells but not endothelial cells are stimulated to divide by PDGF. Growth factors activate cells to divide in the G_1 phase of the cell cycle. The G_1 phase is the stage at which cells become competent to start doubling DNA and other macromolecules. Such competence requires expression of growth factor receptors early in the G_1 stage.

ANSWER:
Question 20: B, D, E
Question 21: B, C, D

22. With regard to tissue ischemia, which of the following statements is/are correct?

A. Prolonged total ischemia followed by reperfusion is a main cause of oxygen-derived free radicals.
B. Oxygen-derived free radicals are highly toxic chemicals that can cause cell death.
C. The deleterious effect of free radicals is worsened by superoxide dismutase.

Ref.: 8

COMMENTS: Because a variety of cells in healing wounds are actively dividing, there is some normal nucleic acid metabolism and catabolism. The enzyme xanthine dehydrogenase type D, is normally used to convert xanthine to uric acid as follows: xanthine + H_2O + nicotinamide-adenine dinucleotide (NAD) → type D uric acid + methemoglobin reductase (NADH) + H^+. This enzyme (dehydrogenase type D) is transformed into type O during ischemia. At the same time, ADP is catabolized to adenosine, inosine, hypoxanthine, and xanthine. In the presence of a reperfusion injury after prolonged ischemia and when oxygen becomes available the following process takes place: xanthine + H_2O + $2O_2$ → uric acid + $2O_2$ + $2H^+$. The superoxide free radicals (O_2) eventually also form hydroxyl free radicals (OH_2). These oxygen-derived free radicals are extremely cytotoxic; superoxide dismutase is a scavenger of superoxide radical and prevents formation of hydrogen peroxide and hydroxyl free radical.

ANSWER: A, B

23. With regard to wound healing, which of the following statements is/are correct?

A. Denervation has no effect on wound contraction or epithelialization.
B. Bacterial count at a level of 100 organisms per square centimeter retards wound healing.
C. Chemotherapy introduced 10–14 days after primary wound closure has little effect on the final status of a wound.
D. Tissue ischemia is the main component of tissue damage after irradiation.

Ref.: 1, 2, 3, 4, 9, 10

COMMENTS: Denervation has no effect on wound contraction or epithelialization; flap wounds in paraplegics heal satisfactorily when other factors, such as nutrition and temperature, are controlled. • Subinfectious bacterial levels appear to accelerate wound healing and the formation of granulation tissue, but when the level reaches 100,000 organisms per square centimeter of wound the healing is delayed because of a decrease in tissue oxygen pressure, increased collagenolysis, and a prolonged inflammatory phase. • Different chemotherapeutic agents have different effects on wound healing. Most antimetabolic agents (e.g., 5-fluorouracil) do not delay wound healing, although agents such as doxorubicin have been shown to decrease it. When chemotherapy begins 10–14 days after wound closure, little effect is noted on its final status despite a demonstrable early retardation in wound strength. • Tissue ischemia may not be the primary factor involved in chronic wound-healing problems associated with irradiation; most likely it is related to the changes within the nuclei and concomitant cytoplasmic malformation.

ANSWER: A, C

24. Normal healing is accelerated by which one or more of the following?

A. Ascorbic acid.
B. Vitamin A.
C. Zinc.
D. Increased local oxygen tension.
E. Scarlet red.

Ref.: 1, 2

COMMENTS: Surgeons have long sought substances with which to accelerate the wound healing process. **Increased local oxygen tension** *stimulates* healing, but it produces only a 15–20% increase in wound strength at 7 days. This increase is not enough to be of clinical significance. Although normal healing requires sufficient quantities of vitamins and minerals such as **vitamin C** or **zinc**, amounts higher than physiologic levels *do not improve* healing. **Vitamin A** may prevent the inhibition of epithelialization resulting from steroid therapy, but it *does not accelerate* the normal healing process. It was once thought that **scarlet red** or other substances incorporated in dressings might stimulate epithelial growth, but they do not. Newer, promising medications are currently being tested.

ANSWER: D

25. If a patient requires reoperation 1 month after a vertical midline abdominal incision has been made, which of the following procedures promote the most rapid gain in strength of the new incision?

A. Separate transverse incision.
B. Midline scar is excised with a 1-cm margin.
C. Midline incision is reopened without scar excision.
D. Rate of strength gained is not affected by incision technique.

Ref.: 1, 2

COMMENTS: When a normally healing wound is disrupted after approximately the fifth day and then reclosed, the return of wound strength is more rapid than with primary healing. This is termed the **secondary healing effect** and appears to be caused by elimination of the lag phase present in normal primary healing. If skin edges more than about 7 mm around the initial wound are excised, so the incision is through essentially uninjured tissue, the accelerated secondary healing does not occur.

ANSWER: C

26. With regard to scar revision, which of the following statements is/are correct?

A. It should be performed within 3 months to minimize fibrosis.
B. It should be performed earlier in children than in adults.
C. It corrects undesirable pigmentation.
D. It should be delayed approximately 1 year to allow maturation.

Ref.: 2

COMMENTS: Changes in pliability, pigmentation, and configuration of a scar are known as **scar maturation**. This process continues for many months after an incision, and it is generally recommended that revision not be carried out for approximately 12–18 months because natural improvement can be anticipated within this period. In general, scar maturation occurs more rapidly in adults than in children. Most erythematous scars show little improvement after revision, and so surgery should not be undertaken for correction of undesirable scar color alone.

ANSWER: D

27. Match the following connective tissue disorders listed on the left with the important characteristic on the right.

A. Osteogenesis imperfecta	a. Can be due to defects in elastin
B. Ehlers-Danlos syndrome	b. Ten types have been characterized
C. Marfan syndrome	c. Defect in gene-protectant collagen
D. Epidermolysis bullosa	d. Phenytoin may be helpful

Ref.: 1, 2

COMMENTS: *Osteogenesis imperfecta* is due to mutations in the genes for type 1 collagen. There are four kinds of osteogenesis imperfecta, and each presents several problems to the surgeon. Bones tend to break with little stress. The dermis is thin, and there is increased bruisability. Scarring usually is normal, and skin has normal extensibility. Children with osteogenesis imperfecta have a higher incidence of inguinal and umbilical hernias. • *Ehlers-Danlos* syndrome is a group of collagen disorders characterized by joint laxity, skin hyperextensibility and fragility, poor wound healing, and vascular rupture. At least 10 types have been identified. • Marfan syndrome patients characteristically have a tall stature, arachnodactyly, lax ligaments, myopia, scoliosis, pectus excavatum, and often dissecting aneurysms of the root of the ascending aorta. It can be due to collagen structure defects or defects in elastin. • *Epidermolysis bullosa* is characterized by blistering and ulcerations. It is thought to have several causes, including excessive fibroblast production of metalloproteases and abnormal adhesion of intracellular matrix to the basement membrane of the epidermis. Gastrointestinal tract wounds are affected often leading to stenosis and stricture. Dermal incisions are associated with blistering. Phenytoin, which can decrease collagenase activity in the skin, has been used to treat these patients.

ANSWER: A-c; B-b; C-a; D-d

REFERENCES

1. Sabiston DC JR: *Textbook of Surgery*, 15th ed. WB Saunders, Philadelphia, 1997.
2. Schwartz SI, Shires GT, Spencer FC: *Principles of Surgery*, 7th ed. McGraw-Hill, New York, 1999.
3. Simmons RL, Steed DL: *Basic Science Review for Surgeons*. WB Saunders, Philadelphia, 1992.
4. Basson MD, Burney RS: Defects in wound healing in patients with paraplegia and quadriplegia. *Surg Gynecol Obstet* 155:9, 1980.
5. Peacock EE: Symposium on biological control of scar tissue. *Plast Reconstr Surg* 41:8, 1968.
6. Barbul A: Immune aspects of wound repair. *Clin Plast Surg* 17: 433, 1990.
7. Folkman J: Angiogenesis. In: Verstraete M, Vermlen R, Lijnan R, Arnout J (eds) *Thrombosis and Hemostasis*. Leuven University Press, Leuven, Belgium, 1987.
8. White MJ, Heckler FR: Oxygen free radicals and wound healing. *Clin Plast Surg* 17:473, 1990.
9. Robson MC, Stenberg BD, Heggers JP: Wound healing alterations caused by infection. *Clin Plast Surg* 17:485, 1990.
10. Rudolph R, Araganese T, Woodward M: The ultrastructure and etiology of chronic radiotherapy damage in human skin. *Ann Plast Surg* 9:282, 1982.

CHAPTER 7

Pharmacology

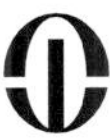

1. With regard to transfer of drugs across cell membranes, which of the following statements is/are true?

A. Passive transport is solely through a process of diffusion, which is governed by concentration gradients across the membrane.
B. The greater the lipid–water partition coefficient of a drug, the faster is its diffusion across a membrane.
C. The transport of ionized compounds or of inorganic ions across membranes is related to the transmembrane potential.
D. Active transport of a drug against an electrochemical gradient is an energy-requiring process.

Ref.: 1

COMMENTS: The crucial step in drug absorption, distribution, biotransformation, and excretion is its passage across a cell membrane. This can occur through either passive or active transport. Cellular membranes are approximately 80 Å thick and are composed of a bimolecular lipid layer in which proteins are embedded and integrated. Aqueous channels of varying size are interspersed throughout the membrane. *Passive* transport can occur by diffusion across the membrane or by passage of the drug through the aqueous channels. In the latter case, the drug must be small enough to pass through unhindered. The size of the channels is site-specific; capillary endothelial cells have large channels (40 Å), whereas red blood cells and intestinal epithelium have smaller channels (4 Å) and therefore permit passage only of water, urea, and other small, water-soluble molecules. Passage through the channels is also governed by transmembrane concentration gradients and transmembrane potentials. Passive diffusion through the membrane (not via the channels) is dictated by concentration gradients and the lipid–water partition coefficient of the drug. The greater the partition coefficient, the more readily a drug diffuses across a membrane. *Active* transport is responsible for the rapid transfer of many organic compounds and occurs against electrochemical gradients. This process is mediated by membrane-based proteins, which form a complex with the drug being transported. Active transport is an energy-requiring process that may be associated with Na-K transport.

ANSWER: B, C, D

2. Which of the following factors may modify drug absorption?

A. Drug solubility.
B. Drug concentration.
C. Circulation to the site of absorption.
D. Area of the absorbing surface.
E. Local pH.

Ref.: 1

COMMENTS: In addition to lipid solubility and molecular size, many variables may influence the absorption of drugs. *Solubility*: Drugs given in aqueous solutions are more rapidly absorbed than those given in oil-like solvents, in suspension, or in solid form. *Concentration*: Similarly, drugs that are ingested or injected in high concentrations are absorbed more rapidly than are drugs in solutions of low concentrations. *Circulation*: Increased blood flow at the site of administration enhances absorption of an administered drug. Increased local blood flow to the site of local injection may be brought about by massage or local application of heat. Decreased blood flow, ischemia, vasoconstrictors, or shock may slow absorption. *Surface area*: The area of the absorbing surface to which a drug is exposed (injected, applied, or administered) is an important determinant of the rate of drug absorption. For example, drugs are absorbed rapidly from a large surface area such as the pulmonary alveolar epithelium. The epithelium of the small bowel is capable of absorbing more drug than can the gastric epithelium. *Local pH*: The pH has a direct bearing on whether a drug is absorbed, especially for weak organic acids and for bases. In an acidic environment, a weak acid is more likely to exist in its nonionized form, which usually is lipid-soluble and likely to diffuse across the cell membrane. In such an environment, a weak base is found in its ionized form. • The distribution of a weak acid or a base is determined by its pKa and the pH gradient. This relation is demonstrated in the following example of an orally administered acid (HA) with a pKa of 4.4. Gastric pH is 2.4, and plasma pH is 7.4. The gastric mucosa is permeable only to the nonionized form (HA) of the acid, whose concentration is arbitrarily designated 1 (see diagram). In the plasma, pH − pKa = 3.0; therefore the ionized form is 1000-fold more likely to be found. Similarly, in gastric juice the nonionized form is more likely to be found, which favors absorption of the weak acid from the stomach.

ANSWER: A, B, C, D, E

3. With regard to the administration of drugs through the gastrointestinal (GI) tract, which of the following statements is/are true?

A. Sublingual administration, in comparison with absorption lower in the GI tract, may yield higher plasma

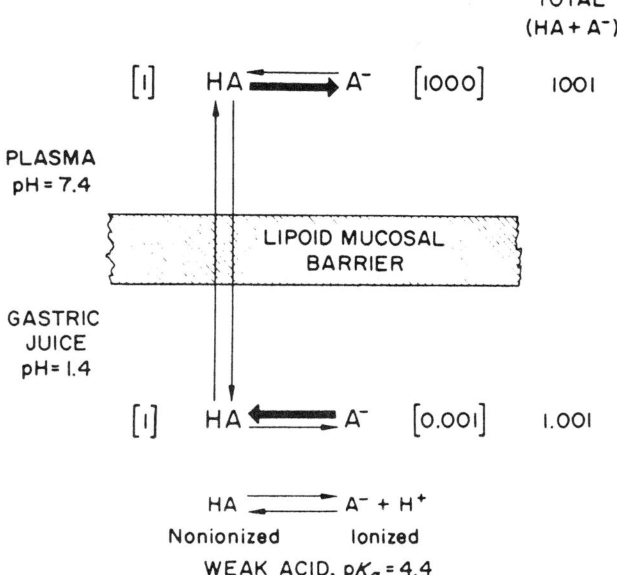

drug levels because it avoids the "first-pass" effect of the liver.

B. Drugs administered through the rectum do not pass through the liver before entry into the systemic circulation.

C. Weak acids are absorbed more easily in the stomach than are weak bases; the converse is true in the small intestine.

D. The gastric absorption of most drugs is improved if gastric emptying is retarded.

E. Altering gastric pH usually has a profound impact on drug absorption.

Ref.: 1

COMMENTS: Absorption of drugs through the GI tract occurs through simple diffusion across the epithelium. The rate of such diffusion is proportional to the lipid solubility of the drug in question. If the drug is a weak acid or a base, its nonionized form is more lipid-soluble, and the pH in the GI tract becomes perhaps the major determinant for diffusion. For example, weak acids, which are predominantly nonionized in the acidic gastric contents, are more readily absorbed from the stomach. In contrast, weak bases are predominantly ionized in the pH of the gastric juice and are therefore not absorbed until they reach the small intestine. If the gastric contents are made more alkaline, acidic compounds become more ionized and may be more slowly absorbed. At the same time, basic drugs become less ionized and may be more rapidly absorbed. Changing the gastric pH, however, may produce a relatively minor effect because the absorption of most drugs occurs primarily from the intestine as a result of its greater surface area. Absorption of drugs from the stomach may be delayed or reduced if gastric emptying is retarded. • "First-pass" metabolism usually occurs in the liver or gut wall after absorption from the oral route and before achieving systemic circulation. When drugs are administered sublingually, absorption from the oral mucosa is rapid, and a higher concentration in the blood may be achieved by this route than by absorption lower in the GI tract. The drug in this instance is not subjected to possible destruction by GI secretions, and thus passage through the liver is minimized as well. The overall result is that drug metabolism or biotransformation is less rapid. • Rectal administration of drugs is useful when any type of ingestion is difficult, as with vomiting or when the patient is comatose. The drug does not pass to the liver (and thus avoids first-pass hepatic metabolism) before its entry into the systemic circulation; for this reason, high serum levels may be obtained. Rectal absorption, however, is often irregular and incomplete; moreover, many drugs cause irritation of the rectal mucosa.

ANSWER: A, B, C

4. Match the route of drug administration in the left column with the correct statements in the right column.

A. Intravenous	a. Not suitable for oily solutions or insoluble substances
B. Subcutaneous	b. Absorption is prompt from aqueous solution and slow from oily or repository preparations
C. Intramuscular	c. Precluded during anticoagulant therapy
D. Oral	d. Most convenient, safe, economical

Ref.: 1

COMMENTS: The major routes of parenteral administration of a drug are intravenous, subcutaneous, and intramuscular. Impediments to absorption are circumvented by the **intravenous** injection of drugs in aqueous solution, and the desired blood concentration is subsequently obtained with accuracy and immediacy. There are many disadvantages with the intravenous route. Unfavorable side effects are more likely to occur than with other routes of administration. As a rule, when administered intravenously, a drug must be injected slowly; and this route is not suitable for oily solutions or insoluble substances. • The **subcutaneous** route of administration can be used only for drugs that are not irritating to tissue; otherwise sloughing may occur. Absorption from a subcutaneously administered drug is prompt but slower than by the intravenous route from aqueous solutions. Absorption is slow and sustained from repository preparations. The parenteral solvent may be oil-like, or the dosage form may be converted to an ester (decanoate or enanthate; i.e., fluphenazine decanoate, haloperidol decanoate, or fluphenazine enanthate). If slow absorption is desired, the drug can be suspended in an insoluble vehicle or incorporated in a vasoconstrictor agent; the latter principle is used when epinephrine is combined with a local anesthetic. In a similar manner, absorption can be even slower when the drug in the form of a pellet is implanted subcutaneously. The subcutaneous route is not suitable for administration of large volumes of a drug. • Drugs in aqueous solution are rapidly absorbed after **intramuscular** injection. Slow, but even, absorption from the intramuscular site results if the drug is injected in an oil-like solvent or is suspended in various repository vehicles. Penicillin is often administered in this manner. Substances that are irritating and cannot be administered subcutaneously can often be given intramuscularly. The intramuscular route is precluded during anticoagulant therapy and may interfere with the interpretation of certain diagnostic tests (e.g., creatinine phosphokinase determination). • The **oral route** of administration is the most convenient, safe, and economical. Absorption, however, is variable and depends on many factors, such as lipid solubility, the pH in the GI tract, and whether the drug is stable in GI fluid.

ANSWER: A-a; B-b; C-b,c; D-d

5. With regard to the administration of drugs through the skin, which of the following statements is/are true?

A. The rate of absorption of a drug is proportional to its lipid solubility in both the epidermis and dermis.
B. Absorption occurs more readily through abraded or denuded skin.
C. Absorption is enhanced by suspending the drug in an oil-like solvent and rubbing the preparation into the skin.
D. Absorption is retarded by occlusive dressings, which accumulate moisture and lower lipid solubility.

Ref.: 1

COMMENTS: Few drugs easily penetrate intact skin. Those that are able to penetrate are absorbed on the basis of their lipid solubility because the epidermis behaves as a lipoid barrier. The dermis, in contrast, is freely permeable to many solutes, and as a result systemic absorption of many drugs occurs through abraded or denuded skin. • Toxic effects can result from absorption through the skin of a highly lipid-soluble substance, as, for example, a lipid-soluble insecticide in an organic solvent. • Absorption can be enhanced by suspending a drug in an oil-like or other enhanced vehicle and rubbing the resulting product into the skin. This method of administration is known as **inunction**. Occlusive dressings enhance absorption through the skin by retaining moisture, which causes maceration of the epidermis and breakdown of the lipoid barrier.

ANSWER: B, C

6. With regard to the distribution of drugs into the central nervous system and the cerebrospinal fluid, which of the following statements is/are true?

A. Ionized and lipid-insoluble drugs are not distributed into the brain.
B. Entry of nonionized organic substrates is dependent on lipid solubility.
C. In a manner similar to that of other capillary endothelial cells, the brain endothelial cells restrict passage of drugs bound to plasma proteins.
D. The cellular barrier between the blood and the extracellular space is composed of capillary endothelial cells, astrocytic processes, and cells of the choroid plexus.

Ref.: 1

COMMENTS: The distribution of drugs into the central nervous system (CNS) generally is restricted in that nonionized and lipid-*insoluble* drugs are largely excluded from entry into the brain. Entry of the nonionized forms of weak acids and bases is somewhat restricted, but these substances can enter in proportion to their lipid solubility. Drugs that are highly lipid-*soluble* enter the brain rapidly. In contrast to other capillary endothelial cells, those of the brain restrict passage of drugs bound to plasma protein. The cellular barrier between the blood and the extracellular space of the CNS is formed by the capillary endothelial cells, glial cell (astrocyte) processes, and cells of the choroid plexus.

ANSWER: A, B, D

7. With regard to the fact that many drugs are bound to plasma protein, which of the following statements is/are true?

A. Albumin is the plasma protein largely responsible for binding drugs.
B. Binding is usually irreversible.
C. Binding to plasma proteins is highly specific; that is, the binding locus is specific for a given drug.
D. Bound drug has enhanced glomerular filtration.

Ref.: 1

COMMENTS: The various body compartments in which a drug accumulates can serve as potential reservoirs for subsequent release of the drug. In this way the pharmacologic effects of the drug are prolonged. The various body compartments include plasma proteins and other extracellular reservoirs such as GI tract secretions, cerebrospinal fluid, the aqueous humor of the eye, endolymph fluids, and joint fluids. Drugs may also accumulate in intracellular reservoirs; an example is the antimalarial agent quinacrine, which may be stored within hepatocytes. Drugs may also be adsorbed into the framework of the bony matrix; examples are tetracycline antibiotics and heavy metals. • Many drugs are bound to plasma proteins, most notably to plasma albumin; binding to other proteins occurs to a much smaller extent. The binding is usually reversible. The degree to which a drug binds to albumin is highly variable; some lipid-soluble organic acids such as penicillins and warfarin are more than 90% bound. A drug that is bound to plasma has limited activity in tissue and at the site of action because only unbound drug is in equilibrium across membranes. Binding therefore also limits glomerular filtration of the drug. Binding of drugs to albumin is nonselective; many drugs with similar physical and chemical properties compete with each other and with endogenous substances for the binding sites. Competition for the binding sites may lead to displacement of one metabolite or parent compound by another. This phenomenon explains why some drugs such as the sulfonamides increase the risk of bilirubin encephalopathy in newborns. These medications displace unconjugated bilirubin bound to albumin. The risk of an adverse effect is highest if the displaced drug has a limited volume of distribution, if elimination of the drug is also reduced, or if the displacing drug is administered in high dosage by rapid intravenous injection. After displacement of a drug from the inactive protein (albumin)-binding site, there may be an increase in the plasma/serum concentration of the free unbound (active) drug, but it is not reflected in the total serum concentration.

ANSWER: A

8. With regard to the hepatic microsomal drug metabolism system, which of the following statements is/are true?

A. Microsomal enzymes are found within the mitochondria.
B. These enzymes catalyze conjugation, demethylation, oxidation, reduction, and hydrolysis of drugs (phase I, or asynthetic phase).
C. Enzyme activity and susceptibility to induction among normal individuals may vary sixfold or more.
D. Lipid solubility is an important requirement for a drug to be metabolized by this system.

Ref.: 1

COMMENTS: The enzyme systems involved in the metabolism of many drugs are located in the hepatic endoplasmic reticulum. When liver homogenates undergo centrifugation, fragments of this enzyme network are isolated in the portion called microsomes. The endoplasmic reticulum resembles a canal system within the cellular cytoplasm and is involved in the intracellular transport of many substances. It is in continuity with the cell membrane and the nuclear membrane, and it contains many small ribonucleoproteins called ribosomes, which render the surface of the reticulum rough. The microsomal enzyme system is capable of catalyzing many chemical reactions, including conjugation, demethylation, oxidation, reduction, and hydrolysis. Thereafter, large water-soluble molecules (glucuronic acid, sulfates) are attached to the drug by a phase II (synthetic phase) reaction, forming a water-soluble metabolite, which is often inactive and ready for renal excretion. The conjugation reaction is with glucuronide. Glucuronides constitute the major proportion of metabolites of many drugs such as phenols, alcohols, and carboxylic acids. Glucuronides usually are inactive and are secreted into the urine and bile. Glucuronides that have been excreted into the bile subsequently may be hydrolyzed by intestinal or bacterial enzymes, and the liberated drug may be absorbed. This enterohepatic cycling may prolong the action of the drug (and is altered when the gallbladder is removed). The activity of the microsomal enzymes can be enhanced by many drugs and chemicals encountered in the environment. A marked variation in enzyme activity can be seen among normal individuals, and these rates may vary sixfold or more. Enzyme activity and susceptibility to induction appear to be genetically determined. • Lipid solubility is an important requirement for the drug to be metabolized by the hepatic microsomal system. A highly lipid-soluble drug penetrates the endoplasmic reticulum more easily, and its binding with cytochrome P-450 is enhanced.

ANSWER: B, C, D

9. With regard to an important group of oxidases in the microsomal system called mixed-function oxidases, which of the following statements is/are true?

A. These enzymes require both reduced nicotinamide adenine dinucleotide phosphate (NADPH) and molecular oxygen.
B. Cytochrome P-450 is a group of proteins constituting the terminal oxidase.
C. Metabolism of many drugs is enhanced by carbon monoxide.
D. The rate of drug metabolism by the mixed-function oxidases is determined solely by the concentration of cytochrome P-450.

Ref.: 1

COMMENTS: The hepatic microsomal system contains an important group of enzymes that catalyze the oxidative reactions; they are called mixed-function oxidases. The reactions catalyzed by these oxidases include N^- and O^- dealkalation, aromatic-ring and side-chain hydroxylation, sulfoxide formation, N oxidation, N hydroxylation, deamination of primary and secondary amines, and replacement of a sulfur by an oxygen atom (desulfuration). These enzymes require both NADPH and molecular oxygen. The NADPH functions as the primary electron donor, and the electron transfer involves the flavoprotein NADPH-cytochrome C reductase. • Cytochrome P-450 is the terminal oxidase of the mixed-function oxidase system. It is so named because it absorbs light at 450 nm when exposed to carbon monoxide. Oxidized cytochrome P-450 binds with a drug, and the resulting complex is reduced by the reductase. The reduced complex then combines with molecular oxygen. NADPH donates an electron and two hydrogen ions, and the subsequent products are the oxidized metabolite: water and regenerated oxidized cytochrome P-450. The metabolism of many drugs can be blocked by carbon monoxide. • The rate of drug biotransformation by the oxidase system is determined by several factors, including the concentration of cytochrome P-450, the proportions of the various forms of cytochrome P-450 and their affinities for the drug, the concentration of the reductase, and the rate of reduction of the drug–cytochrome P-450 complex. The rate of metabolism of the various drugs may be influenced by competing endogenous and exogenous substances. These many factors are therefore responsible for the sometimes marked species, strain, and individual variations in drug metabolism by the microsomal system.

ANSWER: A, B

10. Induction of microsomal enzyme activity is associated with which of the following?

A. Enhanced pharmacologic effects of drugs that are inactivated by the enzyme system.
B. Increased synthesis of cytochrome P-450, NADPH–cytochrome C reductase, and other enzymes.
C. Proliferation of the endoplasmic reticulum and increases in liver weight and hepatic blood flow.
D. Susceptibility to induction, which is highest in individuals who have undergone prior induction.

Ref.: 1

COMMENTS: Many drugs can competitively inhibit microsomal enzymes. Although this has been demonstrated in vitro, such a phenomenon is usually not of clinical significance. Of more importance is the ability of certain drugs to increase the activity, or to *induce the microsomal enzyme system*. When this occurs, metabolism of the administered drug is increased and its pharmacologic effects are subsequently reduced. Induction of microsomal enzyme activity has been associated with proliferation of the endoplasmic reticulum and increases in liver weight, hepatic blood flow, and bile flow. An increase in synthesis of RNA polymerase, cytochrome P-450, NADPH–cytochrome C reductase, and other enzymes involved in drug metabolism has been noted as well. In humans, susceptibility to induction is genetically determined and is the highest for individuals with the slowest drug metabolism before induction. For this reason, the effect of induction may be minimal if the patient has undergone prior induction. After the inducing agent has been discontinued, induction wanes over a period of days or weeks, depending on the time course for accumulation or excretion of the inducing agent. Among the drugs whose activity is altered by mixed-function oxidase inducers are birth control pills, warfarin, disopyramide, metronidazole, doxycycline, mexiletine, theophylline, verapamil, and quinidine. As a group of drugs, the anticonvulsants are enzyme inducers. *Enzyme inhibition*: Some medications eliminated by the liver inhibit certain metabolic pathways and are termed enzyme inhibitors. This decrease/inhibition of enzymes in the liver reduces the rate of metabolism of the other medications, resulting in an elevated serum level and possibly a toxic effect in medications with narrow therapeutic ranges. Saturation of drug-metabolizing enzymes by two or more drugs that use the identical enzyme system results in a decreased metabolic rate of one or more of the competing drugs (e.g., fluoxetine and sertraline). Some drugs bind to an enzyme system (i.e., cimetidine–cytochrome P-450) and inhibit the enzyme system. Such enzyme inhibitors include cimetidine (not ranitidine),

INH, ketoconazole, allopurinol, erythromycin, monoamine oxidase inhibitors, disulfiram, and verapamil.

ANSWER: B, C

11. A deep venous thrombosis develops in a 45-year-old man with a long history of seizures, for which he is taking phenobarbital. In this context, which of the following statements is/are correct?

A. Phenobarbital may induce the microsomal enzyme systems.
B. A higher dose of warfarin is required than if the anticoagulant were administered alone.
C. Cessation of phenobarbital without adjusting the warfarin dose may lead to severe bleeding.
D. Chronic alcohol ingestion should be discouraged because it impairs metabolism of phenobarbital and warfarin.

Ref.: 1

COMMENTS: Several hundred compounds are known to induce the microsomal enzyme system; they are loosely classified into two types: those that resemble *phenobarbital* and those similar to the *polycyclic hydrocarbons*. In the latter category, the increase in drug metabolism is limited to fewer substrates than in the phenobarbital category. Chronic administration of a drug may stimulate not only its own metabolism but that of other drugs as well. Simultaneous administration of phenobarbital and warfarin results in lower plasma concentrations of warfarin and less anticoagulant effect than when warfarin is administered alone. The desired therapeutic effect of the anticoagulant can be obtained if the dosage of warfarin is increased. If the phenobarbital is discontinued after the desired therapeutic effect of the warfarin has been obtained, the plasma concentration and effect of warfarin subsequently increase, and severe bleeding may occur. Thus when drugs are administered simultaneously and involve an agent that stimulates drug metabolism, the effects of the other drugs must be carefully monitored, when the inducing agent is initiated and when it is discontinued. • Environmental factors are also known to induce the microsomal system. Included are some vegetables, alcohol, exposure to insecticides, and chemicals in cigarette smoke. Acute ingestion of alcohol may inhibit the microsomal enzyme system, although during chronic ingestion induction may occur. Ethanol does not appear to stimulate its own metabolism because it is metabolized mainly by nonmicrosomal enzymes. By inducing the microsomal system, however, ethanol could influence the metabolism of other drugs, and so its ingestion should be discouraged in such circumstances.

ANSWER: A, B, C

12. Nonmicrosomal enzymes metabolize fewer drugs than their microsomal counterparts. With regard to nonmicrosomal drug metabolism, which of the following statements is/are true?

A. It occurs primarily in the kidney.
B. These enzymes are capable of catalyzing all conjugations and some oxidations, reductions, and hydrolytic reactions.
C. In contrast to the microsomal enzyme system, nonmicrosomal enzymes do not show interindividual variation in the rate of drug metabolism.
D. None of the nonmicrosomal enzymes is inducible.

Ref.: 1

COMMENTS: Although nonmicrosomal enzymes metabolize fewer drugs than do microsomal enzymes, their function is nevertheless important. Nonmicrosomal enzymes are found primarily in the liver, but they can also be found in plasma and other tissues, such as the GI tract. Nonmicrosomal enzymes are capable of catalyzing all of the major chemical reactions involved in biotransformation of drugs. For example, all conjugations other than glucuronide formation (which is catalyzed by the microsomal enzymes) as well as some oxidation, reduction, and hydrolysis of drugs are catalyzed by nonmicrosomal enzymes. Examples of drugs metabolized by nonmicrosomal enzymes include aspirin, sulfonamides, allopurinol, isoniazid, and hydralazine. Among normal individuals, there is wide variation in the rate of drug metabolism by nonmicrosomal enzymes. As for the microsomal enzymes, this interindividual variation may be sixfold or greater. None of the nonmicrosomal enzymes involved in drug metabolism is known to be inducible.

ANSWER: D

13. With regard to the excretion of drugs, which of the following statements is/are true?

A. The more polar a drug is in its administered state, the more likely it is to be excreted unaltered.
B. The kidney is the most important organ for eliminating drugs and their metabolites.
C. Most metabolites transported into bile are subsequently excreted in the feces.
D. Excretion of drugs can also occur through sweat, saliva, and breast milk, but the proportion of these excretions to the total excretion is quantitatively unimportant.

Ref.: 1

COMMENTS: Drugs are eliminated from the body unchanged or as their metabolites. The more polar a drug is in its administered state, the more likely it is to be excreted unaltered. Lipid-soluble drugs and drugs that are less polar are not readily excreted until they are metabolized to more polar, less lipid-soluble compounds. • The kidney is the most important organ involved in the excretion of drugs. The latter involves three processes: glomerular filtration, active tubular secretion, and passive tubular reabsorption. In addition to the kidney, there are other sites of drug excretion. Drugs may be eliminated in bile and feces, by the pulmonary bronchial tree, and in sweat, saliva, and breast milk. Many drug metabolites formed in the liver are subsequently excreted into the intestinal tract in bile. Although many of these metabolites are excreted in feces, most are reabsorbed into the blood and subsequently eliminated through urine. • Excretion of drugs into sweat and saliva occurs in a manner similar to the process that takes place in the kidney, albeit in clinically small amounts. Drugs pass through the epithelial cells of the glands; active secretion of drugs across the duct of the gland may also occur. Reabsorption of the drug from the secretion has been described as well. Drugs excreted in the saliva enter the mouth, where they are usually swallowed. Their fate thereafter is similar to that of drugs taken by mouth. The same principles apply to the excretion of drugs in breast milk. The amounts excreted within breast milk are important, not because of the quantity but because the eliminated metabolites are possible sources of unwanted medicinal effects in nursing infants.

ANSWER: A, B, D

14. Match each term in the left column with the appropriate definition in the right column.

A. Potency	a. Pattern of effects associated with a drug allergy
B. Efficacy	b. Relation between the effect of a drug and the dose required
C. ED_{50}	c. Ability of a drug to achieve the desired result without untoward side effects
D. LD_{50}	d. Dose of a drug required to produce a specified intensity of effect in 50% of individuals
E. Hyperreactive	e. Condition whereby a drug produces its usual effect at an unexpectedly low dose
F. Tachyphylaxis	f. Drug dose required to cause death in 50% of organisms
	g. Tolerance that develops rapidly after only a few doses of the drug.

Ref.: 1

COMMENTS: An understanding of definitions is important to comprehend the relation between the dose of a drug and its effect. If the intensity of a drug's effect is plotted against the dose of the drug, the location of the appropriate effect of a drug along the dose axis is an expression of the potency of a drug. *Potency*: Dose of a drug required to bring about the desired effect. Potency may be an unimportant characteristic of a drug. Whether the effective dose is 1 μg or 100 mg matters little, so long as the quantity can be reasonably given to a patient and the drug can be administered safely at the appropriate dosage. There is no justification for the view that the more potent of two drugs is clinically superior. *Efficacy*: This is a drug's ability to achieve the desired result without untoward side effects. If undesired effects limit dosage, the drug's efficacy is correspondingly limited, even though it may be inherently capable of producing a greater effect than another drug. *ED_{50}*: Dose of a drug required to produce a specified intensity of effect in 50% of individuals, known as the median effective dose (ED_{50}). *LD_{50}*: If death of the organism is the end sought, the median effective dose (which kills 50% of the organisms) is termed the median lethal dose (LD_{50}). *Hyperreactive*: When a drug produces its customary effect at an unexpectedly low dosage, the patient is said to be hyperreactive. *Hypersensitivity*: This term is used to describe a patient's allergic reaction to a drug. *Tachyphylaxis*: This is tolerance that develops rapidly after only a few doses of a drug have been administered. Reduced sensitivity should be described as immunity only if the acquired tolerance is the result of an immune reaction to that medication.

ANSWER: A-b; B-c; C-d; D-f; E-e; F-g

15. Regarding lipid therapy, match the correct drug on the left with the correct toxicity on the right.

A. Cholestyramine (bile salt resin)	a. Flushing
B. HMG-CoA (3-hydroxy-3-methylglutaryl-coenzyme A) reductase inhibitor	b. Significant drop in high density lipoprotein (HDL)
C. Niacin	c. Rhabdomyolysis
D. Probucol	d. Bleeding

Ref.: 1

COMMENTS: Epidemiologic evidence has shown that elevated low density lipoprotein (LDL) cholesterol and decreased HDL cholesterol are significant risk factors for coronary artery disease. For each 1% lowering of LDL cholesterol there is a 2% reduction in risk. Diet only mildly reduces LDL and exercise only moderately increases HDL. Pharmacologic therapy is far more effective and has been shown to improve survival appreciably in patients with elevated LDL cholesterol. Although all patients with coronary artery disease (CAD) should be undergoing aggressive therapy to reduce LDL to 130 mg/dl or below, pharmacologic therapy has significant toxicity. The bile salt resins such as cholestyramine decrease fat absorption, reducing vitamin K absorption, which can lead to hypoprothrombinemia and cause bleeding. The HMG-CoA reductase inhibitors are the most effective therapy for hypercholesterolemia, although HMG-CoA inhibitors cause hepatic dysfunction and rhabdomyolysis in rare cases. Niacin inhibits hepatic synthesis of cholesterol. Its acute administration can lead to flushing, which can be blocked by the concomitant administration of aspirin. Probucol also inhibits hepatic cholesterol synthesis and is especially effective for treating cholesterol deposits in the skin (xanthelasma) and xanthomas in tendons. However, probucol can significantly reduce HDL, which may worsen CAD progression over time.

ANSWER: A-d; B-c; C-a; D-b

16. Relative to an elevated arterial blood pressure: which of the following statements is/are correct?

A. A patient with an acute rise in blood pressure in the operating room in excess of 220 mm Hg may best be treated with a fast-acting short half-life agent.
B. Short-acting antihypertensive agents are optimal for chronic therapy.
C. The presence of renal artery stenosis can be determined by administration of captopril, an agent that precipitates acute azotemia.
D. In addition to being effective therapy for hypertension, angiotensin-converting enzyme (ACE) inhibitors can reduce proteinuria and prevent renal dysfunction from progressing in patients with type II diabetes.

Ref.: 1

COMMENTS: Hypertension is a highly prevalent disease, with a large portion of the population being untreated or partially treated. Acute hypertensive crises are uncommon, but if untreated they can precipitate an acute myocardial infarction or stroke. Agents should be used that can both control blood pressure and be adjusted quickly for fluctuation in pressure. It is inadvisable to reduce the blood pressure too rapidly in patients with severe hypertensive crises. Sodium nitroprusside (a potent vasodilator), or esmolol (an ultra-short-acting β-blocker) are optimal agents. Another agent, diazoxide, is given as a bolus and thus cannot be titrated to changes in arterial blood pressure. The ACE inhibitors, a frequently used class of antihypertensive agents, have the attribute of preventing congestive heart failure development in the patient who is post-myocardial infarction. In patients with unilateral renal artery stenosis the ACE inhibitors can precipitate acute renal failure; and, in fact, a short-acting ACE inhibitor captopril is used as a test for renal artery stenosis. In addition to being an effective antihypertensive, ACE inhibitors have been reported to prevent progression of renal dysfunction and proteinuria in patients with hypertension and type II diabetes. • For chronic treatment of hypertension, long-acting, once-a-day antihypertensive agents increase patient compliance.

ANSWER: A, C, D

17. Relative to gout, which of the following statements is/are true?

A. Gout is due to underexcretion or overproduction of uric acid.
B. Probenecid is the therapy of choice for underexcretors.
C. Allopurinol should be started in all patients with an acute gouty attack to decrease uric acid production.
D. Colchicine is highly potent uricosuric agent.

Ref.: 1

COMMENTS: Gout is a familial metabolic disease characterized by recurrent episodes of acute arthritis due to depositions of monosodium urate in joints and cartilage. Formation of uric acid calculi in the kidney may also occur. Gout is associated with high serum levels of uric acid, a poorly soluble substance that is the major end-product of purine metabolism. Gout can be due to overproduction of uric acid or underexcretion of uric acid by the kidney. The treatment of gout is aimed at relieving the acute gouty attacks and preventing recurrent gouty episodes and urate lithiasis. Therapy of the acute attack often starts with colchicine, an alkaloid with antiinflammatory properties. It binds to the intracellular protein tubulin, preventing its polymerization into microtubules and leading to inhibition of leukocyte migration and phagocytosis. Colchicine also inhibits the formation of leukotriene B_4. Whereas colchicine is indicated for the acute gouty attack, allopurinol, a zanthine oxidase inhibitor that blocks the oxidation of xanthine or hypoxanthine to uric acid, is indicated for chronic overproducers of uric acid. Allopurinol should never be started during the acute attack because it can worsen it. Allopurinol should follow the administration of colchicine. Probenecid is a uricosuric agent often used to enhance uric acid secretion in patients with elevated uric acid blood levels and undersecretion.

ANSWER: A, B

18. Relative to congestive heart failure (CHF), which of the following statements is/are true?

A. Inotropic therapy is the only way to treat CHF effectively.
B. Unloading therapy decreases cardiac output.
C. Unloading therapy increases cardiac output.
D. β-Blockers are always contraindicated in patients with CHF.
E. Acute heart failure can best be treated by fluids.

Ref.: 1

COMMENTS: Patients can have a decreased ejection fraction (EF), as is often the case following myocardial infarction (MI), or a normal EF and poor left ventricular (LV) compliance, as may be seen in hypertensive patients with LV hypertrophy. Patients with CHF respond best to unloading therapy with ACE inhibitors, which increase cardiac output. Digitalis and diuretics are supportive therapy, but only ACE inhibitors have been shown to reduce mortality. β-Blockers, although acutely decreasing LV function over time, improve the outcome of patients with severe LV failure. Carvedilol, a β-blocker with α-receptor blocking properties causing vasodilation, has also been shown to prolong life in patients with severe LV failure. Patients in acute CHF unresponsive to digitalis and diuretics may need intravenous dobutamine, a β-agonist that is inotropic and a dilator of medium to large arteries, thereby unloading the heart. Fluids in acute CHF would increase the preload, worsening the patient's condition.

ANSWER: C

19. Relative to cardiac arrhythmia, which of the following statements is/are true?

A. Digoxin therapy in atrial fibrillation (AF) increases concealed conduction to the atrioventricular (AV) node and increases AV node refractoriness, slowing the ventricular response.
B. Quinidine if given alone to patients with AF can slow the atrial rate, decreasing concealed conduction at the level of the AV node. This, combined with the vagolytic effect of quinidine, can accelerate AV node conduction and thus permit high ventricular rates.
C. Ventricular premature contractions (VPCs) must always be treated by lidocaine acutely and antiarrhythmic agents chronically.
D. Intravenous amiodarone administration makes no sense, as the half-life of amiodarone is approximately 55 days.

Ref.: 1

COMMENTS: Atrial fibrillation is a frequently encountered supraventricular arrhythmia. The common causes of atrial fibrillation are hypertensive cardiovascular disease, mitral valve disease (mitral regurgitation or stenosis), coronary artery disease, and hyperthyroidism. These conditions should be evaluated in patients presenting in AF. The first aim of therapy for patients with AF is to slow the ventricular response, permitting adequate time for cardiac emptying and filling. Digoxin slows the ventricular response by increasing the AF rate; more impulses bombard the AV node, making the node refractory, and so fewer impulses reach the ventricle, slowing the ventricular response. This is called *concealed conduction*. Digoxin is often given before quinidine to block the AV node, as quinidine alone can cause an increase in the ventricular response by being vagolytic and decreasing concealed conduction by slowing the atrial rate. The Cardiac Arrhythmia Suppression Trial found that antiarrhythmic agents given to suppress VPCs causes higher mortality than placebo therapy. Serious ventricular arrhythmias such as ventricular tachycardia can be treated by intravenous lidocaine, which is effective in 6–10% of cases, or intravenous amiodarone, effective in 30–50% of cases. The long half-life of amiodarone is not relevant to the time to action when given intravenously, which is measured in minutes.

ANSWER: A, B

20. Relative to anticoagulation, match the drug on the left with the correct statement on the right.

A. Coumadin	a. Prolongs the partial thromboplastin time
B. Heparin	b. Antithrombin (thrombolytic)
C. Aspirin	c. Prolongs the prothrombin time
D. Recombinant tissue plasminogen activator (rTPA)	d. Irreversibly blocks the cyclooxygenase enzyme pathway in platelets

Ref.: 1

COMMENTS: Pulmonary embolic and other thrombotic states contribute significantly to patient mortality. Patients with acute ischemic syndromes, those with an acute pulmonary embolus following hip surgery and other orthopedic procedures, or those in chronic atrial fibrillation should be anticoagulated. Depending on the disease process and the underlying pathophysiologic state, various anticoagulants or thrombolytic agents may be employed. Patients with venous disease or chronic prothrombotic states often receive chronic warfarin (Coumadin) therapy monitored by the prothrombin time. Physicians try to keep the INR (international normalized ratio) adjusted to between 2 and 3. The risk–benefit ratio at this range is optimal. Patients who have a repeated thrombotic episode on warfarin should be evaluated for a protein S or protein C deficiency. Heparin is given intravenously for acute ischemic syndromes, immediately following a pulmonary embolism, and occasionally subcutaneously for patients who are placed at bed rest for prolonged periods. The adequacy of anticoagulation with heparin is monitored using the partial thromboplastin time. Aspirin is an antiplatelet agent that irreversibly blocks the cyclooxygenase enzymatic pathway in platelets. Continuing aspirin in patients with coronary artery disease just before and after surgery has been reported to improve outcome. A new group of antithrombin agents are thrombolytic and cause disruption of a newly formed thrombus. rTPA is an antithrombin with proven efficiency during the first 6 hours following an acute myocardial infarction (MI) in patients with an acute pulmonary embolus, or in those with a nonhemorrhagic cerebrovascular accident. The time factor for rTPA administration places considerable urgency on the early detection and diagnosis of MI, stroke, and pulmonary embolus.

ANSWER: A-c; B-a; C-d; D-b

21. Regarding cardiac angina, which of the following statements is/are true?

A. Nitrates as therapy work best when given continuously.
B. β-Blockers should be avoided in patients with a low ejection fraction (< 40%).
C. Nifedipine, a dihydropyridine calcium channel blocker, causes significant vasodilation and reactive tachycardia that may worsen angina.
D. The antiplatelet action of aspirin reduces mortality in patients after myocardial infarction (MI).

Ref.: 1

COMMENTS: Anginal pain develops when the oxygen supply is less than the myocardial oxygen demand. This situation may be due to decreased blood flow secondary to coronary artery disease or increased vasoconstriction, as is found most frequently in young women without coronary atherosclerosis. **Nitrates** are first-line therapy administered sublingually, topically, or intravenously to avoid first-pass hepatic metabolism. Continuous administration of nitrates leads to tolerance and ineffectiveness, so intermittent nitrate therapy is optimal. **β-Blockers** are effective antianginal therapy; they decrease myocardial work and thus oxygen consumption by slowing the heart rate. The best results are seen in patients with a low ejection fraction (< 40%) who show a reduction in mortality post MI on β-blocker therapy. The **calcium channel blockers** are alternative therapy to β-blockers in patients with asthma, severe congestive heart failure, or insulin-dependent diabetes with previous hypoglycemic reactions. However, if the dihydropyridines are used alone, the vasodilation they produce can cause a reactive tachycardia that increases oxygen consumption, worsening the angina. Thus nifedipine is often combined with a β-blocker to slow the heart rate, thereby preventing an increase in oxygen consumption. Whereas angina is due to the imbalance of oxygen supply and demand, an acute MI is due to plaque rupture or platelet thrombus, initiating coagulation. **Aspirin** therapy has been shown to prevent a first MI (primary prevention), or in patients with a prior MI (a recurrence) it can be used as secondary prevention.

ANSWER: C, D

22. Cefazolin 1 gm given intramuscularly or intravenously is used for surgical prophylaxis. Which of the following statements regarding cefazolin is/are true?

A. Cefazolin is used for prophylaxis against infections with gram-negative rods.
B. Cefazolin is used because it penetrates all tissues including the central nervous system (CNS).
C. Cefazolin does not produce a positive Coombs' test.
D. Cefazolin can be given less frequently than other first-generation cephalosporins.
E. Cefazolin can inhibit aldehyde dehydrogenase, and so patients cannot tolerate alcohol.

Ref.: 1, 2

COMMENTS: The spectrum of activity of first-generation cephalosporins is mostly against gram-positive cocci, including some species of β-lactamase-producing *Staphylococcus aureus*. They may have some activity against *Escherichia coli* and *Klebsiella pneumoniae* in vitro. Cefazolin penetrates all tissues well except the CNS, though meningitis increases penetration but not sufficient for clinical use. Cefazolin, like other cephalosporins, can produce a positive Coombs' test. This reaction appears to be nonimmunologic in nature; a cephalosporin–globulin complex forms that coats the erythrocytes and reacts with the Coombs' serum. Cefazolin has the longest half-life of any of the first-generation cephalosporins and therefore can be given less frequently than the other drugs. Only the cephalosporins that have the tetrazole-thiomethyl side chain (cefamandole, cefbuperazone, cefotetan) inhibit aldehyde dehydrogenase.

ANSWER: D

23. Postoperatively a patient develops a low grade fever presumptively due to an infection with *Staphylococcus aureus*. Which of the following would be appropriate therapy before specific laboratory results came back?

A. Penicillin G.
B. Nafcillin.
C. Cefotetan.
D. Vancomycin.
E. Erythromycin.

Ref.: 1, 2

COMMENTS: Staphylococci are gram-positive cocci. Penicillin G, nafcillin, vancomycin, and erythromycin have a spectrum that covers *S. aureus*. Cefotetan, a third-generation cephalosporin, is indicated for gram-negative sepsis. A parenteral first-generation cephalosporin could be used. Most *S. aureus* in a hospital is resistant to penicillin G, so it is not a good antibiotic choice, although it can still be used for community-acquired gram-positive infections. Vancomycin should be saved for methicillin-resistant *S. aureus* (MRSA), and this infection has not been shown to be MRSA. The best choice is a β-lactamase-resistant penicillin, such as nafcillin. If an oral form is acceptable, oxacillin, can be used. Erythromycin could be used but usually is reserved for treatment if nafcillin does not work or if the patient is penicillin-sensitive.

ANSWER: B

REFERENCES

1. Hardman JG, Limbird LE, Molinoff PB, Ruddon RW (eds): *Goodman & Gilman's The Pharmacological Basis of Therapeutics*, 9th ed. McGraw-Hill, New York, 1996.
2. Katzung BG (ed): *Basic and Clinical Pharmacology*, 7th ed. Appleton & Lange, Stanford, CT, 1998, Chap 7.

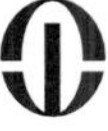

CHAPTER 8

Anesthesia

1. During a tracheostomy, a flash is noted in the surgical field while using electrocautery. Which of the following should be done?

   A. Extinguish flames with saline or H_2O; turn off all anesthetic gases including O_2; hyperventilate with 21% O_2 through the endotracheal tube (ETT).
   B. Extinguish flames with saline or H_2O, turn off all anesthetic gases *except* O_2; hyperventilate with 100% O_2 through the ETT.
   C. Stop ventilation; disconnect all anesthetic gas supply including O_2; extinguish flames with H_2O or saline; remove the ETT; mask-ventilate; and reintubate.
   D. Extinguish flames with saline or H_2O; remove all draping immediately; stop ventilation; disconnect all anesthetic gas supply including O_2; allow patient to awaken; then extubate.

Ref.: 1

COMMENTS: Airway fires occur most often during laser airway surgery but can happen in any O_2-rich environment where igniting stimuli may be produced. Any combustible material, including PVC tubing, surgical drapes, and human tissue, can ignite. The following steps should be taken simultaneously by both the surgeon and anesthesiologist: Stop all gas flow including O_2, extinguish the fire, remove the endotracheal tube or any foreign body present in the airway (e.g., bronchoscope, gauze). Once the airway has been reestablished, bronchoscopy is performed to determine the extent of the airway damage and to remove any foreign bodies that may be present. The patient should be left intubated for at least 24 hours after an airway fire and humidified gases administered through the endotracheal or tracheostomy tube. The use of steroids is controversial and probably of no benefit.

ANSWER: C

2. Effective therapy for gastric acid aspiration includes which of the following?

   A. Tracheal intubation and saline lavage of the lungs.
   B. Prophylactic antibiotic therapy.
   C. Prophylactic steroid therapy.
   D. Tracheal intubation, suctioning, and controlled ventilation with positive end-expiratory pressure (PEEP) therapy.
   E. Diuresis.

Ref.: 1, 2, 3, 4

COMMENTS: Gastric aspiration can be a fatal complication. The severity of the injury is determined by the volume and pH of the gastric fluid aspirated. Fluid with pH less than 2.5 and a volume greater than 0.4 cc/kg (approximately 30 cc in an adult) is associated with a greater degree of pulmonary damage. Initial treatment should begin with intubation, suctioning of aspirated fluid, pH testing of fluid (if readily available), and positive-pressure ventilation with PEEP. The level of PEEP is determined by the ability to adequately oxygenate ($PaO_2 > 60$ mm Hg), ideally with the fractional concentration of oxygen in inspired gas (FiO_2) levels below 60%. Saline lavage is not indicated, as it has been shown to aggravate injury. Prophylactic antibiotic and steroid therapy are also not indicated. With the initiation of positive-pressure ventilation and the loss of fluid into the damaged lung parenchyma, patients are often intravascularly depleted; hence empiric diuretic therapy is not appropriate.

ANSWER: D

3. A 30-year-old man has a hernia repair under spinal anesthesia. He calls the next day complaining of a headache that worsens with moving from a supine to a sitting position. He also has complaints of tinnitus. Initial treatment should include:

   A. Bed rest, increased fluid intake, and analgesics.
   B. Immediate neurology consult.
   C. Immediate anesthesia consult.
   D. Placement of epidural blood patch.

Ref.: 1

COMMENTS: Postdural puncture headaches (PDPHs) are characterized by frontal or occipital pain that worsens with sitting or standing and is usually relieved by assuming a supine position. Initial treatment is conservative with recommendation for bed rest, fluids, and analgesics. PDPH may be associated with neurologic findings; and common complaints are tinnitus, diplopia, and decreased hearing acuity. An epidural blood patch usually gives immediate relief of symptoms and is administered if conservative measure are ineffective in relieving severe symptoms after 24 hours. Factors associated with an increased incidence of PDPH include young age, female gender, large (cutting) spinal needles, and the direction of needle insertion. Insertion in a direction nonparallel to the dural fibers results in a higher incidence of PDPH.

ANSWER: A

4. In a trauma patient with suspected intracranial hypertension, which intravenous anesthetic agent(s) is contraindicated, even when mechanical ventilation is controlled?

A. Midazolam.
B. Methohexital.
C. Thiopental.
D. Ketamine.
E. Morphine.

Ref.: 1, 2

COMMENTS: Benzodiazepenes (midazolam), opioids (morphine), and barbiturates (methohexital and thiopental) decrease cerebral blood flow (CBF) and the cerebral metabolic rate (CMR), which in turn decrease intracranial pressure (ICP). Ketamine is an arylcyclohexylamine structurally related to phencyclidine (PCP). Ketamine increases the CMR and CBF, and therefore the ICP. Hence, ketamine is contraindicated when intracranial hypertension is suspected.

ANSWER: D

5. Intubation of a spontaneously breathing but obtunded patient with a closed head injury is best accomplished by:

A. Awake "blind" nasal intubation.
B. Induction with thiopental, muscle relaxation with succinylcholine, and oral tracheal intubation while maintaining manual in-line axial cervical traction.
C. Awake fiberoptic intubation.
D. Tracheostomy.
E. Awake rigid laryngoscopy.

Ref.: 1, 3, 4

COMMENTS: Securing an airway in a trauma patient can be difficult. Concurrent cervical injury should be suspected in a patient with a head injury. All methods listed are acceptable for intubating this patient, but the best way to reduce rises in intracranial pressure (ICP) is via thiopental induction, which can decrease cerebral blood flow and the cerebral metabolic rate by 40–60%. Succinylcholine causes small transient rises in ICP (approximately 4 mm Hg) that are offset by the ICP-reducing effect of thiopental. In addition, the muscle paralysis induced by succinylcholine prevents coughing, which can increase the ICP by 50–70 mm Hg. Nasal intubation carries the risks of damage to the cribriform plate when preexisting fractures are present, and epistaxis can cause airway compromise in an obtunded patient. Blind intubation under these circumstances therefore is less desirable than other methods for securing an artificial airway. Tracheostomy should be performed whenever airway distortion prevents prompt intubation by other methods. At times, tracheostomy is the appropriate initial approach to securing the airway.

ANSWER: B

6. Use of succinylcholine should be avoided in which of the following patient(s)?

A. Patient with 40% body surface area burn in need of emergency intubation 2 hours after injury.
B. Patient with 40% body surface area burn in need of emergency intubation 5 days after injury.
C. Patient arriving at the emergency room immediately after sustaining an acute spinal cord injury (T4 complete).
D. Children under 2 years of age.

Ref.: 1, 2, 5

COMMENTS: Succinylcholine is a depolarizing muscle relaxant. It causes paralysis by depolarizing the motor endplate via repeated action potential generation. This results in an efflux of potassium ions and a transient rise in extracellular potassium levels. In the normal patient this rise is approximately 0.5 mEq/L. The motor endplates are markedly increased in number 3–5 days after neurologic or muscular injury. Depolarizing muscle relaxants, such as succinylcholine, administered at this time can result in large increases in extracellular potassium, causing cardiac arrest. Therefore succinylcholine should be used only in the acute setting (immediately after injury) in patients with burns or spinal cord injury, where such sensitization is not observed within the first 1–2 days of injury. There are no contraindications to the use of succinylcholine in healthy children.

ANSWER: B

7. Thiopental is accidentally injected into an arterial catheter. Immediate treatment should include:

A. Dilution with saline infusion.
B. Dilution with lidocaine solution.
C. Dilution with phentolamine solution.
D. Any or all of the above.
E. None of the above.

Ref.: 1, 2

COMMENTS: Thiopental exists in solution at pH 8.5. If this basic solution is injected intraarterially, severe vasospasm can develop. Treatment should begin with dilution of the injected thiopental. Saline, local anesthetics, and phentolamine have all been used successfully to minimize the sequelae of accidental intraarterial administration of thiopental. The vasodilatory effects of lidocaine and phentolamine may reduce the risk of arterial vasospasm and the extent of tissue ischemia.

ANSWER: D

8. Which of the following determines spread of local anesthetics in the cerebrospinal fluid?

A. Anesthetic baricity.
B. Patient position.
C. Anesthetic dose.
D. Anesthetic volume.
E. Type of anesthetic agent.

Ref.: 1, 2

COMMENTS: Spinal anesthesia is accomplished by injecting a local anesthetic into the subarachnoid space. The level of spread is determined primarily by the baricity of the solution and patient position. Normal lumbar lordosis and thoracic kyphosis of the spine also play a role in determining the final anesthetic level. The dose and specific type of local anesthetic agent used determine the duration of the resultant blockade, but not spread. Relatively small volumes are utilized for spinal anesthesia and have little effect on the resultant neural blockade.

ANSWER: A, B

9. Which of the following is/are true regarding malignant hyperthermia (MH)?

A. The propensity to develop MH is a genetically transferred trait.
B. It can be triggered by all potent (halogenated) inhalational agents.
C. It can be triggered by succinylcholine.
D. Hyperthermia is an early sign of MH.
E. Testing for elevated creatinine phosphokinase levels is a useful screening tool.

Ref.: 1, 2, 3, 4, 5

COMMENTS: MH is a rare, potentially lethal condition that may manifest in a fulminant episode characterized by muscle rigidity, fever, tachycardia, respiratory and metabolic acidosis, severe hypermetabolism, arrhythmias, and eventual cardiovascular collapse. MH can occur minutes to several hours after the administration of triggering agents such as succinylcholine or potent (halogenated) inhalation agents. The earliest, most sensitive and specific sign of MH is an unexplained rise in end-tidal CO_2 levels (with venous blood gas acidosis) followed by tachycardia, frequently with multifocal premature ventricular contractions (PVCs). Temperature increases are a relatively late finding. Treatment involves cessation of triggering anesthetics, administration of dantrolene, forced cooling of the patient, induction of saline diuresis to avoid renal dysfunction secondary to myoglobinuria from widespread rhabdomyolysis, and monitoring of blood gases and potassium levels. MH is genetically transmitted, probably as an autosomal dominant trait with variable penetrance. Creatinine phosphokinase increases can be seen in MH-susceptible patients, but this test is not useful for screening because of its poor specificity. Avoidance of triggering agents in patients suspected of MH susceptibility is the safest and easiest method of treatment.

ANSWER: A, B, C

10. All the following are benefits of epidural anesthesia *except*:

A. Lower incidence of dural puncture headache compared to spinal anesthesia.
B. Decreased risk for mortality versus general anesthesia in high risk surgical patients.
C. Reduced incidence of deep venous thrombosis during lower extremity surgery.
D. Improved short-term graft patency during lower extremity arterial bypass procedures.
E. Better ability to titrate level of anesthesia compared to spinal anesthesia.

Ref.: 1, 2, 3

COMMENTS: Epidural anesthesia has experienced much greater utilization since the mid-1970s. Injection of local anesthetic into the epidural space and subsequent transfer across the dura produces regional anesthesia and analgesia. Reported benefits include a reduced incidence of deep venous thrombosis during lower extremity surgery, better titratability compared to spinal anesthesia, improved vascular graft patency up to 6 months after surgery, and decreased incidence of spinal headache. Additional benefits include postoperative pain relief via continuous epidural administration of opioids or dilute concentrations of local anesthetics (or both), and the need for less general anesthetic when used intraoperatively as an adjuvant for major thoracic, abdominal, and orthopedic procedures. Mortality in high risk patients has not been shown to be different than that seen with general anesthesia, however.

ANSWER: B

11. Which of the following is/are true with regard to the toxicity of local anesthesia?

A. Neurologic symptoms almost always precede those of cardiac toxicity.
B. Site of injection is an important determinant of toxicity.
C. Addition of 1:100,000 epinephrine solution allows administration of higher doses of local anesthetics without toxicity.
D. Relative toxicity is procaine < lidocaine < bupivacaine < tetracaine.
E. Pregnancy reduces the risk of toxicity because of a hormonally induced resistance to local anesthetics.

Ref.: 1, 2, 3, 5

COMMENTS: Systemic toxicity from local anesthetics primarily involves the central nervous system (CNS) and the cardiovascular system. **CNS toxicity** usually occurs at doses well below those that result in cardiovascular toxicity. It initially manifests as confusion, dizziness, tinnitus, and occasionally somnolence, followed by seizures. The seizures are thought to be due to blockade of inhibitory pathways in the cerebral cortex. **Cardiovascular toxicity** is due to direct blocking effects on both cardiac and vascular smooth muscle; it usually manifests as cardiovascular collapse. Ventricular arrhythmias and asystole are the most common electrocardiographic findings. Systemic absorption of the local anesthetics is highly dependent on vascularity at the site of injection and the presence or absence of epinephrine. Epinephrine causes vasoconstriction and allows a greater maximum dose of local anesthetic to be safely administered without toxicity. Absorption of local anesthetics occurs most rapidly with the highest serum levels from the intercostal space and is slowest with the lowest serum levels from local subcutaneous tissue infiltration. Pregnancy reduces the toxic threshold as well as the dose needed for therapeutic purposes.

ANSWER: A, B, C, D

12. Which of the following statements is/are true regarding propofol?

A. Induction and sedation doses in children are higher than for adults, after adjusting for weight.
B. Propofol is a white, milky emulsion that may be contraindicated in patients with egg allergy.
C. Unlike other induction agents, propofol doses not suppress the respiratory system.
D. The incidence of nausea and vomiting is lower with propofol-based anesthesia than with thiopental/isoflurane anesthesia.
E. Hemodynamic changes seen with equianesthetic doses are less with propofol when compared to thiopental.

Ref.: 1, 2, 6

COMMENTS: Propofol is a nonbenzodiazepene, nonbarbiturate intravenous anesthetic with hypnotic properties. Stemming from its chemical structure as a substituted derivative of phenol, it is insoluble in water and is formulated as a 1% emulsion similar to parenteral lipid formulations. Persons allergic to eggs may have allergies to this formulation. Induction doses are higher in children and adolescents and should be reduced for the elderly, hypovolemic patients, and those with poor cardiac reserve. Propofol produces profound dose-dependent respiratory depression that frequently leads to apnea in patients premedicated with other sedatives. After single-bolus administration, propofol is rapidly redistributed (2–8 minutes) and highly metabolized. For this reason it is most commonly administered by continuous intravenous infusion. Emergence from anesthesia occurs rapidly after discontinuation, making it a particularly suitable agent for short procedures. Nausea and vomiting are seen less frequently with a propofol-based anesthetic than with thiopental/isoflurane anesthesia, but hemodynamic alterations are similar or even greater than those seen with equianesthetic doses of thiopental.

ANSWER: A, B, D

13. Which of the following is/are true about midazolam?

A. Midazolam has no active metabolites, making it ideal for use in outpatients.
B. Midazolam is two to four times as potent as diazepam.
C. Respiratory depression caused by midazolam is usually minor but can be greatly exacerbated by concomitant use of other sedatives or opioids.
D. The degree of anxiolysis, sedation, or hypnosis achieved with midazolam depends on the percentage occupancy of drug at the benzodiazepine γ-aminobutyric acid (GABA) receptor sites in the CNS.
E. Midazolam is safe for use during pregnancy, as it does not cross the placenta.

Ref.: 1, 2, 6

COMMENTS: Midazolam differs from other benzodiazepines in both structure and solubility. An imidazole side ring imparts both stability and ease of rapid hepatic metabolism along with a water-soluble structure that allows painless injection. Two active metabolites of midazolam exist and accumulate when continuous infusions are used. Like other benzodiazepines, it potentiates respiratory depression (often synergistically) when administered with other sedatives or opioids. Benzodiazepines readily cross the placenta and have been associated with an increased incidence of cleft lip and palate formation when administered during the first trimester. Safety later in pregnancy has not been definitively established.

ANSWER: B, C, D

14. All of the following are characteristic of neuromuscular blockade by nondepolarizing agents *except*:

A. Effects are prolonged by aminoglycosides.
B. Vagolytic side effects occur with pancuronium.
C. They are triggering agents for malignant hyperthermia.
D. Vecuronium undergoes mostly hepatic metabolism.
E. Train-of-four monitoring effectively predicts the degree of blockade.

Ref.: 1, 2, 6

COMMENTS: Nondepolarizing muscle relaxants currently in clinical use include pancuronium, vecuronium, atracurium, *cis*-atracurium, mivacurium, rocuronium, doxacurium, and pipecuronium. Nondepolarizing muscle relaxants interfere with transmission at the neuromuscular junction by competing with acetylcholine for available receptor sites. These effects may be reversed by anticholinesterases, which prolong the half-life of acetylcholine to overcome the competitive inhibition of the muscle relaxant. The effect of nondepolarizing agents can be prolonged by aminoglycosides, clindamycin, tetracycline and other antibiotics, hypothermia, hypercarbia, and magnesium. Vagolytic activity is common with pancuronium but not with other agents. Except for mivacurium (which is metabolized by plasma cholinesterase) and atracurium/*cis*-atracurium (which is metabolized by Hoffman elimination and nonspecific ester hydrolysis), metabolism of nondepolarizing agents occurs in the liver with varying amounts of biliary or renal excretion/metabolism. Train-of-four monitoring involves stimuli being administered percutaneously to a peripheral nerve four times over 1 second and noting the muscular response. If fewer than two of the stimuli result in muscle contraction, more than 95% of receptors are blocked.

ANSWER: C

15. Which of the following is/are true with regard to flumazenil?

A. Flumazenil is a benzodiazepine antagonist that acts by competitive inhibition at the benzodiazepine receptor in central nervous system (CNS) tissue.
B. Flumazenil reverses the respiratory depressant actions but not the sedative effects of all benzodiazepines.
C. Flumazenil has been used successfully to reverse the clinical effects of hepatic encephalopathy.
D. Flumazenil is contraindicated in patients with suspected cyclic antidepressant overdoses.
E. Flumazenil antagonizes drugs affecting the γ-aminobutyric acid (GABA)-ergic neurons (barbiturates, ethanol) owing to their close association with the benzodiazepine receptors.

Ref.: 1, 2, 6

COMMENTS: Flumazenil is a benzodiazepine-specific antagonist that competitively inhibits the activity of benzodiazepines at the benzodiazepine–receptor complex. Flumazenil does *not* antagonize the CNS effects of GABAergic-acting drugs (ethanol, barbiturates, or general anesthetics), nor does it antagonize the effects of opioids. Flumazenil antagonizes the sedation, impaired recall, psychomotor impairment, and ventilatory depression produced by all benzodiazepines. Use of flumazenil is contraindicated in patients given benzodiazepines for life-threatening conditions (e.g., control of status epilepticus or increased intracranial pressure), in patients showing serious signs of cyclic antidepressant overdose (due to an increased occurrence of seizures), and individuals with known hypersensitivities. Recent case reports have demonstrated remarkable improvement in encephalopathic changes associated with liver failure. Flumazenil should not be used as the only agent for treating hepatic encephalopathy but may be helpful in patients resistant to conventional medical therapy.

ANSWER: A, C, D

16. Mechanisms of heat loss during general anesthesia include which of the following?

A. Convection.
B. Radiation.
C. Conduction.

D. Evaporation.
E. All of the above.

Ref.: 1, 2, 5

COMMENTS: Heat loss in the operating room (OR) is a complex problem involving all of the above mechanisms. The contribution of each mechanism depends on the surrounding conditions in the OR. **Radiative** losses are often cited as the largest contributor to heat loss in the OR. Radiant energy is emitted by every body having a temperature greater than 0°K. Radiation requires no medium for transport because it is electromagnetic. Heat freely radiates from a body at a temperature of 37°C to a room at 25°C so long as the temperature gradient exists. **Conductive** heat loss requires that bodies be in direct contact with each other. Body heat is conducted to the operating room table and other surfaces that come in contact with the patient. Heat is lost from the body by **convection** when operating room air, which is circulated at a speed of approximately 3 cm/s, passes over the body. Finally, heat losses from latent heat of vaporization (**evaporation**) occur during mechanical ventilation with dry air, during skin preparation with cold cleansing solutions, and via sweating, as well as from large open wounds.

ANSWER: E

17. With regard to pulse oximetry, which of the following is/are true?

A. Pulse oximetry is considered a "standard of care" for all surgical procedures requiring anesthesia.
B. A standard pulse oximeter measures light absorption at four wavelengths.
C. Accuracy of pulse oximetry can be affected by ambient light.
D. Oxygen saturation measurements may be artificially elevated in the presence of carboxyhemoglobin.
E. Methemoglobinemia, sometimes observed with nitroglycerin toxicity, results in a displayed arterial oxygen saturation of 85%.

Ref.: 1, 4, 6

COMMENTS: The use of pulse oximetry has led to marked improvement in the care and safety of patients not only in the operating room but also in the postanesthesia care unit and the intensive care unit. The concept of oximetry is based on **Beer's law**, which relates the concentration of a solute in suspension (in this case hemoglobin) to the intensity of light transmitted through the solution. Pulse oximetry measures the oxygen saturation of only pulsatile blood by using two wavelengths of light (red and infrared). The ratio of the pulse-added absorbances of these two wavelengths is determined by the arterial oxygen saturation. Because both **oxyhemoglobin** and **carboxyhemoglobin** absorb red light similarly, the pulse oximeter reads the sum of the two hemoglobins, producing an artificially elevated reading of the oxygen saturation. A direct measurement of saturation from an arterial blood gas sample is required to confirm the presence of carbon monoxide. **Methemoglobinemia**, a disorder that may occur with nitroglycerin toxicity, results in an oxygen saturation of 85%. This relates to the near-equal absorbance of red and infrared light by methemoglobin, which results in a saturation of approximately 85%. Ambient light can affect pulse oximetry readings and occasionally necessitates covering the probe to avoid artifactual readings.

ANSWER: A, C, D, E

18. While transporting an intubated patient from the OR to the intensive care unit the pressure gauge on a completely filled size E compressed-gas cylinder containing O_2 reads 2200 pounds per square inch (psi). How long can O_2 be delivered at a flow rate of 5 L/min from an E cylinder whose pressure gauge reads 1100 psi?

A. 60 seconds.
B. 5 minutes.
C. 60 minutes.
D. 125 minutes.
E. 220 minutes.

Ref.: 1, 2

COMMENTS: A full E cylinder reading 2200 psi contains approximately 625 liters of O_2. **Boyle's law** states that for a fixed mass of gas at a constant temperature the product of pressure and volume is constant. Boyle's law allows us to estimate the volume of gas remaining in a closed container by measuring the pressure within the container. When the pressure gauge reads 1100 psi it has half the volume of a full cylinder (or about 625 ÷ 2 = 312.5 liters). At a flow of 5 L/min the cylinder in question will last approximately 1 hour. This information is important when using portable sources of oxygen during transport and diagnostic procedures remote from the operating room.

ANSWER: C

19. After administration of epidural anesthesia to the T3 dermatome of a patient with severe lung disease who is undergoing open cholecystectomy, which of the following is/are likely to happen?

A. Heart rate increases.
B. Venous return decreases.
C. Alveolar ventilation decreases.
D. Heart rate decreases.
E. Vagal tone decreases.

Ref.: 1, 2, 5

COMMENTS: Central neuraxial blockade to the T3 **sensory** dermatome is associated with **sympathetic** blockade, on average, two spinal segment levels higher and with **motor** blockade two spinal segments lower. Blockade of the cardiac accelerator nerves (T1–T4) and unopposed vagal activity result in relative bradycardia. This is despite hypotension caused by the reduction in venous return secondary to vasodilation. In addition, motor nerve blockade of intercostal muscle function reduces alveolar ventilation and may precipitate respiratory embarrassment in a patient with underlying pulmonary disease, especially if a significant fraction of intercostal muscle function is impaired.

ANSWER: B, C, D

20. A patient with idiopathic hypertrophic subaortic stenosis (IHSS) becomes hypotensive during general anesthesia for a thyroidectomy. Appropriate treatment includes:

A. Administration of inotropic drugs.
B. Administration of phenylephrine.

C. Administration of ephedrine.
D. Administration of fluids.
E. Administration of atropine.

Ref.: 1, 2, 3

COMMENTS: With IHSS, inotropic drugs including those with indirect effects (e.g., ephedrine) may aggravate left ventricular (LV) outflow obstruction. The hemodynamic consequence of LV outflow obstruction is exacerbated by loss of preload (e.g., hypovolemia, nonsinus rhythm, or tachycardia) as well as by anything producing vasodilation. Fluid administration and administration of a pure vasoconstricting drug are therefore appropriate initial therapies.

ANSWER: B, D

REFERENCES

1. Rogers MC, Tinker JH, Covino BG, Longnecker DE: *Principles and Practice of Anesthesiology*. Mosby-Year Book, St. Louis, 1993.
2. Stoetting RK: *Pharmacology and Physiology in Anesthetic Practice*, 2nd ed. JB Lippincott, Philadelphia, 1991.
3. Sabiston DC Jr: *Textbook of Surgery*, 15th ed. WB Saunders, Philadelphia, 1997.
4. Schwartz SI, Shires GT, Spencer FC: *Principles of Surgery*, 7th ed. McGraw-Hill, New York, 1999.
5. O'Leary JP: *The Physiologic Basis of Surgery*, 2nd ed. Williams & Wilkins, Baltimore, 1996.
6. Greenfield LJ, Mulholland M, Oldham KT, et al: *Surgery: Scientific Principles and Practice*, 2nd ed. Lippincott-Raven, Philadelphia, 1997.

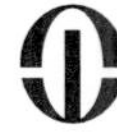

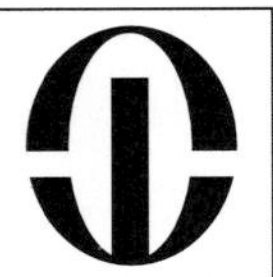

CHAPTER 9

Immunology

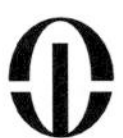

1. With regard to the immune response, which of the following statements is/are true?

A. The primary immune response is more intense and rapid than the secondary immune response.
B. A cell-mediated immune response is mediated primarily by T lymphocytes.
C. B lymphocytes are precursors of plasma cells, which produce antibodies.
D. T lymphocytes develop in the fetal liver and subsequently in the bone marrow.

Ref.: 1, 2, 3, 4, 5

COMMENTS: The immune response is characterized by a series of reactions triggered by an immunogen. An **immunogen** may be defined as any one of a number of substances capable of triggering an immune response. Immunogens include substances recognized as foreign or as non-self (e.g., virus, bacteria, histoincompatible tissues) as well as substances that are "altered-self" or "modified-self" (e.g., most tumor antigens). All immune responses, whether primary or secondary, are characterized by three phases: (1) **cognitive phase** (recognition of non-self antigen); (2) **activation phase** (proliferation of immunocompetent cells or lymphocytes); and (3) an **effector phase** (development of immunologic memory). The **primary** immune response is the result of the first (or primary) exposure to a specific antigen. The **secondary** response results from a second (or third or fourth, . . .) exposure to the same antigen. It is more rapid and more intense than the primary response and is the result of the phenomenon of immunologic memory. • There are two basic types of immune responses: a **cell-mediated** immune response (cellular immunity) mediated primarily by T lymphocytes and a **humoral** immune response mediated primarily by B lymphocytes. There are two major types of lymphocyte. **B lymphocytes**, or **B cells**, differentiate into antibody-producing plasma cells after activation. They develop in the fetal liver and the bone marrow. B lymphocytes are precursors of the plasma cell and can be identified by specific antigen-binding sites on their surface. Plasma cells produce antibodies that are found in serum and that may be transferred passively in the serum. **T lymphocytes**, or **T cells**, mature in the thymus from multipotential cells derived from the bone marrow.

ANSWER: B, C

2. With regard to T lymphocytes (T cells), which of the following statements is/are correct?

A. T cells develop primarily in the thymus and bone marrow, which are referred to as the primary lymphoid organs.
B. T cells subsequently migrate to the spleen, one of the secondary lymphoid organs, and to the lymph nodes, which are considered tertiary lymphoid organs.
C. Helper/inducer T cells may be activated to produce antibodies.
D. Cytotoxic T cells may destroy target cells by recognizing foreign antigens on the target cell surface.
E. The various types of T cells may be identified by the binding of specific monoclonal antibodies to antigens on the T cell surface.

Ref.: 1, 2, 3, 4, 5

COMMENTS: T lymphocytes (T cells) mature in the thymus, and B lymphocytes (B cells) mature in the fetal liver and the bone marrow; those organs are referred to as the **primary** lymphoid organs. The T and B lymphocytes subsequently migrate to the **secondary** lymphoid organs, specifically the spleen, lymph nodes, and dispersed lymphoid tissues found in the bronchus, urogenital tract, and gut (i.e., Peyer's patches). Lymphocytes that differentiate into T cells and B cells express different clusters of antigens on their membranes. All of the T cells express the differentiation antigen cluster designated as CD3, whereas B cells express the differentiation antigen clusters CD19 and CD20. The $CD3^+$ T cells can be distinguished and subdivided further by the expression of additional differentiation antigens on the T cell surface, indicating them to be cytotoxic T cells ($CD3^+/CD8^+$), suppressor T cells ($CD3^+/CD8^+$), helper/inducer T cells ($CD3^+/CD4^+$), and delayed-type hypersensitivity T cells ($CD3^+/CD4^+$). Cytotoxic T cells are capable of destroying a target cell by recognizing a foreign or "modified-self" antigen and class I major histocompatibility complex (MHC) molecules on the target cell surface. Suppressor T cells tend to suppress the activity of other T and B cells. The T-helper cells stimulate B cells to differentiate into plasma cells that produce antibody, facilitate maturation of precytotoxic T cells, and stimulate macrophages to produce a nonspecific, delayed inflammatory response. Delayed-type hypersensitivity T cells bring macrophages and other inflammatory cells to areas in which delayed-type hypersensitivity reactions occur through the production of various chemoattractant molecules known collectively as chemokines.

ANSWER: D, E

3. With regard to the major histocompatibility complex (MHC), which of the following statements is/are correct?

A. The MHC refers to a gene cluster on human chromosome 6 that codes for proteins important to the process of rejection.
B. Part of the MHC codes for some components of the complement cascade.
C. Class I antigens are coded for by the D region of the MHC.
D. Class II antigens are important for presenting antigen to the immune system.
E. Class I antigens are present only on nucleated cells.

Ref.: 1, 2, 3, 4, 5

COMMENTS: The MHC is a cluster of genes located on human chromosome 6. Each person receives copies of chromosome 6 from both the mother and the father. The MHC has many gene loci; the resulting combinations in each successive generation lead to many different haplotypes of MHC. • The products of the MHC are of three basic types or classes: **Class I** MHC products are coded for by genes in the A and B regions of the MHC and are called class I antigens. The class I antigens are glycoproteins found in the plasma membrane of essentially all nucleated cells and in platelets. The class I molecules form a groove that binds antigenic peptides. The complex of class I molecules and antigens can be identified by cytotoxic ($CD8^+$) T cells, leading to lysis of the target cell. **Class II** antigens are also transmembrane glycoproteins but are coded by genes in the D region of the MHC. The class II antigens are expressed on B lymphocytes, macrophages, monocytes, dendritic cells, and activated T cells. Class II molecules also present antigenic peptides to the immune system, but the cell that responds to this is the $CD4^+$ helper-T cell. This leads to activation of the helper-T cell, which can then enhance the development of either cytotoxic T cells or B cells. **Class III** proteins are components of the complement cascade, which are coded for in the MHC. Expression of MHC products in an individual is important in "self" identification and therefore in the process of rejection and intercellular communication.

ANSWER: A, B, D

4. With regard to antibodies, which of the following statements is/are correct?

A. Antibodies are composed of a variable region, which interacts with the host, and a constant region, which interacts with an antigen.
B. Antibody molecules are composed of four polypeptide chains consisting of two heavy chains and two light chains stabilized by interchain and intrachain disulfide bonds.
C. Immunoglobulin A (IgA) is able to bind complement and function as an opsonin.
D. Immunoglobulin G (IgG) is the largest antibody, with a pentameric structure of the basic antibody.
E. Immunoglobulin M (IgM) is the major antibody produced during the primary immune response.

Ref.: 1, 2, 3, 4, 5

COMMENTS: See Question 5.

5. Match each immunoglobulin in the left column with the appropriate statement(s) in the right column.

A. IgA	a. Binds mast cells
B. IgG	b. Major antibody of the secondary immune response
C. IgE	c. Most prevalent serum immunoglobulin
D. IgM	d. May bind complement
E. IgD	e. Found particularly in secretions
	f. Function is essentially unknown
	g. Mediates type I hypersensitivity reactions

Ref.: 1, 2, 3, 4, 5

COMMENTS: Antibodies are a type of serum protein produced by plasma cells. They are made up of a variable region and a constant region. The variable region is able to bind specifically to an antigen, and the constant region is able to interact and mediate functions such as complement fixation and monocyte binding. Genetic recombination allows the diversity of the variable region, enabling the antibodies to bind to many types of antigen. All antibody molecules have the basic structure of four polypeptide chains consisting of two identical heavy chains and two identical light chains stabilized and cross-linked by interchain and intrachain disulfide bonds (see diagram). The protease papain is able to cleave the antibody molecule into two identical fraction antigen-binding (Fab) fragments (variable region) and one fraction crystalline (Fc) fragment (constant region). • The classes of antibodies are distinguished by their heavy chains. The five classes of antibodies include immunoglobulins A, G, M, D, and E. **IgA** is found particularly in secretions, in which it protects mucous membranes. **IgG** is the most prevalent serum immunoglobulin; it is able to bind complement and may function as an opsonin, that is, an antibody that binds antigen to neutrophils and macrophages via the constant region, facilitating antigen phagocytosis. IgG is the major antibody produced during the secondary immune response. **IgM** is a large antibody made up of a pentamer of the basic antibody structure. It is the major antibody produced during the primary immune response. Like

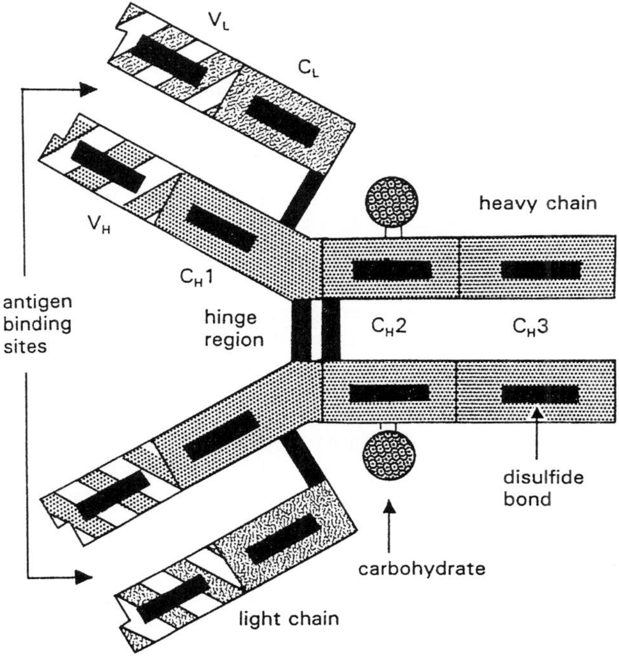

IgG, IgM is able to fix complement efficiently. **IgD** is found only in minimal amounts, and its function is unknown. **IgE** binds to Fc receptors on mast cells and basophils; and after contact with antigen it causes these cells to release histamine and other substances that mediate type I hypersensitivity reactions.

ANSWER:
Question 4: B, E
Question 5: A-e; B-b,c,d; C-a,g; D-d; E-f

6. With regard to immunogens, which of the following statements is/are correct?

A. Immunogens have multiple antigenic epitopes, each of which may react with an antibody or T cell antigen-receptor specific for it.
B. An antigen may be defined as any molecule recognized as foreign by the immune system.
C. Immunogenicity is greater with a xenogeneic antigen than with a syngeneic antigen.
D. A 4000-dalton molecule would be highly immunogenic.
E. Proteins are generally more complex and, as such, are more immunogeneic than are nucleic acids.

Ref.: 1, 2, 3, 4, 5

COMMENTS: An immunogen is any substance that can stimulate an immune response. An antigen may be defined as any molecule recognized by the immune response. • Most immunogens are multivalent; that is, they have multiple antigenic epitopes (one or more molecular structures that can react with the variable region of an antibody or the T cell antigen receptor specific for that individual epitope). • Immunogenicity of an antigen is related to its foreignness, its complexity, and its size. **Foreignness** is greatest with a xenogeneic (different species) antigen, less with an allogeneic (same species, different genotype) antigen, even less with a syngeneic (same species, same genotype) antigen, and least with an autologous (self) antigen. **Complexity** is greatest with proteins, less with carbohydrates, and least with nucleic acids and lipids. **Size** of more than 5000 daltons is generally required for a substance to be immunogeneic. As as example, serum albumin (40,000 daltons) generates a moderate immune response, whereas γ-globulins (160,000 daltons) generate an intense immune response.

ANSWER: A, B, C, E

7. With regard to the process of phagocytosis, which of the following statements is/are true?

A. Monocytes are the major tissue phagocytic cells.
B. A phagolysosome is composed of a membrane-encased foreign particle and collections of enzymes.
C. Lysosomal granules require oxygen to destroy foreign particles.
D. Chronic granulomatous disease results from a flaw in production of superoxide anions and eventually of hydrogen peroxide in neutrophils.
E. Once a monocyte migrates to tissues to become a macrophage, it loses all function except phagocytosis.

Ref.: 1, 2, 3, 4, 5

COMMENTS: There are two groups of phagocytic cells: mononuclear and polymorphonuclear. (1) **Monocytes**, blood-borne mononuclear phagocytes, are derived from bone marrow and migrate to **tissues** in which they mature and are then referred to as macrophages. (2) **Neutrophils** are polymorphonuclear phagocytes; they are the major tissue phagocytic cell, circulate in the blood, and migrate quickly to areas of inflammation or infection. • During phagocytosis a foreign particle is engulfed by a part of the phagocyte to form a vacuole or a phagosome. Cytoplasmic organelles consisting of membrane-bound collections of enzymes called lysosomes bind with the phagosome to form a phagolysosome. • Lysozymal granules within the phagolysosome destroy foreign particles by two methods: One is oxygen-dependent, and the other is oxygen-independent. Oxygen-dependent mechanisms include formation of myeloperoxidase, superoxide anion, hydrogen peroxide, singlet oxygen, and hydroxyl radicals. Oxygen-independent mechanisms include formation of cationic proteins, lysozyme, and proteinases. • A flaw in the production of superoxide anion and eventually of hydrogen peroxide is found in the neutrophils of persons with chronic granulomatous disease. • In addition to phagocytosis, macrophages break down, process, and present antigen to T and B lymphocytes; they also secrete factors that facilitate clonal expansion of the antigen-specific lymphocytes. Macrophages produce a wide variety of cytokines, which are hormone-like glycoproteins with potent biologic activity. Some familiar examples include tumor necrosis factor, interferons, and interleukin-1.

ANSWER: B, D

8. With regard to nonspecific immune reactivity, which of the following statements is/are correct?

A. Natural killer (NK) cells are large granular lymphocytes that do not express the T cell or B cell phenotype and require previous exposure to antigen to express cytotoxicity.
B. Natural killer activity is not restricted by the major histocompatibility complex (MHC).
C. Interferons augment the activity of macrophages, T cells, and NK cells.
D. Interferon γ is produced by fibroblasts in response to trauma.
E. Because NK cells do not express cell surface markers, they can be identified only by their cytotoxicity against a large number of tumor targets.

Ref.: 1, 2, 3, 4, 5

COMMENTS: See Question 9.

9. Match each cell type in the left column with the appropriate statement or statements in the right column.

A. T cells	a. Type of lymphocyte
B. Macrophages	b. May provide some type of antitumor surveillance
C. Natural killer cells	c. Generated from culture in interleukin-2 (IL-2)
D. Lymphokine-activated killer cells	d. Used for anticancer immunotherapy
E. Tumor-infiltrating lymphocytes	e. Produces interferon α

Ref.: 1, 2, 3, 4, 5

COMMENTS: Natural killer cells are large granular lymphocytes that do not express the T cell- or B cell-specific phenotype. They mediate cytotoxicity toward a variety of targets (e.g., tumor cells) despite a lack of previous exposure to antigens from those targets. The cytotoxicity mediated by NK cells is not restricted by the MHC and can be greatly enhanced by different cytokines. As with subsets of T cells, NK cells can be identified by monoclonal antibodies to specific cell surface antigens that are characteristic of the NK cells (e.g., CD16, CD56). • Interferons—glycoproteins synthesized by a variety of cells in response to viral infection—augment the activity of a number of cells, including macrophages and T cells, as well as NK cells. There are three major types of interferon: interferon α, produced by leukocytes, particularly macrophages; interferon β, produced by fibroblasts; and interferon γ, produced by lymphocytes. As is the case with macrophages, NK cells do not require previous exposure to antigen for activation; these cells (NK cells and macrophages) may provide a type of surveillance against foreign cells, including tumor cells. • Culture of NK cells in the cytokine IL-2 (hormone-like glycoprotein molecules other than antibodies that are produced by cells of the immune system and function to regulate the immune system) for several days leads to the generation of lymphokine-activated killer (LAK) cells. The LAK cells possess augmented cytotoxicity against a broad array of tumor targets. In several studies investigators have evaluated the use of LAK cells for adoptive immunotherapy of patients with cancer; although initial results were impressive, more recent results have been far less encouraging. • Tumor-infiltrating lymphocytes are generated by culturing lymphocytes infiltrating tumors in IL-2 for several weeks. These cells may have even greater antitumor activity than LAK cells. Studies regarding their therapeutic potential are ongoing.

ANSWER:
Question 8: B, C
Question 9: A-a,d; B-b,e; C-a,b; D-a,c,d; E-a,c,d

10. With regard to T cell activation, which of the following statements is/are correct?

A. Some antigens are processed and expressed on antigen-presenting macrophages.
B. Antigen recognition is not specific, which allows clonal expansion and differentiation.
C. Antigen recognition requires the T cell to be MHC-compatible with the antigen-presenting cell.
D. T cells produce interleukin-1 (IL-1) in response to antigen presentation.
E. Plasma cells are responsible for the synthesis of interleukin-2 (IL-2).

Ref.: 1, 2, 3, 4, 5

COMMENTS: When antigen enters a lymph node or the spleen, it may first be phagocytized by a macrophage, which processes the antigen and expresses it on its cell surface for presentation to T and B lymphocytes (see diagram). Macrophages that do this are called **antigen-presenting cells**. Other antigen-presenting cells include dendritic cells (a macrophage-like cell found in the skin, in lymph nodes, and in other tissues) and a subset of B lymphocytes. Recognition of the antigen is highly specific and is accomplished only by clones of T lymphocytes that have a receptor specific to that antigen. Presentation of antigen in the context of self (i.e., with MHC compatibility presented by an antigen-presenting cell) leads to the release of IL-1 by the macrophage (see also Question 3). These events, in turn, stimulate synthesis of IL-2 by T cells and an increase in the expression of IL-2 receptor on T cells, which in turn allows full T cell activation. Helper-T cells interact with B cells, leading to blastogenesis and to their differentiation to

MΦ	Macrophage
Ag	Antigen
Self	Major histocompatibility complex
T	Thymocyte
IL-1	Interleukin-1
IL-2	Interleukin-2

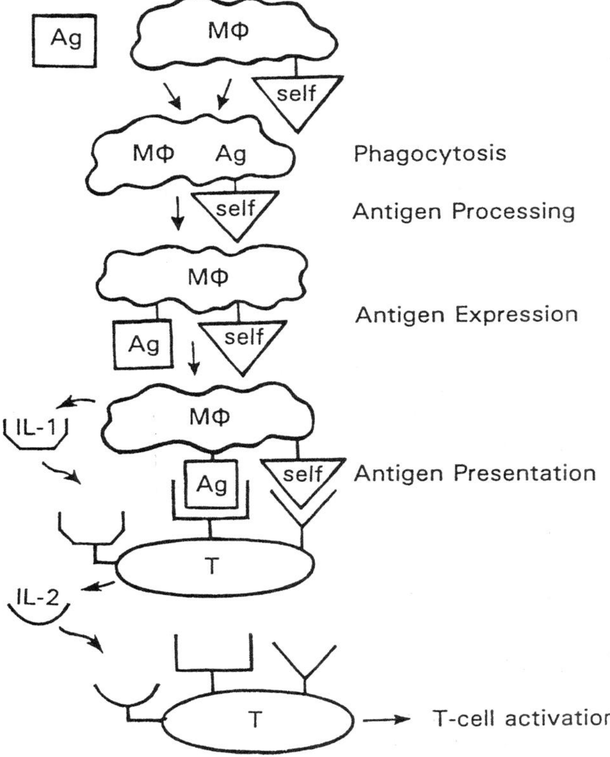

plasma cells. Plasma cells are responsible for antibody synthesis; they do not produce IL-2.

ANSWER: A, C

11. With regard to the cytokine IL-1, which of the following statements is/are true?

A. The major cells producing IL-1 are monocytes and macrophages.
B. IL-1 leads to vasoconstriction and hypertension by directly stimulating the hypothalamus.
C. IL-1 may induce a fever.
D. T lymphocyte production of IL-2 is inhibited by IL-1.
E. IL-1 may augment wound healing by increasing fibroblast proliferation and collagen synthesis.

Ref.: 1, 6

COMMENTS: The cells of the immune system are regulated by a variety of cytokines (soluble substances produced by cells) that have a broad range of interrelated immunologic, inflammatory, and physiologic characteristics. In general, the cytokines are categorized according to their cell of origin (e.g., lymphokines from lymphocytes, monokines from monocytes). One of these cytokines, IL-1, is a key regulator of inflammation, wound healing, and the immune response. There are two forms of IL-1: IL-1α and IL-1β. IL-1β is produced and secreted in 10-fold excess of IL-1α, which for the most part is not secreted but remains associated with the cell membrane. Although IL-1 is produced and secreted principally by cells of the monocyte-macrophage lineage, it is also produced by neutrophils, fibroblasts, natural killer (NK) cells, keratinocytes, endothelial cells, and vascular smooth muscle cells. IL-1 plays an important role in normal inflammatory responses. It may induce endothelial cells to produce prostaglandins, platelet-activating factor, and plasminogen activator; these properties may cause vasodilatation and even hypotension by promoting endothelial leakage and intravascular thrombosis. IL-1 was previously referred to as the "endogenous pyrogen" because of its direct stimulation of the thermoregulatory center in the hypothalamus and, as such, induction of fever. IL-1 stimulates the liver to produce several acute-phase proteins. It plays a key role in joint inflammation through its ability to induce synovial cells to produce prostaglandin E_2, collagenase, and phospholipase. • IL-1 has an important mediator function in wound healing by activating basophils and eosinophils, stimulating neutrophil and macrophage activity, and locally increasing fibroblast proliferation and collagen synthesis. • IL-1 plays a pivotal role in the immune system. It can induce proliferation of T and B lymphocytes, IL-2 production, and expression of the IL-2 receptor. Moreover, IL-1 stimulates release of a variety of other cytokines, including interferon, IL-3, IL-6, and colony-stimulating factors. The effects of IL-1 on immunity are greatly amplified through stimulation of other cytokines.

ANSWER: A, C, E

12. With regard to IL-2, which of the following statements is/are true?

A. The proliferation of T lymphocytes is inhibited by IL-2.
B. IL-2 is produced by activated T lymphocytes.
C. Natural killer (NK) cell cytotoxicity is augmented by IL-2.
D. Cytokine release by macrophages is inhibited by IL-2.

Ref.: 1, 6

COMMENTS: IL-2 was initially referred to as T cell growth factor on the basis of its ability to stimulate the proliferation of T lymphocytes in culture. IL-2 is produced by activated T lymphocytes in response to presentation by antigen or IL-1. It is also produced by NK cells. • IL-2 promotes the proliferation (increase in number) of activated T lymphocytes by binding to receptors on the T lymphocyte surface. IL-2 stimulates B lymphocyte proliferation and differentiation (maturation, i.e., to plasma cells). NK cells stimulated by IL-2 proliferate, and their cytotoxic activity is augmented. IL-2 also activates macrophages, leading to increased production of various cytokines including tumor necrosis factor and colony-stimulating factor.

ANSWER: B, C

13. With regard to the complement cascade, which of the following statements is/are true?

A. Complement is a system of related serum proteins important to the regulation of coagulation.
B. Complement may be activated by immune complexes.
C. The components C3a and C5a are useful for inhibiting mast cell release of granules.
D. The components $C5b_{6,7,8,9}$ form a complex that causes cell lysis.
E. The components C3a and C5a are chemotactic for macrophages and neutrophils.

Ref.: 1, 2, 3, 4, 5

COMMENTS: **Complement** is an interrelated system of serum proteins that are important mediators of inflammation and cell lysis. The system is composed of at least 20 distinct proteins designated by numerals (e.g., C1, C2) that are activated in a cascade mechanism (similar to the coagulation cascade) in such a way that individual components interact so the products of one reaction form the enzyme for the next. The net result is that a small initial stimulus can lead to a greatly amplified effect. Complement is activated (i.e., the cascade is initiated) primarily by immune complexes (an antigen bound to an antibody) binding to the first component called C1 but also by exposure to some microbial products. Activated C3a and C5a (components derived from the activation of C3 and C5) act as chemotactic (chemoattractant) agents for macrophages and neutrophils; they are also referred to as anaphylatoxins in that they stimulate mast cell degranulation, smooth muscle contraction, and increased vascular permeability. Activated C5b initiates formation of a complex of the remaining complement proteins from C6 to C9 (designated $C5b_{6,7,8,9}$) that attach to and lyse cell membranes.

ANSWER: B, D, E

14. With regard to immunizations, which of the following statements is/are correct?

A. Active immunization involves administration of either killed or biologically attentuated but intact organisms or their component parts, so they are antigenic but do not produce disease.
B. Passive immunization involves administration of an exogenous, immunologically active compound.
C. The diphtheria-pertussis-tetanus (DPT) vaccine is an example of passive immunization.
D. The Salk vaccine is an example of active immunization.
E. RhoGAM is an example of specific immunoglobulin administered for passive immunization.

Ref.: 1, 2, 3, 4, 5

COMMENTS: There are two basic types of immunization. **Active immunization** involves administration of intact organisms that are killed or damaged, or their component parts, which are unable to produce disease but are still antigenic and able to induce an immune response. **Passive immunization** involves administration of an exogenous active component that provides immediate but only temporary specific immunity. • Currently used bacterial vaccines for active immunization include the DPT vaccine, which is made up of diphtheria toxoid (toxin treated to render it nontoxic but still immunogenic), pertussis (comprised of heat-killed *Bordetella pertussis* organisms), and tetanus toxoid (a preparation of inactivated *Clostridium tetani* toxin). Other examples include the

Pneumovax vaccine, composed of a pool of capsule polysaccharide material from 23 types of *Streptococcus pneumoniae*. Examples of currently used viral vaccines include the rubella, measles, and mumps vaccines (made up of live attentuated virus grown in tissue culture); poliomyelitis vaccine (Sabin vaccine, which is live, attentuated, and given orally; and the Salk vaccine, which is inactivated polio virus given by injection); rabies vaccine; and hepatitis B vaccine. • There are three basic types of passive immunization: antitoxin, immunoglobulin, and specific immunoglobulin. *Antitoxins* are made up of antiserum or neutralizing antibody specific for a given toxin. An example is tetanus toxin, which is specific for *C. tetani* toxin. *Immunoglobulin* is also referred to as γ-globulin and may be useful for maintenance of immunodeficient individuals. An example of a *specific immune globulin* is RhoGAM, or Rh immunoglobulin, which is administered to Rh-negative women shortly after childbirth. It enables her antibodies to bind the Rh-positive antigen passively acquired from the blood of the fetus, thereby preventing the Rh-negative mother from becoming sensitized and exposing her to possible difficulties with future pregnancies.

ANSWER: A, B, D, E

15. Match each type of hypersensitivity reactions in the left column with the appropriate statement(s) in the right column.

A. Type I	a. ABO incompatibility
B. Type II	b. Contact dermatitis
C. Type III	c. IgE bound to mast cells and basophils
D. Type IV	d. Serum sickness
	e. Anaphylaxis
	f. IgG or IgM antibody reacts with cell-bound antigen
	g. Tuberculin skin test

Ref.: 1, 2, 3, 4, 5

COMMENTS: Gell and Coombs defined four hypersensitivity reactions that were precipitated by both cell-mediated and humoral responses and may lead to inflammation and tissue damage. These reactions are the cause of a wide variety of allergic and autoimmune diseases and conditions. **Type I** (*immediate hypersensitivity*) reactions are initiated by antigens that react with IgE antibody. Immediate hypersensitivity reactions range from food allergy and hay fever to anaphylaxis. Antigens include pollens, mold, danders, and food. Binding of the antigen to IgE bound to mast cells or basophils results in release of a variety of mediators, including histamine, slow-reacting substance of anaphylaxis, serotonin, prostaglandins, and bradykinin. Reactions vary in severity but generally include increased vascular permeability, increased secretions, and smooth muscle contraction. They may clinically manifest as sniffling, sneezing, bronchoconstriction, angioedema, and even convulsions and death. **Type II** reactions, also called *cytotoxic reactions*, are the result of IgG or IgM antibodies reacting with a cell-bound antigen. The most common example is the ABO and Rh incompatibility transfusion reaction, which leads to severe, almost immediate lysis of transfused red blood cells by anti-A or anti-B antibodies in the serum. Rh incompatibility, although not causing immediate complement-mediated intravascular hemolysis, can be serious and is caused by reaction of the Rh antigen with anti-Rh antibodies. Other examples are myasthenia gravis (resulting from autoantibodies to the acetylcholine receptors at the neuromuscular junction), Graves' disease (in which autoantibodies against the thyroid-stimulating hormone receptor actually stimulate the thyroid), and idiopathic thrombocytopenic purpura, which results from antiplatelet antibodies. **Type III**, or *immune complex-mediated*, reactions result from deposition of the antibody–antigen complex from the circulation. Classic immune complex reactions include serum sickness, rheumatoid arthritis, and glomerulonephritis resulting from previous streptococcal infection, deposition of IgG–IgM complexes in the joints, deposition of immune complexes in the kidney, or systemic lupus erythematosus. **Type IV**, or *delayed-type hypersensitivity*, reactions result from antigen stimulation of previously sensitized T cells, primarily the $CD4^+$ helper-T cells. The activated T cells then release cytokines and chemokines (chemoattractants), which result in the attraction and activation of other cells, particularly macrophages. The classic clinical example is demonstrated by the tuberculin skin test characterized by dermal induration due to lymphocyte and macrophage accumulation at the site of antigen injection, which develops over 48–72 hours. Late hypersensitivity may play a role in the rejection of grafted tissues and organs. The classic clinical example is contact dermatitis.

ANSWER: A-c,e; B-a,f; C-d; D-b,g

16. With regard to tumor necrosis factor (TNF), which of the following statements is/are true?

A. It is produced predominantly by monocytes and macrophages.
B. TNF release is stimulated by endotoxin.
C. TNF exerts its effect as an anabolic stimulant of the host, leading to increased deposition of muscle protein and fat.
D. By inducing necrosis in gram-negative bacteria, TNF may be useful in the treatment of gram-negative shock.

Ref.: 1, 6

COMMENTS: Tumor necrosis factor derives its name from its ability to cause hemorrhagic necrosis in methylcholanthrene-induced sarcomas in mice. There are two forms, TNFα and TNFβ. TNFα is produced predominantly by monocytes and macrophages but also by neutrophils and natural killer (NK) cells; TNFβ is produced mostly by T and B lymphocytes. • TNF stimulates the activity of neutrophils, induces endothelial cells to produce interleukin-1 (IL-1), and enhances the production of prostaglandin E_2 and collagenase by synovial cells and fibroblasts. TNF increases the procoagulant activity on endothelial surfaces, increases vascular permeability, degranulates neutrophils, and stimulates release of superoxides and arachidonic acid metabolites. Through its action on a variety of target cells, it plays a major role in gram-negative shock; endotoxin stimulates monocyte and macrophage release of significant amounts of TNF, which leads to fever, metabolic acidosis, hypotension, disseminated intravascular coagulation, and even death. • TNF stimulates a variety of catabolic activities, particularly in muscle and fat cells, leading to an increase in anaerobic glycolysis, protein breakdown, and lipolysis. It is largely responsible for the cachexia associated with malignant disease. Recent studies have shown that TNF receptors on cells, when engaged by the specific TNF cytokine, transmit a cell death signal, leading to programmed cell death or apoptosis.

ANSWER: A, B

17. With regard to interferons, which of the following statements is/are correct?

A. Interferon γ is produced by macrophages.
B. Interferon production is inhibited by infection.
C. Interferons have a direct antiproliferative effect on cells.
D. Interferons stimulate the cytotoxic activity of natural killer (NK) cells and macrophages.
E. The production of cytokines by macrophages is inhibited by interferons.

Ref.: 1, 6

COMMENTS: Interferons are a family of glycoproteins produced by a variety of cells in response to viral infection or other stimulants. The 20 major types of interferons may be broadly classified into three groups on the basis of their cell of origin. Interferon α is produced by leukocytes (primarily macrophages); interferon β is produced by epithelial cells, fibroblasts, and macrophages; and interferon γ is produced by T lymphocytes and NK cells. Interferons are known to have a powerful, direct antiproliferative effect on cells and can also induce cellular differentiation. This is the most likely explanation for their usefulness as anticancer agents, although some of the anticancer effects may also result from stimulation of the cytotoxic activity of macrophages, NK cells, and cytotoxic T lymphocytes. Finally, the interferons stimulate a wide variety of cells to increase production of other mediators, which in turn stimulate the release of other cytokines.

ANSWER: C, D

18. With regard to chemokines, which of the following statements is/are true?

A. Chemokines are high-molecular-weight molecules that are fixed to the tissues.
B. Chemokines bind to specific receptors on leukocytes.
C. Chemokines are increased during an inflammatory event.
D. There is one chemokine for each kind of leukocyte.
E. Some chemokines are able to prevent human immunodeficiency virus (HIV) infections.

Ref.: 7

COMMENTS: A fundamental requirement for an effective immune response is the ability to recruit different kinds of immune cells to the site of an inflammatory or infectious event. Studies conducted during the early 1990s have identified a family of molecules termed "chemokines" that are responsible for this function. Chemokines are low-molecular-weight cytokines that attract specific leukocyte populations to areas of inflammation and effect immune cell activation. All members of the chemokine superfamily have four cysteines linked by disulfide bonding. The chemokines can be further subdivided structurally by whether the first two cysteines are adjacent (i.e., in a C-C sequence) or separated by an amino acid (i.e., in a C-X-C sequence). The first chemokine to be identified was interleukin-8 (IL-8), a cytokine produced by activated monocytes and macrophages with chemoattractant activity for neutrophils. By 1998 at least 30 chemokines had been identified and characterized as belonging to the C-C or C-X-C subgroups. The ability of a chemokine to attract a specific leukocyte population is derived from the expression of a specific receptor for the chemokine on the leukocyte membrane. To date, there are five recognized C-C chemokine receptors (designated CCR1–CCR5) and four recognized C-X-C receptors (CXCR1–CXCR4). For example, the chemokine IL-8 is a C-X-C chemokine that binds to either the CXCR1 or the CXCR2 receptors on neutrophils. The CXCR1 receptor is specific for IL-8, whereas the CXCR2 receptor binds IL-8 and other CXC chemokines. Immune cell stimulation and activation often lead to the increased production of specific chemokines and an increase in the expression of the corresponding chemokine receptor(s) on leukocytes needed at the site of the triggering event. Chemokines for all of the major mononuclear and polynuclear leukocytes have been identified. A highly provocative recent set of studies has also shown that the leukocyte tropism of HIV strains for monocytes and lymphocytes depends on the expression of specific monocyte- or lymphocyte-associated chemokine receptors. Furthermore, specific chemokines have been shown to protect cells against infection with HIV.

ANSWER: B, C, E

REFERENCES

1. Stites DP, Stobo JD, Fudenberg HH, Wells JV: *Basic and Clinical Immunology*. Lange Medical Publications, Los Altos, CA, 1984.
2. Roitt I, Brostoff J, Male D: *Immunology*. CV Mosby, St. Louis, 1986.
3. Toledo-Pereyra LH: *Immunology Essentials of Surgical Practice*. PSG, Littleton, MA, 1988.
4. Myrvik QN, Weiser RS: *Fundamentals of Immunology*. Lea & Febiger, Malvern, PA, 1984.
5. Abbas AK, Lichtman AH, Pober JS: *Cellular and Molecular Immunology*, 3rd ed. WB Saunders, Philadelphia, 1997.
6. Staren ED, Essner R, Economou JS: *Seminars in Surgical Oncology*. Alan R. Liss, New York, 1989.
7. Baggioline M, Dewald B, Moser B: Human chemokines: an update. *Ann Rev Immunol* 15:675–705, 1997.

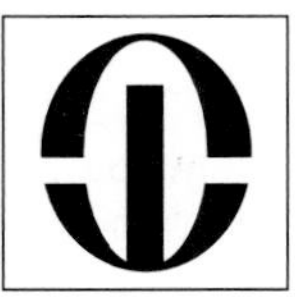

CHAPTER 10

Transplantation

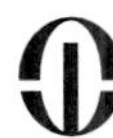

1. Bladder drainage of the transplanted pancreas is associated with:

A. Nongap metabolic acidosis.
B. Recurrent urinary tract infections.
C. Urethral stricture formation in males.
D. Reflux pancreatitis.

Ref.: 1

COMMENTS: Drainage of the transplant pancreas into the bladder previously was believed to be associated with a lesser incidence of anastomotic leaking. This anatomy also allowed collection of urine to determine the urine amylase level, reflecting the functional status of the transplant pancreas. Because of the frequent complications and the ability to diagnose pancreas allograft rejection by biopsy, many have abandoned bladder drainage in favor of enteric drainage; there are fewer complications without compromising graft survival.

ANSWER: A, B, C, D

2. The long term metabolic results of a successful kidney/pancreas transplant is/are:

A. Stabilization of proliferative retinopathy.
B. Reduced risk of diabetic nephropathy.
C. Improvement in nerve conduction velocity.
D. Reversal of peripheral vascular disease.

Ref.: 1

COMMENTS: Successful pancreas transplantation approximates prolonged euglycemia with normalization of glycosylated hemoglobin. Stabilization or improvement in diabetes retinopathy is seen. Renal transplantation in diabetic patients without correction of their glycemic state results in recurrence of diabetic nephropathy as seen in serial renal biopsies. A successful pancreas transplant prevents this recurrence. Diabetic neuropathy, both peripheral and autonomic, is improved following a successful pancreas transplant but requires months to years to be demonstrable.

ANSWER: A, B, C

3. Which of the following patients is *not* an acceptable candidate for liver transplantation because of the probability that the 5-year survival would be less than 20%?

A. A 50-year-old man with cholangiocarcinoma (Klatskin tumor), with no evidence of metastasis on CT and MRI scans, who has normal cardiac, renal, and pulmonary functions.
B. A 48-year-old Hispanic man with advanced cirrhosis from hepatitis C and with a 3 cm hepatoma in the right lobe of the liver.
C. A 48-year-old woman with cirrhosis from hepatitis B who is DNA-negative, surface antigen-positive, and surface antibody-negative.
D. A 50-year-old Caucasian woman given a transplant 6 years ago who had hepatitis C and now has recurrent hepatitis C, cirrhosis, and uncontrollable ascites.
E. A 55-year-old alcoholic man with medically refractory ascites, grade II encephalopathy, prolonged INR of 3, and abstinent from alcohol for 12 months.

Ref.: 2, 3, 4, 5, 6

COMMENTS: Patients with alcoholic liver disease who are abstinent for more than 6 months and have good psychosocial support are considered good candidates for liver transplantation because of the low risk of alcohol recidivism. Their long-term survival may be one of the highest as a group, as they are not as often subject to viral hepatitis and other progressive diseases that may recur in the transplanted liver. • Hepatitis B recurrence can now be prevented, or substantially reduced in its aggressiveness, by postoperative use of antibody treatment [hepatitis B immune globulin (HBIG)], or the protease inhibitor lamivudine. Thus these patients, recently considered poor candidates for liver transplantation because of destructive recurrent disease, can now expect a good chance of long-term survival. • Hepatitis C is known to recur in the transplanted liver of essentially all patients transplanted for this condition. Nevertheless, the disease usually takes an indolent course. If retransplantation becomes necessary for this condition, it also is consistent with good long-term outcome. • Cholangiocarcinoma causing obstruction at the hepatic bile duct confluence was one of the early indications for liver transplantation. Despite the relative ease of the transplant procedure owing to the absence of portal hypertension and coagulopathy, the carcinoma recurs in essentially all patients, usually at the site of the original tumor. More recent variations on the operation, including pancreaticoduodenectomy, have only slightly improved long-term survival. • Hepatocellular carcinoma arising in association with end stage cirrhosis is compatible with prolonged survival when it exists as a single tumor less than 5 cm in diameter or up to three tumors individually less than 3 cm in diameter. Previously reported as "incidental" tumors discovered in the excised liver, these lesions are more frequently detected with improved imaging techniques and recur in fewer than 15% of patients.

ANSWER: A

4. Which, if any, of the following is/are absolute contraindication(s) to orthotopic liver transplantation?

A. History of alcohol abuse.
B. Age greater than 60 years.
C. Portal vein thrombosis.
D. Human immunodeficiency virus (HIV) positivity.
E. Chronic hepatitis C infection.

Ref.: 2, 7, 8, 9

COMMENTS: Alcoholics who have documented abstinence from alcohol and extensive follow-up following transplantation can achieve an acceptable low recidivism rate. Patients over 65 years of age can also expect good results provided the function of vital organs (heart, lungs, kidney) are not compromised. The latest data show that patients older than 65 years have a 75% survival rate at 1 year compared to an overall liver transplants patient survival of 80%. • Portal vein thrombosis previously has been a contraindication to liver transplantation. Identification of it prior to transplantation allows adjustments in techniques that can result in an acceptable survival rate. • HIV positivity has been an absolute contraindication to all solid organ transplantation. Recently, however, the effectiveness of protease inhibitors has resulted not only in an increased life expectancy of those affected by the virus but also essential reduction in their viral load with improvement in their immunocompromised state. Some programs are presently reevaluating this contraindication to organ transplantation. • Hepatitis C is one of the most common indications for liver transplantation. Presently there is no effective antiviral therapy for hepatitis C, so reinfection of the transplanted allograft is expected. Despite reinfection, it is uncommon (i.e., less than 15%) for Rush patients to have early graft loss secondary to hepatitis C.

ANSWER: D

5. Regarding blood transfusions to potential kidney recipients, which of the following is/are true?

A. They should be avoided at all costs.
B. They uniformly decrease graft survival.
C. They result in prolonged graft survival of histocompatibility antigen (HLA)-mismatched grafts, especially if combined with azathioprine therapy.
D. They may sensitize the potential recipient.

Ref.: 13

COMMENTS: Pretransplant blood transfusion to a kidney recipient treated with azathioprine and prednisone is beneficial in that it improves graft survival. Since the emergence of cyclosporine as the mainstay of immunosuppression, the benefits of transfusion have diminished. The risk of sensitizing patients to histocompatibility antigen (HLA) and thus producing a positive crossmatch to potential donor tissue now appears to be a greater issue. Although blood should not be withheld if clinically necessary, widespread random transfusion is falling from favor. Donor-specific transfusion still offers an advantage, however. Many theories have been proposed to explain the mechanism of the effect of blood transfusion, ranging from the removal of "high responders" from the recipient pool to a complex network of idiotypic regulation of the immune response. However, in essence, the mechanism remains unknown.

ANSWER: C, D

6. Of the following, which would exclude a patient from whole-organ pancreas transplantation?

A. History of chronic renal failure with biopsy-proven Kimmelstiel-Wilson's histology.
B. History of coronary artery bypass graft.
C. History of diabetic neuropathy.
D. History of lower extremity peripheral vascular disease.
E. None of the above.

Ref.: 1, 10, 11

COMMENTS: Selection criteria include diabetic patients with secondary complications of diabetes but who do not have complications which would preclude long-term survival. Increasing data have shown that pancreas transplantation is able to arrest further development of early secondary complications of diabetes. After pancreas/kidney transplantation, diabetic renal disease (Kimmelstiel-Wilson's changes) in the transplant kidney does not seem to recur. Diabetic neuropathy is many times reversed and documented by increased nerve conduction velocity studies. However, vascular disease of the lower extremities and of the coronary arteries are not reversed and significantly increase the surgical risk of the procedure.

ANSWER: E

7. Patients with hepatic cirrhosis with concomitant significant portal hypertension should undergo which of the following for the management of recurrent variceal bleeds despite sclerotherapy.

A. Variceal banding therapy.
B. Portosystemic shunt.
C. Trans internal jugular portal system shunt (TIPS).
D. Dependent on the severity of their liver disease and proximity to liver transplantation, either "B" or "C."

Ref.: 12

COMMENTS: The management of portal hypertension should be tailored to each individual patient. All patients should undergo initial scleral therapy or banding to control esophageal varices. Failure of this modality should lead to portosystemic shunt. The TIPS procedure has been shown to be quite successful in the short term, but there is insufficient experience to reliably predict its long-term patency. Patients with Child's A or B cirrhosis therefore should undergo surgical portosystemic shunts while those with Child's C cirrhosis should undergo the TIPS procedure as a prelude to transplantation.

ANSWER: D

8. Which of the following is the most predictive of 1-year patient survival following liver transplantation?

A. Age of the recipient.
B. Severity of the APACHE score prior to transplantation.
C. Presence of an incidental hepatoma less than 4 cm.
D. Use of antilymphocyte globulin.

Ref.: 8

COMMENTS: Patient survival after liver transplantation is directly related to the severity of the illness prior to transplantation. Statistics show that patients who are well enough to be at home with their liver disease at the time of transplantation have a 91.4% one-year survival rate. This is in contrast to that of patients who had been hospitalized, who have an 84.5% survival rate. Those in the intensive care unit (ICU) prior to transplantation had a 79.9% survival rate; those on life support have a 69.7% survival rate.

ANSWER: B

9. FK 506 (Prograf) has a mechanism of action similar to that of:

A. Imuran.
B. OKT3.
C. Cyclosporine.
D. Prednisone.

Ref.: 30

COMMENTS: The main mechanism of action of both cyclosporine and FK506 is inhibition of interleukin-2 (IL-2) and other cytokines produced by the T cell. Both bind with an intracytoplasmic binding protein, a combination that inhibits the action of calcineurin, a phosphatase that participates in activation of specific genes in the T cell. FK506 has good bioavailability orally and seems to enter the lymphocyte more readily than cyclosporine. Both have similar nephrotoxicities, but FK506 produces more gastrointestinal and neurological symptoms. OKT_3 is a mononuclear antibody targeted against T-lymphocytes with the CD_3 receptor. Administration of this commercially available antibody produces near-complete destruction of one of the "kingpins" of allo-immune reaction (i.e., the CD_3 lymphocytes). This agent, therefore, is extremely effective in treating acute rejection. Mycophenolate and azathioprine have the same mechanism of action. Azathioprine inhibits purine synthesis through the metabolite mercaptopurine. Mycophenolate acid (CellCept) also works by purine inhibition but blocks an enzyme in the de novo synthesis pathway only. Lymphocytes are dependent on the de novo pathway for production of purines. Most other cells have a scavenger pathway as an alternative to the de novo pathway for purine synthesis. Therefore mycophenolate has a more specific mechanism of action for immunosuppression than azathioprine.

ANSWER: C

10. Donor organs for pediatric liver transplantation are acquired from the following:

A. Donor of similar size and habitus.
B. Splitting of an adult cadaver liver and transplanting the appropriate segment.
C. Resection of the left lobe or left lateral segment of a liver from an adult living donor.

Ref.: 31

COMMENTS: Over the past 10 years pediatric liver transplantation has experienced a substantial expansion in the availability of donor grafts. Previously, many children died while waiting for an appropriately sized donor to become available. Now with the application of segmental liver resection techniques, full-size cadaver liver grafts can be reduced to the appropriate volume for the pediatric recipient. Also, resection of the left lobe or the left lateral segment from a living adult donor can be done with comparable survival of the recipient and minimal risk to the donor.

ANSWER: A, B, C

11. A patient receiving cyclosporine based immunosuppression presents to the clinic 4 weeks after a cadaveric renal transplant complaining of oliguria, weight gain, and ipsilateral lower extremity edema. His serum creatinine has risen to 2.9 mg/dl from 1.2 mg/dl since his last visit 7 days ago. Ultrasound examination of the graft area reveals a 12 × 18 × 4 cm collection of fluid around the renal allograft. Which of the following statements is/are appropriate?

A. He should undergo immediate percutaneous transplant biopsy to rule out rejection.
B. Biopsy is too risky, and treatment for acute rejection should be promptly begun.
C. The fluid collection should be aspirated, cultured, and evaluated for chemistry.
D. He should be reevaluated in 1 week to give the fluid collection a chance to be absorbed.
E. The dose of cyclosporine should be reduced and reevaluated in 1 week.

Ref.: 10, 13

COMMENTS: The incidence of clinically significant lymphoceles is 0.6–18.0%. Most present within the first 6 months after renal transplantation. They are due either to inadequate ligation of lymphatics transected along the iliac vessels during transplantation or to lymph leakage from the allograft, especially during an episode of rejection. The diagnosis is made by needle aspiration of the fluid under ultrasound guidance, ruling out hematoma or a urinoma by testing the creatinine content and ruling out an infection by Gram stain and culture. Their clinical significance depends on compromise of the kidney, ureter, and adjacent structure. Percutaneous renal transplant biopsy should be avoided in the presence of a large fluid collection, as there are no adhesions to tamponade retroperitoneal bleeding. If percutaneous aspiration does not lead to improvement in renal function, a biopsy should be considered to rule out rejection. Perinephric fluid collections larger than 50–100 ml volume are seen in 20–50% of renal transplant recipients on routine follow-up ultrasound examinations. The treatment is controversial. External drainage or repeated aspiration has an overall success rate of 60–73% but a significant (25–50%) risk of infection. The use of sclerosants such as talc, tetracycline, and other means has a reported success rate above 80%, but there is a risk of chemical peritonitis if the sclerosant leaks into the peritoneal cavity. Intraperitoneal marsupialization, done by removing a wide ellipse of lymphocele wall with omentoplasty to prevent recurrence, is now widely accepted as definitive therapy. This is done through the original incision or laparoscopically. It has a primary success rate near 90% with low risk of recurrence. Because acute rejection can cause a rise in serum creatinine, cyclosporine is not arbitrarily justified, and delay in diagnosis of acute rejection jeopardizes the kidney.

ANSWER: C

12. Six months after renal transplantation, a 56-year-old woman is admitted to the hospital with high fever, elevated serum creatinine, disseminated varicella skin lesions, and bilateral pulmonary infiltrates. Which of the following statements is/are true?

A. Bronchoscopy is unnecessary as the diagnosis is obviously viral pneumonia.
B. At this stage the patient need not be placed in isolation.
C. Immunosuppression should not be changed to avoid rejection.
D. Intravenous acyclovir ± hyperimmune globulin is the treatment of choice.
E. This is a potentially lethal condition.

Ref.: 10, 13

COMMENTS: Reactivation of herpes zoster (shingles) occurs in up to 15–30% of renal transplant recipients, usually during the first 6 months after transplantation. Intravenous, followed by oral, acyclovir usually prevents systemic dissemination and leads to rapid healing of the skin lesions. In the presence of such complications, immunosuppression should be drastically reduced to prevent a mortality. Respiratory isolation is necessary to prevent spread of infection to other patients. Bronchoscopy is advisable to rule out superinfection with bacterial, fungal, or other opportunistic organisms. Intravenous acyclovir ± hyperimmune globulin (varicella zoster immune globulin, or VZIG) is the therapy of choice. The acyclovir analogues famciclovir and valacyclovir are under clinical trials at present.

ANSWER: D, E

13. With respect to de novo post-renal-transplant diabetes mellitus, which of the following statement(s) is/are true?

A. It is more common in African-American recipients.
B. It is a side effect of cyclosporine and FK506 (Prograf) and is reversible after reduction of immunosuppression.
C. Risk factors include weight, age, and family history.
D. It is less common since the introduction of tacrolimus/cyclosporine.
E. There is no association with steroid dosage.

Ref.: 10, 13

COMMENTS: Posttransplant diabetes mellitus (PTDM) is seen in 4–20% of renal transplant recipients. Steroids, cyclosporine, and tacrolimus are diabetogenic. There is a direct relation between steroid dosage and the incidence of PTDM. Tacrolimus-based immunosuppression was associated with an 18% incidence of new-onset PTDM in a recent multicenter trial, and it was decreased to 9% after reduction of steroid and tacrolimus doses. Cyclosporine based immunosuppression resulted in only a 4% incidence of new-onset PTDM. Risk factors include age, obesity, family history of diabetes, and African-American race. The potential mechanisms include decreased insulin secretion, increased insulin resistance, and a toxic effect of tacrolimus and cyclosporine on pancreatic beta cells. Only 25% of patients with PTDM develop persistent hyperglycemia, and 50% of this group require continuous insulin therapy.

ANSWER: A, B, C, E

14. With respect to hepatitis and *renal* transplantation, which of the following statements is/are true?

A. Hepatitis C is an absolute contraindication to organ donation.
B. All hepatitis B surface antigen-positive patients are poor renal transplant candidates.
C. Hepatitis C-positive recipients have an extremely poor prognosis.
D. None of the above.
E. All of the above.

Ref.: 10, 13

COMMENTS: Patients with preexisting hepatitis C who have a moderate viral load measured by polymerase chain reaction (PCR) testing, normal liver function, and minimal chronic active hepatitis on liver biopsy are acceptable recipients for a renal transplant. Donors with a similar profile may be acceptable for such a patient but not for a recipient who does not have hepatitis C. Hepatic disease occurs in 7–24% of patients during the early posttransplant period and is the cause of late death in 8–28% of patients. Hepatitis B and C are responsible for most of these deaths. Hepatitis B surface antigen-positive patients who have stable liver function and are negative for e antigen do fairly well after renal transplantation and low dose immunosuppression. The replacement of Imuran by cyclosporine has reduced the corticosteroid dose and improved the long-term outcome in these patients.

ANSWER: D

15. Of the following liver diseases resulting in end-stage cirrhosis, which one most commonly recurs in the new liver allograft utilizing current prophylactic measures?

A. Chronic excessive alcohol intake.
B. Hepatitis B.
C. Hepatitis C.
D. Primary biliary cirrhosis.
E. Primary sclerosing cholangitis.

Ref.: 4, 14, 15, 16, 17, 18

COMMENTS: Hepatitis C is an RNA virus of the genus *Flavivirus*, which is genetically related to such viruses as those that cause dengue fever and Japanese encephalitis. This virus reinfects essentially all of the liver allograft in hepatitis C-infected persons, producing a "flair" of increased liver enzymes in approximately 60–80% of the liver allograft recipients but without development of significant clinical liver disease. Approximately 10% of the recipients develop marked dysfunction of their liver allograft with marked jaundice, extremely elevated liver enzymes, and clinical signs of liver failure (e.g., ascites, coagulopathy, lethargy). Many of this small group of patients may require retransplantation because of life-threatening liver failure within the first year after transplantation. • Liver transplantation for chronic hepatitis B induced cirrhosis used to result in approximately 80% reinfection of the liver allograft. This reinfection usually resulted in destruction of the liver allograft within the first year, requiring retransplantation. Retransplantation in this clinical situation usually resulted in an even more fulminant course of rejection. With the utilization of monthly doses of hepatitis B immune globulin (HBIG) following transplantation, the incidence of reinfection of the liver allograft has been reduced to approximately 20%, and there is associated excellent long-term patient survival. With the addition of new nucleoside analogues such as lamivudine, alone and in combination with HBIG following transplantation, further prevention of recurrent hepatitis B infection has been noted. • The incidence of recidivism (i.e., drinking any alcoholic beverage) within the first 3–5 years after operation is approximately 20%, with severe, life-threatening liver dysfunction associated with recidivism and drug noncompliance in 2–5% at long-term follow-up. • The recurrence of primary biliary cirrhosis (PBC) and primary sclerosing cholangitis are thought to be rare during the first 5 years following liver transplantation.

ANSWER: C

16. Following transplantation the incidence of primary nonfunction of the liver allograft ranges from 1% to 10%. Immediately following the liver transplant procedure, which of the following is/are associated with this clinical syndrome in the liver allograft recipient?

A. Metabolic alkalosis.
B. Hyperkalemia.
C. Reduced mental status.
D. Marked elevation in liver enzymes.
E. Minimal bile output (if a T-tube biliary drainage catheter is in place).

Ref.: 2

COMMENTS: Primary nonfunction of a liver allograft is a poorly understood clinical syndrome associated with markedly abnormal function of the allograft (i.e., severe coagulopathy, acidosis, hyperkalemia, poor mental status, continued hyperdynamic cardiac function—high cardiac output, low system vascular resistance—liver failure, poor bile output, and usually renal failure). Recipients with a normally functioning graft have marked metabolic alkalosis secondary to the liver graft's metabolism of the citrate component from banked blood replacement to bicarbonate during the immediate posttransplantation period. Within the first 24 hours following liver transplantation, patients with normally functioning grafts normalize their cardiac hemodynamics from a hyperdynamic state. The most specific pretransplantation predictor of this phenomenon is the amount of macrosteatosis (extracellular fat globules) in the liver allograft. With more than 40–50% of the cross-sectional area of liver biopsy being macrosteatotic, the incidence of primary dysfunction may reach 50%. Other purported predictors of this syndrome include high levels of vasopressor support in the donor and cold ischemia time. Usually potential liver donor grafts with these findings are not utilized. The mechanism whereby the fat causes this clinical problem has not been clearly elucidated. Although a variety of strategies have been attempted to ameliorate this syndrome, the only treatment is prompt retransplantation.

ANSWER: B, C, D, E

17. Liver donor allocation for liver transplantation, as administered by the United Network for Organ Sharing (UNOS), is based on which of the following criteria?

A. Medical necessity (the acuity or severity of the candidate's liver disease).
B. Blood type (A, B, O, AB) compatibility between the donor and recipient.
C. Size matching of the donor recipient.
D. Length of time the recipient has been on the waiting list for transplantation compared to other recipients.
E. Human lymphocyte antigen matching between donor and recipient.

Ref.: 19

COMMENTS: All liver transplant candidates are registered with the UNOS waiting list, a private organization of doctors and other health care-related personnel that is overseen by the United States government. The organs are allocated "points" based on the level of liver failure and liver failure-related, life-threatening complications of the candidates (i.e., medical necessity). In almost all instances, the liver recipient's and donor's ABO blood types must match or be compatible (lottery aspect). The donor liver must be able physically to fit inside the recipient. In pediatric recipients the adult donor liver can be "cut down" to size, such that a size-appropriate segment of the donor liver is transplanted (i.e., often the left lateral segment in small children). Finally, candidates accrue a small number of "points" for every month elapsed while they await a donor organ from the UNOS list.

ANSWER: A, B, C, D

18. Regarding chronic rejection (slow loss of graft function due to immunologic mechanisms) of a liver allograft, which of the following statements is/are true?

A. It occurs in approximately 30% during the first year following transplantation.
B. Uncommonly found in patients who have not had an episode of acute rejection.
C. Usually associated with histologic findings of marked hepatitis ("spotty" necrosis of hepatocytes with associated marked microscopic lobular hepatitis).
D. Associated with microscopic disappearance of bile ducts in the portal tracts and arterial thickening.

Ref.: 20, 21, 22

COMMENTS: Chronic rejection of the liver allograft is relatively uncommon (10% within the first 5 years following transplantation). The most common posttransplant predictor is an episode of acute rejection. Excluding recipients with immunosuppressive drug noncompliance, most episodes of chronic rejection are temporally associated with an incompletely resolved episode of acute rejection or multiple treatments of episodes of acute rejection. The histologic findings are distinctive, with complete or nearly complete disappearance of bile ducts on microscopic examination. Indeed, this chronic rejection is often referred to as the "disappearing bile duct syndrome" or "chronic ductopenic rejection." Arterial thickening (transplant vasculopathy) occurs as well but usually is not found in the needle biopsy. Although a variety of medications and medical strategies have been used, retransplantation is the only generally successful treatment. Recurrence following retransplantation is uncommon.

ANSWER: D

19. During donor hepatectomy at the donor harvest procedure, which of the following is/are contraindication(s) to the use of the donor?

A. "Replaced" or accessory *right* hepatic artery (i.e., a hepatic artery usually originating from the superior mesenteric artery).
B. "Replaced" or accessory hepatic *left* hepatic artery (i.e., hepatic artery usually originating from the left gastric artery).
C. Both replaced or accessory *right and left* hepatic arteries.
D. "Fetal lobulation of the liver."
E. Marked atherosclerosis of the aorta.
F. None of the above.
G. All of the above.

Ref.: 23

COMMENTS: In general, there are few anatomic variations in liver anatomy that preclude use of a donor liver for transplantation. A variety of techniques have been used successfully to utilize essentially any variation in the widely variable anatomy of the hepatic artery. In anatomic studies approximately 20% of the donors have a "replaced" or accessory right hepatic artery. Fetal lobulation is persistence of the fetal demarcations of the segments of the liver and has no clinical significance for utilization of the liver as a donor. With the increasing demand for donor organs, increasingly older donor livers are being successfully utilized for transplantation. In anatomic studies, the visceral arteries such as the hepatic artery are often spared significant atherosclerosis despite significant anatomic and clinical atherosclerosis in other parts of the arterial system including the aorta.

ANSWER: F

20. Which of the following is/are the biggest clinical problem(s) associated with transplantation of the small intestine?

A. Inability to safely control acute rejection of the graft.
B. High incidence of fatal lymphoproliferative disease (lymphoma).
C. High incidence of severe cytomegalovirus (CMV).
D. Shortage of donor organs.
E. Severe clinical consequences of chronic graft-versus-host disease (GVHD) inherent to the large amount of lymphoid material associated with transplantation of the small bowel allograft.

Ref.: 24, 25, 26

COMMENTS: Small bowel transplantation is likely the "last frontier" in solid organ transplantation. In most large animal models, control of acute and chronic rejection of the transplanted small intestine has been extremely difficult. The same has been true during the early clinical experience. With the necessary marked increases in short-term and maintenance immunosuppression, the immunologic surveillance for cancerous lymphocytes is markedly degraded, leading to the high incidence of lymphoma (10–20%) in recipients. Additionally, with CMV in the "passenger" lymphoid material of the small bowel allograft, in conjunction with high-dose immunosuppression, fatal, disseminated CMV infections are common despite long-term pharmacological viral prophylaxis. Some surgeons utilize only serologically CMV-negative donor intestine in CMV-negative recipients to avoid this often-fatal complication. With the current low demand for this developing procedure, the potential donors outnumber the candidates currently awaiting transplantation. Because of the marked lymphoid load inherent in small-intestine transplantation and the findings in animal models, problems with GVHD (attack of donor passenger lymphocytes on host tissue, producing skin rashes and hemolysis of red blood cells) were anticipated. A variety of strategies using gamma irradiation of the donor graft and donor administration of a variety of anti-lymphocyte globulins were initially devised for clinical small-intestine transplantation. Surprisingly, with no strategy for donor or recipient modification, GVHD is almost nonexistent.

ANSWER: A, B, C

21. With which of the following is/are acute rejection of the human small bowel allograft associated?

A. Increasing apoptosis of the crypts of the small bowel graft.
B. Increasing lymphocyte infiltration of crypts of the small bowel graft.
C. Increasing high volumes of diarrhea through the ostomy or per rectum.
D. Translocation of bacteria.
E. Endoscopic findings of ulceration of the graft mucosa.

Ref.: 26, 27, 28, 29

COMMENTS: Acute rejection of the small bowel allograft is a clinical and pathologic diagnosis. Usually an episode of acute rejection is heralded by a nonspecific finding of a marked increase of diarrhea through the graft ostomy or per rectum. Serial endoscopic monitoring of the graft demonstrates increasing ulceration and inflammation of the mucosa. Serial endoscopic mucosal graft biopsies usually reveal a fairly distinctive progression of apoptosis of the crypts of the mucosa. Treatment with high-dose immunosuppression is required to preempt complete destruction of the graft or chronic allograft rejection. Although these findings are fairly sensitive for diagnosing acute rejection, a cytomegalovirus infection of the graft may produce similar findings. Only careful review of the small-intestine graft biopsy and serologic monitoring for CMV allow differentiation of these clinical problems. Treatment of a CMV infection of the small-intestine graft is essentially the opposite of acute rejection, namely, some reduction in immunosuppression and treatment with an antiviral agent (e.g., ganciclovir). Acute rejection of the small bowel usually results in severe translocation of bacteria and associated severe bacteremia. These simultaneous events (high-dose immunosuppression and marked bacteremia) lead to a precarious clinical situation associated with septic shock and fatal multiple organ failure. Clinical management of this common occurrence is one of the more difficult ones in solid organ transplantation.

ANSWER: A, B, C, D, E

22. Which of the following statements regarding the process of rejection is/are true?

A. Hyperacute rejection is a cell-mediated immune response.
B. Acute rejection occurs secondary to preformed antibodies, as with ABO blood group incompatibility.
C. Acute rejection is characterized by small lymphocyte and mononuclear cell infiltration.
D. Chronic rejection may occur against minor histocompatibility antigens.

E. Chronic rejection generally occurs within the first month and is easily treated with immunosuppressive therapy.

Ref.: 2, 10, 11

COMMENTS: There are at least three types of rejection: *hyperacute*, *acute*, and *chronic*. **Hyperacute** rejection occurs when the recipient has preformed antibodies; it is the type of rejection that might occur in ABO-incompatible transplants. Hyperacute rejection is characterized by neutrophil infiltration and complement-mediated injury to vascular endothelium. At present, this form of rejection is not reversible and should be treated by graft removal. **Acute** or accelerated rejection is thought to be due to sensitized lymphocytes and generally occurs days to weeks after transplantation. A classic cell-mediated immune response characterized by graft infiltration by small lymphocytes and mononuclear cells occurs, leading to the graft's destruction. Selective immunosuppression using high-dose steroids or antilymphocyte sera usually reverses acute rejection. **Chronic** rejection occurs over a period of months to years and may be due to an antibody response, a cell-mediated response, or a combination of the two. The antigens mediating the response may be minor histocompatibility antigens or weak major histocompatibility antigens. This type of rejection is not reversed by increased immunosuppressive therapy.

ANSWER: C, D

REFERENCES

1. McChesney LP, Martin X, Dubernard JM: Pancreas and islet cell transplantation. In: *Surgical Diseases of the Pancreas*, 3rd ed. Howard JM, Idezuki Y, Ihse I, Prinz RA (eds) Williams & Wilkins, Baltimore, 1998, Ch 86.
2. Williams JW: *Hepatic Transplantation*. WB Saunders, Philadelphia, 1990.
3. Busuttil RW, Klintmalm GB: Patient evaluation: adult. In: *Transplantation of the Liver*. Busuttil RW, Klintmalm GB (eds) WB Saunders, Philadelphia, 1996, Chs 6, 7, 12, and 16.
4. Foster PF, Fabrega F, Karademir K, et al: Prediction of abstinence from ethanol in alcoholic recipients following liver transplantation. *Hepatology* 25:1469–1477, 1997.
5. Frellier L, Mutimer D, Brown D, et al: Lamivudine prophylaxis against re-infection: transplantation for hepatitis B cirrhosis. *Lancet* 348:1212–1215, 1996.
6. Morkowitz JS, Martin P, Conrad AJ, et al: Prophylaxis against hepatitis B recurrence following liver transplantation using combination lamivudine and hepatitis B immune globulin. *Hepatology* 28:585–589, 1998.
7. Campbell D, Lucey M: Liver transplantation for alcoholic cirrhosis. In: *Transplantation of the Liver*. Busuttil RW, Klintmalm GB (eds) WB Saunders, Philadelphia, 1996, Ch 16.
8. United Network for Organ Sharing (UNOS): *1997 Annual Report*, p 147.
9. Olthoff K, Busuttil R: Venous anomalies including portal vein thrombosis and prior portosystemic shunts. In: *Transplantation of the Liver*. Busuttil RW, Klintmalm GB (eds) WB Saunders, Philadelphia, 1996, Ch 46.
10. Morris PJ: *Kidney Transplantation—Principles and Practice*, 4th ed. WB Saunders, Philadelphia, 1994.
11. Flye MW: *Principles of Organ Transplantation*. WB Saunders, Philadelphia, 1989.
12. Hugh G, Labert, Busuttil R: Surgery for portal hypertension in the era of liver transplantation. In: *Transplantation of the Liver*. Busuttil RW, Klintmalm GB (eds) WB Saunders, Philadelphia, 1996, Ch 36.
13. Shapiro R, Simmons RL, Starzl TE: *Renal Transplantation* (1st ed). Appleton & Lange, Stamford, CT, 1997.
14. McGory RW, Ishitani MB, Oliveira WM, et al: *Transplantation* 61:1358–1364, 1996.
15. Sheiner PA, Boros P, Klion FM, et al: The efficacy of prophylactic interferon alfa-2b in preventing recurrent hepatitic C after liver transplantation. *Hepatology* 28:831–838, 1998.
16. Wright TL, Donegan E, Hsu HH, et al: Recurrent and acquired hepatitic C viral infection in liver transplant recipients. *Gastroenterology* 103:317–322, 1992.
17. Goss JA, Shackleton CR, Farmer DG, et al: Orthotopic liver transplantation for primary sclerosing experience. *Ann Surg* 225: 472–483, 1997.
18. Knoop M, Bechstein WO, Schrem H, et al: Clinical significance of recurrent primary biliary cirrhosis after liver transplantation. *Transplant Int* 9(Suppl 1):S115–119, 1996.
19. United Network for Organs Sharing (UNOS): 110 Boulders Parkway, Suite 500, PO Box 13770, Richmond, VA.
20. Lugwig J, Wiesner RH, Batts KP, et al: The acute vanishing bile duct syndrome after orthotopic liver transplantation. *Hepatology* 7:476–483, 1987.
21. Hubscher SG, Buckels JA, Elias, et al: Vanishing bile duct syndrome following liver transplantation: is it reversible? *Transplantation* 51:1004–1010, 1991.
22. Williams JW, Preston PF, Sankary HN: Role of liver allograft biopsy in patient management. *Semin Liver Dis* 12:60–72, 1992.
23. Starzl TE, Iwatsuki S, Esquivel, et al: Refinements in the surgical technique of liver transplantation. *Semin Liver Dis* 5:349–356, 1985.
24. Putman P, Reyes J, Kocoshis S, et al: Gastrointestinal post-transplant lymphoproliferative disease in children after small intestinal transplantation. *Transplant Proc* 28:2777, 1996.
25. Abu-Elmagd K, Reyes J, Todo S, et al: Clinical intestinal transplantation: new perspectives and immunological consideration. *J Am Coll Surg* 186:512–525, 1998.
26. Sigurdsson L, Kocoshis S, Todo S, et al: Severe exfoliative rejection after intestinal transplantation in children. *Transplant Proc* 28:2783–2784, 1996.
27. Lee RG, Tsamandas AC, Abu-Elmagd K, et al: Histological spectrum of acute rejection in human intestinal allografts. *Transplant Proc* 28:2767, 1996.
28. Sigurdsson L, Reyes J, Putman PD, et al: Endoscopies in pediatric small intestinal transplant recipients: five years experience. *Am J Gastroenterol* 93:207–211, 1998.
29. Beuno J, Green M, Kocoshis S, et al: Cytomegalovirus infection after intestinal transplantation in children. *Clin Infect Dis* 25: 1078–1083, 1997.
30. Jain A, Khann A, Molment EP, et al: Immunosupportive therapy. *Surg Clin NA* 79:57–76, 1999.
31. Reyes J, Mazariesos GV: Transplantation. *Surg Clin North Am* 79:163–189, 1999.

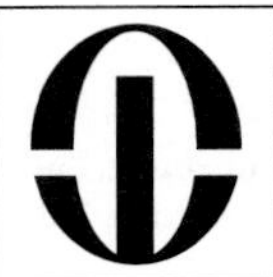

CHAPTER 11

Critical Care

1. With regard to cardiac output (CO), which of the following statements is/are true?

   A. CO alone is not an indicator of myocardial contractility.
   B. Stroke volume (SV) is determined by ventricular end-diastolic volume (EDV), vascular resistance, and myocardial contractility.
   C. Arterial blood pressure alone is an accurate indicator of CO.
   D. CO varies directly with pulse rate up to 160 beats/minute in sinus rhythm, after which it decreases.
   E. Atrial contraction contributes up to 30% of the EDV.

Ref.: 1, 2

COMMENTS: In its simplest terms, CO is equal to the heart rate (HR) multiplied by the SV. In turn, SV is equal to the EDV minus the end-systolic volume (ESV), as shown:

$$CO = HR \times (EDV - ESV)$$

The ejection fraction measures the percentage of EDV ejected during systole.

$$EF = SV/EDV$$

Stroke volume is a function of the extent of shortening of myocardial fiber, which depends on preload (initial volume), afterload (resistance to ventricular emptying), and contractility. The relation between diastolic filling and SV is governed by Starling's law, which states that as muscle fiber length increases so does the force of contraction. Increasing fiber length stretches the sarcomere toward the optimal 2.2 μm length. Therefore, CO alone is not an indicator of myocardial contractility. SV is determined primarily by EDV, vascular resistance, and myocardial contractility. EDV is largely made up of passive ventricular filling during diastole. Diastolic filling time shortens as the pulse rate increases to 160 beats/minute. Beyond this, CO decreases. Ventricular contractility depends on three interdependent variables: velocity of shortening, force of contraction, and length of displacement. Atrial contraction contributes 15–30% of EDV, the so-called atrial kick. Arterial blood pressure alone is not an accurate indicator of CO.

ANSWER: A, B, D, E

2. Which one or more of the following factors determines cardiac output?

   A. End-diastolic volume.
   B. Afterload.
   C. Contractility.
   D. Heart rate.
   E. Ventricular interaction.

Ref.: 3

COMMENTS: The primary goal in the management of the critically ill inpatient is to provide sufficient O_2 delivery to satisfy O_2 demand. Oxygen consumption (VO_2) is initially dependent on oxygen delivery (DO_2); however, when oxygen delivery exceeds that which is necessary (the critical DO_2), VO_2 becomes delivery-independent (see Figure). VO_2 is a reasonable estimate of ATP turnover in the cells. In clinical situations, the co-variation of DO_2 and VO_2 usually represents efforts to deliver more O_2 in response to increased demand rather than "O_2 supply dependence." DO_2 can be optimized by increasing arterial oxygen content, increasing CO, or both. The four factors that determine output are preload, afterload, contractility, and heart rate. *Preload* is defined as end-diastolic sarcomere length, which is linearly related to EDV. Left atrial pressure correlates with left ventricular end-diastolic pressure in normal hearts. Pulmonary capillary wedge pressure (PCWP) is a reflection of left atrial pressure and is commonly used as an index of preload. The relation between PCWP and EDV is not constant but is affected by changes in left ventricular com-

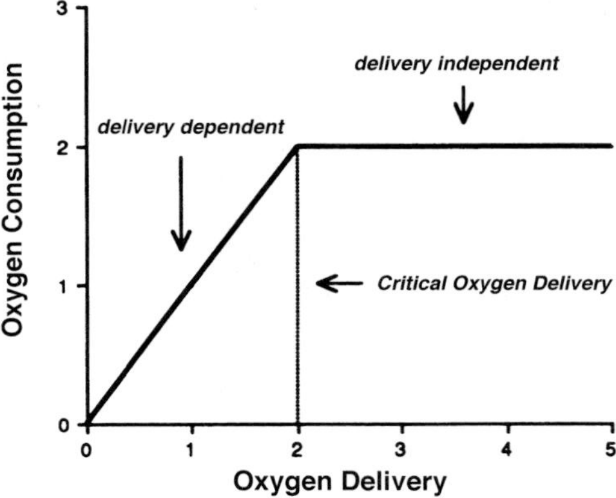

The relation of oxygen consumption to oxygen delivery. As oxygen delivery increases, oxygen consumption becomes independent of delivery. (Adapted from Hill EP, Willford DC, Moore WY, et al: Oxygen transport and oxygen consumption vs. cardiac output at different haematocrits. *Perfusion* 2:39, 1987. Copyright by Edward Arnold/Hodder & Stoughton Educational.)

pliance, wall thickness, heart rate, ischemia, and medications. Ventricular interaction affects CO. Shifts of the interventricular septum, normally slightly convex toward the right ventricle, may compromise ventricular filling. *Afterload* is the impedance to ventricular ejection and is estimated by systemic or pulmonary vascular resistance. An increase in afterload produces an increase in contractility (Anrep effect). *Contractility* is an intrinsic property of the myocardium, which manifests as a greater force of contraction for a given preload. All the available inotropic agents increase contractility by increasing intracellular calcium concentration and availability. *Heart rate* may influence cardiac output in a number of ways; bradycardia and excessive tachycardia should be corrected. An increase in heart rate affects preload; it also increases contractility (Bowditch phenomenon). In general, preload must be optimized before afterload manipulation. Inotropic agents should be used only after the other factors have been optimized.

ANSWER: A, B, C, D, E

3. Which of the following is not a cause of hypoxia?

A. Hypoventilation.
B. Diffusion defects.
C. Changes in lung compliance.
D. Ventilation/perfusion (V/Q) abnormalities.
E. Shunting.

Ref.: 2

COMMENTS: When hypoxia is caused by hypoventilation, it is associated with hypercarbia and decreasing minute ventilation. Minute ventilation is equal to the tidal volume multiplied by the respiratory rate. Hypoxia caused by hypoventilation can be reversed by increasing minute ventilation. Diffusion defects are associated with an increased alveolar-arterial oxygen pressure difference. This condition is responsive to supplemental oxygen therapy. Gas exchange is dependent on the V/Q ratio in each alveolar unit. V/Q mismatch is the most common cause of hypoxemia. Examples are atelectasis (V/Q decreases) and pulmonary embolus (V/Q increases). V/Q mismatch affects oxygen exchange to a greater degree than carbon dioxide exchange. Hypoxemia resulting from V/Q mismatch improves with supplemental oxygen therapy. Shunting describes alveoli that are perfused but not ventilated. Absolute shunts (zero V/Q) are the only cause of hypoxia that cannot be completely corrected by the administration of 100% oxygen. The administration of oxygen should be limited to less than 50% in situations of low V/Q alveoli to prevent denitrogenation atelectasis. Compliance refers to lung expansibility and is defined as volume change per unit pressure ($C = \Delta V/\Delta P$). It is useful for monitoring patients on mechanical ventilators, but changes in compliance are not a primary cause of hypoxia.

ANSWER: C

4. Which one or more of the following mechanisms is/are the body's most important defenses in severe oxygen transport deficiency?

A. Hyperventilation.
B. Reduction of VO_2.
C. Varying the organ distribution of cardiac output.
D. Shift of the oxyhemoglobin dissociation curve.
E. Widening the arterial-venous oxygen content difference.

Ref.: 2

COMMENTS: See Question 5.

5. With regard to tissue utilization of oxygen, which of the following statements is/are true?

A. The brain requires 15% of the resting CO and 20% of the total basal VO_2.
B. The kidneys receive 25% of CO but can tolerate a reduction to one-third of their normal blood flow for up to 1 hour.
C. The heart extracts 70% of available oxygen from its arterial supply.
D. During acute hypoxia, blood is preferentially shunted to the heart and brain.
E. Arterial-venous oxygen difference is a measure of the extent to which blood flow matches the metabolic demand for oxygen.

Ref.: 2

COMMENTS: Increasing the proportion of CO to satisfy the brain's and heart's continuous high requirements for oxygen transport is crucial for survival during states of severe oxygen transport deficiency, such as cardiac arrest. In general, organs with low oxygen extraction ratios tolerate decreased blood flow well. Because the kidneys extract only 10% of oxygen available in the arterial blood supply, they tolerate decreased blood flow far better than does the heart or the brain. Organs other than the heart tend to compensate for decreased blood flow by extracting more oxygen from their blood supply. The extent of this extraction can be estimated by the arterial-venous oxygen content difference. Normally, the blood consumes only 25% of its total oxygen supply. The normal mixed venous blood is 75% saturated, with a partial pressure of oxygen of 40 mm Hg. These values decrease in response to a fall in CO, which can be detected before changes in blood pressure, pulse rate, or central venous pressure (CVP) are noted. Increased extraction is made possible by the relaxation of precapillary sphincters that enlarge the available capillary beds for oxygen exchange.

ANSWER:
Question 4: C, E
Question 5: A, B, C, D, E

6. Which one or more of the following factors can directly affect oxygen delivery?

A. Blood transfusions.
B. Oxygen consumption (VO_2).
C. Cardiac output (CO).
D. Fraction of inspired oxygen (FiO_2).
E. Metabolic alkalosis.

Ref.: 3, 4, 5

COMMENTS: DO_2 is dependent on arterial oxygen content and CO:

$$CaO_2 = ([Hgb] \times 1.39)SaO_2 + (PaO_2 \times 0.0031)$$

where CaO_2 is the arterial oxygen content, [Hgb] is the hemoglobin concentration, SaO_2 is the arterial oxygen saturation, PaO_2 is the partial pressure of oxygen in arterial blood, 1.39

is the amount of oxygen in milliliters carried by each gram of fully saturated hemoglobin, and 0.0031 is the solubility of oxygen in plasma. The factor ($PaO_2 \times 0.0031$) is usually insignificant. DO_2 is calculated with the equation

$$DO_2 = CaO_2 \times CO \times 10$$

where CO is cardiac output. Oxygen consumption (VO_2) is calculated with the equation

$$VO_2 = C(a\text{-}v)O_2 \times CO \times 10$$

where $C(a\text{-}v)O_2$ is the arterial-venous oxygen content. Blood transfusions would affect oxygen delivery by increasing the hemoglobin in blood, thereby increasing the CaO_2. CO would directly affect DO_2 delivery and a change in FiO_2 would change the saturation in arterial blood. VO_2 is dependent on DO_2 because inadequate DO_2 results in suboptimal VO_2 and resultant lactic acidosis. Acid-base abnormalities would not directly affect the DO_2 except in cases in which CO may be impaired by extremes of pH. Changes in acid-base state would have an effect on the P_{50} (described in Question 8) of the oxygen dissociation curve, causing increased or decreased affinity of oxygen at the tissue level. This would affect the VO_2 consumption but would have no bearing on DO_2.

ANSWER: A, C, D

7. In the healthy individual, which of the following is the limiting factor of oxygen consumption (VO_2)?

A. DO_2 to tissue capillaries.
B. Availability of cellular oxygen.
C. Availability of mitochondrial oxygen.
D. Availability of ADP.

Ref.: 2

COMMENTS: Aerobic mitochondrial respiration is a process known as oxidative phosphorylation. The final step of this process involves the passage of two electrons from cytochrome C to an oxygen molecule. This oxygen molecule then combines with hydrogen to form one molecule of water. It is coupled to the conversion of ADP to ATP. When ADP is not available capillary oxygen is not consumed, and it equilibrates with myoglobin, creating a reserve of intracellular oxygen that is released at low oxygen tensions. Normally, the intracellular oxygen tension is 6 mm Hg. Oxygen is not consumed, a gradient is not established, and oxygen does not enter the cell unless ADP is available for oxidative phosphorylation; thus ADP is the rate-limiting factor in healthy individuals. Only at very low mitochondrial oxygen tensions does DO_2 to the tissues become rate-limiting.

ANSWER: D

8. A 70-kg patient is admitted to the intensive care unit (ICU) with a mean arterial pressure (MAP) of 50 mm Hg, central venous pressure (CVP) of 8 mm Hg, pulmonary artery occlusion pressure (PAOP) of 6 mm Hg, cardiac output (CO) of 7.0 L/min, hemoglobin level of 5 gm/dl, pH 7.20, and PCO_2 52 mm Hg. Which one or more of the following values would apply to this patient?

A. $P_{50} > 27$.
B. Systemic vascular resistance (SVR) = 820 dyne·sec/cm^{-5}.
C. $P_{50} < 27$.
D. Shift of the hemoglobin dissociation curve to the left.
E. Oxygen capacity = 8.85 ml/g.

Ref.: 5

COMMENTS: Oxygen (O_2) forms an easily reversible combination with hemoglobin to give oxyhemoglobin: Hgb-O_2. From the hemoglobin dissociation curve, it can be seen that the amount of O_2 carried by hemoglobin increases rapidly up to an oxygen pressure (PO_2) of about 60 mm Hg. Above 60 mm Hg, the hemoglobin dissociation curve flattens out, and there is a much smaller change in hemoglobin saturation for the same change in PO_2 (see Figure). Conversely, in the periphery, hemoglobin can release large amounts of O_2 with decreasing hemoglobin saturation and yet maintain a relatively high PO_2, which is needed to maintain a gradient for diffusion into the peripheral tissues. The maximal amount of O_2 that can combine with hemoglobin is called the O_2 capacity (1.39 ml of O_2 can combine with each gram of hemoglobin). In this patient, the O_2 capacity is $1.39 \times 5 = 6.85$. The O_2 saturation is the actual amount of O_2 combined with hemoglobin divided by the O_2 capacity and then multiplied by 100. Normal O_2 saturation is 97–100%. O_2 content takes into account the amount of O_2 dissolved in plasma, which is 0.0031 ml O_2/dl blood/mm Hg PO_2. This factor is added to the O_2 capacity to give the O_2 content. The position of the hemoglobin dissociation curve is affected by different factors: carbon dioxide pressure (PCO_2), pH, temperature, 2,3-diphosphoglycerate (2,3-DPG) levels, cortisol levels, and aldosterone levels. A shift to the right indicates that there is more unloading of O_2 at a given PO_2 in the tissue capillary; a leftward shift indicates decreased unloading of O_2 at a given PO_2 in the tissue capillary. Elevated PCO_2 and temperature and decreased pH cause a shift to the right. The effect of elevated PCO_2, causing a shift to the right, is known as the Bohr effect and is presumably due to the effect of hypercarbia on pH. ATP and 2,3-DPG lower hemoglobin affinity for O_2, causing a shift to the right. The pH and 2,3-DPG have counterbalancing effects in that elevated pH causes increased formation of 2,3-DPG, and decreased pH causes decreased formation of 2,3-DPG. Elevated cortisol and aldosterone levels cause a rightward shift. The position of the oxyhemoglobin dissociation curve along the horizontal axis is characteristically termed the P_{50} value, which is the PO_2 at which 50% of the hemoglobin is saturated. The normal value is approximately 27 mm Hg. The patient in ques-

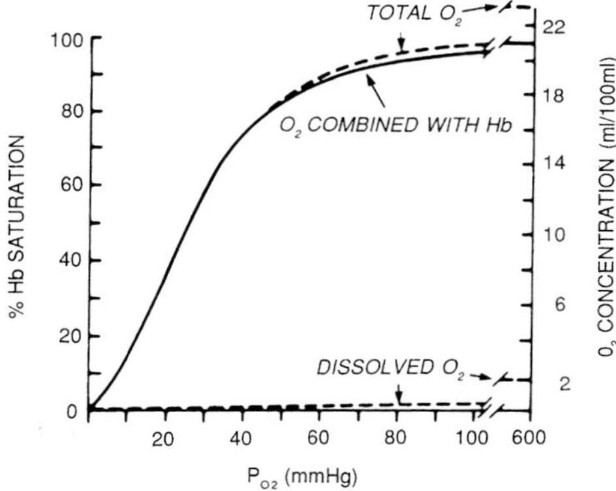

Hemoglobin dissociation curve (*solid line*) for pH 7.4, PCO2 40 mmHg, and 37°C. The total blood O2 concentration is also shown for a hemoglobin concentration of 15 gm/100 ml of blood. (From West JB: *Respiratory Physiology—The Essentials*, 4th ed. Williams & Wilkins, Baltimore, 1990.)

tion not only would have an elevated PCO_2, which would cause a rightward shift, but also metabolic acidosis secondary to low hemoglobin and low perfusion pressure. A rightward shift would be expected, and the resultant P_{50} would be greater than 27. The SVR in this patient is 480 dyne·sec/cm^{-5} as calculated by the formula: SVR = MAP − CVP/CO. This would be compatible with a distributive type of shock in this patient with a low SVR, normal to low PAOP, and a normal CO.

ANSWER: A

9. Which one or more of the following is primarily responsible for increasing the cardiac output in patients with acute mild to moderate normovolemic anemia?

A. Tachycardia.
B. Increased contractility.
C. Increased afterload.
D. Decreased sympathetic nervous activity.
E. Decreased blood viscosity.

Ref.: 6

COMMENTS: Oxygen delivery is maintained in these patients by a higher cardiac output, thereby compensating for a reduction in oxygen carrying capacity. A decreased blood viscosity is primarily responsible for the increase in cardiac output, as it results in improved laminar flow. In blood, viscosity depends on particulate concentration and flow. A reduction in hematocrit by 50% produces an eightfold greater reduction in viscosity in the postcapillary venules compared to the aorta, thus facilitating disruption of cells in rouleaux formation. Because of decreased viscosity in acute normovolemic anemia, decreased afterload, improved preload, and increased contractility are observed. Even though an increased cardiac sympathetic tone is seen during anemia, its direct effect on the heart is not primarily responsible for the increased cardiac output.

ANSWER: E

10. Which of the following statements is/are correct concerning radial artery cannulation?

A. Performance of the Allen test is mandatory.
B. Arterial thrombosis is more common with catheters larger than 20 gauge and those left in place for 4 days or longer.
C. The incidence of infection is higher with catheters placed by surgical cutdown.
D. The catheter should be replaced every 3 days.
E. Intermittent flushing to keep the catheter free of clots is desirable.

Ref.: 5

COMMENTS: The radial artery is the site most frequently used for arterial catheters in the presence of a patent ulnar artery and palmar arterial arch. Therefore the Allen test, which checks for ulnar collateral flow to the palm, should be performed before radial artery catheterization. A normal Allen test consists of a palmar blush within 7 seconds after the ulnar artery is released. The incidence of complications after arterial catheterization seems to be operator-independent, unlike pulmonary artery catheterizations. Known risk factors include intermittent punctures, patients younger than 10 years, prolonged catheterization (lasting more than 4 days), anticoagulant therapy, and catheters larger than 20 gauge or those made out of polypropylene rather than Teflon. Most patients with arterial thrombosis remain asymptomatic. Most thrombi (43%) are present at the time of catheter removal, and another 30% develop within 24 hours. Damping of the arterial waveform may result from thrombosis. If thrombosis is suspected, the catheters should be aspirated and not flushed forcefully. Intermittent manual flushing with as little as 3 ml of fluid has been demonstrated to cause retrograde displacement of emboli from the radial artery cannula to the aortic arch and from there back into the cerebral circulation. A higher incidence of thrombosis occurs within the first 24 hours when a cutdown is performed (48% vs. 23% percutaneously), but the incidence of thrombosis at 1 week is the same for both methods of placement. Brachial artery cannulation has a high incidence of embolic occlusion of the distal arteries (5–41%) and should therefore be avoided. Infection remains the most common complication. Predisposing factors are as follows: prolonged catheterization; surgical cutdown; local inflammation; preexisting bacteremias; and failure to change the saline flush fluid, transducer, and flush tubing every 48 hours. The need for intermittent arterial catheter replacement is not established and indeed is controversial. Infected catheters often grow gram-negative rods, *Enterococcus*, or *Candida*. Povidone-iodine ointment should be used at the insertion site because of the increased risk of *Candida* infection. Median nerve neuropathy has been associated with radial artery catheterizations because of compartment hypertension or nerve compression by blood.

ANSWER: A, B, C

11. Which one of the following statements is/are true concerning arterial catheterization?

A. Aortic systolic pressure is lower than radial systolic pressure.
B. Aortic diastolic pressure is 10 mm Hg higher than radial diastolic pressure.
C. Mean aortic pressure (MAP) is slightly higher than radial MAP.
D. A blunted waveform is caused by small air bubbles in the tubing.
E. Underdamping causes systolic overshoot.

Ref.: 5

COMMENTS: The accuracy of a catheter-tubing-transducer system depends on its resonant frequency and its damping characteristics. In general, a lower damping coefficient requires a higher resonant frequency and vice versa. The best frequency response for arterial pressure monitoring is achieved by using a good quality transducer, the shortest length of noncompliant tubing, and an appropriate-size catheter. A blunted waveform (overdamping) underestimates systolic pressure; it is caused by use of compliant tubing, large bubbles in the tubing, kinking, and blood clots. Underdamping causes systolic overshoot, which is seen with small air bubbles in the tubing and excessive lengths of noncompliant tubing. The aortic mean arterial pressure and diastolic arterial pressure are slightly higher than the mean and diastolic radial ones. However, the systolic pressure is consistently higher in the radial artery than in the aorta. This discrepancy increases with distal progression, smaller arterial caliber, and age. This is explained by the reflection of pressure waves from capillary beds resulting in augmentation of systolic and reduction of diastolic values measured.

ANSWER: A, C, E

12. In which of these circumstances would you expect a central venous pressure (CVP) reading to be a reliable guide in fluid management?

A. Chest radiograph consistent with pulmonary edema.
B. Right ventricular diastolic pressure equal to the CVP.
C. Mitral valve disease.
D. Left ventricular ejection fraction of 0.40.

Ref.: 4

COMMENTS: If CVP monitoring is to be used as a guide to fluid management, the right ventricular function must parallel the left ventricular function for a clinically useful CVP. For readings in the normal patient, right atrial pressure, right ventricular diastolic pressure, and CVP are equal. CVP may be normal in the presence of left ventricular dysfunction and may show increases only after severe left ventricular dysfunction develops with resultant pulmonary congestion and rising right ventricular end-diastolic pressure. CVP has been shown to have little correlation with left atrial pressure or pulmonary capillary wedge pressure (PCWP) in patients with valvar heart disease, pulmonary hypertension, and coronary artery disease with an ejection fraction of less than 0.5. In the critically ill patient, CVP is not well correlated with the PCWP. CVP determination is useful for initial volume resuscitation and diagnosing right ventricular infarction and pericardial tamponade.

ANSWER: B

13. Which one or more of the following noncardiac factors increases central venous pressure (CVP) readings?

A. Transducer positioned too high.
B. Positive-pressure ventilation.
C. Vasodilator drugs.
D. Transducer positioned too low.

Ref.: 2

COMMENTS: It is important to consider the pressure around the heart and great vessels when evaluating CVP because any extrinsic compression increases the intraluminal pressure. Normal values for CVP presume normal values for transmural pressure. Thus CVP readings are elevated when the pleural or mediastinal pressure is elevated, which is the case during positive-pressure ventilation. Correct transducer positioning at the midaxillary line is essential to CVP measurements because the recording pressure is always the pressure above the transducer. Thus a too high position would produce an incorrectly low CVP reading. In general, vasodilators reduce CVP.

ANSWER: B, D

14. With regard to interpretation of central venous pressure (CVP) or wedge pressure (PCWP) measurements, which of the following statements is/are true?

A. They are best and most logically used when observing responses to volume and fluid infusion challenges.
B. Strict adherence to expected normal values is the best guideline for their use.
C. PCWP reflects the pulmonary capillary pressure (Pcap) within 1–2 mm Hg in inflammatory states.
D. In the absence of pulmonary disease, PCWP is a reliable guide to left ventricular end-diastolic pressure.
E. If an acceptable wedge position cannot be obtained, the pulmonary artery systolic pressure is an acceptable indicator of left atrial pressure.

Ref.: 1, 2

COMMENTS: CVP reflects filling pressures of the right ventricle, whereas PCWP reflects those of the left ventricle. Elevated values reflect an inability of either ventricle to handle venous return. Nonmyocardial factors that cause a rise in CVP include mechanical blockage or kinking of the catheter, vasoconstrictor drugs, positive-pressure ventilation, pneumothorax, flail chest, cardiac tamponade, or pulmonary embolism. Nonmyocardial causes of elevated PCWP include pulmonary vascular disease, mitral valve incompetence, increased airway pressure, and increased pleural pressure. Because of the interposed pulmonary vascular system, CVP is not always a reliable index of left ventricular function. Left-sided pressures may rise sharply, and pulmonary edema may occur without a significant rise in CVP. Both measuring devices are best used to assess the response to fluid challenges rather than to measure absolute normal values. In the absence of an acceptable wedge position, the pulmonary artery diastolic pressure, not the pulmonary systolic pressure, can be an alternative indicator of mean left atrial pressure. Pulmonary capillary pressure represents the hydrostatic pressure that drives the formation of edema in the lung. Regardless of serum oncotic pressure and the efficiency of the lymphatic pump, edema occurs beyond a level of Pcap. In normal lungs, with minimal pulmonary vein resistance, PCWP may predict Pcap within 1–2 mm Hg. However, in the presence of acute lung injury, hypoxia, and several vasoactive agents, cytokines have vasoconstrictive effects on either the arterial (serotonin) or the venous (histamine) side. In these cases the Pcap may be higher than the left atrial pressure. Thus PCWP may be used inaccurately as an endpoint during resuscitation of these patients, leading to further deterioration of O_2 transport.

ANSWER: A, D

15. Which one or more of the following criteria indicates correct pulmonary artery catheter positioning?

A. Characteristic wedge pressure (PCWP) waveform.
B. Mean pulmonary artery pressure (MPAP) less than mean PCWP.
C. PO_2 of blood from a catheter in wedge position less than the PO_2 of systemic blood.
D. Amount of air required for balloon inflation less than 0.7 ml.
E. Continuous flush system.

Ref.: 4, 7

COMMENTS: The characteristic waveform of the properly wedged pulmonary artery catheter reveals A and V waves and X and Y descents but no C waves. On the electrocardiogram (ECG), the A wave follows the QRS complex, and the V wave follows the T wave. The absence of this waveform indicates improper pulmonary artery catheter positioning. Because blood flows from the pulmonary artery to the left, the mean PCWP should always be less than the MPAP and less than or equal to the pulmonary artery diastolic pressure. If MPAP were less than the mean PCWP, it would imply reverse flow through the pulmonary circuit. Blood withdrawn through the wedged catheter should be fully oxygenated and have a higher PO_2 and lower PCO_2 than systemic arterial blood. The obstruction to pulmonary blood flow during wedged positioning causes stasis of blood in the pulmonary circuit and allows longer capillary and alveolar exchange. Patients who require high PEEP or have significant shunting of blood do not have as significant capillary-alveolar exchange because shunts cause a decrease in blood flow through the pulmonary capillaries. Three functional lung zones based on the distribution of pulmonary blood flow and ventilation have been described (see Figure below). The position of the catheter tip should be located in zone 3 of the lung fields, which is the most posterior of the lung zones in the supine patient. The importance of zone 3 is based on the dependent flow of blood in the pulmonary circuit when the patient is in the supine position and while venous pressure exceeds alveolar pressure, resulting in increased capillary blood flow. The positioning of the pulmonary artery tip can be determined by a lateral chest radiograph. Hypovolemia and positive end-expiratory pressure (PEEP) or continuous positive airway pressure (CPAP) increase the proportion of zones 1 and 2 in relation to zone 3. Positioning of the catheter in zone 1 or 2 should be suspected when the pulmonary arterial wedge pressure (PCWP) is greater than the pulmonary artery diastolic pressure (PADP), when there are marked respiratory variations in the tracing, and whenever the PCWP increases by more than half of the increase in PEEP. If the catheter tip is located in zone 1 or 2, PCWP reflects alveolar pressure, not left atrial pressure. If less than 0.7 ml of air in the catheter balloon produces a PCWP tracing, the catheter is located too far distally, and complications usually follow. The catheter should never be advanced without the balloon fully inflated (1.5 ml). A continuous flush system is required for accurate pulmonary artery readings but does not indicate correct pulmonary artery catheter positioning.

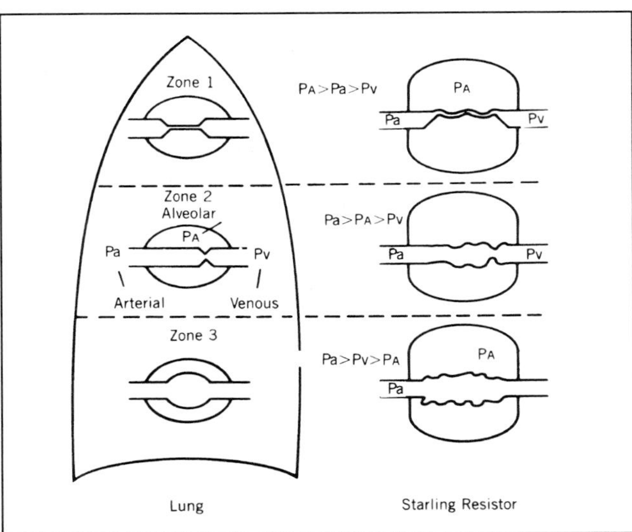

Pulmonary capillary bed has flow characteristics of Starling resistor where, when chamber pressure exceeds downstream pressure, flow is independent of downstream pressure. However, when downstream pressure exceeds chamber pressure, flow is determined by upstream-downstream difference. Alveolar pressure is same throughout lung. Pulmonary arterial pressure increases in the dependent regions of the lung. There may be a region at top of lung (zone 1) where pulmonary arterial pressure falls below alveolar pressure. Thus, zone 1 will occur whenever alveolar pressure exceeds pulmonary arterial pressure. This might occur when pulmonary arterial pressure is decreased, as in hypovolemia, or when alveolar pressure is increased, as with application of positive end-expiratory pressure. Zone 1 produces an alveolar dead space. In zone 2, pulmonary arterial pressure increases and exceeds alveolar pressure. In zone 2, blood flow is determined by the difference between arterial and alveolar pressure. In zone 3, blood flow is determined by arteriovenous difference. (From Bone RC: The treatment of severe hypoxemia due to the adult respiratory distress syndrome. *Arch Intern Med* 140:85, 1980. Copyright 1980, American Medical Association.)

ANSWER: A

16. In which one or more of the following conditions is pulmonary artery diastolic pressure (PADP) not correlated with pulmonary capillary wedge pressure (PCWP)?

A. Acute myocardial infarction.
B. Pulmonary hypertension.
C. Left ventricular dysfunction.
D. Severe chronic lung disease.
E. PADP = 17, left atrial pressure = 10.

Ref.: 4

COMMENTS: PADP has been used to reflect PCWP and left ventricular filling pressures. PADP reflects PCWP with reasonable accuracy in normal patients and in those with acute myocardial infarction, left ventricular dysfunction, or chronic lung disease if no pulmonary vascular changes exist. However, PADP exceeds PCWP in patients with tachycardia or pulmonary hypertension associated with acidosis, hypoxemia, pulmonary embolus, or pulmonary parenchymal disease. PADP also reflects left atrial pressure when no pulmonary vascular hypertension exists. PADP is usually 1–2 mm Hg higher than the PCWP and left atrial pressure. PCWP has always been found to be superior to PADP for estimating left atrial pressure. A difference between PADP and PCWP of more than 4–5 mm Hg is indicative of elevated pulmonary vascular resistance.

ANSWER: B, D, E

17. Which of the following factors are determinants of mixed venous oxygen saturation (SvO_2)?

A. Oxygen consumption (VO_2).
B. Cardiac output (CO).
C. Hemoglobin.
D. Arterial oxygen saturation (SaO_2).
E. Myocardial VO_2.

Ref.: 1, 2

COMMENTS: SvO_2 is a measure of the oxygen saturation of blood in the pulmonary artery. SvO_2 reflects the relation between DO_2 and oxygen consumption (VO_2). When they are balanced, that is, when the critical DO_2 has been achieved, SvO_2 is normal. When VO_2 is greater than DO_2, SvO_2 is decreased owing to increased demand for oxygen by peripheral tissue. Because DO_2 is largely dependent on CO, hemoglobin, and SaO_2, any factor affecting these values must be considered a cause of decreasing SvO_2. Blood returning from the periphery combines with coronary venous blood in the right atrium. Myocardial VO_2 is not a major determinant of SvO_2 because the coronary blood flow is a small part of the total flow through the right heart.

ANSWER: A, B, C, D

18. Which of the following conditions is/are associated with an elevated mixed venous oxygen saturation (SvO_2)?

A. Septic shock.
B. Left-to-right shunt.
C. Pressure venous oxygen (PVO_2) = 40.
D. Lactic acidosis.
E. Right-to-left shunt.

Ref.: 5

COMMENTS: Mixed venous blood represents a perfusion-weighted average of blood draining from all the body's organ systems. Values within the normal range of SvO_2 (0.68–0.77) suggest a balance between DO_2 and VO_2. This balance indicates that the fraction of consumed oxygen delivered to the peripheral tissues is normal. Four factors determine SvO_2: CO, hemoglobin, SaO_2, and VO_2. Causes of elevated SvO_2 indicate an excess of DO_2 and VO_2 and are most commonly associated with septic shock and cirrhosis, in which there are abnormal distributions of blood flow with a low systemic vascular resistance and concomitant high CO. In the septic state, high CO is also a result of the high catecholamine levels associated with sepsis. A left-to-right intracardiac shunt causes an elevated SvO_2 but invalidates SvO_2 as an index of perfusion. Other causes of elevated SvO_2 are hyperbaric oxygen therapy, states of low VO_2 (hypothermia, muscular paralysis, sedation, coma), and cyanide toxicity. In addition, high SvO_2 may indicate improper distal migration of the catheter. Uncompensated changes in any of the four determinants of SvO_2 may result in a decrease in the measured value of SvO_2; however, in the critically ill patient the correlation between a change in an individual factor and a change in the SvO_2 is low. A decrease in SvO_2 of more than 0.10 is likely to be of clinical significance regardless of the initial SvO_2. A sustained decrease in SvO_2 of more than 0.10 does not explain the cause of the disparity in DO_2 and VO_2, and the clinician should analyze the individual factors (CO, hemoglobin, SaO_2, VO_2) that determine SvO_2 and affect the oxygen balance.

ANSWER: A, B

19. With regard to complications associated with pulmonary artery catheterization, which of the following statements is/are true?

A. Prophylactic insertion of a pacing catheter is recommended in patients with preexisting left bundle branch block.
B. Hemoptysis mandates immediate overinflation of the catheter balloon.
C. Inflation of the catheter balloon should not exceed 75% of the balloon capacity to prevent pulmonary artery rupture.
D. Ventricular dysrhythmias occurring while the right atrial pressure is being recorded suggest intracardiac catheter knotting.
E. The rate of catheter-induced sepsis closely parallels the incidence of catheter colonization.

Ref.: 5

COMMENTS: Dysrhythmias occur in 12–67% of catheterizations but are usually self-limited premature ventricular contractions. Complete heart block can develop in patients with preexisting left bundle branch block. Prophylactic pacing wire should be utilized in these patients. Prophylactic lidocaine and full inflation of the balloon may prevent ventricular ectopy. Any hemoptysis in patients with a pulmonary artery catheter suggests the diagnosis of perforation or rupture. Mechanisms involved in pulmonary artery rupture include (1) overinflation of the balloon; (2) incomplete balloon inflation (<75%), forcing the exposed tip through the wall; and (3) pulmonary hypertension. An "overwedge" pattern suggests eccentric balloon inflation, overdistension, or both; the full recommended volume should be used. Should hemoptysis develop, the catheter should be pulled back with the balloon deflated. Massive hemoptysis necessitates placement of a double-lumen endotracheal tube and occlusion of the bronchus on the side of the rupture with a Fogarty catheter; emergency thoracotomy is needed. Intracardiac knotting of the catheter may occur during insertion. Ventricular arrhythmias that occur while the right atrial pressure is being recorded suggest knotting. Insertion of a guidewire into the catheter followed by slow withdrawal of the catheter may help to unknot the catheter. Even though catheter-related sepsis occurs in only up to 2% of insertions, colonization occurs in 5–35% of catheterizations. Infections are more common when the catheter is left in place for more than 72 hours or when it is inserted via an antecubital vein.

ANSWER: A, D

20. True or False: Partial pressure of oxygen in the atmosphere is the same as that which reaches the alveoli and ultimately appears on the left side of the heart.

Ref.: 1, 2

COMMENTS: The partial pressure of oxygen in the atmosphere is 160 mm Hg. As this air is humidified in the upper airways, the partial pressure drops to 149 mm Hg as a result of the effect of water vapor pressure at body temperature. Ultimately, arterial blood leaves the pulmonary capillaries with an oxygen tension of 100 mm Hg. This blood is diluted by unsaturated blood from the bronchial and coronary circulation that empties into the left side of the heart. The volume of this shunt is 3% of the output of the right side of the heart and results in an arterial partial pressure of 95 mm Hg as blood enters the left ventricle.

ANSWER: False

21. True or False: The normal pulmonary capillary bed can tolerate a two- to threefold increase in blood flow without a sacrifice in oxygenation.

Ref.: 2

COMMENTS: Only 90 ml of the right ventricular output is in the pulmonary capillaries at any one time. It takes approximately 0.8 second for a red blood cell to pass through the alveolar capillaries. As flow rate increases, the time spent in the capillaries is reduced. Only when this time is reduced to below 0.35 second does arterial desaturation occur, a phenomenon known as the "speed shunt."

ANSWER: True

22. True or False: The alveolar-arterial oxygen gradient, or $P(A\text{-}a)O_2$, is useful as an early indicator or incipient respiratory failure.

Ref.: 1, 2, 5

COMMENTS: The $P(A\text{-}a)O_2$ is the difference between calculated alveolar and arterial oxygen pressures. Assuming normal CO, an alveolar-arterial oxygen tension difference below 350 mm Hg corresponds to a shunt fraction of less than 15–20% at $FiO_2 = 1$. When the inspired oxygen concentration is 100%, the normal $P(A\text{-}a)O_2$ is 25–65 mm Hg. In circumstances causing serious venous admixture, this gradient may be more than 600 mm Hg, resulting in a PaO_2 of 60 mm Hg or less. When the PaO_2 falls below 60 mm Hg in a patient without previous lung disease or intracardiac defects, acute respiratory failure is diagnosed. A PaO_2 below 30 mm Hg is incompatible with life if allowed to continue for more than a few hours. Several factors can cause this drop in oxygen tension: Perfusion of sections of the lung containing closed or nonventilated airways or alveoli causes shunting of unsaturated blood into the arterial circulation. Injuries to pulmonary capillary endothelium or pulmonary vascular congestion leads to an increased diffusion distance for oxygen and collapse of alveoli. Pulmonary surfactant is depleted by the resultant hypoxemia, furthering the insult. As alveoli collapse, the lung volume is reduced, and there is an accompanying loss of compliance that contributes to further shunting. A number of insults can lead to this series of events, which is commonly known as adult respiratory distress syndrome (ARDS). The use of PEEP helps correct this deficit by increasing the functional residual capacity of the lung, increasing compliance and leading to alveolar reexpansion. Nonrespiratory causes of an increased alveolar-arterial oxygen pressure difference include right-to-left intracardiac shunt and hyperthermia. A decrease in PaO_2 with normal $P(A\text{-}a)O_2$ is seen with high altitude, decreased respiratory quotient, and central hypoventilation.

ANSWER: True

23. With regard to the measurement of arterial blood gases and alveolar-arterial oxygen tension gradients, which of the following statements is/are true?

A. The Clark polarographic oxygen electrode uses a platinum probe to detect current that is proportional to the number of diffusing oxygen molecules.
B. The Severinghaus potentiometric carbon dioxide electrode detects changes in pH caused by the diffusion of carbon dioxide.
C. Iced arterial blood gas samples exhibit a 50% drop in oxygen tension within 1 hour.
D. In normal individuals breathing room air, the alveolar arterial pressure differential of oxygen [$P(A\text{-}a)O_2$] varies between 10 and 15 mm Hg.
E. Radiographic changes usually precede abnormalities in $P(A\text{-}a)O_2$.

Ref.: 2, 5

COMMENTS: The development of the Clark and Severinghaus electrodes during the 1950s made routine measurement of arterial and venous blood gases a standard procedure in the care of acutely ill patients. Iced heparinized blood samples can be kept for 1 hour with only a 1% drop in oxygen tension. In patients breathing room air, the $P(A\text{-}a)O_2$ represents an admixture of true shunting of blood and desaturation caused by a V/Q imbalance. When 100% oxygen is breathed, this gradient is caused by true shunting and perfusion of total nonventilated alveoli, eliminating the effects of alveolar-capillary diffusion barriers and V/Q imbalances. When 100% oxygen is breathed, PaO_2 is slightly higher than 600 mm Hg. When mixed venous blood passes through the lung but does not come into contact with the alveoli, an absolute shunt exists, which is minimally improved by 100% oxygen. A relative shunt results from reduced ventilation that is less than the corresponding perfusion. This shunt is a common cause of hypoxemia in acute and chronic respiratory insufficiency and can be corrected when a patient inspires 100% oxygen. Increases in CO tend to minimize hypoxia and the alveolar-arterial gradient that results from right-to-left absolute-relative shunt. PEEP is used to improve lung function, but by virtue of its potentially deleterious effect on cardiac function it can accentuate hypoxemia. Hence pulmonary and cardiac function must always be assessed to evaluate arterial blood gases. An increase in the $P(A\text{-}a)O_2$ on 100% oxygen is an early warning sign of deteriorating lung function. This increase in gradient usually occurs before radiographic changes are evident.

ANSWER: A, B, D

24. Which of the following conditions is/are usually associated with elevated deadspace ventilation?

A. Low cardiac output (CO).
B. Pulmonary embolism.
C. Pulmonary hypertension
D. Adult respiratory distress syndrome (ARDS).
E. Excessive positive end-expiratory pressure (PEEP).

Ref.: 5

COMMENTS: Minute ventilation is determined by carbon dioxide production and the deadspace/tidal volume ratio (VD/VT). Patients whose VD/VT exceeds 0.6 are usually not weanable from ventilatory support. Small increases in DV/VT above 0.6 require large increases in minute ventilation to maintain a given arterial carbon dioxide pressure ($PaCO_2$). The anatomic deadspace includes the volume of the airways to the level of the bronchiole (150 ml). The physiologic deadspace includes, in addition, alveoli that are well ventilated but poorly perfused. The most common causes of elevated deadspace in critically ill patients are decreased CO, pulmonary embolism, pulmonary hypertension, ARDS, and excessive PEEP. In deadspace ventilation, there is decreased blood flow to ventilated areas, which primarily affects carbon dioxide elimination. Deadspace ventilation is defined as a high V/Q ratio. Low CO, pulmonary embolism, and pulmonary hypertension directly cause decreased blood flow to the pulmonary vasculature. In ARDS, some areas of lung are perfused but not ventilated; alveoli may be filled with secretions, exudate, blood, or edema, thereby increasing the shunt fraction. Other areas of lung may be ventilated but not perfused, which accounts for the deadspace ventilation. PEEP can cause deadspace ventilation by decreasing CO and by stenting open alveoli, which cause a collapse of surrounding capillaries, thereby decreasing alveolar perfusion.

ANSWER: A, B, C, D, E

25. With regard to ventilatory mechanics, which of the following statements is/are true?

A. The work of breathing at rest consumes 2% of total body oxygen consumption.
B. The work of breathing may increase to 50% of total body oxygen consumption in postoperative patients.

C. Chronic obstructive pulmonary disease (COPD) is associated with an increase in the work of breathing resulting from hindered inspiration.
D. Airway pressure reflects the compliance of the chest wall and diaphragm as well as that of the lungs.
E. Compliance is measured as the change in volume divided by the change in pressure.

Ref.: 2

COMMENTS: The work of breathing at rest consumes 2% of total body VO_2. The work of breathing can be markedly increased, up to 50% of the total VO_2, in postoperative patients because of increased airway resistance and decreased compliance of lung, chest wall, and diaphragm. In patients with COPD, the work of breathing is increased because of increased expiratory work. It can be assessed by preoperative pulmonary function testing and optimized by preoperative chest physical therapy, bronchodilators, and antibiotics if infection is present. The proper use of volume-cycled ventilators and pressure support ventilation can take over most of the work of breathing during the postoperative period. Measuring airway pressure reflects the compliance of the chest wall and diaphragm as well as that of the lungs. In the relaxed patient this is of little importance, but in restless patients intraesophageal or intrapleural pressures provide a more accurate measure of compliance. Compliance is defined as the change in pressure associated with each milliliter increase in lung volume. Changes in blood pH and carbon dioxide tensions reflect changes in patients' ventilation requirements. The most useful variable in this regard is the end-expiratory carbon dioxide tension.

ANSWER: A, B, D, E

26. Which one or more of the following suggests the need for ventilatory support?

A. Respiratory rate greater than 35 breaths per minute.
B. $PaCO_2$ greater than 60 mm Hg.
C. Alveolar-arterial oxygen difference greater than 350 mm Hg.
D. Deadspace/tidal volume ratio (VD/VT) greater than 0.6.
E. Shunt fraction greater than 5%.

Ref.: 1, 2

COMMENTS: The indications for respiratory support include inadequate parameters of ventilation (respiratory rate greater than 35, VD/VT greater than 0.6, $PaCO_2$ greater than 60 mm Hg), oxygenation (A-a O_2 difference, PaO_2), and respiratory mechanics (vital capacity, inspiratory force). In the absence of metabolic alkalosis or chronic hypercarbia, $PaCO_2$ greater than 60 mm Hg is abnormal. The pulmonary venous admixture (shunt fraction) can be defined as the amount of blood shunted around the lung as a fraction of the CO. Shunt fraction is measured at the inspired oxygen concentration required to maintain adequate oxygenation (PO_2 60–70 mm Hg). A shunt fraction greater than 20% requires respiratory support.

ANSWER: A, B, C, D

27. Which of the following characterizes adult respiratory distress syndrome (ARDS)?

A. Pure hypoxemia that is relatively unresponsive to elevations of inspired oxygen concentration.
B. Increased deadspace ventilation and increased pulmonary compliance.
C. Hypoxemia with hypercarbia.
D. Interstitial changes on chest radiograph, that usually precede clinical abnormalities.
E. Hypocarbia with hypoxemia.

Ref.: 2, 5

COMMENTS: Because the lung has a limited response to injury, it is now recognized that there are many similarities in the pathophysiology and clinical presentation of acute lung injury after a variety of insults. ARDS is seen with the systemic inflammatory syndrome (SIRS) and the multiple organ failure (MOF). The lung response can be divided into an *exudative phase* (24–96 hours), with leakage of proteinaceous fluid into the pulmonary interstitium and corresponding damage to the alveolar–capillary interface; an *early proliferative phase* (3–10 days), with proliferation of alveolar type II cells, cellular infiltration of the septum and organization of hyaline membranes; and a *late proliferative phase* (7–10 days), with fibrosis of alveolar septum, ducts, and hyaline membranes. The major criteria for the diagnosis of ARDS include hypoxia, which is relatively unresponsive to an increase in the inspired oxygen concentration; decreased pulmonary compliance (stiff lung); decreased functional residual capacity; increased deadspace ventilation; and a diffuse interstitial pattern seen on the chest radiograph. Of note is that the clinical and arterial blood gas abnormalities associated with ARDS may occur well before the radiographic changes are appreciated. Similarly, clinical improvement may occur at a time when the radiograph is still grossly abnormal. In contrast to the classic picture of pulmonary failure, these patients are usually hypocarbic rather than hypercarbic. To rule out other causes of pulmonary edema resulting from cardiogenic or hydrostatic causes, measurement of filling pressures is often required.

ANSWER: C, E

28. Which of the following is/are thought to represent the common mechanisms in adult respiratory distress syndrome (ARDS)?

A. Neutrophil and macrophage activation.
B. Injury to the alveolar-capillary interface.
C. Endotoxemia.
C. Platelet aggregation.
D. Leukocyte–endothelial cell interaction.

Ref.: 2, 5

COMMENTS: See Question 29.

29. Which of the following may be associated with ARDS?

A. Gram-negative sepsis.
B. Pulmonary aspiration.
C. Excessive oxygen administration.
D. Pancreatitis.
E. Multiple trauma.

Ref.: 1, 2

COMMENTS: ARDS is a form of pulmonary pathology, the exact understanding of which is still in evolution. It may be seen after a number of events, including major trauma, sepsis, and aspiration. All the aforementioned etiologic factors may be associated with ARDS. Although a number of ventilatory and gas-exchange abnormalities coexist in ARDS, the final common pathophysiologic pathway is thought to relate to injury to the alveolar–capillary interface, which would allow intravascular fluid to leak into the interstitium and alveoli, resulting in increased extravascular lung water. The exact mechanisms of acute lung injury (ALI) are not known. The macrophage plays an important role in the release of cytokines and modulation of the host response. Neutrophils accumulate in the pulmonary microvasculature in most patients with ALI because of various chemotaxins: C5a, lymphokines, leukotrienes, immunoglobulins. Neutrophils release granular substances, species of reduced oxygen and arachidonic metabolites. Disseminated intravascular coagulation (DIC) and platelet aggregation often are found in these patients. The fibrotic reaction may be due to endotoxin stimulation of connective tissue synthesis and alveolar macrophages. Activation of endothelial cells in inflammatory states is divided into an early phase that leads to release of P-selectin causing leukocyte adhesion and a late phase, induced by tumor necrosis factor (TNF) and interleukin-1 (IL-1), causing expression of adhesion molecules [E-selectin and interstitial and vascular (ICAM and VCAM) adhesion molecules] and the conversion of the endothelial cell to a procoagulant phenotype.

ANSWER:
Question 28: A, B, C, D, E
Question 29: A, B, C, D, E

30. Which one or more of the following treatment modalities would be appropriate in the management of virtually all cases of adult respiratory distress syndrome (ARDS)?

A. Mechanical ventilation.
B. Moderate-dose loop diuretics.
C. PEEP.
D. Steroids.
E. Broad-spectrum antibiotics.

Ref.: 5

COMMENTS: Because the principal physiologic problem in ARDS is hypoxemia refractory to increasing FiO_2, the therapy is centered on the provision of mechanical ventilation. The latter nearly always includes the application of PEEP, which should be optimized with the help of pressure/volume curves, to facilitate the maintenance of open alveoli and the diffusion of oxygen into the pulmonary capillaries. For a given FiO_2, the PaO_2 usually increases upon administration of PEEP in cases of ARDS. Excessive PEEP (>15 cm) can be hazardous because it may result in pneumothorax (barotrauma) and cause decreased venous return to the heart. Newer ventilatory methods attempt to enhance alveolar recruitment, maintain alveolar patency throughout the respiratory cycle, maintain an SaO_2 of more than 90%, avoid dynamic hyperinflation ("volutrauma"), and reduce the risk of oxygen toxicity. Spontaneous, augmented, low volume ventilation, using pressure support ventilation (PSV) as a primary ventilatory support mode, directs flow to regions of low ventilation/perfusion. It is supplemented by intermittent mandatory ventilation (IMV) and PEEP. The tidal volumes used are lower (6–8 ml/kg), accepting a lower PaO_2. These newer modes of ventilation allow iatrogenic permissive hypercapnia. At times, inverse-ratio ventilation is used to prolong the inspiratory phase. Diuretics (in cases of obvious fluid overload and cardiac decompensation) and broad-spectrum antibiotics (in the case of established pulmonary infection or other sources of sepsis) may be useful in patients with ARDS. Methylprednisolone in doses of 2–20 mg/kg/day has been used during the fibroproliferative phase of ARDS or in cases where eosinophilia is found in the blood or bronchoalveolar aspirates. However, the routine use of these drugs in the absence of these complicating factors has not been shown to be beneficial and should be avoided.

ANSWER: A, C

31. With regard to functional residual capacity (FRC), which of the following statements is/are true?

A. FRC = residual volume (RV) + tidal volume (TV).
B. Atelectasis occurs when the FRC is less than the closing volume (CV).
C. FRC = expiratory reserve volume (ERV) + RV.
D. FRC is increased by positive end-expiratory pressure (PEEP).

Ref.: 1, 2

COMMENTS: FRC is the volume of air in the lungs at the end of quiet exhalation. It is equal to the sum of ERV and RV. If the FRC falls too low, alveolar collapse ensues. This is called the CV. Early ambulation and incentive spirometry are used to support FRC above the CV in postoperative patients. PEEP can increase the FRC in mechanically ventilated patients.

ANSWER: B, C, D

32. With regard to long-term ventilator patients, which of the following statements is/are true?

A. Most long-term ventilator patients have COPD, sepsis, ARDS, or refractory heart failure.
B. Spontaneous ventilatory measurements do not predict an ability to wean.
C. Correction of underlying pulmonary and nonpulmonary complications best predicts successful weaning.
D. An effective static compliance of more than 50 ml/cm H_2O and a dynamic compliance of more than 40 ml/cm H_2O are associated with an improving gas exchange.
E. Vital capacity (VC) of 12–15 ml/kg and peak inspiratory pressure (PIP) less than −25 cm H_2O are appropriate guidelines for weaning.

Ref.: 3, 8, 9

COMMENTS: Most surgical patients (90%) are weaned from mechanical ventilation in less than 1 week. Conventional weaning criteria include (1) measurements of oxygenation by pulse oximetry (best by arterial blood gases; an SaO_2 greater than 90% on any FiO_2 is usually adequate for weaning); and (2) measurements of ventilation, such as a respiratory rate less than 24/min, a $PaCO_2$ less than 50 mm Hg, a peak inspiratory pressure (PIP) below −30 cm H_2O, a tidal volume (TV) of at least 5–8 ml/kg, and a vital capacity (VC) double the TV value. These conventional criteria are associated with unsuccessful weaning in as many as 63% of patients. Clinical judgment and correction of underlying pulmonary and nonpulmonary complications continue to be the best guides to successful weaning. In addition, helpful ventilation scores include an FiO_2 less than 40%, CPAP 3 cm H_2O, effective static compliance greater than 50 ml/cm H_2O, dynamic compliance greater than 40 ml/cm H_2O, ventilator minute ventilation less than 10 L/min, and triggered ventilatory rate less than 20/min. The duration of ventilatory support is not correlated with survival rates at discharge; 41% of long-term ventilated patients survive. Because of muscle atrophy, progressive ventilatory withdrawal designed to restore muscle function should be used. IMV, pressure support ventilation, and weaning by T-piece have been used effectively.

ANSWER: A, B, C, D, E

33. Which of the following is an appropriate definition of the shock state?

A. Low blood pressure.
B. Low cardiac output (CO).
C. Low circulating volumes.
D. Inadequate tissue perfusion.
E. Abnormal vascular resistance.

Ref.: 1, 2

COMMENTS: The clinical state of shock can result from several mechanisms. Cardiogenic shock, involving the heart, may decrease CO. Furthermore, the fluid that is pumped (i.e., the blood volume) may be decreased. In addition, alterations in the vessels—either arteriolar resistance vessels or venous capacitance vessels—may also produce a distributive state, as is seen in septic shock. Cardiogenic shock can be brought about by primary myocardial events such as myocardial infarction or cardiac dysrhythmias. Reduction in blood volume may be caused by bleeding, reduction of extracellular fluid, or loss of plasma. Changes in the blood vessels may be brought about by neurogenic reflexes, spinal anesthesia, the end-stage of hypovolemic shock, or septic shock. The final common pathway in all forms of shock, however, appears to be related to inadequate tissue perfusion. Alterations in blood pressure may not adequately reflect the shock state. High CO can be seen in many septic shock states.

ANSWER: D

34. In which one or more of the following physiologic variables may alterations independently result in a state of shock?

A. Cardiac pumping action.
B. Circulating blood volume.
C. Arteriolar resistance.
D. Venous capacitance.

Ref.: 1, 2

COMMENTS: Shock has also been considered in many categories (e.g., cardiogenic, extracardiac, obstructive, distributive, hypovolemic). These are useful considerations because they deal with the proposed etiology of the shock state. It is also useful, however, to consider shock in terms of the physiologic abnormalities that are actually occurring to produce shock. Abnormalities in any of the physiologic parameters listed above may produce shock independently or in combination. Neurogenic shock, for example, may result from many causes, including spinal trauma, severe pain, or spinal anesthesia; however, its final common pathophysiologic pathway is that of reduced peripheral vascular resistance, leading to relative hypovolemia as a secondary event. Septic shock may be caused by altered myocardial contractility or by primary vascular events, including increased venous capacitance, decreased peripheral arterial resistance, and peripheral arteriovenous shunting. In such circumstances, CO may actually be increased. However, the effective circulating volume and tissue perfusion are clearly diminished.

ANSWER: A, B, C, D

35. An 83-year-old man becomes hypotensive (systolic pressure 85 mm Hg) after repair of an inguinal hernia. Urine output is low and unresponsive to fluid administration, although the blood pressure increases to 110 mm Hg. A pulmonary artery catheter is inserted; CO is 3.0, systemic vascular resistance is 2140, mixed venous oxygen saturation is 0.55, and PCWP is 24. Which of the following single agents is/are adequate for administration?

A. Dopamine.
B. Epinephrine.
C. Nitroprusside.
D. Milrinone.
E. Dobutamine.

Ref.: 3, 4, 5

COMMENTS: Patients with cardiac failure may have symptoms of backward failure with congestion, forward failure with hypoperfusion, or a combination of the two. An increase in systemic vascular resistance typically occurs with left ventricular failure. An increase in the compliance of the large arteries or a decrease in arteriolar resistance decreases systemic vascular resistance. The patient described has an elevated systemic vascular resistance, which should be treated for the purpose of increasing the CO. Nitroprusside dilates both arterial and venous systems; however, best results are achieved in patients with severe hypertension accompanied by reduced CO and high systemic vascular resistance. The best agent listed above, which has inotropic properties and vasodilatory effects, is milrinone. This agent causes relaxation of vascular smooth muscle, which induces a decrease in systemic pressure and pulmonary arterial occlusion pressure with a reflex increase in heart rate. Other agents that could be used are nitroglycerin, phentolamine, and trimethaphan, all of which would cause a decrease in systemic vascular resistance. As vascular resistance is decreased by these vasodilators, systolic blood pressure decreases unless there is a corresponding increase in CO. CO is usually augmented by a reflex tachycardia. However, in patients with myocardial dysfunction, the stroke volume, not the heart rate, increases in response to decreased systemic vascular resistance. Another option is to decrease this resistance with a vasodilating agent and simultaneously augment CO with a β-adrenergic agent such as dopamine or dobutamine. Dopamine is not a good choice as a single agent because it does not decrease systemic vascular resistance and increases it at higher doses. Dopamine augments the CO, but the patient described has cardiogenic shock secondary to left ventricular failure with a resultant elevated systemic vascular resistance. Lowering by itself usually raises the CO. It must be remembered that adequate filling pressures must be present (PCWP > 18) before afterload reduction is initiated. Dobutamine increases CO and may cause a drop in systemic vascular resistance; peripheral vascular resistance is usually unchanged because of the balanced α-adrenergic effects and weak β_2-adrenergic effects. Norepinephrine, like dopamine, has inotropic effects but would be expected to increase the systemic pressure due to its α-agonist properties; the heart rate remains the same. Epinephrine would not be indicated in this patient as a single agent because it does not lower systemic vascular resistance, it predisposes to arrhythmias, and it increases myocardial oxygen demand, which can induce myocardial ischemia.

ANSWER: D, E

36. Match each clinical situation in the left column with the most appropriate treatment in the right column.

A. Adequate volume status; hypotension refractory to inotropic agents
B. Distended neck veins, distant heart sounds, equalization of pressures across the myocardium
C. Hypotension, appropriate volume, atrial fibrillation with ventricular response rate of 40
D. Hypotension, low right and left atrial pressures
E. Adequate volume, no mechanical defects, hypotension

a. Inotropic agents
b. Cardiac pacing
c. Pericardiocentesis
d. Fluid administration
e. Intraaortic balloon counterpulsation

COMMENTS: Cardiogenic shock may occur as a result of several mechanisms. Before assuming, however, that hypotension is caused by a cardiogenic mechanism, one must be sure that there is adequate blood volume. Therefore a patient who is hypotensive with low right and left atrial pressures should undergo fluid administration as the initial management. If cardiac performance improves with fluid administration, cardiogenic shock is probably not present. If adequate filling pressures are attained and hypotension persists in the absence of mechanical defects, arrhythmia, and sepsis, a primary pump problem probably exists and should be managed with inotropic agents. One form of cardiogenic shock seen in traumatized patients, postoperative cardiac patients, and patients suffering from uremia and certain malignancies is cardiac tamponade. It manifests clinically with evidence of venous hypertension; and on Swan-Ganz pressure determinations, there appears to be a trend toward equalization of pressures in the right and left sides of the heart. Appropriate treatment is initial pericardiocentesis to relieve the intrapericardial pressure and allow adequate heart filling. Abnormal heart rate and rhythm may alone produce cardiogenic shock, even if the myocardium contracts normally. Tachyarrhythmias are frequently caused by atrial fibrillation or flutter and respond well to digitalis. In the patient who is overdigitalized or hypokalemic, a very low ventricular rate in response to atrial fibrillation or flutter may result in hypotension and should be managed with cardiac pacing. If—despite adequate blood volume, an appropriate heart rate, absence of a mechanical or valvular defect, appropriate administration of inotropic agents, and restoration of pressure and coronary blood flow—a patient remains in cardiogenic shock, support via intraaortic balloon counterpulsation may be needed. Ballon counterpulsation is most beneficial in severe left ventricular dysfunction. Patients with hemodynamic compromise secondary to right ventricular myocardial infarction require fluid resuscitation and inotropic support (dobutamine). Any preload reducers must be avoided; afterload reducers in the presence of hypotension are not warranted.

ANSWER: A-e; B-c; C-b; D-d; E-a

37. Match each clinical and ECG finding (A–E) with the most appropriate drug therapy on the right (see Figure).

A. Chest pain and dizziness; heart rate, 100; blood pressure, 140/70.

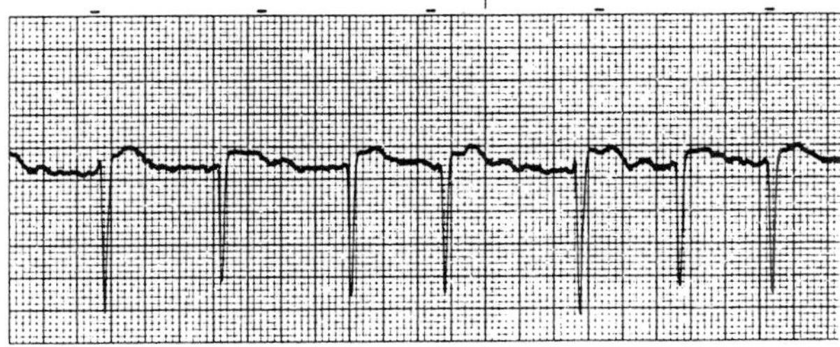

B. Asymptomatic.

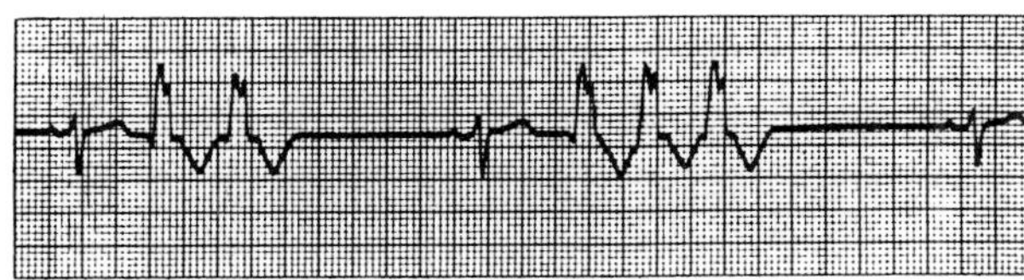

LEAD MCL

C. Patient confused; heart rate, 50; pressure, 90/65.

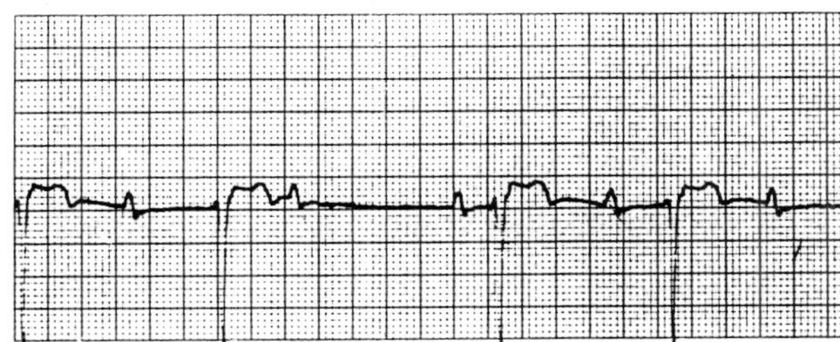

D. Dizziness; heart rate, 160; blood pressure, 155/70.

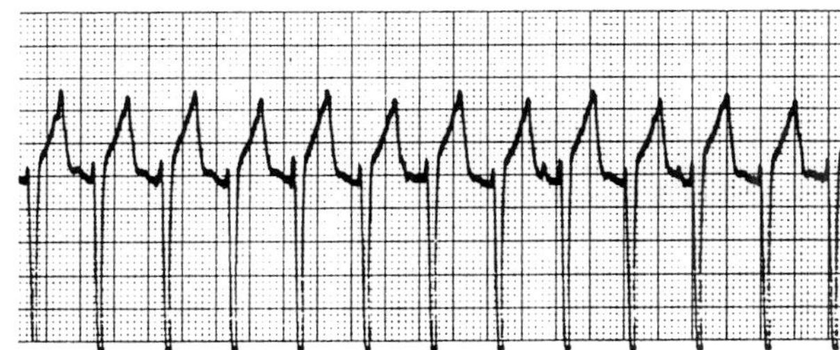

E. Sudden onset of coma.

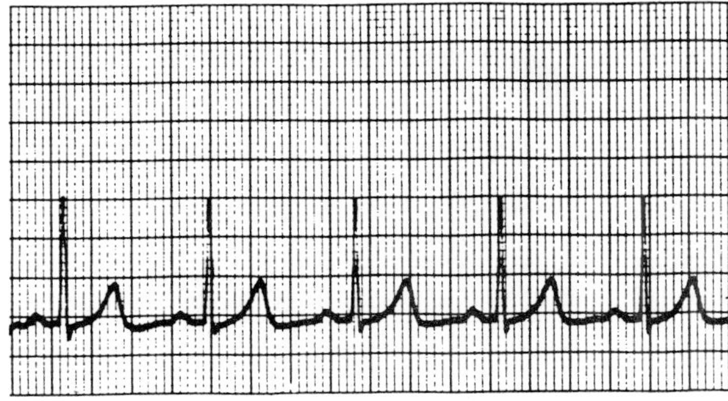

LEAD 2

Drug Therapy

a. Adenosine
b. Lidocaine
c. Digoxin intravenously followed by quinidine or procainamide (Pronestyl)
d. Atropine intravenously
e. Quinidine followed by digoxin orally
f. No specific cardiac therapy

Ref.: 1, 2

COMMENTS: Atrial fibrillation: The rhythm is irregularly irregular without P waves and narrow QRS complexes. The treatment is intravenous digoxin initially to control the ventricular rate, followed by quinidine or procainamide (Pronestyl) to convert the patient to sinus rhythm. Giving quinidine first followed by digoxin orally is incorrect, because the rate may accelerate with quinidine if digoxin is not given first. Lidocaine and atropine are not used in the treatment of atrial fibrillation. Adenosine is not used as a primary treatment of atrial fibrillation, although it is occasionally used as an adjunct to digoxin for rate control. **Ventricular tachycardia**: Isolated premature ventricular contractions may not require treatment; however, runs of more than three beats should prompt a search for treatable causes of arrhythmia. Runs of six beats or more are more significant and can be treated with lidocaine pending evaluation of potentially treatable causes of arrhythmia, such as hypokalemia, hypoxia, perioperative myocardial infarction, ischemia, and congestive heart failure. Adenosine, atropine, and digoxin do not have a role in the treatment of ventricular tachycardia. **Second-degree atrioventricular (AV) block (Mobitz type I or Wenckebach)**: Second-degree AV block is characterized by intermittently nonconducted P waves (a P wave without a QRS complex). This tracing shows a gradual PR interval prolongation followed by a nonconducted P wave. Such prolongation of the PR interval is characteristic of Mobitz type I (or Wenckebach) second-degree block. It is most often caused by excess vagal tones and responds to treatment with atropine. If the patient is stable hemodynamically (i.e., stable blood pressure, no evidence of congestive heart failure), no treatment is necessary. In this case, however, the low systolic blood pressure and confusion indicate that therapy is warranted. **Supraventricular tachycardia**: A rapid, regular rate with narrow QRS complexes and absent or retrograde P waves suggests supraventricular tachycardia. Adenosine usually provides rapid conversion to sinus rhythm. The primary side effect is hypotension, which may be managed by placing the patient in a Trendelenburg position. Lidocaine and atropine have no role in supraventricular tachycardia. Although digoxin can be used a chronic or subacute therapy, adenosine is superior for immediate conversion. The rhythm is **normal sinus**, and the patient does not require any specific cardiac therapy. However, other causes of coma should be sought and treated. For example, empiric therapy such as intravenous glucose to treat possible hypoglycemia or naloxone (Narcan) to treat narcotic overdose might be appropriate. Other causes may be stroke, drug ingestion (intentional or accidental), and respiratory events causing some hypoxia or hypercarbia.

ANSWER: A-c; B-b; C-d; D-a; E-f

38. Match each inotropic agent on the left with one or more of its properties on the right.

A. Epinephrine	a. Phosphodiesterase inhibitor
B. Dobutamine	b. Stimulates α_2-receptors
C. Milrinone	c. Stimulates β_1-receptors
D. Norepinephrine	d. Stimulates β_2-receptors
E. Dopamine (2 μg/kg)	e. Stimulates α_1-receptors

Ref.: 3, 5

COMMENTS: See Question 39.

39. Match each receptor on the left with one or more of its actions on the right.

A. α_1	a. Relaxes renal vascular smooth muscle
B. Dopamine$_1$	b. Stimulates myocardial contractility
C. β_2	c. Relaxes bronchial and vascular smooth muscle (skeletal muscle)
D. α_2	d. Inhibits uptake of norepinephrine at the sympathetic nerve terminal
E. Dopamine$_2$	e. Constricts venous vessels
F. β_1	f. Constricts vascular smooth muscle

Ref.: 3, 5

COMMENTS: Inotropic agents increase cardiac contractility by increasing the concentration and availability of intracellular calcium. The **phosphodiesterase inhibitor** (milrinone) blocks conversion of cyclic adenosine monophosphate (cAMP) to 5′-AMP. The higher concentration of cAMP results in increased calcium flux and increased calcium uptake by endoplasmic reticulum, which improves cardiac contractility and relaxation following contraction. In vascular smooth muscle, the calcium uptake by the endoplasmic reticulum results in relaxation and subsequent vasodilatation. This effect limits its use in hypovolemic shock unless it is combined with a vasopressor. **Catecholamines** act by binding to adrenergic receptors. Each type of receptor controls a particular cardiovascular function. Epinephrine, norepinephrine, dopamine, and dobutamine are all catecholamines. Alpha$_1$ mediates arterial vasoconstriction by causing contraction of vascular smooth muscle; alpha$_2$ induces constriction of venous capacitance vessels; beta$_1$ stimulates myocardial contractility; and beta$_2$ causes relaxation of bronchial smooth muscle and relaxation of vascular smooth muscle in skeletal muscle beds. The dopamine receptors cause relaxation of vascular smooth muscle: The dopamine$_1$ receptor causes relaxation of renal and splanchnic vascular smooth muscle, and the dopamine$_2$ receptor inhibits uptake of norepinephrine at the sympathetic nerve terminal, resulting in prolonged action of norepinephrine at the mother end-plate. Response to catecholamines is different in normal individuals from that in critically ill patients. Receptor populations change over short periods of time; up-regulation and down-regulation occur depending on the disease state. Because the receptor numbers and affinities are different in each clinical setting, different and unexpected responses are seen. What is important in the use of catecholamines is that they should be administered for a predetermined effect. If the effect is not attained with the particular catecholamine chosen, the dose should be adjusted or another agent used. **Dopamine** stimulates dopamine receptors at infusion rates less than 5 μg/kg/min, and α_2-receptors at infusion rates as low as 2 μg/kg/min. As the plasma concentration increases, dopamine selectively stimulates β-adrenergic receptors (5–10 μg/kg/min); further increases in the dopamine concentrations result in progressive α-adrenergic stimulation (10 μg/kg/min). **Dobutamine** is a synthetic catecholamine that is a β_1-receptor stimulant at the usual dosage of 5–15 μg/kg/min; at higher doses, tachycardia and vasodilation of vessels in skeletal muscle bed occur as a result of β_2 stimulation. Dobutamine increases CO, DO_2, and VO_2 in septic shock. **Epinephrine** at low doses has β_1- and β_2-receptor activity (<0.02 μg/kg/min), whereas at higher doses it has α_1- and α_2-receptor activity (>0.02 μg/kg/min). Epinephrine increases cardiac ectopic pacemaker activity, leading to dysrhythmias, and increases cardiac oxygen demand. Its metabolic effects include increased renin production, hyperglycemia, and free fatty acid production. **Norepinephrine** at low doses is a β_1- and β_2-receptor agonist and a potent chronotrope. At higher doses, α_1- and α_2-receptor activity predominates and the chronotropic effect diminishes. Norepinephrine is a potent splanchnic and renal vasoconstrictor.

ANSWER:
Question 38: A-b,c,d,e; B-c,d; C-a; D-b,c,d,e; E-b
Question 39: A-f; B-a; C-c; D-e; E-d; F-b

40. In cases of hemorrhagic shock, what initial alteration in blood pressure is seen?

A. Increase in systolic pressure.
B. Decrease in systolic pressure.
C. Increase in diastolic pressure.
D. Decrease in diastolic pressure.

Ref.: 10

COMMENTS: Hemorrhagic shock is defined as being caused by an acute loss of the circulating blood volume. In normal adults, the circulating blood volume is approximately 7% of the body weight, or approximately 5 liters in a normal 70-kg man. The response to hemorrhage has been divided into four classes. *Class I* hemorrhagic shock consists of the loss of up to 15% of the circulating volume. No measured changes occur with blood losses of this magnitude. In *class II* hemorrhagic shock, which is defined as the loss of 15–30% of the circulating blood volume, tachycardia is noted, as is a decrease in the pulse pressure. This decrease in pulse pressure is generally related to an increase in the diastolic component, which in turn is related to elevation of catecholamines produced by the neurohormonal response to shock. *Class III* hemorrhagic shock is the loss of 30–40% of the total circulating volume. It is at this stage that a consistent drop in systolic blood pressure occurs. It is also in class III hemorrhagic shock that the degree of blood loss requires a blood transfusion. *Class IV* hemorrhagic shock consists of the loss of more than 40% of the circulating volume. Symptoms include marked tachycardia and profound depression of the systolic blood pressure. At this stage, tissue perfusion is significantly altered, urinary output is negligible, and the skin is cold and pale.

ANSWER: C

41. Which one or more of the following statements accurately characterize(s) fluid shifts that occur during hemorrhagic shock?

A. The loss of intravascular volume is usually fully compensated by movement of extravascular interstitial fluid into the vascular space.
B. Intracellular fluid volume decreases as fluid shifts from the intracellular to the extracellular fluid compartment to compensate for the intravascular loss.
C. There is movement of interstitial fluid into the intracellular space even though full compensation of intravascular losses has not yet occurred.
D. There is a decrease in the transmembrane potential, resulting in increased sodium permeability and influx of sodium into the cell.

Ref.: 1, 2

COMMENTS: After acute hemorrhage, the extracellular fluid is depleted by two mechanisms. The first mechanism consists of transcapillary refill, wherein the extracellular fluid replaces the circulating blood volume. This transcapillary refill ultimately results in a reduction in the hematocrit. In addition, however, the cell in shock is deprived of its energy-dependent moieties. With severe hemorrhagic shock, there is an alteration in the transmembrane potential of cells (particularly muscle cells) associated with an alteration of the sodium-potassium pump, which is one of the energy-dependent moieties. Because of a decrease in the efficiency of the sodium pump, sodium and fluid from the extracellular space leaks into the interior of the cell, and potassium leaks from the intracellular space into the extracellular space. The cells thus become swollen with extracellular fluid. The net effect of both of these mechanisms, therefore, is a profound reduction in the functional extracellular fluid. Thus even though the fluid that is lost in hemorrhagic shock is blood, the initial volume deficit experienced by the patient is a reduction in extracellular fluid.

ANSWER: C, D

42. Which one or more of the following may be commonly seen as clinical manifestations of shock?

A. Decreased core temperature.
B. Thirst.
C. Restlessness.
D. Apathy.
E. Vomiting.
F. Diarrhea.

Ref.: 1, 2

COMMENTS: The clinical manifestations of shock are many and varied, depending on the cause and severity of the shock state. The more obvious clinical manifestations relate to the sequelae of decreased circulating volume and include hypotension, tachycardia, and pale, cool skin. A fall in the body's core temperature possibly caused by a lowered metabolic rate, is also seen. In the injured patient suffering from hemorrhagic hypovolemia, thirst is commonly seen. Obviously, administration of water by mouth in such circumstances may be hazardous. Also, in patients with hemorrhagic hypovolemic shock, states of anxiety and restlessness resulting from tissue hypoxia may be seen initially and give way to apathy and somnolence as central nervous system perfusion falls. Nausea and vomiting from hypovolemic shock are commonly seen. However, diarrhea is uncommon, and in fact intestinal ileus may be a common sequela of shock.

ANSWER: A, B, C, D, E

43. Which one or more of the following biochemical changes may be seen in patients in shock?

A. Hyperglycemia.
B. Negative nitrogen balance.
C. Hyperlacticacidemia.

D. Metabolic alkalosis.
E. Hyperkalemia.

Ref.: 2

COMMENTS: Shock almost invariably produces stimulation of the adrenal medullary output of epinephrine, stimulation of the pituitary-adrenocortical axis, induction of a low-flow state, and occasionally specific organ failure. These events in turn result in the relatively common biochemical changes seen in states of hemorrhagic shock. Increased circulating levels of epinephrine and cortisol result in glycogenolysis and frequently sustained hyperglycemia, as well as a change to a catabolic state, resulting in a negative nitrogen balance. The low-flow state caused by hypovolemia results in decreased oxygen delivery to skin and muscle, among other organs, and an obligatory change in the metabolism of those organs from aerobic to anaerobic. This is usually associated with significant metabolic acidosis, resulting in part from the excess production of lactic acid. One of the compensatory mechanisms in hemorrhagic shock is the renal retention of sodium and water at the expense of increased potassium excretion. However, the intracellular stores of potassium are sufficient that hypokalemia is virtually never seen, even during maximal renal compensation. If hypoperfusion of the kidney persists for any significant length of time, the characteristic biochemical findings of renal failure, including metabolic acidosis and hyperkalemia, are seen.

ANSWER: A, B, C, E

44. Regarding indexes of tissue perfusion, which one or more of the following is/are false?

A. Normal cardiac index precludes tissue hypoxia.
B. Normal mixed venous oxygen saturation (SvO_2) precludes tissue hypoxia.
C. High plasma lactate levels always reflect hypoxia.
D. Supernormal oxygen delivery (DO_2) reverses tissue hypoxia.
E. There is pathologic dependence of oxygen consumption (VO_2) on oxygen delivery.

Ref.: 11

COMMENTS: When the oxygen needs of the body are not being met, oxidation of pyruvate is carried out anaerobically, leading to the creation of lactic acid. Acidosis and elevated lactate levels can be detected in arterial blood only if capillary perfusion is sufficient to wash these products into the venous circulation. Moreover, hypoxic and nonhypoxic mechanisms of lactic acid should be considered. Gastric tonometry, measurement of intramucosal pH, can assess regional perfusion before a generalized low flow state manifests. This is why in some shock states peripheral arterial pH may not accurately reflect intracellular pH. Oxygen consumption is physiologically dependent on DO_2 below the critical DO_2 (4 ml/kg/min). VO_2 is maintained constant as DO_2 decreases by progressive increases in the oxygen extraction ratio (O_2ER).

$$O_2ER = VO_2/DO_2$$

The critical O_2ER (0.6) is that at the critical DO_2 below which the VO_2 decreases as the DO_2 decreases. Incomplete reversal of tissue hypoxia and occult tissue hypoxia (gut) have been suggested as mechanisms of multiple organ failure. One proposed reason for this is the concept of pathologic dependence of VO_2 on DO_2, characterized by a greater critical DO_2, a lower critical O_2ER, and a greater VO_2 of the plateau phase. However, when independent measurements are used, pathologic dependence is not found. Randomized trials of supernormal delivery suggest that supernormal DO_2 could prevent but not reverse tissue hypoxia.

ANSWER: A, B, C, D, E

45. What is the correct management of the most common acid-base imbalance seen in long-standing or severe hemorrhagic shock?

A. Intravenous sodium bicarbonate.
B. Administration of additional blood products.
C. Increased fluid administration.
D. No treatment required.

Ref.: 2

COMMENTS: See Question 46.

46. With regard to fluid therapy in hemorrhagic shock, which of the following statements is/are correct?

A. Fresh whole blood is probably the best fluid to be administered for hemorrhagic shock.
B. With early acute hemorrhage, the hematocrit may be used as a reliable indicator of the total volume of blood loss and the requirements for transfusion.
C. Lactated Ringer's solution should be avoided in the management of shock because the lactate present within it worsens the already existing lactic acidosis.
D. Albumin is an excellent volume expander when blood is not available because most of it stays within the vascular space for relatively long periods of time.
E. Low-molecular-weight dextran is of use as a volume expander but may be associated with increased bleeding.

COMMENTS: Although the earliest acid-base balance during shock tends to be respiratory alkalosis due to tachypnea, it rapidly gives way to an increasingly severe metabolic acidosis as the hemorrhagic shock phase continues. The underlying cause of this metabolic acidosis is inadequate tissue perfusion, which results in anaerobic metabolism and the liberation of lactic and pyruvic acids. Thus the appropriate treatment is to restore tissue perfusion by increasing intravenous fluids. Treatment with intravenous sodium bicarbonate is not indicated in the normothermic shock patient unless the pH is less than 7.1. When available, properly crossmatched fresh whole blood and a balanced electrolyte solution are the ideal replacement fluids in a patient in hemorrhagic shock. It not only replenishes the intravascular volume but does so with red blood cells, thereby preserving the oxygen-carrying capacity of the blood. In the absence of type-specific blood, type O Rh-negative (preferably with a low anti-A titer) can be administered as the "universal donor" blood. Preparation of blood does require some time; and in an emergency when the vascular volume must be replenished quickly, lactated Ringer's solution may be administered at a rate as high as 2000 ml over a 45-minute period. Failure of the patient to stabilize despite this rapid crystalloid administration is usually a sign of life-threatening, ongoing hemorrhage. Many patients, however, do stabilize for variable periods during crystalloid administration, allowing proper preparation of type-specific blood. In the normal patient with an average hematocrit, the sudden massive loss of blood that is characteristic of hemorrhagic shock does not immediately produce a drop in the hematocrit. The drop in hematocrit is caused by the transcapillary refill of extracellular fluid that replaces the blood loss. It is clear, therefore, that during the acute hemorrhagic shock process the initial hematocrit is not indicative of the total blood loss or of the need to transfuse blood. Although lactic acidosis clearly occurs in states of hypoperfusion, the additional lactate present in lactated Ringer's solution does not appear to aggravate this metabolic situation. Much work has been done looking at the relative value of other "volume expanders." Albumin has the theoretic advantage of being a protein and therefore more likely to stay within the intravascular space; however, it has been found to rapidly equilibrate with all of the extracellular fluid compartment, and its value as a blood volume substitute is transient. Low-molecular-weight dextran is probably more effective as a pure volume expander, but it has been shown to interfere with the clotting mechanism and may worsen the hemorrhage.

ANSWER:
Question 45: C
Question 46: A, E

47. Match the ventilator modes on the left with the appropriate characteristics on the right.

A. Intermittent mandatory ventilation (SIMV)
B. Pressure support ventilation (PSV)
C. Airway pressure release ventilation (APRV)
D. Pressure-targeted assist control ventilation (A/C)
E. Inverse ratio ventilation (IRV)
F. High frequency ventilation (HFV)

a. Bronchopleural fistulas
b. Limits peak airway pressures
c. Muscle atrophy
d. Decreases total work of breathing
e. Delivered breath is high volume, high pressure
f. Excessive gas trapping

Ref.: 5, 9

COMMENTS: IMV combines a preset number of mandatory breaths of predetermined tidal volume (Vt) and spontaneous breaths. Minute ventilation is the sum of patient-initiated (high pressure/low volume) and ventilator-generated (high pressure/high volume) breaths. This combination has been associated with dynamic hyperinflation (volutrauma) and barotrauma. Addition of PEEP, often more than 15 cm H_2O, increases the potential for barotrauma. IRV has been primarily used in patients with acute lung injury or neonatal respiratory distress syndrome. The inspiratory time is extended beyond the normal inspiratory/expiratory (I:E) ratio of 1:2 to as high as 4:1, potentially reducing risk of barotrauma by improving gas exchange at lower levels of peak distending pressures. Yet no benefit has been demonstrated in ARDS patients. Furthermore, IRV can seriously compromise hemodynamics, it requires heavy sedation and may lead to muscle atrophy. Extending the I:E ratio can be accomplished with PCV or with volume-controlled ventilation. With PCV the maximal airway pressure is preset, the Vt may not remain constant throughout the cycle due to variable resistance in contrast to volume-controlled ventilation, and the inspiratory flow is initially high but then decreases as alveolar pressure rises. This decelerating flow pattern generates greater shear forces than a constant inspiratory flow at the beginning of inspiration. At the end, it generates lesser shear forces. PSV is used during stable support periods and for weaning. It decreases the total work of breathing. The patient must have an intact respiratory drive. PSV can be used alone or in combination with IMV. APRV is a pressure-controlled, time-triggered, pressure-limited, time-cycled ventilation that allows spontaneous breathing during the cycle and minimizes lung expansion. CPAP is maintained until the time release valve opens, allowing the pressure in the system to fall to a lower level (FRC). The goal of APRV is to reduce peak airway pressures, thus minimizing barotrauma and volutrauma. However, APRV has potential drawbacks in cases of severe airway obstruction. It needs further evaluation in patients with low compliance. HFV uses a small Vt at high frequencies. It is useful during airway endoscopy and in cases of tracheobronchial fistula. This technique has shown no advantages over conventional ventilation in cases of acute RDS. With A/C ventilation, every patient breath is supported. Excessive work of breathing occurs in cases of inadequate peak flow or inspiratory sensitive setting. Pressure-targeted A/C ventilation may result in inadequate minute ventilation; when properly functioning, the patient on A/C performs no work, leading to muscle atrophy.

ANSWER: A-e; B-d; C-b; D-c; E-f; F-a

48. Concerning pressure support (PS), which one or more of the following statement(s) is/are false?

A. The inspiratory pressure is terminated when a certain inspiratory flow minimum is reached.
B. Pressure-support ventilation controls the ultimate inspiratory flow and tidal volume.
C. Pressure-volume (P-V) characteristics with pressure-supported breathing improves muscle efficiency during weaning.
D. High level PS (5–50 cm H_2O) can be used as a stand-alone ventilatory support mode.
E. PS makes spontaneous breathing more comfortable for ventilator-dependent patients.

Ref.: 12

COMMENTS: Pressure support is a pressure-triggered, pressure-targeted, flow-cycled mode of ventilation. It is used as a ventilatory mode during stable ventilatory support and for weaning. PS can shift the work of breathing from the patient to the ventilator. The flow delivery pattern of a PS-assisted breath synchronizes with spontaneous breathing patterns better than the fixed pattern of a volume-assisted breath. The inspiratory pressure is held consistent through servo control of delivered flow and is terminated when an inspiratory flow minimum is reached. The patient controls ventilatory timing and sets the inspiratory flow and tidal volume. During the weaning process, PS changes muscle work characteristics to a more normal P-V configuration, thereby facilitating gradual load return to patients during the weaning process. During weaning, patient pressure support facilitates synchronization with ventilatory pattern reflexes, hence producing more physiologic muscle reloading as a stand-alone mode. High level PS (5–50 cm H_2O) provides ventilatory support to patients who have a reliable ventilatory drive and stable or improving lung mechanics.

ANSWER: B, D

49. Which one or more of the following is/are associated with inaccurate estimation of hemoglobin saturation of oxygen (SaO_2) by pulse oxymetry?

A. Carboxyhemoglobin.
B. Dark pigmentation.

C. Septic syndrome.
D. Nail polish.
E. Nitrite intoxication.

Ref.: 5

COMMENTS: Pulse oximetry is based on placing a pulsating arterial vascular bed between a diode and a light detector (spectrophotometer with plethysmographic characteristics). It detects the oxygenated part of hemoglobin **available** for carrying oxygen (SaO_2) as opposed to the percent of **total** hemoglobin that is oxygenated (% $HgbO_2$). An elevated carboxyhemoglobin level causes overestimation of SaO_2 by pulse oximetry because its absorption coefficient is similar to that of oxygenated hemoglobin. Inaccurate readings are associated with the following: dark pigmented skin, low-flow states, nail polish, vital dyes, ambient light, anemia, changes in oxyhemoglobin dissociation curve, and cardiac arrhythmias.

ANSWER: A, B, C, D, E

50. With regard to the use of vasopressors and vasodilators in the management of hemorrhagic shock, which of the following statements is/are true?

A. Vasopressors usually result in an elevation of the blood pressure.
B. Vasopressors achieve their goal of blood pressure support primarily through inotropic effects.
C. Dopamine given in low to moderate doses may provide inotropic and chronotropic support to the heart as well as enhance renal blood flow.
D. In general, the use of vasopressors in hemorrhagic shock is discouraged.
E. Vasodilators should be employed early in the management of hemorrhagic shock to promote tissue perfusion.

Ref.: 1, 5

COMMENTS: The use of vasopressors in the management of hemorrhagic shock has been somewhat controversial, but the general tendency is toward avoidance of their use. Although they are effective in raising the blood pressure in patients in hemorrhagic shock, they do it primarily through increasing peripheral vascular resistance, which further reduces tissue perfusion (thus aggravating the principal problem in hemorrhagic shock). Different vasopressors work through different mechanisms, depending on their relative α- and β-receptor stimulation effects. Dopamine is an attractive vasopressor in that it provides beneficial inotropic and chronotropic support to the heart while selectively enhancing renal blood flow through its peripheral β-adrenergic effects. Even so, dobutamine, dopamine, and the other vasopressors should probably be avoided during the initial management of hemorrhagic shock because the principal deficit is one of effective circulating blood volume and poor tissue perfusion. There is some evidence suggesting that after a proper circulating blood volume has been restored or if volume correction does not correct hypotension the positive inotropic and chronotropic effects of vasopressors on the heart may lead to further improvement in a patient's status. Because dopamine is not always successful, even at high doses, norepinephrine in combination with volume expansion is indicated initially, particularly if the mean systemic pressure is less than 60 mm Hg or there is evidence of organ dysfunction. Vasodilators have a theoretic advantage of promoting tissue perfusion by reducing peripheral vascular resistance. However, this would be appropriate only once an effective circulating blood volume had been established, and the use of vasodilators for initial management of hemorrhagic shock should be avoided.

ANSWER: A, C, D

51. Match each drug in the left column with one of the statements in the right column.

A. Intravenous morphine	a. Torsades de pointes
B. Haloperidol	b. Requires analgesic for pain
C. Diazepam	c. Pain management in shock
D. Propofol	d. Choice for hepatic failure
E. Lorazepam	e. Short-term sedation

Ref.: 13

COMMENTS: Perhaps paradoxically, pain is not a common problem among patients suffering from hypovolemic shock. When significant pain is present, however, administration of small intravenous doses of morphine is probably the preferred method of management. Haloperidol has been associated with torsades de pointes, particularly in patients with a prolonged QTc (>500 msec) on the electrocardiogram. Diazepam is a short-acting sedative, but it is metabolized in the liver. Lorazepam does not require extensive hepatic metabolism. Propofol possesses anxiolytic, sedative, and hypnotic activities, but it is not an analgesic.

ANSWER: A-c; B-a; C-e; D-b; E-d

52. A 24-year-old woman undergoes a laparotomy for a stellate injury to the liver and during the procedure undergoes transfusion with 12 units of cold, stored, packed red blood cells. Despite appropriate treatment of the liver injury, there is persistent bleeding from the raw surface of the parenchyma. In addition to aggressive resuscitation, administration of which of the following is initially most appropriate?

A. Calcium chloride.
B. Fresh-frozen plasma.
C. Platelets.
D. Correction of hypothermia if present.
E. Heparin.

Ref.: 1, 14

COMMENTS: Massive transfusion is defined as the administration of more than 10 units of blood or more than one blood volume of the patient within 24 hours. The known associated complications include electrolyte and acid-base abnormalities, changes in hemoglobin-oxygen affinity, hypothermia, coagulopathy, and dysfunction of various organs. A number of studies have documented a drop in the platelet count after massive transfusion. Also, platelet aggregation with ADP and collagen are noted to be depressed for up to 4 days after the transfusion. Further studies analyzing the effect of routine prophylactic platelet transfusions in such patients have failed to document any advantage unless the patient has nonmechanical bleeding. Also, platelet transfusion is not harmless; it results in ultrastructural pulmonary lesion–platelet aggregates within microcapillaries, degeneration of endothelial and alveolar cells, and protein exudate in the interstitium. Despite low levels of factors V and VIII in blood stored for 14–21 days, dilutional coagulopathy is rare. In some patients, dilutional effects of massive transfusion can lead to bleeding complications. Recommendations to combat this situation have included prophylactic administration of 1 or 2 units of fresh-frozen plasma for every 2–10 units of transfused blood. Actually, the continued bleeding is often secondary to the underlying disease process. Initially, a transient dilutional coagulopathy may be related to the duration of hypotension. No correlation has been demonstrated between the coagulation factors and the incidence or degree of bleeding complications. It can reasonably be concluded, therefore, that the routine administration of fresh-frozen plasma is of little value in patients undergoing massive transfusions. The indications for administration of calcium should be based on hemodynamic considerations because lowering the ionized calcium by citrate to a level that blocks coagulation could lead to death from myocardial dysfunction and decreased peripheral vascular resistance. Hypothermia decreases clearance of citrate from the blood, thereby allowing a marked reduction in ionized calcium. Because blood products are stored between 1° and 6°C, rapid transfusion of these products leads to hypothermia, which in turn brings about a decrease in citrate metabolism, the hepatic clearance of drugs, and synthesis of acute-phase reactive proteins. The clotting system is impaired because of a decreased ability to form stable clots and a decreased production of clotting factors. Blood warmers, warm saline lavage, blankets, and heated inspired gases are useful adjunctive measures to prevent hypothermia. Heparin is not indicated as the initial step in such a situation.

ANSWER: D

53. With regard to renal function during states of hemorrhagic shock, which of the following statements is/are true?

A. The kidneys, like the brain and heart, are "favored" organs during hemorrhagic shock, to which adequate blood flow is usually preserved until late in the clinical picture.
B. Renal ischemia for as long as 10 minutes produces irreversible renal damage in most patients.
C. Most patients tolerate renal ischemia for up to 100 minutes.
D. Alteration in the blood urea nitrogen (BUN) is as sensitive a measure of renal function as is osmotic, creatinine, or urea clearance.
E. Furosemide does not effectively protect against renal failure.

Ref.: 1

COMMENTS: Although the kidneys are clearly "vital" organs, blood flow to them is quickly diminished in states of hypovolemia and hemorrhagic shock in favor of flow to the brain and heart. Thus a compensatory reduction in blood flow to the kidneys, like that to the skin and liver, is an early finding in hemorrhagic shock. Most kidneys tolerate ischemia for up to 15 minutes with full return of function; ischemia for 15–90 minutes leads to varying degrees of chronic renal failure; beyond 90 minutes of ischemia, irreversible renal damage develops in virtually all patients. Numerous physiologic parameters can be followed when monitoring the extent of renal damage sustained during hemorrhagic shock, including urine output, BUN, serum creatinine, and clearance of creatinine and urea. BUN does not appear to be a particularly sensitive parameter to follow. BUN may be normal even in states of significant renal parenchymal loss (e.g., unilaterally nephrectomized patients), or it may rise in response to prerenal azotemia even though there may be no significant parenchymal renal damage. The clearance of creatinine, urea, and osmotic particles is a more sensitive indicator of renal function. The simplest calculation compares fractional excretion of sodium with creatinine in oliguric patients.

$$\text{Renal failure index} = \text{UNa} \times \text{PLcr/Ucr}$$

where UNa is urine sodium, PLcr is plasma creatinine, and Ucr is urine creatinine. An index of less than 1 usually indicates prerenal oliguria. Because these clearances are calculated on the basis of the ratio of urine/plasma concentrations, it takes into account alterations caused by diminished urine output and therefore is a better measure of the physiologic activity of the kidneys. Obviously, the ideal initial management of the renal manifestations of hemorrhagic shock relate to restoration of a proper, effective circulating blood volume. Furosemide (a loop diuretic) alone, although increasing urine flow in many circumstances, is not effective in redistributing blood flow to the renal cortex and, in the absence of effective renal blood flow, may worsen renal function by producing hypovolemia.

ANSWER: E

54. Which of the following is not consistent with acute tubular necrosis (ATN)?

A. Oliguria.
B. Fractional excretion of sodium (FeNa) greater than 4.
C. Urine osmolality (Uosm) less than 300 mOsm/L.
D. Creatinine clearance (Ccr) greater than 125 ml/min/1.73 m^2.

Ref.: 1, 2

COMMENTS: The prevention and early diagnosis of ATN are extremely important. Although oliguria is a feature of ATN, it can result from other prerenal, renal, and postrenal etiologies. Urine chemistry and osmolality are the earliest measurable changes in tubular function. FeNa greater than 3 and Uosm less than 350 mOsm/L represent the inability of the renal tubule to reabsorb sodium and concentrate urine. Ccr greater than 125 ml/min/1.73 m^2 is normal. It should be remembered that 70% of the nephron mass is damaged before the BUN and creatinine levels begin to rise.

ANSWER: D

55. Which one or more of the following may occur in a patient with normal to elevated urine output following hemorrhagic shock?

A. Dehydration.
B. Hyperkalemia.
C. Progressive azotemia.
D. Need for hemodialysis.
E. Death from renal failure.

Ref.: 2

COMMENTS: Although the classic clinical presentation of renal failure is that of oliguria, possibly followed by a diuretic phase, it must be recognized that "high-output renal failure" may occur with no antecedent oliguric phase. Excretion of water is only one of the kidneys' numerous functions, and the ability to put out large volumes of urine in no way ensures the appropriate clearance of solutes. Thus most of the characteristic findings of oliguric renal failure may be seen in the patient with high-output renal failure. The exact mechanism of high-output renal failure is not fully understood but is thought to be an intermediate form of renal failure, representing a response to a form of ischemic renal injury that is less severe than that required to produce oliguric renal failure. Microscopic examination of renal tissue shows damage principally to the distal nephron and regenerating patchy tubular necrosis. Potassium should be carefully monitored. A typical course shows an increasing urea nitrogen level, which parallels an increasing urine volume, mild metabolic acidosis, and acute hyperkalemia that is frequently precipitated by administration of potassium salts. Hypernatremia is seen whenever fluid restriction is instituted. Replacement of isotonic salt losses with lactated Ringer's solution corrects the hypovolemia and low carbon dioxide combining power. When serum potassium reaches 6 mEq/L, exchange resins should be used. Hemodialysis may be required.

ANSWER: A, B, C, D, E

56. A 62-year-old diabetic patient with rest pain is admitted for evaluation of his peripheral arterial system. He has chronic renal failure (BUN 70 mg/dl, creatinine 5.0 mg/dl). Which one or more of the following is/are *not* indicated to avoid contrast-related injury?

A. Calcium channel blockers.
B. Mannitol.
C. Volume expansion.
D. Diuretics given after the angiogram.
E. Theophylline.

Ref.: 15

COMMENTS: Contrast agents can cause renal failure in patients with preexisting azotemia, diabetes, and left ventricular failure. Volume expansion with crystalloid solutions prior to angiography is the best prevention. Theophylline, calcium channel blockers, and nonionic agents have proved to be beneficial.

ANSWER: B, D

57. With regard to the systemic inflammatory response syndrome, which of the following statements is/are true?

A. Invariably associated with infection.
B. Body temperature above 38°C or under 36°C.
C. Tachypnea (>20 breaths/minute) or hyperventilation ($PaCO_2$ < 32 mm Hg).
D. Leukocytosis (>12,000 cells/mm^3) or leukopenia (<4000 cells/mm^3).
E. Heart rate greater than 90 beats/minute.

Ref.: 16, 17

COMMENTS: Sepsis is a clinical response arising from infection, although similar responses can arise in the absence of infection and are termed the systemic inflammatory response syndrome. All of the characteristics listed above may be present in the systemic response to a wide variety of insults, not only to infection. Noninfectious causes include pancreatitis, ischemia, multiple trauma, hemorrhagic shock, immune-mediated organ injury, burns, and the exogenous administration of mediators of the inflammatory process [tumor necrosis factor, cytokines: interleukins (e.g., IL-1, IL-6, IL-8)]. When this syndrome is the result of confirmed infection, it is termed sepsis. Septic shock is defined as sepsis-induced hypotension, persisting despite adequate fluid resuscitation, along with manifestations of organ dysfunction and hypoperfusion abnormalities. Septic shock is a distributive form of shock that results in a severe decrease in systemic vascular resistance associated with a normal or elevated CO. In addition, abnormalities of cardiac performance—decreased ejection fraction ventricular dilatation—are characteristic of septic shock.

ANSWER: B, C, D, E

58. Which one or more of these cytokines are known mediators of systemic inflammatory response syndrome?

A. IL-1.
B. IL-4.
C. Transforming growth factor-beta (TGF-β).
D. IL-2.
E. Tumor necrosis factor-alpha (TNF-α).

Ref.: 5

COMMENTS: See Question 59.

59. Which one of the following is correct regarding cytokines in the pathophysiology of sepsis?

A. Elevated circulating phospholipase A_2 (PLA_2) is not predictive of lethal multiple organ failure (MOF).
B. Serum levels of cytokines have greater biologic meaning than tissue levels.
C. Elevated IL-6 levels most consistently correlate with mortality in severe sepsis.
D. Circulating protein C levels are not predictive of outcome in septic patients.
E. Nitric oxide (NO) synthase inhibition improves survival in models of sepsis.

Ref.: 5

COMMENTS: Experimental and clinical studies have demonstrated that the physiologic and metabolic effects of TNF and endotoxin [lipopolysaccharide (LPS)] are nearly identical. IL-1 has been shown to have metabolic effects similar to those of TNF. However, TNF-α, IL-1, and other cytokines have dual beneficial and adverse effects depending on the amount, timing, and anatomic locus of production. TNF is thought to play an important role, but it is variably detected in the blood of patients with sepsis. Cytokines are low-molecular-weight proteins produced by activated monocytes or macrophages. Cytokines are involved in the differentiation, proliferation, and immunoregulatory function of various cells, including lymphocytes and macrophages. MOF is a systemic disorder of immunoregulation, inflammatory damage, endothelial dysfunction, and hypermetabolism. Stimulation of mononuclear cells, neutrophils, and endothelial cells leads to an inappropriate regulation of endogenous inflammatory mediators such as cytokines (IL-1, IL-6, IL-8), platelet-activating factor, nitric oxide, and eicosanoids. One source of cytokines is the tissue macrophage, where these substances may have local paracrine effects; cytokines at tissue levels may be of greater importance than the variable serum levels. Antiinflammatory cytokines (TGF-β, IL-4, IL-10, granulocyte colony-stimulating factor) and IL-1 receptor antagonist constitute some of the host effort to limit excessive reaction to endotoxemia. TNF and IL-1 activate PLA-1. Circulating PLA-1 is highly predictive of death in patients with peritonitis. Endotoxin may damage the endothelium, but most of its effects can be facilitated by its association with an acute-phase reactant lipopolysaccharide (LPB) leading to activation of nuclear factors and increased cytokine production. The physiologic responses of TNF are nearly identical to the responses of LPS. TNF can cause fever or hypothermia, tachycardia, elevated cardiac output, and decreased systemic vascular resistance. In higher concentrations, TNF can cause hypotension, circulatory collapse, and acidosis. Hormonal response from elevated TNF concentrations includes elevations in catecholamines, cortisol, and glucagon. Oxygen consumption and carbon dioxide production also increase in response to elevated TNF. IL-1 can cause fever and leukocytosis, increased production of acute-phase reactants, increased muscle catabolism, and other events that occur in sepsis. Reciprocal interaction among cytokines, complement, and coagulation systems occur in MOF. TNF down-regulates thrombomodulin in the endothelial cell, which impairs activation of protein C; this may explain the strongly predictive value of this protein serum level. There is a strong correlation between elevated levels of IL-6 and mortality in MOF patients. NO plays an unclear role in sepsis.

ANSWER:
Question 58: A, E
Question 59: C

60. Which one or more of the following treatment modalities may be appropriate in the management of a patient in severe septic shock?

A. Interleukin (IL-1) receptor antagonist.
B. Aggressive volume administration.
C. Vasopressor therapy.
D. Mechanical ventilation.
E. Steroids.

Ref.: 1, 2

COMMENTS: Of the various forms of "shock," septic shock is probably the most difficult to manage. In many instances the source of sepsis may not be immediately apparent, and therefore correction of the underlying infectious process may be delayed. Appropriate antibiotic therapy of recognized or presumed infections is obviously central to the ultimate resolution of septic shock. While this is occurring, support of the patient's cardiopulmonary status is frequently warranted. In most cases of septic shock there is peripheral vasodilatation leading to pooling of the blood volume and a need for aggressive fluid administration initially. Toxins produced in many infections are inhibitory to myocardial contractility; thus once adequate volume has been achieved, inotropic agents (e.g., dobutamine) may be warranted. Dopamine is one of the preferred agents in that it provides inotropic and chronotropic support for the heart while augmenting renal blood flow when given in low to moderate doses. Norepinephrine has been used with success, provided volume restoration has been started. Sepsis is one of the common predisposing factors in the development of acute RDS, and as a consequence many patients in septic shock require mechanical ventilation. The use of pharmacologic doses of corticosteroids is somewhat controversial, but large prospective trials have shown no benefit and possible detriment. Clinical trials conducted with agents that target the initiating toxins and mediators have shown no change in outcome.

ANSWER: B, C, D

61. With regard to multiple organ failure (MOF), which of the following statements is/are true?

A. Sepsis is the major risk factor.
B. Injury to the microvascular endothelium is uniformly present.
C. Neutrophil-mediated injury is dependent on adherence to the microvascular endothelium.
D. The high concentration of xanthine oxidase present in ischemic endothelial cells prevents generation of toxic oxygen radicals.
E. Increase in the gastrointestinal barrier is often present.

Ref.: 3

COMMENTS: Sepsis is the major risk factor in the development of MOF. Injury to the microvascular endothelium causes a generalized inflammatory state; early recognition and adequate treatment are essential if serious ischemia-reperfusion injury and MOF are to be prevented. Several components of the immune defense system are involved. Neutrophil-mediated injury is dependent on adherence to the endothelium and neutrophil aggregation; both are mediated by the glycoprotein complex CD11/CD18, to which monoclonal antibodies can be directed. The endothelial cell exposed to ischemia is subject to a depression of ATP levels accompanied by an increased xanthine oxidase/xanthine dehydrogenase ratio, which generates toxic oxygen radicals upon reperfusion. Arachidonic acid metabolites are leukotrienes and prostacyclines. Platelet-activating factor, produced by various inflammatory cells, causes microvascular injury through ischemia and stasis. Breakdown of the intestinal mucosal barrier may allow the ongoing bacterial translocation and stimulation of the immunoinflammatory reaction. Measurement of intragastric pH by tonometry may facilitate early detection of regional tissue hypoxia and optimization of resuscitation.

ANSWER: A, B, C, D

62. Which one or more of the following factors decreases the rate of bacterial translocation in the gastrointestinal tract?

A. Parenteral nutrition.
B. Glutamine-enriched TPN.
C. Septic shock.
D. Addition of fiber to an elemental diet.
E. Prolonged ileus.

Ref.: 18

COMMENTS: Several investigators have shown an increase in intestinal mucosal permeability to bacteria and bacterial products (bacterial translocation) following hemorrhagic shock, sepsis, or lipid A infusion, although the gastrointestinal tract is grossly intact. This breakdown of the mucosal barrier has been implicated in the pathophysiology of multiple organ failure; the susceptibility of the splanchnic circulation to hypoperfusion, the high concentration of xanthine oxidase, and the presence of enteric flora enhance this theory. Several factors are known to increase the rate at which bacterial translocation occurs: hemorrhagic shock, septic shock, bacterial overgrowth, prolonged ileus, bowel manipulation, parenteral nutrition (TPN), and antibiotic use. Prolonged ileus and antibiotic use are probably predisposing factors to bacterial overgrowth. It has been demonstrated that enterocytes of the gut mucosa preferentially use the amino acid glutamine and ketone bodies as respiratory fuel. Furthermore, enteral and parenteral formulas that contain glutamine and/or ketone bodies (β-hydroxybutyrate, acetoacetate) promote bowel mucosal growth and probably decrease the rate of bacterial translocation. Villous atrophy, decreased secretion of immunoglobulin A (IgA), decreased cellular immunity, bacterial overgrowth, and decrease in barrier function with bacterial translocation have been associated with parenteral rather than enteral nutrition.

ANSWER: B, D

63. A patient involved in a motor vehicle accident is found to have a thoracic spine fracture and paraplegia. The patient is hypotensive with a systolic blood pressure of 70 mm Hg and is bradycardic. The patient is breathing comfortably. Which one or more of the following would be appropriate treatment?

A. Fluid administration.
B. Steroid administration.
C. Immediate intubation.
D. Ephedrine administration.
E. Nasogastric tube placement.

Ref.: 2, 5, 19

COMMENTS: Neurogenic shock results from a loss of balance between vasodilatory and vasoconstrictor influences in the arterioles and venules. Common causes include sensory stimulation, such as severe pain, exposure to unpleasant events or sights, high spinal anesthesia, and traumatic spinal cord injury. Clinical characteristics include a blood pressure that is often low, as in other forms of shock; however, the pulse rate is usually slower than normal, and the skin is flushed, warm, and dry. A reduction in cardiac output is found secondary to decreased blood return to the heart because of the increased capacitance of the arterioles and venules. Bradycardia is caused by the sympathectomy of spinal insult if above the level of T4 with no capacity for compensatory tachycardia. The treatment of milder forms of neurogenic shock consists of removing the nociceptive stimulus. Neurogenic shock resulting from high spinal anesthesia can usually be treated with a vasopressor such as ephedrine or phenylephrine, each of which increases CO by direct effects on the heart and by increasing peripheral vasoconstriction. The treatment of neurogenic shock secondary to spinal cord injury is usually more complicated, not only because of more prolonged hypotension but also because of the question of coincident hypovolemic shock resulting from associated injuries. Such patients often require ventilatory support because of decreased spontaneous respiration and loss of accessory muscles for breathing. Aggressive fluid therapy should be instituted early under continuous cardiovascular monitoring; persistent hypotension necessitates recognition of possible hemorrhagic shock. A vasopressor such as ephedrine or phenylephrine may be needed. A nasogastric tube should be inserted because these patients develop gastric atony, dilatation, and hypersecretion. Although the administration of steroids remains controversial, their usefulness for a blunt spinal cord injury has been supported. Continued cardiac monitoring is necessary in patients with sinus bradycardia because the patient may develop cardiac pause, sinus arrest, asystole, and ventricular dysrhythmias.

ANSWER: A, B, D, E

64. Match the nutritional components in the left column with the corresponding immunologic characteristics in the right column.

A. Arginine	a. Decrease in prostaglandin (PG) E_2 and leukotriene B
B. Nucleotides	b. Diet free of this nutrient leads to decrease in T cell-mediated immunity, decreased IL-2 production, and increased susceptibility to infections
C. ω-3 Fatty acids	c. Gut major fuel source
D. Glutamine	d. Nitric oxide (NO) production

Ref.: 18

COMMENTS: All the above-mentioned nutrients play an important role in the process of modifying immune function. **Arginine** increases protein synthesis and IL-2 production, induces secretion of anabolic hormones, enhances guanyl and adenyl cyclase activity, enhances total CD-4 cells, and is responsible for NO production essential for optimal lymphocyte DNA synthesis. Animals fed diets without purines and pyrimidines (**nucleotides**) showed a decrease in T cell-mediated immune response, decreased IL-2 production, and increased susceptibility to *Staphylococcus* and *Candida* infections. Administration of **ω-3 fatty acids** is thought to reverse the immunosuppression caused by excessive production of PGE_2 and leukotriene B. **Glutamine** is a nonessential amino acid involved in the production of ammonia and ketoglutarate; it contributes an amide group for nucleotide synthesis. Enterocytes use it as a preferential fuel source. Glutamine deficiency in the stressed state is thought to result in an alteration of the gut mucosal barrier, which in turn may continue the systemic inflammatory response.

ANSWER: A-d; B-b; C-a; D-c

65. Which one or more of the following statements concerning nosocomial sinusitis is/are true?

A. Conventional radiographs of the sinuses are as sensitive and specific as are computed tomography (CT) scans.
B. Ventilated patients with orotracheal and orogastric tubes have an increased risk over that of nonventilated patients.
C. The presence of nasal tubes is not an independent risk factor in the nonventilated patient.
D. *Haemophilus influenzae* is the most common pathogen in hospitalized patients.
E. Headache, purulent discharge, and pain are frequently present.

Ref.: 5

COMMENTS: Diagnosis of nosocomial sinusitis is best accomplished by CT scan, showing air-fluid levels and opacification of one or more sinuses. Gram-negative organisms and *Staphylococcus* are the predominant organisms isolated. The presence of nasal tubes, mechanical ventilation, and oral tubes in ventilated patients are risk factors. Classic findings of sinusitis are frequently absent.

ANSWER: B

66. A 38-year-old baseball player undergoes chemotherapy for a lymphoma. He presents in shock. Laboratory abnormalities include hyperphosphatemia, hypocalcemia, and azotemia. An ECG shows peaked T waves, PR prolongation, and diminished P wave amplitude. Which one of the following is/are indicated for the prevention and therapy of this syndrome?

A. Hydration.
B. Allopurinol.
C. Prednisone.
D. Diuretics.
E. Alkalinization of urine.

Ref.: 2, 5

COMMENTS: Renal and metabolic complications result from acute tumor lysis as a consequence of dissolution of bulky tumors (lymphomas and leukemias) by irradiation and chemotherapy. Hyperuricemia, hyperphosphatemia, and hypocalcemia with or without renal failure are characteristic findings. The mainstay in prophylaxis is hydration. If this is not successful, dopamine, mannitol, and diuretics should be used. Allopurinol is given to control hyperuricemia. While the patient remains hyperuricemic, the urine should be alkalinized. Phosphate-binding antacids should be started before the onset of therapy.

ANSWER: A, B, D, E

67. A 45-year-old man is recovering from multiple organ failure (MOF) following an operation for a perforated gastric ulcer. He has been afebrile for 48 hours and is off antibiotics. His white blood cell count is normal. Renal failure has resolved. His encephalopathy is improving, and his oxygenation is adequate on 30% oxygen and 5 cm PEEP. Attempts at weaning him off the ventilator have been unsuccessful. His negative inspiratory pressure is −10 cm H_2O. Neurologic examination shows a symmetric quadriparesis with facial sparing and depressed deep tendon reflexes. A spinal tap fluid is normal. Select the most likely diagnosis:

A. Guillain-Barré syndrome.
B. Myasthenia gravis.
C. Neuromuscular blockade.
D. Primary myopathy.
E. Critical illness polyneuropathy (CPU).

Ref.: 20

COMMENTS: See Question 68.

68. Which of the following statements is/are true concerning the condition described in Question 67.

A. A nerve biopsy often shows demyelinization or inflammation.
B. Failure to wean from the ventilator is due to phrenic nerve involvement.
C. Corticosteroids are the treatment of choice.
D. Serum antibodies against acetylcholine receptor are always present.
E. Plasmapheresis is the initial treatment of choice.

Ref.: 20

COMMENTS: CPU is an axonal motor sensory neuropathy that accompanies sepsis with encephalopathy. It is due to primary axonal degeneration, affecting motor fibers more than sensory fibers. Frequently, it presents as failure to wean a patient from the ventilator, due to phrenic nerve involvement despite clinical improvement. Symmetrical quadriparesis with facial sparing and depressed deep tendon reflexes is characteristic. Electromyography confirms the diagnosis. Spinal fluid is normal, unlike in Guillain-Barré syndrome. Facial involvement and detection of antibodies against acetylcholine is characteristic of myasthenia gravis. Nerve biopsy shows axonal degeneration without demyelination or inflammation. Treatment is supportive. Corticosteroids are contraindicated.

ANSWER:
Question 67: E
Question 68: B

69. Which of the following statements is/are true concerning hemodynamic monitoring in critically ill patients?

A. Right ventricular end-diastolic volume index (RVEDVI) correlates better than wedge pressure (PAWP) with cardiac output.
B. PAWP is a better predictor of effective pulmonary capillary pressure than RVEDVI.
C. RVEDVI correlates well with both right ventricular stroke wave index and left ventricular stroke work index.
D. Ejection fraction is not a good index of ventricular contractility.
E. At moderate to high levels of ventilatory support (PEEP 10–50 cm H_2O) there is a good correlation between PAOP and the cardiac index.

Ref.: 21

COMMENTS: Critically ill patients show great differences in right (RV) and left (LV) ventricular function. PAWP has been considered a clinically relevant measure of LV preload. Yet measurement and interpretation of PAWP in mechanically ventilated patients in whom PEEP or inverse ratio ventilation is used is difficult, particularly when variable LV compliance exists. The stroke volume index, calculated by dividing the cardiac index by the heart rate, can be divided by the ejection fraction, yielding the RV end-diastolic volume index. Furthermore, a RVEDVI value of less than 140 ml/m^2 is a better predictor of the cardiac index response to volume loading than either CVP or PAWP whenever PEEP is used. The RV ejection fraction depends greatly on the RV afterload, so increases in the pulmonary vascular resistance index reduce the ejection fraction. Ejection fraction is not a good index of RV contractility. End-diastolic volume is a more reliable indicator of ventricular preload than is filling pressure, especially in patients who require PEEP.

ANSWER: A, B, C, D

70. In regard to adult respiratory distress syndrome (ARDS), which one or more of the following statements is/are true?

A. Sepsis and gastric aspiration are most commonly associated with ARDS.
B. Presence of more than 10% bands found on a peripheral smear increases mortality.
C. Duration of mechanical ventilation is predictive of mortality.
D. Persistent acidemia is not predictive of mortality.
E. ARDS following cardiopulmonary bypass has a better prognosis than that following bone marrow transplant.

Ref.: 5, 22, 23

COMMENTS: ARDS was first described by Ashbaugh in 1967. Sepsis and gastric aspiration are most commonly associated with ARDS; but shock, major trauma, multiple transfusions, pancreatitis, drug overdose, pneumonia, and near drowning are also associated. Fowler found four variables associated with increased mortality in the setting of ARDS: presence of more than 10% bands, persistent acidemia, calculated bicarbonate level less than 20 mEq/L, and BUN greater than 65 mg/dl. Neither duration of mechanical ventilation nor level of static compliance is predictive of mortality. Severity scoring and prognostic estimates are difficult. Because death from ARDS is frequently due to nonrespiratory causes, measuring the severity of ARDS to predict mortality as an outcome may not be practical. The severity of nonpulmonary organ dysfunction provides an additional estimate of prognosis: the more organ systems failing, the greater the mortality.

ANSWER: A, B, E

71. Which one or more of the following statements is/are true concerning the incidence of nosocomial pneumonia in mechanically ventilated patients?

A. The development of pneumonia is directly related to the length of ventilatory support.
B. The gastropulmonary route of bacterial contamination exists, and the source of bacteria is the duodenum.
C. Selective gut decontamination reduces the incidence of nosocomial pneumonia.
D. The incidence of nosocomial pneumonia is lower when sucralfate is used for prophylaxis of stress ulcer bleeding rather than intensive antacid or H_2-blocker therapy.
E. Bacterial translocation has proved to play an important role in the development of nosocomial pneumonia patients in the intensive care unit (ICU).

Ref.: 5

COMMENTS: The development of pneumonia appears to be directly related to length of ventilatory support; the risk is highest during the first 2 weeks of therapy. The incidence is in the 20–25% range, and the mortality is in excess of 30%. Patient risk for development may be reduced by avoidance of antacid therapies, nasogastric tube suctioning, supine position, and ventilator circuitry changes every 24 hours. Nosocomial aspirates with colonized gastric secretions by duodenal bacteria plays a major etiologic role in the development of pneumonia. Selective gut decontamination reduces the likelihood of colonization, but it does not reduce the incidence of nosocomial pneumonia. Bacterial translocation via the portal system has not proved to be an etiologic factor in the clinical setting. Gastroenteral feedings do not appear to predispose patients to a higher risk of pneumonia than do jejunostomy feedings.

ANSWER: A, B, D

72. In regard to lactic acidosis, which of the following statements is/are true?

A. Type A lactic acidosis (Woods classification) is always a consequence of tissue hypoxemia associated with tissue hypoperfusion.
B. Type B lactic acidosis is always a consequence of tissue hypoxia associated with tissue hypoperfusion.
C. Lactate per se does not cause lactic acidosis.
D. The treatment of lactic acidosis requires administration of bicarbonate.
E. Serial lactate determination may be a useful preoperative indication of circulatory shock.

Ref.: 1

COMMENTS: With the Cohen and Woods classification, lactic acidosis is divided into two major types: A and B. Type A lactic acidosis is a consequence of tissue hypoxia associated with tissue hypoperfusion (abnormal vascular permeability, left ventricular failure, decreased cardiac output) or of reduced arterial content ($PaO_2 < 35$ mm Hg, CO poisoning, severe anemia). Type B acidosis is not associated with tissue hypoxemia and may be the result of liver disease, diabetes mellitus, drugs (acetylsalicylic acid, ethanol), and inborn errors of metabolism. Anaerobic glycolysis produces lactate, ATP, and water; it does not produce lactic acidosis. The acidosis associated with hyperlacticacidemia is caused by hydrolysis of ATP, with release of hydrogen ions. Gluconeogenesis from lactate produces hydrogen ions directly. The treatment of lactic acidosis should be directed toward correction of the cause of acidosis. Sodium bicarbonate has failed to improve the acid-base or hemodynamic state of these patients. The presence of lactic acidosis represents the best objective determination of the presence and severity of circulatory shock. In addition, both hypoxia and hypercapnia are important in this scenario.

ANSWER: A, C, E

73. In regard to pulmonary embolism (PE), which one or more of the following is/are false?

A. Symptoms of early small to medium PEs are usually pulmonary in nature.
B. Ventilation perfusion (V/Q_2) abnormalities are present early after embolism, and shunt becomes the predominant mechanism for hypoxemia later.
C. Chest radiographic abnormalities are rarely present in most patients with PE.
D. More than one-third of patients with angiographic PE have negative leg studies for deep vein thrombosis (DVT).
E. Thrombolytic therapy has been shown to reduce mortality in comparison with heparin in patients with PE.

Ref.: 5

COMMENTS: The incidence of pulmonary embolism in the United States exceeds 500,000, with the prevalence for nonfatal PE approaching 20 per 1000 inpatients. As many as two-thirds of these cases go undiagnosed. Iliofemoral thrombosis appears to be the source of most clinically apparent emboli. Predisposing factors include (1) prior embolism; (2) factors promoting stasis; (3) lower extremity and pelvic operations and pelvic trauma; (4) hypercoagulable states. Many emboli are silent. Symptoms of small to medium emboli are usually pulmonary (i.e., dyspnea, chest pain, and cough); tachypnea and tachycardia are present as well. Massive PEs often produce cardiovascular findings. Pulmonary artery pressure tends to be increased but correlates poorly with the size of the embolus and may even be normal. Even without infarction, radiographic abnormalities appear as diaphragmatic elevation, atelectasis, and effusion. Even though noninvasive leg studies for determination of DVT are negative in up to one-third of patients, its addition to clinical suspicion and lung screening, could reduce the need for pulmonary angiography. Angiography, however, is the definitive diagnostic technique for this disease. Heparin therapy over 5–7 days with 4–5 days overlap with warfarin (Coumadin) constitutes the therapy of choice. Coumadin should be continued for 6–12 weeks for calf vein and large vein thrombosis. Thrombolytic therapy has not been shown to reduce mortality in comparison with heparin in large prospective series.

ANSWER: A, C, E

74. Concerning auto-PEEP, which one or more of the following is/are true?

A. Auto-PEEP can be caused by increased airway resistance and expiratory flow limitations.
B. Auto-PEEP is easily detected by the ventilator manometer.

C. Auto-PEEP is best managed by prolonging the expiratory time.
D. Auto-PEEP can be offset by applying external PEEP up to 50% of the auto-PEEP.
E. Auto-PEEP is best managed by increasing the tidal volume.

Ref.: 5

COMMENTS: Auto-PEEP is due to gas trapping at the end of expiration. This increases the work of breathing, decreases effective alveolar ventilation, and subjects the patient to a higher risk of volutrauma and compromised hemodynamics. In mechanically ventilated patients, increased expiratory resistance can cause auto-PEEP. Risk factors include obstructive airway disease, minute ventilation requirements greater than 10 L/min, high ventilator rates with lower tidal volume, or low inspiratory flow rates. Auto-PEEP is more reliably detected by graphic flow displays. Alternatively, auto-PEEP can be measured by the end-expiratory occlusion technique or by an esophageal balloon pressure reading. Even if intrinsic PEEP exists, the ventilator water manometer cannot detect it. Auto-PEEP is best treated by prolonging the expiratory time and reducing the inspiratory time. In the volume-cycled ventilatory mode, expiration can be prolonged by decreasing the respiratory rate, decreasing the tidal volume, or increasing the flow rate. Minute ventilation should be minimized and bronchodilator therapy optimized. Application of PEEP up to 10–15 cm H_2O but not exceeding 80–85% of auto-PEEP can decrease the work of breathing needed to initiate inspiratory flow. Switching the patient from pressure triggering to flow triggering can be helpful as well.

ANSWER: A, C

75. Which one or more of the following preclude(s) a diagnosis of brain death?

A. Uremia.
B. Body temperature less than 30°C.
C. Systemic blood pressure of 70/40 mm Hg.
D. Normal plantar reflex.
E. Desaturation during an apnea test.

Ref.: 24

COMMENTS: Brain death is the irreversible cessation of all functions of the brain, including the brain stem. This condition must persist for a minimum of 6–12 hours unless there is no identifiable structural abnormality, in which case more prolonged observation is advisable. The diagnosis is mainly clinical in a patient unresponsive to painful stimuli and with absent oculovestibular reflexes to ice-water calorics and a positive apnea test. A confirmatory test—blood flow study, electroencephalography, or angiogram—is not obligatory. Reversible causes of brain dysfunction that may confound the diagnosis must be identified and corrected: drug intoxication, hypothermia (≤32°C), hepatic encephalopathy, severe electrolyte disorder, hyperglycemia, uremia, hypotension (mean arterial pressure <60 mm Hg). The corneal reflex and gag response should be absent. The apnea test requires the following prerequisites: core temperature of 97.8°F (36.5°C) or more, systolic pressure of 90 mm Hg or more, euvolemia, apnea, and normal oxygenation. The patient is disconnected from the respirator while maintaining a supply of 100% oxygen. If respiratory movements are absent and the $PaCO_2$ is more than 60 mm Hg or there is a 20 mm Hg increase in PaCO above the baseline (if starting with more than 40 mm Hg), the test is positive. If the mean arterial pressure drops below 60 mm Hg or the patient desaturates, the test is terminated and the patient is connected to the ventilator. If the PaCO is less than 60 mm Hg or if the increase is less than 20 mm Hg, the patient should be given vasopressors and the test repeated later. Up to 30% of brain death patients have a normal plantar response to pain.

ANSWER: A, B, C, E

REFERENCES

1. Sabiston DC Jr: *Textbook of Surgery*, 15th ed. WB Saunders, Philadelphia, 1997.
2. Schwartz SI, Shires GT, Spencer FC: *Principles of Surgery*, 7th ed. McGraw-Hill, New York, 1999.
3. Weigelt JA: Surgical critical care. *Surg Clin North Am* 71:683, 1991.
4. Sprung CL: *The Pulmonary Artery Catheter: Methodology and Clinical Applications*. University Park Press, Baltimore, 1983.
5. Civetta JM, Taylor RW, Kirby RR: *Critical Care*. Lippincott-Raven, Philadelphia, 1997.
6. Tuman KJ: Tissue oxygen delivery: the physiology of anemia. *Anesth Clin North Am* 8:451, 1990.
7. West JB: *Respiratory Physiology: The Essentials*, 4th ed. Williams & Wilkins, Baltimore, 1990.
8. Morganroth ML, Morganroth JL, Nett LM, Petty JL: Criteria for weaning from prolonged mechanical ventilation. *Arch Intern Med* 144:1012, 1984.
9. Tharratt RS (ed): Mechanical ventilation. *Crit Care Clin* 14:563, 1998.
10. American College of Surgeons: *Advanced Trauma Life Support. Instructor Manual*. Chicago, 1989.
11. Levy MM (ed): Monitoring cardiac function and tissue perfusion. *Crit Care Clin* 12:4, 1996.
12. MacIntyre NR: Pressure support: coming of age. *Sem Respir Med* 14:293–298, 1993.
13. Society of Critical Care Medicine: *Practice Parameters for Systemic Intravenous Analgesia and Sedation for Adult Patients in the ICU*. Anaheim, CA, Society of Critical Care Medicine, 1995, p 1.
14. Patt A, McCroskey BL, Moore EE: Hypothermia-induced coagulopathies in trauma. *Surg Clin North Am* 68:775, 1988.
15. Porter GA: Radiocontrast induced nephropathy. *Nephrol Dial Transplant* 9:146, 1994.
16. Parrillo JE (moderator): Septic shock in humans: advances in the understanding of pathogenesis, cardiovascular dysfunction, and therapy. *Ann Intern Med* 113:227, 1990.
17. Bone RC (conference chairperson): American College of Chest Physicians Society of Critical Care Medicine consensus conference: Definitions for sepsis and organ failure and guidelines for the use of innovative therapies in sepsis. *Crit Care Med* 20: 1992.
18. Hickey MS: Nutritional management of the critically ill patient. In: Weigelt JA, Lewis FR (eds) *Surgical Critical Care*. WB Saunders, Philadelphia, 1996.
19. Bracken MB, Shepard MJ, Collins WF, et al: A randomized, controlled trial of methylprednisolone or naloxone in the treatment of acute spinal cord injury: results of the second National Acute Spinal Cord Injury Study. *N Engl J Med* 322:1207, 1990.
20. Leijten FS, et al: Critical illness polyneuropathy: a review of the literature, definition and pathophysiology. *Clin Neurol Neurosurg* 96:10, 1994.
21. Nelson LD: The new pulmonary arterial catheters. *Crit Care Clin* 12:795–818, 1996.
22. Ashbaugh DG, Bigelow DB, Petty TL, et al: Acute respiratory distress in adults. *Lancet* ii:319, 1967.
23. Fowler AA, Hamman RF, Good JT, et al: Adult respiratory distress syndrome: risk with common predispositions. *Ann Intern Med* 98:593, 1983.
24. Wijdicks EFM: Determining brain death in adults. *Neurology* 45: 1003, 1995.

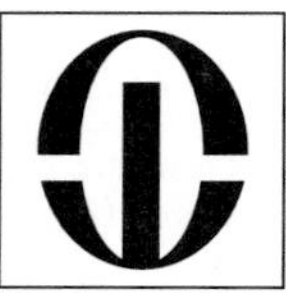

CHAPTER 12

Trauma

1. A 22-year-old man is brought to the emergency room after being involved in a motorcycle crash. He is combative, pale, is bleeding profusely from the nose and mouth, and has a sizable scalp laceration. There is an obvious deformity of his right thigh. Vital signs are blood pressure 80/40; pulse 130; respiratory rate 40 and noisy. Which of the following initial management choices is correct?

   A. Endotracheal intubation, rapid infusion of lactated Ringer's solution through a central venous catheter, traction splint of extremity, and rapid suture of scalp laceration.
   B. Endotracheal intubation, rapid infusion of lactated Ringer's solution through percutaneous large-bore catheters, traction splint of extremity, rapid suture of scalp laceration, and exposure of patient.
   C. Oxygen by mask, rapid infusion of lactated Ringer's solution through percutaneous large-bore catheters, pressure dressing on scalp wound, and exposure of patient.
   D. Cricothyroidotomy, rapid infusion of lactated Ringer's solution through percutaneous large-bore catheters, pressure dressing on scalp wound, traction splint of extremity, and exposure of patient.
   E. Open airway with chin-lift or jaw-thrust maneuver, rapid infusion of lactated Ringer's solution through percutaneous large-bore catheters, rapid suture of scalp laceration, traction splint of extremity, and exposure of patient.

Ref.: 1, 2

COMMENTS: In the trauma patient, there are several injuries that are immediately life-threatening. Upon arrival in the emergency room, a primary survey is performed on all injured patients to identify and treat these life-threatening conditions. The mnemonic "**ABCDE**" defines the specific, ordered, prioritized initial evaluation. A = airway and cervical spine control, B = breathing, C = circulation, D = disability or neurologic status, and E = exposure. **Airway**: Because of its urgency, assessment of the airway should be clinical. Digital exploration and clearance of the mouth followed by the chin-lift or jaw-thrust maneuvers often eliminate the need for tracheal intubation and are the first maneuvers performed. Simple mechanical adjuncts such as nasal or oral airway can prevent passive airway occlusion. When this is not effective, orotracheal or nasotracheal intubation is performed without delay. Cricothyroidotomy is indicated when the trachea cannot be intubated. **Breathing**: After the airway is secured, ventilation and oxygenation must be assessed. Physical examination should identify conditions such as tension pneumothorax, flail chest, open pneumothorax, and massive hemothorax. In a patient with tension pneumothorax, a 14- to 16-gauge catheter inserted into the thorax at the 2nd intercostal space, midclavicular line, can be life-saving. Defects in the chest wall greater than two-thirds the diameter of the tracheal lumen require occlusive dressing of the defect and a tube thoracostomy. In unstable patients, rapid performance of tube thoracostomy is indicated based on clinical grounds alone. Pulse oximetry is used for continuous monitoring of hemoglobin oxygen saturation (SaO_2), and arterial blood samples to measure gases are drawn as soon as possible. All injured patients are given supplemental oxygen initially. There should be a low threshold for instituting mechanical ventilation in patients with severely depressed mental status, unstable vital signs, or respiratory distress. **Circulation**: Hemorrhagic shock is the most common preventable cause of death in trauma patients. The pulse is checked for quality, rate, regularity, and paradox. A palpable distal pulse indicates a blood pressure of at least 80 mm Hg. Skin color and level of consciousness are indirect indicators of tissue perfusion. Ashen gray coloring or mottling of the skin and agitation or decreased level of consciousness are indications of at least 30% total blood volume (TBV) loss. Additionally, the systemic blood pressure usually remains normal due to compensatory mechanisms, until about a 30% TBV loss. Two large-bore intravenous catheters are instituted immediately. When percutaneous placement is difficult, cutdowns are necessary. The preferred site is the saphenous vein at the ankle. Central venous catheters can be inserted quickly and safely, especially when the femoral vein is used, but it should not be the first option. **Bleeding**: Rapid inspection for external sites of bleeding is performed. Direct pressure can control hemorrhage in most circumstances. However, this rarely works on large scalp lacerations; rapid suturing or stapling of the scalp without concern about cosmesis is usually effective. Grossly deformed limbs are gently straightened, and the vascular status of the limb is noted before and after its manipulation. The human thigh is a cylinder about 40 cm in length and 8 cm in radius; an increase in the radius of the cylinder by 1 cm represents a change in volume of 2 liters. Thus bleeding into the thigh can be a source of substantial hemorrhage. Unstable fractures of long bones are reduced and splinted. **Disability**: A brief neurologic examination assessing pupillary reaction, level of motor and sensory responsiveness, and level of consciousness is performed. **Exposure**: Complete disrobement of the patient is performed to facilitate thorough examination and assessment.

ANSWER: E

2. A 32-year-old woman leaps from the 10th floor of her apartment building in an apparent suicide attempt. Upon presentation, the patient has obvious head and extremity injuries. Primary survey reveals that the patient is totally apneic. By which method is a definitive airway in this patient best provided immediately?

A. Orotracheal intubation.
B. Nasotracheal intubation.
C. Cricothyroidotomy.
D. Intubation over a bronchoscope.
E. Needle cricothyroidotomy.

Ref.: 1, 2

COMMENTS: During the initial assessment of a multiple traumatized patient, the airway takes precedence over all other interventions. In a patient who is totally apneic, an appropriate airway must be restored as rapidly as possible. **Fiberoptic intubation** with a bronchoscope or laryngoscope, although appropriate in certain circumstances, cannot be performed in a sufficiently rapid time frame to fulfill the requirements of this patient. **Nasotracheal intubation**, although operator-dependent, is more than 90% successful. Visualization of the vocal cords via direct laryngoscopy is unnecessary so there is no manipulation of the neck, making it the method of choice for patients with confirmed or suspected cervical spine injury. However, it is mandatory that the patient have some spontaneous respirations. In this case of a totally apneic patient, blind nasotracheal intubation would be contraindicated. It is also contraindicated in patients with instability of the midface or suspected fracture of the cribriform plate. **Orotracheal intubation** can be accomplished rapidly and effectively. Because all patients with altered mental status or incomplete radiographic evaluation are assumed to have a cervical spine injury, the two-person technique with inline manual cervical immobilization is mandatory. **Needle cricothyroidotomy** with jet insufflation is a useful technique for obtaining direct control of the airway in small children. In adults, however, carbon dioxide retention occurs quickly because of the limited size of the catheter that can be placed with this technique. **Cricothyroidotomy** is reserved for emergency airway control in the patient with significant maxillofacial trauma and for those in whom attempts at orotracheal intubation have failed.

ANSWER: A

3. A 24-year-old obese man is involved in an automobile fire. He shows evidence of inhalation injury with carbonaceous sputum, an edematous oropharynx, tachypnea, and stridor. After attempted nasotracheal intubation, the patient remains hemodynamically stable with oxygen saturation of 97%. Before attempting orotracheal intubation, which of the following maneuvers is/are correct?

A. Oxygenation via high-flow oxygen face mask.
B. Cricoid pressure.
C. Axial stabilization of the neck.
D. Administration of paralyzing agents.
E. Preparation for cricothyroidotomy.

Ref.: 1, 2

COMMENTS: When a patient presents to the emergency room needing intubation, initial care of the airway must include adequate suction and oxygenation with a face mask at high flow (10–12 L/min) for spontaneously breathing patients or a bag-valve mask for others. Positive-pressure ventilation should be administered before intubation to elevate the SaO_2 to near 100%. It should be assumed that all trauma patients have a full stomach, so cricoid pressure (Sellick maneuver) should be applied before and during intubation to compress the esophagus and prevent regurgitation. It must also be assumed that patients who have sustained blunt trauma above the clavicles have a cervical spine injury, and the neck must be stabilized with in-line axial immobilization during intubation. If nasotracheal intubation fails or if the patient is not a candidate for nasotracheal intubation, orotracheal intubation is the next mode of airway management. It is not necessary to paralyze a patient to establish airway control via endotracheal intubation. For a patient who has blunt facial trauma or penetrating injuries to the face or upper airway and for any patient in whom intubation may be difficult, the initial intubation attempt should be made with sedation alone. Midazolam, etomidate, and thiopental are the agents most commonly used. When a paralyzing agent is needed, it is imperative that a cricothyroidotomy tray be at the bedside as well as a surgeon who is capable of performing the procedure. The most common neuromuscular blocking agent used is succinylcholine, at a dose of 1.0–1.5 mg/kg, because of its rapid onset (30–60 seconds) and short duration of action (3–10 minutes).

ANSWER: A, B, C, E

4. A 56-year-old man hit by a car presents with multiple face lacerations, profuse bleeding from the nose and mouth, palpable deformity of the mandible, and left periorbital swelling and ecchymosis with impaired upward gaze. His respiratory rate is 40 per minute, he is stridorous and anxious. Which of the following represent the correct order of initial valuation and management?

A. Supplemental oxygen/CT of the face/suturing of facial lacerations/lateral cervical (C)-spine radiograph.
B. Nasotracheal intubation/posterior nasal packing/lateral C-spine radiograph/CT of the face.
C. Endotracheal intubation/posterior nasal packing/lateral C-spine radiograph/CT of the face.
D. Posterior nasal packing/endotracheal intubation/lateral C-spine radiograph/CT of the face.
E. Endotracheal intubation/posterior nasal packing/lateral C-spine radiograph/plain films of the face.

Ref.: 1

COMMENTS: As for all injured patients, those with facial trauma require a systematic primary survey to secure the airway, breathing, and circulation. Airway obstruction is the foremost life-threatening complication of facial trauma. Multiple mandibular fractures or combined maxillary, mandibular, and nasal fractures predispose the patient to developing acute airway obstruction due to posterior displacement of the tongue or soft tissue swelling of the oropharynx (or both). The attending physician should have a low threshold of suspicion regarding the need to control the airway. Clinical signs such as stridor or profuse bleeding, decreased mental status, and low oxygen saturation are signs of impending airway compromise. Nasotracheal intubation is contraindicated in these patients. Orotracheal intubation may be attempted with cervical spine immobilization; however, a surgical airway via cricothyroidotomy is occasionally necessary. Profuse bleeding through the nares or facial wounds may occur after massive facial trauma and should be controlled in the primary survey. Direct pressure is applied to open wounds. Posterior packing or Foley balloon tamponade are usually successful in controlling nasopharyngeal bleeding and should be instituted early to control life-threatening hemorrhage. All patients with facial trauma must be assumed to have a cervical spine injury. Portable lateral cervical spine radiographs should be obtained after the secondary survey. Patients with neck pain or tenderness should undergo a complete cervical spine series with flexion and extension views or CT, if the cervical spine series cannot be adequately performed. Patients with altered mental status should remain in a cervical collar as though they have an injury. Once the patient is stabilized and life-threatening injuries are controlled, CT of the face taken at 1.5- or 3.0-mm intervals in **both axial and coronal views** is performed as the diagnostic test of choice. Standard facial roentgenograms add little to the management and are not indicated if CT is available.

ANSWER: C

5. In regard to the patient in Question 4, which of the following is/are true?

A. Repair of the facial fractures should be performed within 2–3 days, after the edema is decreased.
B. If CT is performed, Panorex of the mandible is not indicated.
C. In general, if a patient's mandibular fracture is reduced with a compression plate and screw fixation, the patient can resume eating sooner than if the fracture had been immobilized by intermaxillary fixation (IMF).
D. Most fractures of the mandibular ramus, coronoid, and condyle are treated with IMF alone.

Ref.: 1

COMMENTS: Periorbital swelling and ecchymosis should alert the physician to the possibility of orbital fractures. A thorough evaluation of vision, pupillary reaction, and extraocular movements is crucial if permanent eye damage is to be avoided. Impaired upward gaze and diplopia on upward gaze signify orbital floor fracture with herniation of orbital contents into the maxillary sinus and associated inferior rectus entrapment. This orbital "blowout" is well demonstrated on coronal views of the CT scan. This finding mandates emergent surgical liberation of the herniated tissues and restoration of the orbital floor by plating the bone fragments or autogenous bone grafting. If entrapment is ruled out clinically and by CT scan, facial bone fractures may be repaired on a semielective basis after the patient has been stabilized and life-threatening injuries have been dealt with. With regard to mandibular injury, swelling and tenderness are usually present, but malocclusion is the most sensitive indicator of mandibular fracture. Panorex provides a complete view of the body, angle, ramus, and condyles; it is used as an adjunct to CT scanning. The technique of IMF involves application of metal arch bars to the upper and lower dental arches; these are joined by wires or rubber bands to immobilize the fracture. Most mandibular fractures require immobilization in this manner for 6–8 weeks. Frequent complaints by the patient include discomfort and weight loss. Compression plating systems have been used increasingly often in the management of mandibular fractures. Compression plates are technically unforgiving and necessitate precise alignment of fracture fragments, but their advantage is that the patient can resume eating at a much earlier stage. Most fractures of the ramus, coronoid, and condyle are treated with IMF alone.

ANSWER: C, D

6. A 47-year-old woman is brought to the trauma unit after a motor vehicle crash. She is alert but confused; her eyes open to command, and she moves all extremities to command. She complains of headache and neck and left leg pain. Her airway, breathing, and vital signs are intact. She has a large frontal scalp hematoma. Portable cervical spine, chest, pelvic, and left femur radiographs are normal. While cervical spine series is being performed, she is noted to become much more lethargic, moving only to pain. Which of the following pathologic conditions is most likely to be present?

A. Subdural hematoma.
B. Epidural hematoma.
C. Cerebral contusion.
D. Intracerebral hematoma.
E. Diffuse axonal injury.

Ref.: 1, 2

COMMENTS: Acute **epidural hematoma** is characteristically associated with arterial bleeding from the middle meningeal artery. There is commonly a lucid interval followed by sudden neurologic deterioration. Immediate CT of the head is indicated to identify the site of the lesion and assess the degree of mass effect. Operative evacuation of the hematoma is indicated if significant mass effect is noted, if there is a midline shift of more than 5 mm, or if there is neurologic deterioration. **Subdural hematoma** is the most common traumatic mass lesion of the head, occurring in approximately 20–40% of severely head-injured patients. This lesion is usually due to tearing of venous sinuses and occurs between the dural and arachnoid layers. Operative evacuation is necessary if significant mass effect is present. **Intracerebral hematomas** most commonly occur in the subfrontal and anterior temporal regions of the brain. They have the potential to cause significant mass effect requiring evacuation. Intraoperative ultrasonography is useful for localizing the clot and ensuring complete removal. **Cerebral contusions** occur when blunt trauma causes cerebral parenchymal injury and microvascular disruption. They may occur at the site of impact (coup lesion) or at a point opposite (contrecoup lesion) owing to a rebound effect of the brain. These lesions may create considerable mass effect. **Diffuse axonal injury** is generally a diagnosis of exclusion. Severely head-injured patients without significant lesion on CT or those who remain vegetative or severely disabled despite rapid evacuation of mass lesions are given this diagnosis. Presently, the only treatment is supportive care and optimization of cerebral perfusion pressure.

ANSWER: B

7. A 27-year-old man is brought by ambulance after sustaining a blow to the head. Upon arrival in the emergency room he is breathing spontaneously, has stable vital signs, opens his eyes only to pain, mumbles his words, and withdraws only to painful stimulus. His pupils are equal, round, and reactive to light. Which of the following is/are indicated in the initial evaluation and stabilization period?

A. CT of the head.
B. Endotracheal intubation and hyperventilation.
C. Intracranial pressure monitoring.
D. Emergency burr hole on the right side.

Ref.: 1, 2,

COMMENTS: Brain injury is the most common cause of death in trauma victims, accounting for about half of the deaths at the scene. A neurologic assessment is performed by assessing pupillary response and the Glascow Coma Scale (GCS). The GCS, which evaluates eye opening, verbal response, and motor response objectively measures the severity of injury and guides therapeutic interventions. A score of 13–15 reflects mild head injury. A score of 9–12 indicates moderate head injury. These patients require urgent CT scan of the head and admission with frequent neurologic evaluations. A score of 8 or less reflects a severe head injury. This patient requires early intubation to stabilize the airway. **Hyperventilation**, which causes cerebral vasoconstriction and a reduction in intracranial pressure (ICP) was popular during the 1970s. However, it may also exacerbate cerebral ischemia, and its effects are transient. Thus it is no longer recommended as a first-line treatment for the head-injury patient. The current recommendation is that mild hyperventilation, producing a PCO_2 of 30–35, should be used only when necessary to control the ICP and for as short a duration as possible. **Computed tomography** of the head should be performed as soon as the cardiopulmonary status of the patient has been stabilized. CT scans can accurately identify intracranial hematomas and contusions, subarachnoid and intraventricular hemorrhage, and skull fractures. If the CT scan identifies a surgically correctable lesion, as discussed in the prior question, it is treated accordingly. Nonsurgical management of these patients involves supportive care in an intensive care unit (ICU) and aggressive maintenance of cerebral perfusion pressure (CPP), which is the mean arterial pressure minus the intracranial pressure. **Intracranial pressure monitors** are routinely inserted in patients with severe head injuries and no surgically correctable lesion. Ventriculostomy allows drainage of cerebrospinal fluid and cerebral compliance measurements; it may be performed in the emergency room or ICU. The normal ICP is about 10 mm Hg, and most authorities initiate treatment when the level reaches about 20 mm Hg. Initial therapy includes intravenous sedation and possibly paralysis. When this fails, mild hyperventilation and osmotic diuretics may be used. The purpose of osmotic diuretics is to dehydrate and shrink the normal brain tissue where the blood-brain barrier is intact, reducing the ICP. Serum sodium levels and serum osmolality should be checked regularly; optimal sodium levels are 140–145 mEq/L, and optimal serum osmolality is 295–310 mOsm/L. The typical loading dose for mannitol is 1 gm/kg and then 0.25 gm/kg intravenously every 4 hours. Recently emphasis has been placed on aggressive colloid and isotonic crystalloid fluid infusion and vasopressor therapy to maintain a CPP of at least 60–70 mm Hg. Despite aggressive efforts, the mortality rate for patients with severe head injuries is 30–50%, and a large proportion of the survivors have serious neurologic defects. Emergency **burr holes** are undertaken only in exceptional circumstances and only with the advice and consent of a neurosurgeon. The burr hole should be placed on the side of the largest pupil in comatose patients with decerebrate or decorticate posturing whose condition does not respond to medical therapy.

ANSWER: A, B, C

8. With regard to cervical spine injury, which of the following is/are true?

A. C1 (atlas) fractures are usually caused by an axial load and involve a blowout of the ring.
B. Hangman's fractures are unstable and are best treated by operative spinal fusion.
C. Type II odontoid fractures are considered stable.
D. Anterior spinal subluxation with bilateral facet dislocation is rarely associated with a complete spinal cord injury.

Ref.: 1, 2

COMMENTS: Any patient sustaining an injury above the clavicles, an injury produced by a high speed motor vehicle crash, or a head injury resulting in an unconscious state must be suspected of having a cervical spine injury and be immobilized with a cervical collar and backboard until screening roentgenograms are obtained and fractures or dislocations are excluded. **C1 burst fractures** (or Jefferson's fractures) are caused by axial loading and often result in widening of the spinal canal. When isolated, they are considered stable and are treated with a rigid cervical collar. **Hangman's fractures** involve the posterior elements of C2 and are usually caused by extension and distraction. This is an unstable fracture, and the treatment is traction for displacement followed by a halo vest for 3 months. **Odontoid fractures** are divided into three types. *Type I* involves the odontoid above the base and is considered stable. *Type II* fractures occur at the base and are usually unstable. Fractures with less than 5 mm of displacement can be treated with 3 months of immobilization in a halo jacket, whereas those with greater displacement generally require posterior fusion of C1 and C2 or screw fixation of the anterior odontoid process. *Type III* odontoid fractures extend into the vertebral body and are treated with rigid orthosis or a halo jacket. Anterior subluxation of the cervical spine can occur with **facet fracture**, unilateral or bilateral **facet dislocation**, or bilateral perched facets. Most bilateral facet fractures or **perched facets** result in complete cord injury, whereas unilateral dislocations can produce incomplete injury or no neurologic deficits.

ANSWER: A

9. A 22-year-old man presents with a stab wound along the anterior border of the sternocleidomastoid muscle 1 cm superior to the cricoid cartilage with penetration of the platysma; there are no other findings. The vital signs are normal. Which of the following management choices is/are correct?

A. Admit the patient to the intensive care unit (ICU) to observe closely for airway obstruction and expanding hematoma.
B. Perform a carotid arteriogram; if it is normal, observe the patient.
C. Perform carotid arteriography, barium swallow, and rigid esophagoscopy; if these are normal, observe the patient.
D. Formally explore the neck.
E. Perform carotid arteriography, barium swallow, and flexible esophagoscopy; if these are normal, observe the patient.

Ref.: 1, 3, 4, 5, 6

COMMENTS: For purposes of managing penetrating neck trauma, the neck is divided into three zones (see Figure). **Zone I** extends from the clavicle to the cricoid cartilage, **zone II** from the cricoid cartilage to the angle of the mandible, and **zone III** from the angle of the mandible to the base of the skull. Zone II neck injuries may involve major vascular, laryngotracheal, or pharyngoesophageal structures. A careful history and physical examination are essential, even though the physical examination may be found to be normal in as many as 30% of patients with such injuries. Management of the unstable or symptomatic patient with penetrating zone II neck injuries should include securing of the airway, avoidance of nasogastric intubation, and mandatory operative exploration. Absolute indications for formal exploration of anterior neck

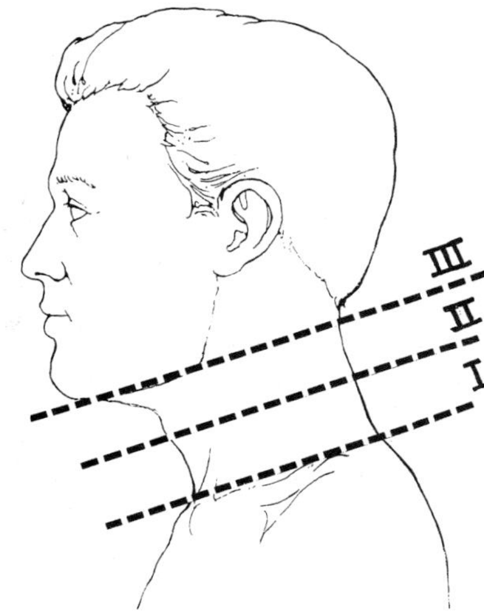

wounds penetrating the platysma can be divided according to the organ systems affected. Vascular indications are persistent hemorrhage, pulsatile or expanding hematoma, coma, and stroke. Respiratory indications are crepitance, dysphonia, palpable laryngeal injury, stridor, hemoptysis, and tracheal tenderness. Digestive indications are dysphagia, hematemesis, crepitation, and odynophagia. The management of asymptomatic zone II neck injuries is the subject of long-standing controversy. Mandatory exploration of zone II injuries, which penetrate the platysma, is safe, economical, and time-honored. Selective management requires a thorough diagnostic workup, including arteriography, esophagraphy, rigid esophagoscopy, and possibly bronchoscopy to rule out injury; thus it can be more costly and time-consuming than mandatory exploration. Neither has been shown to be superior to the other in numerous clinical trials. Four-vessel arteriography is the gold standard for assessing the carotid and vertebral arteries in the neck. If an injury is identified, cerebral blood flow should additionally be assessed to ensure perfusion from the contralateral side in case arterial ligation is necessary. Injury to the larynx and/or trachea usually manifests with physical findings. If respiratory tract injury remains a question, laryngoscopy and bronchoscopy can be performed. CT scanning is also excellent for diagnosing laryngeal injury. The most difficult diagnosis to establish is that of esophageal injury. In one study, investigators estimated the sensitivity of physical examination, esophagram, and rigid esophagoscopy to be 80%, 89%, and 89%, respectively. However, the combination of esophagraphy and rigid esophagoscopy identified all esophageal injuries. Thus complete workup of esophageal injury involves performance of both barium swallow and rigid esophagoscopy. Flexible esophagoscopy is associated with a false-negative rate of more than 50%, so it should not be included as part of the evaluation.

ANSWER: C, D

10. A 27-year-old woman presents to the emergency room awake and alert after sustaining a gunshot wound to the neck. The wound is located anterior to the origin of the sternocleidomastoid muscle at the angle of the mandible. She is asymptomatic. Which of the following management choices is/are correct?

A. Cervical spine radiography.
B. Mandatory neck exploration.
C. Four-vessel angiography.
D. Contrast esophagography.
E. Rigid esophagoscopy.

Ref.: 1, 7, 8

COMMENTS: See Questions 9 and 11

11. Soon after the patient in Question 10 arrives in the emergency room, a left hemiparesis and aphasia develop. At this time, which one or more of the following treatments should be used?

A. Continued observation and implementation of selective management protocol.
B. Repair of carotid artery injury.
C. Ligation of injured carotid artery.
D. Repair of vertebral artery injury

Ref.: 1, 7, 8

COMMENTS: Zone I and Zone III injuries represent difficult problems for the surgeon because of the difficulty of making a preoperative clinical diagnosis and choosing the proper approach to the injury to obtain adequate exposure. For this reason, selective management of asymptomatic patients is the accepted approach for these types of injury. Aortic arch and four-vessel arteriography should be routinely performed to rule out major vascular injury. Evaluation of the respiratory and aerodigestive structures are performed based on clinical suspicion. Zone III injuries, as in this case, pose difficult problems with exposure. Anterior subluxation of the jaw and vertical ramus osteotomy are two techniques used to enhance exposure to distal common carotid artery injuries. Neurologic deficit associated with carotid artery trauma is an interesting circumstance. Controversy exists as to whether repair of the injured vessel converts an ischemic cerebral infarct into a hemorrhagic infarct or neurologic improvement occurs. Several reviews of the literature and individual studies have concluded that if a patient has a neurologic deficit less than coma and is not in shock repair of the artery produces a better outcome than ligation. Vertebral artery injuries may lead to fatal hemorrhage but almost never cause neurologic sequelae. Angiography can accurately localize the side of injury. If there is a patent vertebral artery on the contralateral side, proximal and distal embolization may be performed safely and effectively by invasive radiology. If this is unsuccessful or unavailable, surgical exploration is performed, and the proximal portion is exposed at the C1–2 interspace and ligated.

ANSWER:
Question 10: A, C, D, E
Question 11: B

12. With regard to neck injuries, which of the following states is/are true?

A. The internal jugular vein may be ligated unilaterally without unfavorable sequelae.
B. Unilateral ligation of the common carotid artery results in a neurologic deficiency in 80% of cases.
C. Esophageal injuries should be drained externally only when extensive devitalization is present.
D. Tracheostomy is indicated when dealing with most laryngeal or tracheal injuries.
E. Injuries to the thyroid gland must be drained externally.

Ref.: 1

COMMENTS: The management of patients with penetrating trauma to the neck requires the skills of a surgeon capable of performing vascular, general surgical, and otolaryngologic procedures. The management of **carotid artery injuries** is somewhat controversial. Physical examination alone cannot be relied on to diagnose carotid artery injuries. In the patient who has no neurologic deficit preoperatively, every effort should be made to repair a carotid artery injury. This may include the use of a temporary shunt and vein grafting. Patients with mild neurologic deficit, as defined by paresis of an extremity, also should undergo repair of the carotid artery. Carotid artery ligation might also be employed in patients who are unstable or in whom the repair is technically impossible. It has been shown that a neurologic deficit develops in only 20% of adults as a result of carotid artery ligation. Injuries to the **internal jugular vein** should be repaired if the patient's condition allows and the injuries are amenable to repair. The internal jugular vein can be ligated unilaterally without adverse consequences, and this treatment is advised in unstable patients. **Esophageal** and **hypopharyngeal** injuries should be débrided and repaired primarily if possible. If the damage is extensive or the injury has been present for more than 12 hours, it may be advisable to perform cutaneous esophagostomy for purposes of feeding and drainage, with a planned second-stage procedure once sepsis subsides. All esophageal repairs must be adequately drained externally because anastomotic leakage occurs in an many as 20% of patients. Simple **laryngeal** or **tracheal** injuries can be repaired with mucosal-to-mucosa apposition. Cartilage fragments should be sutured in place to provide support for the airway. If cartilage is lost or shattered, a flap created from strap muscles can be used to provide airway support. A tracheostomy is performed in most patients with these injuries to allow edema to subside and to assess for stricture formation. **Thyroid gland** injuries can be managed by débridement, hemostasis, and adequate external drainage with expected excellent results.

ANSWER: A, D, E

13. A 30-year-old man suffers a stab wound to the right mid-infraclavicular region. He had a weak pulse in the ambulance 10 minutes ago, and now presents to the emergency room with no palpable pulse or obtainable blood pressure, but his pupils are reactive. The initial surgical approach involves which of the following?

A. Median sternotomy.
B. Right-sided cervical incision.
C. Right-sided clavicular incision.
D. Right-sided anterolateral thoracotomy.
E. Left-sided anterolateral thoracotomy.

Ref.: 1, 9, 10

COMMENTS: Approximately 5% of patients admitted to level I trauma units are either in extremis or without signs of life. Patients in extremis are in profound shock with respiratory depression and mental obtundation. **Emergency department thoracotomy** is not indicated for patients in arrest after blunt trauma owing to extremely low success rates. However, it may be lifesaving in patients for extremis or arrest after penetrating trauma. Clear indications include (1) severe postinjury hypotension with suspicion of cardiac tamponade or thoracic hemorrhage; (2) cardiac arrest but still with signs of life; (3) recent arrest after penetrating trauma (within 20 minutes) followed by performance of cardiopulmonary resuscitation. Relative indications include severe hypotension or arrest secondary to intraabdominal vascular injury or pelvic bleeding. Even if the suspected bleeding site is the right chest or abdomen, the first procedure performed is a left anterolateral thoracotomy. Once the chest is entered, the aorta is cross-clamped to preferentially perfuse the heart, lungs, and brain. Next, the pericardium is opened to release potential tamponade, and open cardiac massage is instituted. Internal defibrillation may be necessary. The left-sided thoracotomy can then be carried across the sternum to the right side to gain control of the suspected injury. Combined salvage rates from several series are 37% if the patient had vital signs upon admission, 6.5% if the patient had signs of life, and 3% if the patient had neither. Emergency department thoracotomy permits the salvage of 40–53% of adult patients presenting with signs of life following isolated penetrating cardiac trauma.

ANSWER: E

14. Assume that the patient in Question 13 is hemodynamically stable but that no pulse can be obtained in the right upper extremity. Angiography shows a midclavicular right subclavian thrombosis. The initial surgical approach may involve which of the following?

A. Median sternotomy.
B. Right-sided clavicular incision.
C. Right-sided cervical incision.
D. Right-sided anterolateral thoracotomy.
E. Left-sided anterolateral thoracotomy.

Ref.: 1, 9, 10

COMMENTS: If a patient is hemodynamically stable and is suspected of having a great vessel injury, an angiogram should be obtained. The choice of incision is based on the site of injury. The patient in Question 14 has suffered a subclavian thrombosis on the right side. The optimal approach for repair of this vessel would be a **right-sided clavicular incision** with subperiosteal resection of the medial half of the clavicle. Extension to a **median sternotomy** may be necessary to expose the innominate artery. The right common carotid artery can be entirely exposed through a **right cervical incision**. The distal left common carotid artery can be exposed through a **left cervical incision**. Proximal exposure requires extension to a median sternotomy. The distal left subclavian artery can be approached via a horizontal clavicular incision; proximal control requires a **left anterolateral thoracotomy** or "**trapdoor**" **incision**, which would expose the proximal left carotid and left innominate vein. Trapdoor incisions are formed by combining the horizontal clavicular, median sternotomy, and anterolateral thoracotomy incisions. In unstable patients with suspected mediastinal injury, median sternotomy is the incision for best exposure. If subclavian artery injuries are suspected and there is active hemorrhage, control is most easily obtained via **anterolateral thoracotomy** on the side of injury.

ANSWER: B

15. You are called to the emergency room to evaluate a 47-year-old man who has been involved in a high-speed, head-on motor vehicle crash. His vital signs are stable; he has multiple rib fractures and a femur fracture. A portable frontal view of the chest has been obtained (see Figure). Which of the following is/are more appropriate for further evaluation?

A. Admit for observation and a second chest radiograph at 6–8 hours.

B. Immediate aortography.
C. CT scan of the chest with contrast infusion.
D. Immediate left anterolateral thoracotomy.
E. Transthoracic echocardiography.

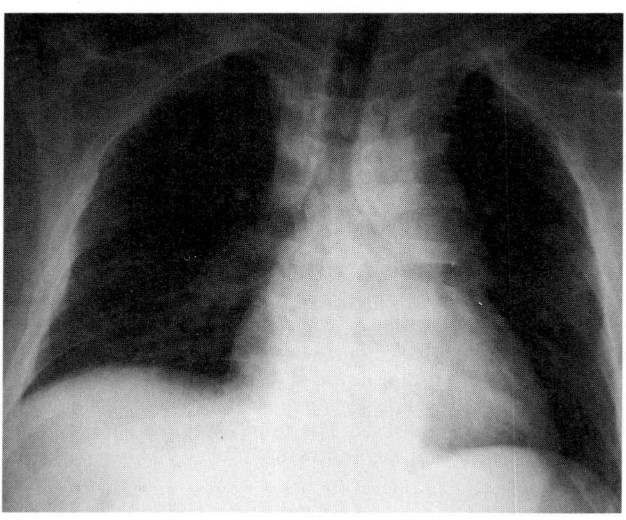

Ref.: 1, 11, 12, 13, 14

COMMENTS: Ninety percent of **aortic transections** are fatal at the accident scene. Most of the patients who arrive at the hospital with vital signs have few or no signs or symptoms indicating the presence of aortic transection. Thus a high index of suspicion is necessary. The mechanism of injury is a sudden deceleration that leads to the development of shear forces between the mobile aortic arch and the fixed descending aorta. These shear forces lead to intimal disruption at the ligamentum arteriosum distal to the left subclavian artery, which is the first point of fixation. Any patient who has sustained a significant deceleration injury, such as a car crash at more than 30 mph or a fall of more than 30 feet, should be considered at risk for an aortic transection. Physical findings of chest injury or tenderness should heighten the suspicion. The most reliable finding on a chest radiograph indicating a potential aortic transection is widening of the superior mediastinum more than 8 cm. Other radiographic findings in approximate decreasing order of frequency include indistinct or obscured aortic arch, rightward nasogastric tube and tracheal deviation, depressed left mainstem bronchus, apical pleural cap, abnormal aortic contour, left hemothorax, wide left and right paraspinal line. Because only 20% of patients with a positive chest radiograph have an aortic injury, further diagnostic testing is required to establish the diagnosis. The new rapid helical CT scanners with intravenous contrast have sensitivities and specificities of 100% and 90% for mediastinal hematoma, respectively, and 87% and 99% for aortic injury. However, arch aortography remains the most reliable test for diagnosing and localizing aortic injury and should be performed liberally based on clinical suspicion. Either routine aortography or a screening CT scan followed by aortography if the CT scan is positive should be performed. Transesophageal echocardiography (TEE) also can effectively and expediently assess the thoracic aorta. TEE has a sensitivity of 63% and a specificity of 84% for definitively diagnosing ruptured aorta. It should be considered when angiography cannot be performed. Operation on an emergency basis is indicated to repair this injury because about half the patients suffer rupture of the contained injury and die within the first 24 hours after the accident if it is not repaired. Operative treatment of thoracic aortic injury carries an approximate 15% mortality and 8% incidence of paraplegia. Immediate thoracotomy without diagnostic tests is not indicated in a stable patient.

ANSWER: B, C

16. A 22-year-old woman presents with a single stab wound to the left 5th intercostal space in the midclavicular line. She is anxious, with a systolic blood pressure of 70 mm Hg, a pulse of 130, and a respiratory rate of 34. There is no jugular venous distension, the trachea is in the midline, and there are muffled heart tones and decreased breath sounds on the left. Which of the following is/are possible diagnoses?

A. Pericardial tamponade.
B. Massive left hemothorax.
C. Tension pneumothorax.
D. Open pneumothorax.
E. Flail chest.

Ref.: 2, 15

COMMENTS: See Question 17.

17. With regard to the patient in Question 16, which of the following initial management choices is/are correct?

A. Pericardiocentesis.
B. Subxiphoid pericardial window.
C. Needle decompression of the left chest in the 2nd intercostal space, midclavicular line.
D. Left tube thoracostomy.
E. Emergency department thoracotomy.

Ref.: 2, 15

COMMENTS: All of the possible thoracic injuries listed above are life-threatening and must be identified and treated during the primary survey of the trauma victim. The triad of systemic hypotension, distended neck veins, and muffled heart tones is known as Beck's triad and is useful for diagnosing **pericardial tamponade**. However, these findings often are not evident even in the presence of severe, acute tamponade particularly if the patient is hypovolemic. Other signs of pericardial tamponade include pulsus paradoxus and the "water-bottle" sign on the chest radiograph. If the diagnosis of pericardial tamponade is suspected, diagnostic maneuvers should be selected on the basis of test availability and stability of the patient. For patients with hypotension unresponsive to fluid infusion, *pericardiocentesis* is the procedure of choice, as it can be both diagnostic and temporarily therapeutic. As little as 20–30 ml of blood aspirated may decrease intrapericardial pressure sufficiently to allow ventricular filling. For patients in extremis, an *emergency department thoracotomy and pericardotomy* may be lifesaving. For relatively stable patients in whom the diagnosis is in question, transthoracic echocardiography can quickly and accurately diagnose the presence of pericardial fluid. Creation of a *subxiphoid pericardial window* is also a useful maneuver that can be performed in the emergency or operating room under local anesthesia. Once pericardial tamponade has been diagnosed, the patient should receive vigorous fluid resuscitation and expedient operative intervention. A **massive hemothorax** is defined as more than 1500 ml of blood within the pleural space. Massive hemothorax, which may cause hypotension and decreased breath sounds over the affected side, requires prompt tube thoracostomy. **Tension**

pneumothorax may mimic pericardial tamponade because both conditions inhibit filling of the right heart. Pericardial tamponade inhibits filling by elevating intrapericardial pressure, whereas tension pneumothorax causes shifting of the mediastinum and obstruction of venous return. Before placement of a left tube thoracostomy, a temporizing maneuver to relieve the tension is to place a 14-gauge needle in the 2nd intercostal space at the midclavicular line. Patients with **open pneumothorax** are in respiratory distress secondary to total collapse of the affected lung and have an obvious "sucking" chest wound, which is not present in this patient. Likewise, patients with **flail chest** present with paradoxical motion of the chest wall and respiratory failure. Systemic hypotension is not usually associated with isolated flail chest; endotracheal intubation and mechanical ventilation are the initial measures taken to circumvent this life-threatening condition.

ANSWER:
Question 16: A, B, C
Question 17: A, B, C, D

17. Which of the following modalities is the most important for identifying a patient who will suffer complications from myocardial contusion?

A. Serial creatine phosphokinase (CPK) isoenzymes.
B. Electrocardiography (ECG).
C. Echocardiography.
D. Gated ventricular angiography.
E. Sternal films to rule out sternal fracture.

Ref.: 15, 16, 17, 18

COMMENTS: The reported incidence of myocardial contusion ranges from 1% to 76%; this range exemplifies the lack of a widely acceptable definition for myocardial contusion and lack of a reliable standard for its diagnosis. Myocardial contusion results from extravasation of blood and edema into the myocardium, which causes reduced local coronary microcirculation. Diminished perfusion in these localized areas may lead to tissue necrosis and infarction, although circulation through major coronary arteries may be intact. Hypotension or hypovolemic shock may further compromise coronary perfusion. Classic symptoms of significant myocardial contusion are limited to angina-like pain. The most common cause of early death after myocardial contusion is arrhythmia, usually ventricular tachycardia or ventricular fibrillation. Serious arrhythmias can be produced by conduction abnormalities, which consist of premature ventricular contractions, bundle branch block, supraventricular tachycardia, junctional rhythm, and first, second, and third degree heart block. The first 24 hours after injury is the time period when patients are at greatest risk for the occurrence of these arrhythmias. Late development of ventricular arrhythmias due to endocardial scars is also possible. CPK isoenzymes have been advocated as useful in the diagnosis of myocardial contusion. However, there is a poor correlation between elevated CPK levels and conduction abnormalities. Echocardiography has never been shown to be superior to ECG as a predictor of arrhythmia. Gated ventricular angiography is a nuclear medicine study that calculates right- and left-sided ventricular ejection fractions and quantification of ventricular function. This test deserves further evaluation. A number of investigations have shown that most "clinically significant" cardiac contusion injuries are revealed via ECG changes obtained in the emergency room setting.

ANSWER: B

19. A 52-year-old bank manager is an unrestrained driver involved in a high-speed motor vehicle crash against a bridge abutment. The paramedics report a bent steering wheel. Upon presentation, the patient has multiple fractures on both the right and left sides of his chest. The patient is profoundly tachypneic and confused, and pulse oximetry shows marked hypoxia. Paradoxical motion of the central portion of his chest is noted. Which of the following initial management choices is/are correct?

A. Stabilization of the flail segment by supporting it with sandbags.
B. Stabilization of the flail segment by taping or strapping.
C. Stabilization of the flail segment by means of internal fixation.
D. Use of a pressure-controlled ventilator.
E. Use of a volume-controlled ventilator.

Ref.: 1, 2

COMMENTS: In patients with flail chest, the bony and cartilaginous continuity of the thoracic cavity has been disrupted. The loose segment therefore creates a paradoxical motion as the patient attempts to breathe. The most significant injury in these patients is not the flail itself but rather the underlying pulmonary contusion. Therefore treatment of patients with flail chest should be directed toward the underlying pulmonary contusion. In patients who are unable to maintain satisfactory ventilation or who have significant hypoxia, intubation and mechanical ventilation are the appropriate treatment. Because of the presence of pulmonary contusion and associated decreased lung compliance, pressure-controlled ventilation may not deliver sufficient tidal volume. Volume-controlled ventilation, however, ensures that adequate tidal volumes are delivered to the patient and thus alleviates the underlying hypoxia. Vigorous respiratory therapy and pain control can obviate the need for routine intubation. Thoracic epidural anesthesia and intercostal nerve blockade are useful adjuncts. Few patients present with a localized fracture amenable to direct operative stabilization.

ANSWER: E

20. With regard to open pneumothorax wounds, which of the following statements is/are true?

A. If the chest wall opening is one-third the diameter of the trachea, inspired air passes preferentially through the chest wall defect into the pleural cavity.
B. A flutter-valve type of dressing may be used temporarily if formal surgical closure is not immediately available.
C. Tube thoracostomy is not indicated for such an injury because the pleural cavity already freely communicates with the atmosphere.
D. Ventilation by the contralateral lung is unaffected by this injury because the two sides are separated by the mediastinum.

Ref.: 1, 2

COMMENTS: An open pneumothorax, or "sucking" chest wound, occurs when major chest trauma produces a defect in the chest wall through the parietal pleura. If the defect is more than two-thirds the diameter of the trachea, on inspiration air passes preferentially through the chest wall with each respiratory effort, resulting in ineffective ventilation and hypoxia.

The initial management includes covering the defect with an occlusive dressing taped on three sides to allow a flutter-valve effect. This type of dressing theoretically acts as a barrier to entry of air into the pleural cavity during inspiration but allows air to escape on expiration. If the air does not escape freely, it may turn an open pneumothorax into a tension pneumothorax. Thus tube thoracostomy at a site remote from the wound is mandatory. Most of these wounds then require operative closure of the chest wall defect. Intermittent shifts of the mediastinum during respiration can cause ineffective ventilation in the contralateral lung, impaired venous return because of bending of the vena cava, and cardiac arrhythmias.

ANSWER: B

21. A 24-year-old man is an unrestrained driver in a motor vehicle crash. The patient remains hypoxic after administration of oxygen. He has bilateral chest tenderness. A chest roentgenogram shows bilateral infiltrates. Which of the following is the most likely diagnosis?

A. Bilateral pneumonia.
B. Adult respiratory distress syndrome (ARDS).
C. Aspiration of gastric contents.
D. Atelectasis.
E. Pulmonary contusion.

Ref.: 15, 19

COMMENTS: Pulmonary contusion can be defined as direct damage to the lung parenchyma from external trauma and can be caused by penetrating wounds, blunt trauma to the chest wall, or blast injury. Pulmonary contusion appears on the chest radiograph as an infiltrate that represents diffuse parenchymal hemorrhage in the involved lobe or segment of lung. As a rule, the infiltrate of pulmonary contusion is apparent on the initial chest film. The subsequent appearance of an infiltrate is usually not caused by pulmonary contusion, and the diagnosis of aspiration, atelectasis, or pneumonia should be considered. The hemorrhage of pulmonary contusion can continue for several hours after the injury, with progression of the infiltrate on radiograph. Hemoptysis is a common but not constant finding with contusion. When pulmonary contusion is caused by a penetrating injury, the pulmonary infiltrate surrounds the site of lung perforation and spreads circumferentially around the injury site. If a major vasculature structure is injured near the hilum, massive hemorrhage into the lung and the bronchial tree may occur, resulting in substantial hemoptysis. Most pulmonary contusions are benign because pulmonary blood flow is under low pressure in the right side of the heart circuit and bleeding generally stops by itself, with flow diverted to normal lung channels. Blunt thoracic trauma is often associated with serious lacerations of the lung parenchyma secondary to direct injury of the chest wall, fracture of ribs, and tearing of the visceral pleura when the lung is compressed against a closed larynx, similar to popping a balloon. Manifestations of these injuries are pneumothorax, hemothorax, or hemopneumothorax. Aspiration of gastric contents usually does not produce immediate radiographic changes and is manifested by abundant tracheobronchial secretions or bile in the tracheobronchial tree. Pneumonia, ARDS, and atelectasis are not apparent on chest radiographs in the initial trauma room setting.

ANSWER: E

22. A 40-year-old man presents with a single stab wound to the left chest in the 7th intercostal space in the anterior axillary line. His vital signs are normal, and he has bilaterally normal breath sounds. On abdominal examination, there is no tenderness or mass. An upright chest radiograph shows no sign of hemothorax or pneumothorax. With regard to this patient's further management, which of the following statements is/are true?

A. The absence of a hemothorax or pneumothorax on a chest radiograph indicates that the pleural cavity was not entered during injury.
B. The absence of a hemothorax or pneumothorax effectively rules out significant intraabdominal injury.
C. If this patient is to have general anesthesia, he must first undergo a left-sided tube thoracostomy.
D. Further evaluation must be carried out for a possible intraabdominal injury.

Ref.: 1, 20, 21

COMMENTS: Patients with penetrating trauma can have violation of the pleural cavity without the development of a hemothorax or pneumothorax. Also a hemothorax or pneumothorax may develop later as a complication of penetrating injuries to the chest, especially if the patient is given positive-pressure ventilation during general anesthesia. It is therefore advisable to perform prophylactic left-sided tube thoracostomy in these patients before general anesthesia is induced if the life-threatening complication of a tension pneumothorax is to be avoided. Additionally, for asymptomatic patients with a stab wound to the chest and normal initial chest radiograph, an additional upright film should be obtained 6 hours after the first to rule out delayed hemothorax or pneumothorax. If this additional film is normal, it can be safely concluded that no injury has occurred, and the patient may be discharged home. On moderate expiration, the diaphragm rises to the level of the 5th intercostal space on the left and to the 5th rib on the right. As a consequence, injury to intraabdominal organs or to the diaphragm alone can occur with any penetrating injury to the lower chest. In a wound medial to the midaxillary line and below the level of the nipples, a diagnostic peritoneal lavage should be performed to rule out penetration of the diaphragm. Although there is disagreement, most centers use a cutoff of 10,000 RBC/ml as an indication for laparotomy. Patients with wounds lateral to the anterior axillary line are best managed by observation.

ANSWER: C, D

23. A 28-year-old woman is an unrestrained driver in a motor vehicle crash. She has stable vital signs and left upper quadrant tenderness, but no signs of peritonitis. What is the next step in management?

A. Exploratory laparotomy.
B. Diagnostic peritoneal lavage.
C. Admission to the hospital for observation.
D. Computed tomography (CT) of the abdomen and pelvis.
E. Abdominal ultrasonography.

Ref.: 1, 22, 23

COMMENTS: For evaluation of the blunt abdominal trauma patient, the physical examination is neither sensitive nor specific for injury. However, signs of peritonitis are an absolute indication for exploratory laparotomy. Further testing to rule out intraabdominal injury should be performed on all patients with abdominal pain or tenderness, those with an altered level of consciousness [Glascow Coma Score (GCS) < 14], spinal cord injury, or unexplained hypotension. Intraabdominal injury should also be excluded in all patients undergoing general anesthesia for surgery of extraabdominal injuries within the observation period. The diagnostic modalities available to the physician include diagnostic peritoneal lavage (DPL), CT, and abdominal ultrasonography. **Diagnostic peritoneal lavage** was introduced by Root in 1965 and has been the standard for evaluating blunt abdominal trauma. Peritoneal lavage has an accuracy rate as high as 98% and a complication rate of less than 1%. The pitfalls are lack of specificity, leading to high rate of nontherapeutic laparotomy, and an inability to evaluate the retroperitoneum. For these reasons, **CT scanning** with intravenous and oral contrast has become the diagnostic test of choice to evaluate *stable* patients after blunt abdominal trauma. It can identify specific solid-organ injuries, allowing nonoperative management. It also provides excellent assessment of renal perfusion and the retroperitoneum and pelvis. Caveats include the difficulty of diagnosing hollow-viscus injury, increased time required, and higher cost. In *unstable* patients the danger of transportation and the time required to perform the scan preclude its use. Peritoneal lavage should be performed for rapid screening of intraabdominal hemorrhage in unstable patients. A positive tap or aspirate indicates the need for emergent laparotomy. Otherwise, other sources of blood loss should be sought. **Abdominal ultrasonography** can be used for the initial evaluation of trauma patients. Early data in the United States on the initial evaluation of trauma patients by ultrasonography revealed a sensitivity of 70% and specificity of 96% for detecting intraabdominal fluid and pericardial effusion. As more surgeons become familiar with the techniques of ultrasonography, its use should continue to increase in the trauma setting.

ANSWER: D

24. A 25-year-old woman is the driver of an automobile involved in a high-speed motor vehicle accident. She is 30 weeks pregnant. She complains of abdominal pain but does not have peritoneal signs. Her vital signs are stable. Which one or more of the following should be included in the workup of this patient?

A. CT scan.
B. Ultrasonography.
C. Diagnostic peritoneal lavage.
D. Arteriography.

Ref.: 1, 2

COMMENTS: Trauma is the leading cause of death in women of childbearing age. The most common cause of fetal death in such situations is maternal death. For this reason, all initial resuscitative efforts are directed toward the mother. The approach to an injured pregnant patient is the same as to a nonpregnant one. Knowledge of the physiologic processes throughout the progression of pregnancy is needed to best understand a pregnant patient's response to trauma. During the second trimester, the mother's cardiac output reaches 7 L/min and remains at that level for the term of pregnancy. Blood volume may increase by as much as 50%, a normal hematocrit being 32–36%. Because of the elevated blood volume, pregnant patients can have a 30–35% blood volume loss without clinical signs of hypovolemia. During pregnancy, systolic and diastolic blood pressures are 5–15 mm Hg lower than normal because of the drop in systemic vascular resistance normally found in pregnancy. If blood pressure is elevated, eclampsia and preeclampsia must be considered. Diagnostic procedures for the seriously injured pregnant patient must be performed aggressively because cardiovascular resuscitation and stability are essential for fetal survival. The fetus should also be assessed by physical examination as well as by continuous fetal monitoring. Ultrasonography is a valuable adjunct for assessing not only the fetal/intrauterine contents but also the intraperitoneal contents. Peritoneal lavage should be performed using the open technique, cephalad to the uterine fundus. Indications for laparotomy are similar for the pregnant and nonpregnant patient. CT scanning is generally not indicated for the workup of pregnant trauma patients because of the increased radiation exposure. Arteriography exposes the patient to even higher doses of radiation and is indicated only when hemodynamic instability secondary to pelvic fractures warrants its use.

ANSWER: B, C

25. With regard to the diagnosis and treatment of injuries in the pregnant patient, which of the following statements is/are true?

A. As pregnancy progresses the blood volume increases, and the blood pressure, hematocrit, and calculated bicarbonate concentration decrease.
B. Pregnant patients are at high risk for development of disseminated intravascular coagulation (DIC).
C. Amniotic fluid analysis is a reliable test for determining the viability of the fetus.
D. A pregnant patient should be positioned on her right side when transported and evaluated.
E. Patients who require celiotomy for intraabdominal injuries should undergo cesarean section even if the uterus is uninjured.

Ref.: 1, 2

COMMENTS: Pregnancy causes physiologic and structural changes that are sufficiently major; they may alter the signs and symptoms of injury as well as the results of diagnostic laboratory tests. The blood volume increases by 50%; and there is a decrease in the blood pressure, hematocrit, and calculated bicarbonate concentration and an increase in the pulse and the plasma volume. Pregnant patients are at risk for DIC because of premature separation of the placenta or amniotic fluid embolism, which necessitates termination of the pregnancy. Because the pregnant uterus pressing on the vena cava reduces venous return to the heart, it is best if these patients are kept on their left side if possible. If the patient needs to be supine, the right hip should be elevated and the uterus manually displaced to the left side. Aspiration of amniotic fluid enables determination of the lecithin/sphingomyelin ratio (2:1) and detection of the phosphatidylglycerol level, both of which indicate fetal pulmonary maturity. In most cases of direct uterine trauma, a cesarean section is required. Other indications include worsening fetal distress, DIC, inability to deliver vaginally because of thoracolumbar spine fractures, and the need to decompress the uterus to address major abdominal vessel injuries. In general, the noninjured uterus should be left intact during celiotomy for other conditions; the mother can usually deliver vaginally even in the presence of pelvic fractures.

ANSWER: A, B, C

26. A 30-year-old man is ejected from his automobile after a head-on collision at high speed. He has sustained a pelvic fracture and undergoes exploratory laparotomy because of a grossly positive supraumbilical open peritoneal lavage. On exploration, a contained pelvic hematoma and an expanding central abdominal hematoma are noted. Which of the following is/are included in the appropriate management of this patient?

A. Observation of both hematomas.
B. Exploration of both hematomas to clarify the underlying pathology.
C. Exploration of the central hematoma after obtaining proximal and distal vascular control; observation of the pelvic hematoma.
D. Observation of the central hematoma and exploration of the pelvic hematoma after application of external fixators.

Ref.: 24

COMMENTS: The hallmark of retroperitoneal injury is the retroperitoneal hematoma, which may be visualized on CT scan or encountered upon surgical exploration. **Retroperitoneal hematomas** are classified into three zones, depending on their location. *Zone I* is defined as the central medial portion of the retroperitoneum and includes the duodenum, pancreas, and major abdominal vascular structures. In general, all zone I hematomas require exploration, regardless of the mechanism of injury (blunt or penetrating). Zone I hematomas can be classified as supramesocolic and inframesocolic. *Supramesocolic hematomas* should be explored after obtaining proximal and distal vascular control by reflecting all left-sided viscera to the midline (Mattox maneuver). Injury to the aorta or the celiac, mesenteric, or proximal renal arteries should be suspected. *Inframesocolic* midline hematomas most commonly result from injuries to either the infrarenal aorta or the infrarenal vena cava. Exposure is obtained by opening the midline retroperitoneum or reflecting the right-sided viscera cephalad (Cattell maneuver). *Zone II* is lateral to the psoas muscle, above the iliac crest and below the diaphragm, incorporating the kidneys and retroperitoneal portion of the colon and its mesentery. Hematomas caused by penetrating trauma should be explored. There is no consensus on whether control of renal hilar vessels before opening the hematoma leads to improved morbidity and mortality. Zone II hematomas after blunt trauma need not be opened if they are nonexpanding or nonpulsatile and if there are no urologic indications, such as nonvisualization of the kidney or extravasation of urine. In stable patients with hematuria or suspected renal injury, preoperative CT scanning should be performed to define the hematoma and assess renal excretion. Up to 95% of patients with blunt perirenal hematomas can be treated without operation. *Zone III* hematomas arise in the pelvis and are the most common retroperitoneal hematoma associated with blunt trauma. In patients with blunt trauma, the hematoma is not explored. Those caused by penetrating injury often expand rapidly as a result of iliac vessel damage. Control of the infrarenal abdominal aorta and inferior vena cava proximally and the iliac vessels distally should be obtained before the hematoma is opened. Patients with pelvic fractures who are exsanguinating may need immediate operation. However, operative control of pelvic bleeding is seldom successful, and pelvic packing is usually necessary. Ligation of the hypogastric vessels has only occasionally been effective. In summary, all retroperitoneal hematomas caused by penetrating trauma should be explored, whereas only zone I hematomas caused by blunt trauma should be routinely explored.

ANSWER: C

27. A 30-year-old man undergoes an exploratory laparotomy for a gunshot wound to the right upper quadrant. A hematoma is present in the area of the portal triad. An injury to the common bile duct (CBD) is discovered with a loss of more than 50% of the circumference of the wall of the duct. Further exploration reveals incomplete transection of the portal vein. Which one of the following is the appropriate management of these injuries?

A. Ligation of the portal vein. Débridement of the duct and primary anastomosis with stent.
B. Resection of the portal vein with end-to-end anastomosis. Débridement of the duct and primary anastomosis with stent.
C. Venous interposition repair of the portal vein. Roux-en-Y choledochojejunostomy without stent.
D. Lateral venorrhaphy. Roux-en-Y choledochojejunostomy with stent.
E. Lateral venorrhaphy. Ligation of the CBD with formation of a cholecystojejunostomy.

Ref.: 1, 24

COMMENTS: Hematomas in the portal triad must be explored. Injuries to the extrahepatic biliary tract are uncommon; most are penetrating. Associated intraperitoneal injuries are the rule and determine the surgical treatment and eventual outcome of patients with bile duct injury. Most associated injuries involve the liver (78%) and major vascular structures (32%). **Extrahepatic bile duct**: Repair of this injury depends on the condition of the patient. Stenting of the duct rather than repair might be appropriate in the unstable patient. In this situation, a second operation in a difficult, scarred field is necessary. Should the injury to the duct involve less than 50% of the circumference of the wall, primary repair with a stent brought out and away from the anastomosis is indicated. Construction of a Roux-en-Y choledochojejunostomy with a stent brought out and away from the anastomosis is indicated for more complex injuries. If the diagnosis cannot be established on the basis of exploration, which may be the case with injuries to the intrapancreatic portion of the bile duct, an intraoperative cholangiogram should be performed via a needle into either the gallbladder or the bile duct. The danger of repairing injuries to the bile duct is the development of a stricture at the site of repair, as the blood supply to the bile duct comes primarily from vessels that run parallel to the duct. The key principles in the management of ductal injuries, therefore, are débridement, repair without tension, mucosal apposition of the edges, and knowledge of the duct blood supply. Stents, although not mandatory, provide decompression and ready access for cholangiography. All anastomoses to the bile duct should be drained externally because 10% of them leak. **Portal vein**: Injuries to a portion of the portal vein are treated by lateral venorrhaphy. If it is necessary to expose the retropancreatic vein, transection of the pancreas may be performed. However, the surgeon may then be committed to performing a distal pancreatectomy and splenectomy. On occasion, resection with end-to-end anastomosis, grafting, and even portosystemic shunt may be indicated even though the success rate has been poor. Ligation of the portal vein is compatible with survival in up to 50% of patients and can be appropriate in an unstable, hypothermic patient with extensive destruction of the vein. Postoperatively, these patients need massive fluid replacement because of bowel edema and sequestration of fluid in the splanchnic bed.

ANSWER: D

28. With regard to duodenal injuries, which of the following statements is/are true?

A. The most frequent site of injury is the second portion of the duodenum.
B. During abdominal exploration for blunt trauma, a retroperitoneal hematoma in the area of the duodenum does not need to be explored, provided it is small and the peritoneum overlying the hematoma is intact.
C. Approximately 75–85% of all duodenal injuries can be managed by simple débridement and closure.
D. When dealing with associated pancreatic injuries, it is not possible to resect the entire head of the pancreas without significant risk of devascularization of the remaining duodenum.
E. Some form of tube decompression after repair of complex duodenal injuries is advisable to reduce the incidence of duodenal leak and fistulization.

Ref.: 1, 24, 25, 26, 27

COMMENTS: Duodenal injuries are associated with a high rate of morbidity and mortality (13–28%). Blunt injuries have a higher mortality rate as a result of diagnostic delays. The most common site of injury is the second portion of the duodenum, followed in decreasing order by the third, fourth, and first portions. The preoperative diagnosis of duodenal injury is challenging. The early signs and symptoms are nonspecific, so blunt duodenal injuries often manifest late with signs of peritonitis and sepsis. CT scans may identify the injury by subtle findings of retroperitoneal air or fluid, duodenal thickening, or contrast extravasation. Intraoperatively, the lesser sac should be opened and the periduodenal tissues inspected for blood or bile. All central medial retroperitoneal hematomas should be explored and the duodenum mobilized by the Kocher maneuver and inspected for injury. Approximately 75–85% of all duodenal injuries can adequately be dealt with by simple débridement and closure. Segmental resection with end-to-end anastomosis is possible in all parts of the duodenum but the second portion. In cases of duodenal injuries involving 75% of the circumference of the second portion, large tissue loss, devascularization, or delayed repairs in inflamed tissues, the following techniques are available to aid in protecting the repair. Buttressing the repair may be accomplished with omentum or a serosal patch from a loop of jejunum. Diversion of gastric contents is accomplished by pyloric exclusion or duodenal diverticulization. The addition of tube decompression to simple closure or to gastric diversion is controversial. An overall mortality of 19.4% and fistula rate of 11.8% without decompression is seen, compared to 9% mortality and 2.3% fistula rate with decompression. Retrograde jejunostomy is preferred over lateral tube duodenostomy because of lower fistula rates. Other clinical reviews suggest that decompression does not lessen and in fact may increase complications following duodenal injury. Pancreaticoduodenectomy is reserved for cases that involve massive tissue destruction and devascularization of the pancreaticoduodenal complex and is necessary in less than 3% of pancreaticoduodenal injuries.

ANSWER: A, C, D, E

29. With regard to duodenal hematomas, which of the following statements is/are true?

A. The common presentation is that of a high small bowel obstruction occurring 12–72 hours after abdominal trauma.
B. Patients with duodenal hematomas generally present with peritonitis.
C. An upper gastrointestinal series can demonstrate extravasation of contrast into the retroperitoneum.
D. Associated injuries must be ruled out before conservative management is undertaken.
E. Nonoperative management with nasogastric decompression and parenteral nutrition is usually successful.

Ref.: 1

COMMENTS: Duodenal intramural hematomas generally result from blunt upper abdominal trauma. The mechanism of injury is thought to be a force that crushes the third portion of the duodenum against the vertebral column. This causes disruption of submucosal vessels and the development of an enlarging hematoma that occludes the duodenal lumen. In general, the patient presents with signs of high small bowel obstruction, including nausea, vomiting, and upper abdominal pain with significant tenderness. The signs and symptoms usually develop during the 12–72 hours after the trauma episode. Once associated injuries are ruled out by physical examination or CT scanning with infusion (or both), a barium swallow should be administered. The demonstration of a "coiled spring" or "stacked coins" sign confirms the diagnosis. This study must be obtained to ensure that there is no extravasation. Conservative management, including nasogastric decompression, electrolyte repletion, and parenteral nutrition, is likely to be successful in 80–90% of cases. The process of resorption of the hematoma may take as long as 2–3 weeks. If no resolution occurs over this period of time, surgical intervention is almost certainly necessary. The operation can include evacuation of the intramural hematoma with careful inspection of the mucosa for areas of disruption and reapproximation of the seromuscular coat, or the performance of a gastrojejunostomy. The overall prognosis for this injury is excellent.

ANSWER: A, D, E

30. The upper abdomen of a 42-year-old man strikes the steering wheel during a motor vehicle accident. Because of positive peritoneal lavage, he undergoes an exploratory laparotomy, at which time transection of the pancreas at the neck is found. Which of the following is the most appropriate management of this injury?

A. Distal pancreatectomy with oversewing and drainage of the proximal pancreatic stump.
B. Primary repair and drainage of the pancreatic duct.
C. Roux-en-Y pancreaticojejunostomy to the distal pancreas with oversewing and drainage of the proximal pancreatic stump.
D. Loop pancreaticojejunostomy to both proximal and distal pancreatic stumps.
E. Total pancreatectomy.

Ref.: 1

COMMENTS: Blunt pancreatic injuries are usually associated with liver, spleen, and/or duodenal injuries and are quite difficult to **diagnose** preoperatively. Initially, these patients have nonspecific signs and symptoms. With time, they may develop nausea, vomiting, abdominal distension, upper abdominal pain, and increased fluid requirement. Although the initial amylase level is unreliable, even if elevated, demonstration of persistent or rising hyperamylasemia signifies pancreatic injury. Computed tomography of the abdomen with contrast is poor at diagnosing pancreatic injury initially. However, delayed scans may identify free abdominal fluid, pancreatic edema, or even necrosis. High suspicion of pancreatic injury warrants operative exploration. Eighty percent of pancreatic injuries are secondary to penetrating trauma, almost all being diagnosed during exploratory laparotomy. Care must be taken to thoroughly explore all hematomas within the lesser sac or at the root of the small bowel mesentery to identify pancreatic injury. The **operative management** of pancreatic injuries centers on débridement of devitalized tissue, hemostasis, assessment and treatment of the pancreatic duct, and adequate *external drainage*. Soft closed suction drains are preferred to Penrose or sump drains. Lacerations of the capsule can be repaired with nonabsorbable sutures without compromising the duct. For pancreatic wounds with an intact duct, drainage of the area suffices. Careful exploration of the duodenum requires searching for bile staining, swelling, or edema in the retroperitoneal region; a Kocher maneuver is essential for this exploration. If the main pancreatic duct is injured to the left of the mesenteric vessels, the standard treatment is to perform *distal pancreatectomy and splenectomy*, with adequate drainage of the proximal stump. The remaining proximal duct stump is closed with suture ligatures. Nonabsorbable mattress sutures are placed across the free edge of the parenchyma to minimize leaking. Stapling devices, such as the TA55, may also be used across the parenchyma. The injury described in this question is the typical blunt pancreatic injury that results from a crushing abdominal blow against the vertebral body. This, likewise, may be treated by distal pancreatectomy. Concern about postsplenectomy sepsis has prompted interest in *splenic preservation during distal pancreatectomy*, which requires isolation and ligation of splenic branch vessels and can be technically challenging. One report found that distal pancreatectomy without splenectomy added an average of 50 minutes to the operating time. Therefore, this measure should be attempted only when the patient is hemodynamically stable, is normothermic, and has only minor or no associated injuries. Some surgeons have advocated *Roux-en-Y pancreaticojejunostomy* to the distal pancreas and oversewing of the proximal pancreas in an effort to preserve as much functioning pancreatic tissue as possible. However, this technique has rarely been performed since 1971 due to associated complications. Internal drainage of the proximal pancreas is not indicated because the proximal pancreatic duct is not obstructed. Injuries of the main pancreatic duct to the right of the mesenteric vessels are unusual but can be handled by internal drainage, diverticulization, or subtotal pancreatectomy. Major pancreatic resection such as *total pancreatectomy* or *pancreaticoduodenectomy* (Whipple's operation) are reserved for injuries that involve extensive devitalization of the duodenum and head of the pancreas.

ANSWER: A

31. Which of the following is/are indications for resection of a segment of injured small bowel?

A. Loss of more than 75% of the bowel wall.
B. Multiple injuries in a short segment.
C. Compromise of the blood supply of a segment.
D. Injuries within 3 feet of the ileocecal valve.
E. Injuries within 3 feet of the ligament of Treitz.

Ref.: 1, 24

COMMENTS: Small bowel injuries can be surprisingly lethal if not dealt with promptly. There is a 3–7% mortality rate when blunt small bowel injuries are treated more than 24 hours after the trauma. Most small bowel injuries are secondary to **penetrating trauma** and are found during the routine abdominal exploration. During a laparotomy for abdominal trauma, the small bowel and its mesentery must be inspected segment by segment, from the ligament of Treitz to the ileocecal valve. **Blunt trauma** can give rise to small bowel injuries by one of three mechanisms: a sudden deceleration that causes shear forces to develop near a point of fixation (e.g., ileocecal valve, ligament of Treitz, adhesion from previous surgery); a crushing force that traps the small bowel against the vertebral body; or a blow to a fluid-filled loop of small bowel that causes a burst injury. Isolated jejunal or ileal injuries frequently do not cause peritonitis immediately because the succus entericus that is spilled is chemically neutral and relatively sterile. It is only after bacterial growth occurs, over a period of hours, that peritoneal signs develop. Aggressive use of peritoneal lavage may help diagnose the presence of these injuries. A white blood cell count (WBC) of more than 500 WBC/dl indicates the need for surgery, but lavage may be negative in the presence of a small bowel injury if performed less than 4 hours from the injury. The findings on CT scan are often subtle and nonspecific. The presence of intraperitoneal fluid not associated with a solid organ injury, bowel wall thickening, and a mesenteric hematoma warrant surgical exploration. Most small bowel injuries are managed by **débridement and primary closure** in one or two layers, oriented transversely to avoid stricturing. The indications for **segmental resection** include (1) loss of more than 50% of the bowel wall, in which case primary closure leads to stricture; (2) multiple injuries in a short segment, in which case a great deal of operative time can be saved by resection with one reanastomosis; and (3) any compromise of the blood supply to a segment of small bowel. Mesenteric hematomas require exploration whenever they are large (>2 cm), expanding, uncontained, or near the root of the mesentery.

ANSWER: A, B, C

32. With regard to colon injuries, which of the following statement is/are true?

A. They are reliably diagnosed by CT scanning.
B. Exteriorization of the repaired segment is recommended.
C. Colon lacerations are preferentially treated by resection.
D. Hematomas of the colonic mesentery should not be opened unless expanding.
E. They are associated with an intraabdominal abscess rate of 5–15%.

Ref.: 1, 29, 30

COMMENTS: Colon injuries occur in about 18% of penetrating abdominal trauma cases and remain an important source of morbidity and mortality. There continues to be a 5–15% rate of abscess formation, regardless of the operation performed and about a 1–2% fistula rate, which is most often associated with primary repair. Colon injury may be suspected in patients with abdominal trauma and peritoneal signs or positive lavage. However, most are discovered during routine abdominal exploration for gunshot or stab wounds. Free air can be demonstrated on chest radiographs in only 10% of these patients. Computed tomography of the abdomen with intravenous, oral, and rectal contrast is advocated to rule out colon injury in patients with stab wounds to the flank. However, the accuracy is only about 85%, so these patients must also be followed clinically for at least 24 hours. During the trauma laparotomy, care must be taken to explore all hematomas involving the wall of the colon or the mesocolon to identify relatively occult perforations. The surgical options for repair of colon injury include primary repair; resection, and primary anastomosis; resection and end colostomy with mucous fistula or Hartmann's pouch; and exteriorized repair. Colostomy formation has been the standard of care since the 1950s, although primary repair has assumed an increasing role during the last 15 years. Exteriorized repair (which includes closure of the perforation, mobilization of the colon, and exteriorizing that segment) is associated with increased wound complications and fistula formation and is seldom used today. Early studies advocated primary repair for colon injury only when patients were explored within 6 hours of injury, were hemodynamically stable, had minimal soilage, required less than 6 units of blood transfusion, and had no medical problems. More recent data suggest that *all* colon injuries may be repaired primarily without an increase in morbidity or mortality, yet this method is still controversial. Most agree that primary repair should be performed on colonic lacerations not necessitating resection. For injuries of the right colon requiring resection, ileocolostomy can be performed with an anastomotic leak rate of less than 5%. For descending and sigmoid colon injury requiring resection, end colostomy should be considered, as colocolostomy in this setting has resulted in anastomotic leak rates of up to 20%.

ANSWER: E

33. Which of the following is/are appropriate steps in managing rectal injuries?

A. Presacral drainage.
B. Proximal, completely diverting colostomy.
C. Irrigation of the distal segment with saline solution.
D. Débridement and primary repair of the rectal injury if it is accessible.
E. Insertion of a rectal tube if the injury cannot be repaired.

Ref.: 1, 24

COMMENTS: Rectal injuries continue to be a challenging problem facing the trauma surgeon. The mortality rates average 10–15% and are a reflection of the particularly dangerous soilage that occurs in the pelvis, which is a relatively hypovascular area and thus poor in combating sepsis. A high index of suspicion and prompt performance of proctoscopy are necessary for diagnosing these injuries in a timely manner. Any blood on the examining finger and any penetrating injury that cross the midline in the pelvis warrants rigid proctoscopy. There are three principles in the management of rectal injuries: (1) Formation of a proximal, completely **diverting colostomy**. Classic teaching is to form a double-barrel colostomy, although a generously opened loop colostomy probably functions just as well. (2) Insertion of **presacral drains**. This is done through a curvilinear incision midway between the anal verge and the coccyx. The surgeon must take care to dissect the entire retrorectal space and ensure that the drains are placed high enough to communicate with the rectal injury. For most civilian injuries, passive drains suffice; however, if there is extensive contamination or devitalization, active suction-drainage is preferable. Drains are removed after 5 days in the absence of significant drainage. Most rectal fistulas that develop close spontaneously. (3) **Débridement and primary repair** of the rectal injury itself, it it is accessible. This can be accomplished transperitoneally for high rectal injuries (i.e., 9 cm or more above the anal verge) or transanally for low rectal injuries (i.e., 5 cm or less above the anal verge). Midrectal injuries are sometimes inaccessible. **Distal irrigation** was found to be beneficial in treating victims in the Vietnam War. Studies in which this modality was used in civilians, however, have failed to demonstrate any effect on mortality or morbidity. Distal irrigation should be used for wounds caused by high-velocity missiles, for those associated with extensive contamination and/or devitalization, and whenever the rectal vault is full of stool. Insertion of a rectal tube can enlarge existing wounds and is of no benefit if the colostomy is completely diverting.

ANSWER: A, B, D

34. With regard to splenic trauma, which of the following statements is/are true?

A. Splenorrhaphy should be considered as the first line of operative treatment for all patients with blunt splenic injury.
B. The risk of postsplenectomy sepsis increases each year after removal of the spleen.
C. Splenic wound breaking strength is identical to that of uninjured splenic tissue 3 weeks after splenorrhaphy.
D. A major disadvantage of splenic salvage is increased need for blood transfusion.
E. Nonoperative management of blunt injury is successful in 70% of eligible adult patients.

Ref.: 1, 31, 32, 33

COMMENTS: The spleen is the most commonly injured organ after blunt trauma. Splenic injuries are classified as follows: class I, capsular tear; class II, lacerations not extending to hilum; class III, open lacerations extending into the hilum; class IV, shattered spleen. **Splenectomy** is the gold standard for definitive management of splenic injury, although the splenectomized state has been shown to predispose patients to overwhelming sepsis from encapsulated organisms, which carries a mortality of more than 50%. **Postsplenectomy sepsis** occurs more frequently during the first 5 years of life, and the risk is greatest during the first 2 years after removal of the spleen. To avoid this risk of overwhelming infection and death, which occurs in 0.026–1.0% of postsplenectomy patients, emphasis has been placed on splenic salvage. **Operative salvage** of the injured spleen is successful in at least 50% of patients after either blunt or penetrating trauma and should be considered on *stable* patients with few other injuries. The highest success rate is in patients with class I or II injuries, which require only direct pressure, hemostatic agents, and simple splenic suture. Suturing of splenic parenchyma, mesh wrapping, and anatomic resection are used for grade III and IV injuries. Wound healing studies of class II splenic injuries show that the wound breaking strength equaled that of uninjured splenic tissue by 3 weeks after splenorrhaphy. The wound strength of injured splenic tissue healed by second intention equaled that of intact splenic tissue by 6 weeks. Compared to splenectomy, splenorrhaphy results in an increased need for blood transfusion, with its associated infectious complications and transfusion reactions. This point must be taken into consideration when choosing the operation. Splenorrhaphy should not be undertaken when there is life-threatening hemorrhage from the spleen, when there are multiple injuries in an unstable patient, or when the surgeon is not familiar with the appropriate techniques. **Nonoperative observation** is indicated in stable patients without associated hollow viscus or other injuries and who do not require more than 2 units of blood during the initial 48 hours to maintain a hemoglobin of 8 gm/L. After blunt trauma, nonoperative splenic salvage is successful in 85% of eligible children and 70% of eligible adults. None of the class IV and only 7% of the class III splenic injuries can be treated successfully by nonoperative means.

ANSWER: C, D, E

35. Which of the following is/are contraindications to nonoperative management of splenic injury?

A. Blunt splenic trauma.
B. Penetrating splenic trauma.
C. Unconscious patient.
D. Associated intraabdominal injuries.
E. Pediatric patient.

Ref.: 1, 31, 32

COMMENTS: Preservation of all or most of the injured spleen rather than splenectomy has become the preferred treatment in many patients with splenic trauma. Splenic preservation may take the form of splenorrhaphy, partial splenectomy, or nonoperative management of splenic injury. Nonoperative therapy for splenic trauma is the preferred management in most pediatric patients and has been successful in approximately 90% of cases. Nonoperative management of adult patients with recognized splenic injury has been more controversial, but in appropriately selected patients success rates approach those seen in the pediatric population. Nonoperative management of splenic injury is appropriate only in certain patients with blunt trauma. It is not indicated in those with penetrating trauma because of the exceedingly high incidence of associated injuries, such as to the colon and diaphragm, necessitating operative repair. According to strict selection criteria, more than 40% of adult patients may be eligible for nonoperative management. The first and foremost contraindication to nonoperative management is hemodynamic instability. Hemodynamic instability in the presence of abdominal trauma indicates the need for emergent laparotomy. Those who are hemodynamically stable should also have minimal transfusion requirements: less than one-half of the total blood volume in children and 2–3 units of packed red blood cells in an adult. The patient should have a documented splenic injury on CT scan and no other organ injuries. Most agree that grade I and II injuries may be observed, and some advocate observation of stable grade III injuries. There is also no consensus on whether the age of the patient affects the success rate of nonoperative management. However, because elderly patients may not handle the stress of hemorrhage as well, some centers attempt nonoperative management only in patients less than 55 years of age. Unconscious patients who cannot be followed clinically should not be considered for nonoperative management.

ANSWER: B, C, D

36. A 22-year-old man has an exploratory laparotomy for a gunshot wound to the abdomen, at which time a through-and-through injury to the infrarenal inferior vena cava is encountered. Which of the following is/are included in the appropriate management of this patient?

A. No specific repair is necessary because venous injury tamponade will occur spontaneously.
B. Primary repair of the injuries if the resultant stenosis will not exceed 50% of the lumen.
C. Synthetic patch graft.
D. Saphenous vein patch graft.
E. Ligation of the infrarenal inferior vena cava.

Ref.: 1

COMMENTS: Injuries to the inferior vena cava most often result from gunshot wounds to the abdomen. A major determinant of survival is hemorrhagic shock, which, if present, is associated with a mortality rate as high as 80%. Inferior vena caval injuries are most reliably diagnosed by a thorough exploration of retroperitoneal hematomas. The Cattell maneuver, involving mobilization of the right colon and small bowel mesentery provides rapid exposure of the entire infrarenal inferior vena cava. Proximal and distal control of bleeding is most easily achieved by direct pressure on the inferior vena cava above and below the injury. Complete encirclement and application of vascular clamps frequently make repair difficult because they lead to complete collapse of the vessel on itself. Primary venorrhaphy is the simplest, quickest method of repair and can be accomplished with a running nonabsorbable monofilament suture. Sometimes repair of injuries to the posterior wall can be accomplished through the anterior injury; more often it is accomplished by mobilizing the inferior vena cava sufficiently to "roll it over." A resultant stenosis of up to 50% of the cross-sectional area is acceptable; a saphenous vein patch graft should be used if more than 50% stenosis will result from a primary venorrhaphy. The use of a prosthetic graft should be avoided because of the potential for infection, especially when there are associated gastrointestinal injuries. In patients who are unstable, the infrarenal inferior vena cava can be ligated, although the incidence of late complications with this treatment exceeds 50%. Therefore this technique should be used only as a life-saving measure. Ligation must never be used to treat suprarenal inferior vena caval injuries.

Ref.: B, D, E

37. During laparotomy in a trauma patient, an actively bleeding injury in the right lobe of the liver is found. Which of the following five sequences of maneuvers to control the bleeding is correct?

Maneuver	***Sequence***
1. Perihepatic packing and closure of abdomen	A. 3, 5, 4, 2, 1
2. Pringle maneuver	B. 5, 3, 2, 4, 1
3. Temporary compression and packing	C. 3, 4, 2, 5, 1
4. Hepatotomy and selective vascular ligation	D. 2, 3, 4, 5, 1
5. Right hepatic artery ligation	E. 3, 2, 4, 5, 1

Ref.: 1, 34, 35

COMMENTS: See Question 38.

38. With regard to liver trauma, which of the following is true?

A. Nonoperative management is considered the treatment of choice for stable patients with isolated hepatic trauma.
B. Temporary compression of the hepatoduodenal ligament may be performed for up to 90 minutes without causing ischemic damage.
C. Contained subcapsular hematomas discovered in the operating room should not be explored.

D. For deep lacerations that are actively bleeding, the finger-fracture technique is rarely successful.
E. Liberal use of intraoperative packing, rapid abdominal closure, and secondary resuscitation in the intensive care unit (ICU) has led to increased mortality rates in patients with grade IV and V hepatic injuries.

Ref.: 1, 34, 35

COMMENTS: More than two-thirds of liver injuries are simple (grade I and II). More than half of these have stopped bleeding by the time exploration is performed. This finding and the widespread use of CT scanning in stable patients has prompted a growing interest in nonoperative management of isolated hepatic trauma. Numerous reports have documented its success, and currently nonoperative management of stable patients with isolated hepatic trauma is considered the treatment of choice. **Minor liver injuries** found on operative exploration can be effectively controlled by electrocautery, topical hemostatic agents, and simple suture hepatorrhaphy. Contained subcapsular hematomas discovered in the operating room should not be explored. **Complex injuries** not involving the vena cava are almost always controlled by incorporating a variety of techniques. Upon entering the abdomen, temporary compression and perihepatic packing with laparotomy pads are performed to stop hemorrhage. The addition of temporary occlusion of the hepatoduodenal ligament (Pringle maneuver) may be necessary at this time. Studies have documented that a warm ischemic time of up to 60 minutes may be performed without untoward effects. Once hepatic bleeding is temporarily controlled, the rest of the abdomen is inspected. The packs are then removed from the liver, and any superficial bleeding vessels are point-ligated with absorbable suture. For deep lacerations, the finger-fracture technique is successful on all but the most severe cases. Nonviable tissue is then débrided, and a viable omental graft is placed in the defect. This aids in combating sepsis, decreasing deadspace, and sealing small bile leaks. The use of closed suction drains allows the elimination of blood, perihepatic fluid, and bile; and drains should be placed after repair of grade III, IV, and V injuries. Right or left hepatic artery ligation is used on rare occasions when previous techniques fail to control hemorrhage. Although ligation of one branch of the hepatic artery appears to be associated with minimal long-term morbidity, its use in hypotensive patients may produce hepatic ischemia. Enthusiasm for hepatic lobectomy has waned since the early 1970s because of the associated high mortality rate and because hemostasis can usually be obtained by less aggressive techniques. For patients who are in extremis or those with exsanguinating liver hemorrhage that cannot be controlled with other maneuvers, perihepatic packing may be lifesaving. It may be necessary in up to 5% of liver injuries. Omental graft or steridrape is placed over the liver, followed by rolled laparotomy pads placed on either side of the liver defect and inferior to the liver to provide vector forces to approximate tissue planes. The abdomen is then rapidly closed, preferably with towel clips, and the patient is transferred to the ICU for secondary resuscitation, maximization of oxygen delivery, and correction of hypothermia and coagulopathy. Once the patient is stabilized, usually within 24–48 hours, he or she is returned to the operating room for definitive repair and closure. Liberal use of intraoperative packing has decreased the mortality from more than 80% to under 50% in these patients.

ANSWER:
Questin 37: E
Question 38: A, C

39. A 37-year-old man presents after a motorcycle crash. His airway is intact; his respiratory rate is 35, heart rate 130, and blood pressure 90/55 after 2 liters of crystalloid solution. He has a tender abdomen, clear chest radiograph, and butterfly type pelvic fracture. Which one of the following is the most appropriate next step?

A. CT scan of abdomen.
B. Infraumbilical percutaneous peritoneal lavage.
C. Supraumbilical open peritoneal lavage.
D. Application of external pelvic fixator.
E. Emergent exploratory laparotomy.

Ref.: 1, 24, 38

COMMENTS: Pelvic fractures may be a source of exsanguinating hemorrhage. A systematic approach with simultaneous evaluation and resuscitation is necessary. The most common pelvic fractures associated with hemorrhage are the **butterfly or straddle fracture**, which is fracture of all four pubic rami; the **open book fracture**, which is diastasis of the symphysis pubis of more than 2.5 mm; and the **vertical shear fracture**, a fracture of both anterior and posterior elements with vertical displacement of one hemipelvis by 1 cm or more. In all cases of hypotension and significant pelvic ring fractures, intraabdominal bleeding must be ruled out. Computed tomography is contraindicated in unstable patients. Diagnostic peritoneal lavage (DPL) should be performed using a supraumbilical open approach. Grossly positive aspiration signifies significant intraabdominal hemorrhage and the need for emergent laparotomy. If the lavage is negative, angiography should be considered for evaluation and possible embolization of pelvic bleeding. Hypotensive patients with microscopically positive DPL should first undergo angiography for potential embolization of arterial bleeding in the pelvis, followed by exploratory laparotomy. Likewise, an unstable patient with a complex pelvic fracture who continues to show signs of bleeding after laparotomy should be taken emergently to angiography. Placement of an external fixation device is considered early in patients with pelvic ring fractures and hemodynamic instability. Studies have shown that the use of anterior pelvic external fixation during the resuscitation period decreases transfusion requirements and mortality. Anterior pelvic fixation acts by decreasing pelvic volume, allowing tamponade to occur, and decreasing movement of the fractured elements, allowing hemostasis to occur. The fixation is ideally used for temporary stabilization for 5–7 days, followed by definitive internal fixation. Exsanguinating hemorrhage unresponsive to resuscitation or angiographic control requires immediate exploration and surgical control of the bleeding. Pelvic packing is an effective last resort but requires a return trip to the operating room for pack removal.

ANSWER: C

39. Which of the following is/are indications for emergent angiography in hemodynamically unstable patients with a pelvic ring fracture?

A. Patients with grossly negative diagnostic peritoneal lavage (DPL).
B. Patients with microscopically positive DPL.
C. Patients with grossly negative DPL and continued bleeding necessitating more than 8 units of packed red blood cells during the first 24 hours.
D. Patients with a pelvic hematoma on CT scan.

E. Unstable patients who are noted to have an expanding pelvic hematoma during exploratory laparotomy.

Ref.: 1, 24, 28

COMMENTS: In hemodynamically unstable patients with no other intraabdominal injury, control of pelvic retroperitoneal bleeding takes priority. Aggressive resuscitation and blood and factor replacement is mandatory. Most pelvic bleeding is self-limiting. However, when the patient continues to be hemodynamically unstable, angiography is considered the diagnostic and therapeutic modality of choice. Approximately 20% of patients with high-risk pelvic fractures who require more than 4 units of blood have pelvic arterial bleeding, which can be managed by embolization. Indications for angiography in patients with pelvic fractures also include those who are hemodynamically unstable with grossly negative DPL or microscopically positive DPL (this situation would not account for enough blood loss to produce hemodynamic instability) and those who remain unstable after exploration and control of intraabdominal bleeding, especially if a pelvic hematoma is identified intraoperatively. If a rapidly expanding hematoma is found at the time of operation, and resuscitation requirements preclude closing the abdomen and taking the patient to angiography, intraoperative angiography may be considered. If it is not available, the hematoma should be opened, and ligation of arterial and major venous bleeding attempted. Pelvic packing may be lifesaving.

ANSWER: A, B, C

40. Which of the following is/are appropriate management of an open pelvic fracture with a perineal wound?

A. Diverting colostomy and distal irrigation only if there is an associated rectal injury.
B. Diverting colostomy and distal irrigation, regardless of the presence of a rectal injury.
C. Parenteral nutrition and strict enforcement of no oral feeding.
D. Frequent débridement and irrigation of the open wound and cleansing of the perineum.
E. Primary suture closure of the open perineal wound after débridement and irrigation.

Ref.: 1

COMMENTS: The mortality rate associated with an open pelvic fracture is reported to be as high as 50%. Early mortality is largely the result of uncontrollable hemorrhage or concomitant head and thoracic injuries. Late mortality usually is caused by sepsis. Steps designed to avoid perineal and pelvic sepsis include diversion of the fecal stream by a colostomy and washout of any stool that is present in the distal colon and rectum. A concomitant rectal injury must be examined and dealt with appropriately by a diverting colostomy. The rectal tear may be repaired if exposure does not require extensive mobilization of the proximal rectum, and the distal rectum is irrigated until free of all feces. Presacral drains should be placed if the injury is associated with a perineal laceration. The perineal wound should be adequately débrided and irrigated frequently, with the patient under general anesthesia if necessary, and packed open for continued wound care.

ANSWER: B, D

41. A 30-year-old man is brought into the emergency room after being involved in a jet ski crash. His vital signs are stable. He is found to have bilateral pubic rami fractures on portable pelvic roentgenogram. He is unable to void urine freely. Which of the following should be the next step?

A. Wait for the patient to void urine freely before attempting transurethral bladder catheterization.
B. Initially attempt gentle transurethral bladder catheterization, but stop if resistance is encountered.
C. Obtain a urethrogram before attempting transurethral bladder catheterization.
D. Insert a suprapubic cystostomy tube.
E. Obtain a CT scan of the pelvis with three-dimensional reconstruction.

Ref.: 1

COMMENTS: Genitourinary injuries are frequently associated with pelvic fractures, especially bilateral pubic rami fractures. The membranous portion of the urethra is particularly at risk for transection in the male patient. Inability to void is one of the classic signs of urethral transection. Other signs are blood at the urethral meatus, a freely movable or high-positioned prostate on rectal examination, and scrotal or perineal hematoma. If any of these signs are present or there is a significant anterior pelvic fracture, a urethrogram should be obtained to exclude an injury before transurethral catheterization is attempted. If no injury is identified, a Foley catheter is inserted, and a cystogram may be obtained if bladder injury is suspected. If a complete urethral injury is present, suprapubic cystostomy is necessary to provide urinary drainage in the acute setting, followed by delayed repair. Likewise, a partial urethral tear, as indicated by contrast extravasation along with bladder filling on the urethrogram, is managed by a bridging catheter left in place for at least 3 weeks, or suprapubic cystostomy, followed by delayed repair. If the tear is allowed to heal over a catheter, a voiding cystourethrogram is obtained upon removal.

ANSWER: C

42. With regard to ureteral injuries, which of the following statements is/are true?

A. A significant ureteral injury from penetrating abdominal trauma can safely be excluded if no red blood cells are seen on microscopic urinalysis.
B. An intravenous pyelogram is indicated in any patient with penetrating abdominal injury near the course of the ureter.
C. The procedure of choice for injuries of the lower third of the ureter near the bladder is primary repair over a stent with external drainage.
D. An excretory urogram after ureteral repair may be omitted only if the patient is asymptomatic.

Ref.: 1, 39

COMMENTS: Hematuria is an unreliable indicator of ureteral injury, as it is absent in up to 30% of cases. Multiple-film **intravenous pyelography** (IVP) accurately establishes the diagnosis more than 90% of the time and should be performed in patients with suspected ureteral injury who are managed nonoperatively. A "one-shot" large-bolus IVP may be obtained in the emergency department preoperatively or in the operating room to give some clues to the extent of renal injury and, more importantly, document function of the contralateral kidney. It does not evaluate the ureters. Most ureteral injuries are found on routine abdominal exploration for concomitant intraabdominal injuries. Any missile tract through the retroperitoneum must be explored, and the ureter should be mobilized and inspected for injury. A questionable injury may be assessed intraoperatively by injection of contrast medium through a catheter inserted in the urethral orifice via the bladder or by injection of indigo carmine dye intravenously. Principles of repair include adequate mobilization and débridement. It should be noted that the blood supply to the ureter is medial in the upper two-thirds and lateral below the pelvic brim. Most injuries to the proximal two-thirds of the ureter are amenable to **ureteroureterostomy** incorporating spatulation and oblique anastomosis with fine absorbable interrupted sutures. Renal mobilization may be added to obtain a tension-free anastomosis. Injuries to the lower one-third of the ureter are best treated by **reimplantation** into the bladder. Boari flap and psoas bladder hitch are techniques that aid in obtaining a tension-free ureterocystostomy. **Ileal interposition** and **renal autotransplantation** are more advanced techniques that are rarely necessary. Unstable patients may be managed by **ligation** of the ureter proximal to the injury and insertion of a nephrostomy tube. This may be followed by delayed reconstruction. Retrograde ureterograms should be obtained in all patients for proper follow-up.

ANSWER: B

43. Which of the following statement is/are true regarding renal trauma?

A. CT scan is inferior to IVP for evaluating renal function.
B. Any extravasation after blunt renal injury is an indication for surgical exploration.
C. On routine exploration of a patient with splenic rupture after blunt trauma, if a nonexpanding perinephric hematoma is encountered it should not be opened.
D. Before opening a perirenal hematoma, vascular control of the renal artery and vein must be obtained.

Ref.: 1, 21, 22, 36

COMMENTS: The diagnosis and management of renal trauma varies, depending on the mechanism of injury: blunt or penetrating. The most sensitive indicator of renal injury after blunt trauma is hematuria. In hemodynamically stable patients without gross hematuria the incidence of renal injury is less than 1%. The presence of gross hematuria should prompt further radiologic evaluation. Intravenous pyelography and CT scanning with intravenous infusion reliably demonstrate major renal injury, specifically extravasation of contrast (indicating collecting system disruption) and nonfunction (implying thrombosis, vascular disruption, or shattered kidney). CT scanning clearly defines the extent of minor renal injuries and the degree of hemorrhage. **Indications for operation** on isolated blunt renal trauma include clinical or CT evidence of ongoing hemorrhage, major collecting system disruption, unresolving extravasation, or severe hematuria. Renal parenchymal injuries and minor lacerations of the collecting system generally heal without complications. The presence of extravasation is not an absolute indication for surgical exploration. Up to 95% of blunt renal trauma can be successfully managed nonoperatively. Penetrating renal trauma is generally identified upon routine exploration. All **perinephric hematomas** secondary to penetrating trauma should be opened. Conversely, after blunt trauma only expanding or pulsatile hematomas should be opened, unless preoperative testing revealed major collecting system disruption or nonfunction. There is disagreement on whether **vascular control** should be obtained before opening Gerota's fascia, the argument being that early vascular control decreases the rate of nephrectomy and minimizes bleeding while the injured kidney is inspected. In fact, initial vascular control has no bearing on the rate of nephrectomy; the nephrectomy rate is dependent on the severity of renal injury. Opening Gerota's fascia before obtaining vascular control does not increase the nephrectomy rate, has no bearing on overall blood loss, and decreases operative time by approximately 1 hour. Furthermore, if a rapidly expanding hematoma is encountered intraoperatively, a hematoma is crossing the midline, or the patient is hemodynamically unstable, the swiftest maneuver to gain control of the renal pedicle is via the lateral approach. Upon exploration of the kidney, all hematomas should be evacuated and the kidney evaluated for venous, arterial, and collecting system injury. If a collecting system injury is in question, methylene blue dye may be given intravenously and its excretion in the defect sought approximately 10 minutes after infusion. All nonviable tissue is removed, all bleeding points secured with a 4-0 absorbable suture, and the collecting system closed with 4-0 absorbable suture so it is watertight. Hemostatic agents may be used. The parenchyma is then covered with capsular coaptation or omental packing. Retroperitoneal drains are placed, especially if a collecting system injury is present.

ANSWER: C

44. Which one or more of the following has the strongest influence on the pattern of injury and the probability of survival of a patient injured from a free fall?

A. The material on which he or she landed.
B. Body orientation at the time of impact.
C. Impact velocity.
D. Age of patient.
E. Direction and velocity of the wind.

Ref.: 27, 37

COMMENTS: Although all of the items listed above are important determinants of the pattern of injury and probability of survival, body orientation and age strongly influence the ultimate outcome. Some patients suffer severe injuries from short falls, whereas others survive falls from great heights. Deformable materials allow dissipation of kinetic force, thereby decreasing the impact force. Children have a larger proportion of subcutaneous fat and more flexible skeletons and relaxed muscles and so are more tolerant of high-energy impact or falls from great heights. The most favorable survival is associated with feet-first vertical impacts regardless of surface. The probability of death is much higher in falls from heights of seven stories or higher onto a solid surface. When landing is on water from a height of about 130 feet or more, there is a significant risk of death. The direction and velocity of the wind may be factors to the extent that they influence body orientation during the impact. The most common findings at autopsy are intracranial injuries (42%) and massive thoracic and abdominal injuries. With shorter falls, injuries to the head, thoracic cage, pelvis and spine, and long bones are the common causes of morbidity and death. Falls from heights of more than 30 feet are associated with a significant risk of aortic transection. The most common injury to a hollow viscus is disruption at the junction of its fixed and mobile portions. Massive pulmonary contusion with progressive respiratory distress is also an important cause of death.

ANSWER: B, D

45. A 19-year-old man presents to the emergency room after sustaining a gunshot wound to the left thigh. The path of the projectile is in proximity to the superficial femoral artery and vein. The patient shows no sign of active bleeding and has normal pulses, no sign of ischemia, and no bruits or thrills. Which of the following is/are acceptable management of this patient?

A. Exploration of the left thigh.
B. Angiogram to exclude arterial injury.
C. Observation for 24 hours.
D. Venogram to exclude venous injury.
E. Discharge to home.

Ref.: 1, 40, 41

COMMENTS: The evaluation of penetrating extremity injury starts with the history and physical examination. A penetrating wound over the course of a major artery and vein should arouse immediate concern about vascular injury. "Hard" signs of arterial injury include hemorrhage, distal pulse deficit, large expanding or pulsatile hematoma, distal ischemia, and bruit or thrill. Patients with penetrating injury of an extremity who exhibit hard signs on physical examination should be explored without further testing unless the injury is secondary to a shotgun injury or the point of injury cannot be reconstructed by the trajectory of the bullet. "Soft" signs that arouse suspicion of an arterial injury include a history of hemorrhage, deficit of an anatomically related nerve, history of hypotension, small stable nonpulsatile hematoma, and proximity of an injury to the arterial blood supply. The presence of soft signs generally warrants angiography. There is controversy over care of penetrating injuries that are in proximity to major vessels but do not exhibit any signs of injury. Methods of diagnosis and treatment in such a situation are exploration, arteriography, and observation. Surgical exploration of the extremity vessels at risk from penetrating trauma was routinely performed from the 1950s to the 1970s. However, this approach resulted in a 60–80% rate of unnecessary exploration. This approach has been generally abandoned with the emergence of routine angiography, which can be performed with a complication rate of less than 1%. Angiography is less costly, less invasive, and equal in accuracy to surgical exploration in asymptomatic patients. Recent studies have shown that angiography performed for proximity injuries are positive in only 5% of patients. Thus most experts currently are not using proximity to a major vessel as the sole indication for angiography. All patients with proximity injuries who do not undergo angiography should be observed for 24 hours and reevaluated for signs of vascular injury.

ANSWER: B, C

46. With regard to peripheral arterial injuries, which of the following statements is/are true?

A. All patients with peripheral arterial injuries have diminished or no pulses distal to the injury.
B. If the injury cannot be primarily repaired, prosthetic material should be used.
C. All patients with posterior knee dislocations should undergo popliteal arteriography.
D. Evidence of compartmental hypertension is a contraindication to arteriography.
E. After insertion of an interposition graft, completion angiography is unnecessary if distal pulses are present.

COMMENTS: Peripheral arterial injuries may be a source of substantial morbidity and disability if not appropriately managed. About 20% of patients with serious arterial injuries have normal pulses distal to the site of the injury. Consequently, any penetrating injury that threatens the path of a major artery should be carefully evaluated. The ankle brachial index (ABI) should be determined bilaterally for lower extremity injuries. An ABI of less than 0.9 on the injured side raises suspicion of injury and should prompt further workup. Most peripheral arterial injuries are caused by penetrating trauma, and, certain blunt injuries are associated with a high incidence of vascular damage. The latter include posterior knee dislocation, supracondylar femoral or humeral fractures, and 1st or 2nd rib fractures. These injuries traditionally indicate the need for arteriography. The only contraindications to arteriography are exsanguinating hemorrhage, limb-threatening ischemia, and compartmental hypertension. In these cases, immediate surgical intervention must be undertaken. The **principles of surgical repair** of major vascular trauma include proximal and distal control of the injured vessel and repair of major venous and arterial injuries, as ligation of major draining veins can increase venous pressure and cause decreased arterial inflow, leading to thrombosis. Venous repair should be attempted first in these cases. An intraluminal shunt is placed in the artery to avoid limb ischemia during the venous repair. This procedure is also frequently necessary to allow stabilization of associated fractures. The damaged vessel is sharply débrided, mobilized, and reanastomosed end-to-end if possible. Otherwise, an interposition graft is placed. Autogenous greater saphenous vein is the conduit of choice. When autogenous vein is not available, a synthetic graft may be used for both arterial or venous repair, although long-term patency rates are lower. Synthetic grafts should be avoided in contaminated wounds if possible. About 75% of local repairs and 50% of interposition grafts are patent during the early postoperative period. Completion arteriography should be performed to evaluate the repair, visualize the runoff, and ensure that there are no concomitant injuries. Finally, adequate soft-tissue coverage is required to protect the site of vascular repair.

ANSWER: C, D

47. A 25-year-old man sustains a gunshot wound to the right thigh and complete transection of the superficial femoral artery. His injury was repaired with an interposition graft within 5 hours of the injury. Postoperatively, he complains of persistent pain in the right calf and foot, with decreased sensation. His distal pulses are normal, and his calf is firm. Which of the following is/are the appropriate next step(s)?

A. Continue observation and neurovascular checks.
B. Measure the compartment pressures.
C. Perform emergent fasciotomy in the operating room.
D. Perform emergent angiography.

Ref.: 27

COMMENTS: Compartment syndrome is a condition in which increased tissue pressure in a confined anatomic space causes progressive venous hypertension followed by decreased perfusion, which leads to ischemia and possible permanently impaired function. The development of compartment syndrome requires a relatively inflexible envelope and a cause for increased pressure in that envelope. Causes include blunt and penetrating soft tissue injury with or without fractures, reperfusion after prolonged (> 4–6 hours) ischemia, ligation of a major artery or vein, and popliteal vessel injury. The most common symptoms are pain out of proportion to the injury, intense pain on passive stretch of the muscle, and paresthesias followed by loss of sensation and motor weakness. Decreased arterial pulses is a late finding and usually indicates irreversible nerve damage and tissue necrosis. If there is substantial clinical suspicion, prompt surgical decompression is performed without delay. In equivocal cases, compartment pressures may be directly measured using a solid-state transducer intracompartmental catheter pressure monitoring system. Normal pressures range from 5 to 15 mm Hg. Pressures above 30 to 40 mm Hg generally indicate the need for surgical intervention. Angiography is not indicated when the diagnosis of compartment syndrome is considered. The definitive treatment of compartment syndrome is expedient surgical decompression of the involved compartments by liberal incision of the investing fascia or fasciotomy. The most commonly used technique for the lower leg is the double-incision four-compartment fasciotomy.

ANSWER: C

48. An 18-year-old factory worker suffers a traumatic amputation of all four digits of his dominant hand in a bacon slicer. Which of the following methods should be used to transport the amputated fingers with the patient?

A. Placed in a clean plastic bag and packed in Dry Ice.
B. Placed in a plastic bag, sealed, and placed in a larger plastic bag filled with water at 37°C.
C. Wraped in sterile gauze.
D. Placed in a sealed plastic bag in a cooling chest filled with crushed ice and water.

Ref.: 26

COMMENTS: Successful reattachment of amputated parts depends on a number of factors. Upper extremity reattachments are more successful than lower extremity reattachments, and younger patients are better candidates than older ones. In addition, sharp amputations are more likely to prove successful than amputations caused by blunt mechanisms. It is important, therefore, that the amputated part be recovered, if possible, and transported with the patient. Such parts may well remain viable for 4–6 hours at room temperature but can remain viable for up to 18 hours if they are cooled. Because it is important not to allow the amputated part to freeze, it should not be placed in Dry Ice. The recommendation therefore is that the amputated part be placed in a sterile, sealed plastic bag and transported in an insulated cooling chest filled with crushed ice and water.

ANSWER: D

REFERENCES

1. Moore EE, Mattox KL, Feliciano DV: *Trauma*, 3rd ed. Appleton & Lange, Stamford, CT, 1996.
2. Alexander RH, Proctor HJ: *Advanced Trauma Life Support Course for Physicians*. American College of Surgeons, Chicago, 1993.
3. Shuck JM, Gregory J, Edwards WS: Selective management of penetrating neck wounds. *Ann Emerg Med* 12:159, 1983.
4. Metzdorff MT, Lowe DK: Operation or observation for penetrating neck wounds? A retrospective analysis. *Am J Surg* 147:646, 1984.
5. Wood J, Fabian TC, Mangiante EC: Penetrating neck injuries: recommendations for selective management. *J Trauma* 29:602, 1989.
6. Weigelt JA, Thal ER, Snyder WH III, et al: Diagnosis of penetrating cervical esophageal injuries. *Am J Surg* 154:619, 1987.
7. Liekweg WG Jr, Greenfield LJ: Management of penetrating carotid arterial injury. *Ann Surg* 188:587, 1978.
8. Ledgerwood AM, Mullins RJ, Lucas CE: Primary repair vs. ligation for carotid artery injuries. *Arch Surg* 115:488, 1980.
9. Cogbill TH, Moore EE, Millikan JS, Cleveland HC: Rationale for selective application of emergency department thoracotomy in trauma. *J Trauma* 23:453, 1983.
10. Feliciano DV, Bitondo CG, Cruse PA, et al: Liberal use of emergency center thoracotomy. *Am J Surg* 152:654, 1986.
11. Cohen AM, Crass JR: Traumatic aortic injuries: current concepts. *Semin Ultrasound CT MR* 14:71, 1993.
12. Harris JH, Harris WH, Novelline RA: *The Radiology of Emergency Medicine*, 3rd ed. Williams & Wilkins, Baltimore, 1993.
13. Mirvis SE, Shanmuganathan K, Miller BH, et al: Traumatic aortic injury: diagnosis with contrast-enhanced thoracic CT—five year experience at a major trauma center. Radiology 200:413, 1996.
14. Vingnon P, Lagrange P, Boncoeur MP, et al: Routine transesophageal echocardiography for the diagnosis of aortic disruption in trauma patients without enlarged mediastinum. *J Trauma* 40:422, 1996.
15. Blaisdell, T: Cervicothoracic trauma In: *Trauma Management*. Thieme, New York, 1986.
16. Miller FB, Shumate CR, Richardson JD: Myocardial contusion: when can the diagnosis be eliminated? *Arch Surg* 124:805, 1989.
17. Fabian TC, Mangiante EC, Patterson CR, et al: Myocardial contusion in blunt trauma. *J Trauma* 28:50, 1988.
18. Frazee RC, Mucha P Jr, Farnell MB, Miller FA Jr: Objective evaluation of blunt cardiac trauma. *J Trauma* 26:510, 1986.
19. Wagner RB, Jamieson PM: Pulmonary contusion. *Surg Clin North Am* 69:31, 1989.
20. Kerr TM, Sood R, Buckman RF Jr, et al: Prospective trial of the six hour rule in stab wounds of the chest. *Surg Gynecol Obstet* 169:223, 1989.
21. Marx JA: Penetrating abdominal trauma. *Emerg Med Clin North Am* 11:125, 1993.
22. Rozycki GS, Ochsner MG, Jaffin JH, Champion HR: Prospective evaluation of surgeons' use of ultrasound in the evaluation of trauma patients. *J Trauma* 34:516, 1993.
23. Rozycki GS: Abdominal ultrasonography in trauma. *Surg Clin North Am* 75:175, 1995.
24. Morris JA Jr, Eddy VA, Rutherford EJ: The trauma celiotomy: the evolving concepts of damage control. *Curr Probl Surg* 33: 611, 1996.
25. McAnena OJ, Moore EE, Mark JA: Initial evaluation of the patient with blunt abdominal trauma. *Surg Clin North Am* 70:495, 1990.
26. Cogbill TH, Moore EE, Feliciano DV, et al: Conservative management of duodenal trauma: a multicenter perspective. *J Trauma* 30:1469, 1990.
27. Cameron. *Current Surgical Therapy*, 5th ed. Mosby-Year Book, St. Louis, 1995.
28. Hasson JE, Stern D, Moss GS: Penetrating duodenal trauma. *J Trauma* 24:471, 1984.
29. Stone HH, Fabian TC: Management of perforating colon trauma: randomization between primary closure and exteriorization. *Ann Surg* 190:430, 1979.
30. Chappuis CW, Frey DJ, Dietzen CD, et al: Management of penetrating colon injuries: a prospective randomized trial. *Ann Surg* 213:492, 1991.
31. Trunkey L: *Current Therapy of Trauma*, 3rd ed. Mosby-Year Book, St. Louis, 1991.
32. Lucas CE: Splenic trauma: choice of management. *Ann Surg* 213: 98, 1991.
33. Feliciano DV, Spjut-Patrinely V, Burch JM, et al: Splenorrhaphy: the alternative. *Ann Surg* 211:569, 1990.
34. Pachter HL, Hofstetter SR: The current status of nonoperative management of adult blunt hepatic injuries. *Am J Surg* 169:442, 1995.
35. Croce MA, Fabian TC, Menke PG, et al: Nonoperative management of blunt hepatic trauma is the treatment of choice for he-

modynamically stable patients: results of a prospective trial. *Ann Surg* 221:744, 1995.
36. Atala A, Miller FB, Richardson JD, et al: Preliminary vascular control for renal trauma. *Surg Gynecol Obstet* 172:386, 1991.
37. Buckman RF, Buckman PD: Vertical deceleration trauma: principles of management. *Surg Clin North Am* 71:331, 1991.
38. Poka A, Libby EP: Indications and techniques for external fixation of the pelvis. *Clin Orthop* 329:54, 1996.
39. Baniel J, Schein M: The management of penetrating trauma to the urinary tract. *J Am Coll Surg* 178:417, 1994.
40. Frykberg ER: Advances in the diagnosis and treatment of extremity vascular trauma. *Surg Clin North Am* 75:207, 1995.
41. Frykberg ER, Dennis JW, Bishop K, et al: Reliability of physical examination in the evaluation of penetrating extremity trauma for vascular injury: results at one year. *J Trauma* 31:502, 1991.

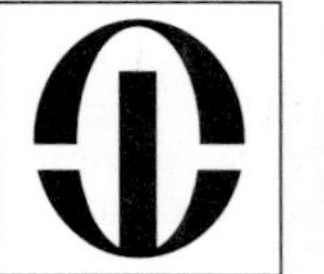

CHAPTER 13

Burns

1. Select the true statements regarding the epidemiology of a burn injury.

A. Scald burns are the most frequent forms of burn injury.
B. Flame burns are the most frequent forms of burn injury admitted to burn centers.
C. Burn injuries are most common among adults.
D. About 15% of pediatric burn injuries are attributed to abuse or neglect.
E. Burn-related deaths are highest among adults.

Ref.: 1, 2, 3

COMMENTS: Scald burns are the most frequent forms of burn injury. Flame burns, most often caused by a house fire or ignition of clothing, is the predominant type of injury in patients admitted to burn centers. The incidence of burn is highest among children under 6 years of age. During adolescence the incidence falls, and occupational burn injuries produce a secondary peak incidence among adults before a gradual decline with advancing age. Child abuse may present as thermal injury. About 15% of pediatric burn injuries are attributed to child abuse or neglect. Burn-related deaths are highest among young children and the elderly, who have difficulty escaping from a fire.

ANSWER: A, B, D

2. Select the true statements regarding the depth of burn.

A. First-degree burns are physiologically important and therefore considered when calculating the total body surface area burned.
B. Second-degree burns always affect the epidermis and dermis of the skin.
C. Third-degree circumferential burns of the extremities always require escharotomy.
D. Third-degree burns are very painful.
E. All first-degree burns heal within 2 to 3 days.

Ref.: 1, 2, 3

COMMENTS: Burn depth is important when evaluating a patient for surgical procedure and long term rehabilitative care. **First-degree** burns involve only the epidermis (see Figure), most commonly result from prolonged exposure to ultraviolet (UV) light or minor flashes, and are characterized by painful blanching erythema without blisters. They usually heal within 2–3 days. These burns are physiologically unimportant and not considered when calculating the total body surface area burned. **Second-degree** (partial-thickness) burns involve the epidermis and the varying depths of dermis (see Figure). They most commonly result from contact with hot liquids, flashes of flame, or exposure to chemicals. These burns are divided into three subtypes: *superficial*, *deep*, and *indeterminate*. *Superficial partial-thickness* burns affect the epidermis and superficial level of the dermis and are recognized by severe pain, moist erythema, and characteristic bullae formation. These burn wounds heal within 2 weeks by reepithelialization from the skin appendages (hair follicles and sweat glands). *Deep partial-thickness* burns affect the deeper layer of dermis and destroy most of the skin appendages. They are recognized by their dark-red or mottled yellow-white appearance and decreased pinprick sensation. These burn wounds usually require skin grafting because reepithelialization is unlikely or occurs slowly. In *indeterminate partial-thickness* burns, the depth of burn is difficult to assess at the time of admission. A variety of techniques to determine depth have been used including fluorescein and indocyanine green fluorometry, laser Doppler flowmetry, thermography, ultrasonography, nuclear magnetic resonance imaging, and light reflectance, but none of these methods is accurate. These burns should be observed over a period of 10 days to 2 weeks to predict the need for skin grafting. **Third-degree** (full-thickness) burns involve coagulation necrosis of all skin elements down to the subdermal plexus (see Figure). They are usually caused by flame, immersion scalds, high voltage electricity, or exposure to concentrated chemicals. The burns are anesthetic, pearly white, charred, or parchment-like; and thrombosed veins may be seen through the eschar. These wounds necessitate excision of eschar and skin grafting. Circumferential full-thickness burns in the extremities do not always require escharatomy. Use of Doppler ultrasonography has increased the accuracy of perfusion assessment in these circumferential burns and has reduced the need for escharatomy by as much as 50%.

ANSWER: B, E

3. A 50-year-old man sustains a flame burn involving the entire left upper extremity, entire anterior trunk, genital area, and half of the left lower extremity. Approximately what percentage of the total body surface area is burned?

A. 24%
B. 28%
C. 37%
D. 45%
E. 30%

Ref.: 1, 2

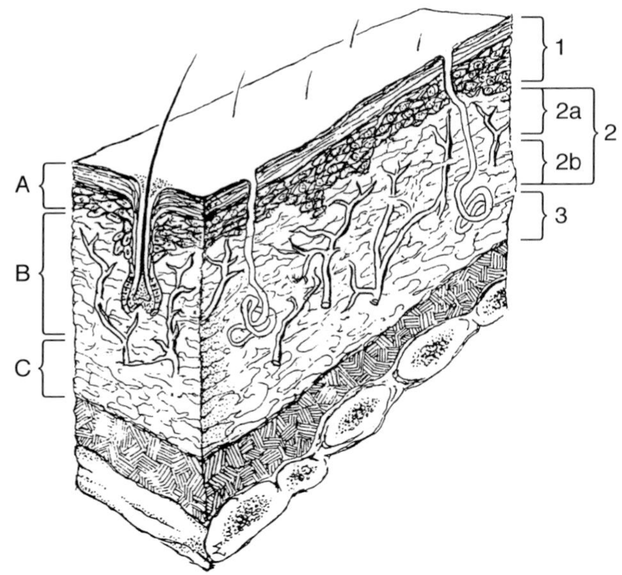

Various depths of burns. Layers of skin: A = epidermis; B = corium (dermis); C = subcutaneous fat. Depth of burn: 1= first degree; 2 = second degree (2a = superficial; 2b = deep); 3 = third degree. (Adapted from Greenfield LJ: *Surgery: Scientific Principles and Practice*, 2nd ed., 1997, chapter 12, reproduced with kind permission.)

COMMENTS: Estimation of the extent of the burn is important when determining the fluid requirements, calorie requirements, and outcome (mortality and morbidity). The initial triage to the appropriate level of medical care is determined primarily by the extent of injury. It is usually described in terms of the percentage of total body surface area (TBSA) involved. The "rule of nines" (see Figure), developed as a guideline to estimate the size of burn injuries in adults, describes the percentage of body surface represented by various anatomic areas as follows: the entire head and neck 9%; each entire upper extremity 9%; the anterior trunk 9% for the upper part and 9% for the lower part; the posterior trunk 9% for the upper part and 9% for the lower part; each lower extremity 9% for the anterior part and 9% for the posterior part; the perineum and genitalia 1%. For small burns, the area defined by patient's hand represents approximately 1% of the TBSA. It is not applicable to infants and children because they have proportionally larger heads and smaller legs than adults.

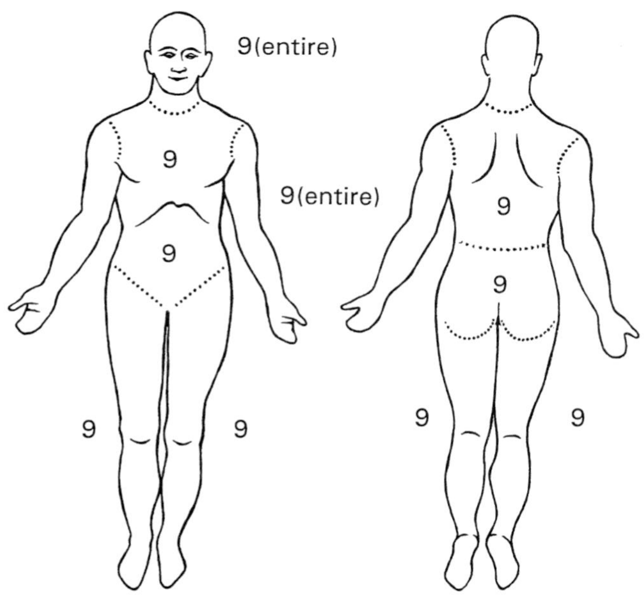

Rule of nines.

ANSWER: C

4. According to American Burn Association criteria, which of the following patients should be referred to a burn center?

   A. Second- and third-degree burns involving more than 20% of the total body surface area (TBSA) in patients younger than 10 or older than 50 years of age.
   B. Full-thickness burns that involve 2% of the TBSA in patients of any age.
   C. Significant burns of the face, hands, feet, genitalia, perineum, or skin overlying major joints.
   D. Burn injury in children with suspected or actual child abuse or neglect.
   E. Acute massive skin loss syndromes (e.g., Stevens-Johnson syndrome/toxic epidermal necrolysis, large traumatic degloving injuries).

Ref.: 1, 2

COMMENTS: The American Burn Association has prepared the following guidelines for burn center referral following burn injuries: (1) second- and third-degree burns involving more than 10% of the TBSA in patients younger than 10 or older than 50 years of age; (2) second- and third-degree burns involving more than 20% of the TBSA in other age groups; (3) burns of the face, hands, feet, genitalia, perineum, or the skin overlying major joints; (4) full-thickness burns that involve more than 5% of the TBSA in patients of any age; (5) electrical injury including lightning injury; (6) chemical injury; (7) burn injuries with associated inhalation injury, concomitant mechanical trauma, or significant preexisting medical disorders; (8) burn injuries in patients who will require special social, emotional, or long-term rehabilitative support, including cases of suspected or actual child abuse and neglect; (9) acute massive skin loss syndromes requiring burn center quality of care (e.g., Stevens-Johnson syndrome/toxic epidermal necrolysis, large traumatic degloving injuries).

ANSWER: A, C, D, E

5. All of the following are true regarding the pathophysiology of thermal injury, *except*?

   A. Increased capillary permeability is due to the direct effect of heat and the liberation of vasoactive mediators.
   B. Increased pulmonary vascular resistance occurs during the immediate postburn period.
   C. Elevated thyronine (T_3) and thyroxine (T_4) levels.
   D. Elevated interleukin-6 (IL-6) level.
   E. Decreased immunoglobulin G (IgG) level.

Ref.: 1, 2, 3

COMMENTS: Immediately following thermal injury, loss of fluid from the vascular compartment has been attributed to an increase in microvascular permeability due to the direct effect of heat and liberation of humoral factors and cytokines such as histamine, thromboxane A_2, free oxygen radicals, leukotrienes, platelet-activating factor (PAF), and interleukins (IL-1, IL-6, IL-8) from damaged tissues. Pulmonary vascular resistance increases during the postburn period, and pulmonary edema is rare during fluid resuscitation, even when large volumes of fluid are infused. The early postburn period shows elevated levels of glucagon, cortisol, and catecholamines and decreased levels of thyronine (T_3) and thyroxine (T_4). The IgG level is decreased after burn injury and gradually returns to normal within 2–4 weeks.

ANSWER: C

6. A 60-year-old, 80-kg man has sustained a second-degree burn to 40% of the total body surface area (TBSA) with a significant inhalation injury. He was admitted to the burn unit 30 minutes after the accident. According to the Parkland formula, resuscitation was started with lactated Ringer's solution at 800 ml/hr. Six hours later the patient was found to be oliguric. What should be the next step in resuscitation of this patient?

A. Swan-Ganz catheter placement and measurement of pulmonary wedge pressure.
B. Trial of small dose of furosemide.
C. Low doses of dopamine (2–3 μg/kg/min).
D. Increase in volume of the lactated Ringer's solution infusion.
E. Bolus of colloid solution.

Ref.: 1, 2

COMMENTS: The Parkland formula provides an initial estimate of fluid requirements, but the patient's response should determine the actual volumes administered. Urine output is the most reliable indicator of the adequacy of burn resuscitation during the first 24 hours. A urine output of 0.5–1.0 ml/kg/hr in adults and 1 ml/kg/hr in children up to 30 kg is considered appropriate. The Parkland formula is based on surface area and may grossly underestimate the volume of the resuscitation fluid in some situations (i.e., inhalation injury, electrical injury, postescharatomy, and alcohol intoxication). In burn patients with concomitant inhalation injury, the fluid requirement may increase by 40–50%. Oliguria during the first 24 hours is secondary to hypovolemia, and fluid replacement should be the most essential element of therapy before any other mode of therapy is instituted. Diuretics are almost never indicated during resuscitation. Plasma volume changes are independent of plasma colloid content during the first 24 hours after the burn, and therefore colloid-containing fluid resuscitation is of little benefit during this time.

ANSWER: D

7. Which of the following statements is/are true regarding resuscitation of patients with burn injury during the first 24 hours?

A. Parkland formula uses a balanced electrolyte solution and the fluid requirement is calculated as 3 ml/kg body weight per percent of total body surface area (TBSA) burned.
B. Patients with 15% or more TBSA burn require intravenous fluid resuscitation.
C. Adequate urine output implies hemodynamic stability and adequate organ perfusion.
D. Crystalloid resuscitation restores cardiac output more rapidly than colloid alone.
E. Late pulmonary morbidity and mortality are higher in colloid-resuscitated patients.

Ref.: 1, 2

COMMENTS: Thermal injury results in loss of fluid from the intravascular compartment to the extravascular compartment due to an increase in capillary permeability and is proportional to the extent of burn injury. The fluid lost from the intravascular compartment resembles plasma in its protein and electrolyte content. Because of this similarity a balanced electrolyte solution, such as lactated Ringer's, is considered an effective resuscitation fluid in burn patients. Fluid resuscitation should be started in all patients with 15% or more of TBSA burn. The amount of fluid required during the first 24 hours postburn using the Parkland formula is calculated as 4 ml of lactated Ringer's solution per kilogram of body weight for each percent of the TBSA with second- and third-degree burns. Half of the 24-hour requirement is administered during the first 8 hours and remainder over the next 16 hours from the time of injury. The kidney is the most poorly perfused organ after thermal injury. With resuscitation, restoration of renal perfusion returns to normal only after the perfusion in other organs has been restored. Therefore, adequate urine output implies hemodynamic stability and adequate organ perfusion and is considered the most reliable indicator of the adequacy of burn resuscitation. Restoration of cardiac output is more rapid with colloid fluid than with crystalloid fluid alone during the early postburn period, but by the end of the first 48 hours crystalloid and colloid resuscitation have proved to be equally effective in terms of restoring cardiac output and intravascular volume. The major disadvantage of colloid resuscitation is an associated increase in extravascular lung water resulting in a high incidence of late pulmonary morbidity and mortality. Therefore, colloid resuscitation should be avoided in burn patients until capillary integrity is restored.

ANSWER: B, C, E

8. Match the items in two columns.

Topical Agents	Characteristics
A. Sodium mafenide (Sulfamylon)	a. Limited eschar penetration, resistant organisms, neutropenia, thrombocytopenia
B. Silver nitrate 0.5% solution	b. Painful application, hyperchloremic acidosis, hypersensitivity reactions, good eschar penetration
C. Silver sulfadiazine (Silvadene)	c. Hyponatremia, hypokalemia, hypocalcemia, methemoglobinemia

Ref.: 1, 2

COMMENTS: The use of clinically effective topical antimicrobial agents has significantly decreased the incidence of invasive burn wound infection and improved the survival of burn patients. Topical antimicrobial agents act by limiting the microbial proliferation in the burn wound until burned tissue can be surgically excised. **Sodium mafenide (Sulfamylon)** cream, an 11.1% suspension of mafenide acetate, is bacteriostatic and readily diffuses through the eschar. This agent has the broadest spectrum of activity against *Pseudomonas* organisms in particular and gram-negative organisms in general. The main disadvantage of this agent is its strong carbonic anhydrase inhibition resulting in hyperchloremic acidosis. Other disadvantages include pain on application and hypersensitivity reactions in 7% of patients. **Silver sulfadiazine (Silvadene)** cream, a 1% suspension of silver sulfadiazine, is bacteriostatic, poorly penetrates the eschar, and is not painful on application. The limitation of this agent includes development of neutropenia, thrombocytopenia, bacterial resistance, and ineffectiveness against certain gram-negative organisms (some *Pseudomonas* strains and virtually all *Enterobacter cloacae*). **Silver nitrate 0.5% solution** has a broad antibacterial activity and causes no pain on application; its limitations include discoloration of unburned skin of the patient and attending personnel, development of hyponatremia, hypokalemia, and hypocalcemia. Methemoglobinemia may occur in patients whose burns are colonized by nitrate-reducing bacteria.

ANSWER: A-b, B-c, C-a

9. Which of the following statements is/are true regarding metabolism in the burn patient?

A. Postburn hypermetabolism is mediated by catecholamine release.
B. IL-1 and IL-6 are elevated in burn injuries and enhance the hypermetabolic response by increasing oxygen consumption.
C. Elevated core and skin temperature and lower core-to-skin heat transfer are manifested in postburn hypermetabolism.
D. Increased blood flow to the muscles in the burned limb.
E. The burn wound preferentially utilizes glucose by anaerobic glycolytic pathways despite increased blood flow to the wound.

Ref.: 1, 2, 3

COMMENTS: The metabolic response after burn injuries is related to the extent of burn and is manifested as a biphasic response. The **ebb** phase begins immediately after injury and is characterized by hypotension, decreased intravascular volume, poor tissue perfusion, and generalized hemodynamic instability. Histamine, activated complement factors, oxidants, and prostanoids appear to be the major mediators of this phase of the injury response. During this phase of hypometabolism, metabolic expenditure is decreased and total body oxygen consumption is below normal levels. Following resuscitation, the **flow** phase of physiologic response starts, wherein cardiac output is restored to normal, usually 24–48 hours after the burn injury. The metabolic rate begins to rise between the 5th and 10th postburn days and plateaus at levels of 2.0–2.5 times that for an uninjured individual; this is known as postburn hypermetabolism. Postburn hypermetabolism is manifested by increased oxygen consumption, elevated cardiac output and minute ventilation, increased core temperature, wasting of lean body mass, and increased urinary nitrogen excretion. Catecholamines (principally norepinephrine) are the major endocrine mediators of hypermetabolic response. Recent studies implicate interleukin-1 (IL-1) and interleukin-6 (IL-6), tumor necrosis factor (TNF), and probably interferon γ in postburn hypermetabolism. The core temperature, skin temperature, and core-to-skin heat transfer are higher during postburn hypermetabolism due to increased heat production. Blood flow to the wound increases markedly, exceeding by more than 10 times the blood flow to an equivalent area of uninjured skin. Blood flow to the muscle in the burned area remains unchanged. The burn wound utilizes glucose mainly by the anaerobic glycolytic pathway with no significant change in oxygen consumption compared with that in unburned tissue.

ANSWER: A, B, E

10. Which of the following can minimize metabolic expenditure in burn patients?

A. Nursing the patients at ambient temperature below 30°C.
B. Adequate analgesia and sedation.
C. Early excision of the burn and complete wound closure.
D. Early diagnosis and treatment of infection.
E. Use of β-adrenergic blockers.

Ref.: 1, 2

COMMENTS: Metabolic expenditure can be minimized by modifying the stressful stimuli. Central thermoregulation is altered in burn patients, with an upward shift of the temperature of maximal comfort and least metabolic expenditure; this zone of thermal neutrality is approximately 31–33°C. Nursing of burn patients at ambient temperature above 30°C to minimize cold stress has been shown to diminish the metabolic rate. Pain accentuates metabolic expenditure, and controlled administration of analgesics and sedatives reduces the metabolic rate. Laboratory studies have shown that early excision and complete wound closure reduces postburn hypermetabolism. Systemic infection accentuates erosion of body mass, and metabolic expenditure in burn patients can be minimized by early diagnosis and treatment of infection. Catecholamines comprise the major endocrine mediator of postburn hypermetabolic response. It has been shown experimentally, but not clinically, that pharmacologic blockade of β-receptors, but not α-receptors substantially reduces the intensity of hypermetabolism.

ANSWER: B, C, D, E

11. Select the correct statements regarding nutrition in burn patients.

A. The optimal calorie/nitrogen ratio varies between 150:1 and 160:1.
B. Fat is the best source of nonprotein calorie.
C. Glutamine deficiency results in atrophy of gut mucosa.
D. Long-chain triglycerides are much more effective than medium-chain triglycerides for maintaining lean body mass.
E. Overfeeding is associated with hyperventilation.

Ref.: 1, 2

COMMENTS: The addition of nonprotein calories to the source of nitrogen further improves nitrogen balance and enables more calories to be utilized for restoration of nitrogen equilibrium. The optimal calorie/nitrogen ratio varies between 150:1 and 160:1. Glucose is the best source of nonprotein calories in burn patients. Certain tissues, including the burn wound, neural tissues, and the formed elements of blood, utilize glucose in an obligatory fashion. Glucose is provided to these tissues at the expense of lean body mass if adequate nutrition is not provided. After severe injury, including burns, gut mucosa utilizes glutamine as a respiratory energy source, thereby sparing glucose and allowing it to be utilized for tissues with an obligatory glucose requirement. In the absence of glutamine administration, gut mucosa becomes atrophic. For extensive burns, carbohydrate maintains body protein more effectively than fat when each food source is used alone. If fat emulsion is administered parenterally, reduced nitrogen excretion is due to the glycerol in the emulsion. Emulsions of medium-chain triglycerides are much more effective than long-chain triglycerides for maintaining lean body mass. Accurate nutritional support is essential because overfeeding is associated with hepatic steatosis, hepatic dysfunction, and increased carbon dioxide production resulting in hyperventilation. Underfeeding results in continued loss of lean body mass and poor wound healing.

ANSWER: A, C, E

12. Which of the following statements is/are true for invasive burn wound infection?

A. Common in burns larger than 30% total body surface area.
B. Characterized by conversion of a partial-thickness burn to a full-thickness burn.
C. Definitive diagnosis can be made if quantitative culture of the biopsy recovers more than 10^5 organisms per gram of tissue.
D. Incidence of *Candida* wound infection has increased owing to topical antimicrobial chemotherapy.
E. Topical antimicrobial agents have markedly decreased the incidence of invasive burn wound infection.

Ref.: 1, 2

COMMENTS: All burn wounds become contaminated with a patient's endogenous flora or with the organisms resident in the treatment facility. Bacterial proliferation may occur underneath the eschar at the viable–nonviable interface, resulting in subeschar suppuration and separation of the eschar. In a few patients microorganisms invade the underlying viable tissue, producing invasive burn wound sepsis. The incidence of invasive burn wound infection is higher in patients with multisystem organ failure or burns over more than 30% of the total body surface area. Gram-negative bacteria, primarily *Pseudomonas* species, are the most common causative organisms. Topical chemotherapy has markedly decreased the incidence of invasive bacterial burn wound infection, but the incidence of fungal wound infection has increased. *Candida* species is the most common fungus colonizing burn wounds but rarely causes burn wound sepsis. Invasive burn wound infection is characterized by conversion of a second-degree burn to a full-thickness burn, focal dark-brown to black discoloration of the wound, and unexpectedly rapid eschar separation. Invasive burn infection can be definitively diagnosed by wound biopsy, and the single most important criterion is the presence of microorganisms in unburned viable tissue. The presence of more than 10^5 organisms per gram of tissue is highly suggestive but not diagnostic of invasive burn wound infection.

ANSWER: A, B, D, E

13. Select the true statements regarding infection in the burn patient.

A. Infection is the most frequent cause of death in burn patients.
B. Cell-mediated immunity is not altered in major burn injuries.
C. Hematogenous pneumonia is the most common pulmonary infection in burn patients.
D. Diminished granulocyte chemotaxis is an important factor in burn infection.
E. Suppurative thrombophlebitis can be a major source of sepsis.

Ref.: 1, 2, 3

COMMENTS: The incidence of invasive burn wound infection has been significantly reduced owing to topical antimicrobials, but infection in other organs and tissues is still common and is the most frequent cause of death in burn patients. Bronchopneumonia has replaced hematogenous pneumonia as the most common form of pulmonary infection in burn patients. The decrease in the incidence of invasive burn wound infection has significantly reduced the incidence of hematogenous pneumonia. Suppurative thrombophlebitis is also a major source of sepsis in burn patients and can occur in any previously cannulated peripheral or even central vein. In major burns, a high incidence of infection is due to destruction of the mechanical barrier of the skin and global immunosuppresion. Circulating phagocytes, principally neutrophils and macrophages, demonstrates major alterations in function. Granulocytes show diminished chemotaxis and decreased bactericidal activity due to intracellular elevation of 3,5-cyclic AMP. Cell-mediated immunity is also impaired after major burn injury as evidenced by prolonged skin allograft survival.

ANSWER: A, D, E

14. Which of the following statements is/are true regarding administration of antibiotics to burn patients?

A. Prophylactic systemic antibiotics are indicated in patients with extensive burns.
B. With invasive burn wound sepsis, systemic antibiotics should not be instituted before culture and sensitivity results are available.
C. Positive wound cultures should be treated with systemic antibiotics.
D. Antibiotics effective against anaerobic organisms are always indicated for burn wound sepsis.
E. Subtherapeutic serum antibiotic levels are common in burn patients.

Ref.: 1, 2

COMMENTS: Prophylactic antibiotics have no role in the treatment of burns, and their use results in emergence of multiple antibiotic-resistant organisms. Antibiotics should be used only for a documented infection or presumed sepsis. Positive wound cultures do not necessarily indicate infection but reflect the organism likely responsible if infection is present. In patients with invasive burn wound sepsis, systemic antibiotics should be instituted before culture and sensitivity results are available, with the choice of antibiotics based on the sensitivity patterns of microbial flora resident in the burn center as determined by the microbial surveillance program. Antibiotics are adjusted as necessary when culture and sensitivity results are available. Anaerobic infection almost never occurs in burned patients, but anaerobic coverage is indicated rarely in patients with severe muscle necrosis or associated intraabdominal infection. Burn patients have altered pharmacokinetics of antibiotics, especially among those predominantly excreted by the kidney, resulting in lower serum levels, when the usual recommended dosage is employed.

ANSWER: E

15. Which of the following statements is/are true regarding burn wound excision?

A. Excision is indicated for deep partial-thickness and full-thickness burn wounds.
B. Early excision and closure of burn wounds has been shown to reduce the incidence of invasive burn wound infection, shorten the hospital stay, reduce pain, and improve functional recovery.
C. Excision should be performed after successful fluid resuscitation.
D. Tangential excision involves sequential excision of the eschar down to bleeding, viable tissue.
E. Excision of more than 10% of the total body surface area (TBSA) as a single procedure is associated with significant morbidity.

Ref.: 1, 2

COMMENTS: Excision of the burn wound is indicated for deep partial-thickness and full-thickness burn wounds. Early excision and closure of burn wounds decreases the incidence of invasive burn wound infection, shortens the hospital stay, reduces pain, and improves functional recovery. Excision should be performed after successful fluid resuscitation. The two most common techniques of excision include tangential excision and fascial excision. Tangential excision involves sequential excision of the eschar down to bleeding, viable tissue using a guarded dermatome. Intraoperative hemorrhage may be profuse with tangential excision, so the excision should be limited to a maximum of 20% of the TBSA, 2 hours of operating time, or blood loss equivalent to the patient's blood volume. Fascial excision is usually performed for very deep full-thickness burns and involves excision of eschar above the deep fascia.

ANSWER: A, B, C, D

16. Which of the following statements is/are true regarding burn wound closure?

A. Split-thickness autograft is contraindicated if wound culture is positive for β-hemolytic streptococci.
B. Xenograft is the most frequently used and effective biologic dressing when an autograft is not available.
C. Allograft dressings promote bacterial proliferation.
D. Cultured autologous keratinocyte sheets can be used for permanent wound coverage with good results.
E. Dermal substitutes provide better temporary wound coverage than biologic dressings.

Ref.: 1, 2, 3

COMMENTS: The goal of burn wound care is timely, definitive closure. After excision the wound is immediately covered with a split-thickness autograft. A split-thickness autograft is contraindicated if the surface bacterial count is more than 10^5 organisms per square centimeter of wound surface or β-hemolytic streptococci are cultured from the wound. For large burns, closure of the wound is limited by available autograft, so a biologic dressing such as cadaver cutaneous homograft (also called allograft) and xenograft (commonly porcine skin) are used for temporary wound closure. The homograft is the dressing of choice when an autograft is not available and is the most frequently used biologic dressing. Cutaneous homograft limits bacterial proliferation in the burn wound, prevents wound desiccation, promotes maturation of granulation tissue, prevents exudative protein and red blood cell loss, decreases wound pain, diminishes evaporative water loss thus decreasing heat loss, and promotes maturation of granulation tissue. Xenograft is less effective as a biologic dressing and allows survival of greater numbers of subgraft bacteria, presumably because such tissue is not vascularized by the host. Cultured autologous keratinocytes sheets have been used for definitive coverage of extensive burn wounds, but these wounds are susceptible to microbial lysis, mechanical trauma, and development of wound contraction and scar formation. Clinical experience with dermal subsitutes such as Biobrane (collagen gel dermal analogue plus a Silastic epidermal analogue) and acellular allodermis has been limited, and their beneficial effects over biologic dressing have not been established.

ANSWER: A

17. Select the true statements regarding inhalation injury.

A. Presence of carbonaceous sputum is a specific sign of inhalation injury.
B. Normal carbon monoxide level on admission excludes inhalation injury.
C. Chest radiography is sensitive for diagnosing inhalation injury.
D. Combined fiberoptic bronchoscopy and ^{133}Xe ventilation-perfusion lung scan has a diagnostic accuracy of more than 96%.
E. Pulmonary infection is the most frequent cause of morbidity and mortality with inhalation injury.

Ref.: 1, 2, 3

COMMENTS: Inhalation injury is defined as a chemical tracheobronchitis and acute pneumonitis caused by inhalation of smoke and other irritative products of combustion. The extent of injury depends on the composition of inhaled gases, size of particulates, duration of toxicant exposure, and quantity of concomitant fluid administration. The pathophysiology of inhalation injury includes (1) carbon monoxide poisoning leading to functional anemia, (2) upper airway obstruction secondary to progressive edema, (3) reactive bronchospasm from aerosolized irritants, (4) small airway occlusion initially from edema and subsequently from sloughed endotracheal debris and loss of ciliary clearance mechanism, (5) microatelectasis from loss of surfactant and alveolar edema, and (6) interstitial and alveolar edema secondary to loss of capillary integrity. The main physiologic consequences are upper and lower airway obstruction, increased airway resistance, decreased compliance, an increase of the deadspace/tidal volume ratio, and intrapulmonary shunting. It should be suspected in any patient with burn in a closed space or burn during a period of impaired mentation. Head and neck burns and singed nasal vibrissae are commonly present but are nonspecific. The presence of carbonaceous sputum is the most specific sign of inhalation injury. Other signs include hoarseness, stridor, bronchorrhea, and wheezing. A baseline carbon monoxide level should be determined in all fire victims. A normal carbon monoxide level does not exclude inhalation injury, but a high level reflects significant inhalation injury. The ^{133}Xe ventilation-perfusion lung scan has an accuracy of more than 90% and can be used in patients suspected of inhalation injury. Fiberoptic bronchoscopy is the most reliable modality for the diagnosis and management of inhalation injury and can be performed at the bedside after the patient has been stabilized; combined with a ^{133}Xe ventilation-perfusion lung scan, it provides a diagnostic accuracy of more than 96%. Positive findings of inhalation injury in bronchoscopy include erythema of mucosa, blebs, ulceration, bronchorrhea, or carbonaceous material in the infraglottic airway. Pulmonary infection is the most frequent cause of morbidity and mortality after an inhalation injury.

ANSWER: A, D, E

18. Select the correct statements regarding electrical injury.

A. Depth of tissue injury is related to density and duration of the current flow.
B. High-voltage electric injury results in more severe injury to the trunk than the extremities.
C. Risk of acute renal failure is relatively high with an electrical injury due to myoglobinuria and underestimation of fluid needs.
D. Incidence of cholelithiasis is high in patients after electrical injury.
E. With a lightning injury cardiopulmonary arrest is common, and burns are characteristically superficial.

Ref.: 1,2, 3

COMMENTS: Electrical and lightning injuries cause more than 1000 deaths each year in the United States. Tissue damage is due to conversion of electrical energy to thermal energy. Electricity causes injury by direct contact, conduction, arc, and secondary ignition. Injury by line voltage above 1000 volts is designated as high voltage injury. The depth of tissue damage is related to the density and duration of current flow through the tissues. Current density is higher in the body part with smaller cross-sectional areas (e.g., an extremity) than with larger cross-sectional areas (e.g., the trunk), resulting in more severe tissue injury to the extremity than the trunk in high-voltage injuries. Patients with high-voltage injury require a complete trauma evaluation, cardiac monitoring because of the high frequency of cardiopulmonary arrest and arrhythmia, serial evaluation of extremities involved for compartment syndrome, and urine monitoring for myoglobinuria. The risk of acute renal failure is high in electrical burn patients because of myoglobinuria from muscle injury and underestimation of the fluid requirement due to misleadingly small cutaneous lesions overlying an area of devitalized tissue. Complications following electrical injury include polyneuritis, quadriplegia, hemiplegia, transverse myelitis, cataracts, liver necrosis, intestinal perforation, focal pancreatic necrosis, and focal gallbladder necrosis. An increased incidence of cholelithiasis has been reported to occur within 2 years of electrical injury. Lightning injury, an unusual form of electrical injury, commonly produces immediate cardiopulmonary arrest due to electrical paralysis of the brain stem, and burns are characteristically superficial and present with a serpiginous and arborizing pattern.

ANSWER: A, C, D, E

19. Which of the following statements is/are true regarding chemical injuries?

A. Immediate wound care involves application of a neutralizing agent.
B. Acid burns cause liquefaction necrosis.
C. Alkali burns produce deeper injuries than acid burns.
D. Hydrofluoric acid burn is treated with local calcium gluconate gel.
E. Coal tar burn is best treated with immediate application of a petroleum-based ointment.

Ref.: 1, 2

COMMENTS: Chemical burns are produced by thermal energy released during the reaction of strong acids or strong bases with viable tissues. Other mechanisms of local tissue damage include liquefaction necrosis caused by strong alkalis, depilation caused by petroleum products, and vesicle formation by vesicant gases. Immediate wound care is the most important aspect in chemical injuries and includes copious irrigation with water or saline to remove or dilute the chemical agents to prevent further skin damage or absorption. For ordinary acids, irrigation should be performed for at least 30–60 minutes, whereas for alkali burns prolonged irrigation is required. Application of neutralizing agent is not indicated because it may accentuate the tissue damage by generating heat. An acid burn causes coagulation necrosis of tissue and the coagulated tissue acts as a barrier for further acid penetration. In contrast, an alkali burn causes liquefaction necrosis; thus there is no barrier of coagulated tissue resulting in more invasive injury. Hydrofluoric acid, an occupational hazard, is a highly corrosive acid that produces deep tissue injury. The hydrogen ions of hydrofluoric acid produce coagulation necrosis, and free fluoride ions cause liquefaction and penetrate deeply to form salts with calcium and magnesium. Administration of calcium gluconate is the most effective treatment for relieving pain and terminating the invasive tissue destruction. It reacts with hydrofluoric acid to form inactive calcium fluoride and can be used by local application as a gel, a local injection, or regional intravenous perfusion. Hot coal tar causes direct thermal injury. Immediate cooling of tar with cold water is the most important treatment, and any attempt to remove the adherent tar may accentuate the cutaneous injury. After cooling, adherent tar should be covered with petroleum-based ointment to solubilize the tar and facilitate removal.

ANSWER: C, D

20. Select the true statements regarding postburn sequelae.

A. All second- and third-degree burns produce permanent scarring.
B. The incidence of hypertrophic scar formation is less after excision and skin grafting than with wounds that heal spontaneously.
C. Hypertrophic scars are best treated by early excision and wound closure.
D. Burn scar hypopigmentation and irregularities can be significantly improved by dermabrasion and thin split-thickness skin grafting.
E. Basal cell carcinoma is the most common carcinoma in an old burn scar.

Ref.: 1, 2

COMMENTS: All second- and third-degree burns produce permanent scarring. Hypertrophic scar formation, one of the most troublesome sequelae of cutaneous burns, typically develops in deep partial-thickness and third-degree burns that heal spontaneously. Hypertrophy after excision and skin grafting occurs less frequently and is dependent on the time from injury to excision, the involved anatomic part, and the surgical technique employed. Hypertrophic scars are best treated with elastic garments until the scar matures (3–6 months in adults and up to 4 years in children), followed by excision and skin grafting of the residual scar. Many burn wounds heal with hypopigmentation and irregular scar formation, which can be significantly improved by dermabrasion and thin split-thickness skin grafting. Malignancy is a rare complication in unstable burn scars and is referred as a Marjolin ulcer. The latent period for malignant change ranges from 1 to 75 years, with a mean of approximately 35 years. Although basal cell carcinoma has been described in old burn scars, they are exceedingly rare, and most Marjolin's ulcers are squamous cell carcinomas.

ANSWER: A, B, D

REFERENCES

1. Schwartz SI, Shires GT, Spencer FC: *Principles of Surgery*, 7th ed. McGraw Hill, New York, 1999.
2. Sabiston DC Jr: *Textbook of Surgery*, 15th ed. WB Saunders, Philadelphia, 1997.
3. Greenfield LJ: *Surgery: Scientific Principles and Practice*, 2nd ed. Lippincott-Raven, New York, 1997.

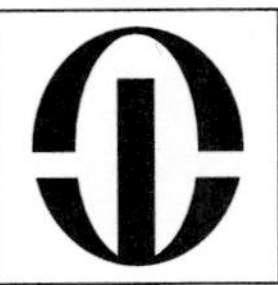

CHAPTER 14

Surgical Infections

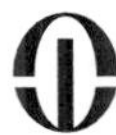

1. Bacterial factors that aid in the development of infection in surgical wounds include which of the following?

A. A thick capsule around certain bacteria that inhibits phagocytosis.
B. Surface components on gram-negative bacteria (endotoxin or lipopolysaccharide) that are toxic.
C. The ability of a microbe to produce an exotoxin.
D. The presence of *Staphylococcus epidermidis* from a clean wound at the time of closure.
E. All of the above.

Ref.: 1

COMMENTS: Although the presence of bacteria in a wound is a prerequisite for infection, most clean wounds usually contain skin bacteria such as *Staphylococcus epidermidis* at the time of closure. A thick microbial capsule (*Klebsiella* and *Streptococcus pneumoniae*) can inhibit phagocytosis and resist intracellular destruction. Surface components in gram-negative bacteria can be toxic (endotoxin and lipopolysaccharide) by inhibiting phagocytosis. Other bacteria (*Clostridium* and streptococci) produce exotoxins, which require smaller inocula and shorter incubation times (within 24 hours) before becoming severe life-threatening infections.

ANSWER: A, B, C

2. With regard to bacteremia, which of the following statements is/are true?

A. Bacteremia seldom, if ever, occurs in the absence of a preexisting clinical infection.
B. Bacteria usually persist in the bloodstream for several hours, allowing colonization of numerous organs and subsequent disseminated sepsis.
C. Bacteremic patients who are not receiving appropriate antibiotics show clinical signs of toxemia or septicemia.
D. Bacteremia from an occult source is a possible etiologic factor in the development of isolated infections in internal organs.

Ref.: 2

COMMENTS: Bacteremia is defined simply as the presence of bacteria in the circulating blood. Although the release of bacterial toxins or bacteria in sufficiently large numbers may produce signs of septicemia, it is likely that most bacteremia episodes are asymptomatic. Normal individuals probably have frequent episodes of asymptomatic bacteremia. In immunocompetent patients, humoral and cellular immune mechanisms are quite effective in ridding the blood of bacteria within a short time. Occult sources, such as dental procedures, insignificant traumatic wounds, and even breaks in the anal skin during defecation, may lead to transient episodes of bacteremia that usually have no clinical significance. On occasion, blood-borne bacteria colonize and infect internal organs, causing serious clinical infections (e.g., osteomyelitis, brain abscess, pyelonephritis, bacterial endocarditis).

ANSWER: D

3. Review of a patient's clinical course reveals that at approximately 4 o'clock every afternoon the patient develops an abrupt temperature elevation to 39.5°C and a chill. Which of the following times would be the best time to draw blood for culture from this patient?

A. During the febrile period.
B. One hour before the anticipated temperature elevation and chill.
C. One hour after the return of the temperature to normal.
D. At random.

Ref.: 1, 2

COMMENTS: Systemic manifestations of bacteremia, which include abrupt temperature elevations and chills, may occur as much as 30–90 minutes after bacteria enter the bloodstream. Because circulating phagocytes usually are quite effective in removing these bacteria, blood drawn during the chill are frequently culture-negative. If there is a time pattern to the chill and fever, the likelihood of obtaining a positive blood culture increases if it is obtained approximately 1 hour before the anticipated fever.

ANSWER: B

4. With regard to the role of immunotherapy in the treatment of septic shock, which of the following statements is/are true?

A. Endotoxin is the lipopolysaccharide component of gram-positive bacterial cell walls.
B. Endotoxin triggers the release of interleukin-1 (IL-1), IL-6, and tumor necrosis factor (TNF) from macrophages.
C. The lipid A region of endotoxin is primarily responsible for the initiation of sepsis.

D. Antibodies directed against TNF may be beneficial in the treatment of septic shock.

Ref.: 1, 2, 3, 4, 5

COMMENTS: Gram-negative bacterial septic syndrome is caused principally by endotoxin, the lipopolysaccharide component of gram-negative bacterial cell walls. Endotoxin binds to an acute-phase protein manufactured by the liver, forming a complex that binds to macrophages and initiates the release of cytokines IL-1, IL-6, and, most important, TNF. TNF/cachectin is an important mediator in the severe systemic effects seen in septic patients: fever, cardiac depression, acute respiratory distress syndrome, and hypotension. Endotoxin is composed of an "O" side chain, a polysaccharide core, and a lipid A region. The lipid A region of endotoxin plays a central role in sepsis and is highly conserved (identical) among gram-negative bacteria. Current immunotherapeutic phase II and III trials are directed at inactivation of the lipid A region of lipopolysaccharides or the initial mediators of sepsis, such as TNF. At present, results of phase III trials examining antiendotoxin monoclonal immunoglobulin M (IgM) antibodies (E5 or HA-1A) for treatment of patients with gram-negative sepsis suggest beneficial effects; however, these antibodies have not conclusively improved survival rates. The mainstay of support and therapy for septic shock remains removal of the septic focus, administration of antibiotics, and cardiopulmonary support.

ANSWER: B, C, D

5. With regard to anaerobic bacterial infections, which of the following statements is/are true?

A. Anaerobic bacteria are common inhabitants of skin and mucous membranes.
B. *Bacteroides* species are the most common isolates in anaerobic infections.
C. If appropriate cultures are obtained, anaerobes are found in only 20% of intraabdominal abscesses.
D. Proper treatment of anaerobic infections consists of surgical drainage, débridement of necrotic tissue, and appropriate antibiotic therapy.

Ref.: 1, 2

COMMENTS: Anaerobic bacteria are found as normal flora on the skin and mucous membranes and, in fact, outnumber aerobic organisms by more than 10:1 in the oral cavity and by more than 1000:1 in the colon. It is not surprising, therefore, that anaerobes are cultured from up to 90% of intraabdominal abscesses. The most common pathogens in this group are the *Bacteroides* species. *Bacteroides fragilis* is an important copathogen in the pathogenesis of intraabdominal abscess. As with most serious infections, proper treatment involves appropriate drainage of abscesses and débridement of devitalized tissue when present, as well as appropriate antibiotic therapy.

ANSWER: A, B, D

6. With regard to methicillin-resistant *Staphylococcus aureus*, which of the following statements is/are true?

A. Methicillin-resistant *S. aureus* (MRSA) is a common nosocomial pathogen.
B. Treatment of choice is vancomycin.
C. MRSA is more virulent than methicillin-sensitive *S. aureus*.
D. Hospitalized patients colonized with MRSA require glove isolation.
E. All the above.

Ref.: 1, 2, 6, 7

COMMENTS: The pyogenic cocci, staphylococci, are the most common cause of nosocomial infections in surgical patients. Both *S. aureus* and *S. epidermidis* are facultative anaerobes; those producing coagulase are termed *S. aureus*. The virulence of MRSA is identical to that of methicillin-sensitive *S. aureus*, but treatment with vancomycin is required. There is no significant increase in mortality rates from infections caused by MRSA. Hospitalized patients colonized with MRSA require glove isolation to avoid spreading the bacteria to other patients.

ANSWER: A, B, D

7. Match each statement in the left column with the appropriate description in the right column.

A. All microorganisms are killed	a. Antiseptic
B. Pathogenic organisms on the body are killed or their is growth inhibited	b. Disinfectant
C. Pathogenic organisms on inanimate objects are killed	c. Sterilization

Ref.: 2

COMMENTS: The safety of modern surgery is enhanced by the ability to reduce the number of bacteria in the vicinity of the operative field. An **antiseptic** is a chemical agent that either kills or inhibits the growth of pathogenic organisms. By custom and law, this term refers only to agents applied to the body. A **disinfectant** is a chemical used on inanimate objects to kill pathogenic organisms. Not all organisms are necessarily killed by antiseptic and disinfectant chemicals. **Sterilization**, on the other hand, is the process of killing all microorganisms (bacteria, viruses, parasites, fungi, and spores). This can be achieved through pressurized steam, dry heat, chemicals, or radiation.

ANSWER: A-c; B-a; C-b

8. Match each antiseptic agent in the left column with the affected microorganism in the right column.

A. Hexachlorophene	a. Effective against gram-positive and gram-negative bacteria and fungi
B. Iodophors	b. Effective against gram-positive pathogens only
C. Chlorhexidine gluconate	c. Effective against gram-positive and gram-negative bacteria.

Ref.: 1, 2

COMMENTS: Antiseptics, which are incorporated into soaps, are used for both preoperative skin preparation and surgical hand scrubs. **Hexachlorophene** leaves on the skin an active film that is effective against gram-positive pathogens and is renewed with each scrubbing. **Iodophores** are organic complexes of iodine and synthetic detergents that are effective against both gram-positive and gram-negative bacterial cells but not spores. They do not maintain adequate residual activity as does hexachlorophene. **Chlorhexidine gluconate** (Hibiclens) is effective against gram-positive and gram-negative bacteria, fungi, and bacterial spores at higher temperatures.

ANSWER: A-b; B-c; C-a

9. Match each clinical situation in the left column with the appropriate tetanus prophylaxis in the right column.

A. A previously unimmunized child under 5 years of age without wounds	a. No treatment
B. Previously unimmunized adult without wounds	b. Absorbed toxoid 0.5 ml
C. Previously immunized patient, booster 7 years ago, non-tetanus-prone wound.	c. Absorbed toxoid 0.5 ml and 250 units of human tetanus immune globulin; two additional injections of toxoid over the next year
D. Previously immunized patient, booster 7 years ago, tetanus-prone wound	d. Three injections of toxoid over approximately 1 year with booster every 10 years
E. No prior immunization, non-tetanus-prone wound	e. Series of four injections of tetanus toxoid with diphtheria and pertussis vaccine
F. No prior immunization, tetanus-prone wound	

Ref.: 1, 2

COMMENTS: Tetanus is a severe, progressive syndrome caused by the neurotoxin released by *Clostridium tetani*. Even in ideal therapeutic circumstances, the mortality rate exceeds 30%. As with most diseases, the best treatment is prevention. Fortunately, active immunization with adsorbed tetanus toxoid and passive immunization with human tetanus immunoglobulin have been effective in preventing this clinical syndrome.

ANSWER: A-e; B-d; C-a; D-b; E-d; F-c

10. Prophylactic antibiotics reduce infection in which of the following circumstances?

A. Elective cholecystectomy.
B. Vaginal or abdominal hysterectomy.
C. Implantation of prosthetic material.
D. Colon resection with anastomosis.
E. Gastrostomy tube placement.

Ref.: 1

COMMENTS: The use of prophylactic antibiotics is recommended when a brief period of contamination by organisms can be predicted or when a foreign body is being placed. High risk biliary procedures (common bile duct exploration, biliary bypass procedures, and acute inflammatory processes) are indicators for prophylactic antibiotics, but elective cholecystectomy without manipulation of the bile duct does not require prophylaxis. Gastric operations when gastric acid production has been suppressed or operations for cancer, bleeding, or obesity require prophylaxis, but placement of a feeding tube does not. Obviously, crossing the vagina or colon during hysterectomy or colon resection is associated with wound contamination and therefore requires prophylaxis. Other recommended circumstances for antibiotic prophylaxis are (1) cardiac procedures requiring sternotomy; (2) vascular procedures of the abdominal aorta or lower extremities; (3) amputation of an extremity for ischemia; (4) cesarean section; and (5) oral pharyngeal procedures with neck dissections.

ANSWER: B, C, D

11. With regard to vascular catheter sepsis, match each clinical statement in the left column with the appropriate incidence of sepsis in the right column.

A. Long-term vs. short-term catheter	a. Increased incidence of catheter-caused sepsis
B. Multiple-lumen vs. single-lumen catheter	b. Decreased incidence of catheter-caused sepsis
C. Swan-Ganz catheter vs. subclavian hemodialysis catheter	c. No effect on incidence of catheter-caused sepsis
D. Plastic occlusive dressings over catheter at insertion site	
E. Routine periodic changing of catheter over guidewire	
F. Insertion site: femoral vs. internal jugular vein	

Ref.: 8, 9

COMMENTS: The incidence of sepsis resulting from indwelling vascular catheters is less than 1%. Several factors increase the risk of infection and sepsis substantially. The length of time the catheter is in place is the most important risk factor for infection via vascular access; it has been determined that the risk of infection is heightened for each day the catheter is in place. Additional factors that **increase** the risk of infection include (1) the use of *multilumen catheters*, rather than single lumen ones (indeed, the incidence of infection at 6 days is three times greater with Swan-Ganz catheters than with hemodialysis catheters; (2) the *number of catheter manipulations*; and (3) *plastic occlusive dressings*, which seem to increase the risk of infection two- to fourfold in comparison with traditional gauze dressings. Factors that do **not change**, in and of themselves, the incidence of catheter-related sepsis include (1) routine periodic changing of vascular catheters over a guidewire and (2) femoral lines, for which the incidence of line sepsis is similar to that for subclavian or internal jugular lines (provided proper skin preparation is performed). • Three organisms are responsible for most vascular access infections: *Staphylococcus epidermidis*, *Staphylococcus aureus*, and yeast. Because of the cost of treatment, prevention of vascular access infection should remain the surgeon's goal. In addition to meticulous technique of insertion and the appropriate maintenance of indwelling vascular catheters, the use of antimicrobially impregnated catheters to prevent biofilm development and the use of antimicrobial cuffs to prevent migration of skin organisms along the catheter may lower the incidence of catheter-related infections.

ANSWER: A-a; B-a; C-a; D-a; E-c; F-c

12. With regard to intestinal antisepsis, which of the following statements is/are true?

A. In the presence of adequate systemic antimicrobial prophylaxis, mechanical bowel cleansing does little to reduce the incidence of postoperative infection.

B. In the presence of adequate mechanical cleansing of the bowel, oral antibiotic bowel preparation does little to reduce the incidence of postoperative infection.
C. Mechanical bowel preparation effectively reduces the number of bacteria per gram of stool.
D. There is as yet no general agreement as to the ideal oral antibiotic agent or agents.
E. Appropriate intestinal antisepsis allows some added measure of protection against infection should there be an anastomotic leakage.

Ref.: 1, 2, 9

COMMENTS: It is generally agreed that proper intestinal antisepsis involves a combination of mechanical cleansing of the bowel and intraluminal antibiotic therapy. This procedure has resulted in a decrease in the incidence of postoperative wound infections. Mechanical cleansing may be achieved by a combination of appropriate cathartics and enemas or by the oral administration of large volumes of balanced salt solutions to effectively flush the colonic contents. Whatever stool remains, however, continues to contain large numbers of bacteria (approximately 10^{11} per gram of stool). Although there is no general agreement as to which antibiotic agents are most effective, a commonly employed regimen includes oral neomycin/erythromycin base the afternoon before surgery. Regardless of the method of achieving mechanical or antibiotic preparation of the bowel, neither alone appears to result in the same reduction in postoperative wound infections as the two combined. The mechanical cleansing must be completed before antibiotic preparation of the bowel. The timing of the oral antibiotic preparation of the colon should account for the time of operation. The familiar regimen of cleansing at 1 p.m., 2 p.m., and 11 p.m. the day before surgery achieves high concentrations of antibiotic in the left colon (where bacterial concentration is highest) by 8 o'clock the next morning. If there is no interference with normal transit of intestinal contents and bowel length is normal, the operation should take place at or near this time; otherwise the cleansing time should be adjusted accordingly. All this discussion notwithstanding, proper mechanical and antimicrobial bowel preparation does not protect against infections resulting from technical operative errors. Although done commonly, the addition of systemic antibiotic therapy to mechanical preparation has not been shown to further reduce the incidence of postoperative infection.

ANSWER: D

13. With regard to antibiotic interactions, which of the following statements is/are true?

A. High concentrations of carbenicillin or ticarcillin decrease the effectiveness of aminoglycosides.
B. Bacteriostatic agents (tetracyclines) interfere with the mechanism of action of β-lactam antibiotics on cell wall synthesis.
C. Cephalosporins decrease the nephrotoxicity of aminoglycosides.
D. Amphotericin B increases the nephrotoxicity of aminoglycosides.

Ref.: 9, 10

COMMENTS: The interactions between various antibiotics and their intended target pathogens can create a variety of situations ranging from synergism to antagonism. A decrease in the effectiveness of aminoglycosides in the presence of high concentrations of carbenicillin or ticarcillin has been shown in vitro, although no clinical significance has been demonstrated. The mechanism of action of β-lactam antibiotics involves inhibition of cell wall synthesis. Bacteriostatic agents such as tetracyclines interfere with this action. In contrast, β-lactam antibiotics facilitate cell wall penetration by aminoglycosides, aiding in the treatment of enterococcal and *Pseudomonas* infections. The nephrotoxicity potential of aminoglycocides is sometimes increased with the use of other antibiotics, including amphotericin B and vancomycin. Cephalothin may also lead to increased nephrotoxicity.

ANSWER: A, B, D

14. Match each agent in the left column with one or more mechanisms of antimicrobial action in the right column.

A. Amphotericin B	a. Inhibition of cell wall synthesis
B. Penicillin	b. Disruption of membrane barrier function
C. Cephalosporins	c. Disruption of ribosomal protein synthesis
D. Aminoglycosides	d. Impairment of bacterial DNA synthesis
E. Quinolones	e. Calcium homeostasis disruption

Ref.: 9

COMMENTS: All of the antimicrobial agents listed are bactericidal or fungicidal (i.e., their associated mechanism of action results in bacterial or fungal death). Bacteriostatic agents (e.g., tetracyclines, chloramphenicol, erythromycin, clindamycin) act by preventing bacterial growth but do not result in bacterial death; they work primarily through inhibition of ribosomal protein synthesis. • Amphotericin B is a polyene antibiotic that binds to the cytoplasmic cellular membrane, altering the selective permeability. The ability of an organism to bind amphotericin B depends on the presence of ergosterol in the cytoplasmic membrane. Bacterial cell walls contain no sterols and are therefore unaffected by amphotericin B. • Both penicillin and cephalosporins are β-lactam antibiotics and hence have a similar mode of activity. Enzymes located within the bacterial cytoplasmic membrane are responsible for peptide cross-linkage. These enzymes are called penicillin-binding proteins (PBPs) and are the site at which β-lactam drugs bind. This binding interferes with bacterial cell wall synthesis, eventually resulting in cell lysis. Gram-negative bacteria contain a variable number of different PBPs; each β-lactam antibiotic has different affinities for the various PBPs. • Aminoglycosides bind irreversibly to the 30S bacterial ribosome and interfere with protein synthesis. For this to take place they must penetrate the cell wall, which occurs only under aerobic conditions. Unlike other antibiotics that inhibit protein synthesis, aminoglycosides are bactericidal. This feature is secondary to their disruptive effect on calcium homeostasis. • Quinolones inhibit the enzyme DNA gyrase, impairing DNA synthesis in bacteria. Appreciation of the mechanism of action of antimicrobials may have a bearing on the selection of alternative therapies when bacterial resistance to the drug of choice develops.

ANSWER: A-b; B-a; C-a; D-c,e; E-d

15. Match each cephalosporin generation in the left column with the appropriate susceptibility of the bacterial groups in the right column.

A. First-generation cephalosporin	a. Aerobic gram-positive (+++); aerobic gram-negative (+); anaerobic (*Bacteroides fragilis*) (−)
B. Second-generation cephalosporin	b. Aerobic gram-positive (++); aerobic gram-negative (++); anaerobic (*B. fragilis*) (+)
C. Third-generation cephalosporin	c. Aerobic gram-positive (+); aerobic gram-negative (+++); anaerobic (*B. fragilis*) (+)

Ref.: 1, 2, 9

COMMENTS: The first cephalosporin was derived from a fungus discovered in the sewer systems in Italy in 1948. The basic cephalosporin structure consists of a dihydrothiazine ring fused to a β-lactam ring. Different pharmacologic activity is achieved by the substitution of various side chains at different places within the cephalosporin nucleus. The varied pharmacologic activity results in a division into "generations," which are based on the antimicrobial spectrum of the antibiotics. However, each cephalosporin may have significant differences within each generation. The **first-generation** cephalosporins are active against the gram-negative species: *Escherichia coli, Klebsiella pneumoniae*, and *Proteus mirabilis*. Resistance is common, however: currently in as many as 30% of cases. They also are active against most anaerobic cocci and bacilli (except *B. fragilis*). In addition, the first-generation cephalosporins have excellent activity against gram-positive bacteria. Thus the best use of first-generation cephalosporins is in surgical prophylaxis. **Second-generation** cephalosporins have expanded activity against gram-negative organisms, and there is less resistance to them than to the first-generation cephalosporins. Their activity against gram-positive organisms is similar to that of the first generation, except for some decrease in activity against *S. aureus*. Of note, cefoxitin and cefotetan are cephamycins with good activity against *B. fragilis*. **Third-generation** cephalosporins expand on the gram-negative coverage of the first- and second-generation cephalosporins at the expense of activity against gram-positive bacteria. They have variable activity against *Pseudomonas aeruginosa*, with the specific cephalosporin ceftazidime demonstrating the greatest activity against this organism. Despite their inherent resistance to β-lactamase hydrolysis, all third-generation cephalosporins demonstrate an inoculum effect; that is, their mean inhibitory concentrations are significantly increased when larger bacterial inocula are tested in vitro. Third-generation cephalosporins often are indicated for treatment of hospital-acquired infections in lieu of or in combination with other antibiotics.

ANSWER: A-a; B-b; C-c

16. Match each gram-positive coccus in the left column with one or more of the antibiotics that would be therapeutic choices in the right column.

A. β-Lactamase-producing *S. aureus*	a. Methicillin
B. Non-β-lactamase-producing *S. aureus*	b. Penicillin G
C. *Staphylococcus pyogenes*	c. Ampicillin
D. *Streptococcus pneumoniae*	d. Oxacillin
E. *Streptococcus faecalis*	
F. *Clostridium perfringens*	

Ref.: 1, 2

COMMENTS: Penicillins are classified into subgroups according to their structure, β-lactamase susceptibility, and spectrum of action. Most gram-positive cocci (e.g., *S. pyogenes, S. pneumoniae*, and non-β-lactamase-producing *S. aureus*) are sensitive to penicillin G, a natural penicillin that is the drug of choice if the patient has no history of allergy to it. Exceptions to this general rule include β-lactamase-producing *S. aureus* (> 95% of today's isolates), which is able to destroy penicillin G. Alterations in penicillin structure have led to a number of penicillinase-resistant penicillins (methicillin, nafcillin, oxacillin) that are highly effective against these species of *Staphylococcus*. *S. faecalis* is, on occasion, resistant to penicillin G. Because ampicillin, an aminopenicillin, is more active than penicillin G on a weight basis, it is preferable for treating this organism. These organisms have recently been recategorized as *Enterococcus faecalis* and have a significant resistance pattern. Vancomycin is an alternative to ampicillin, although recently vancomycin resistance has started to emerge in many hospital settings. The gram-positive bacillus *C. perfringens* is highly sensitive to penicillin G, and large doses are required for effective treatment.

ANSWER: A-a,d; B-a,b,c,d; C-a,b,c,d; D-a,b,c,d; E-c; F-b

17. With regard to the relation of the penicillins to the cephalosporins, which of the following statements is/are true?

A. Both are bactericidal.
B. Both are effective against almost all strains of *Staphylococcus*.
C. Cephalosporins are recommended for management of streptococcal infections in patients who have had anaphylactic reactions to penicillin.
D. Although the biochemical structures of the cephalosporins and penicillins are similar, their mechanisms of action against bacteria are different.

Ref.: 1, 2, 9

COMMENTS: The cephalosporins and penicillins share many properties. In addition to their similar biochemical structures, they both produce their bactericidal effects by binding to and inhibiting the penicillin-binding protein enzymes that synthesize the bacterial cell wall. Both antibiotics are effective against pneumococci and most streptococci; however, cephalosporins are more effective than penicillin against staphylococci that produce β-lactamases. Semisynthetic isoxazolyl penicillins that are effective against these strains of *S. aureus* and actually are more active on a weight basis than cephalosporins have been developed. There is significant cross-resistance of these strains of staphylococci to the penicillins and the cephalosporins. Cephalosporins do not bind well to enterococcal penicillin-binding proteins; thus the mean inhibitory concentration of cephalosporins is 64–128 times that of ampicillin for *Enterococcus*. Approximately 10–15% of patients with allergy to penicillin are also allergic to cephalosporins, which should be taken into account before patients allergic to penicillin are treated with cephalosporins.

ANSWER: A

18. Which one or more of the following is/are characteristic of tetracyclines?

A. Bactericidal.
B. Activity against *Mycobacterium tuberculosis*.
C. Discoloration of teeth.

D. Risk of superinfection.
E. Narrow spectrum of activity.

Ref.: 1, 2

COMMENTS: The tetracyclines are a family of closely related antibiotics that exert their bacteriostatic effect by altering ribosomal protein synthesis. These antibiotics have a broad spectrum of activity against most gram-positive species and many gram-negative species, as well as *Treponema pallidum* and atypical *Mycobacterium* species. Tetracycline may be deposited in developing teeth during the early stages of calcification, which results in yellowish brown discoloration of the teeth. For this reason these drugs should be avoided in children younger than 8 years. As with most broad-spectrum antibiotics, alteration in the normal flora may result in superinfection by a number of other organisms, including *Candida*, *Staphylococcus*, *Proteus*, and *Pseudomonas*.

ANSWER: C, D

19. Which one or more of the following is/are characteristic of aminoglycosides?

A. Active against a broad spectrum of gram-negative aerobes.
B. Emergence of resistant bacterial strains does not occur.
C. Narrow margin between therapeutic and toxic blood levels.
D. Nephrotoxicity.
E. Ototoxicity.

Ref.: 1, 2, 9

COMMENTS: Aminoglycosides were, until the mid-1980s, the only reliable empiric treatment for serious gram-negative infections. The introduction of third-generation cephalosporins, extended-spectrum penicillins, carbapenems, and quinolones, however, has reduced the frequency of use of aminoglycosides. The aminoglycoside mechanism of action involves irreversible binding to the 30S bacterial ribosome. However, aminoglycosides must first penetrate the cell wall, and this step is oxygen-dependent; hence it does not occur under anaerobic conditions. For this reason, aminoglycosides have no activity against anaerobic bacteria or facultative bacteria in an anaerobic environment. • Resistance to aminoglycosides, particularly by *Pseudomonas*, does occur; and specific hospital recommendations as to specific aminoglycoside patterns of resistance should be routinely observed. Aminoglycosides are difficult to use clinically because of their low therapeutic level/toxic level ratio (approximately 2:3). • The two major toxic side effects are nephrotoxicity and ototoxicity. The ototoxicity, both auditory and vestibular, is potentially more significant because it is nonreversible and cumulative. The auditory toxicity affects response to the higher frequencies, making early detection difficult. The nephrotoxicity usually is a dose-dependent, reversible acute tubular necrosis. • If serum concentrations of aminoglycosides are determined in an appropriate and timely manner, safe and therapeutic aminoglycoside levels should be achievable.

ANSWER: A, C, D, E

20. Which of the following statements is/are true with regard to secondary peritonitis?

A. Usually occurs as a result of perforation of an intraabdominal viscus.
B. Monomicrobial infection.
C. Increased age, cancer, cirrhosis, and systemic illness are factors that increase the mortality rate.
D. Sequestration of bacteria within fibrin clots leads to intraabdominal abscess formation.
E. The most common anaerobe cultured from the abdomen is *Clostridium welchii*.

Ref.: 11

COMMENTS: Secondary peritonitis usually occurs as a result of a perforation of an intraabdominal viscus: perforated peptic ulcer, appendix, diverticula, or gastrointestinal (GI) penetrating trauma. The infection is polymicrobial, with facultative aerobes and anaerobes acting synergistically. *Bacteroides* species are the most common anaerobes cultured from abdominal infections. About 10^{12} bacteria reside in the colon per gram of feces, with 90% of these bacteria being anaerobic organisms. Any process that impairs immunologic function or is associated with general debilitation increases mortality. Age, cancer, hepatic cirrhosis, and the presence of a systemic illness have been shown to increase mortality. One of the defense mechanisms of the peritoneal cavity is the production of fibrin to sequester bacteria to limit systemic spread. This sequestration leads to the formation of intraabdominal abscesses that require radiologic or open surgical drainage.

ANSWER: A, C, D

21. Treatment of secondary peritonitis includes which of the following?

A. Treatment of the source of infection.
B. Eradication of residual bacteria with antimicrobial therapy.
C. Continuous antimicrobial therapy until both fever and white blood cell (WBC) count have returned to normal.
D. Carbapenems, aminoglycosides and fourth-generation cephalosporins have equal efficiency in treatment studies.
E. Requires only perioperative (12 hours) antimicrobial therapy if initiated within 4 hours of penetrating GI injuries.

Ref.: 11

COMMENTS: Treatment of secondary peritonitis relies on three principles of management: (1) removal of the source of infection; (2) eradication of residual bacteria with antimicrobial agents; and (3) metabolic and hemodynamic support for the critically ill patient. Broad-spectrum coverage of facultative aerobes and anaerobes is required to eradicate residual bacteria. Carbapenems cover both aerobes and anaerobes, but aminoglycosides and fourth-generation cephalosporins lack antianaerobic activity. An antianaerobic antimicrobial agent is necessary when using aminoglycosides or fourth-generation cephalosporins for severe secondary peritonitis. Antimicrobial therapy should be continued until fever and the WBC count are normal. Patients with fever after discontinuation of antibiotics have as high as a 50% infection rate. Patients who are afebrile but have an elevated WBC count have a 20–33% recurrent infection rate. With penetrating GI trauma, perioperative antibiotics are needed only if started within 4 hours of injury; otherwise, 3–7 days of therapy is necessary.

ANSWER: A, B, C, E

22. Match each wound classification in the left column with the appropriate surgical example in the right column.

A. Clean	a. Perforated appendix
B. Clean-contaminated	b. Traumatic colon perforation and repair
C. Contaminated	c. Mastectomy
D. Dirty	d. Elective cholecystectomy

Ref.: 1, 2

COMMENTS: Clean wounds (e.g., mastectomy) are nontraumatic and do not enter the digestive, respiratory, or genitourinary tract. Antibiotic prophylaxis is not needed except for immunocompromised patients. In **clean-contaminated** cases (e.g., elective cholecystectomy), the digestive, respiratory, or genitourinary system is entered, without visible contamination and without obvious infection. Perioperative antibiotics are usually required. **Contaminated** wounds (e.g., traumatic colon perforation and repair) are those in which there is visible contamination from a hollow viscus or there is a fresh wound with contamination less than 3 hours old. **Dirty** wounds (e.g., perforated appendix) are clinically infected. Both contaminated and dirty wounds necessitate antibiotic treatment for a length of time that must be clinically determined.

ANSWER: A-c; B-d; C-b; D-a

23. Which of the following is/are appropriate times to begin administration of prophylactic antibiotic therapy for abdominal surgery?

A. Two days before the operation.
B. Immediately before the operation.
C. As the incision is being closed.
D. When and if contamination is found during the operation.
E. After closure of the abdomen.

Ref.: 1, 2, 12

COMMENTS: Debate persists over the optimal choice of antibiotics for perioperative chemoprophylaxis and the length of time during the postoperative period that antibiotics should be administered. There has been general agreement that the effective use of perioperative antibiotics depends on the presence of tissue levels of the drug when the opening incision is made. This is best achieved by administering the drug just before the operation. However, evidence indicates that intravenous antibiotics, started when and if contamination is discovered, achieve results similar to those seen with immediate preoperative antibiotic prophylaxis so long as they are administered within 4 hours from the time of injury. This procedure reduces the use and expense of antibiotics in many patients. Beginning antibiotic therapy after the operation is completed does not appear to alter the risk of postoperative wound infection.

ANSWER: B, D

24. Match each form of infection in the left column with one or more appropriate characteristics in the right column.

A. Cellulitis	a. Suppuration
B. Lymphangitis	b. Erythematous streaking
C. Abscess	c. Antibiotics almost always indicated
	d. Surgical treatment alone frequently sufficient

Ref.: 1, 2

COMMENTS: It is useful to consider surgical infections in terms of their being suppurative or nonsuppurative. **Abscesses** are localized suppurative collections that may or may not be associated with surrounding cellulitis. In the absence of cellulitis, surgical drainage alone is frequently sufficient treatment. **Cellulitis** is a nonsuppurative, poorly localized infection of soft tissues that in its late stages may progress to necrosis and abscess formation. Group A β-hemolytic streptococci and *Staphylococcus aureus* are the most common bacteria causing nonnosocomial cellulitis. Appropriate initial treatment involves antibiotic therapy, which usually results in significant improvement within 48–72 hours. Lack of improvement mandates search for an associated abscess, resistant organism, unusual pathogen, or failure of drug delivery to the site of infection. **Lymphangitis** is an infection of the lymphatic vessels and usually occurs in association with another focus of cellulitis or abscess. It is characterized by erythematous streaking of the skin and is appropriately managed with rest and antibiotics. Lymphadenitis (inflammatory swelling of the lymph nodes) may be seen in association with any of these forms of surgical infection.

ANSWER: A-c; B-b,c; C-a,d

25. Match each form of superficial infection in the left column with one or more appropriate characteristic in the right column.

A. Furuncle	a. Primarily cellulitis
B. Carbuncle	b. Primarily abscess
C. Erysipelas	c. Usually group A β-hemolytic streptococci
D. Impetigo	d. Usually staphylococci
	e. Surgery is primary therapy

Ref.: 2

COMMENTS: A **furuncle**, or boil, is an abscess that begins in the area of a hair follicle or sweat gland. There usually is an intense inflammatory response that leads to central necrosis and a peripheral zone of cellulitis. A **carbuncle** is a furuncle that has extended into the surrounding subcutaneous tissues in a multilocular fashion. Both furuncles and carbuncles are usually caused by staphylococci; and because they represent localized areas of suppuration they are treated primarily by surgical drainage. Antibiotic therapy is indicated for management of furuncles and carbuncles when the associated cellulitis is severe. **Erysipelas** is an acute cellulitis, usually caused by group A β-hemolytic streptococci. Its onset may be abrupt, and it is usually associated with systemic symptoms of chills, fever, and prostration. It is usually effectively treated with appropriate antibiotics. **Impetigo** is a contagious skin infection characterized by small intraepithelial abscesses. Both streptococci and staphylococci are commonly cultured from them. Although they are considered small abscesses, appropriate treatment usually involves systemic or topical antibiotics (or both).

ANSWER: A-b,d,e; B-b,d,e; C-a,c; D-c,d

26. Match each clinical characteristic in the left column with the correct streptococcal infection in the right column.

A. May be polymicrobial
B. Often significant overlying skin involvement
C. Seen after trauma and abdominal surgery for peritonitis
D. Treatment consists of appropriate surgical drainage, débridement, and antibiotics

a. Necrotizing fasciitis
b. Myonecrosis
c. Both
d. Neither

Ref.: 1, 2

COMMENTS: These severe infections are distinguished by whether the infection involves primarily the superficial fascia or the underlying muscle. Both infections may be polymicrobial. **Necrotizing fasciitis** usually is caused by β-hemolytic streptococci, which may be found in association with coagulase-positive staphylococci or gram-negative enteric pathogens. Necrotizing fasciitis involves superficial and widespread fascial necrosis; the overlying skin is frequently pale red and may progress to a distinct purple, in association with the development of blisters and bullae. **Myonecrosis** is caused by clostridia, aerobic streptococci, and anaerobes that may be found in association with *S. aureus* or gram-negative rods. Although both of these entities may appear following operation, they are most often seen in traumatic wounds. Both necrotizing fasciitis and myonecrosis are potentially life-threatening infections that must be treated immediately with wide surgical débridement and appropriate antibiotic therapy.

ANSWER: A-c; B-a; C-c; D-c

27. With regard to clostridial infections, which of the following statements is/are true?

A. The presence of clostridial organisms in a surgical or traumatic wound warrants immediate antibiotic administration and surgical intervention.
B. The oxidation-reduction potential in contaminated tissues is a significant factor in the development of a clostridial infection.
C. Despite the potentially fulminant course of clostridial infections, the skin overlying clostridial cellulitis may not be discolored or edematous.
D. Clostridial myonecrosis (gas gangrene) should be treated with immediate surgical débridement, antibiotics, clostridial antitoxin, and hyperbaric oxygenation.

Ref.: 1, 2

COMMENTS: Clostridial organisms are ubiquitous and are a common contaminant of traumatic wounds. In most wounds, however, the high oxidation-reduction potential of the surrounding healthy tissues prevents colonization and invasion of these tissues. In such cases, the presence of clostridia is clinically insignificant. When colonization with clostridia occurs in the presence of necrotic tissue, their proliferation and invasion of other tissue can occur, leading to clostridial cellulitis. This form of clostridial infection is confined to the superficial fascial planes; and although it may spread rapidly, systemic effects may be mild and the skin of normal color. Clostridial myonecrosis occurs when the deeper muscular compartments are invaded, usually by *C. perfringens*. The inaccessibility of systemic antibiotics to this ischemic, necrotic tissue coupled with the low oxidation-reduction potential of such wounds permits rapid dissemination of the clostridia through the muscular compartments. Symptoms of clostridial myonecrosis are variable: pain out of proportion to the physical examination findings, systemic toxicity, rapidly spreading zone of cellulitis, bronzing of the skin, and a thin, watery, brown discharge. Gram staining reveals large numbers of gram-positive rods and no neutrophils. In the appropriate clinical setting, an innocuous appearance of the postoperative wound does not exclude the possibility of clostridial sepsis. Therapy should be immediate surgical débridement and antibiotic therapy (penicillin G). Adjunctive hyperbaric oxygenation may be helpful; horse antitoxin therapy is of no proven value and may be followed by serum sickness.

ANSWER: B, C

28. With regard to diabetic foot infections, which of the following statements is/are true?

A. Foot infection occurs more frequently in diabetic than in nondiabetic patients.
B. The saline injection-aspiration method is the preferred method for obtaining reliable cultures.
C. Diabetic foot infections are commonly polymicrobial.
D. Osteomyelitis of the foot is frequently encountered in patients with a long history of diabetes and associated neuropathy.

Ref.: 1, 2

COMMENTS: The factors that predispose diabetic patients to infections of the lower extremity include decreased blood flow, diabetic neuropathy, hyperglycemia, and impairment of the immune system, particularly neutrophil dysfunction. • The most reliable results of culture are obtained by deep tissue biopsy of the infected foot. • Diabetic foot infections commonly are polymicrobial. Although gram-positive aerobic cocci are the most commonly isolated species, anaerobic bacteria and aerobic gram-negative bacilli are also frequently isolated. These various microorganisms act synergistically in initiating and perpetuating infection. Because of this synergy and the decreased perfusion secondary to vascular impairment, these infections may necessitate higher than normal doses of antimicrobial agents to achieve therapeutic antibiotic tissue levels. The choice of antimicrobial therapy should be directed against gram-positive cocci, gram-negative anaerobes, and aerobes, including *Bacteroides fragilis*, with the use of either a combination of agents or a single broad-spectrum antibiotic. In addition to antibiotics, early incision and drainage of abscess with débridement of devitalized tissue, immobilization, and supportive care are important in the total management of the diabetic foot. • Radiographs of the infected limb and even bone scan should be routinely obtained because osteomyelitis of the foot is typically encountered in patients with a long history of diabetes and associated neuropathy and, if present, may significantly extend the duration of antibiotic therapy. An assessment of the vascular supply of the foot is important because surgical correction of impaired blood flow in the affected limb has increased the incidence of healing and has decreased the need for amputation in diabetic patients with foot infections.

ANSWER: A, C, D

29. Which one or more of the following clinical situations or laboratory results require systemic antifungal therapy?

A. A single positive blood culture obtained from an indwelling intravascular catheter.
B. *Candida*-caused endophthalmitis.
C. Oral candidiasis.
D. *Candida* isolated from more than three sites with negative blood cultures.
E. None of the above.

Ref.: 8

COMMENTS: The decision to treat a presumed invasive fungal infection is difficult, and the physician must rely on the clinical setting in conjunction with laboratory results. • When blood cultures from a vascular catheter are positive for fungus, the catheter should be exchanged over a guidewire and the midportion and tip sent for culture. The most recent evidence supports therapy with systemic antifungal agents for *all* patients with even one blood culture positive for *Candida*. Parenteral amphotericin B or fluconazole should be administered. For patients with negative blood cultures but with cultures from three sites (e.g., wound, abdominal abscess, urinary tract, respiratory tract, mouth) that are positive for *Candida*, parenteral amphotericin B or fluconazole should be instituted for presumed disseminated candidiasis. • Clinical evaluation should always include funduscopic examination; if endophthalmitis is present, systemic therapy must be instituted. • Oral and esophageal candidiasis can be treated with oral nystatin, ketoconazole, or fluconazole. Prophylaxis against oral candidiasis is best performed with oral nystatin or clotrimazole. • With candidal urinary tract infections, indwelling catheters are removed if possible. If the catheter cannot be removed or if a symptomatic candidal urinary tract infection remains after catheter removal, treatment consists of bladder irrigation with amphotericin B or oral fluconazole.

ANSWER: A, B, D

30. Match each clinical statement in the left column with the appropriate antifungal agent or agents in the right column.

A. Best available antifungal agent for the treatment of serious systemic mycotic infections	a. Amphotericin B
B. Effective against systemic candidiasis	b. Fluconazole
C. May cause fever and chills	c. Griseofulvin
D. May cause permanent renal damage	

Ref.: 1, 2

COMMENTS: **Amphotericin B** currently is the best, most predictable antifungal agent for the treatment of systemic mycotic infections, including candidiasis, mucormycosis, cryptococcosis, histoplasmosis, coccidioidomycosis, sporotrichosis, and aspergillosis. Its numerous potential toxic effects include fever, chills, vomiting, anemia, hypokalemia, and renal impairment. A number of antifungal antibiotics (griseofulvin, nystatin, flucytosine, imidazole derivatives) are available for oral or topical administration (or both) for treatment of superficial fungal infections. Ketoconazole has some activity against certain systemic fungi, particularly *Histoplasma*, *Blastomyces*, *Coccidioides*, and *Paracoccidioides*. It possesses minimal toxicity except for occasional hepatic toxicity and is active against *Candida albicans*, *Cryptococcus*, and coccidioidal meningitis. **Fluconazole** is a highly selective inhibitor of the fungal cytochrome P-450 system utilized in the production of sterols for cell wall synthesis. It is effective against systemic candidiasis and *Cryptococcus neoformans*. **Griseofulvin** is active against dermatophytic fungi and is associated with occasional gastrointestinal upset, syncope, and leukopenia.

ANSWER: A-a; B-a,b; C-a; D-a

31. Match each clinical characteristic in the left column with the correct infecting organism or organisms in the right column.

A. Not a true fungus	a. *Actinomyces israelii*
B. Amphotericin B is the drug of choice for severe infection	b. *Nocardia asteroides*
C. Common inhabitant of oral cavity	c. *Histoplasma capsulatum*
D. Pulmonary manifestations are common	d. *Cryptococcus neoformans*
E. Central nervous system manifestations are common	e. *Candida albicans*

Ref.: 1, 2

COMMENTS: Pseudomycotic infections, actinomycosis, and nocardiosis are caused by organisms that are true bacteria but behave morphologically and clinically like fungi. ***Actinomyces israelii*** is an inhabitant of normal oral flora and causes burrowing, tortuous abscesses in the cervicofacial, thoracic, and abdominal areas. Appropriate treatment includes surgical drainage and penicillin G as the preferred drug. **Nocardiosis**, an opportunistic infection caused by *Nocardia asteroides*, occurs as either a pulmonary infection or subcutaneous and brain abscesses. It is difficult to treat. Sulfonamides are used in combination with other antimicrobial agents. **Histoplasmosis** is predominantly a pulmonary infection caused by *Histoplasma capsulatum*, which is endemic to the Mississippi and Ohio River valleys and along the Appalachian Mountains. Infection may be mild or may progress to a severe form with pulmonary cavitation; pulmonary and extrapulmonary manifestations may mimic tuberculosis. **Cryptococcosis** is caused by the yeast *Cryptococcus neoformans*. Its most frequent form of disseminated disease is meningitis, although cavitary and nodular pulmonary disease is also seen. ***Candida albicans*** is a common inhabitant of the mucous membranes and the gastrointestinal tract. In debilitated patients or those whose normal flora has been altered by antibiotic therapy, superficial candidal infections (e.g., thrush) may develop. They usually are effectively treated with topical agents (e.g., nystatin). Severe systemic candidiasis is a life-threatening infection commonly associated with severe debilitation, immunosuppression, other chronic infections, and the use of intravenous catheters. The foundation of therapy for systemic candidiasis and the other true systemic mycotic infections is amphotericin B.

ANSWER: A-a,b; B-c,d,e; C-a,e; D-a,b,c; E-b,d

32. Which of the following statements is/are correct regarding spontaneous bacterial peritonitis (SBP) in a cirrhotic patient?

A. Polymicrobial infection.
B. Ascitic cultures are always positive.
C. Due to transmucosal migration of a gut flora.

D. Ascitic protein concentration of less than 1 gm/dl is a risk factor.
E. Mortality approaches 50%.

Ref.: 13

COMMENTS: Spontaneous bacterial peritonitis has an incidence of 8–22% and a hospital mortality of 48–57% in cirrhotic patients. It is a monomicrobial infection (*Escherichia coli* 46%, streptococci/group D streptococci 30%, *Klebsiella pneumoniae* 9%) that results from the combination of prolonged bacteremia secondary to abnormal host defense mechanisms, intrahepatic shunting, and impaired bactericidal activity in ascites rather than transmucosal migration of gut flora. Patients with ascitic protein concentrations less than 1 gm/dl are 10 times more likely to develop SBP. Ascitic fluid cultures are negative in many cases. Blood and urine cultures should be done to isolate the organism in all suspected cases. Ascitic polymorphonuclear neutrophil (PMN) count of greater than 500 cell/mm^3 with negative cultures is also diagnostic for SBP.

ANSWER: D, E

33. Treatment of spontaneous bacterial peritonitis (SBP) should include which of the following?

A. Ten-day course of antimicrobial agent effective against aerobic gram-positive and gram-negative organisms.
B. Repeat paracentesis 48 hours after initiation of antibiotics.
C. Long-term oral antibiotic prophylaxis to prevent recurrence.
D. Search for intraabdominal source of infection if patient does not respond to the initial antibiotic regimen.
E. Liver transplantation.

Ref.: 13

COMMENTS: Initial antimicrobial treatment should include coverage against aerobic gram-positive and gram-negative organisms. A third-generation cephalosporin such as cefotaxime is the antibiotic of choice. If the patient is penicillin-allergic, aztreonam and an agent with gram-positive coverage are used. Superinfection with gram positive organisms is prevalent (15–20%) during an episode of SBP. Repeat paracentesis is performed 48 hours after initiation of antimicrobial therapy. If the PMN count is decreased and cultures are negative, 5 days of antimicrobial therapy is sufficient. If the PMN count is increased or cultures are positive, either resistance to the antibiotic is present requiring an alternative antibiotic or secondary peritonitis is present from an unsuspected intraabdominal source. Oral prophylaxis with norfloxacin has been shown to be effective for short-term prophylaxis in high risk patients, but the cost-effectiveness of long-term prophylaxis has yet to be determined. Liver transplantation is not an option in a patient with active infection.

ANSWER: B, D

REFERENCES

1. Sabiston DC Jr: *Textbook of Surgery*, 15th ed. WB Saunders, Philadelphia, 1997.
2. Schwartz SI, Shires GT, Spencer FC: *Principles of Surgery*, 7th ed. McGraw-Hill, New York, 1999.
3. Simmons RL, Kispert PH: Infection and host defenses. In: Simmons RL, Steed DL (eds): *Basic Science Review for Surgeons*, WB Saunders, Philadelphia, 1992, pp 56–83.
4. Zeigler EJ, Fisher CJ, Sprung CJ, et al: Treatment of gram-negative bacteremia and septic shock with HA-IA human monoclonal antibody against endotoxin. *N Engl J Med* 324:429–436, 1991.
5. Greenberg RN, Wilson KM, Kunz AY, et al: Observations using antiendotoxin antibody (E5) as adjuvant therapy in humans with suspected, serious, gram-negative sepsis. *Crit Care Med* 20:730–735, 1992.
6. Muder RR: Control of methicillin resistant *Staphylococcus aureus*. *Infect Med* 9:19–23, 1992.
7. McManus AT, Mason AD Jr, McManus WF, Pruitt BA Jr: What's in a name? Is methicillin-resistant *Staphylococcus aureus* just another *Staphylococcus aureus* when treated with vancomycin? *Arch Surg* 124:1456–1459, 1989.
8. Howard RJ (ed): Surgical infections. *Surg Clin North Am* 68:1–232, 1988.
9. Christou NV, Solomkin JS: Antibiotics. In: Wilmore DW, Brennan MF, Arken AH (eds): *Care of The Surgical Patient: Infection*. Scientific American, New York, 1993, pp 1–34.
10. Lyerly HK, Gaynor JW: *The Handbook of Surgical Intensive Care*, 3rd ed. Year Book, St. Louis, 1992.
11. Sawyer MD, Dunn DL: Antimicrobial therapy of intra-abdominal sepsis. *Infect Dis Clin North Am* 6:545–570, 1992.
12. Bates T, Siller G, Crathern BC, et al: Timing of prophylactic antibiotics in abdominal surgery: trial of a pre-operative versus an intra-operative first dose. *Br J Surg* 76:52–56, 1989.
13. Bhuva M, Ganger G, Jensen D: Spontaneous bacterial peritonitis: an update on evaluation, management, and prevention. *Am J Med* 97:169–175, 1994.

CHAPTER 15

Infectious Diseases in Surgery

1. Which of the following markers is the most clinically useful for following the course of a person infected with the human immunodeficiency virus (HIV)?

A. Plasma viremia.
B. CD4 cell count.
C. Serum neopterin.
D. Serum β_2-microglobulin.
E. p24 antigen level.

Ref.: 1

COMMENTS: The CD4 cell count, although somewhat imperfect, is the most useful determination for following the course of an HIV infection. The normal CD4 cell count is approximately 800–1200 cells/mm^3. Symptomatic disease usually begins when the CD4 cell count falls below 300–400 cells/mm^3. Opportunistic infections begin to occur when the CD4 cell count is less than 200 cells/mm^3. The time course of this CD4 cell count decline is prolonged and may take more than 10 years. Direct quantitation of virus load with **plasma viremia** shows increasing viral titers as the disease progresses. **β_2-Microglobulin is** shed into the serum in HIV-infected patients and reflects increased lymphocyte turnover. **Neopterin** is produced by macrophages stimulated by interferon. Although both are found in increasing amounts as HIV infection progresses, neither of these two determinations is specific for HIV infection and generally is used only in the research setting. The determination of **p24 antigen** is specific for HIV but not very sensitive.

ANSWER: B

2. Therapy of a person infected with HIV consists of which one or more of the following?

A. Zidovudine (AZT) therapy when the patient's CD4 cell count falls below 500 cells/mm^3.
B. Prophylactic therapy with trimethoprim/sulfamethoxazole to prevent *Pneumocystis carinii* pneumonia in patients with CD4 cell counts less than 200 cells/mm^3.
C. Didanosine (ddI) therapy in patients who are intolerant to AZT.
D. Combination therapy consisting of AZT and zalcitabine (ddC) in patients who have had disease progression.
E. Protease inhibitors for patients with CD4 counts less than 500 cells/mm^3.

Ref.: 1, 2

COMMENTS: The therapy of an HIV infection consists of antiviral therapy beginning at the time the CD4 cell count falls below 500 cells/mm^3 and prophylaxis to prevent the most common opportunistic infection, *Pneumocystis carinii* pneumonia, when the CD4 cell count falls below 200 cells/mm^3. AZT is the most extensively used antiviral agent at this time. In patients who either become intolerant to AZT (usually the development of anemia or leukopenia) or have disease progression (onset of repeated opportunistic infections), didanosine (ddI) or zalcitabine (ddC) is used. The viral protease enzyme is an HIV protein essential for viral application. Protease inhibitors, first approved by the Food and Drug Administration (FDA) in 1995, have the distinct advantage of the potential ability to inhibit replication in chronically infected cells. Studies have shown the ability of the protease inhibitors to increase the CD4 count while decreasing the viral load in combination therapy with other antiviral agents. Protease inhibitors have become as common as AZT in antiviral therapy since their release.

ANSWER: A, B, C, D, E

3. Match the type of exposure in the left column with the appropriate risk of seroconversion in the right column.

A. Blood transfusion of HIV-positive blood	a. 0%
B. Gamma globulin injection	b. 0.1%
C. Needle stick from a known HIV-positive patient	c. 0.3%
D. Infant born from an HIV-positive mother	d. 30%
E. Mucous membrane exposure	e. >70%

Ref.: 1, 3, 4

COMMENTS: *Blood transfusions* of HIV-positive blood virtually ensure seroconversion. It is estimated that approximately 1 in 40,000 to 1 in 200,000 units of blood are contaminated with HIV in the United States. *Gamma globulin* preparations are free of HIV and pose no risk for transmission. *Needle stick* exposures pose a risk to health care workers. It is estimated that up to 40% of needle-stick exposures are preventable. The most common situation in which a needle stick occurs is recapping needles after use. Individual cases of HIV transmission after mucous membrane exposure have been reported. The incidence of seroconversion after mucous membrane exposure in prospective studies is approximately 0.1%. Similarly, there are few well described cases of seroconversion following cutaneous contact with HIV-infected blood, but no prospective study has reported a seroconversion secondary to cutaneous contact with blood. It is estimated that approximately 30% of infants born of HIV-infected mothers are HIV-infected.

ANSWER: A-e; B-a; C-c; D-d; E-b

4. What is/are the proper procedure following a parenteral exposure to HIV in the hospital setting, such as a needle stick?

A. HIV serology as soon as possible after the exposure and at 6 weeks, 12 weeks, 24 weeks, and 1 year.
B. Persons exposed should follow guidelines for preventing HIV transmission, including safe sexual practices, refraining from blood or organ donation, and avoidance of breast feeding.
C. Zidovudine (AZT) should be given immediately to all persons who have a parenteral exposure.
D. Immediate administration of HIV vaccine.

Ref.: 1

COMMENTS: A person exposed to HIV by a parenteral contact should follow the guidelines as outlined in answers A and B. The use of AZT in such circumstances is controversial. There are no data showing that this is effective therapy. There are several case reports of AZT failure in this situation. However, because AZT is relatively nontoxic, some authorities do recommend giving AZT 100–200 mg orally every 4 hours for 6–8 weeks. The drug should be started as soon as possible after exposure. At present there is no effective vaccine for HIV.

ANSWER: A, B

5. Which of the following is the most frequent type of pathology leading to laparotomy in HIV-infected patients?

A. Opportunistic infection.
B. Kaposi's sarcoma.
C. Gastrointestinal (GI) lymphoma.
D. Immune thrombocytopenia.
E. Non-HIV-related illness.

Ref.: 5

COMMENTS: Approximately 10–20% of HIV-infected patients develop abdominal or GI symptoms that warrant surgical evaluation. A wide array of pathology may be encountered in these patients, and the illness may or may not be related to HIV infection. An emergency laparotomy may be indicated for GI bleeding, obstruction, perforation, peritonitis, or trauma. Elective procedures may have a diagnostic, therapeutic, or supportive intent. Approximately two-thirds of known HIV-infected patients undergoing laparotomy are found to have HIV-related disease, among them, opportunistic infections (e.g., cytomegalovirus, *Mycobacterium avium intracellulare*) are the most common, followed by neoplastic disease (lymphoma, Kaposi's sarcoma) and HIV-related thrombocytopenia. The general surgeon must be mindful, however, that acute surgical conditions unrelated to HIV infection (acute appendicitis, calculous cholecystitis, perforated duodenal ulcer) are present in one-third of patients with known HIV disease and a surgical abdomen.

ANSWER: A

6. Which one or more of the following pathogens has been associated with acalculous cholecystitis in HIV-infected patients?

A. *Pneumocystis carinii.*
B. *Mycobacterium avium intracellulare.*
C. Cryptosporidia.
D. Cytomegalovirus.

Ref.: 1

COMMENTS: Biliary infection due to several opportunistic organisms may cause acute acalculous cholecystitis, papillary stenosis, biliary stricture, or sclerosing cholangitis. The organisms generally implicated in these cases include cytomegalovirus, cryptosporidia, and *Candida*. Infection with *Mycobacterium avium intracellulare* may result in hepatitis, ileitis, intraabdominal abscess, intestinal obstruction, or intraabdominal or retroperitoneal adenopathy. The mechanism by which these various opportunistic pathogens produce GI injury may involve vasculitis and end-vessel thrombosis. *Pneumocystis carinii* is a common cause of opportunistic pneumonia.

ANSWER: C, D

7. Which of the following statements is/are true concerning the anorectal manifestations of acquired immunodeficiency syndrome (AIDS)?

A. Cytomegalovirus (CMV) proctitis is the most common nongonococcal proctitis in sexually active homosexual men.
B. Ulcerative herpes simplex virus (HSV) perianal infection, which has been present for longer than 1 month in an HIV-positive patient, is diagnostic of AIDS.
C. Idiopathic anal ulcers are typically located in either the anterior or posterior midline.
D. The rectum is the second most common site within the GI tract for AIDS-related lymphoma.
E. Anal carcinoma is found more frequently in homosexual and bisexual men than in heterosexual men.

Ref.: 6

COMMENTS: CMV is the most frequently found infectious organism in AIDS patients. CMV enterocolitis is the most common intestinal manifestation of AIDS; it may produce inflammation, hemorrhage, ulceration, or perforation. The diagnosis is confirmed by endoscopic visualization of erythematous, hemorrhagic patches with or without ulcers, or by biopsy, which reveals intranuclear cytomegalic viral inclusions. Surgery may be necessary for persistent bleeding or perforation. If operative intervention is necessary, abdominal colectomy and ileostomy is the appropriate operation. For less severe cases, medical treatment with intravenous ganciclovir can produce responses in approximately 85% of patients. • HSV is the most common cause of nongonococcal proctitis in sexually active homosexual men. The treatment usually has been symptomatic with oral analgesics, lidocaine ointment locally, and sitz baths. Acyclovir administered orally and topically has been effective in lengthening the asymptomatic period, promoting healing, and shortening the period of virus shedding. If chronic HSV infection lasts 1 month or longer in an HIV-positive patient who otherwise is asymptomatic, immunoincompetence is suggested. The Centers for Disease Control has declared this phenomenon diagnostic for AIDS. • Idiopathic anal ulcers are easily distinguishable from anal fissures; the latter usually are located in the anterior or posterior midline and are associated with edematous skin tags. HIV-related anal ulcers frequently are multiple, lateral in location, deep, and not always associated with skin tags. Biopsy is advised for histologic examination, as is viral culture and acid-fast stain. The pathogens sought are CMV, HSV, *Mycobacterium avium intracellulare*, and HIV. A darkfield examination should be done to exclude the presence of syphilis. Biopsy is also done to exclude malignancy. • Within the GI tract, the rectum is the second most common site for lymphoma, following the stomach. Most lesions are non-Hodgkin's lymphomas, 70% of which are high-grade B cell type. They usually present as extraluminal, diffuse processes initially diagnosed incorrectly as abscesses. Treatment consists of multiagent chemotherapy with a median survival of less than 12 months. • Anal carcinoma occurs more frequently in homosexual and bisexual men than in heterosexuals. This phenomenon is thought to be due to infection with the human papilloma virus.

ANSWER: B, D, E

8. Concerning anorectal surgery in patients infected with the human immunodeficiency virus (HIV), which of the following statements is/are true?

A. Wound healing is dismal in both asymptomatic and symptomatic HIV-positive patients.
B. Up to one-third of wounds in patients with symptomatic AIDS may take longer than 6 months to heal.
C. Most symptomatic AIDS patients undergoing sphincterotomy are rendered partially incontinent by the operation.
D. Surgical morbidity rates correlate with CD4 counts.

Ref.: 6

COMMENTS: Anorectal surgery in HIV-positive patients should be approached with caution and concern regarding wound healing during the postoperative period. A distinction should be made between HIV-negative patients, asymptomatic HIV-positive patients, and patients with symptomatic HIV disease. In the first two categories, wound healing can be expected to occur within the usual 6 weeks following the operation. Patients with symptomatic HIV disease, particularly those with less than 200 CD4 cell counts, may experience dismal healing; only 12% are healed within the first month, and 34% may take longer than 6 months to heal. Furthermore, if a sphincterotomy is performed, most have some impairment of continence postoperatively. In light of the above, a thorough evaluation of potential risk factors and, if possible, determination of HIV status are advised before proceeding with anorectal surgery in groups at high risk of being infected. CD4 counts have been shown to correlate with morbidity; 65% morbidity rates have been seen in patients with CD4 counts of less than 200, compared with only 7% morbidity in patients with counts greater than 200. In summary, withholding cautiously performed appropriate therapy in an asymptomatic HIV-positive patient is unnecessary. Anorectal surgery in a symptomatic HIV-positive patient, however, may be followed by prolonged wound healing and functional impairment.

ANSWER: B, C, D

9. Acute pancreatitis has been associated with which one or more of the following medications used in HIV-infected patients?

A. Ganciclovir.
B. Pentamidine.
C. Zidovudine (AZT).
D. Didanosine.

Ref.: 5, 7

COMMENTS: The interpretation of abdominal symptoms in patients with HIV disease involves many considerations. Abdominal pain may be due to a surgical or nonsurgical condition; it may be related or unrelated to HIV infection; and it may result from either therapeutic or illicit drug use. Pentamidine used for the treatment and prophylaxis of *Pneumocystis* pneumonia may cause acute pancreatitis. The antiviral agent ganciclovir, used for treatment of cytomegalovirus, has not been associated with pancreatitis. AZT and didanosine are nucleoside analogues that inhibit HIV replication. The most serious adverse effect of AZT is hematologic toxicity. The most serious adverse effects of didanosine are pancreatitis and peripheral neuropathy. Pancreatitis has also been described in patients receiving zalcitabine (ddC), particularly if they are receiving concomitant intravenous pentamidine. Pancreatitis has occurred in 3–13% of patients in clinical trials and can be fatal. The incidence of hyperamylasemia with these medications is two to three times higher than the rate of clinical pancreatitis.

ANSWER: B, C, D

10. Which of the following is/are true concerning splenectomy in patients with HIV infection?

A. Most common indication is opportunistic splenic abscess.
B. Indicated for HIV-related thrombocytopenia unresponsive to corticosteroids.
C. Not indicated for HIV-related thrombocytopenia because the mechanism differs from that of classic idiopathic thrombocytopenic purpura (ITP).
D. Associated with 30% risk of overwhelming postsplenectomy sepsis.

Ref.: 5

COMMENTS: HIV infection may be associated with immune thrombocytopenia and increased peripheral platelet destruction, although the process is not immunologically identical to that seen in typical ITP. When the process is unresponsive to steroids, splenectomy has yielded a favorable response in most patients. The procedure has been accomplished with low morbidity, and the risk of overwhelming postsplenectomy sepsis has not been exceptional. Splenic abscess due to mycobacterial infection may be another indication for splenectomy in HIV-infected individuals.

ANSWER: B

11. The operative mortality of laparotomy in HIV-infected patients has most closely been associated with which one of the following?

A. Total lymphocyte count less than 1200.
B. CD4 cell count less than 500.
C. Active opportunistic infection.

D. Duration of HIV infection.
E. Emergency operation.

Ref.: 5

COMMENTS: Prognostic factors in HIV patients undergoing abdominal operations have not been extensively analyzed. Cumulative operative mortality following major abdominal procedures is approximately 20%; most deaths are related to the patient's underlying disease and not to specific operative complications. Emergency operations have been associated with higher mortality rates than elective procedures. Specific demographic, hematologic, and other clinical factors that correlate with operative mortality have not been established.

ANSWER: E

12. A 32-year-old HIV-positive intravenous drug user is admitted following a seizure. Examination reveals a pronator drift. A computed tomography (CT) scan with intravenous contrast shows two ring-enhancing lesions. Which of the following statements is/are true?

A. Neurologic symptoms are extremely unusual as a first manifestation of AIDS.
B. Toxoplasmosis is the most common cause of focal-enhancing lesions on CT in HIV-infected patients.
C. Biopsies should be performed on all enhancing lesions in HIV patients.
D. Primary central nervous system (CNS) lymphoma is less common in HIV-infected patients than in immunosuppressed transplant patients without HIV.

Ref.: 1

COMMENTS: Ten percent of AIDS patients present with a neurologic symptom as a first sign of their illness, and 40% of AIDS patients eventually develop one or more neurologic deficits. Major HIV-related CNS diseases include HIV encephalopathy, meningitis, myelopathy, opportunistic infections (progressive multifocal leukoencephalopathy caused by papova virus JC, cytomegalovirus, herpes, toxoplasmosis, cryptococcosis), neoplasms (primary CNS lymphoma), and cerebrovascular complications. *Toxoplasma gondii*, the protozoan that causes toxoplasmosis, accounts for 50–70% of focal brain lesions in these patients. Ten to twenty-five percent of focal lesions are CNS lymphomas. Primary CNS lymphoma is a rare intracranial tumor, accounting for 1.5% of all primary brain tumors. However, it is significantly more common in HIV patients, even compared to that in other immunosuppressed populations. Current management recommendations for HIV patients with focal brain lesions include 2–3 weeks of empiric treatment for toxoplasmosis, followed by biopsy if the radiologic or clinical condition deteriorates.

ANSWER: B

13. Which statements are correct about HIV-positive patients with gastrointestinal (GI) bleeding?

A. Gastrointestinal bleeding is usually related to a complication of HIV infection.
B. Lower GI bleeding is more common than upper GI bleeding.
C. Colitis from cytomegalovirus (CMV), bacteria, or herpes simplex is the most common source of lower GI bleeding.
D. Upper GI bleeding is usually from an infectious source (CMV-induced ulcers).
E. Colonoscopy is the initial diagnostic test of choice for the stable patient.

Ref.: 8

COMMENTS: Gastrointestinal bleeding is an unusual occurrence in HIV-infected individuals, but when it does occur it is usually related to a complication of HIV infection. Lower GI bleeding is twice as common as upper GI bleeding. Lower GI bleeding is usually caused by localized colitis of infectious origin (CMV, bacteria, or herpes simplex). Upper GI bleeding, on the other hand, can be related to Kaposi's sarcoma or lymphoma approximately 50% of the time. CMV-induced ulcers do occur in the upper GI tract but not as frequently as in the lower GI tract. In the stable patient colonoscopy is the initial procedure of choice for lower GI bleeding to obtain biopsy specimens for special infectious stains and culture material.

ANSWER: A, B, C, E

14. The classic diagnostic modalities for active microbacterium tuberculosis include which of the following?

A. Mantoux tuberculin test intradermally.
B. Chest radiograph.
C. Sputum smear and culture for acid-fast bacilli (AFB).
D. Chest computed tomography (CT).
E. Bronchoscopy.

Ref.: 9

COMMENTS: Once tuberculosis (TB) is suspected, the three classic tests for tuberculosis should enable the clinician to make a definitive diagnosis. First a Mantoux tuberculin test is placed intradermally. If positive within 48–96 hours, chest radiography is performed. A chest film compatible with TB should initiate sputum smears and cultures. A positive smear then initiates immediate therapy; otherwise treatment is held until culture results are obtained. A negative PPD has a 10–25% false-positive rate. If TB is still suspected, a chest film is obtained. Patients with a negative chest film and suspected of having TB (regardless of their PPD status) should receive INH prophylaxis (6–12 months) if they are at high risk or are less than 35 years old. A patient with a positive chest film and a negative culture and smear should receive INH prophylaxis for 12 months.

ANSWER: A, B, C

15. Which statements about tuberculosis during the last decade are true?

A. Fewer than 50% of the new cases are in persons infected several to many years ago.
B. Approximately 25% of new cases are found in the immunocompromised HIV-positive population.
C. Extrapulmonary tuberculosis is rarely infectious and poses no public health threat.
D. The infectious source for most persons at risk are the patients with adult pulmonary tuberculosis (i.e., those with positive sputum cultures).
E. The mode of transmission of infection is by hand-to-hand (skin) contact.

Ref.: 9

COMMENTS: The mode of transmission is by airborne droplet nuclei when in the same room as a patient with adult pulmonary tuberculosis (TB). Adult pulmonary TB is defined as a patient with a positive sputum culture, and they often also have smears positive for acid-fast bacilli (AFB) especially if the disease is cavitary. About 90% of the 25,000 new cases in 1990 arose from persons infected several to many years ago. Ten million people in the United States harbor *Mycobacterium tuberculosis*; 90% of these PPD-positive people never develop clinical TB. These numbers reflect the large number of cases occurring in the elderly. The largest growing new population of TB patients is occurring in the HIV-infected population, and in urban settings 25% of the new cases occur in the HIV-infected population. Extrapulmonary TB makes up about 15% of all clinical cases; it is rarely infectious and therefore poses no public health threat.

ANSWER: B, C, D

16. Which statements about *Mycobacterium tuberculosis* treatment and prophylaxis are true?

A. Two-drug therapy with isoniazid (INH) and rifampin (RIF) for 12 months is the standard regimen recommended by the Centers for Disease Control (CDC) for active TB.
B. The standard regimen of treatment for active TB should be extended in immunocompromised hosts.
C. Patients should be considered drug-resistant if they have been previously treated or inadequately treated.
D. Isoniazid prophylaxis should be given to all persons who convert from PPD-negative to PPD-positive.
E. INH prophylaxis should continue for at least 12 months.

Ref.: 9

COMMENTS: The standard regimen recommended jointly by the CDC and the American Thoracic Society is triple-drug therapy with isoniazid, rifampin, and pyrazinamide for an intensive phase over 2 months followed by a 2-month continuation phase. The duration of standard therapy should be extended in immunocompromised hosts. The continuation phase is extended to 9 months or for at least 6 months after cultures become negative, whichever is longer. Drug resistance is considered when a patient has been treated previously or inadequately. An additional drug, usually ethambutol, is added for the drug-resistant patient. All patients with a positive conversion of PPD and less than 35 years old should be treated with INH prophylaxis. Patients over age 35 should be treated if a high risk condition exists. High risk factors include HIV infection, intravenous drug users, recent contact with an active infectious person, an abnormal chest radiograph, foreign-born persons, and residents of long-term care facilities or medically underserved low-income populations. INH prophylaxis consists of 300 mg daily for 6 months. Duration of prophylaxis should be extended to 12 months in patients with HIV infection and those with abnormal findings on chest films consistent with past tuberculosis.

ANSWER: B, C

17. The prevalence of hepatitis C infection in the United States is greater than that of the general population in which of the following groups?

A. Military personnel.
B. Heath care workers.
C. Injecting-drug users.
D. Chronic hemodialysis patients.
E. Patients currently receiving blood transfusions.

Ref.: 10

COMMENTS: Currently hepatitis C virus (HCV) is rarely transmitted by blood transfusion. During the late 1980s screening policies for HIV and surrogate markers for non-A, non-B hepatitis lowered the transfusion-associated risk of HCV to 1.5% per recipient. Routine testing of donors for evidence of HCV infection was initiated during 1990, and multiantigen testing was implemented during 1992, reducing the risk for infection to 0.001% per unit transfused. Injecting-drug use currently accounts for most HCV transmission in the United States. Injecting-drug use leads to HCV transmission through transfer of HCV-infected blood by sharing syringes and needles directly or through contamination of drug preparation equipment. The prevalence of HCV infection among health care workers, including orthopedic, general, and oral surgeons, is no greater than that in the general population, averaging 1–2%. The average incidence of anti-HCV seroconversion after unintentional needle sticks or sharps exposures from an HCV-positive source is 1.8%. There are no reports of an increased incidence of HCV transmission among military personnel. Prevalence of antibody to HCV positivity among chronic hemodialysis patients averages 10%, with some centers reporting rates greater than 60%.

ANSWER: C, D

18. Which statements about hepatitis C virus (HCV) infection are true?

A. Fulminant hepatic failure following acute hepatitis C is common.
B. Chronic HCV infection occurs in 75–85% of patients after acute infection.
C. Cirrhosis develops in 10–20% of patients with chronic infections within 10 years.
D. Factors predicting severity of liver disease include male gender, alcohol abuse, and age less than 40 at the time of infection.
E. Postexposure prophylaxis with interferon is recommended.

Ref.: 10

COMMENTS: Persons with acute HCV infection typically are either asymptomatic (60–70%) or have a mild clinical illness. Fulminant hepatic failure following acute hepatitis C is rare. After acute infection without subsequent sequelae, chronic HCV infection develops in 75–85% of persons. Most studies have reported that cirrhosis develops in 10–20% of persons with chronic hepatitis C over a period of 20–30 years and hepatocellular carcinoma in 1–5%. Recent data indicate that increased alcohol intake, being aged over 40 years at infection, and being male are factors that predict increased severity of liver disease. No studies have been undertaken regarding the use of antiviral agents (i.e., interferon) to prevent HCV infection after exposure. Antiviral therapy is recommended for patients with chronic hepatitis C who are at increased risk for progression to cirrhosis i.e., anti-HCV-positive patients with persistently elevated liver function tests, detectable HCV RNA, or a liver biopsy that indicates moderate degrees of inflammation and necrosis or the presence of portal or bridging fibrosis.

ANSWER: B

REFERENCES

1. Wyngaarden JB, Smith LH Jr, Bennett JC: *Cecil Textbook of Medicine*, 19th ed. WB Saunders, Philadelphia, 1992, pp 1908–1965.
2. Threlkeld SC, Hirsch MS: Antiretroviral therapy. *Med Clin North Am* 80:1263–1282, 1996.
3. Henderson DK, Fahey BJ, Willy M, et al: Risk for occupational transmission of HIV-1 associated with clinical exposure. *Ann Intern Med* 113:740–746, 1990.
4. Chamberland ME, Ciesielski CA, Howard RJ, et al: Occupational risk of infection with human immunodeficiency virus. *Surg Clin North Am* 75:1057–1070, 1995.
5. Deziel DJ, Hyser MJ, Doolas A, et al: Major abdominal operations in acquired immunodeficiency syndrome. *Am Surg* 56:445–450, 1990.
6. Beck DE, Wexner SD: *Fundamentals of Anorectal Surgery*. McGraw-Hill, New York, 1992, pp 423–439.
7. Kahn JO, Lagakos SW, Richman DD, et al: A controlled trial comparing continued zidovudine with didanosine in human immunodeficiency virus infection. *N Engl J Med* 327:581–587, 1992.
8. Sabiston DC Jr: *Textbook of Surgery*, 15th ed. WB Saunders, Philadelphia, 1997.
9. Pust RE: Tuberculosis in the 1990's: resurgence, regimens, and resources. *South Med J* 85:584–593, 1992.
10. CDC: Recommendations for prevention and control of hepatitis C virus infection and HCV-related chronic disease. *MMWR* 47(RR-19):1–39, 1998.

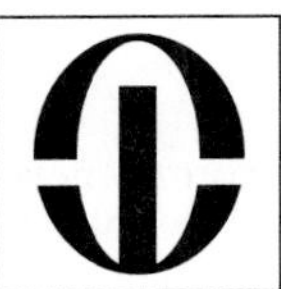

CHAPTER 16

Surgical Technology and Techniques

1. Regarding tissue expansion, which of the following statements is/are true?

   A. A stress load applied to human skin causes the collagen fibers to become aligned parallel to the stretching force.
   B. Skin, subcutaneous tissue and muscle all adapt well to slow stretching.
   C. During the first few weeks of expansion, the dermis thins rapidly by approximately 30%.
   D. The epidermis, dermal appendages, sensory nerves, and blood vessels of expanded skin undergo little change.
   E. The excess skin created by tissue expansion is the result of recruitment and thinning of adjacent skin, as well as increased epidermal mitotic activity and dermal collagen synthesis.

Ref.: 1, 2, 3

COMMENTS: Human tissue responds readily to expansion, both physiologic (e.g., pregnancy) and pathophysiologic (e.g., subcutaneous tumors). The ability of skin to stretch and then return to its original position is primarily dependent on the collagen and elastin within the dermis. The normally randomly oriented collagen fibers become more parallel in response to a stretching force and lose their twisted configuration. Elastin fibers function to return collagen to its relaxed state. Although muscle tissue appears to be more sensitive to rapid or overexpansion, muscle expands without loss of power or excursion. Histologically, the dermis undergoes the most change during tissue expansion, thinning rapidly during the first 3 weeks of expansion. The epidermis and specialized organs of the skin undergo little or no histologic change; slow expansion allows these structures to adapt without harm. It is for that reason that expansion techniques have been used to lengthen nerves and blood vessels as well. The excess skin created by tissue expansion is due to at least three factors: local recruitment, thinning, and increased epidermal mitotic activity and dermal collagen synthesis. Donor tissue usually is expanded from areas adjacent to the defect because they offer color match and hair-bearing characteristics superior to those offered by other reconstructive techniques.

ANSWER: A, B, C, D, E

2. In this illustration of the shoulder area, match the lettered arteries with their anatomic name.

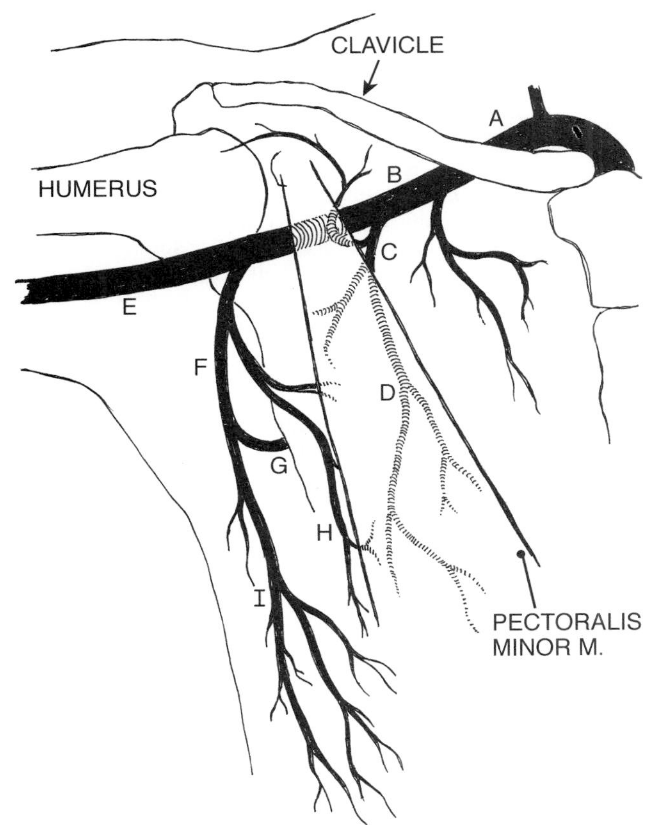

Artery	*Anatomic Name*
A	a. Thoracodorsal a.
B	b. Thoracoacromial a.
C	c. Pectoral branch of thoracoacromial a.
D	d. Subclavian a.
E	e. Axillary a.
F	f. Subscapular a.
G	g. Circumflex scapular a.
H	h. Lateral thoracic a.
I	i. Brachial a.

Ref.: 4

COMMENTS: See Question 3.

3. During a modified radical mastectomy on a patient for whom immediate reconstruction with a pedicled latissimus dorsi flap is planned, bleeding occurs requiring you to electrocoagulate and then ligate and divide the subscapular artery just proximal to the takeoff of the thoracodorsal artery. To proceed with the breast reconstruction you should:

A. Convert to a free latissimus dorsi flap reconstruction.
B. Try to reanastamose the severed artery and proceed with reconstruction of the latissimus dorsi muscle as planned.
C. Explain to the patient's family that the blood supply to the latissimus dorsi has been compromised and that after consultation with the plastic surgeon you believe reconstruction with a tram flap is the best alternative.
D. Proceed with plastic surgical wound closure and perform breast reconstruction at a later date.

Ref.: 5, 6

COMMENTS: A pedicled latissimus dorsi flap is based on the thoracodorsal artery and vein. The thoracodorsal artery is a branch of the subscapular artery, which is a branch of the axillary artery. The thoracodorsal artery sends a branch to the serratus anterior muscle and to the latissimus dorsi muscle. In this particular situation the artery is divided proximal to the serratus anterior and latissimus dorsi branches, which allows retrograde flow through the serratus anterior branch into the thoracodorsal artery and then on into the latissimus dorsi muscle. In most cases this flow can well support the latissimus dorsi muscle, so converting it to a free flap is most likely not necessary. On a delayed basis, the latissimus dorsi muscle can even be used if its nerve supply has been severed; however, once radiation is added it is no longer reliable, even if this retrograde flow is intact. The tram flap is an excellent myocutaneous flap for breast reconstruction but requires a more complex operation with a longer operative and recovery time; it is also associated with greater morbidity. This flap with its higher morbidity related to increased flap necrosis, ventral hernia, or abdominal wall weakness, as well as increased bleeding and infection, must be discussed and planned well in advance. Consideration should strongly be made for proceeding with reconstruction at a later date if this arterial repair is unsuccessful or the latissimus dorsi muscle is not supported by retrograde flow.

ANSWER:
Question 2: A-d; B-e; C-b; D-c; E-e, F-f; G-g; H-h; I-a
Question 3: B

4. In well-studied animal models of the arterial response to balloon injury, what is the basic sequence of events leading to intimal hyperplasia following balloon distension of the vessel wall?

A. Vessel spasm, local thrombosis, scarring.
B. Smooth muscle cell (SMC) death, leukocyte infiltration, fibrosis.
C. Local extravasation of growth factors due to increased permeability, SMC hypertrophy.
D. Platelet degranulation, migration of adventitial fibroblasts, collagen deposition.
E. Platelet degranulation; SMC proliferation, migration, and matrix deposition.

Ref.: 7, 8

COMMENTS: Balloon distension injury of a normal muscular artery sets in motion a complex response. The delicate endothelium is denuded, exposing the underlying collagenous tissue to the blood. A carpet of platelets adheres and their degranulation releases a host of local mitogens including serotonin, transforming growth factor β, and platelet-derived growth factor (PDGF). These compounds have many local effects, the most important of which may be to direct migration of SMCs from the media across the internal elastic lamina (IEL) in the area of subintimal damage. Thrombocytopenic animals develop little intimal hyperplasia (IH) following balloon injury. The medial SMCs themselves are directly activated by the balloon injury. Both mechanical stretching and release of intracellular and matrix-derived factors, including those of the fibroblast growth factor (FGF) family, are released. The normally quiescent SMCs undergo a wave of cell division. Proliferation peaks at 48 hours and declines to near baseline at 4 weeks. Migration into the inner portion of the artery also takes place during this period and is essential for development of IH. Proliferation and deposition of matrix material in the intima by SMCs that have left the arterial media is the final step in generation of a thick, potentially obstructive neointima. It should be noted that the muscular artery of a young animal is different from a diseased, plaque-laden, stenotic vessel in an aged human. Although a variety of pharmacologic treatments reduce IH following balloon injury in animal models, only platelet adherence blockade (a monoclonal antibody against glycoprotein IIb/IIIa) has been shown to reduce restenosis rates in human clinical trials following percutaneous transluminal coronary angioplasty.

ANSWER: E

5. What are the mechanisms of the immediate increase in diameter of the flow channel following balloon dilatation in atherosclerotic arteries?

A. Molding of soft atheroma to the "imprint" of the balloon.
B. "Stretching" the nondiseased portion of the artery around the plaque.
C. A dissection of artery wall and plaque with subsequent distension and late healing.
D. Displacement of plaque radially, partially through the vessel wall.
E. Displacement of the plaque axially into a less diseased portion of the artery, where obstruction is no longer critical.

Ref.: 9, 10

COMMENTS: The mechanism of action of balloon angioplasty probably varies from lesion to lesion depending on the physical characteristics of the plaque and artery locally. However, in a study of iliac angioplasty in humans using intravascular ultrasonography to assess mechanisms, dissection of the plaque away from the artery wall, creating a new extension and enlarging the previous flow channel occurred in each case. To a lesser extent, stretching the free wall and compression of the plaque itself also played a role in luminal enlargement in that study. Subsequent studies using intravascular ultrasonography have differed mainly in terms of the proportional enlargement due to dissection versus plaque compression and arterial wall stretching. It may be that "plaque fracture," as it is termed, with creation of an expanded flow channel in the area of dissection between plaque and vessel wall, is necessary for a good result. In clinical terms, this is likely in larger arteries with plaques that are focal and concentric rather than diffuse and eccentric.

ANSWER: B, C

6. The diagram below is a capnogram in an anesthetized, mechanically ventilated patient. Match the letters in the capnogram (in the left column) with the statements in the right column.

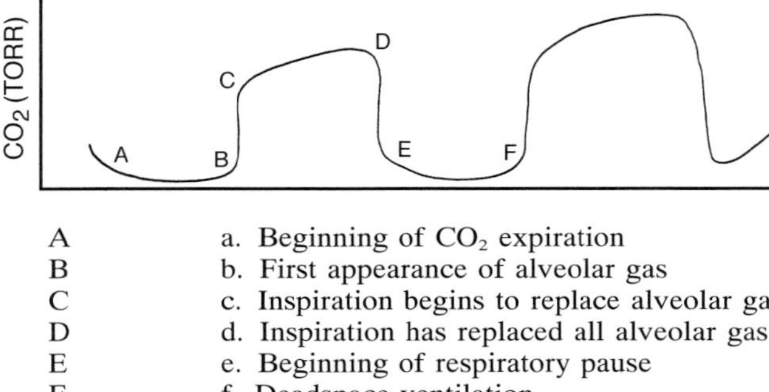

A	a. Beginning of CO_2 expiration
B	b. First appearance of alveolar gas
C	c. Inspiration begins to replace alveolar gas
D	d. Inspiration has replaced all alveolar gas
E	e. Beginning of respiratory pause
F	f. Deadspace ventilation

Ref.: 11

COMMENTS: See Question 7.

7. The "lazy slope" pattern of segment C–D in the above capnogram could be the result of which one or more of the following?

A. Wheezing.
B. Endotracheal tube kinking.
C. Herniation of endotracheal tube cuff.
D. Injection of sodium bicarbonate.

Ref.: 11

COMMENTS: The capnogram is a graphic display of the concentration of CO_2 in both inspired and expired air. End-expired concentrations of CO_2 are measured as a reflection of alveolar CO_2. Normally, the correlation between end-tidal CO_2 and alveolar CO_2 is good, with a normal difference of 4–6 mm Hg, the alveolar CO_2 being lower. There are many factors other than ventilation and perfusion that can affect the end-tidal CO_2. These factors should be considered when evaluating a capnogram and assessing a patient. The trachea must be intubated to produce a normal capnogram; end-tidal CO_2 value has become the standard to confirm successful intubation. Rate is the first variable to be evaluated by observing the number of waves per unit of time. To ensure accuracy, the rate of respiration as determined by the capnogram should be the same as the rate measured by examining the patient. With a patient who is breathing irregularly and "fighting" the ventilator, the rhythm of the capnogram is irregular with numerous fluctuations in the waveform (i.e., a patient who is ineffectively sedated or in need of increased pain medication). An irregular rhythm might also be seen in a patient with inadequate muscle relaxation. The contour of the capnogram, which is essentially horizontal in the normal state, can provide significant information about both the diagnosis and subsequent treatment of difficulties. Absence of a plateau immediately renders a capnogram nondiagnostic. The lazy slope demonstrated in the capnogram above can be produced by any factor that delays release of CO_2 over time, as is typically seen with obstructive airway disease, kinking of the endotracheal tube, or a foreign object that impedes flow of exhaled gases. Any outside source of acid may be converted to CO_2 via the carbonic anhydrase system. This CO_2 must be eliminated as well as the CO_2 produced by normal metabolic activity. Likewise, CO_2 administered during laparoscopy diffuses into the bloodstream, is delivered to the pulmonary circulation, and adds to expired gases, thereby affecting the measurement of end-tidal CO_2; states of increased metabolism such as fever are associated with increased CO_2 production. Inadequate flow of blood via the pulmonary vessels is associated with decreased CO_2 delivery and decreased end-tidal CO_2. Embolic phenomenon, both air and particulate in nature, can be responsible for sudden, persistent drops in end-tidal CO_2. Finally, following cardiac arrest the quality of resuscitation can be judged by the appearance of CO_2 in expired gases.

ANSWER:
Question 6: A-f; B-a; C-b; D-c; E-d; F-e
Question 7: A, B, C

8. An 80-year-old man undergoes cardiac catheterization through the right femoral artery. Two days later he complains of pain and swelling in the right groin, where a tender, pulsatile mass is palpable. His condition is stable. Which one or more of the following is/are indicated?

A. Arteriography.
B. Needle aspiration.
C. Surgical exploration.
D. Observation.
E. Color duplex scan.

Ref.: 12

COMMENTS: See Question 9.

9. In the patient in Question 8, a 3 cm pseudoaneurysm of the common femoral artery is detected. Initially, which one or more of the following is/are indicated?

A. Observation with restriction of activity.
B. Surgical repair.
C. Apply sandbag to site.
D. Ultrasound (US)-guided compression.
E. US-guided thrombin injection into the pseudoaneurysm.

Ref.: 12

COMMENTS: Localized swelling and hematoma are not infrequent complications of arterial catheterization, especially when anticoagulants and thrombolysins are used. The diagnostic aim is to differentiate a false aneurysm from hematoma. **Color Duplex scanning** is the ideal diagnostic procedure here. **Arteriography** can be helpful for evaluating for possible endovascular therapy if peripheral edema is present. **Blind needle aspiration** of the mass is hazardous, as bleeding may ensue. **Surgical exploration** can be successful but should be reserved for patients who do not respond to more conservative means or in whom massive bleeding or instability develops. **Observation** only may be appropriate in a patient with a small lesion who is stable; restricted activity may allow spontaneous thrombosis of the aneurysm. **Local sandbag** application may limit hematoma formation but rarely affects the aneurysm. **Compression** of the aneurysm under ultrasound guidance is successful in 90% of cases, but often it is time-consuming and fatiguing as well as uncomfortable for the patient. Sedation is usually required. Recently, ultrasound-guided **injection of 500–1000 units of thrombin** into the pseudoaneurysm has been successful in 90% of cases, with thrombosis of the aneurysm occurring within seconds.

ANSWER:
Question 8: D, E
Question 9: D, E

10. The neck anatomy of a 69-year-old man about to undergo carotid endarterectomy is shown in the diagram below. Match any one or more of the clinical statements (A–C) with the appropriate labeled anatomic structures.

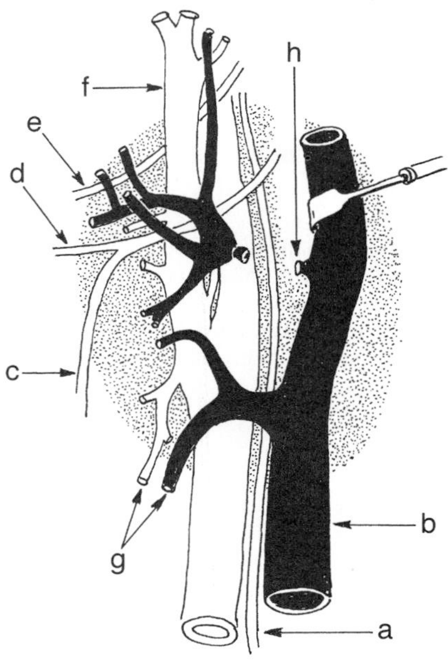

A. Injury causes deviation of tongue toward injured side.
B. Injury causes minor swallowing difficulty with ipsilateral vocal cord paralysis.
C. No discernible dysfunction follows its interruption.

Ref.: 4

COMMENTS: The rich supply of vessels, nerves, and conduits in the neck requires a thorough knowledge of the anatomy of this area and careful, precise operative technique if the possible serious consequences of injury are to be avoided in the course of performing carotid endarterectomy. The **hypoglossal nerve (d)** has a curvilinear path crossing the carotid bifurcation 1–2 cm cephalad to its bifurcation. Mobilizing this nerve to gain greater access to the internal carotid artery should be done with care. Injury to it results in deviation of the tongue to the side of the operation and subsequent difficulty with speech and mastication. The **ansa hypoglossi (c)** innervates the strap muscles; it can be sacrificed without serious dysfunction. The **vagus (a)** is large enough that inadvertent division is unlikely. It can, however, be injured by injudicious handling with the thumb forceps or even an errant clamp. Also, its close association with the carotid vessels necessitates dissection from them, which can lead to neurapraxia. However caused, this injury is manifested by minor swallowing difficulty, cord paralysis (recurrent laryngeal nerve), and temporary or permanent hoarseness. The **glossopharyngeal nerve (e)** is encountered in the upper reaches of the operative field. Sectioning this nerve is almost unheard of; more commonly, strong retraction in this area can injure it, resulting in difficulty swallowing. The common **facial vein (h)** or its branches (or both) are almost routinely divided to obtain better exposure of the carotid bifurcation; this operation is harmless. The **external carotid artery (f)** has an almost constant number of branches; they rarely require ligation, but if they do it can be done without consequences, as is true of the external carotid itself. The **superior thyroid artery and vein (g)** comprise a similar example. Even the **internal jugular vein (b)** can be divided unilaterally (which is extremely unlikely) with no important adverse consequences.

ANSWER: A-d; B-a, e; C-b, c, f, g, h

11. Regarding sentinel lymph node biopsy, which of the following is/are true?

A. This technique has been applied to the treatment of malignant melanoma, neuroendocrine carcinoma of the skin, penile and vulvar carcinoma, and breast cancer.
B. A sentinel lymph node is defined as the first lymph node (or nodes) to receive lymphatic drainage from a tumor at a given site. The histologic status of the sentinel lymph node is hypothesized to be representative of the entire lymph node basin.
C. Sentinel lymph node biopsy is an acceptable alternative to level I and II axillary lymph node dissection in breast cancer patients with clinically negative nodes and a tumor less than 3 cm in size.
D. Preoperative lymphoscintigraphy is not advisable prior to sentinel lymph node biopsy for melanomas of the head and neck.
E. Unfiltered ^{99m}Tc sulfur colloid is retained preferentially in the sentinel lymph node(s).

Ref.: 13, 14, 15, 16

COMMENTS: Although much effort has been directed toward employing molecular, cellular, and biochemical markers to determine the prognosis and treatment of solid tumors, the presence or absence of lymph node metastasis remains the most powerful predictor of outcome for both malignant melanoma and breast cancer. The concept of sentinel lymph node biopsy is that there is a primary, or "sentinel," lymph node (or nodes) through which tumor cells from a primary tumor in a particular location must first travel to spread to a given regional lymph node basin. A tracer substance injected at the primary tumor site provides a road map to identify the sentinel lymph node(s). In addition, careful examination of the sentinel lymph node(s) is hypothesized to represent the status of the entire lymph node basin. The objectives of employing sentinel lymph node biopsy in clinical practice include both decreasing the extent of operation for selected patients (decreasing the number of nontherapeutic lymphadenectomies) and increasing the identification rate of occult lymph node metastases (increasing the accuracy of staging). Evidence of a survival benefit for elective lymph node dissection in selected melanoma patients and immunohistochemical and reverse transcriptase–polymerase chain reaction (RT-PCR) based detection of metastases in lymph nodes deemed negative by standard histopathology imply that some patients are understaged by conventional techniques. Similar findings have been observed in studies of micrometastatic nodal disease in breast cancer. Sentinel lymph node biopsy as an alternative to elective node dissection in melanoma was first proposed by Morton et al., who used blue dye injected around the primary melanoma site to identify the sentinel node. Since then, others have advocated the use of radioactive colloid and a hand-held gamma counter with or without the use of blue dye. Either technique, or in combination, is generally acceptable at the present time for staging melanoma patients. Although a variety of radiocolloids have been employed successfully, unfiltered technetium 99m (^{99m}Tc) sulfur colloid diffuses out of the sentinel lymph node(s) (to second echelon lymph nodes) less rapidly than smaller particle tracers. Not all surgeons advocate the use of preoperative two-view lymphoscintigraphy in all melanoma patients, but most agree that it is necessary to identify the sentinel nodes in patients with head and neck melanoma. In these cases, not only is it common to find multiple sentinel lymph nodes, but finding multiple cervical sentinel lymph nodes or intraparotid lymph nodes may make a modified neck dissection or superficial parotidectomy (or both) advisable. Sentinel lymph node biopsy for breast cancer has not yet been established as the standard of care. The true false-negative rate, rather than the sensitivity of the test (as most patients studied have negative axillary lymph nodes), needs to be scrutinized. The technique of sentinel node localization varies widely among investigators, and the exclusion criteria in the reported studies have not been uniform. There is also disagreement on what to do about the nonaxillary sentinel lymph node. Some investigators are performing biopsies of internal mammary nodes—but to unclear benefit. Also, the technique of sentinel lymph node examination is demanding of the pathologist. There is no consensus on whether frozen section examination should be performed or on the number of sections that should be obtained from the sentinel lymph node. Multicenter trials are needed to confirm that a negative sentinel lymph node is an accurate indication that nodal metastases are not present before this approach can be proposed as the standard of care for clinically node-negative breast cancer patients.

ANSWER: A, B, E

12. Concerning the use of electrosurgical units during surgical incisions, which one or more of the following is/are true?

A. Coagulation current causes a higher risk of infection than does the scalpel.
B. Coagulation current causes greater necrosis than does cutting current.
C. Cutting current is based on the use of alternating current between 100 kHz and 10 MHz with a dampened sine wave.
D. Bipolar applicator limits tissue destruction to the area between electrodes.
E. The type of tissue destruction caused by alternating currents depends on the power level and the specific waveform utilized.

Ref.: 17, 18

COMMENTS: See Question 13.

13. Concerning the effect of lasers, electrocautery, and scalpel on wound healing, which one or more of the following is/are true?

A. Electrocautery requires less time to construct cutaneous flaps than the other modalities.
B. Bursting strength of flaps created using the scalpel is greater than that of those constructed using electrocautery but not greater than of those constructed using an Nd:YAG or CO_2 laser.
C. Better hemostasis is achieved using electrocautery than achieved using the scalpel.
D. Less drainage is observed at 48 hours for flaps created using the scalpel compared with that using other modalities.
E. Electrocautery significantly increases the risk of infection.

Ref.: 17, 18

COMMENTS: In 1928 W.T. Bovie, in collaboration with Harvey Cushing, developed the first commercially feasible electrosurgical unit. Cushing warned "that the new instrument adds a complication to already complicated procedures." The advantages of rapid and meticulous hemostasis should be balanced against the hazards of tissue destruction. Electrosurgical units develop local heat by electrical resistance to alternating current between 100 kHz and 10 MHz. Tissue destruction depends on the power level and the specific waveform utilized. A continuous sine wave produces temperatures exceeding 1000°C in an arc, leading to instant vaporization and rapid dissipation of heat; this provides little conduction of heat for coagulation. In contrast, a dampened sinusoidal wave, applied in short bursts, heats more slowly and facilitates charring coagulation of surrounding tissue. A bipolar applicator produces tissue destruction nearly limited to the area between the electrodes, using any waveform. Coagulation current causes more inflammation, necrosis, and abscesses than the scalpel, but it provides a tool for constructing cutaneous flaps and achieving hemostasis more rapidly. Cutting current is less destructive than coagulation current but less hemostatic. Drainage is less and bursting strength greater for flaps created using sharp dissection compared with those achieved by other modalities. Significantly less drainage is observed after 48 hours for flaps constructed using electrocautery than those created with a CO_2 laser.

ANSWER:
Question 12: A, B, D, E
Question 13: C, D, E

14. Concerning the cardiopulmonary effects of pneumoperitoneum during laparoscopy, which one or more of the following is/are true?

A. Cardiopulmonary dysfunction occurs when the intraabdominal pressure (AP) reaches 20 or more mm Hg in normovolemic patients.
B. Positive end-expiratory pressure (PEEP) offsets the hemodynamic effects of pneumoperitoneum.
C. Hypovolemia lowers the level of IAP needed to cause deleterious hemodynamic effects.
D. Laparoscopic surgery prevents diaphragmatic dysfunction during the postoperative period of patients with chronic obstructive pulmonary disease (COPD).
E. Increased IAP leads to increased concentrations of plasma renin, decreased venous return, and decreased intracavitary atrial pressures.

Ref.: 19, 20

COMMENTS: See Question 15.

15. Concerning carbon dioxide (CO_2) pneumoperitoneum, which one or more of the following is/are true?

A. CO_2 directly vasodilates peripheral arterioles and depresses myocardial contractility.
B. CO_2 indirectly evokes sympathoadrenal activation.
C. CO_2 can cause cardiac arrhythmias because of gas emboli.
D. CO_2 pneumoperitoneum can result in persistent postoperative hypercapnia.

E. CO_2 causes a decrease in gastric mucosal pH.

Ref.: 19, 20

COMMENTS: Intraabdominal hypertension can cause pulmonary and cardiovascular compromise when the IAP reaches 20–40 mm Hg of pressure in normovolemic patients. PEEP and IAP have additive effects on preload. IAP hypertension results in elevated peak airway pressures, decreased pulmonary compliance and vital capacity, and increased alveolar deadspace. Even though laparoscopic surgery has been associated with lesser derangement of pulmonary function and a lower incidence of postoperative pulmonary complications when compared to laparotomy, its use in patients with COPD may be deleterious. The hemodynamic effects of increased IAP seem to be due to a decreased cardiac output caused by a decreasing preload, an increasing systemic vascular resistance, and an abrupt increase in mean arterial pressure. Therefore myocardial oxygen demand is increased and coronary perfusion is decreased. Indirectly, CO_2 activates the sympathoadrenal axis, increasing myocardial contractility and causing tachycardia and hypertension. During CO_2 pneumoperitoneum, the indirect effects of CO_2 seem to dominate. Renal function deteriorates at an IAP of 10 mm Hg because of lower renal cortical perfusion, which results in activation of the renin system. In addition, insufflation of cold CO_2 may cause renal vasoconstriction. Avoiding high IAP and the use of warm CO_2 may be beneficial in patients with limited renal function. Profound hypercarbia and respiratory acidosis during CO_2 pneumoperitoneum may occur, leading to prolonged postoperative mechanical ventilation. The minute volume ventilation must be increased by 35% to avoid acidosis. End-tidal CO_2 concentrations increase progressively, reaching a plateau at 40 minutes. Thereafter, CO_2 begins to accumulate in the body, the bone being the largest reservoir. The stored CO_2 must be exhaled postoperatively. Gastric tonometry measures the mucosal CO_2 concentration and permits calculation of the mucosal pH, which is lower in cases of splanchnic ischemia. As perfusion decreases, the concentration of hydrogen ions increases. The cellular buffer system produces CO_2, which accumulates in the mucosa.

ANSWER:
Question 14: A, C
Question 15: A, B, C, D, E

16. Concerning the use of ultrasonography in clinical practice, which one or more of the following is/are false?

A. Ultrasound has a frequency equal to human hearing, that is, 20 kHz.
B. A 10 MHz transducer is ideal for scanning deep abdominal structures.
C. The speed of ultrasound waves in blood is slower than that of ultrasound through air.
D. Hypoechoic tissues are less echoic or darker than surrounding tissue.
E. Acoustic shadowing is due to the ultrasound wave being reflected back to the transducer.
F. B-mode ultrasonography refers to amplitude mode.

Ref.: 21

COMMENTS: Ultrasonography is highly operator-dependent. Ultrasound is mechanical energy, generated by the piezoelectric crystal and transmitted through a medium. The higher the frequency, the greater is the resolution and the lesser the penetration. Thus deep structures require lower frequencies. Ultrasound has a frequency higher than human hearing (20 MHz).

The propagation velocity in tissue depends on the mechanical properties of the medium through which it travels. In general, the more stiff and less compressible the medium, the faster is the propagation velocity. Ultrasound travels more slowly through air (343 m/s) and faster through bone (3000 m/s). For soft tissue, the speed of ultrasound is approximately 1540 m/s.

As ultrasound interacts with tissue, energy is lost by reflection, scattering, refraction, and absorption. Refraction and absorption divert sound energy from the receiving transducer. Most common causes of artifacts include air, calcium and reverberation.

A-mode refers to the amplitude mode and is used primarily for ocular imaging and echoencephalography. B-mode refers to brightness mode; for real-time imaging B-mode ultrasonography is the most common mode used in clinical practice. M-mode, which refers to motion mode, is designed to study the myocardium.

ANSWER: A, B, C, F

17. Which of the following provides the best image resolution?

A. Human eye.
B. Photographic film 35 mm.
C. Computer-enhanced high-definition television (HDTV).
D. National Television Systems Committee (NTSC) video format.
E. Phase alternating line (PAL) video format.

Ref.: 22

COMMENTS: Video technology converts the optical image from a laparoscope or endoscope into an electronic signal that can subsequently be used for a variety of purposes, such as display, recording, or transmission. Video systems originated from television analogue formats that capture and send an image using scanning lines. More scanning lines can store more information and hence provide better resolution. Digital systems use a row of silicon elements on a CCD chip instead of scanning lines. The NTSC format used in North America has 525 lines at a rate of 30 frames per second. The PAL format, used in some other parts of the world, has 625 lines at 25 frames per second. HDTV may provide more than 1000 scan lines. The human eye can detect about 1600 scan lines, whereas the resolution of 35 mm photographic film is about 2300 scan lines. The best-quality still images are thus 35 mm photographs. However, attaching a camera to the ocular lens of a scope during a procedure is less convenient than capturing lower quality stills from current video systems.

ANSWER: B

18. Which of the following types of video signals provides the highest quality recording?

A. Composite signal.
B. Super VHS component signal.
C. RGB component signal.
D. Digitally processed signal.

Ref.: 22

COMMENTS: Video signals can be categorized as composite signals or component signals. **Composite** signals, which are used in standard video and television, have a single channel for all of the information. Higher quality images are obtained with **component** systems that carry the information over separate channels. Super VHS (S-VHS or S-video) divides the signal into brightness (luminance = Y) and color (chrominance = C) components. RGB signals split the color into red, green, and blue over three separate channels with a fourth channel for brightness. When connecting the cameras, recorders, and monitors during endoscopic or laparoscopic procedures, the operator should ensure that compatible outlets are used. Also, whether the monitor and recorder are arranged in a parallel or serial configuration with the camera unit affects image quality. Digital processing of the CCD signal currently provides the highest quality image for recording and subsequent duplication or modification. The analogue image is converted to a binary code, which is not subject to the same distortion (as a continuous electronic waveform) during transmission or reconstruction. Most systems in current use are not completely digital, however, and are limited by the analogue components.

ANSWER: D

19. Fiberoptic light cables have which of the following characteristics?

A. Fiberoptic cables are more flexible than fluid cables.
B. Fiberoptic cables transmit a more accurate light spectrum than fluid cables.
C. Fiberoptic cables must be soaked for sterilization.
D. Fiberoptic cables can be gas-sterilized.

Ref.: 22

COMMENTS: Cables transmit high intensity light from the light source to the viewing scope during laparoscopic or endoscopic procedures. Light transmission to and through the scope is critical to visualization and documentation. Fiberoptic cables are flexible but do not transmit as precise a light spectrum as fluid cables. Fluid cables transmit more light and a complete spectrum but are more rigid and require soaking for sterilization.

ANSWER: A, D

20. Which of the following statements is/are true with regard to the ultrasonically activated harmonic scalpel?

A. The active blade vibrates at a frequency of 100,000 Hz.
B. The time required for advanced laparoscopic procedures has been reduced when using the harmonic scalpel.
C. Electrical energy generated by the scalpel is the mechanism for coagulation.
D. Use of the harmonic scalpel is more cost-effective than the use of clip appliers for dividing medium-sized blood vessels.

Ref.: 23

COMMENTS: The harmonic scalpel uses mechanical energy rather than electrical energy to achieve hemostasis. A transducer in the handpiece vibrates at a frequency of 55,000 Hz; and a laparoscopic extender carries the energy to the tissue. The blade couples with the tissue and mechanically denatures protein by disrupting hydrogen bonds within the protein structure. The disorganized protein forms a sticky coagulum that coats the vessel walls. Time required for procedures such as short gastric vessel division has been reduced, resulting in a shortened operating time for advanced laparoscopic procedures. If one considers the shortened time for a procedure when using the harmonic scalpel and the cost of clip appliers when they are used for vessel ligation and division, the harmonic scalpel has also been shown to reduce the overall cost of advanced laparoscopic procedures.

ANSWER: B, D

21. With regard to expanded polytetrafluoroethylene (Gore-Tex) and polypropylene mesh (Marlex) which of the following statements are true?

A. Expanded polytetrafluoroethylene contains spaces smaller than 10 μm and may harbor bacteria.
B. Expanded polytetrafluoroethylene and polypropylene mesh are well tolerated without significant evidence of rejection.
C. Polypropylene mesh and expanded polytetrafluoroethylene incorporate into host tissue at equal infiltration rates.
D. Polypropylene mesh and expanded polytetrafluoroethylene come in both absorbable and nonabsorbable forms.

Ref.: 24

COMMENTS: Absorbable synthetic mesh materials include polyglycolic acid (Dexon), polyglactin (Vicryl), and carbon fiber mesh. Nonabsorbable meshes include tantalum, stainless steel, polyester cloth (Dacron), polyester sheeting (Mylar), nylon mesh, Dacron mesh (Mersilene), acrylic cloth (Orlon), polyvinyl sponge (Ivalon), polytetrafluoroethylene (PTFE: Teflon mesh and cloth), expanded PTFE (Gore-Tex), polyvinyl cloth (Vinyon-N), and polypropylene mesh (Marlex and Prolene). Polypropylene mesh, PTFE, Dacron, and Teflon mesh are well tolerated without significant evidence of rejection. Any biomaterial that contains pores or spaces less than 10 μm in size cannot allow ingress of granulocytes to clear infection. Consequently, they are associated with an increased chance of infection and sinus tract formation. Expanded PTFE contains spaces smaller than 10 μm. In contrast, polypropylene is made of widely spaced monofilament fibers. Expanded PTFE has been shown to allow penetration of fibroblasts at a depth of only 10% at 3 years, whereas polypropylene mesh has complete incorporation of host tissue throughout the thickness of the biomaterial at 3 years.

ANSWER: A, B

22. Which of the following insufflation gases for a laparoscopic pneumoperitoneum has the greatest solubility in water?

A. Carbon dioxide.
B. Nitrous oxide.
C. Helium.
D. Argon.

Ref.: 22

COMMENTS: see Question 24.

23. Which of the following insufflation gases for a laparoscopic pneumoperitoneum supports combustion?

A. Carbon dioxide.
B. Nitrous oxide.
C. Helium.
D. Argon.
E. None of the above.

Ref.: 22

COMMENTS: see Question 24.

24. Which of the following insufflation gases for a laparoscopic pneumoperitoneum can cause hypercarbia and acidosis?

A. Carbon dioxide.
B. Nitrous oxide.
C. Helium.
D. Argon.
E. None of the above.

Ref.: 22

COMMENTS: The gas used for laparoscopic pneumoperitoneum should be colorless, inert, nonexplosive, and nontoxic, with high solubility in water (blood) and low solubility in tissue; also, it should be available and inexpensive. Gases that rapidly dissolve in blood have a lower risk of venous air embolus, which can be fatal. CO_2, the most commonly used insufflating gas, is highly soluble in water but can cause hypercarbia and acidosis. CO_2 can also be associated with increases in arterial pressure, pulmonary vascular resistance, and pulmonary arterial pressure and with decreased cardiac contractility. Usually these changes are not clinically significant, but they can be important in patients with underlying cardiac or respiratory problems. The other gases listed do not affect acid-base balance but have their own disadvantages. Nitrous oxide supports combustion, so it could be hazardous when electrocautery or laser is used. Helium is less water-soluble than CO_2 (although more diffusible) and may therefore result in subcutaneous emphysema of longer duration and theoretically a higher risk of gas embolism. Argon is more water-soluble than nitrogen but is still much less soluble than CO_2. Argon has been associated with significant cardiac depression in experimental settings and has not been widely used clinically.

ANSWER:
Question 22: A
Question 23: B
Question 24: A

25. Laparoscopic splenectomy is performed for idiopathic thrombocytopenic purpura (ITP). The specimen should be removed by:

A. Extending one of the port site incisions to accommodate the specimen.
B. Fragmenting the specimen and removing the pieces through a 12 mm port.
C. Placing it in a retrieval bag, fragmenting it, exteriorizing the bag through a port site and removing it piecemeal.
D. Placing it in a retrieval bag and removing intact specimen through a separate incision.

Ref.: 22

COMMENTS: Laparoscopic surgery must contend with the need to remove specimens that are larger than the laparoscopic port sites. There are a variety of techniques by which this may be accomplished, depending on the nature and size of the specimen and whether there is a need to preserve the specimen intact. Potential routes for specimen removal include port sites, extension of port site incisions, separate abdominal wall incisions, and transanal and transvaginal routes. Use of a retrieval bag can minimize contamination and specimen loss and is particularly important if the specimen is infected, friable, or malignant. Fragmentation of large solid specimens is appropriate to preserve the advantage of small laparoscopic incisions, provided an intact specimen is not required for pathologic evaluation. Fragmentation is contraindicated if the lesion is potentially malignant. When laparoscopic splenectomy is performed for ITP, it is standard to place the spleen in a sturdy retrieval bag, externalize the bag orifice at a port site, and then remove the spleen piecemeal. Great care must be taken to avoid internal rupture of the spleen or of the bag, which could result in splenosis.

ANSWER: C

26. The ultrasound images displayed below illustrate anatomic structures **routinely** seen during the performance of a breast ultrasound examination as well as a number of commonly encountered **artifacts** related to the real-time performance of a breast scan. Match the answer that most closely corresponds to the images shown.

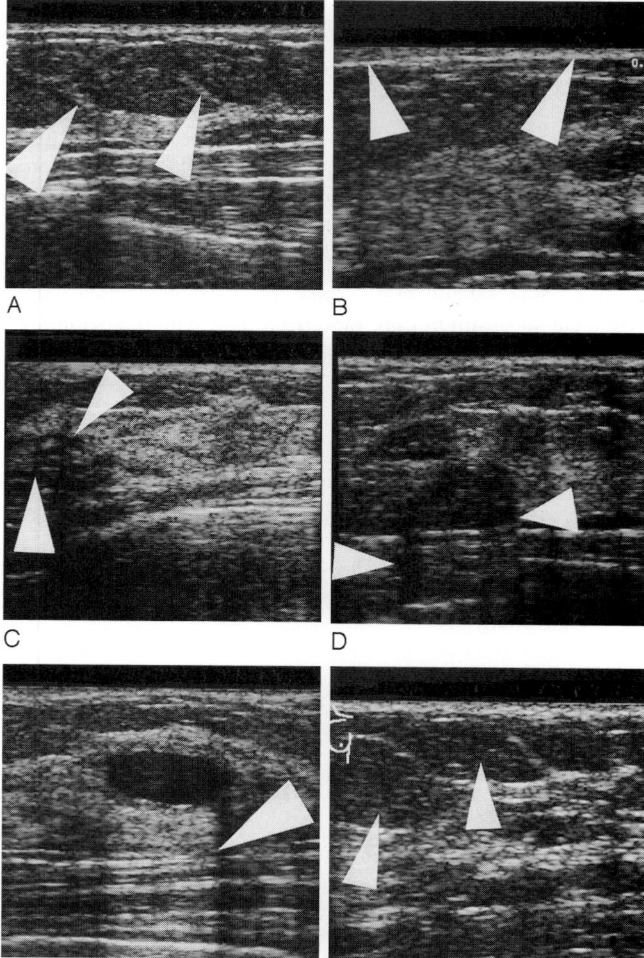

Image	*Demonstrates*
A	a. Subareolar ducts
B	b. Shadowing
C	c. Adipose tissue
D	d. Enhancement
E	e. Skin illustrating variable thickness
F	f. Cooper's ligaments

Ref.: 25

COMMENTS: Cooper's ligaments: During its formation the breast develops within an envelope of connective tissue. This envelope of fascia splits into an anterior and posterior layer within which the parenchyma resides. Cooper's, the suspensory ligaments of the breast, tether the breast tissue to this bilaminar fascial envelope. They are most clearly seen as bright, hyperechoic linear extensions arching toward and away from the anterior leaf of the superficial fascia at the dermal boundary. **Skin of variable thickness**: The skin appears as a hyperechoic (bright) line at the top of the image. It has a variable thickness that can be seen on the image. The skin is thickest at the nipple–areolar junction (approximately 4 mm in depth) and thinnest at the periphery of the breast (approximately 2 mm in depth). Careful assessment of the skin line during breast scanning can provide important clues (i.e., a localized area of thickness) that may be reflective of changes in the parenchyma deep to the area. A light touch on the transducer preserves these subtle differences. **Subareolar duct**: A scan of the nipple–areolar area delineates multiple hypoechoic (dark) structures in a rich connective tissue lattice work that is hyperechoic (bright). The hypoechoic areas are ducts. Depending on the orientation of the transducer to the scanned area, the ducts may appear in cross section, tangentially, or parallel to the ducts. The ducts converging at the nipple–areolar junction are larger than those located peripherally. Nipple discharge is often associated with an ectatic (i.e., markedly enlarged) duct and ultrasound can be used effectively to locate and analyze an area that is often clinically difficult to detect. **Shadowing**: Shadowing is an artifact generated by the interaction of tissue with the ultrasound beam. The ultrasound pulse generated by the transducer travels in a straight line from this source into the tissue being scanned and receives the returning pulse echo as well. The amplitude (strength of signal) of the returning echo is then displayed on the monitor in varying shades of gray that are dependent for their intensity on the strength of the returning signal. The returning signal may be diminished by the number of pulse–tissue interactions and can result in shadowing. Shadowing is seen as a hypoechoic (dark) area immediately underneath the area of interest. The shadowing itself results from a lack of return signal to the transducer. The loss of signal is accounted for by a number of interactions: The signal may be deflected away from the transducer, scattered within the focal lesion with resultant diminution of the return echo, or simply converted to heat and dissipated. Shadowing is seen in both benign and malignant conditions. **Enhancement**: Enhancement is another useful artifact. Often it is called through-transmission and is seen on the monitor as a bright band extending below the area of interest. Because of the lack of impedance to the ultrasound signal (i.e., reflection, scatter) in and through the area of interest, there is increased signal reception deep to the focal lesion. The area of through-transmission appears correspondingly brighter than the areas immediately adjacent to this point. Ultrasound pulses are reflected back to, or away from, the transducer by slight differences in acoustic impedance between one tissue type and another. If an area is composed of tissue or fluid with the same acoustic properties, the strength of the returning ultrasound signal is greater than the returning signal from the area adjacent to it. Enhancement results. **Adipose tissue**: Adipose tissue appears hypoechoic (darker) in relation to stromal tissue (hyperechoic). Adipose tissue can appear around the breast parenchyma as well as within it. It is seen immediately underneath the skin and is traversed by Cooper's ligaments. By virtue of the contrast between the darker adipose tissue and brighter stromal network of the parenchyma, the anterior lobar contour is easily seen. Additionally, there is a layer of adipose tissue deep to the posterior surface of the breast lobe. This retromammary fat pad is not commonly well developed and often is poorly developed or not seen.

ANSWER: A-f; B-e; C-a; D-b; E-d; F-c

27. Breast ultrasonography is used as a clinical tool to evaluate *mammographic* abnormalities, *clinically detected* abnormalities, and as an *adjunctive* means to evaluate "dense breasts" noted on mammography. Evaluation of an ultrasonically detected focal lesion includes an assessment of a lesion's contour, margins, internal echo characteristics, and the presence or absence of shadowing and enhancement. Match the lettered image with the most likely diagnosis.

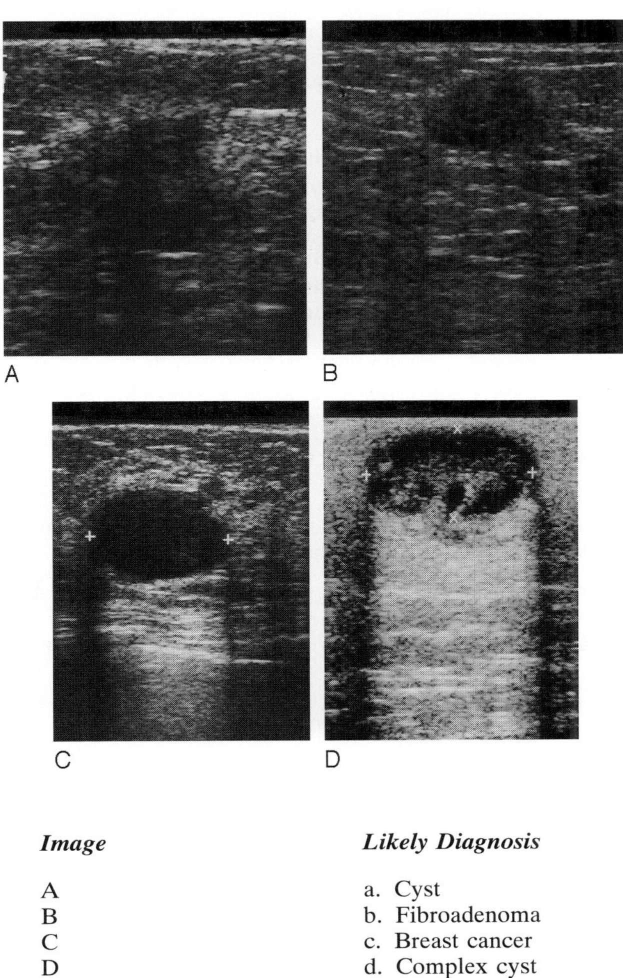

Image	*Likely Diagnosis*
A	a. Cyst
B	b. Fibroadenoma
C	c. Breast cancer
D	d. Complex cyst

Ref.: 25

COMMENTS: **Cyst**: Depending on the fluid characteristics within a cyst and the tension exerted on the cyst wall by hydrostatic pressure, the contours and internal echo pattern of a cyst may vary. If tense, cyst contours are round; if not, the cyst may appear ovoid or even elongated. The margins, however, are always sharp and smooth with bilateral edge shadowing. If the fluid within the cyst is uniform, the cyst appears anechoic (black); and because of nonimpedance of the ultrasound pulse, through-transmission (posterior enhancement) is present. **Complex cyst**: The classic picture of a fluid-filled cyst is an anechoic (black) lumen. However, the presence of internal echoes in what would otherwise appear to be a simple cyst may be due to more viscous liquid. This is most commonly seen in long-standing cysts where proteinaceous material has been secreted into the cyst lumen. Internal echoes within the cyst may also be generated by an intracystic papilloma and, on occasion, by reverberation artifact. Because of the indeterminate nature of the internal echoes, fine-needle aspiration is required for diagnosis. **Fibroadenoma**: Fibroadenomas have many of the characteristics of a cyst. Their smooth contour can result in bilateral edge shadowing; the homogeneity of the tissue comprising a fibroadenoma often produces posterior enhancement because of the low impedance to the ultrasound pulse. These internal characteristics produce a homogeneous internal echo pattern that is hypoechoic. Its appearance may mimic that of a complicated cyst. Focal lesions thought to be potentially solid on ultrasound scans should be subjected to histologic or cytologic evaluation. Medullary carcinoma, a solid lesion, may appear indistinguishable from a fibroadenoma. **Carcinoma**: Breast carcinoma displays characteristic features on ultrasound examination. Typically, the contour of most cancers is jagged and irregular. Because of the desmoplastic response generated by the malignancy, the internal echo pattern seen is markedly heterogeneous and irregular. Because of the great degree of scattering and attenuation caused by the mixed tissue components, the area corresponding to the body of the tumor is hypoechoic. Posterior shadowing, when present, is irregular and does not disappear with a change of transducer angulation or increased transducer pressure. Remember, some breast cancers can have smooth contours, posterior enhancement, and other findings associated with benign conditions. Careful and thoughtful analysis of each focal lesion encountered is required.

ANSWER: A-c; B-b; C-a; D-d

28. Which of the following statements is/are true with regard to the argon beam coagulator?

A. The coagulator delivers a laser beam that coagulates tissue by a light reaction.
B. The depth of necrosis is related to the power setting of the argon beam.
C. The coagulator is useful for minimizing bleeding from raw surfaces of intestine.
D. The coagulator can be a useful adjunct to laparoscopic surgery.

Ref.: 26, 27, 28

COMMENTS: The argon beam coagulator (ABC) uses a radiofrequency range of energy across a jet of inert gas (argon) that provides a noncontact monopolar zone of necrosis. It is most useful for aiding hemostasis with solid organs such as the liver, spleen, and kidney. The depth of injury is proportional to the duration and energy delivered and the organ treated. The depth of thermal injury to the spleen and liver ranges from 2 to 7 mm. The absence of smoke and the no-touch technique makes it particularly useful for laparoscopic application. The argon has demonstrated a clear advantage in the reduction of hyperplastic nasal turbinates, telangiectatic lesions in the nasal mucosa, and progressive papillomatosis of the larynx. When used properly and with an understanding of its potential for inadvertent thermal injury, ABC can be safely used with improved hemostasis; minimal depth of thermal injury; shortened duration of the procedure; decreased blood loss, edema, and ecchymosis; and the ability to more safely coagulate around neural tissue.

ANSWER: B, D

29. Which of the following statements regarding the physics of laser light is/are true?

A. When atoms become excited, electrons move to lower energy states.
B. Return of electrons to a ground state leads to release of energy as photons or heat.
C. All stimulated photons are amplified and released as laser light.
D. Laser light is coherent.
E. Laser light is multichromatic.

Ref.: 29

COMMENTS: The word laser is an acronym for *l*ight *a*mplification *s*timulated for the *e*mission of *r*adiation. The development of the laser was based on theories first proposed in 1917 by Einstein on the existence of stimulated emission of energy from atoms. When atoms become excited (stimulated) by an energy source, they absorb energy. This leads to the electrons of these atoms moving to higher orbits (higher energy states) around the nucleus. The excited electron spontaneously returns to a lower orbit (ground state) with release (emission) of the absorbed energy in the form of a photon (light) or as heat. It was not, however, until 1960 that Theodore Maimon invented the first laser that produced visible light. The laser energy source (or pump) generally is an electrical current, but other energy sources may also lead to stimulated emission of light. The stimulated light is amplified in an optical resonator composed essentially of two opposing mirrors. The light exits through a partially transmissive mirror at one end and may be focused through lenses placed in the path of the laser beam. Only photons traveling back and forth between the two opposing mirrors become amplified and are released as laser light. The photons that move out of this plane are lost as heat and are the reason most lasers need an efficient cooling system. This process of stimulated emission results in light with three unique properties. Laser light is **coherent**; the laser light waves are in phase, analogous to waves landing on a beach. This results in the ability to focus a laser beam into a small spot with high power. Laser light is **collimated**; the laser light beams remain tightly together over a long distance without significant loss of this high power. Finally, laser light is **monochromatic**; that is, laser light produces a pure-color light, which allows targeting of molecules with strong absorption of a specific wavelength.

ANSWER: B, D

30. Match each type of laser in the left column with the appropriate medium in the right column.

A. Carbon dioxide (CO_2)
B. Neodymium:yttrium aluminum garnet (Nd:YAG)
C. Argon
D. Potassium titanyl phosphate (KTP)
E. Diode

a. Solid
b. Gaseous
c. Electronic

Ref.: 29

COMMENTS: Increasing types of lasers have found application in medicine. Primarily, they include the CO_2 laser, argon laser, KTP laser, and Nd:YAG laser. Lasers are named for the medium used to produce light, that is, the medium stimulated by the energy source leading to release of the stored energy as photons (light). These media may be **gasseous**, as in the case of the CO_2 and argon; **solid**, as in the case of the KTP or Nd:YAG laser; and even **electronic**, as in the case of the diode laser. The wavelength of laser light produced depends on the medium used; lasers of different wavelength have dramatically different abilities to cut, coagulate, or vaporize tissue.

ANSWER: A-b; B-a; C-b; D-a; E-c

31. Which of the following characteristics affect the energy generated in tissue by the laser?

A. Laser power.
B. Laser beam diameter.
C. Duration of exposure.
D. Tissue color.
E. Color of the laser light.

Ref.: 29

COMMENTS: Lasers produce their effect on tissue through absorption; therefore laser energy is absorptive energy. The absorbed light generates heat, resulting in tissue effects, which include cutting, coagulation, and vaporization. There are a variety of factors that regulate the effect of laser light on tissue: (1) the **power** of the laser machine as measured in watts; (2) the **spot size**, or diameter, of the laser beam contacting the tissue; (3) the **duration** of laser exposure; and (4) the degree of **absorption** of laser light, which is a function of tissue **color** and the laser light color (which is a function of the laser's wavelength). Power (watts) divided by spot size (cm^2) equals the *power density*. This, plus an increase in time of exposure or increased tissue absorption, increases the local tissue effect. Generally, to **cut** with a laser, one uses a higher power with a small spot size (focused beam) for a short duration. For optimal **coagulation**, one uses a somewhat lower power but with a larger spot size (defocused beam) and for a longer duration.

ANSWER: A, B, C, D, E

32. Concerning the characteristics of the CO_2 laser, which of the following statements is/are true?

A. It produces a relatively short wavelength of 500 nm.
B. It has a wide scatter, making it an excellent instrument for coagulation.
C. It produces visible red light, which minimizes the risk of inadvertent eye injury.
D. It is excellent for treating pelvic endometriosis and adhesions.
E. It is transmitted via a flexible fiber.

Ref.: 29

COMMENTS: The CO_2 laser produces a long wavelength of 10,600 nm, which results in nonvisible light in the infrared range. Inadvertent eye injury is avoided by using an accompanying aiming beam laser of low power and a visible light (i.e., helium/neon) and by the mandatory routine use of protective eyewear. The CO_2 laser is quite precise with scant penetration, or scatter, resulting in minimal adjacent tissue injury of approximately 0.5 mm and a histologic zone of necrosis of approximately 0.1 mm. As such, the CO_2 laser is a particularly effective cutting instrument, but it has minimal coagulative ability. The CO_2 laser has been the workhorse of lasers in clinical medicine and has demonstrated its utility in procedures involving the skin, eye, and upper aerodigestive and female genital tracts. Because of its excellent vaporization ability, it has been the preferred laser of gynecologists for treating pelvic endometriosis for lysing of adhesions, and of dermatologists for treating verrucae. It is also quite effective for the débridement of decubitus ulcers. The CO_2 laser cannot, however, be transmitted through flexible optic fibers and therefore is somewhat limited by its requirement for a rigid, articulated arm delivery system, which directs the laser beam with the aid of angled, mounted mirrors.

ANSWER: D

33. Match each type of laser in the left column with the appropriate statement(s) in the right column.

A. Nd:YAG
B. Argon
C. KTP

a. Fiberoptic laser
b. Deep coagulation
c. Superficial coagulation
d. Useful for treating neovascular lesions in diabetic retinopathy
e. Treatment of obstructing, nonoperable rectal cancer

Ref.: 29

COMMENTS: The Nd:YAG, argon, and KTP lasers are deliverable via optical fibers. When used as a free beam, the Nd: YAG laser generates significant coagulation. The argon and KTP lasers are considered superficial photocoagulators but may also cut and vaporize without the extensive damage characterized by the free-beam Nd:YAG laser. In contrast to the CO_2 laser, there is fair divergence of the Nd:YAG, argon, and KTP laser beams, which results in minimal tissue effect 2 inches or more from the tip. When the tip is quite near (1–2 mm) the tissue, cutting results; several millimeters from the tip, vaporization results; and at 1–2 cm from the tip, coagulation occurs. Whereas the depth of tissue injury with the argon and KTP laser varies between 0.5 and 2.0 mm, the free-beam YAG is highly absorbed in dark tissue and may result in tissue injury at 2–6 mm depth. The argon laser is absorbed by pigments (i.e., hemoglobin, melanin), making it useful for procedures such as treatment of neovascular lesions in diabetic retinopathy and superficial vascular lesions such as telangiectasias or port-wine stains, but limiting its ability to coagulate a frankly bleeding lesion. Because the Nd:YAG laser causes deep tissue penetrance and coagulation, it has become the laser of choice for endoscopic palliation of nonoperable obstructing tumors of the respiratory and gastrointestinal tracts and for the treatment of a bleeding lesion (i.e., ulcer).

ANSWER: A-a, b, e; B-a, c, d; C-a, c

34. The absorption time for chromic catgut suture is approximately:

A. 1 week.
B. 2 weeks.
C. 2 months.
D. 6 months.
E. It is nonabsorbable.

Ref.: 1

COMMENTS: Surgical sutures are broadly characterized as absorbable or nonabsorbable. Suture materials can also be braided or monofilament. Knowledge of the specific characteristics of suture material is important for selecting the type of suture for a particular clinical application. Plain catgut suture, derived from sheep or cattle intestine, absorbs in about a week. Treatment of catgut with chromium delays proteolytic digestion. All catgut suture incites more inflammatory reaction than the various synthetic absorbable sutures (polyglycolic acid, polyglyconate, polyglactic acid, polydiaxanone), which are dissolved by hydrolysis and last 60–90 days or longer. Nonabsorbable suture materials include silk, polyester, nylon, and polypropylene. Monofilament sutures are more resistant to infection than braided materials but do not handle as easily.

ANSWER: B

35. Which of the following is the most appropriate type of central catheter for a patient requiring long-term home parenteral nutrition?

A. Tunneled, single-lumen catheter.
B. Tunneled, double-lumen catheter.
C. Single-lumen catheter with implanted port.
D. Double-lumen implanted port.
E. Peripherally inserted central venous catheter.

Ref.: 1

COMMENTS: A number of catheter devices are available for the purpose of providing long-term central venous access. These catheters are typically indicated for administration of parenteral nutrition, chemotherapeutic agents, antibiotics, or other medications. Selection of the most appropriate device must take into account the specific therapeutic needs, the estimated duration of therapy, and the concerns and capabilities of the individual patient. The goal is to provide durable access for the necessary length of treatment with the lowest risk of complications, particularly catheter sepsis. Multilumen catheters in general have been associated with higher infection rates than single lumen catheters. Implanted ports are designed for intermittent cannulation and have been particularly useful for patients receiving cytotoxic chemotherapy for malignant disease. They are convenient for patients because there is no externalized portion that requires attention. However, implanted ports have been associated with higher rates of sepsis when used for home hyperalimentation.

ANSWER: A

36. Which one of the following infectious complications of an implanted central venous catheter (Hickman type) require(s) catheter removal?

A. Exit site infection.
B. Subcutaneous tunnel infection.
C. Bacteremia without local signs of catheter infection.
D. Septic thrombophlebitis.
E. All of the above.

Ref.: 1

COMMENTS: The seemingly obvious response to a possibly infected central venous catheter would be to remove the catheter and treat the patient with antibiotics. In clinical practice, the solution is often not so simple, as many patients have important ongoing needs for central vascular access and often do not have other readily available access sites. There is also a spectrum of clinical severity of catheter infection and infection sources other than the catheter that may be responsible for the patient's symptoms. Local infection at the catheter exit site can frequently be resolved without catheter removal. Infections involving the subcutaneous tunnel are more problematic and necessitate removal more often, although catheter salvage may still be possible. If there is bacteremia without local evidence of infection, other sources should be sought. Gram-positive bacteria infect a vascular catheter more easily than gram-negative bacteria. Septic thrombophlebitis mandates catheter removal. Obviously, if the patient does not have a pressing need for the catheter it should be removed.

ANSWER: D

37. A patient with a subclavian Hickman catheter develops pain and swelling of the arm and neck. The catheter still functions, and ongoing vascular access is required. The most appropriate management is:

A. Intravenous antibiotics and catheter removal.
B. Infusion of thrombolytic agents through the catheter.
C. Systemic anticoagulation and catheter removal.
D. Systemic anticoagulation without removing catheter.
E. Catheter removal.

Ref.: 30

COMMENTS: Venous thrombosis is an important complication of long-term central vascular access catheters. The diagnosis can often be confirmed by noninvasive ultrasonographic Doppler evaluation or venography. Because the thrombosis typically forms in the vein distal to the catheter tip it is not unusual for the catheter to continue to function. Treatment requires systemic anticoagulation. The catheter can be left in place, particularly for patients who require continued access and who may have limited alternative access sites. If there is evidence of infected thrombosis, catheter removal and antibiotics are indicated.

ANSWER: D

38. Which of the following is/are true regarding cryosurgical ablation of liver tumors?

A. A treatment goal of −40° to −50°C is needed to ensure cellular death.
B. Tissue freezing produes a hypertonic environment.
C. Tissue thawing produces a hypotonic milieu.
D. Ultrasonography is an integral tool for this procedure.
E. Complications include myoglobinuria, abnormalities of coagulation, pleural effusion.

Ref.: 31

COMMENTS: Cryosurgical ablation is the destruction of tissue by a process of freezing and thawing. It has recently become a widely accepted method for treating unresectable liver metastases. Unresectability may be due to the number of lesions, the ability of the patient to tolerate a major resection, or the limited reserve of the remaining liver, as in the case of cirrhosis. It has been established that a treatment goal of −40° to −50°C or below is necessary to maximize cellular necrosis. To achieve this goal, liquid nitrogen is supercooled and circulated through cryoprobes at a temperature of −196°C. Tissue in contact with the tip of the probe is then quickly frozen. Freezing the tissue results in formation of ice crystals from pure water in both the intracellular and extracellular spaces. This creates a hypertonic environment of the extracellular space that draws additional water from within the cell, leading to cell shrinkage and membrane damage. Tissue thawing is also a damaging process; and as warming progresses, remaining intact cells are exposed to a now hypotonic environment. These cells may then rupture from osmotic forces and volume expansion. Intraoperative cryotherapy of the liver is aided by ultrasonography whereby the probe is inserted under ultrasound guidance into the tumor nodule. The effect of freezing is then directly visualized by the appearance of an "ice ball" on the ultrasound monitor. Untreated tumor can be visualized by ultrasonography; and if it is present, the probe can be repositioned or a second probe inserted into the untreated area. Complications of hepatic cryotherapy include hypothermia, myoglobinuria, abnormalities of the coagulation pathway, and pleural effusions. Myoglobinuria can be prevented by osmotic diuresis and alkalinization of the urine.

ANSWER: A, B, C, D, E

REFERENCES

1. Sabiston DC Jr: *Textbook of Surgery*, 15th ed. WB Saunders, Philadelphia, 1997.
2. Schwartz SI, Shires GT, Spencer FC: *Principles of Surgery*, 7th ed. McGraw-Hill, New York, 1999.
3. Aston S, Beasly R, Thome C (eds): *Grabb & Smith's Plastic Surgery*, 5th ed. Lippincott-Raven, Philadelphia, 1997.
4. Netter FH: *Atlas of Human Anatomy*, 2nd ed. Novartis, East Hanover, NJ, 1997.
5. Serafin D: *Atlas of Microsurgical Composite Tissue Transplantation*. WB Saunders, Philadelphia, 1996.
6. Strauch B, et al: *Atlas of Microvascular Surgery: Anatomy & Operative Approaches*. Thieme, New York, 1993.
7. Clowes AW, Kohler TR: Anatomy, physiology and pharmacology of the vascular wall. In: Moore W (ed). *Vascular Surgery, A Comprehensive Review*, 5th ed. WB Saunders, Philadelphia, 1998, Chap 3.
8. LeBoretin H, Plow EF, Topol EJ: Role of platelets in restenosis after percutaneous coronary revascularization. *J Am Coll Cardiol* 28:1643–1651, 1996.
9. Losordo DW, Rosenfield K, Pieczek A, et al: How does angioplasty work? Serial analysis of human iliac arteries using intravascular ultrasound. Circulation 86:1845–1858, 1992.
10. VanLankeren W, Gussenhoven EJ, vanderLugt A, et al: Intravascular sonographic evaluation of iliac artery angioplasty: what is the mechanism of angioplasty and can intravascular sonography predict clinical outcome? *Am J Roentgenol* 166:1355–1360, 1996.
11. Jubran A, Tobin MJ: Noninvasive respiratory monitoring. In: Parillo JE, Bone RC (eds). *Critical Care Medicine*. Mosby-Year Book, St. Louis, 1995, p 157.
12. Pilcher DB, Ricci MA: Vascular ultrasound. *Surg Clin North Am* 78:273–293, 1998.
13. Morton DL, Wen DR, Wong JH, et al: Technical details of intraoperative lymphatic mapping for early stage melanoma. *Arch Surg* 127:392–399, 1992.
14. McMasters KM, Giuliano AE, Ross ML, et al: Sentinel lymph node biopsy for breast cancer: the standard of care. *N Engl J Med* 339:990–995, 1998.
15. Leong SPL: The role of sentinel lymph nodes in human solid cancer. In: *Principles & Practice of Oncology Update* 12(4), 1998.
16. Kuhn JA, McCarty TM: Malignant melanoma and the sentinel node biopsy. *Cancer Invest* 17:39–46, 1999.
17. Gelman CL, Parroso EG, Britton CT, et al: The effect of lasers, electrocautery, and sharp dissection on cutaneous flaps. *Plast Reconstr Surg* 94:829–833, 1994.
18. Soballe PW, Nimbkar NV, Hayward I, et al: Electric cautery lowers the contamination threshold for infection of laparotomies. *Am J Surg* 175:263–266, 1998.
19. Koivvusalo AM, Kellokumpu I, Sheenin M, et al: A comparison of gasless mechanical and conventional carbon dioxide pneumoperitoneum methods for laparoscopic cholecystectomy. *Anesth Analg* 86:153–158, 1998.
20. Kraut EJ, Anderson JT, Safwat A, et al: Impairment of cardiac performance by laparoscopy in patients receiving positive end-expiratory pressure. *Arch Surg* 134:76–80, 1999.
21. Case TD: Ultrasound physics and instrumentation. *Surg Clin North Am* 78:197–217, 1998.
22. *The SAGES Manual: Fundamentals of Laparoscopy and GI Endoscopy*. Springer, New York, 1999.
23. Laycock WS, Tru TL, Hunter JG: New technology for the division of short gastric vessels during laparoscopic Nissen fundoplication. *Surg Endosc* 10:71–73, 1996.
24. Amid PK, Shulman AG, Lichtenstein IL: Selecting synthetic mesh for the repair of groin hernia. *Postgrad Gen Surg* 4:150–155, 1992.
25. Staren ED: *Ultrasound for the Surgeon*. Lippincott-Raven, Philadelphia, 1997, pp 65–84.
26. Dowling RD, Ochoa J, Yousem SA, et al: Argon beam coagulation is superior to conventional techniques in repair of experimental splenic injury. *J Trauma* 31:717–720, 1991. Discussion 720–721.
27. Gale P, Adeyemi B, Ferrer K, et al: Histologic characteristics of laparoscopic argon beam coagulation. *J Am Assoc Gynecol Laparosc* 5:19–22, 1998.
28. Go PM, Goodman GR, Bruhn EW, Hunter JG: The argon beam coagulator provides rapid hemostasis of experimental hepatic and splenic hemorrhage in anticoagulated dogs. *J Trauma* 31:1294–1300, 1991.
29. Joffe SW: *Lasers in General Surgery*. Williams & Wilkins, Baltimore, 1989.
30. Greenfield LJ, Mulholland M, Oldham KT, Zeleneck GB, Lillemoe KD: *Surgery: Scientific Principles & Practice*, 2nd ed. Lippincott-Raven, Philadelphia, 1997.
31. Yeh KA, Fortunato L, Hoffman JP, Eisenberg BL: Cryosurgical ablation of hepatic metastases from colorectal carcinomas. *Am Surg* 63:63–68, 1997.

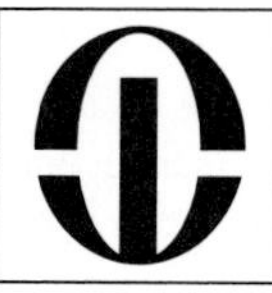

CHAPTER 17

Oncology

A. Principles

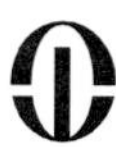

1. With regard to neoplastic disease in general, which of the following statements is/are true?

A. Neoplasms are populations of cells that have undergone extensive proliferation and have escaped normal control mechanisms.
B. By definition, all neoplasms are malignant tumors.
C. Malignant neoplasms are those capable of local tissue invasion and metastatic spread to distant sites.
D. Benign neoplasms do not spread to distant sites.

Ref.: 1, 2, 3

COMMENTS: Neoplasms are abnormal growths of tissue characterized by excessive cell division unresponsive to normal control mechanisms. Malignant neoplasms may be differentiated from benign neoplasms in that the former impair normal function by local tissue invasion and destruction and by metastatic spread to distant sites. Benign neoplasms do not invade locally; they may displace, or push aside, local tissue; and they do not metastasize to distant sites.

ANSWER: A, C, D

2. Which of the following statements is/are true?

A. Neoplastic disease is the leading cause of death in the United States.
B. Nearly one-third of persons living today develop some form of cancer.
C. The incidence of a given cancer parallels the death rate from the same cancer.
D. The incidence of cancer is decreasing in all populations.

Ref.: 2

COMMENTS: Cancer is second only to cardiovascular disease as a cause of death in the United States for people older than 40 years of age. Approximately 30% of Americans living today eventually develop cancer. The incidence of cancer is rising in nearly all populations. No one cause for this increased incidence can be identified, although longer life expectancy and environmental factors likely play a role. There have been significant changes in the incidence of various cancers and in cancer death rates over the past 50 years. The incidence and mortality rates of lung cancer have increased to such an extent that it is currently the leading cause of death from cancer for both sexes. The death rate from pancreatic cancer is two to three times what it was in 1930. Conversely, the death rate from stomach and uterine cancer is less than half of what it was at that time. Early detection has decreased the incidence and mortality of some cancers, such as cervical cancer by the widespread use of Papanicolaou (Pap) smears. Because different forms of cancer are not equally lethal, the incidence of a malignancy differs from its death rate. Approximately 40% of people who develop cancer survive at least 5 years.

ANSWER: B

3. With regard to carcinogenesis, which of the following statements is/are true?

A. The latency period begins before initiation.
B. Exposure to asbestos has been associated with the development of nasopharyngeal cancer.
C. Promotion is an irreversible process.
D. Benzene exposure has been associated with the development of acute leukemia.

Ref.: 2

COMMENTS: Carcinogenic agents may be chemical, physical, viral, or genetic and have in common the ability to induce malignant neoplasms. **Chemical carcinogens**: The first description of a causal relation between a carcinogen and the development of cancer was made in 1775, when Pott described cancer of the scrotum in chimney sweeps. Aromatic hydrocarbons isolated from coal tar were ultimately shown to be the causative agents. Coal tar has been associated with cancer of the skin, larynx, and bronchus. Exposure to β-naphthylamine, an aromatic amine used in the dye industry, has been associated with tumors of the urinary tract. Benzene exposure has been associated with the development of acute leukemia and asbestos exposure with the development of mesothelioma. Chemical carcinogens act via a multistep process. The first step is **initiation**, during which the carcinogen reacts irreversibly with DNA to form a covalent adduct. The reaction is nonenzymatic and therefore nonspecific. The second step is **promotion**, which is a slow, reversible process in which initiated cells are stimulated by promoting agents to develop into cancer cells. Promotion occurs during the latency period. The third and final step is **progression**, which involves the maturation of cancer cells into a fully malignant tumor. There is a characteristic **latency period** between the first exposure to a carcinogen and the development of a tumor. The latency period is dose-dependent. **Physical carcinogens** include ionizing and ultraviolet radiation. Both are associated with the development of skin cancer, and ionizing radiation may lead also to the development of neoplasms of the thyroid, bone, and blood. **Viral carcinogens**: There is clear-cut evidence that both RNA and DNA viruses are carcinogenic in several animal species. In humans, only RNA viruses have been clearly linked with malignant neoplasms; the Epstein-Barr virus has been associated with the development of Burkitt's lymphoma and nasopharyngeal cancer.

ANSWER: A, D

4. With regard to the progression of cells from normal to cancerous, which of the following is/are true?

A. Metaplasia describes cells that have altered size, shape, and organization.
B. Hyperplasia in the absence of atypia or dysplasia confers only modest, if any, risk of cancer in that tissue.
C. All dysplastic tissues eventually progress to frank carcinoma.
D. Metaplastic changes may be reversible.

Ref.: 1, 2

COMMENTS: The development of cancer is a multistep process where cells develop dysregulated growth. Malignancy is characterized by unregulated growth and dissemination of cells. Malignant transformation occurs through a series of alterations in a number of genes within a cell. The progression of a cell from normal to malignant can be seen in a series of histologic "plasias." **Hyperplasia** is an increase in cell number with rapid growth rates above normal. It rarely progresses to the development of cancer unless associated with atypia or dysplasia. Hyperplastic colonic polyps, for example, do not progress to cancer like their adenomatous counterparts do. Hyperplastic breast tissue may have a slight association with increased breast cancer risk but not nearly that which is seen with atypical hyperplasia. **Metaplasia** is the reversible replacement of one mature cell type with another in an area of tissue where it is not normally found. It can be caused by chronic inflammation, such as squamous cell metaplasia to gastric columnar-type cells in the lower esophagus in a patient with chronic reflux. **Dysplasia** is a term used for epithelial tissues that contain cells altered in size, shape, and organization. Dysplasia can be mild, moderate, or severe depending on the degree of cell dedifferentiation. Although there is an association of dysplastic tissues with the development of invasive cancers, not all dysplastic tissues progress to carcinoma.

ANSWER: B, D

5. With regard to the biology of malignant neoplasms, which of the following statements is/are true?

A. Most malignant neoplasms arise from a single cell that has undergone transformation to form a malignant clone.
B. Cancer cells proliferate faster than normal cells, and the rate of proliferation increases as the tumor mass increases.
C. Malignant cells are characterized by reversion to more primitive cell types, cellular pleomorphism, and loss of contact inhibition.
D. Tumors double in size at least every 20 days; thus essentially all human neoplasms are clinically detectable within 1 year after the inception of neoplastic transformation.

Ref.: 1, 2, 3

COMMENTS: Most cancers are believed to arise from a single cell that has undergone transformation to form a malignant clone, although some cancers (e.g., neurofibrosarcomas in von Recklinghausen's disease) may develop from multiple clones of cells. • With the possible exceptions of leukocytes and intestinal mucosa cells, cancer cells generally proliferate faster than normal cells. As such, the bone marrow and intestinal mucosa are often affected by anticancer therapies designed to take advantage of the rapid proliferative rate of malignant tissue. A tumor's proliferative rate tends to decrease as the tumor size increases. • Changes characteristic of malignant cells include the production of various polypeptides and hormones not normally produced, reversion to a more primitive cell type, cellular pleomorphism, frequent mitoses, hyperchromatism, and the loss of contact inhibition. Tumor doubling time may be used to assess the aggressiveness of a tumor and therefore the patient's prognosis after therapy. A clinically detectable 1 cm tumor represents approximately 30 divisions and 1 billion cells. Most tumors double in volume every 20–100 days, although this rate can vary from every 8 days to every 600 days. Most tumors therefore are present at least 1 year (and many for as long as 10–15 years) before they are clinically detectable.

ANSWER: A, C

6. With regard to the spread of neoplasms, which of the following statements is/are true?

A. Lymph node metastases permeate the sinusoids of the node and later spread throughout it to involve the subcapsular space.
B. Carcinoma in situ is a lesion with histopathologic characteristics of malignancy but without detectable invasion beyond the basement membrane.
C. Lymphatic involvement is common with sarcomas, whereas most epithelial neoplasms metastasize hematogenously.
D. The metastatic process is highly inefficient, as evidenced by the fact that tumors that shed into the bloodstream have a variable incidence of metastasis.

Ref.: 2

COMMENTS: Carcinoma in situ is a neoplasm with cytologic characteristics of malignancy but without detectable invasion through the basement membrane of the epithelial layer. • There are essentially four mechanisms by which cancer cells disseminate: **tissue infiltration**, **lymphatic invasion**, **vascular invasion** (capillaries and veins frequently and arteries rarely), and **direct implantation**. • Metastatic cells generally enter lymph nodes via the subcapsular space. Only later do the tumor cells permeate the sinusoids and gradually replace the parenchyma of the node. Lymph nodes are commonly involved in epithelial neoplasms, whereas sarcomas rarely metastasize to them. The **metastatic process** is highly inefficient. In some animal tumor models tumors shed as many as 100 million viable cells into the bloodstream during their growth and yet produce fewer than 100 lung metastases. To metastasize, a malignant cell must go through a complex multistep process that some investigators have likened to a decathlon. This process is referred to as the **metastatic cascade**. The elements of this cascade are the same whether the cell begins its journey by passing into the lymphatics or the capillaries. The first step is **detachment and invasion**: Before a malignant cell can invade, it must detach from the parent tumor and pass into the lymphatic or venous system. The second step is **transport**: once in the lymphatic or venous system, the cell must be transported to the distant site of growth. During this transport, the cell must survive a number of host defense mechanisms, such as destruction by antibodies, complement, natural killer cells, or macrophages. In addition, these cells must survive a multitude of mechanical stresses, including turbulence in small blood vessels, poor nutrition, and widely variable oxygen levels. The next step is **arrest and extravasation**: surviving tumor cells are arrested in the small blood vessels of the organ in question. Precisely how the tumor cells attach to endothelial cells and then invade surrounding tissue is unknown; aggregation with platelets may be one method. Attachment to the endothelial cells is mediated by cellular adhesion molecules (CAM), which include the I-CAM and M-CAM family (cadhedrins), cell surface lectins, and lectin-binding glycoproteins. Endothelial cells from small vessels of different organs express different levels of such molecules. Such organ differences may help explain different patterns of organ preference seen in different metastasizing tumors. After arrest, the tumor cells must move through the subendothelial basement membrane to invade the surrounding tissue. To accomplish this, the basement membrane is digested by various proteolytic enzymes (plasminogen activator, metalloproteinases, and cathepsins) produced by the tumor cells. Study of these molecules may facilitate the understanding, prediction, and prevention of metastases. An example is the use of cathepsin D as a prognostic indicator in breast cancer. The final step is **establishment of a new growth**: the more primitive and autonomous a tumor, the less dependent it is on normal growth factors and the more capable it is of forming tumors in the interstitial space.

ANSWER: B, D

7. With regard to oncogenes and proto-oncogenes, which of the following statements is/are true?

A. Proto-oncogenes are proteins capable of inhibiting oncogenes.
B. Oncogenes are nucleic acid sequences unique to the viral genome.
C. Exposure to carcinogens causes insertion of oncogenes into the human genome.
D. Proto-oncogenes may be activated by mutation, amplification, or translocation.

Ref.: 1, 2

COMMENTS: A number of gene types may be altered during the development of cancer. **Oncogenes** are genes that, when expressed, contribute to the development of malignancy. **Proto-oncogenes** are genes found in normal tissues that, when activated by mutation, amplification, or translocation (to become oncogenes), may lead to transformation of the cell to a malignant phenotype. **Mutator genes** are responsible for improving the fidelity of the DNA replication process. When these genes do not function properly, an increase in the number of mutations is seen and an underlying predisposition to cancer may now be expressed. **Tumor suppressor genes** differ from oncogenes in that it is the loss of their expression that contributes to the development of cancer. Unlike oncogenes, a tumor suppressor gene must develop mutations in both alleles before it can lead to a malignant phenotype.

ANSWER: D

8. With regard to monoclonal antibodies, which of the following statements is/are true?

A. A monoclonal antibody is defined as an antibody with specificity against only one set of antigenic determinants.
B. Monoclonal antibodies have the ability to react with an indefinite number of antigenic determinants.
C. Monoclonal antibody hybridomas are made by fusing a plasma cell to a myeloma cell.
D. Because a given monoclonal antibody reacts with many antigenic specificities, its usefulness as a diagnostic or therapeutic tool is limitless.
E. An idiotype is the antigenic determinant in the variable region of an antibody.

Ref.: 1, 2, 3

COMMENTS: Hybridomas are created by fusing a plasma cell to a myeloma cell, thereby conferring the immortality of the myeloma cells on the plasma cell population. Because the initial plasma cell is capable of synthesizing a monoclonal antibody with specificity against only one set of antigenic determinants (epitopes), the resulting hybridoma cell line produces an essentially limitless amount of that monoclonal antibody. Because immunoglobulins are proteins they may have antibodies against themselves. The antibody against the immunoglobulin may bind specifically to an antigenic determinant in the variable region (a so-called idiotype). An anti-idiotype is an antibody to the idiotype, which may suppress or augment the host's response to different antigens. The potential applications of monoclonal antibodies seem limitless and include immunodiagnosis, immunotherapy, tests for the follow-up after cancer treatment, and research.

ANSWER: A, C, E

9. Which of the following statements is/are true?

A. The enzymes prostatic acid phosphatase, alkaline phosphatase, neuron-specific enolase (NSE), and CA 125 are useful tumor markers.
B. Lactic dehydrogenase (LDH) has little value as a tumor marker.
C. M protein is a nonspecific protein of inflammation.
D. Prostatic acid phosphatase is an important parameter when staging prostatic cancer.
E. Prostate-specific antigen (PSA) is highly specific for prostate cancer and therefore is a useful screening marker for the disease.
F. None of the above.

Ref.: 1, 2, 3

COMMENTS: Prostatic acid phosphatase, alkaline phosphatase, LDH, and NSE are enzymes that may be elevated in association with certain malignancies. **Prostatic acid phosphatase** is secreted by the normal prostate. Elevation in patients with prostate cancer indicates extension of tumor beyond the capsule, but the correlation between elevated levels and total body tumor burden is poor. Therefore it is not helpful for staging prostatic tumors. **Alkaline phosphatase** is, in fact, a number of isoenzymes produced by the liver, bone, and placenta. Elevation in patients with malignancy usually indicates involvement of liver or bone by metastatic disease. It is nonspecific for malignancy because it is elevated in a number of benign disorders, including choledocholithiasis. **Placental alkaline phosphatase** is a nonspecific marker that is normally made in the placenta. It is elevated in a few patients with ovarian cancer and testicular seminomas. **LDH** is an isoenzyme found in a number of normal organs. It has proved valuable for observation of patients with lymphoma. Elevated levels reflect tumor bulk. **NSE** is occasionally elevated in patients with small-cell neuroendocrine carcinoma of the lung. Measuring the polypeptide chains of immunoglobulins has been valuable in patients with multiple myeloma or B cell lymphoma. In these cases, there is often asynchronous production of the polypeptide chains, the light chains being produced in excess of the heavy chains; these proteins can be detected in blood or urine. Electrophoresis demonstrates a distinct peak, indicating the presence of an **M protein**. The presence of an M protein in association with abnormal plasma cells is considered specific for multiple myeloma. **CA 125** is a tumor-associated antigen. Its major use is in patients with ovarian cancer. CA 125 can be useful for monitoring treatment but is not useful as a diagnostic screening tool because it is produced by other tumors, or lung and colon cancer, and in some patients with benign processes such as gynecomastia and cirrhosis. **CA 15.3** is another tumor-associated antigen that can be elevated in patients with breast, ovary, and lung cancer. It has been used as a guide for monitoring treatment of breast cancer. **CA 19.9** is a tumor-associated antigen whose usefulness seems to be in detecting pancreatic cancer. **PSA** is elevated in patients with prostatic disease. Although it is sensitive for the presence of prostatic disease, it is not specific for prostate cancer; elevations can also be seen in patients with benign prostatic hypertrophy. PSA levels do correlate with the tumor burden in patients with prostate cancer, so the test is useful for monitoring these patients, especially those who have undergone total prostatectomy.

ANSWER: F

10. Match the molecular genetic technique on the left with its definition on the right.

A. PCR (polymerase chain reaction)	a. Used to reattach fragments of DNA
B. DNA ligase	b. Used to separate DNA into small fragments
C. DNA polymerase	c. Used to multiply the number of copies of a gene
D. Restriction endonuclease	

Ref.: 2

COMMENTS: As cancer is rapidly becoming understood on a molecular level, an understanding of basic molecular genetic technology is necessary. The **PCR (polymerase chain reaction)** technique was developed during the mid-1980s. Since its development it has revolutionized molecular genetics by making possible a new approach to the study and analysis of genes. The major problem associated with analyzing genes is that they are rare targets in a complex genome; in mammals this genome may contain as many as 100,000 genes. PCR allows production of enormous numbers of copies of a specified DNA sequence without resorting to cloning. Single-stranded DNA templates are used with a DNA polymerase directed to synthesize a specific region of DNA. The starting material for a PCR is DNA that contains the sequence to be amplified. It is not necessary to isolate this sequence because it is defined by the primers used in the reaction. One advantage to PCR techniques is that the amount of DNA needed for a PCR is small; in fact, PCR may be used to amplify sequences from a single DNA molecule. The technique has been used to aid in screening for mutations found in cancers and inherited disorders. It can be used to monitor the response to cancer therapy, such as determining whether a patient being treated for leukemia is free of malignant cells. It can also be used to monitor bacterial or viral infection, particularly in the detection of human immunodeficiency virus (HIV) infection. **Restriction enzymes** are nucleases that break the phosphodiester bonds of nucleic acids. Specific restriction nucleases cleave DNA at specific sites, recognizing specific sequences of bases. The ability to cleave DNA in a predictable way has made gene mapping possible. **DNA ligases** and **polymerases** are enzymes that may be used to seal together restriction fragments. The use of this recombinant DNA technology has made gene cloning gene therapy possible.

ANSWER: A-c; B-a; C-a; D-b

11. With regard to metastatic carcinoma, which of the following statements is/are true?

A. Axillary lymph node dissection is essential for staging a sarcoma of the breast.
B. Melanoma tends to metastasize to lung, brain, and the gastrointestinal tract.
C. Bone is frequently the site of metastasis for cancer of the breast and prostate.
D. Primary brain cancers have a predilection for metastasis to the lung.

Ref.: 2

COMMENTS: It is necessary to understand the routes by which particular cancers spread to make rational decisions concerning therapy. In general cancers are able to spread thorough four main routes: **direct invasion of adjacent tissues, lymphatic spread, hematogenous spread** via vascular embolization, and **implantation** in a serous cavity. Metastasizing tumors often have a predilection for selected organ sites. The reasons for this are not clearly understood and are being studied by many investigators. Some theories include the presence of essential growth factors in certain tissues needed for a particular tumor's growth and the interaction of tumor surface adhesion molecules with certain tissues, leading to the establishment of metastatic disease. Understanding the behavior of a particular tumor is important for treatment planning. Systemic therapy may play a significant role in the treatment of a cancer with a propensity for hematogenous spread, such as breast, colon, or lung cancers. Systemic therapy may have a limited role in cancers that spread primarily by local invasion, such as brain neoplasms and tumors of the oral pharynx. With tumors with a low proclivity for metastasizing to lymph nodes, lymph node dissection may not improve outcome or aid in staging, such as with sarcoma. It is also necessary to understand the patterns of metastatic spread to make rational decisions concerning surveillance testing. For example, there is little sense in obtaining serial bone scans for surveillance of a tumor that does not tend to metastasize to bone.

ANSWER: B, C

12. With regard to unknown primaries presenting as metastatic disease, match the site of metastasis on the left with the more likely possible site(s) of the primary tumor on the right.

A. Supraclavicular node
B. Axillary lymph node
C. Ovarian metastasis
D. Bone metastasis
E. Skin metastasis

a. Breast cancer
b. Melanoma
c. Prostate cancer
d. Colon cancer
e. Stomach cancer
f. Ovarian cancer

Ref.: 2

COMMENTS: Usually the site of a primary tumor is known, although some cancers present as metastatic disease with the primary tumor not being readily apparent. In fact, sometimes the site of the primary tumor may never be identified. This may be due to a primary too small to be detected by standard methods or to regression of the primary lesion prior to identification of the metastases (i.e., malignant melanoma). Knowledge of likely sites of origin can direct the evaluation of metastasis of unknown origin.

ANSWER: A-a,d,e,f; B-a,b; C-d,e; D-a,c; E-a,b

13. Which of the following statements are true:

A. Granulocyte colony-stimulating factor (G-CSF) is used to ameliorate the neutropenic effects of chemotherapy agents.
B. Interleukin-2 (IL-2) is produced by natural killer (NK) cells.
C. Tumor necrosis factors (TNF-α and TNF-β) are produced by NK cells.
D. G-CSF, granulocyte/macrophage colony-stimulating factor (GM-CSF), and erythropoietin exert their effects on bone marrow.

Ref.: 1, 2

COMMENTS: The underlying principle of biologic therapy (biologic response modifiers) for treatment of cancer is to augment the host's native immune responses and intensify tumor rejection responses. A number of proteins have been found to be responsible for the growth and development of cells within the hematopoietic and lymphoid systems. **Cytokines** are proteins produced and secreted by a cell. Several of the key regulatory cytokines (i.e., interleukins and interferon α) have been isolated, and some are in clinical use currently; others are undergoing further investigation. **IL-2**, a lymphokine produced by activated T cells, can bind to a specific cell surface receptor on activated T lymphocytes. In addition to being a key factor in T cell proliferation, it also activates **natural killer (NK) cells**. IL-2 has been used extensively in clinical trials in patients. It has single-agent activity (i.e., against melanoma and renal cell cancer) and is being studied in combination with other chemotherapeutic agents. **Interferon alpha (IFN-α)** has immune modulatory effects including activation of the NK cell, modulation of antibody production by B lymphocytes, and induction on the tumor cell surface of major histocompatibility complex (MHC) antigens. **Tumor necrosis factors (TNF-α and TNF-β)** are produced by activated macrophages and serve a wide variety of biologic effects. They activate osteoclasts, act as growth factors for fibroblast, and have antiviral activity. They also exert immunomodulatory effects, interacting with other cytokines and inducing surface MHC antigens. TNF may have direct cytotoxic effects on cells and may have a role in the development of cancer cachexia. Hematopoietic growth factors are playing an increasing role in modulating the hematologic effects of chemotherapy. **Granulocyte colony-stimulating factor (G-CSF)** and **granulocyte/macrophage colony-stimulating factor (GM-CSF)** have proliferative effects on bone marrow progenitor cells from which neutrophils are derived, modulating the effects of chemotherapy-induced neutropenia. **Erythropoietin** promotes the proliferation of committed erythroid precursors, ameliorating anemia.

ANSWER: A, D

14. With regard to radiation therapy, which of the following statements is/are true?

A. Malignancies such as leukemias and prostate cancer are relatively radioresistant, whereas those such as melanoma are more radiosensitive.
B. Placement of intracavitary radiation sources plays a role in the treatment of uterine cancer.
C. Pancytopenia, telangiectasias, pericarditis, and nephropathy are possible sequelae of radiation therapy.
D. Combination neoadjuvant treatment with chemotherapy and radiation is increasing the surgeon's ability to perform conservative surgery, resulting in organ preservation.

Ref.: 1, 2

COMMENTS: Radiation therapy is another method of locoregional control in cancer care. It makes use of **ionizing radiation**, which is energy sufficiently strong to remove an orbital electron from an atom. This radiation may have a particulate form, such as electrons, protons, or neutrons; or it may have an electromagnetic form, such as high-energy photons. **Radiosensitivity** is the measure of susceptibility of cells to injury by ionizing radiation. In general, the more frequently the cells divide, the more sensitive they are to the effects of radiation. The effects of radiation in achieving cell damage may occur through impairing the cells' ability to replicate (reproductive death). Radiation may also cause structural damage or injure cells through metabolic incapacitation independent of a cell's reproductive cycle (interphase death). **Radioresistance** is when a cell becomes impervious to the damaging effects of ionizing radiation. Radiation-induced cell kill can be modified by several factors, including oxygenation of the tumor, hyperthermia, and concomitant administration of chemotherapeutic agents. The basic unit of radiation, known as the **gray (Gy)**, is the amount of energy absorbed (joules) per unit mass (kg). This terminology has replaced the unit **rad** used in the past (100 rad = 1 Gy; 1 rad = 1 cGy). Normal tissues are able to tolerate specified amounts of radiation before short-term or long-term injury occurs. Irradiation causes progressive changes in small vasculature and interstitial connective tissues. **Early radiation-induced toxicity** may include fatigue, diarrhea, esophagitis, skin and mucosal reactions, and hematopoietic suppression. **Late sequelae of irradiation** may appear months or years after treatment and may include chronic skin changes, strictures of the gastrointestinal tract, bone necrosis, nephritis/renal insufficiency, pulmonary fibrosis, and chronic pericarditis with the exception of fatigue, these sequelae develop as a consequence of the specific organs being irradiated. Careful planning of radiation therapy and its delivery is necessary to minimize such sequelae. Radiation therapy may be used as single-modality therapy (e.g., prostate cancer therapy), adjuvant therapy following surgical resection (e.g., for treatment of early-stage breast cancer), neoadjuvant treatment prior to definitive surgical resection (e.g., combined-modality treatment of esophageal or rectal cancers), or in combination with chemotherapy without the addition of surgical resection (treatment of some head and neck cancers). **Brachytherapy** is a term used to describe radiation treatment in which the radiation source is in contact with the tumor. Common examples of the use of brachytherapy include **low-dose-rate sources (LDR)** used for treatment of uterine cancer and the **high-dose-rate sources (HDR)** used for treatment of esophageal and lung cancers.

ANSWER: B, C, D

15. With regard to chemotherapy agents, which of the following statements is/are true?

A. Alkylating agents exhibit a linear dose-response curve.
B. Fluorouracil is an example of a purine analogue antimetabolite.
C. Anthracyclines exert their antitumor effects by inhibiting microtubule formation.
D. Antibiotics derived from certain bacteria and fungi may have antitumor effects.

Ref.: 2

COMMENTS: Most chemotherapy agents currently used exert their effects by affecting cell multiplication and tumor growth. Chemotherapy agents may be classified according to the phase of the cell cycle on which they act. **Cell cycle-specific agents** exhibit a plateau in cell killing ability; cell kill does not increase with increases in the dosage given. In contrast, **cell cycle-nonspecific drugs** exhibit a linear dose-response curve: the greater the dose of drug, the greater the fraction of cell kill. Drugs work by affecting the cell cycle in different ways and at different points in the cell cycle. **Alkylating agents** (i.e., cyclophosphamide, ifosfamide, melphalan, thiotepa, streptozocin) act by forming covalent bonds to amino, carboxyl, sulfhydryl, and phosphate groups in biologically important molecules such as DNA, RNA, and proteins. Alkylating agents are not cell cycle-specific, although they require cell proliferation for activity. Antimetabolites are structural analogues of naturally occurring metabolites involved in DNA and RNA synthesis. They exert their cytotoxic activity by competing with the normal metabolites for a site on a key enzyme or substituting for a metabolite normally incorporated in DNA or RNA. They are most active when cells are in S phase, making them most effective in tumors with a high growth fraction. **Antimetabolites** can be divided into **folate analogues** (methotrexate), **purine analogues** (fludarabine, mercaptopurine), **adenosine analogues** (cladribine), **pyrimidine analogues** (cytarabine, fluorouracil), and **substituted ureas** (hydroxyurea). Another group of compounds possessing antitumor activity has been isolated from natural substances such as bacteria, fungi, and plants. These agents are **antitumor antibiotics**, including bleomycin and dactinomycin, anthracyclines (doxorubicin, idarubicin), and mitomycin. A number of plant derivatives exert their effects through inhibiting microtubular formation, such as **vinca alkyloids** (vincristine, vinblastine, vinorelbine) and **taxanes** (paclitaxel, docetaxel).

ANSWER: A, D

16. Which of the following treatment options is/are reasonable for treatment of advanced (metastatic) cancer?

A. A Whipple procedure to relieve obstructive jaundice in a patient with adenocarcinoma of the head of the pancreas and multiple metastatic lesions in the liver.
B. Resection of three liver lesions metastatic from a colorectal primary and no other metastatic sites identified.
C. Radiation therapy to a painful hip lesion in a patient with diffuse bony metastases from prostate cancer.
D. Pain medication and antiemetics for a patient with diffuse carcinomatosis from a pancreatic primary.

Ref.: 2

COMMENTS: Treatment of advanced (metastatic) cancer varies widely. In most circumstances the goal of treatment for metastatic disease is palliation, as cure is unlikely. Decisions concerning appropriate treatment of metastatic disease must take into account multiple factors, including the natural history of the disease, number of metastatic sites, rate of tumor growth, history of prior response to therapy, the patients overall physiologic condition, toxicity of the proposed treatment, likelihood of achieving a response to therapy, the quality of life with and without therapy, and the patient's desires. Whereas aggressive therapy may be indicated for limited metastatic foci, such as surgical resection for a hepatic metastasis from colorectal carcinoma in a patient with an otherwise good performance status, it may be reasonable simply to provide supportive care for a patient with multiple metastatic sites, a history of failing multiple prior therapeutic regimens, or who is in a debilitated condition. The two overriding goals of treatment for advanced cancer are to palliate symptoms and prolong life. When evaluating options for palliation of symptoms, the side effects of the treatment should be less than the severity of the symptom it is supposed to palliate. Attempts to prolong life have generally been less than successful. There are few circumstances where our current therapeutic modalities (surgery, chemotherapy, biologic therapy, and radiation therapy) have been shown to improve survival. However, there is a clear survival advantage with the resection of a solitary metastasis to the lung or brain for treatment of melanoma and a survival advantage with the resection of fewer than four lesions in the liver when this is the sole site of metastatic colorectal carcinoma.

ANSWER: B, C, D

17. With regard to clinical trials, which of the following statements is/are true?

A. Phase II trials establish the maximum tolerated dose of an experimental agent.
B. Comparing one group of patients receiving a given treatment with another receiving a different treatment 10 years ago introduces observational bias into a study.
C. Randomization into trials is done to ensure that each group of patients has a similar chance of achieving the desired outcome.
D. An example of a phase I trial would be studying whether herceptin + docetaxel is effective in decreasing the size of metastasis from breast cancer.

Ref.: 1, 2

COMMENTS: Clinical trials in oncology are an important method for bringing new therapies into clinical use in a rational and scientific way. The essence of a clinical trial is the idea that by examining how a given treatment affects a small representative group of patients generalizations can be made as to the applicability of the treatment to a broader group of patients who will have similar disease in the future. The results are examined (**statistical analysis**) to determine the probability that, with a certain level of confidence in the observed outcome (**confidence interval**), the results could have been achieved by random variation or chance alone (***p* value**). The surgeon must understand the basic premises of clinical trial designs to be able to analyze critically the data that comes out of these studies, evaluate the strength of the evidence the study reports, and use it to make rational clinical decisions. **Phase I trials** ask the question: "Is the new treatment safe and at what dose?" **Phase II trials** ask the question: "Is the new treatment effective in treating the disease in question?" **Phase III trials** ask the question: "Is the new treatment any better than our standard treatment?" It is phase III trials that often take the form of randomized, controlled clinical trials to minimize the chance that variations in treatment outcome are related to factors other than differences in treatment (**bias**). Minimizing the sources of bias introduced into a study helps to strengthen the study design and the evidence for its conclusions. Avoiding bias is achieved by: **Having comparative control groups**: To assess the efficacy of a new treatment it is compared with a control group receiving standard therapy. The control group established the *expected rate* of outcome in the null hypothesis of no effect of the investigational intervention, and the intervention group gives the *observed rate* of this outcome with investigational treatment. **Randomizing patients into treatment arms**: This measure ensures that patients in the treatment arms are equally likely to achieve a given outcome. It is accomplished by randomizing patients into treatment arms and stratifying for known prognostic factors. **Blinding investigators and patients**: This removes the possibility of observational bias that may occur with differences in how outcome observations are made in the control and intervention arms of a trial. Observational bias can be minimized by blinding patients and investigators to which treatment was received, documenting all outcome observations for later verification by an independent blinded observer, and ensuring similar follow-up for the groups of patients. **Concurrent comparison of intervention and control groups:** This eliminates the possibility of a chronologic bias, which can occur because therapeutic and diagnostic capabilities can change over time and can affect the quality of the observations of outcomes. **Analyzing data on an "intention to treat" basis**: An analysis that examines the treatment the patient actually received rather than the treatment they were supposed to receive no longer is comparing the randomly assigned groups, which were supposed to ensure that each group has a similar chance of achieving the desired outcome. There are multiple reasons why patients assigned to a particular treatment group may not actually receive the intended therapy. These factors that affect failure to receive therapy are an important part of evaluating the experimental and control therapies.

ANSWER: C

18. Which of the following statements is/are true?

A. Mutations in the *RET* proto-oncogene are found in 90% of patients with medullary thyroid carcinoma from multiple endocrine neoplasia type II (MEN-II) kindreds and 70% from non-MEN familial medullary thyroid carcinoma kindreds.
B. All women who carry a *BRCA1* mutation develop breast cancer at some point in their life.
C. Mutations in *BRCA2* are found on the long arm of chromosome 17.
D. All familial adenomatous polyposis patients with the 5q21 mutation go on to develop cancer of the colon if left untreated.

Ref.: 1, 2

COMMENTS: Over the past 10 years a number of cancer-susceptibility genes have been identified. It is now possible to test for the presence of mutations on genes associated with susceptibility for the development of malignancy. *BRCA1*, located on the long arm of chromosome 17 (17q21), was identified in 1994. In 1995 a second susceptibility locus, *BRCA2*, was mapped to chromosome 13. Together they account for approximately 75% of highly penetrant hereditary breast cancers. Several genes are associated with a predisposition to the development of colon carcinoma, including the *APC* gene (**A**denomatous **P**olyposis **C**oli genes located on the long arm of chromosome 21; 5q21) in familial adenomatous polyposis patients and mutations of *hMSH2*, *hMLH1*, *hPMS1*, and *hPMH2* in hereditary nonpolyposis colorectal cancer (HNPCC) patients. Mutations in the *RET* proto-oncogene, located on the centromeric region of chromosome 10, have been found to be associated with the development of medullary thyroid cancer in MEN-II kindreds and familial medullary thyroid carcinoma kindreds. The decision to perform genetic testing is made by the patient after consultation with the physician and a genetic counselor to evaluate the risks and benefits of doing such a test. Many questions are still unanswered in this developing field, including who exactly should undergo testing, what recommendations should be made to those who are found to be carriers, the psychological impact of a positive or a negative test, the implications of testing with regard to insurability and employment, and other legal, ethical, and financial issues.

ANSWER: A, D

REFERENCES

1. Sabiston DC Jr: *Textbook of Surgery*, 15th ed. WB Saunders, Philadelphia, 1997.
2. Schwartz SI, Shires GT, Spencer FC: *Principles of Surgery*, 7th ed. McGraw-Hill, New York, 1999.
3. Tannock IF, Hill RP: *The Basic Science of Oncology*, 2nd ed. McGraw-Hill, New York, 1992.

Oncology

B. Surgical Therapy

1. Which one or more of the following historical characteristics of a mass suggests malignancy?

A. Sudden development of a painful, tender mass.
B. Slow, progressive, painless growth of a mass.
C. Sudden dramatic enlargement of a previously stable-sized mass.
D. A mass that waxes and wanes in size with or without associated tenderness.
E. Slow development of pain without tenderness in the area of a slowly enlarging mass.

Ref.: 1, 2

COMMENTS: The age of the patient and the location of a mass are obviously important characteristics that raise or lower one's index of suspicion that a mass may be malignant. However, those factors excluded, one's level of concern that a mass may be malignant is affected by the growth characteristics of the mass, the presence or absence of pain, and the presence or absence of associated inflammatory symptoms. The growth characteristic most suggestive of malignancy is that of slow, progressive enlargement. The sudden and dramatic enlargement of a previously stable-sized mass is usually caused by spontaneous or trauma-induced hemorrhage into the mass. This is commonly seen in thyroid nodules. A mass that waxes and wanes in size or is painful, especially when associated with tenderness, warmth, and erythema, usually suggests an inflammatory process. The rapid onset of pain likewise suggests inflammation, whereas a more gradual onset of pain in a slowly enlarging mass suggests malignant invasion of adjacent structures, especially nerves. There are, of course, many exceptions to these broad generalizations (e.g., inflammatory carcinoma of the breast; hemorrhage into a small thyroid cancer).

ANSWER: B, E

2. Which one or more of the following physical characteristics of a mass suggests malignancy?

A. Hard texture.
B. Soft texture.
C. Fixation to deeper structures.
D. Pulling inward of overlying skin.
E. Matting together of contiguous masses.
F. Associated warmth.
G. Associated erythema.
H. Paralysis of muscles innervated by nearby motor nerves.
I. Well circumscribed mass.

Ref.: 1, 2

COMMENTS: Malignancies characteristically invade surrounding structures and, in many instances, incite a scirrhous host response within and around the tumor. This leads to the hard texture characteristic of most epithelial malignancies and to the fixation of locally advanced cancers to deeper structures or overlying skin, the matting of contiguous lymph nodes, and the invasion of nerves. Neural invasion causes pain or functional loss (e.g., vocal cord paralysis from recurrent laryngeal nerve invasion by thyroid cancer, or facial nerve paralysis from parotid malignancies). A rubbery feel can indicate a benign (breast fibroadenoma) or malignant (solitary or matted lymphoma nodes) process. Well-circumscribed masses are usually benign because the invasiveness of malignancies usually makes their borders somewhat indistinct. In most cases, warmth or erythema (or both) associated with a mass suggests a benign inflammatory condition.

ANSWER: A, C, D, E, H

3. Which of the following eponyms is/are used to describe a physical finding suggestive of metastatic or locally advanced malignancy?

A. Blumer.
B. Trendelenburg.
C. Virchow.
D. Grey Turner.
E. Krukenberg.
F. Horner.
G. Sister Mary Joseph.
H. Kussmaul.

Ref.: 1, 2

COMMENTS: Part of the physical evaluation of a patient with a suspected malignancy involves the search for signs that suggest invasion of surrounding structures or distant spread. **Blumer's shelf** (rectal shelf) is a hard, nodular ridge anteriorly on digital rectal examination between the rectum and the uterus in a female or the rectum and the bladder in a male. It signifies transcoelomic spread of an intraabdominal cancer with implants in the deep pelvic peritoneal sulcus. **Virchow's node** is a left, medially located supraclavicular lymph node metastasis from an intraabdominal primary site (most often gastric or pancreatic). **Krukenberg's tumor** is an ovarian mass detectable on bimanual pelvic examination, ultrasonography, or computed tomography (CT) scan and signifies a "drop metastasis" or transcoelomic implantation of tumor on the ovary from another intraabdominal primary site (classically gastric). **Horner syndrome** (ptosis, miosis, anhidrosis) is caused by disruption of the cervical sympathetic chain, which in the absence of an iatrogenic cause suggests cervical or upper mediastinal involvement with an invasive malignancy. **Sister**

Mary Joseph's sign is a periumbilical deposit of tumor within the abdominal wall secondary to an underlying intraabdominal malignancy. The precise pathophysiology of such tumor nodules is not agreed on but may be due to direct invasion through the abdominal wall by peritoneal seeding or retrograde lymphatic or hematogenous spread via the umbilical ligament. **Trendelenburg's sign** (rapid filling of venous varicosities as a result of incompetent valves in the lower extremities), **Grey Turner's sign** (flank ecchymosis classically secondary to hemorrhagic pancreatitis), and **Kussmaul's respirations** (labored rhythmic respirations seen in diabetic ketoacidosis) are important clinical signs but are unrelated to neoplasia.

ANSWER: A, C, E, F, G

4. With regard to the biopsy of a tumor mass, which of the following statements is/are true?

A. Fine-needle aspiration biopsy enables definitive diagnosis of a malignancy only rarely and runs the significant risk of leaving tumor deposits along the needle tract.
B. Excisional biopsy is the favored procedure for large soft-tissue sarcomas of the extremities.
C. Incisional biopsy involves removal of a small portion of a tumor and is useful for thyroid nodules so as not to compromise curative resection.
D. Biopsy incisions for suspected cancers need not always be oriented in natural skin creases.

Ref.: 1, 2, 3

COMMENTS: Interpreting the results of **fine-needle aspiration (FNA) biopsy** of a tumor, a simple office procedure with minimal risk, requires the expertise of a cytopathologist. Results positive for malignancy are highly accurate. Negative results, especially from clinically suspicious lesions, should be viewed with caution and may warrant further investigation, usually with open biopsy. Reports of needle-tract seeding from FNA biopsy are rare, and the clinical significance of the possibility of seeding is lessened by the fact that the area in question will likely be definitively resected or irradiated as part of the local therapy for the cancer. **Incisional biopsy**, best used for large tumors, involves removing of a small portion of a tumor through an open incision. Negative results of an incisional biopsy of a clinically worrisome lesion must be viewed with caution because of the possibility of sampling error. Biopsy incisions for suspicious lesions should be oriented in a manner that allows them to be easily encompassed in the planned resection incision, not necessarily in the natural skin lines. Incisional biopsy is usually inappropriate for thyroid nodules because of the risks of bleeding and of seeding the neck wound with tumor cells. Biopsy of thyroid nodules is generally performed preoperatively with FNA or core biopsies, or intraoperatively with total excision (usually by thyroid lobectomy). **Excisional biopsy** is used for total removal of small masses (e.g., breast or subcutaneous nodules), frequently with a margin of normal tissue to avoid the need for reexcision. It is usually inappropriate to perform a biopsy of large suspicious masses by marginal excision because the definitive wide reexcision might be unnecessarily debilitating, both cosmetically and functionally.

ANSWER: D

5. With regard to the staging of cancer, which of the following statements is/are true?

A. Assessment of the degree of local growth and regional (lymphatic) and distant (hematogenous) involvement of a cancer is mandatory when planning therapy.
B. Open sampling of clinically suspicious regional lymph nodes before definitive surgical therapy is advisable to stage tumors adequately preoperatively.
C. Computed tomography (CT) or magnetic resonance imaging (MRI) of the brain, chest, abdomen, and pelvis, along with radionuclide bone scans, should be performed preoperatively in most patients with epithelial malignancy.
D. Staging laparotomy for Hodgkin's disease remains an appropriate staging technique in selected cases and can influence therapy in up to 30% of patients.

Ref.: 1, 2, 3, 4

COMMENTS: The proper choice of therapy in cancer management depends on adequate knowledge of the local, regional, and distant extent of disease. Therefore, all cancers must be clinically, radiographically, or surgically staged before definitive therapy. The degree to which the oncologist relies on radiographic imaging techniques and surgical staging depends on the natural history of the cancer in question, the likelihood of metastasis to specific sites, and the cost, risk, and accuracy of the staging technique under consideration. Careful clinical evaluation and routine laboratory testing to include a chest radiograph and chemistry profile constitute the minimal accepted staging workup for most cancers. Additional imaging techniques are of variable benefit, depending on the natural history of the cancer in question. Total body scanning occasionally detects distant disease not previously suspected; however, the prohibitive cost makes it unwise to use such an approach as a routine staging strategy. Hodgkin's disease, when it presents confined to supradiaphragmatic or upper abdominal sites, remains an appropriate indication for a staging laparotomy in selected cases but only when therapy will be altered by the outcome. This procedure, which involves splenectomy, liver biopsy, and sampling of intraabdominal lymph nodes at multiple sites, can lead to changes in the staging of the disease that would influence therapeutic strategy in up to 30% of cases. The risk of inappropriately treating these patients if surgical staging is not performed is thought to justify the small but acceptable risk of laparotomy. The risk can be lessened further with the use of minimally invasive laparoscopic techniques. In cases of cancers likely to spread to cervical, axillary, or groin lymph nodes, clinically suspicious nodes in the expected lymph drainage site generally warrant formal dissection of the area without prior surgical staging. Preliminary open biopsy of these areas might compromise the subsequent definitive surgery, risk tumor spillage within these relatively poorly defined fascial compartments, and increase the likelihood of injury to the neurovascular structures in the area.

ANSWER: A, D

6. Performing which one or more of the following operations would be inappropriate without first obtaining a biopsy confirming the presence of cancer?

A. Radical right hemicolectomy for an "apple core" narrowing of the ascending colon.
B. Modified radical mastectomy for a clinically and mammographically obvious breast cancer with overlying skin puckering.
C. Partial glossectomy and neck dissection for an ulcerated tumor of the middle third of the tongue with clinically suspicious ipsilateral cervical lymphadenopathy.

D. A pancreaticoduodenectomy for a large, hard mass in the head of the pancreas that produces painless jaundice.
E. Resection of a highly vascular painful mass deep in the proximal thigh abutting but not invading bone, nerve, or major vessels by radiographic assessment and with no evidence of metastatic disease.
F. Parotidectomy for a 2 cm, slowly growing solid parotid mass without evidence of facial nerve dysfunction.

Ref.: 1, 2, 3, 4

COMMENTS: Ideally, tissue confirmation of malignancy is obtained before radical surgical extirpation is performed. In cases in which the tumor is easily accessible, either directly or endoscopically (e.g., breast tumors and tumors of the upper aerodigestive tract), it would be improper to perform radical surgery without tissue confirmation. On occasion, however, biopsy is not easily obtained, carries unacceptable risk, complicates subsequent extirpative therapy, or would not alter the extent of the operation. In such cases, it may be proper to proceed with definitive, curative surgical excision in the absence of a confirming biopsy. Colon lesions that are radiographically worrisome but colonoscopically inaccessible should be resected without histologic confirmation because colotomy and biopsy at the time of laparotomy risk both tumor spillage and stool contamination of the peritoneal cavity. Even multiple transduodenal needle aspiration biopsies may fail to prove the presence of pancreatic carcinoma because of sampling error. If the surgeon believes that pancreaticoduodenectomy is an appropriate therapy for cancer of the head of the pancreas, and if the clinical index of suspicion is high enough, proceeding without tissue confirmation may be appropriate. The large extremity mass described in case E, apparently resectable without loss of bone or major neurovascular structures, requires excision regardless of its histologic features. A preliminary biopsy would complicate the subsequent resection by necessitating enveloping the skin, subcutaneous tissue, and muscle traversed to obtain the biopsy. A marginal resection of this lesion followed by radiation therapy, once the malignant nature is confirmed, would likely be preferable to amputation. Parotid tumors, whether benign or malignant, are generally resected with preservation of uninvolved branches of the facial nerve, with radiation therapy given postoperatively for malignant lesions with close margins. Preoperative histologic confirmation of malignancy in such cases would not alter the extent of resection. In all of these cases, clinical judgment, enhanced by thorough knowledge of the tumor's natural history, enables the surgeon to make a proper risk-benefit assessment regarding the need for biopsy.

ANSWER: B, C

7. Rank the following tumors in terms of the margin of normal tissue around the clinically obvious tumor that should be resected to achieve an acceptable likelihood of control at the *local primary* site. Assume that no other treatment modalities will be used, and rank the following from the narrowest to the widest margin.

A. Adenocarcinoma of the colon.
B. Basal cell carcinoma of the skin.
C. Invasive breast cancer.
D. Squamous carcinoma of the distal esophagus.
E. Squamous carcinoma of the skin.

Ref.: 1, 2, 3

COMMENTS: See Question 8.

8. When determining how widely to resect a primary malignancy, which one or more of the following factors should be considered?

A. Location of tumor.
B. Capacity for implantation of tumor cells.
C. Capacity for contiguous spread through tissue planes.
D. Capacity for hematogenous dissemination.
E. Capacity for lymphatic dissemination.
F. Capacity for embolic interstitial spread.
G. Tendency for multifocal disease to be present within the organ in question.
H. Blood supply to the organ to be resected.

Ref.: 1, 2, 3

COMMENTS: Proper surgical therapy of solid tumors (excluding myeloproliferative malignancies) requires careful consideration of the tumor's *local* growth behavior and invasiveness, as well as its capacity for and pattern of *regional* (lymphatic) and *distant* (hematogenous) spread. Cancers are known to spread by one or more of five pathways: (1) direct invasion through tissue planes; (2) interstitial emboli; (3) via lymphatic channels to regional nodes; (4) systemically via lymphovenous connections or hematogenous (venous and occasionally arterial) routes; and (5) implantation within serosa-lined cavities (peritoneal, pleural, and pericardial spaces). The extent of excision around a primary tumor is determined by the tumor's ability to invade locally through contiguous tissues or to spread embolically within the interstitium in the vicinity of the tumor but in a noncontiguous manner. Pathophysiologically, the capacity of a tumor to invade and spread locally relates to its capacity for cellular multiplication, cellular migration, alteration of cellular adhesiveness, phagocytosis, and elaboration of cytotoxic and lytic substances. The location of a tumor also has a bearing on the breadth of excision. Risk-benefit considerations suggest that in certain circumstances tumors close to functionally or cosmetically important organs should be resected with a narrower margin to avoid injury to or loss of that organ, even if this adds slightly to the risk of local recurrence (e.g., a skin cancer close to the eye, in contrast to one in the middle of the back). Proximity to bone, major motor nerves, or major vessels may also influence the decision for closer margins. The breadth of local excision (e.g., mastectomy for breast cancer) is influenced by the multifocal or multicentric nature of some tumors. Finally, the blood supply to the organ in question may have an impact on the extent of local excision. Much more colon, for example, is resected than is needed to achieve free margins around the primary tumor because the mesenteric dissection requires ligation of the blood supply to large sections of the colon. • The local invasiveness of a tumor influences the breadth of excision needed to achieve local control. *Basal cell carcinoma* rarely invades more than a few millimeters beyond its clinically evident border; *squamous cell carcinoma* of the skin spreads slightly wider. *Carcinoma of the colon* requires only a 1- to 2-cm margin around the primary site to achieve local control, although much more colon is usually resected to encompass regional nodes. *Breast cancer* requires a significant margin of normal tissue around the primary site if local control is to be achieved without the use of radiation therapy. *Esophageal and gastric cancers* have a propensity to spread in the submucosal plane as far as 10 cm from the primary site, and extremely wide margins are therefore required to clear the suspected areas of tumor infiltration. The capacity of tumors to implant locally or to spread via lymphatics on blood vessels influences the ultimate disease-free survival rate, but the breadth of excision of the primary tumor is not likely to affect such aspects of tumor biology.

ANSWER:
Question 7: B, E, A, C, D
Question 8: A, C, F, G, H

9. In which one or more of the following cases would regional lymph node dissection be appropriate as part of the initial definitive surgical therapy?

A. A T1 (<2 cm in diameter) squamous carcinoma of the anterior one-third of the tongue.
B. A small (approximately 2 cm in diameter) exophytic adenocarcinoma of the cecum not associated with obstruction or bleeding.
C. A nonpalpable, mammographically detected infiltrating duct carcinoma of the breast, 1.2 cm in diameter, with clinically negative axillary nodes.
D. An adenocarcinoma of the head of the pancreas, 4 cm in diameter, producing jaundice and duodenal obstruction.
E. A Clark level IV, 1.6 mm thick, superficial spreading melanoma of the proximal anterior right thigh with a single firm, enlarged right inguinal lymph node.
F. A high-grade pleomorphic liposarcoma, 5 cm in diameter, of the deep anterior proximal thigh.

Ref.: 1, 2, 3

COMMENTS: See Question 10.

10. With regard to regional lymphadenectomy, which of the following statements is/are true?

A. Anatomic lymph node dissection adversely affects the host's immune response and should be performed only in cases of clinically suspicious adenopathy.
B. Regional lymph nodes act as a fairly effective barrier to the spread of epithelial malignancies beyond the local or regional site.
C. A pathologically negative regional node dissection confers an approximately 95% likelihood that there has been no distant spread of the tumor.
D. The rationale for regional lymph node dissection is primarily therapeutic rather than prognostic.
E. The risk of swelling and propensity for infection in an extremity must be considered when elective axillary or groin dissections are recommended.
F. Resection of regional nodes en bloc with the primary tumor should generally be avoided because of excessive disruption of uninvolved interposed tissue.

Ref.: 1, 2, 3

COMMENTS: The rationale for performing regional lymphadenectomy for epithelial malignancies is based on the desire to remove all tumor that may be present and to determine the metastatic potential of the tumor so as to predict prognosis and direct subsequent systemic therapy more accurately. Risk-benefit decisions in this regard relate to the morbidity of the regional dissection contemplated, the likelihood (based on the characteristics of the primary tumor) that nodes are positive, and the degree to which prognosis or subsequent therapy will be altered by the information provided by the dissection. From the standpoint of morbidity, removal of axillary and groin lymph nodes disrupts collateral venous and lymphatic channels and confers an increased risk of swelling in the associated extremity. The propensity for infection after minor breaks in the skin in these extremities may be increased as a result of inadequate processing of antigenic information because of the absence of regional lymph nodes. There is no clear evidence, however, that the patient's overall systemic immune response is adversely affected. It was originally believed that regional lymph nodes acted as barriers to further spread of cancer, and that systemic disease would be seen only after the regional nodes had become "choked" with tumor. It is now recognized that this "barrier function" of regional lymph nodes is performed poorly; and from a biologic standpoint, it is more appropriate to consider involvement of regional lymph nodes as a measure of the metastatic potential of the tumor. Thus regional lymph node dissections are as much for prognostic purposes and subsequent treatment planning as for therapeutic purposes, increasingly so in this era of broadening indications for adjuvant systemic therapy. For example, in breast cancer, clinical trials (e.g., NSABP B-04) have shown that axillary lymph node dissection may be of prognostic value only insofar as survival does not appear to be influenced by whether the axillary lymph nodes are resected, irradiated, or observed until clinically positive and then removed. A negative regional node dissection is not a guarantee against systemic disease, and the predictive value of a negative dissection varies tumor by tumor. For example, systemic disease in those with breast cancer develops relatively commonly (in up to 30% of patients) after negative regional lymph node dissections. In cancers of the upper aerodigestive tract, however, systemic disease is rarely seen without previous cervical lymph node involvement. The rationale for performing regional lymph node dissections en bloc with the primary tumor is based on the desire to avoid cutting across the intervening lymphatic channels, thereby more effectively enveloping the primary tumor and its suspected lymph node involvement. Such an approach is preferred when the tumor is close to the regional nodal basin and when undue morbidity is not caused by incontinuity dissections. This principle is exemplified in the performance of a modified radical mastectomy, which removes the breast en bloc with the regional axillary nodes. • The decision to proceed with regional node dissection in the clinical cases presented in Question 9 is based on consideration of all of the aforementioned concepts. (A) *Small cancer, anterior oral cavity*: The likelihood of nodal disease in such a small cancer is sufficiently low that it does not warrant the morbidity associated with a neck dissection. (B) *Small exophytic colon cancer*: Proper staging of colon carcinoma requires mesenteric lymphadenectomy, which can be done with minimal additional risk. (C) *Small breast cancer*: Axillary dissection is warranted for this invasive cancer because of the minimal additional morbidity and the information gained that will direct possible adjuvant systemic therapy. (D) *Obstructing pancreatic cancer*: The regional nodes that drain the head of the pancreas are so widely scattered (e.g., celiac, mesenteric, subhepatic, paraduodenal) that the added dissection to remove them would not be warranted in the absence of data supporting improved survival by doing so. (E) *Advanced melanoma*: Clinically positive primary lymph node drainage areas should be dissected for melanoma (and other malignancies) in the absence of systemic disease. Elective lymph node dissection for melanoma remains controversial. (F) *Pleomorphic liposarcoma*: Knowledge that liposarcomas, even aggressive ones such as that described in case F, rarely metastasize to regional lymph nodes makes dissection of the nodes inappropriate, despite the relatively high likelihood that distant disease will develop in this case.

ANSWER:
Question 9: B, C, E
Question 10: E

11. Assuming that there is no other evidence of disease, which one or more of the following cases of distant metastatic disease would be appropriately treated by surgical resection of the metastasis?

A. A solitary 6 cm right lobe liver metastasis from a sigmoid cancer resected 1 year earlier.
B. Three right-sided and one left-sided pulmonary metastases from a chondrosarcoma of the pelvis successfully treated 18 months earlier.
C. Three small metastases easily resectable with a left lateral segmentectomy from a node-negative infiltrating lobular carcinoma of the breast treated by mastectomy 3 years earlier.
D. Three small (<2 cm in diameter) superficial liver metastases (two in the right lobe and one in the left lobe) from a previously resected cecal cancer.
E. A solitary left lobe liver metastasis, 3 cm in diameter, with associated involvement of a single periaortic lymph node from a splenic flexure colon carcinoma resected 2 years earlier.

Ref.: 1, 2, 3

COMMENTS: See Question 12.

12. With regard to the surgical management of distant metastases, which of the following statements is/are true?

A. Liver resection for metastatic colon carcinoma should be reserved for solitary lesions less than 5 cm in diameter, with a long (>3 years) disease-free interval from the time of the initial surgery.
B. The 5-year survival after liver resection for selected cases of metastatic colon carcinoma is approximately 25%.
C. Pulmonary resection for metastatic sarcoma is not warranted because of the propensity for sarcomas to disseminate widely and subclinically to other organ systems.
D. Resection of metastatic cancer is warranted if all gross disease from all sites of metastasis can be removed.
E. A solitary lung nodule in a patient with a history of melanoma successfully resected 2 years earlier should be treated with systemic therapy because of the high likelihood of additional subclinical systemic metastases.

Ref.: 1, 2, 3

COMMENTS: Until the mid-1960s, surgical resection of distant metastatic disease was considered surgical heresy because of the generally held belief that patients so afflicted were incurable. It has become clear, however, that in many instances distant metastatic disease is not necessarily a harbinger of widespread dissemination and that successful surgical resection may in fact lead to cure or at least long-term disease-free survival. The decision to proceed with resection of distant metastases depends on the following factors: the likelihood that the true extent of disease is confined to what is clinically or radiographically apparent, the morbidity of the proposed operation, and the unavailability of more effective nonsurgical methods of controlling the disease. Successes have generally been confined to cases with relatively limited metastatic disease to a single organ site (usually liver or lung). Metastases to skin and subcutaneous tissue, bone, or mediastinal or retroperitoneal lymph nodes generally suggest a more disseminated process and are a relative contraindication to surgical therapy. The clinical situations most successfully managed by surgical resection of metastatic disease have been colon cancer metastatic to the liver and sarcoma metastatic to the lung. With colon cancer, liver resection should be considered when there is no extrahepatic metastatic disease and all of the apparent disease can be resected with free margins, preserving sufficient functional liver volume. This may necessitate a formal lobar resection or may be accomplished by multiple wedge resections, depending on the size and location of the lesions. A short disease-free interval between primary therapy and development of the metastases may reflect the biologic aggressiveness of the tumor but is not in and of itself a contraindication to liver resection. Disease-free survival rates of 40% at 3 years and 25% at 5 years have been reported in a series of selected cases. With the mortality rate for major liver resection in the range of 5% in competent hands, liver resection for limited metastatic colon cancer confined to the liver could be considered standard therapy. Liver resection for metastases from other tumors has been reported, but successes are anecdotal, and such procedures are not considered standard therapy. In the case of sarcomas, distant metastases are so frequently confined to the lungs that resection of the pulmonary involvement is reasonable, even in cases of multiple and bilateral metastases. A solitary lung nodule appearing in a patient with a history of cancer is not necessarily a metastasis. If the patient is a smoker, the likelihood that the solitary nodule represents a primary lung cancer (rather than a solitary metastasis) is approximately 50% and warrants careful evaluation and potentially curative resection.

ANSWER:
Question 11: A, B, D
Question 12: B

13. With regard to en bloc multiorgan resection for cancer, which of the following statements is/are true?

A. En bloc resection of the breast, axillary nodes, pectoralis muscles, and internal mammary nodes improves survival from breast cancer but should not be done because of the morbidity associated with the procedure.
B. Total pelvic exenteration for extensive invasive rectal carcinoma can provide cure in up to 25% of selected cases.
C. Colon cancer invading the abdominal wall should be treated by limited resection of the colonic portion of the tumor and irradiation of the abdominal wall portion.
D. A large gastric cancer invading the diaphragm should be irradiated because large defects of the diaphragm cannot be adequately reconstructed.
E. A large right adrenal tumor invading the kidney and liver should be resected en bloc with the involved contiguous organs if technically possible.

Ref.: 1, 2, 3, 4

COMMENTS: Many patients have probably been denied the opportunity for cure by surgeons unwilling to perform en bloc multiorgan resections when indicated. The reluctance to proceed with such an operation is frequently based on the assumption that a large tumor invading contiguous organs has likely already metastasized distantly and is therefore incurable. On occasion, this assumption is erroneous because some tumors grow to a large size without evidence of distant metastasis as a result of their limited biologic potential to spread hematogenously. The issues to consider before undertaking large multiorgan resections include the presumed distant metastatic potential of the tumor; the functional (or in some cases cosmetic) importance of the organs requiring resection; the capability of reconstructing the defects in soft tissue, bone, blood vessels, or hollow viscus; the ability of the patient to withstand the magnitude of the procedure contemplated; and the unavailability of other equally or more effective but less invasive modalities of therapy. Cutting across gross tumor to avoid resection of contiguous involved organs and relying on radiation therapy or systemic therapy to control gross residual disease are rarely successful and should be avoided in potentially curable situations. The Urban procedure for breast cancer (case A) represents an appealing operative strategy from the standpoint of en bloc resection of the primary site and its major regional lymph node basins, but it has never been shown to enhance survival and is no longer recommended. Total pelvic exenteration (en bloc resection of the rectum, the uterus in females, and the bladder: case B) is moderately disabling functionally because construction of both a colostomy and a urinary conduit is required. However, it has been shown to provide long-term disease-free survival and cure in up to 25% of selected cases and offers the best opportunity (especially when supplemented with pelvic irradiation) to achieve local control of extensively invasive rectal carcinoma. Bulky but locally confined colon cancers are potentially curable if treated by en bloc multiorgan resection, including the abdominal wall (case C). Because of the generally poor prognosis of patients with gastric cancer, the likelihood of cure in case D is remote, but local control is certainly best achieved by removing all gross disease, including the attached diaphragm, large portions of which can easily be reconstructed while adequate pulmonary mechanics are maintained. In case E (adrenal carcinoma), the only opportunity for cure would be with a resection that included an appropriate portion of the attached liver and the kidney. In this location, it would likely be involvement of the vena cava that would limit resectability.

ANSWER: B, E

14. With regard to cytoreductive (debulking) surgery, which of the following statements is/are true?

A. Adequate debulking of diffuse intraabdominal ovarian adenocarcinoma followed by systemic chemotherapy offers the best opportunity for cure or long-term survival.
B. After subtotal resection of a retroperitoneal sarcoma attached to the aorta, conventional radiation therapy is more effective if only 2 gm rather than 10 gm of tumor remains.
C. The effectiveness of radiation therapy in sterilizing residual tumor after incomplete resection is linearly and inversely related to the volume of tumor remaining.
D. In selected cases, cytotoxic chemotherapy is capable of sterilizing deposits of clinically detectable gross residual tumor.

Ref.: 1, 2, 3, 4

COMMENTS: The effectiveness of radiation therapy or chemotherapy (or both) for enhancing local control or improving survival after complete surgical resection of a solid tumor has been demonstrated in a number of clinical trials investigating a number of tumor sites. It is generally believed that the less residual tumor there is to be treated by these adjunctive therapies, the more effective are the therapies. This is not, however, a linear relationship. In fact, effectiveness is frequently not seen unless the tumor has been reduced to microscopic residual volume. One notable exception to this generalization is ovarian cancer, which frequently tends to disseminate widely to the visceral and parietal peritoneal surfaces of the abdominal cavity. It has been shown that if the tumor can be "debulked," leaving no nodules longer than 2 cm, cytotoxic chemotherapy in many instances is effective in sterilizing the remaining tumor load, leading to long-term survival and potential cure.

ANSWER: A, D

15. Partial or complete resection of which of the following organs could be justified to *prevent* a future cancer?

A. Colon.
B. Stomach.
C. Breast.
D. Testicle.
E. Pancreas.
F. Thyroid.

Ref.: 1, 2, 3

COMMENTS: On occasion, the risk that cancer will develop in an organ is sufficiently high that consideration is given to the prophylactic removal of part or all of that organ. Risk-benefit considerations when proceeding to resection include the likelihood that cancer will develop, the functional or cosmetic disability caused by loss of the organ, the morbidity of the surgical procedure itself, and the likelihood that the cancer will be disseminated and incurable at the time of diagnosis if the organ is not prophylactically removed. Unfortunately, the last consideration applies to most solid tumors insofar as subclinical lymphatic or hematogenous spread can occur before the primary tumor becomes clinically evident. Although gastric and pancreatic cancers are highly aggressive and usually incurable, prophylactic resection of these organs is not appropriate. In the colon, however, the polyposis syndromes (e.g., Gardner's syndrome and familial polyposis), as well as longstanding pancolonic involvement with ulcerative colitis, confer such a high risk of future colon cancer that in patients so afflicted prophylactic proctocolectomy or a sphincter-preserving variation of that procedure should be considered. A strong family history of breast cancer, especially when coupled with the presence of a mutation in the *BRCA1* or *BRCA2* gene, can be associated with a future risk of breast cancer that approaches 90%. In such high-risk individuals, bilateral mastectomy reduces the risk by more than 90%, usually with an acceptable cosmetic result if reconstruction is performed. Undescended testicles have a known association with subsequent development of testicular carcinoma, and many oncologists believe that if the testicles cannot be repositioned into the scrotum they should be resected. Identification of the *RET* proto-oncogene in patients with a family history of medullary thyroid cancer or multiple endocrine neoplasia type II (MEN-II) syndrome is associated with a nearly 100% likelihood of development of medullary thyroid cancer. Total thyroidectomy is being performed in patients as young as 5 years old with this proto-oncogene.

ANSWER: A, C, D, F

16. In which one or more of the following circumstances would *palliative* surgery be indicated?

A. Carcinoma of the body of the pancreas that produces severe back pain.
B. A large gastric cancer obstructing the gastroesophageal junction, associated with two small liver metastases.
C. A bleeding cecal cancer, 5 cm in diameter, with multiple liver and lung metastases.
D. Adenocarcinoma of the head of the pancreas with celiac nodal involvement that produces jaundice.
E. Breast carcinoma metastatic to the lungs that produces cough and shortness of breath after appropriate management of the primary tumor.
F. An ulcerated chest wall recurrence from breast cancer that invades the ribs and sternum and is associated with metastatic involvement of the iliac wing.

Ref.: 1, 2, 3, 4

COMMENTS: All of these clinical scenarios represent disabling symptoms caused by cancers that are incurable. In many instances, however, surgical resection may offer the best means of palliation for the patient. Consideration of surgery as a palliative measure depends on the pathophysiologic mechanism of the symptom being produced, the likelihood that resection would be effective in alleviating the symptom, the likelihood of morbidity from the proposed surgical procedure, the availability of effective but less invasive palliative measures, and the life expectancy of the patient. As a rule, tumors within a hollow viscus produce symptoms by obstruction or bleeding. These are most effectively alleviated by resection or, in the case of obstruction, surgical bypass. Radiation therapy can be effective in controlling bleeding and relieving obstruction, but the benefits are usually short-lived. Mechanical stenting of obstructions such as those at the gastroesophageal junction and within the biliary tree can be effective, but it often requires multiple stent changes, can be associated with infection, and is generally not recommended for long-term use of the cases described above; those cases of the gastroesophageal obstruction and the bleeding cecal cancer would be best managed by resection, whereas that of biliary obstruction would be best bypassed with a biliary-enteric anastomosis. Skin ulcerations caused by recurrent cancer are effectively managed with radiation therapy if bone invasion is not present. For the patient with an ulcerated chest wall recurrence from breast cancer, the most effective palliative treatment would be a full-thickness chest wall resection. The back pain associated with pancreatic cancer is usually due to ingrowth of tumor into the parietal retroperitoneal nerves and somatic structures and would not be relieved by pancreatectomy. The patient with breast cancer associated with shortness of breath likely has endobronchial metastases, lymphangitic spread, or associated pleural effusion and would not be effectively treated by resection.

ANSWER: B, C, D, F

17. With regard to improved survival or reduced morbidity of therapy, planned primary multimodality therapy has made a major impact on which one or more of the following tumors?

A. Locally advanced squamous carcinoma of the pharynx.
B. Adenocarcinoma of the pancreas.
C. Infiltrating carcinoma of the breast.
D. Wilms' tumor.
E. Melanoma.
F. Sarcoma of the extremities.

Ref.: 1, 2, 3, 4

COMMENTS: Although all of the major treatment modalities (surgery, radiation therapy, chemotherapy, and immunotherapy) have individually contributed to improved results in cancer therapy, the greatest impact on the management of cancer since the early 1970s has probably been the evolution of multimodality therapy, which involves using two or more of the listed modalities in a planned primary attack on the tumor. In some cases it has led to improved survival, exemplified dramatically by Wilms' tumor, which in the past was considered a highly lethal tumor but now is associated with cure rates (when treated with combinations of chemotherapy, surgery, and irradiation) exceeding 80%. In other cases, multimodality therapy has reduced morbidity while maintaining equivalent cure rates. Locally and regionally advanced carcinoma of the pharynx, for example, has successfully been treated with combined modalities involving radiation therapy and chemotherapy, thereby avoiding the functional and cosmetic disabilities attendant to major resections in this area. Lumpectomy, axillary detection, and radiation therapy provide the same cure rate as modified radical mastectomy for many breast cancers but with preservation of the breast. The cure rates are further improved by the addition of adjuvant chemotherapy or hormonal therapy. Limb preservation surgery (marginal resection of the tumor followed by radiation therapy) for sarcoma of the extremities offers, in selected cases, the same opportunity for local control and cure as does amputation. Surgery remains the sole curative therapy for melanoma. This is also true for carcinoma of the head of the pancreas, although the results remain relatively poor.

ANSWER: A, C, D, F

18. Which one of the following statements concerning sentinel lymph node biopsy is/are true?

A. The technique utilizes blue dye and/or radioactive tracer to identify the sentinel node.
B. The sentinel node is the first draining node, from a particular location, in each basin.
C. There is only one sentinel node in each basin.
D. The technique is particularly useful in patients with palpable adenopathy.

Ref.: 1, 2, 4

COMMENTS: See Question 19.

19. In which of the following patients would sentinel node biopsy be a reasonable option?

A. A 1.5 mm melanoma of the right thigh with a clinically negative groin.
B. A 2 cm infiltrating ductal carcinoma of the right breast with a clinically negative axilla.
C. A 1 cm infiltrating ductal carcinoma of the right breast with a 1.5 cm firm node in the right axilla.
D. A 2.5 cm basal cell carcinoma overlying the right scapula.

Ref.: 1, 2, 4

COMMENTS: Sentinel lymph node biopsy is a technique first widely utilized for melanoma but more recently used also for invasive breast cancer. Some investigators are also employing it for other malignancies that characteristically metastasize to regional lymph nodes. The technique was first described utilizing injection of a vital blue dye at the primary tumor site, but radioactive tracers have now also been used as effective localizing agents. Some surgeons use a combination of the two techniques for more accurate detection of the nodes. The sentinel lymph node, by definition, is the first draining node in a given regional lymph node basin, although often up to three sentinel lymph nodes can be found in a given basin. Different lymph nodes within the same nodal basin may represent sentinel nodes depending on the location of the primary tumor within the anatomic area served by that particular basin. For instance, a breast cancer in the upper, outer quadrant may drain to a different sentinel node in the axilla than a cancer in the lower, inner quadrant. Sentinel node biopsy is likely best utilized in patients with early cancers that may not yet have lymph node metastases, thereby sparing patients a full lymph node dissection. It therefore currently has no role in the patient with palpable suspicious adenopathy. This would benefit the patient with a 1.5 mm melanoma, considered an intermediate-thickness lesion, and the patient with a 2 cm breast cancer; both of these patients have relatively low chances of metastasis to lymph nodes. It would not be useful in the breast cancer patient with a suspicious palpable node in the axilla. It also would not be useful in a patient with a basal cell carcinoma because such cancers have a negligible rate of metastasis to lymph nodes.

ANSWER:
Question 18: A, B
Question 19: A, B

REFERENCES

1. Sabiston DC Jr: *Textbook of Surgery*, 15th ed. WB Saunders, Philadelphia, 1997.
2. Schwartz SI, Shires GT, Spencer FC: *Principles of Surgery*, 7th ed. McGraw-Hill, New York, 1999.
3. Economou SG, Witt TR, Deziel DJ, et al: *Adjuncts to Cancer Surgery*. Lea & Febiger, Philadelphia, 1991.
4. DaVita VT, Hellman S, Rosenberg SA: *Cancer: Principles & Practice of Oncology*, 5th ed. JB Lippincott, Philadelphia, 1998.

Oncology

C. Radiation Therapy

1. Which part of the cell is thought to be the target of radiation damage?

A. Mitochondria.
B. Nucleus.
C. Nucleolus.
D. Cytoplasm.

Ref.: 1

COMMENTS: In most cell types, radiation causes the cells to lose reproductive integrity. Experimental data are most consistent with the nucleus being the critical target in the cell, specifically in the DNA of the chromosomes. There is some evidence that the cell membrane may be another target by which irradiation may cause cell death, but the most critical target appears to be the nucleus.

ANSWER: B

2. Which one or more of the following beams would be appropriate for treating a skin cancer?

A. Superficial (100 kV).
B. Cobalt 60 (1.25 MV).
C. X-rays from a linear accelerator (20 MV).
D. Electrons (6 MeV).
E. X-rays from a linear accelerator (6 MV).

Ref.: 2, 3

COMMENTS: See Question 3.

3. Which one or more of the following beams would be appropriate for treating a rectal cancer?

A. Superficial (100 kV).
B. Cobalt 60 (1.25 MV).
C. X-rays from a linear accelerator (20 MV).
D. Electrons (6 MeV).
E. X-rays from a linear accelerator (6 MV).

Ref.: 2, 3

COMMENTS: For treating superficial lesions, low-energy x-rays or electrons are most commonly used. Superficial x-rays and electrons deposit most of their energy close to the surface, with the maximum dose at the skin surface with superficial x-rays and within several millimeters of the skin surface with electrons. Higher-energy x-rays, such as cobalt 60 or megavoltage x-rays, have a "skin-sparing" effect, where the maximum dose is 0.5–5.0 cm below the skin surface, and much of the energy is deposited in deeper tissues. Electrons have a limited range in which their energy is deposited, with higher-energy electrons having a greater depth of penetration. Nearly all of the energy from a 6-MeV electron beam is deposited within the first 3 cm of tissue, making it an ineffective treatment of deeper tumors. The dose from a superficial x-ray beam is also deposited near the skin surface, with a rapid drop in dose past the first few millimeters. The megavoltage x-ray beams have a much greater depth of penetration and are useful for treating deep-seated tumors. Cobalt 60 and a 6 MV photon beam would be as effective for treating a deep tumor as would a higher-energy beam (such as 20 MV photons), but the higher-energy beam may spare more of the normal tissues, especially in a large patient.

ANSWER:
Question 2: A, D
Question 3: B, C, E

4. Which of the following patients would have the most radioactivity in his or her body?

A. A 47-year-old woman treated with 6 MV photons from a linear accelerator for a rectal cancer, 10 minutes after daily treatment.
B. An 82-year-old man treated with 10 MV photons for a prostate cancer, 1 hour after daily treatment.
C. A 52-year-old woman undergoing a bone scan, 30 minutes after injection with radioactive technetium (^{99m}Tc).
D. A 75-year-old man treated with cobalt 60 x-rays for a larynx cancer, 10 minutes after daily treatment.
E. A 73-year-old man treated with 13 MeV electrons for a lymphoma in the left neck.

Ref.: 4

COMMENTS: Patients receiving external beam irradiation are not made radioactive by treatment. Once the daily treatment is completed, there is no radioactivity in the patient's body. A bone scan is performed by measuring the relative amounts of radioactivity in different areas of the body. The radioactive technetium is preferentially taken up in bone and remains there until it undergoes radioactive decay.

ANSWER: C

5. With regard to the deposition of energy from radiation into cells, which of the following statements is/are true?

A. Occurs in a random fashion.
B. Continues to occur long after the radiation beam is turned off.

C. Causes histologically apparent changes in most cells.
D. Is greater with increasing oxygen concentration in the cells.

COMMENTS: Energy deposition from radiation occurs by random interactions of charged particles with targets in the cells. The energy deposition and subsequent chemical changes are almost instantaneous, occurring within seconds. These changes are not always clinically important or apparent. Affected cells may have lost reproductive integrity but still often appear viable histologically. Oxygen is an important modifier of radiation damage but does not affect the amount of energy absorbed by tissues.

ANSWER: A

6. With regard to cells damaged by radiation, which of the following statements is/are true?

A. They are killed immediately.
B. They may be able to struggle through one or two mitoses before dying.
C. They may be able to divide with minimal alterations in cellular fashion.
D. They may be unable to divide but remain physiologically functional, although reproductively sterile.

Ref.: 1, 2

COMMENTS: Although some cells may die an intermitotic death following irradiation, most cells do not die until the time of cell division. If there is enough time between doses of irradiation, some of the damage is repaired (this is called sublethal or potentially lethal damage). Irradiation causes a delay in division, even in cells that are not lethally damaged.

ANSWER: B, C, D

7. With regard to irradiation of normal tissues, the risk of long-term injury (late complications) depends on which one or more of the following?

A. Type and amount of tissue treated.
B. Total dose of radiation.
C. Amount of dose given with each daily fraction.
D. Whether a short treatment break is given during the course of therapy.
E. Severity of acute reactions during treatment.

Ref.: 2

COMMENTS: Late complications occur more often with high total doses of radiation and with high doses per fraction of treatment. Small areas of normal tissue can tolerate relatively high doses of radiation, but the doses to large volumes or entire organs are limited. For example, if both entire lungs are treated with doses of 2 Gy per fraction, the risk of fatal pneumonitis is high even with total doses of only 15–20 Gy; however, small areas of lung can be safely treated with total treatment doses of 70 Gy or more. Some organs or tissues (kidney, liver, lungs, lymphocytes) are much more sensitive to radiation than others (e.g., muscle, bone, peripheral nerve). Protracting the treatment course over a long time or giving breaks from treatment during a course of irradiation decreases the acute reactions but has little impact on the late normal tissue complications. The amount and severity of acute reactions do not predict the appearance of late normal-tissue injury. In general, acute reactions occur in a different population of cells (rapidly dividing cells) than do late reactions (slowly dividing cells).

ANSWER: A, B, C

8. Which one or more of the following methods decreases the risk of long-term injuries from radiation therapy when compared with a standard course of treatment?

A. Using large doses for each treatment but to a slightly lower total dose.
B. Using small doses for each treatment but to the same total dose.
C. Using small doses for each treatment multiple times per day (at least 4–6 hours between doses) to a slightly lower total dose.
D. Using only one or two large doses to a slightly lower total dose.

Ref.: 2

COMMENTS: The risk of long-term injuries depends more on dose per fraction and total treatment dose than it does on duration or protraction of treatment. Using large doses per fraction to a slightly lower total dose likely yields the same rate of tumor cure as a more standard course of therapy but at the expense of late complications. Using small doses of radiation per fraction spares normal tissues from late complications. The use of one or two large doses of radiation is associated with a high risk of late normal-tissue injury, especially such devastating complications as spinal cord injury (transverse myelitis). This is less of a problem with palliative treatment when the patient may not live long enough to develop long-term injury.

ANSWER: B, C

9. Which of the following is/are reasons for dividing treatment with radiation therapy into multiple small doses?

A. Tumors are able to repopulate between treatments.
B. Normal cells are able to repair damage between treatments.
C. Tumor cells are redistributed through the cell cycle.
D. Tumors become less hypoxic.
E. Normal cells become less hypoxic.

Ref.: 1, 2, 5

COMMENTS: The primary reasons for dose fractionation of radiation therapy are repair, redistribution, reoxygenation, and repopulation. Cells can recover from some damage caused by radiation, with 90% of the repair occurring within 2–6 hours. Cells are more sensitive to radiation during the M and G_2 phases of the cell cycle and are more resistant during S and G_1. Fractionation of the treatment allows more of the cells to progress through the cell cycle to more sensitive phases of the cell cycle. Tumors often contain hypoxic areas, which are relatively resistant to radiation. With divided doses, some hypoxic tumor cells become more oxygenated as other tumor cells die and are removed. Radiation causes some delay in repopulation; although during a period of protracted radiation both tumor cells and normal cells eventually begin repopulating. There appears to be accelerated repopulation of tumors, which may become a clinical problem when the total treatment course lasts more than 30 days (which is one of the problems of fractionated irradiation).

ANSWER: B, C, D

10. With regard to planning a course of radiation therapy, which one or more of the following factors determines the total dose of treatment?

A. Type of surrounding normal tissues.
B. Histologic tumor type.
C. Size of the tumor.
D. Gender of the patient.
E. Total volume of tissue irradiated.

Ref.: 2

COMMENTS: When a course of radiation therapy is given, the usual factors limiting the dose are the type and amount of normal tissue included in the treatment volume. The general principle is to give a large enough dose to have a chance of curing the tumor but a low enough total dose to limit the risk of complications. The type of tumor also influences the total dose because some tumors (seminoma, lymphomas) are much more sensitive to radiation and can be cured with lower doses than other histologic types (epithelial tumors, sarcomas). Because a dose of radiation kills only a proportion of cells, a large dose of radiation is required for large tumor burdens. To control microscopic amounts of epithelial tumors, a total dose on the order of 45–50 Gy is required; for tumors 2–3 cm in size, a dose of 70 Gy or more is necessary.

ANSWER: A, B, C, E

11. With regard to radiation absorbed dose (rad), which of the following statements is/are true?

A. One rad is equal to 1 gray (Gy).
B. One rad is equal to 1 cGy.
C. One gray of neutrons is equivalent in effectiveness to 1 Gy of x-rays.
D. A single dose of 10 Gy of photons is equivalent in effectiveness to 10 Gy given in five fractions of 2 Gy each.

Ref.: 1, 3

COMMENTS: The old unit of measure for the absorption of energy per unit of matter or tissue was the rad. Currently, the unit used internationally is the gray, which is defined as 1 joule of absorbed energy per kilogram of tissue. The gray (Gy) is equivalent to 100 rad (thus 1 rad = 1 cGy). The biologic effects of radiation depend not only on the total dose but also on the type of radiation and the relative biologic effectiveness (RBE). Neutrons have a higher RBE than photons (x-rays) by a factor of approximately 3. One gray of neutrons causes three times the damage as 1 Gy of photons. Fractionated doses of radiation are not biologically equivalent to the same dose given in a single fraction. When the dose is fractionated, some of the damage caused by the radiation can be repaired before the next dose is given.

ANSWER: B

REFERENCES

1. Hall EJ: *Radiobiology for the Radiologist*, 3rd ed. JB Lippincott, Philadelphia, 1988.
2. Hendrickson FR, Withers HR: Principles of radiation oncology. In: Holleb AI, Fink DJ, Murphy GP (eds) *Clinical Oncology*. American Cancer Society, Atlanta, 1991.
3. Khan FM: *The Physics of Radiation Therapy*. Williams & Wilkins, Baltimore, 1984.
4. Johns HE, Cunningham JR: *The Physics of Radiology*. Charles C Thomas, Springfield, IL, 1983.
5. Withers HR: Biologic basis of radiation therapy. In: Perez CA, Brady LW (eds) *Principles and Practice of Radiation Oncology*, 2nd ed. JB Lippincott, Philadelphia, 1992.

Oncology

D. Systemic Therapy

1. With regard to small-cell lung cancer, which of the following statements is/are true?

A. In general, small-cell lung cancer is not treated by surgical resection because it has often spread systemically at the time of diagnosis.
B. Patients with limited stage small-cell lung cancer, in whom the disease is confined to the chest and can be encompassed with radiotherapy, can be cured with a combination of chemotherapy and radiotherapy.
C. Patients who have limited stage disease and a complete clinical response to chemotherapy should receive prophylactic cranial irradiation (PCI) to treat occult metastatic disease and prolong overall survival.
D. The syndrome of inappropriate antidiuretic hormone secretion (SIADH) and the Eaton-Lambert syndrome (a myasthenia-like syndrome) are paraneoplastic syndromes associated with small-cell lung cancer.

Ref.: 1

COMMENTS: Small-cell carcinoma of the lungs is associated with the early development of distant metastases. A study of patients with small-cell lung cancer who underwent curative surgical resection and died within 30 days of surgery from non-cancer-related causes showed that at autopsy 70% had metastatic cancer. • Patients with limited-stage small-cell lung cancer can be cured with a combination of chemotherapy and radiotherapy although the 5-year survival rate is only about 7%. • The role of PCI remains controversial. Only patients who have a complete response to therapy at other sites of disease should be considered for PCI. PCI decreases from 20% to 6% the likelihood that patients will later develop brain metastases, but such therapy does not increase overall survival. • SIADH and the Eaton-Lambert syndrome are strongly associated with small-cell lung cancer. The presence of SIADH does not correlate with the stage of disease or prognosis. The Eaton-Lambert syndrome is a myasthenia-like syndrome characterized by muscle weakness and fatigue that is most pronounced in the pelvic girdle and thighs. In contrast to true myasthenia gravis, muscle strength improves with exercise. Often the symptoms of the Eaton-Lambert syndrome are alleviated following chemotherapy for small-cell lung cancer, but sometimes they worsen. Guanidine can also be used as therapy.

ANSWER: A, B, D

2. With regard to prostate cancer, which of the following statements is/are true?

A. In patients with metastatic prostate cancer, hormonal therapy with leuprolide—a luteinizing hormone-releasing hormone (LH-RH) agonist—and flutamide is clearly more effective than orchiectomy.
B. In patients who have progression of disease following hormonal therapy, the administration of combination chemotherapy using a mitoxantrone and prednisone regimen can result in improved quality of life.
C. Patients with stage A-1 prostate cancer, in which a small amount of disease is found incidentally on transurethral resection, require no further treatment.
D. The prostate-specific antigen (PSA) assay is a sensitive serum test for detecting prostatic carcinoma, but it may also be elevated in those with benign prostatic hypertrophy (BPH).

Ref.: 1, 5

COMMENTS: Currently, no form of hormonal therapy for prostate cancer is clearly superior to orchiectomy. LH-RH agonists combined with flutamide give response rates and survival rates that are similar to those with orchiectomy. Response rates with chemotherapy are modest, although 36% of patients treated with mitoxantrone and prednisone had a decrease in their requirement for pain medication. No study has shown an increase in overall disease-free survivals with any chemotherapy. Patients with stage A-1 prostate cancer have small amounts of well-differentiated disease that is usually discovered incidentally during transurethral resection or by needle biopsy. These patients require no further immediate treatment because the disease may not become a clinical problem for many years. One review reported a cancer-related mortality rate of 1.9% in patients with stage A-1 cancer. The PSA may be elevated in the presence of BPH, but the elevation is only moderate; a marked elevation in the PSA level is more likely to be due to prostate cancer.

ANSWER: B, C, D

3. With regard to testicular cancer, which of the following statements is/are true?

A. Metastatic, nonseminomatous testicular cancer can be cured with chemotherapy.
B. Several effective chemotherapy regimens have been used for testicular cancer, all of which include doxorubicin (Adriamycin), the most effective drug against testicular cancer.
C. With metastatic, nonseminomatous germ cell tumors, if the elevated markers fail to return to normal following chemotherapy, persistent disease is almost certainly present.
D. Primary mediastinal seminomas have a high cure rate with radiotherapy or chemotherapy.

Ref.: 1

COMMENTS: Metastatic testicular cancer is curable in 70–80% of patients using a regimen of cisplatin, VP-16, and bleomycin. Adriamycin does not have significant activity against testicular cancer. Human chorionic gonadotropin-beta (β-hCG) or α-fetoprotein levels (or both) are elevated in 85% of patients with metastatic nonseminomatous germ cell tumors. About 40% of patients have an elevation of the α-fetoprotein, and 75% have an elevation of β-hCG. Embryonal carcinomas can secrete both β-hCG and α-fetoprotein. Choriocarcinomas are associated specifically with an elevation of β-hCG. Yolk sac (endodermal sinus) tumors are associated with elevated α-fetoprotein and normal β-hCG; β-hCG is elevated in about 10% of apparently pure seminomas, but the α-fetoprotein should not be elevated in a pure seminoma. If patients with a seminoma have elevated α-fetoprotein levels, they should be managed as having nonseminomatous disease. Failure of these elevated tumor markers to return to normal strongly suggests the presence of residual or persistent disease. In young men with midline tumors (retroperitoneal or mediastinal), the diagnosis of an extragonadal germ cell tumor should always be considered because this is a potentially curable disease. Although primary mediastinal seminomas have a high cure rate, the cure rate for nonseminomatous extragonadal germ cell tumors is less than 50%.

ANSWER: A, C, D

4. With regard to the treatment of metastatic malignant melanoma, which of the following statements is/are true?

   A. Dacarbazine (DTIC) is the most effective single chemotherapeutic agent.
   B. Interferon-α gives objective response rates of about 50%, with a 20–25% rate of long-term remission.
   C. Interleukin-2 (IL-2) combined with lymphokine-activated killer (LAK) cells has demonstrated antitumor effects against advanced disease, but the toxic side effects can be severe.
   D. Patients having surgical resection for cutaneous malignant melanoma but who have a high risk of recurrence benefit from adjuvant treatment with IL-2b.

Ref.: 1

COMMENTS: DTIC is the most active single chemotherapeutic agent for metastatic melanoma, with response rates of 15–25%. As adjuvant chemotherapy, however, DTIC has not been shown to be beneficial. • The response rates to interferon-α are between 10% and 20% and are partial and short-lived. • IL-2 and LAK cell therapy has demonstrated antitumor activity, but the toxicities include hypotension, oliguria, a capillary leak syndrome, confusion, and arrhythmias. • IL-2b has been shown to improve the rates of disease-free survival and overall survival when used in the adjuvant setting for patients with positive lymph nodes. Ongoing studies are trying to determine the optimal dose and schedule.

ANSWER: A, C, D

5. Which of the following solid tumors is/are generally considered to be curable with chemotherapy?

   A. Hodgkin's disease.
   B. Testicular cancer.
   C. Intermediate-grade non-Hodgkin's lymphoma.
   D. Low-grade non-Hodgkin's lymphoma.

Ref.: 1

COMMENTS: **Hodgkin's disease** can be cured by a number of regimens of combination chemotherapy, including Adriamycin, bleomycin, vinblastine, and dacarbazine (ABVD); nitrogen mustard, vincristine (Oncovin), procarbazine, and prednisone (MOPP); or MOPP/ABV (Adriamycin, bleomycin, and vinblastine). ABVD is the regimen used most commonly because of the high risk of developing myelodysplasia or acute myelogenous leukemia with MOPP. Most metastatic **testicular cancers** are highly curable when treated with cisplatin-based regimens such as the Einhorn regimen, which contains cisplatin, VP-16, and bleomycin. **Intermediate-grade non-Hodgkin's lymphomas**, such as diffuse large-cell lymphoma, are curable with several regimens, including CHOP [cyclophosphamide, doxorubicin (Adriamycin), vincristine (Oncovin), and prednisone]. • The **low-grade non-Hodgkin's lymphomas** are highly responsive to chemotherapy, and patients can have a prolonged survival, often of many years. In general, however, these diseases are not curable with chemotherapy.

ANSWER: A, B, C

6. With regard to epithelial ovarian cancer, which of the following statements is/are true?

   A. Elevation of the serum CA 125 level may precede the appearance of clinically obvious recurrence by 2–7 months.
   B. Patients who are clinically free of disease following chemotherapy and then have a negative second-look surgical reassessment have a subsequent recurrence rate of approximately 5%.
   C. Taxol, a chemotherapeutic agent that disrupts mitosis, is extracted from the bark of the Pacific yew tree. It has shown significant antitumor activity in ovarian cancer.
   D. Cisplatin given intraperitoneally is in direct contact with the local disease and results in better response rates and more prolonged survival than when administered systemically.

Ref.: 1

COMMENTS: Elevation of CA 125 levels can precede by months the appearance of detectable recurrent ovarian cancer. At present, however, CA 125 is not specific enough to be used as a screening diagnostic test for ovarian cancer. • Following a negative second-look operation for ovarian cancer, the recurrence rate is generally 15–20% or even higher in some groups of patients. Some have questioned the value of second-look operations because of the associated high recurrence rates despite "negative" findings and the poor prognosis in those with "positive" findings. • Taxol has demonstrated significant activity in ovarian cancer, even in platinum-resistant disease. • Cisplatin can be given intraperitoneally, but there is no convincing evidence that this route of administration has any therapeutic advantage over systemic administration. For the present, therefore, intraperitoneal chemotherapy should be considered experimental.

ANSWER: A, C

7. Patients who are positive for the human immunodeficiency virus (HIV) have an increased risk of developing which one or more of the following malignancies?

   A. Hodgkin's disease.
   B. Kaposi's sarcoma.
   C. High-grade non-Hodgkin's B-cell lymphomas.
   D. Acute nonlymphocytic leukemias.

Ref.: 1

COMMENTS: The incidence of **Hodgkin's disease** does not appear to be increased in patients who are positive for HIV. However, in such patients who simultaneously develop Hodgkin's disease, the malignancy may have an atypical presentation or distribution. HIV-positive patients with Hodgkin's disease more frequently present with advanced stages of the disease and with systemic (B) symptoms. **Kaposi's sarcoma** is clearly seen more often in HIV-positive patients and is an "AIDS-defining" illness. Interestingly, the percentage of acquired immunodeficiency syndrome (AIDS) patients who develop Kaposi's sarcoma has been declining for several years. **High-grade non-Hodgkin's B cell lymphomas** also are "AIDS defining"; that is, patients who are HIV-positive and develop these lymphomas are defined as having AIDS by the Centers for Disease Control. The prognosis for these patients is much poorer than for patients who have the same lymphomas but do not have HIV infection. **Acute nonlymphocytic leukemia** is not seen more frequently in HIV-positive patients.

ANSWER: B, C

8. Patients with Hodgkin's disease who are cured by chemotherapy can later develop which one or more of the following side effects or complications?

A. Infertility in men.
B. Acute nonlymphocytic leukemia.
C. Non-Hodgkin's lymphomas.
D. Hyperthyroidism.

Ref.: 1

COMMENTS: More than 80% of men treated with MOPP chemotherapy (see Question 5) develop azospermia and testicular atrophy. The ABVD regimen [Adriamycin, bleomycin, vinblastine, and DTIC (dacarbazine)] appears to be less toxic, with only about 35% of the patients developing azospermia. • The incidence of secondary malignancies such as leukemia or non-Hodgkin's lymphoma is increased in patients who have been treated for Hodgkin's disease. The combination of radiation therapy and alkylating agents increases the risk of developing leukemia even further than chemotherapy alone. At the National Cancer Institute, patients treated with MOPP alone had a 10-year actuarial risk of developing leukemia of less than 2%, whereas those who received chemotherapy and radiation therapy had a risk of 17%. • Hypothyroidism is seen more frequently in patients treated for Hodgkin's disease, but it is not thought to be due to chemotherapy but rather to radiation scatter during radiotherapy.

ANSWER: A, B, C

9. In the United States, most malignant lymphomas are of B cell origin, although several subtypes of non-Hodgkin's lymphomas do originate from T cells. Which of the following is/are T-cell lymphomas?

A. Human T cell lymphotropic virus type 1 (HTLV-1)-related leukemia lymphoma.
B. Mycosis fungoides.
C. Burkitt's lymphoma.

Ref.: 1

COMMENTS: HTLV-1-related leukemia lymphoma is caused by the HTLV-1 retrovirus. The disease is endemic in Japan and in the Caribbean and presents with skin lesions and hypercalcemia. Many patients have circulating cells with a characteristic cloverleaf appearance of the nucleus. The prognosis is poor. **Mycosis fungoides** is one manifestation of cutaneous T cell lymphomas. Patients often present with erythematous skin changes that may be misdiagnosed as eczema or some other dermatosis. Indurated plaques may form, or patients may develop generalized erythroderma. Circulating malignant cells with convoluted nuclei are called Sézary cells. Often cutaneous T cell lymphoma has an indolent course. Treatments include radiation therapy, topical chemotherapy, photochemotherapy, systemic chemotherapy, and interferon. **Burkitt's lymphoma** is a B cell malignancy. It is most common in Africa, is nearly always associated with the Epstein-Barr virus, and has a characteristic chromosomal translocation (8:14). Involvement of the mandible as well is more commonly seen in Africans.

ANSWER: A, B

10. Which of the following is/are effective treatment for hairy-cell leukemia?

A. Splenectomy.
B. Interferon-α.
C. 2′-Deoxycoformycin (pentostatin).
D. 2-Chlorodeoxyadenosine (CdA).

Ref.: 1

COMMENTS: Hairy-cell leukemia causes neutropenia, with the most common associated complication being infection. Splenectomy is an established therapy, with blood counts returning to normal in about half of patients. Responses are short, however, and all patients should be considered for systemic therapy. Spleen size alone is not an accurate predictor of response to splenectomy. Interferon-α given daily or three times a week produces partial remission in 80–90% of patients, with complete remission in 5%. The purine analog 2′-deoxycoformycin (pentostatin) is an inhibitor of adenosine deaminase and can induce complete remission in more than 60% of patients. Another purine analogue, 2-chlorodeoxyadenosine (CdA), is now considered the treatment of choice for hairy-cell leukemia. More than 80% of patients treated with a single 7-day course of 2-CdA enter remission. The responses are doubled as well with one study showing a 97% disease-free survival at 3 years of follow-up.

ANSWER: A, B, C, D

11. Match each malignancy in the left column with its available systemic therapy in the right column.

A. HER-2 positive metastatic breast cancer
B. Colon cancer, stage III (node-positive)
C. Node-positive, estrogen receptor (ER)-negative breast cancer
D. Postmenopausal, node-negative, ER-positive breast cancer
E. High-grade sarcoma
F. Small-cell lung cancer
G. Invasive bladder cancer
H. Prostate cancer
I. Testicular cancer

a. Carboplatin and etoposide
b. Cisplatin, etoposide, and bleomycin
c. Doxorubicin (Adriamycin) and cisplatin
d. 5-Fluorouracil (5-FU) and leucovorin
e. Trastuzumab (Herceptin)
f. Methotrexate, vinblastine (Velban), doxorubicin, and cisplatin (MVAC)
g. Methotrexate, doxorubicin, ifosfamide, and dacarbazine (DTIC) (MAID)
h. Tamoxifen
i. Flutamide

Ref.: 1

COMMENTS: The range of active chemotherapeutic agents available for use has increased considerably during the past decade. The treatment of a number of tumor types, of which the above are a few, has been enlarged by chemotherapy/hormone/monoclonal antibody therapy either as an adjuvant regimen or in the setting of metastatic disease. • Herceptin is a monoclonal antibody against the growth factor receptor HER-2/*neu*. This receptor is overexpressed in approximately 25% of all breast cancers. The receptor is also present on other epithelial malignancies including lung, prostate, colon, ovarian, head and neck, and pancreatic cancers. Studies are underway to determine the efficacy of Herceptin in the treatment of other cancers. • The effectiveness of 5-FU against metastatic colon cancer is significantly enhanced when it is given with folinic acid (leucovorin): 5-FU and folinic acid (leucovorin) are better than 5-FU alone against metastatic (stage IV) colon cancer, and this combination reduces the rate of recurrence by one-third when used as adjuvant therapy for node-positive (stage III) *colon cancer*. • Patients with node-positive, ER-negative *breast cancer* should be treated with adjuvant chemotherapy, no matter what the menopausal state of the patient. Doxorubicin (Adriamycin) and cyclophosphamide comprise one of several effective adjuvant regimens. • Survival of postmenopausal women with node-negative breast cancer is improved when they are treated with adjuvant tamoxifen alone. • The combination of carboplatin and etoposide (VP-16) is probably as good as any of the other combinations for *small-cell lung cancer*; it is also a useful combination for non-small-cell lung cancer, although newer agents such as paclitaxel may replace VP-16. • Metastatic high-grade *sarcomas* are highly responsive to combination chemotherapy such as the MAID program. Some studies even suggest a usefulness for this program in an adjuvant setting. • A similar situation has been found with cisplatin-based programs such as MVAC for *invasive bladder cancer*. • Flutamide (Eulexin) is an antiandrogen utilized with luteinizing hormone-releasing hormone (LH-RH) antagonist [goserelin or leuprolide (Lupron)] in place of orchiectomy for advanced *prostate cancer*. • *Testicular cancer* is highly curable with a combination of surgery and the Einhorn combination chemotherapy regimen of cisplatin, etoposide, and bleomycin.

ANSWER: A-e; B-d; C-c; D-h; E-g; F-a; G-f; H-i; I-b

12. In which one or more of the following ways can chemotherapy be effectively used in the treatment of cancer?

A. As induction or salvage treatment for advanced disease.
B. As an adjuvant to the local/regional methods of treatment.
C. As the primary treatment of patients presenting with localized cancer.
D. By direct installation or site-directed perfusion of specific organs or body regions.

Ref.: 1

COMMENTS: Induction chemotherapy describes drug therapy given as a primary treatment to patients who present with advanced or widespread cancer and, in most cases, when no alternative treatment exists. This treatment can be *curative* (leukemia, non-Hodgkin's lymphomas, Hodgkin's disease, and germ cell neoplasms) or *palliative*, as for most solid tumors. **Salvage** treatment is used for patients whose tumors fail to respond to the initial chemotherapy program and who are generally less likely to respond to alternative regimens. • **Adjuvant** chemotherapy is a systemic drug treatment after the primary tumor has been treated by surgical excision, irradiation, or both with intent to cure. The selection of appropriate regimens is based on experience in the treatment of patients with advanced stages of the same tumor type. Success of this treatment probably depends on the sensitivity of "micrometastases" (clinically undetectable cancer) to the drug or drugs being given. Adjuvant chemotherapy is considered the standard for improving the cure rate for many patients with colorectal and breast cancer and is being investigated in many other tumor types. • **Primary** chemotherapy, also referred to as neoadjuvant, prototherapy, or up-front chemotherapy, utilizes cytotoxic drugs to minimize or localize the cancer and thus improve the effectiveness of surgery and radiation therapy. Such therapy has been shown to be beneficial in lung cancer, locally advanced breast cancer, bladder cancer, and head and neck cancer. Preliminary studies have shown benefit in stomach and rectal cancer. The treatment benefits may result from the destruction of micrometastases, thereby leading to downstaging of the tumor. In addition, response implies a decrease in the size and extent of the local tumor mass, influencing the extent of the subsequent surgical procedure or the necessary radiation field. It has not been shown conclusively, however, if such systemic therapy can indeed permit a diminution of local/regional therapy with maintenance of the cure rate. • Special uses of chemotherapy include the *perfusion* of organs (e.g., infusion for metastatic cancer in the liver, for primary hepatic tumors, or, limb perfusion for sarcomas). *Intrathecal* chemotherapy, via a lumbar puncture needle or into an Ommaya reservoir, can be used to treat carcinomatous meningitis or meningeal leukemia and lymphoma. *Installation* chemotherapy into the pleural or pericardial space can control malignant effusion. *Intraperitoneal* chemotherapy may be effective treatment for intraperitoneal carcinomatosis.

ANSWER: A, B, C, D

13. With regard to the testing of new anticancer drugs, which of the following statements is/are true?

A. Phase II drug trials determine the effectiveness of a National Cancer Institute (NCI) group A drug in specific human tumors.
B. Phase I drug testing utilizes laboratory animals exclusively.
C. Group C drugs are those with proven effectiveness within a tumor type and are available for use, but they require special application for release by the NCI on an individual basis.
D. Phase III trials are usually randomized, comparing experimental therapeutic regimens with standard treatment.

Ref.: 1

COMMENTS: The average time from discovery of a new anticancer agent to its marketing is 10–12 years. Preclinical trials utilize laboratory assays or animal studies exclusively. Three or four phases of clinical testing or trials are utilized before a new agent is released for clinical use. **Phase I** determines the maximally tolerated dose (MTD) and outlines a toxicity profile. Patients with any histologically confirmed, advanced malignancy not amenable to conventional forms of treatment are eligible. **Phase II** utilizes the MTD from phase I studies to determine the effectiveness in patients with various tumor types. **Phase III** utilizes agents that have demonstrated (variable) benefit against a particular tumor type in phase II trials and compares them in a randomized fashion with standard programs. This may involve a combination of drugs rather than just single agents. **Phase IV** is the integration of drug therapy with the primary therapy (surgery, radiation, or both).

ANSWER: A, C, D

14. With regard to the chemotherapy of urothelial tract malignancies, which of the following statements is/are true?

A. Cisplatin and methotrexate are considered the most effective single agents.
B. Combination chemotherapy has not been proved to be superior to single agents and is significantly more toxic.
C. For metastatic disease, responses to chemotherapy are reported in up to 70% of patients, with 10–15% achieving a prolonged disease-free interval.
D. Studies investigating "neoadjuvant" chemotherapy (given prior to definitive surgery) report a complete response (no tumor in the surgical specimen) in more than 25% of cases.
E. Adjuvant chemotherapy (given during the immediate postoperative period) has not shown statistically significant improvement in tumor-free survival.

Ref.: 1, 2

COMMENTS: Responses of metastatic bladder cancer to single agents are usually partial and brief. The most active agents are cisplatin and methotrexate, with combinations based on cisplatin with or without methotrexate. Other active available agents include vinblastine, doxorubicin (Adriamycin), 5-fluorouracil (5-FU), and gallium nitrate. Prior to 1990 no combination of agents had been shown to be superior to single agents. Subsequent randomized trials, however, have clearly demonstrated the response to MVAC [methotrexate, vinblastine (Velban), doxorubicin (Adriamycin), cisplatin] as being superior to cisplatin alone or to other combinations. Other studies have suggested survival advantage in patients treated with chemotherapy before or after operation. A combination of chemotherapy and radiation may be equal to radical cystectomy, allowing the bladder to be spared in some patients.

ANSWER: A, D

15. Which of the following chemotherapeutic agents is/are known to cause nephrotoxicity?

A. Cisplatin.
B. Carboplatin.
C. Ifosfamide.
D. Methotrexate.
E. Cyclophosphamide.
F. 5-Fluorouracil (5-FU).

Ref.: 1

COMMENTS: Cisplatin is found to improve the outcome in a number of solid tumors, including cancer of the lung, head and neck, ovary, bladder, and germ cell tumors. The nephrotoxicity that has been associated with its use can be prevented or minimized with diuretics and vigorous saline hydration. **Carboplatin** is better tolerated than cisplatin and is being substituted for it in many of these diseases. Whether it is as effective remains controversial. Renal impairment is infrequent with carboplatin. **Ifosfamide** and **cyclophosphamide** cause hemorrhagic cystitis but do not cause nephrotoxicity. **Methotrexate**, a folate antagonist, can cause dose-dependent renal toxicity from tubular deposition of the drug. **5-FU** toxicity usually manifests as stomatitis or diarrhea.

ANSWER: A, D

16. Match each chemotherapeutic agent in the left column with its appropriate characteristic and mode of action in the right column.

A. Methotrexate	a. Acts as an alkylating agent
B. Cyclophosphamide	b. Is a plant alkaloid
C. Doxorubicin (Adriamycin)	c. Is an antimetabolite
D. Vincristine	d. Is an antitumor antibiotic

Ref.: 1

COMMENTS: Methotrexate, an antimetabolite that inhibits dihydrofolate reductase, maintains the intracellular pool of reduced folates. This causes folate to accumulate intracellularly in an inactive form. Purine nucleotide synthesis is ultimately inhibited. This effect can be reversed by administering a reduced folate such as leucovorin. Other commonly used antimetabolites include 5-fluorouracil (5-FU), 6-thioguanine, and cytosine arabinoside. **Cyclophosphamide** is an alkylating agent that interacts with DNA, causing continuing single- and double-strand breaks and a misreading of the DNA code. The alkylating agents as a group form positively charged carbonium ions that attach to electron-rich sites on nucleic acids and proteins. The primary cytotoxic effect is due to interaction with DNA. The original alkylating agent is nitrogen mustard, which is still used to treat Hodgkin's disease. Other alkylating agents include **melphalan**, which is used to treat multiple myeloma, and **chlorambucil**, which is used to treat chronic lymphocytic leukemia. **Doxorubicin (Adriamycin)** is an antibiotic that has been found to have several antitumor mechanisms of action, including intercalation between DNA basepairs and the formation of free radicals. Doxorubicin-induced cardiomyopathy is thought to be due to free radical formation in the heart muscle. **Vincristine** and **vinblastine** are plant alkaloids derived from the periwinkle plant, *Vinca rosea*. Both drugs arrest mitosis in metaphase by binding to tubulin. Vincristine causes minimal myelosuppression but can cause peripheral neuropathy. Another commonly used plant alkaloid, **VP-16 (etoposide)**, is derived from the mandrake plant and inhibits a DNA structure enzyme, topoisomerase II.

ANSWER: A-c; B-a; C-d; D-b

17. With regard to bone marrow transplantation, which of the following statements is/are true?

A. Bone marrow transplantation requires an architecturally intact organ.
B. Immunosuppressive therapy is always necessary after bone marrow transplantation.
C. Graft rejection occurs in about 30% of allogeneic bone marrow transplantations.
D. ABO blood group compatibility is necessary for a successful allogeneic bone marrow transplantation.
E. Graft-versus-host disease is not observed after syngeneic (identical twin) bone marrow transplantation.
F. Patients older than 50 years of age are eligible for bone marrow transplantation.

Ref.: 3, 4

COMMENTS: Bone marrow transplantation is achieved by intravenous infusion of a small subset of hematopoietic cells called stem cells that can proliferate, differentiate, and mature after administration to the recipient. The stem cells are always obtained from a living donor, either from the bone marrow using needle aspirations or from peripheral blood by apheresis. There are three sources of stem cells: *autologous* (patient's own marrow), *syngeneic* (identical twin), and *allogeneic* (the donor is not genetically identical to the recipient). Allogeneic bone marrow donors are selected on the basis of identity of the HLA typing. Immunosuppressive therapy is not used for autologous and syngeneic transplantation, but it is required after allogeneic bone marrow transplantation because here a tissue mismatch exists between donor and recipient. Immunosuppression is achieved by administration of total-body irradiation, chemotherapy, or both prior to transplantation and by the use of immunosuppressive agents after transplantation. With adequate immunosuppression, the risk of graft rejection is less than 5% in recipients of marrow from HLA-identical siblings and is about 5–15% in patients receiving a T-cell-depleted marrow graft. ABO incompatibility does not constitute a barrier to allogeneic bone marrow transplantation. However, because a severe hemolytic reaction can be induced following marrow reinfusion from an ABO-incompatible donor, all erythrocytes should be removed from the graft before transplantation. Graft-versus-host disease, resulting from the presence of immunocompetent cells in the graft that react against the recipient's tissue, is the most serious complication of allogeneic bone marrow transplantation. It is not seen with autologous or syngeneic bone marrow transplantation, in which donor and recipient are genetically identical. Patients older than 50 years are frequently treated with an autologous marrow transplant. Allogenic transplant carries a higher morbility and mortality due to graft-versus-host disease with increasing age. However, as immunosuppresive therapy and supportive care techniques improve, age limits are rising, especially at centers that perform many transplants.

ANSWER: E, F

18. With regard to autologous marrow transplantation, which of the following statements is/are true?

A. It is not used for treatment of acute leukemia.
B. Autologous marrow must be used within 1 year of being harvested.
C. The stem cells can be obtained from the bone marrow or from the peripheral blood.
D. Bone marrow collection is always performed under general anesthesia.
E. The risk of severe complications is less than with allogeneic bone marrow transplantation.

Ref.: 3, 4

COMMENTS: The first studies demonstrating the benefit of autologous bone marrow transplantation were in patients with acute myeloid and acute lymphoblastic leukemia in their second or third remission. Up to 30% of such patients were cured with the use of high-dose therapy and autologous bone marrow support, compared with less than 5% survival with conventional-dose chemotherapy. The bone marrow is collected when the patient is in first or second remission and purged ex vivo to decrease the risk of reinfusing residual tumor cells. The purging process is performed with cytotoxic agents or monoclonal antibodies directed against specific markers present on the surface of tumor cells. • Marrow cells can be refrigerated for up to 1 week without serious damage to the proliferative capacity. For longer storage, cryopreservation in liquid nitrogen is required. There have been successful engraftments with marrow that has been cryopreserved for up to 10 years. • Currently autologous hematopoietic stem cells are generally obtained from the peripheral blood by apheresis after mobilization with growth factors, chemotherapy, or both. If these collections are insufficient, stem cells can be harvested from bone marrow. • Bone marrow harvest from the iliac crest can be performed under general, regional, or local anesthesia, albeit it is most often done under general anesthesia. • The rate of fatal complications following allogeneic bone marrow transplantation is higher than that following autologous bone marrow transplantation as a result of histocompatibility differences between donor and recipient and the need for posttransplant immunosuppression.

ANSWER: C, E

19. With regard to the current indications for bone marrow transplantation in the treatment of cancer, which of the following statements is/are true?

A. The complete remission rate of patients with metastatic breast cancer is similar to that achieved with conventional-dose chemotherapy, but the disease-free interval is longer.
B. The use of high-dose systemic therapy and bone marrow transplantation is often curative in metastatic melanoma.
C. Because of the high frequency of bone marrow involvement, bone marrow transplantation is not used for neuroblastoma.
D. Bone marrow transplantation has been proven effective in the treatment of recurrent or persistent malignant lymphoma.
E. Bone marrow transplantation in the management of solid tumors is generally reserved for use in advanced stages of malignancies already known to be sensitive to conventional-dose chemotherapy.
F. Bone marrow transplantation is not used for chronic myeloid leukemia because of the chronic nature of the disease.

Ref.: 3, 4, 6

COMMENTS: Essentially, two categories of disease are treated with bone marrow transplantation. About 15% of all allogeneic bone marrow transplantations are performed to treat congenital or acquired marrow failures such as aplastic anemia. Here the purpose of transplantation is to replace the defective marrow with a healthy one. Eighty-five percent of allogeneic bone marrow transplantations and virtually all autologous bone marrow transplantations are performed for the treatment of cancer. Administration of an intensive cytoreductive therapy (combination chemotherapy with or without total body irradiation) and bone marrow support takes advantage of the steep dose-response curve seen with many tumors. Bone marrow transplantation allows up to a 10-fold increase in the intensity of the cytoreductive therapy, resulting in higher complete remission rates and sometimes cure of malignancies that are invariably fatal when treated with conventional-dose therapy. • Most reports on the use of high-dose therapy with bone marrow transplantation for the treatment of stage IV melanoma failed to demonstrate an improved disease-free interval or survival advantage compared with treatment with conventional-dose therapy. • The use of high-dose therapy and bone marrow transplantation is an accepted form of treatment for patients with stage IV neuroblastoma. Patients with marrow involvement are candidates for an allogeneic transplant if a donor is identified or for an autologous bone marrow transplant using a purged autograft. In the latter instance, the marrow is harvested only after bone marrow involvement is controlled with conventional-dose cytoreductive therapy. • Patients with malignant lymphoma who fail to achieve a complete remission or relapse after initially achieving complete remission have virtually no chance of cure with a second attempt with conventional-dose chemotherapy. On the other hand, up to 50% of such patients can be cured with the early use of high-dose therapy and bone marrow transplantation. • Although the use of high-dose therapy and bone marrow transplantation carries a high risk of morbidity and fatal complications, several clinical trials are in progress investigating the use of myeloablative therapy and marrow support in patients with newly diagnosed stage II or III breast cancer with 10 or more lymph nodes involved. Such patients have a high relapse rate (over 75%) following conventional-dose adjuvant chemotherapy. Ongoing clinical trials are attempting to determine whether the use of high-dose chemotherapy and bone marrow support in the adjuvant setting can decrease the rate of relapse. • Tumors that are known to be poorly responsive to conventional-dose chemotherapy (e.g., colon, stomach, non-small-cell lung, or pancreas cancer) have virtually no chance of responding to high-dose therapy and bone marrow transplantation. The current indications for bone marrow transplantation include malignancies that are sensitive to conventional-dose chemotherapy (i.e., breast, ovarian, and testicular cancer and hematologic malignancies). Whether transplant is superior to conventional therapy is controversial. • Chronic myeloid leukemia is incurable with conventional-dose chemotherapy; high-dose therapy and allogeneic bone marrow transplantation is curative in more than 50% of patients treated during the first 3 years after diagnosis.

ANSWER: D, E

20. With regard to monoclonal antibody therapy, the following is/are true:

A. Monoclonal antibodies cannot be used with chemotherapy.
B. Commercially available monoclonal antibodies have been chimerized to allow a patient to be treated more than once without the formation of a human anti-mouse antibody (HAMA) response.
C. Responses to monoclonal antibody therapy are inferior to responses to chemotherapy.
D. Monoclonal antibodies exhibit antitumor activity by multiple mechanisms.
E. Treatment with monoclonal antibodies is palliative in nature.

Ref.: 7, 8

COMMENTS: Two monoclonal antibodies have been recently approved for use in the systemic treatment of cancer. Trastuzumab (Herceptin), a monoclonal antibody against the epidermal growth factor receptor HER-2/*neu*, was approved for treatment of metastatic breast cancer. Rituximab (Rituxan), an antibody against the B-cell marker CD20, has been approved for treatment of low grade non-Hodgkin's lymphoma. These antibodies can be used with chemotherapy; in the case of Herceptin, it has been shown to increase response rates to both paclitaxel (Taxol) and cis-platinum. Both Rituxan and Herceptin are derived from mouse antibodies but have been chimerized to decrease the immunogenicity of the molecules. The active regions of the antibodies have been grafted onto human immunoglobulins. This is necessary because pure mouse antibodies evoke a HAMA response from the host. Retreatment with murine antibodies can be ineffective due to rapid clearing of the agents from the circulation by host defense mechanisms. Responses to monoclonal antibodies have been as good or better than standard chemotherapy in patients with similar treatment histories. The response rate to Rituxan in patients with low grade lymphomas has been 50–100%. The response rate to Herceptin has been 11–15% in pretreated patients and 24% in chemotherapy naive patients. Furthermore, an additional 20–25% of patients treated with Herceptin have attained stable disease. Historically, these numbers compare favorably with the results of chemotherapy. Response duration seems better with monoclonal antibodies as well. However, phase III studies randomizing chemotherapy against monoclonal antibody therapy have yet to be done. Although the exact mode of in vitro antitumor activity is not completely understood, several mechanisms have been postulated. Complement-dependent cytotoxicity (CDC), antibody-dependent cell-mediated cytotoxicity (ADCC), direct cytotoxicity, and competitive receptor binding displacing or obstructing the receptor's ligand have been observed with these agents. Thus far, antibodies have been used only for palliation, but studies are underway to determine if Rituxan can increase the cure rate of intermediate grade non-Hodgkin's lymphoma in combination with chemotherapy. Similarly, Herceptin has been proposed as adjuvant treatment for breast cancer and adjuvant or curative treatment of other diseases.

ANSWER: B, D, E

REFERENCES

1. DeVita VT, Hellman S, Rosenberg S: *Cancer, Principles and Practice of Oncology*. JB Lippincott, Philadelphia, 1997.
2. Scher HI: Chemotherapy for invasive bladder cancer; neoadjuvant versus adjuvant. *Semin Oncol* 17:555–565, 1990.
3. Ayash L, Antman K, Cheson B: A perspective on dose-intensive therapy with autologous bone marrow transplantation for solid tumors. *Oncology* 5:25–33, 1991.
4. Armitage J, Gale R: Bone marrow autotransplantation. *Am J Med* 86:203–206, 1989.
5. Tannock I, Osaba D, Stockler M, et al: Chemotherapy with mitoxantrone plus prednisone or prednisone alone for symptomatic hormone refractory prostate cancer: a Canadian randomized trial with palliative end points. *J Clin Oncol* 14:1756–1764, 1996.
6. Hoffman R, Benz E, Shattil S, et al: *Hematology, Basic Principles and Practice*. Churchill Livingstone, New York, 1995.
7. Hortobagyi G, Hung M: The role of the *HER-2* gene and its product in the management of primary and metastatic breast cancer. In: *American Society of Clinical Oncology 1998 Fall Educational Book*. American Society of Clinical Oncology. Alexandria, VA, 1998, pp 146–154.
8. Horning S: Targeted therapy for B cell lymphoma. In: *Hematology 1998. American Society of Hematology Education Program Book*. Washington, DC, 1998, pp 89–95.

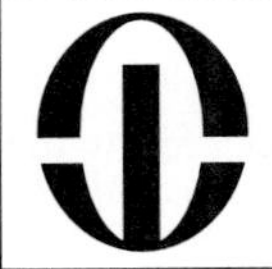

CHAPTER 18

Skin

1. Which of the following statements about skin structure is/are true?

   A. The epidermis is composed mainly of cells that provide specialized barrier functions.
   B. The Langerhans cells located in the dermis mainly provide a mechanical barrier to ultraviolet radiation.
   C. The basal cells in the basement membrane of the epidermis represent the least-differentiated form of keratinocyte.
   D. The number of melanocytes in the epidermis is constant among individuals of different skin color.
   E. Type II collagen represents 50% of the dry weight of the dermis.

Ref.: 1

COMMENTS: The skin consists of two layers, the predominantly cellular **epidermis**, separated by the basement membrane from the deeper **dermis**, which is largely composed of structural proteins. **Keratinocytes**, the main cell type in the epidermis, originate as the rapidly dividing, less-differentiated basal cells in the basal layer of the epidermis; they travel upward, differentiate, and acquire keratohyalin granules. These cells provide a protective mechanical barrier. **Melanocytes**, of neuroectodermal origin, are present in the basal layer of the epidermis. These cells have dendritic processes that transfer melanin pigment to neighboring keratinocytes via melanosomes. The density of melanocytes is the same among people of various races; differences in the rate of melanin production, transfer, and degradation lead to variations in skin color. **Langerhans cells**, which originate from the bone marrow and express class II major histocompatibility antigens, are the immunologic cells of the epidermis and act as antigen-presenting cells. Collagen is responsible for the tensile strength of the skin and for about 70% of the dry weight of the dermis. Type I collagen is the predominant type in adults, whereas early fetal dermis consists mostly of type III collagen.

ANSWER: A, C, D

2. True statements regarding the physical properties of skin include:

   A. Tension enables skin to regain its original shape after distortion.
   B. Elasticity is the property that resists stretching.
   C. The striae of Cushing syndrome are caused by loss of tensile strength and elasticity.
   D. Langer's lines indicate the direction of elastic forces in the skin.
   E. None of the above.

Ref.: 1, 2

COMMENTS: Tension is the property of skin that resists stretching. It is reduced in infants, the elderly, and patients with collagen disorders such as Ehlers-Danlos syndrome. Elasticity is the property that allows skin to regain its original shape after distortion. It is decreased in the elderly and as a result of sun damage. Elastic fibers in the skin are composed of branching proteins that can be stretched to twice their resting length. The direction of the lines of tension varies anatomically. In 1861 Langer described the direction of these lines of tension in the skin, a concept useful today; skin incisions are placed along these lines to reduce tension and the width of the resultant scar.

ANSWER: C

3. With regard to percutaneous absorption of some materials, which of the following statements is/are true?

   A. The major barrier to diffusion is the stratum corneum.
   B. Electrolytes applied to the skin in aqueous solution are rapidly absorbed.
   C. Lipid-soluble substances are rapidly absorbed.
   D. Substances in gaseous form cannot penetrate the skin.
   E. Only trace amounts of drugs can enter the bloodstream from a patch application.

Ref.: 1

COMMENTS: The skin allows selective absorption of some materials, enabling them to appear in detectable amounts in the blood; this is the physiologic basis for skin patch pharmaceuticals. Water is absorbed in vapor or liquid form. Electrolytes applied in aqueous form are not absorbed except in small quantities that enter via skin appendages. Iodine may enter the blood by skin appendage absorption or by causing an increase in the negative charge of skin. Lipid-soluble substances, particularly those that are partially water-soluble, are rapidly absorbed. Phenol and steroid hormones rapidly penetrate the skin, whereas protein hormones do not. Lipid-soluble vitamins, but not water-soluble vitamins, are rapidly absorbed. With the exception of carbon monoxide, substances in gaseous form (oxygen, nitrogen, carbon dioxide) easily penetrate the skin.

ANSWER: A, C

4. Match each item in the left column with the appropriate item in the right column.

A. Contributes to the color of skin	a. Sympathetic nervous system
B. Arteriovenous shunts	b. Glomus bodies
C. Causes vasoconstriction of cutaneous arteries and arterioles	c. Subpapillary plexus
D. Prolonged exposure to cold water	d. Trench foot

Ref.: 1

COMMENTS: The blood supply to the skin is complex and capable of multiple vascular reactions. Skin color and temperature depend on the amount of blood flowing through the subpapillary plexus, flow increasing as ambient temperature rises. Vertical vascular channels connect the subpapillary plexus to another horizontal plexus at the dermal–subcutaneous junction. Cold produces vasoconstriction and pallor. Prolonged cold causes paresis of skin capillaries and arteriolar dilatation, producing livid discoloration. If after prolonged exposure to ice-cold water the skin is rapidly brought to normal temperature, reactive hyperthermia and even blistering may result (trench foot). Arteriovenous anastomoses in the digital skin (glomus bodies) contribute to temperature regulation. Dissipation of large amounts of body heat can occur via increased flow through these shunts. Sympathetic stimulation of skin vessels causes vasoconstriction, whereas sympathectomy results in dilatation of small cutaneous arteries and arterioles, forming the basis of the therapeutic usefulness of sympathectomy.

ANSWER: A-c; B-b; C-a; D-d

5. Match each item in the left column with the appropriate item in the right column.

A. Modulate cold sensation	a. Ruffini's endings
B. Modulate sensitivity to warmth	b. Krause's end-bulbs
C. Modulate sensation of pressure	c. Meissner's corpuscles
D. Modulate tactile sensation	d. Pacinian corpuscles
E. Modulate thermoregulation	e. Autonomic nerve fibers

Ref.: 1, 3

COMMENTS: A variety of highly specialized structures are responsible for modulating the skin's various sensory functions. The numbers of these structures vary with the region of the body. **Pacinian corpuscles** are found in subcutaneous tissue, in the nerves of the palm of the hand and the sole of the foot, and in other areas. Each of these corpuscles is attached to and encloses the termination of a single nerve fiber. They are involved in the sensation of pressure. **Ruffini's endings** are a variety of nerve endings in the subcutaneous tissue of the fingers and modulate sensitivity to warmth. **Krause's end-bulbs** are formed by expansion of the connective tissue sheath of medullated fibers and are involved in the sensation of cold. **Meissner's corpuscles** occur in the papillae of the corium of the hands, the feet, the skin of the lips, and other areas concerned with tactile sensation. **Autonomic fibers** that synapse to sweat glands and receptors in the vasculature govern thermoregulation.

ANSWER: A-b; B-a; C-d; D-c; E-e

6. With regard to sweat secretion, which of the following statements is/are true?

A. There are three types of sweat gland: apocrine, eccrine, and holocrine.
B. The highest concentration of sweat glands is in the axilla.
C. Direct application of heat is the major stimulus for sweat formation.
D. Eccrine sweat is an ultrafiltrate of plasma.
E. Eccrine sweat glands are distributed over the entire body and produce aqueous sweat for thermal regulation.

Ref.: 1

COMMENTS: There are two types of sweat glands: eccrine glands and apocrine glands. The **eccrine** glands secrete aqueous sweat, and the **apocrine** glands secrete a milk-like substance. Sweat glands are distributed over the entire body, the highest concentration per square inch being on the palms and soles. Most sweat is the result of nervous stimulation carried over sympathetic nerves and mediated by acetylcholine; it is inhibited by atropine. Hyperhidrosis is a condition of increased sweating that can be corrected by direct surgical excision or sympathectomy performed at the appropriate level. The production of sweat is an active process. Normally, sweat is hypotonic but can approach isotonic concentrations during high rates of production. It is not a simple ultrafiltrate of plasma. Sodium secretion in sweat parallels that of chloride, the concentration being less than that in plasma. Potassium concentration in sweat approaches that in plasma. Urea and ammonia are excreted in concentrations much higher than those in plasma. Lactic acid is actively secreted and provides the skin with an acidic mantle. With evaporative water loss no electrolytes are lost, and the process is insensitive to atropine. Total cutaneous water loss as the result of evaporation at rest without visible sweating is about 500–700 ml/day.

ANSWER: E

7. With regard to hidradenitis suppurativa, which of the following statements is/are true?

A. It is an infection of apocrine glands, subcutaneous tissue, and fascia.
B. Staphylococci and streptococci are the predominant organisms isolated.
C. The axilla, areola, groin, perineum, and perianal and periumbilical areas are usually involved.
D. The lesions begin with slight subcutaneous induration and progress to suppuration and cellulitis.
E. Treatment can vary from improved hygiene to curettage and primary wound closure to radical excision with split-thickness skin grafting or open wound packing.

Ref.: 1, 2

COMMENTS: Hidradenitis suppurativa is an acneiform infection involving the apocrine glands in several areas. The presenting symptoms are suppuration and cellulitis or a chronic condition characterized by coalescing cutaneous nodules surrounded by fibrous reaction. Treatment is individualized. In some patients, cure is achieved with improved hygiene. Some patients respond to high doses of tetracycline or topical antibiotics; in occasional extensive chronic cases, radical excision and reconstruction with split-thickness skin grafts, flaps, or open wound packing is required.

ANSWER: A, B, C, D, E

8. Match each item in the left column with the appropriate item in the right column.

A. Cystic mass occurring over a tendon sheath	a. Epidermal inclusion cyst
B. Epidermal cell-lined cysts filled with keratin	b. Ganglion
C. Congenital lesion occurring in the midline	c. Dermoid cyst
D. Congenital coccygeal sinus	d. Pilonidal cyst
E. Cyst found most commonly on the scalp	e. Trichilemmal cyst

Ref.: 1, 2

COMMENTS: A number of cystic lesions occur in the skin. Complete excision of each of the lesions listed above is curative; otherwise recurrence is common. When infection is present, primary incision and drainage with secondary excision is preferred. The diagnosis often can be determined from the history and location of the cyst. **Epidermal inclusion cysts**, the most common type of cutaneous cyst, have a completely mature epidermis with a granular layer. The creamy material in the center of these cysts is keratin from desquamated cells. The wall of a **trichilemmal cyst**, the second most common type, does not have a granular layer and is often found on the scalp. A **ganglion** consists of a wall of connective tissue filled with a collagenous material; ganglions commonly occur over the tendons of the wrist, hands, and feet and may be congenital, related to trauma, or a result of arthritic conditions. **Dermoid cysts** are found along the body fusion planes and usually occur over the midline abdominal and sacral regions, over the occiput, and on the nose. Malignant degeneration has not been reported. **Pilonidal cysts** result from penetration of a congenital coccygeal sinus by an ingrown hair, which sets the stage for infection and cyst formation. They are more common in males.

ANSWER: A-b; B-a; C-c; D-d; E-e

9. Match each lesion in the left column with the appropriate clinicopathologic statement in the right column.

A. Wart	a. Hypertrophy of epidermis
B. Keratosis	b. Viral etiology, contagious, autoinoculable
C. Keloid	c. Dense accumulation of fibrous tissue
D. Lipoma	d. Occurs commonly on the back, between the shoulders, and on the back of the neck
E. Neuroma	e. Can be associated with von Recklinghausen's disease

Ref.: 1, 2, 4

COMMENTS: **Warts** (verruca vulgaris) can occur anywhere on the body but are most common on the hands and feet. Those occurring on the plantar surface of the foot can become highly painful. Treatment options include cryotherapy, laser ablation, caustic agents (salicylic acid), and electrodesiccation. Surgical excision is associated with a high incidence of recurrence. There are several types of **keratosis**, some considered premalignant, others not. *Actinic* keratoses may be premalignant, although at least 25% spontaneously regress; these occur in areas of sun-damaged skin. Suspicious lesions should be examined by biopsy before treatment. *Seborrheic* keratoses are not premalignant and develop mainly on the trunk in older persions. They can be darkly pigmented and may be mistaken for melanomas. Treatment consists of complete surgical excision, electrodesiccation, shave excision, or curettage. A third type of keratosis, *arsenical* keratosis, is associated with dedifferentiation to squamous cell carcinoma. **Keloids** are the result of exuberant scar formation outgrowing its original dimensions. They can occur after trauma and have a predilection for the skin on the back, sternum, neck, face, ears, and feet. They are more common in dark-skinned individuals. Treatment includes excision with primary closure combined with pressure dressings, application of silicone gel sheets, intradermal steroids, or low-dose radiation therapy. **Lipomas** are extremely common, often encapsulated, and cured by excision. Malignant degeneration is uncommon. **Neuromas** can be either neurilemmomas or neurofibromas. The latter may be associated with von Recklinghausen's disease, which is actually two distinct heritable disorders of neuroectoderm (NF-1 and NF-2). NF-1, the more common form, is an autosomal dominant disorder, affecting 1 in 5000 people and characterized by café au lait spots, axillary freckling, Lisch nodules of the iris, optic nerve gliomas, and cutaneous, subcutaneous, and visceral plexiform neurofibromas. The *NF-1* gene, located on 17q11.2, encodes a protein, neurofibromin, that is important in neuroectodermal differentiation and cardiac development. Children with NF-1 have an increased risk for the development of central nervous system (CNS) tumors, Wilms' tumor, and lymphoma; and 10–30% develop malignant schwannomas. NF-1-associated malignant schwannomas may be multiple and tend to occur at a younger age than their sporadic counterparts. There is also an increased incidence of other soft tissue sarcomas among these patients.

ANSWER: A-b; B-a; C-c; D-d; E-e

10. With regard to keloids and hypertrophic scars, which of the following statements is/are true?

A. There are no histologic differences between the two.
B. The differences between hypertrophic scar and keloid are clinical, not pathologic.
C. Hypertrophic scars outgrow their original borders.
D. Hypertrophic scars and keloids have been treated successfully with intralesional injection of steroids.
E. Keloids are seen in dark-skinned individuals, whereas hypertrophic scars are seen in fair-skinned individuals.

Ref.: 1

COMMENTS: Histologically, keloids and hypertrophic scars appear the same. Hypertrophic scars are thick, red, raised scars that do not outgrow their original borders, whereas keloids do. Keloids are dense accumulations of fibrous tissue that form at the surface of the skin. The defect appears to result from a failure in collagen breakdown rather than an increase in its production. Keloids and hypertropic scars have been successfully treated with intralesional steroid injection, radiation, pressure, and the use of silicone gel sheets.

ANSWER: A, B, D

11. Match each lesion in the left column with the appropriate clinicopathologic feature in the right column.

A. Atypical nevus
B. Congenital nevus
C. Compound nevus
D. Freckle
E. Hutchinson's freckle

a. Precancerous melanosis of the face
b. Pigments located in the basal layer of the epidermis and upper dermis
c. Often familial
d. May contain hair
e. Epidermal and intradermal melanocytes

Ref.: 1, 2, 5

COMMENTS: Melanocytic nevi have been classified as congenital or acquired. **Congenital** nevocellular nevi occur in 1% of newborns. For small congenital nevi (< 10 cm) the lifetime risk for the development of melanoma is about 5%. Classification of acquired melanocytic nevi into intradermal, compound, and junctional nevi is based on the location of melanocytes within the skin. Initially most acquired nevi begin in the epidermis (junctional), extend partially into the dermis (compound), and then come to rest intradermally. **Compound** nevi are smooth, usually slightly raised, and hairless. **Atypical** (dysplastic) nevi are melanocytic nevi whose occurrence may be familial. These nevi confer an increased risk for melanoma. In some individuals the nevi represent true precursors of malignant melanoma. They are usually reddish to brown, have scalloped edges and variegated pigmentation, are usually larger than 6 mm in diameter, and often appear on areas not exposed to the sun. **Hutchinson's freckle**, or lentigo maligna, occurs most often in the elderly and generally does not behave aggressively. Most melanomas arise de novo or from preexisting "nondysplastic" nevi. **Freckles** pose no threat and are found mostly in persons with light complexions. The pigment is in the basal layer and upper dermis.

ANSWER: A-c; B-d; C-e; D-b; E-a

12. With regard to basal cell and squamous cell carcinomas, which of the following statements is/are true?

A. Basal cell carcinomas grow more slowly than squamous cell carcinomas; they can be darkly pigmented, resemble melanomas, and produce few signs of inflammation or induration.
B. Basal cell carcinomas grow more rapidly and metastasize to regional lymph nodes more readily than do squamous cell carcinomas; and they induce significant induration.
C. Ulceration without induration or inflammation is characteristic of the squamous cell carcinoma, which has been referred to as a "rodent ulcer."
D. Squamous cell carcinomas induce induration, may be surrounded by satellite nodules, can lead to ulceration with rolled edges, and metastasize more frequently than do basal cell carcinomas.
E. Squamous cell carcinomas can develop in postradiation dermatitis or in old burn-scar ulcers (Marjolin's ulcer).

Ref.: 1, 2

COMMENTS: **Basal cell** carcinomas grow slowly and rarely metastasize, but they are capable of extensive local invasion. Although most common in the head and neck, they can occur in any location. They are often waxy or translucent with underlying telangiectasia, but with time they can produce a flat ulcer with little induration or reaction that can become quite deep ("rodent ulcer"). Superficial nonrecurrent basal cell carcinomas can be treated with topical 5-fluorouracil (5-FU), curettage, cryosurgery, or electrodesiccation, but surgical excision is preferred (to confirm the diagnosis and because of higher cure rates). **Squamous cell** carcinomas grow more rapidly and can metastasize. They are common at the vermilion border, paranasal areas, and maxillary skin. They tend to occur in persons with blond hair and light, thin, dry, irritated skin. Central ulceration with marked induration is common. These carcinomas arise often in patients with actinic keratosis, xeroderma pigmentosum, and atrophic epidermis and in persons exposed to arsenicals, nitrates, and hydrocarbons. Excision of both types of lesion should be accompanied by a frozen section evaluation of the surgical margins. Both lesions are radiosensitive, and in some cases radiotherapy offers better cosmetic results. Operation is preferred in areas that have a burn scar or that have been irradiated. Large lesions may require adjuvant radiotherapy after surgical excision. Mohs' chemosurgery involves application of zinc chloride paste followed by histologic examination of excised tissue; this regimen is repeated until all tumor margins are clear. Regional lymph node dissection for squamous cell carcinoma should be performed for clinically evident (palpable) disease.

ANSWER: A, D, E

13. True statements regarding melanoma include which of the following?

A. The most common histologic type is superficial spreading.
B. Depth of invasion (measured in millimeters), ulceration, and patient gender are important prognostic criteria.
C. Nodular melanomas carry a poorer prognosis than do superficial spreading melanomas of the same thickness.
D. Melanomas in dark-skinned people are frequently subungual or appear on the palms and soles.

Ref.: 1, 2, 6

COMMENTS: The incidence of melanoma is increasing and may be related to increased exposure of fair-skinned people to solar radiation. Melanomas are uncommon in dark-skinned people. Superficial spreading melanoma accounts for about 70% of all melanomas. Nodular and acral lentiginous melanomas tend to carry a poorer prognosis than do superficial spreading melanomas but only because they are thicker. Ulcerated melanomas and melanomas in men carry a poorer prognosis. Two-thirds of melanomas arise from a preexisting mole with junctional activity, and one-third arise de novo.

ANSWER: A, B, D

14. With regard to the classification of malignant melanoma, which of the following statements are true?

A. Stage I melanoma refers to melanoma in situ.
B. Clark's level IV denotes a melanoma extending as deeply as the papillary dermis.
C. Clark's level I implies melanoma in situ.

D. A T4 melanoma is one with invasion of the subcutaneous tissue or that is more than 4.0 mm in thickness.
E. Stage III melanoma refers to those with involved lymph nodes or in-transit metastases.

Ref.: 1, 2, 5

COMMENTS: Microstaging—by level of invasion (Clark) or tumor thickness in millimeters (Breslow)—is used to predict prognosis and the likelihood of regional and distant metastasis. Breslow's measurements are considered more precise for predicting biologic behavior. **Clark's** levels are defined as follows: I, above the basement membrane (i.e., melanoma in situ); II, into the papillary but not the reticular dermis; III, to an ill-defined interface between papillary and reticular dermis; IV, in reticular dermis; V, into subcutaneous fat. **Breslow's** method makes use of an oculomicrometer to determine maximal tumor thickness as defined from the top of the granular layer of the epidermis to the deepest point of tumor invasion. In ulcerated lesions the base of the ulcer over the deepest point of penetration is used instead of the granular layer. The American Joint Committee on Cancer (AJCC) staging system classifies melanoma by a TNM system. T1 tumors are Clark's level II, or less than 0.76 mm in thickness; T2 are Clark's level III, or 0.76–1.5 mm in thickness; T3 are Clark's level IV, or 1.51–4.0 mm in thickness; and T4 are Clark's level V, or more than 4.0 mm thick. The N0 classification implies no nodal involvement, N1 implies metastasis of 3 cm or less in regional nodes, and N2 refers to metastasis of more than 3 cm or in-transit metastases. Stage grouping is such that stage I disease is T1 or T2, N0, M0; stage II is T3 or T4, N0, M0; stage III is any T, N1 or N2, M0; and stage IV refers to patients with distant metastatic disease.

ANSWER: C, D, E

15. Select the treatment option(s) in the right-hand column that is/are most appropriate for the melanoma case summaries outlined in the left-hand column.

A. Level III superficial spreading melanoma (0.4 mm thick), with clinically negative regional lymph nodes
B. Level IV nodular melanoma (2 mm thick), with satellitosis and clinically negative regional lymph nodes
C. Level IV superficial spreading melanoma (1.5 mm thick), with palpable regional lymph nodes
D. Level IV acral lentiginous melanoma (2 mm thick), with clinically negative regional lymph nodes
E. Level II lentigo maligna melanoma (0.3 mm)

a. Moh's micrographic surgery
b. Wide local excision with 0.5 cm margins
c. Wide local excision with 1.0 cm margins
d. Wide local excision with 2.0 cm margins
e. Wide local excision with 4.0 cm margins
f. Sentinel lymph node biopsy
g. Regional lymph node sampling
h. Radical regional lymphadenectomy

Ref.: 1, 5, 7

COMMENTS: Virtually all melanomas are best treated by wide excision. The excision margin that minimizes the risk of local recurrence depends on the thickness of the tumor. Melanoma in situ and thin lentigo maligna melanomas of the face are treated adequately by margins of 0.5 cm. For melanomas less than 1.0 mm thick, 1 cm excision margins are appropriate. For intermediate-thickness melanomas (1.0–4.0 mm) a 2 cm margin is sufficient. Margins of 3–5 cm are generally employed for melanomas more than 4 mm in thickness and for those with associated satellitosis. Moh's chemosurgery is not appropriate for the treatment of any melanomas. The indications for elective lymph node dissection remain controversial. Recently, the technique of sentinel lymph node biopsy to pathologically stage patients with clinically negative nodes has become widely accepted. This technique may be of benefit to patients with melanomas more than 1 mm in thickness, but the value of this procedure in terms of prolonged survival (versus wide excision and observation) has not been established and is the subject of an ongoing randomized clinical trial. Patients with clinically positive lymph nodes should undergo radical regional lymphadenectomy. The extent of operation may be modified to suit the individual situation (e.g., modified radical neck dissection for patients without bulky disease or gross involvement of the posterior triangle). Random lymph node sampling or "cherry-picking" is never indicated for treatment of melanoma.

ANSWER: A-c; B-e,f; C-d,h; D-d,f; E-b

16. Match the lesion in the left column with the appropriate characteristic in the right column.

A. Cutaneous horn
B. Keratoacanthoma
C. Squamous cell carcinoma
D. Bowen's disease
E. Actinic keratosis

a. Rapidly growing benign lesion that can mimic squamous cell carcinoma or basal cell carcinoma
b. Often seen after radiation exposure or extensive sun exposure
c. Premalignant lesion of skin
d. Squamous cell carcinoma in situ of the skin

Ref.: 1

COMMENTS: **Squamous cell carcinoma** has been related to several premalignant conditions and environmental factors. Chronic excessive sun exposure has been implicated as a cause; lesions appear on exposed ears, the lower lip, and the dorsum of the hands. These cancers can metastasize, this potential being related to etiology, location, and size of the lesion. **Actinic (solar) keratosis** and **cutaneous horns** are premalignant lesions found on the sun-exposed areas of skin in fair-skinned individuals, more commonly in those with prolonged exposure to the sun or to carcinogens. These lesions can be treated topically (e.g., cryotherapy or topical 5-fluorouracil). Lesions resistant to this treatment should be excised. **Bowen's disease** is squamous cell carcinoma in situ; about 10% of these lesions progress to invasive squamous cell carcinoma. These lesions should be completely excised with negative margins. **Keratoacanthoma**, characterized by rapid growth, rolled edges, and a crater filled with keratin, can be confused with squamous and basal cell carcinoma. Keratoacanthomas involute spontaneously over a period of several months. A biopsy to include adjacent normal tissue is always necessary. When the diagnosis is established, large lesions can be observed; small lesions can be excised in their entirety.

ANSWER: A-b,c; B-a; C-b; D-d; E-b,c

17. With regard to ultraviolet radiation, which of the following statements is/are true?

A. Most of the ultraviolet radiation that reaches the earth is type B (290–320 nm).
B. Type A ultraviolet radiation is responsible for most of the sun damage to human skin.
C. Type A ultraviolet radiation is within the photoabsorption spectrum of DNA, whereas type B is not.
D. Melanin content of skin is the single best intrinsic factor for protecting skin from the harmful effects of ultraviolet radiation.
E. Ultraviolet radiation is both a tumor initiator and promoter.

Ref.: 5

COMMENTS: Ultraviolet (UV) radiation comprises the middle of the electromagnetic spectrum and is further divided into type A (UVA: 320–380 nm), type B (UVB: 290–320 nm), and type C (UVC: 240–290 nm). Visible light is 700–400 nm. Type C is virtually eliminated by stratospheric ozone. Only 5% of solar ultraviolet light is type B, but it is responsible for much of the chronic sun damage and carcinogenic degeneration of the human skin. UVB is partially eliminated by stratospheric ozone, and a 1% decrease in stratospheric ozone increases UVB flux at the earth's surface by about 3%. Whereas UVB and UVC are within the photoabsorption spectrum of DNA, UVA is not. There is increasing evidence that UVA radiation contributes to the development of skin cancers via non-DNA targets. Melanin is the most important factor in protecting the skin from the harmful effects of ultraviolet light. Tightly woven clothing, sunscreen use, and sun avoidance also offer protection against the harmful effects of ultraviolet radiation. UV light acts by both directly damaging DNA and other mechanisms such as altering cellular immunity and DNA repair mechanisms.

ANSWER: D, E

18. With regard to basal cell carcinoma, which of the following statements is/are true?

A. It originates from the deep dermal appendages.
B. It can be produced experimentally with ultraviolet light energy.
C. The aggressive behavior of morpheaform basal cell carcinoma is related to collagenase production.
D. The tumor metastasizes primarily through the hematogenous route.

Ref.: 1, 2

COMMENTS: Basal cell cancer is the most common malignancy in the United States, accounting for about 70% of all skin cancers and one-third of malignant tumors. Basal cell carcinoma originates from the pluripotential basal epithelial cells of the epidermis and from hair follicles, not from the dermis. The most common type of basal cell carcinoma is the nodular form, accounting for 70% of cases. The morpheaform type is the most aggressive clinically. This aggressive behavior may be related to the ability of this tumor to produce type IV collagenase, which facilitates local spread. Other types of basal cell carcinoma include superficial and pigmented lesions. Basal cell carcinomas rarely metastasize; but if they are unattended or are repeatedly recurrent, they can be locally destructive and problematic.

ANSWER: C

19. Which of the following is/are appropriate treatment for in-transit metastasis from cutaneous malignant melanoma?

A. Excision.
B. Injection.
C. Laser treatment.
D. Heated limb perfusion.
E. Amputation.

Ref.: 1, 5, 7

COMMENTS: In-transit metastases are a specialized form of locoregional recurrence of cutaneous melanoma. These lesions may be treated by local excision or ablation, although the recurrence rate is high. Intralesional injection with immune modulators such as BCG (bacille Calmette-Guérin) has led to complete regression of both injected and neighboring lesions in some cases. In patients with extensive in-transit metastases, limb perfusion with various cytotoxic agents [most commonly melphalan or tumor necrosis factor α (TNF-α)] results in complete response rates of 30–90% and a limb salvage rate of more than 80% in most series. The overall 5-year survival after limb perfusion in these patients averages 50%, although it is lower (about 30%) for patients with concomitant regional lymph node metastases. Major amputation may be performed for control of disease or palliation, although the indications for this have diminished since the advent of limb perfusion.

ANSWER: A, B, C, D, E

20. Select the *true* statements regarding genetic predisposition to skin cancer.

A. About 10% of cases of malignant melanoma are familial.
B. Familial melanoma is characterized by an earlier age of onset of disease, multiple primary tumors, and a frequent association with multiple dysplastic nevi.
C. The *p16/CDKN2A* tumor suppressor gene located on chromosome 9 has been implicated in 90% of cases of inherited melanoma.
D. Mutations of *PTC*, a tumor suppressor gene, are responsible for most cases of basal cell nevus syndrome.

Ref.: 5, 8, 9, 10

COMMENTS: About 1 in 10 cases of melanoma are familial. Described initially as the familial mole and melanoma syndrome, these patients frequently present at a young age, have multiple primary tumors, and have multiple (>40) characteristic large dysplastic nevi. Although linkage studies have implicated a number of candidate sites (including loci on chromosome 1, 6, 7, and 9) in the etiology of familial melanoma, recent studies have shown that mutations of the *MTS1* (*p16/ CDKN2A*) gene on chromosome 9 is implicated in a number of kindreds. Multiple mutations of this gene have been observed, and current data suggest that such mutations account for about one-fourth of all familial cases of melanoma. Mutations of the *CDK4* gene have been identified in a few melanoma families. Although commercial testing for *p16* mutations is available, uncertainties regarding interpretation of the results of this genetic testing, as well as discrimination concerns, mitigate against the clinical use of this test at this time. Mutations in *PTC*, the human homologue of the *Drosophila* patched gene, have been identified in most patients with the basal cell nevus (Gorlin) syndrome. Mutations have also been identified in a few sporadically occurring basal cell carcinomas. The most common are frameshift mutations resulting in premature termination. Determination of the functional significance of *PTC* may lead to innovative treatments (and prevention strategies) for basal cell carcinoma.

ANSWER: A, B, D

REFERENCES

1. Schwartz SI, Shires GT, Spencer FC, et al: *Principles of Surgery*, 7th ed. McGraw-Hill, New York, 1999.
2. Sabiston DC Jr: *Textbook of Surgery*, 15th ed. WB Saunders, Philadelphia, 1997.
3. Williams PL, Warwick R, Dyson M, Bannister LH: *Gray's Anatomy*, 37th ed. Churchill Livingstone, Edinburgh, 1989.
4. Das Gupta TK, Chaudhury P: *Tumors of the Soft Tissues*, 2nd ed. Appelton-Century-Crofts, Norwalk, CT, 1998.
5. Lejeune FJ, Chaudhuri PK, Das Gupta TK: *Malignant Melanoma: Medical and Surgical Management*. McGraw-Hill, New York, 1994.
6. Ridgeway CA, Hieken TJ, Ronan SG, et al: Acral lentiginous malignant melanoma. *Arch Surg* 130:88–92, 1995.
7. Coit D, Wallack M, Balch C: Melanoma surgical practice guidelines. *Oncology* 11:1317–1323, 1997.
8. Hahn H, Wicking C, Zaphiropoulous PG, et al: Mutations of the human homolog of *Drosophila* patched in the nevoid basal cell carcinoma syndrome. *Cell* 85:841–851, 1996.
9. Johnson RL, Rothman AL, Xie J, et al: Human homolog of patched, a candidate gene for the basal cell nevus syndrome. *Science* 272:1668–1671, 1996.
10. Huska FG, Hodi FS: Molecular genetics of familial cutaneous melanoma. *J Clin Oncol* 16:670–682, 1998.

CHAPTER 19

Breast

1. A thin, 35-year-old woman with no family history of breast cancer visits you after her initial (and normal) mammogram. Her menarche was at age 13, and her first child was born when she was 20. She has never taken contraceptives and drinks an occasional glass of wine. She wants to know what the chance is that she will develop breast cancer in her lifetime. What would you tell her the chance is, approximately?

   A. 1%.
   B. 4%.
   C. 11%.
   D. 15%.
   E. 20%.

Ref.: 1, 2

COMMENTS: The incidence of breast cancer has been steadily increasing worldwide in recent decades for unclear reasons. Also poorly understood are the large geographic variations in its prevalence, with the United States, United Kingdom, and Scandinavian countries having high rates and Japan a low rate. About 180,000 cases of breast cancer are diagnosed annually in the United States, and 45,000 patients die of the disease, making it the most common malignancy (other than skin cancer) in American women. Approximately 11% of women in the United States can expect to develop breast cancer in their lifetime, but that figure assumes a longevity of more than age 80 years and includes those who are at high risk (in some cases >50%) because of multiple factors. It is important when counseling patients to remember that a woman with no risk factors has closer to a 4% chance of developing breast cancer.

ANSWER: B

2. With regard to risk factors for breast cancer, which of the following statements is/are true?

   A. Incidence does not appear to be age-related among those older than age 35 years.
   B. Family history is a major predictor of risk for developing breast cancer.
   C. Late first pregnancy increases the risk of breast cancer.
   D. Diet and weight have no association with breast cancer risk.

Ref.: 1, 2

COMMENTS: Breast cancer is clearly age-related, with its incidence being extremely low in women younger than 20 years of age. In all countries, the age-specific incidence then increases steadily up to menopause. In high-risk countries such as the United States, the incidence continues to increase with advancing age. In intermediate-risk countries such as those of central Europe, the rate plateaus at menopause. In low-risk countries such as Japan, the rate declines after menopause. Family history is a major risk factor for the development of breast cancer, particularly among first-degree relatives (mother, sister, daughter). The risk is further increased if the relative developed cancer at a premenopausal age and if it was bilateral. A patient's risk increases slightly if an aunt or grandmother develops unilateral, postmenopausal breast cancer, whereas it increases to as high as 50% if a first-degree relative develops bilateral, premenopausal breast cancer. The length of time a patient menstruates prior to her first pregnancy influences the risk; therefore an early menarche and a late first pregnancy both increase the risk, particularly if the time span between these two events is more than 20 years. Obesity, exposure to ionizing irradiation, a high-fat diet, and excess alcohol ingestion have all been implicated as risk factors. The data on the role of estrogen replacement therapy and oral contraceptives are conflicting, but retrospective studies suggest that prolonged (>10 years) use of estrogen and the use of contraceptives prior to the first pregnancy may increase the risk of subsequent breast cancer.

ANSWER: B, C

3. With regard to the natural history of breast cancer, which of the following statements is/are true?

   A. On average, a 1 cm breast cancer has been subclinically present for approximately 1 year.
   B. Dimpling of the skin occurs as a result of glandular fibrosis and shortening of Cooper's ligaments.
   C. Skin edema in breast cancer results only from direct skin invasion by tumor.
   D. Vertebral metastases result from arterial dissemination of cancer cells.
   E. Ipsilateral lung involvement occurs most often as a result of direct lung invasion.

Ref.: 2

COMMENTS: Most breast cancers are estimated to have volume-doubling times of 2–9 months, suggesting that the average 1 cm tumor has been present for at least 5 years prior to clinical detection. Neither skin dimpling nor edema requires direct skin invasion; these conditions result from fibrosis (with shortening of Cooper's ligaments) and lymphatic blockage, respectively, in the subdermal tissues. The axial skeleton is a favored site for distant metastases from breast cancer, which is thought to be due to access of cancer cells to the paravertebral venous plexus by way of intercostal veins. All other forms of distant metastases, including ipsilateral lung involvement, are due to hematogenous spread.

ANSWER: B

4. With regard to the natural history of breast cancer, which of the following statements is/are true?

   A. Virtually all patients with untreated breast cancer die within 2 years of their diagnosis.
   B. The likelihood of distant metastasis is related to primary tumor size and involvement of axillary nodes.
   C. The most common initial site of metastasis is bone.
   D. Liver and bone metastases occur with essentially equal frequency throughout the time course of a given cancer.
   E. Appropriate surgical therapy for breast carcinoma has been shown to increase overall survival.

Ref.: 1, 2

COMMENTS: Breast cancer is a disease of wide biologic variability; and although the median survival among untreated patients is 2.7 years, nearly 20% of patients survive 5 years and some as long as 15 years without treatment. The increased likelihood that distant metastases will occur in the presence of axillary nodal metastases and (to a lesser extent) large tumors has led, through the results of clinical trials, to the current recommendations of adjuvant systemic therapy in these high-risk patients. Among patients dying of disseminated breast cancer, lung is the most common site of distant disease. However, as the initial site of distant metastasis, bone predominates, followed by lung, soft tissues, liver, and the central nervous system. Appropriate local/regional therapy, including surgery and radiation therapy, has definitely improved both disease-free and overall survival.

ANSWER: B, C, E

5. Each of the patients depicted in the accompanying figure has a breast cancer and a normal chest radiograph and blood chemistries; none has bone pain. What is the preoperative clinical TNM designation and the stage of each cancer?

Ref.: 3

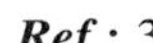

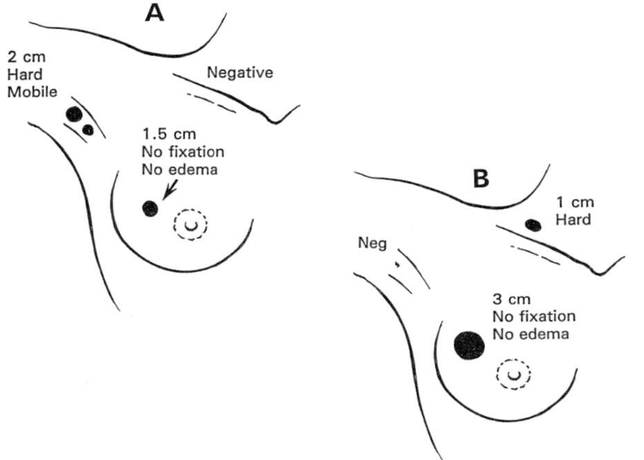

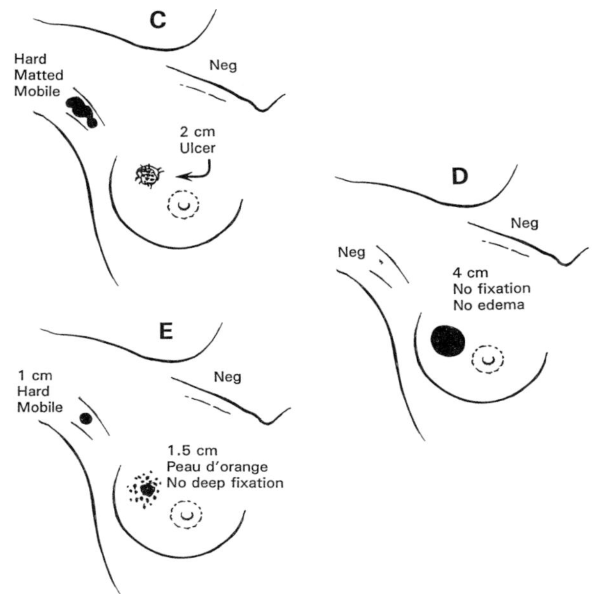

COMMENTS: The correct staging of breast cancer is important as a prognostic indicator. **T** is for **tumor size**: T1 is for tumors less than 2 cm; T2 between 2 and 5 cm; T3 larger than 5 cm. Chest wall or direct skin involvement (T4) should also be assessed. **N** is for **lymph nodes**; suspicious mobile axillary nodes (N1), matted or fixed axillary nodes (N2), and ipsilateral internal mammary nodes (N3) should be specifically described. **M** is for **metastases**. Evidence of lung (chest radiograph) or liver or bone involvement (serum chemistries or scans) (M1) should be sought in each patient. Supraclavicular nodes (formerly considered to be N3) are now thought to represent distant metastases (M1).

ANSWER: A-T1,N1,M0, stage IIA; B-T2,N0,M1, stage IV; C-T4,N2,M0, stage IIIB; D-T2,N0,M0, stage IIA; E-T4,N1,M0, stage IIIB

6. A 58-year-old woman presents with a chronic, erythematous, oozing, eczematoid rash involving the left nipple and areola. There are no breast masses palpable, and her mammogram is normal. Which of the following recommendations is appropriate?

   A. Referral to a dermatologist.
   B. Oral vitamin E and topical aloe and lanolin.
   C. Biopsy.
   D. Advise patient to wear a nonallergenic brassiere.
   E. Topical 5-fluorouracil (5-FU).

Ref.: 1, 2

COMMENTS: Paget's disease of the breast, unrelated to Paget's disease of the bone, is generally considered to be a primary ductal carcinoma that secondarily invades the epithelium of the nipple and areola, although lobular carcinomas have been reported. The eczematoid rash described in this patient is a typical presentation. Biopsy of any chronic nipple rash is mandatory and, in Paget's disease, shows distinctive pagetoid cells. Depending on the chronicity, Paget's disease may present with an intraductal carcinoma or an infiltrating carcinoma with or without a palpable mass. The treatment is dictated by the extent of the underlying tumor. Because of the rich network of lymphatics underneath the nipple–areolar complex and the proximity of the cancer to this plexus in Paget's disease of the breast, mastectomy is usually indicated; however, breast-conserving therapies may be considered in selected cases. Local treatment with ointments is not helpful and only delays diagnosis.

ANSWER: C

7. Match each histologic type of breast cancer in the left column with its associated features in the right column.

A. Infiltrating duct carcinoma
B. Ductal carcinoma in situ
C. Lobular carcinoma in situ
D. Malignant cystosarcoma phylloides
E. Medullary carcinoma
F. Inflammatory carcinoma

a. Lymphocytic infiltrate and better-than-average prognosis
b. Often large but quite mobile
c. Highest likelihood of multicentric ipsilateral disease
d. Highest likelihood of bilateral disease
e. Dermal lymphatic invasion
f. Most common carcinoma presenting as a breast mass.

Ref.: 1, 2

COMMENTS: The clinical presentation, natural history, and biologic aggressiveness of breast cancer depend in large part on the histologic type. **Lobular carcinoma in situ**, often called lobular neoplasia to emphasize that it is a risk marker rather than a true malignancy, usually presents as an incidental histologic finding at biopsy of another lesion in premenopausal women. Its significance is that it portends an approximately 20–25% chance of developing an invasive carcinoma within 15 years of diagnosis, with both breasts being at essentially equal risk. **Ductal carcinoma in situ** (DCIS; intraductal carcinoma) frequently presents as an area of clustered microcalcifications on the mammogram but uncommonly presents as a palpable mass. The outlook for localized noncomedo DCIS treated with total excision alone is excellent. Early results from clinical trials suggest that radiation after total excision may be preferable. The comedo pattern, in contrast, is associated with a high incidence of multicentricity; and when it is treated conservatively, there is a correspondingly high recurrence rate, with half of these recurrences being invasive carcinoma. **Medullary carcinoma** usually presents as a palpable mass with smooth mammographic borders that can mimic benign conditions. Indeed, the appearance of this cancer on ultrasound scans can closely mimic the sonographic findings seen with fibroadenoma; these findings include smooth contour, homogeneous interior echogenicity as well as posterior enhancement. Histologically, it is characterized by a lymphocytic infiltrate and carries a better-than-average prognosis. **Inflammatory carcinoma**, a variant of infiltrating ductal carcinoma, is characterized by the clinical appearance of inflammation (peau d'orange, warmth, and erythema) secondary to dermal lymphatic invasion. Although the overall prognosis is poor, it has recently improved with the addition of preoperative chemotherapy followed by mastectomy and irradiation. **Cystosarcoma phylloides** resembles a giant fibroadenoma clinically and histologically, and it occurs in both benign and malignant forms. If benign, adequate treatment consists of total excision with adequate (2–3 cm) margins. Long-term follow-up is mandatory, as recurrences are not uncommon and can be of the malignant variety. If malignant, its primary mode of metastasis is vascular, and lymph node involvement is uncommon. The malignant variety usually necessitates mastectomy to achieve local control.

ANSWER: A-f; B-c; C-d; D-b; E-a; F-e

8. A 34-year-old woman underwent wide local excision, axillary dissection, and radiation therapy (5000 cGy over a 5-week period) to her left breast for a node-positive, 2-cm infiltrating duct carcinoma 3 years earlier. She received 6 months of adjuvant chemotherapy with Cytoxan, methotrexate, and 5-fluorouracil (5-FU) at that time. You now perform a biopsy of a new 2-cm mass in the same breast, and it shows infiltrating duct carcinoma. She has no other evidence of local, regional, or distant disease. Which of the following treatment plans is most appropriate?

A. Reexcision to free margins, second axillary dissection, and a 5000-cGy "boost" to the breast.
B. Adriamycin-based combination chemotherapy alone.
C. Left total mastectomy.
D. Left modified radical mastectomy.
E. 5000-cGy "boost" to the breast and combination Adriamycin-based chemotherapy.

Ref.: 1, 2, 4

COMMENTS: Local recurrence of cancer in the breast occurs in approximately 10% of patients who are treated with wide local excision (lumpectomy), axillary dissection, and irradiation. "Salvage" mastectomy is usually required and results in long-term survival approaching that seen when mastectomy is done for a first primary lesion. In the absence of palpable nodes, a second axillary dissection is unnecessary and hazardous. The effects of ionizing irradiation are cumulative and do not diminish with time. Treatment with an additional 5000 cGy would therefore lead to serious dermal complications in the irradiated area. Treatment with chemotherapy alone would be inappropriate and would deny the patient the best chance for long-term survival and local control.

ANSWER: C

9. With regard to the management of patients with metastatic breast cancer that is estrogen receptor (ER)-positive, which of the following treatments is/are appropriate?

A. Bilateral oophorectomy.
B. Antiestrogen drugs (tamoxifen).
C. High-dose estrogen or progesterone.
D. Androgenic steroids.
E. Aromatase inhibitors.

Ref.: 1, 2

COMMENTS: For incompletely understood reasons, a variety of sometimes seemingly conflicting hormonal manipulations may cause a therapeutic response in patients with metastatic breast cancer, particularly in those who have significant amounts of estrogen receptor (ER) and progesterone receptor (PR) protein on their cells (ER-positive and PR-positive). Patients with high ER and PR levels also have a better prognosis than those with low or absent values when other discriminants are comparable. The most common hormonal manipulation is estrogen withdrawal, usually with the receptor-blocking agent tamoxifen (Nolvadex); however, bilateral oophorectomy in premenopausal women is still a reasonable option, particularly since the advent of laparoscopic oophorectomy. Paradoxically, approximately 40% of patients respond to the addition of estrogen in the form of diethylstilbestrol, conjugated estrogens (Premarin), or synthetic estrogen (ethinyl estradiol). Progestational agents such as megestrol acetate (Megace) are associated with about a 30% response rate and androgenic agents such as testosterone with a 15% response rate. Surgical hypophysectomy and adrenalectomy were at one time common forms of hormonal manipulation, but they have been all but totally replaced by "medical adrenalectomy" with drugs such as anastrozole and letrozole, which inhibit the production of adrenal steroids and the conversion of androgens to estrogens in the adrenal gland and peripherally. Other blocking agents are under investigation.

ANSWER: A, B, C, D, E

10. A 29-year-old woman presents with an ill-defined 2 cm mass in the outer quadrant of her breast. Mammography shows very dense tissue but no discrete lesion. Ultrasound examination shows a solid lesion. An ultrasound-guided fine-needle aspiration (FNA) is performed, and the aspirate is plated, fixed, and sent for cytology. A highly cellular, monomorphic pattern is seen, with poorly cohesive intact cells, nuclear "crowding" with a variation in nuclear size, radial dispersion and clumping of the chromatin, and prominent nucleoli. Which of the following management choices is/are appropriate?

A. Modified radical mastectomy.
B. Reassuring the patient that the process is benign.
C. Lumpectomy, axillary dissection, and irradiation.
D. Excision of a fibroadenoma with narrow margins.
E. Follow-up examination in 1 month.

Ref.: 4

COMMENTS: Aspiration biopsy with a 22-gauge needle is an effective and safe way of assessing palpable breast lesions. Performing the aspiration under ultrasound guidance ensures that the lesion has been sampled thoroughly while under direct vision. Although a smaller volume of tissue is obtained than with needle core biopsy, FNA frequently yields results that are equal or superior to core biopsy if read by an experienced cytopathologist. A fibroadenoma would show broad sheets of cohesive cells with nuclei that are uniform in size and shape. The chromatin pattern would be finely granular, and large numbers of bare nuclei would be present. The cytologic findings described in the question are diagnostic for carcinoma. Appropriate management includes either a modified radical mastectomy or lumpectomy, axillary dissection, and whole breast irradiation. Because of the small (<1%) possibility of a false-positive cytology reading, many surgeons perform a confirmatory histologic biopsy prior to proceeding with mastectomy. Either an ultrasound-guided core biopsy performed in an office setting or an open biopsy frozen section performed intraoperatively is appropriate under these circumstances.

ANSWER: A, C

11. A 39-year-old woman underwent a lumpectomy and axillary dissection for a 2 cm moderately differentiated, ER-negative infiltrating duct carcinoma. Margins around the primary tumor were free, and 1 of 19 lymph nodes was positive for carcinoma. Which of the following treatment plans is most appropriate?

A. Radiation therapy alone.
B. Radiation therapy and single-drug chemotherapy for 1 year.
C. Radiation therapy and single-drug chemotherapy for 3–6 months.
D. Radiation therapy and multiple-drug chemotherapy for 1 year.
E. Radiation therapy and multiple-drug chemotherapy for 3–6 months.
F. Radiation therapy, multiple-drug chemotherapy for 6 months and tamoxifen.
G. Completion mastectomy and multiple-drug chemotherapy for 6 months without irradiation.

Ref.: 1, 2, 4

COMMENTS: Most prospective, randomized studies have shown both disease-free and overall survival benefit for adjuvant chemotherapy in node-positive premenopausal women, the greatest advantage being among those with one to three positive nodes. Postmenopausal node-positive women have generally shown a more modest benefit. Multiple-drug therapy has consistently been more effective than single-drug therapy, and a 3- to 6-month regimen (depending on the drugs selected) has been shown to be as effective as a 12-month regimen. Adding tamoxifen to chemotherapy for node-positive premenopausal patients (regardless of receptor status) is not yet considered standard therapy but is under study. Proper sequencing of the irradiation and chemotherapy is controversial and awaits further clinical trials, but preliminary results show a survival benefit if chemotherapy precedes whole breast irradiation. Converting the local management of this tumor to mastectomy in the presence of free margins is not necessary and would not improve the survival rate.

ANSWER: E

12. With regard to adjuvant radiotherapy following mastectomy, which of the following statements is/are true?

A. Local recurrence rate is reduced.
B. Disease-free survival is improved.
C. There are few, if any, significant side effects from irradiation of the chest wall.
D. It should be offered routinely to all patients whose primary tumors are larger than 2 cm.

Ref.: 1, 2, 4, 5, 6

COMMENTS: Adjuvant radiation therapy does decrease the local recurrence rates; however, this has not been generally found to translate into longer overall or relapse-free survival except in two recent reports involving node-positive patients. Although relatively uncommon with modern techniques, skin ulceration, arm edema, rib fracture, radiation pneumonitis, radiation-related chest wall sarcomas, and increased incidence of contralateral breast cancer represent some of the potential side effects from chest wall irradiation. Therefore adjuvant radiotherapy should be reserved for patients who are at high risk for local recurrence (large tumors, skin involvement, more than four axillary lymph nodes involved).

ANSWER: A

13. Which of the following 5-year survival rates by stage for treated breast cancer is/are correct?

A. Stage I: 90–95%.
B. Stage II: 50–80%.
C. Stage III: 30–50%.
D. Stage IV: 15–20%.

Ref.: 1, 2, 4

COMMENTS: The wide range in rates of survival among patients with the same stages of breast cancer reflects the wide range of staging criteria used by various investigators as well as the variability in biologic behavior among the differing subtypes of breast cancer. Historically, there has been nonconformity among investigators in the criteria used to assign a cancer a particular stage, which has led to overlap in the staging designations. Additionally, over time, new histologic and cytologic means have emerged that are providing investigators the markers to define these groups more precisely. Any period of follow-up shorter than 10 years is considered inadequate because of the ability of breast cancer to recur even after long disease-free intervals. When reporting breast cancer follow-up data, one must differentiate between "survival" and "disease-free interval." Because of these factors, therefore, all of the survival rates given are appropriate for their respective stages.

ANSWER: A, B, C, D

14. Match the ER/PR value of the recurrent cancer in the left column with its expected rate of response to hormonal therapy in the right column.

A. ER-positive/PR-negative	a. 80%
B. ER-positive/PR-positive	b. 45%
C. ER-negative/PR-positive	c. 35%
D. ER-negative/PR-negative	d. 10%

Ref.: 2

COMMENTS: Because they are lipids, steroid hormones circulating in the blood move passively across membranes into cells. For them to influence the growth or function of the cell, highly specific receptor proteins must be present in the cell to bind with the hormone. The activated steroid–receptor complex associates with chromatin in the nucleus and stimulates the synthesis of nucleic acids and proteins that subsequently govern the growth and differentiation of the cell. Normal breast cells have receptors for estrogen, progesterone, androgens, and glucocorticoids. Many breast cancers retain these receptors. ER and PR assays can be performed quantitatively if enough tumor is present (approximately 300–500 mg) or, if not, by immunohistochemical techniques. In general, if the receptors are present, the tumor has to some degree retained the regulatory mechanisms operating in normal breast epithelium. Their absence therefore implies less controlled growth and a poorer overall prognosis. The increased response rate seen in some breast cancer subtypes with positive receptors provides the basis for endocrine manipulation, both additive and ablative. Approximately 90% of breast cancers in males are ER-positive, accounting for the frequent response in males to tamoxifen and orchiectomy. The most responsive receptor status is ER-positive/PR-positive followed by ER-negative/PR-positive, ER-positive/PR-negative, and ER-negative/PR-negative.

ANSWER: A-c; B-a; C-b; D-d

15. With regard to chronic cystic mastitis, which of the following statements is/are true?

A. It is a well defined abnormality of the breast with specific and consistent histologic features.
B. It is of primarily bacterial etiology.
C. It is rarely seen in women younger than 45 years of age.
D. Cysts must measure at least 1 cm to make the diagnosis.
E. None of the above.

Ref.: 1, 2

COMMENTS: See Question 16.

16. Which of the following forms of breast pathology does not belong to the chronic cystic mastitis group?

A. Papillomatosis.
B. Blunt duct adenosis.
C. Sclerosing adenosis.
D. Apocrine metaplasia.
E. Mondor's disease.

Ref.: 1, 2

COMMENTS: Chronic cystic mastitis, commonly referred to as chronic cystic mastopathy, is a catchall phrase that refers to a poorly defined group of histopathologic processes in the breast of rather obscure etiology. Indeed many modern investigations now refer to this group of histologic findings as fibrocystic change because of its widespread prevalence in the breast. The various alterations in the stromal and epithelial architecture of the breast are unrelated to trauma or bacterial infection. Pathologic changes commonly referred to by this name include fibrosis, mammary duct ectasia, apocrine metaplasia, blunt duct adenosis, sclerosing adenosis, epithelial hyperplasia, and papillomatosis. Mondor's disease, which does not belong in this group, is a superficial thrombophlebitis presenting as a characteristic painful, tender cord along the lateral aspect of the breast and inframammary chest wall.

ANSWER:
Question 15: E
Question 16: E

17. A 42-year-old woman with no family history of breast cancer presents with an ill-defined lump in the upper outer quadrant of her left breast. Her mammogram shows only minimal increase in the fibroglandular markings in that area. Because the mass seems slightly more prominent when you see her at follow-up 1 month later, you perform an excisional biopsy. The pathologic diagnosis is "fibrocystic disease," with the comments describing increased fibrosis, duct ectasia, periductal inflammation, and microcyst formation with no epithelial hyperplasia. What is the increase in likelihood that she will subsequently develop breast cancer?

A. Essentially none.
B. Three times.
C. Five times.
D. Ten times.

Ref.: 4

COMMENTS: It is widely cited in both the surgical literature and the lay press that there is a threefold increase in the incidence of breast cancer among women with fibrocystic disease, but this figure is misleading. When the changes are "nonproliferative" (i.e., no epithelial hyperplasia), there is no significant increased risk. The presence of proliferative lesions, such as papillomatosis (multiple tiny ductal papillomas) or hyperplasia of the usual variety, minimally increases the risk of breast cancer. Atypical hyperplasia increases the risk fourfold unless it accompanies a strong family history of breast cancer, in which case the risk is increased ninefold.

ANSWER: A

18. With regard to breast infections, which of the following statements is/are true?

A. Acute bacterial infections occur most often as a result of preexisting chronic dermatitis.
B. Bacterial infections are usually indolent, taking up to several weeks to become clinically apparent.
C. Surgical drainage, once suppuration has occurred, is the treatment of choice for acute infections.
D. Tuberculosis is a rare cause of breast infection.

Ref.: 1, 2

COMMENTS: Acute bacterial breast infection most often occurs during lactation within the first several months following delivery. Because the lactating breast is such an excellent culture medium, these infections usually develop rapidly, and their size is often underestimated on clinical examination. If cellulitis without abscess formation is encountered, antibiotics may abort the infection. Once suppuration has occurred, however, surgical drainage is required. Ultrasonography can be used diagnostically to identify the presence of one or more abscess cavities; additionally, it can be used to guide catheters for closed drainage and, if required, for precise placement of an incision for open drainage. Depending on the extent of suppuration, local or general anesthesia can be used. Chronic bacterial subareolar abscesses and fistulas occasionally occur and require surgical therapy. Tuberculosis, at one time a not uncommon cause of breast infection, is now rare.

ANSWER: C, D

19. With regard to breast development, which of the following statements is/are true?

A. Breast enlargement in male neonates is indicative of an underlying estrogen-secreting adrenal tumor.
B. Accessory nipples can be found anywhere from the axilla to the groin.
C. Extramammary breast tissue is not under the influence of the hormonal status of the patient.
D. Inverted nipples in children suggest underlying breast cancer.

Ref.: 1, 2

COMMENTS: If the embryologic mammary ridge extending from the axilla to the groin fails to involute fully, accessory nipples (polythelia) can appear along this route. Accessory breast tissue (polymastia) is also seen frequently in the axilla and may enlarge during pregnancy and lactation as well as during the response to normal fluctuations in the patient's hormonal status during her menstrual cycle. Indeed, accessory breast tissue is detected on mammography and may present differential diagnostic difficulties for both mammographer and clinician. Shortly after birth, both males and females may exhibit unilateral or bilateral breast enlargement, which is attributed to high levels of circulating maternal estrogens; these changes regress spontaneously during the neonatal period. In female infants, failure of one or both nipples to evert following birth and into adulthood leads to functional problems related to future breast-feeding, but is unrelated to future breast cancer.

ANSWER: B

20. With regard to mammography for evaluation of breast disease, which of the following statements is/are true?

A. It can detect many cancers too small to be palpated.
B. It accurately detects lesions in breasts regardless of patient age or glandular architecture.
C. It delivers 2 cGy to the middle of the breast being studied and therefore should not be used for routine screening.
D. Although it occasionally misses small cancers, a positive reading for carcinoma on mammography is virtually always accurate.

Ref.: 1, 2, 4

COMMENTS: Mammography is an important aid in the overall evaluation of breast disease, frequently identifying carcinomas before they become palpable and, in many instances, before they become invasive. The accuracy of mammography declines as breast density increases, and it increases as the breast parenchyma is replaced by adipose tissue as involution occurs with advancing age. The overall false-negative and false-positive rates encountered in mammography screening are approximately 10%. Current technology allows as little as 0.1 cGy to the midbreast per study, making it safe for routine annual mammography in women older than 35 years of age. Because the harmful effect of radiation is greatest in the breasts of younger women (i.e., those under age 35), because of the low incidence of breast cancer in younger women, and because of the inherent limitations of mammography in dense breasts often encountered within this age group, screening mammography is not performed routinely until age 40. High-risk individuals are an exception to this rule. Breast ultrasonography, devoid of any harmful effect on the parenchyma of the breast, is an ideal imaging modality for younger patients with breast complaints regardless of the degree of breast density encountered. It is also useful for breast evaluation of the pregnant patient in whom radiation exposure is avoided if possible.

ANSWER: A

21. With regard to the current therapy of stage I and stage II breast cancer, which of the following statements is/are true?

A. The Halsted radical mastectomy has resulted in a cure rate superior to that of other treatment options.
B. The modified radical mastectomy involves preservation of the nipple to improve cosmesis following reconstruction.
C. Wide local excision with axillary dissection and radiation therapy to the remainder of the breast is reserved for patients too debilitated to undergo the more radical mastectomy.

D. Clinical trials have shown equivalent disease-free survival for selected patients randomized to receive either modified radical mastectomy or wide local excision, axillary dissection, and breast radiation therapy.

Ref.: 1, 2, 4

COMMENTS: The two most commonly employed modalities of definitive therapy for stage I and stage II breast cancer are (1) modified radical mastectomy, which preserves the pectoralis major muscle while excising all breast tissue, including the nipple, and the axillary nodal basin; and (2) a wide local excision of the breast tumor (lumpectomy) and axillary dissection in conjunction with postoperative whole-breast irradiation. Studies with long-term follow-up have shown no significant disease-free survival advantage for the more radical (pectoralis-removing) Halsted mastectomy. The National Surgical Adjuvant Breast Project (NSABP) has conducted a multiinstitutional study with more than 1800 patients with stage I or II breast cancer randomized to undergo modified radical mastectomy or wide local excision (lumpectomy) with axillary dissection with and without breast radiation therapy. At an average of 10 years from treatment, there appear to be no statistically significant differences in disease-free survival between the mastectomy group and the breast preservation group. Those undergoing wide local excision with axillary dissection but *without* radiotherapy had a higher local recurrence rate. Patients too debilitated to undergo general anesthesia are not candidates for either a mastectomy or axillary dissection. Elderly, high-risk patients are sometimes managed with lumpectomy or partial mastectomy under local anesthesia followed by tamoxifen, irradiation, or both. Studies to date have shown that introduction of the sentinel node biopsy performed under local/intravenous sedation may well provide an accurate, minimally invasive axillary staging procedure that can be used in even high-risk stage I and II breast cancer patients.

ANSWER: D

22. Which of the following physical characteristics of breast masses are more suggestive of carcinoma than of benign disease?

A. Indistinct borders blending into the surrounding breast tissue.
B. Hardness.
C. Excessive mobility within breast tissue.
D. Tethering to underlying muscular structures.

Ref.: 1, 2

COMMENTS: Although there are many exceptions to the classic physical findings of breast cancer, the typical breast carcinoma is hard and has fairly distinct borders. Fixation to deeper structures is highly suggestive of malignancy. A smooth, rubbery, mobile mass is more suggestive of fibroadenoma. Fibrocystic disease may present as a disc-like or polynodular thickening, with one or more of the borders blending indistinctly into the surrounding breast tissue.

ANSWER: B, D

23. With regard to subcutaneous mastectomy, which of the following statements is/are true?

A. It involves removal of all breast tissue.
B. It includes removal of the lower axillary lymph nodes.
C. The best reconstruction results are associated with this type of mastectomy.
D. It is the treatment of choice for early (<1 cm) microinvasive cancers with clinically negative nodes.

Ref.: 1, 2

COMMENTS: Subcutaneous mastectomy is removal of the breast with preservation of the rim of the nipple. When performing this operation, the incision line has been classically described as submammary. In reality the incisional line is within the breast compartment and by necessity must transect Cooper's ligaments as they attach to the anterior sheath of the superficial fascia. Terminal ductal lobular units (TDLUs) are considered by many respected investigators as the site of development of both ductal and lobular carcinoma. They are often in close proximity to these fascial sheaths (Cooper's ligaments) and are perforce transected during operation; thus remnants of TDLUs can be left attached to the dermis. Additionally, TDLUs are found sprouting from the ductal system at or near the nipple–areolar junction. Axillary nodes are not removed as part of this operation; in fact, exposure of the axilla to remove the entire tail of the breast is at times difficult. Consequently, it is estimated that at least 1–2% of breast tissue remains after subcutaneous mastectomy. Because of preservation of some of the nipple and most of the "subcutaneous fat," and because of the more cosmetic incision, "subcutaneous mastectomy" offers the opportunity for reconstruction with the most favorable cosmetic result. However, there have been reports of cancer developing in the remaining nipple and small amount of remaining breast parenchyma. In fact, there is no evidence that removal of 98% of the breast tissue decreases the risk of developing cancer by an equivalent amount. For this reason, many surgeons do not consider it a good "prophylactic" operation. It is clearly not recommended for therapeutic management of breast cancer.

ANSWER: C

24. With regard to cystosarcoma phylloides, which of the following statements is/are true?

A. It bears a histologic relation to fibroadenoma.
B. Ten percent are malignant.
C. As with ductal carcinoma, it has a high incidence of multicentricity within the breast.
D. Axillary lymph nodal metastases are uncommon.
E. Wide local excision or total (simple) mastectomy usually suffices for treatment.

Ref.: 1, 2, 4

COMMENTS: Although only approximately 10% of all cystosarcomas are malignant, cystosarcoma is still the most common primary sarcoma of the breast. The benign variant of cystosarcoma is considered by many to be a "giant fibroadenoma" and, as such, usually presents clinically as a solitary, discrete, mobile mass within the breast (usually quite a bit larger than the average fibroadenoma). The diagnosis of malignancy in phylloides tumor is at times difficult because of the poor correlation between histology and clinical behavior. Differentiation between the benign and malignant varieties is, among other features, determined by counting the number of mitoses seen per high power field. If the tumor is histologically benign, wide local excision is considered adequate treatment. Even though benign, phylloides tumors have a high frequency of local recurrence, so careful long-term follow-up is essential.

If the malignant variety is encountered, total mastectomy without axillary dissection is usually indicated. The malignant cystosarcoma has no significant incidence of multicentricity within the breast (unlike ductal or lobular carcinoma).

ANSWER: A, B, D, E

25. With regard to breast carcinoma in men, which of the following statements is/are true?

A. It accounts for approximately 1% of all breast cancers.
B. The prognosis is poorer in affected men than it is in affected women.
C. Radical mastectomy is utilized for treatment of breast cancer in a higher percentage of cases in men than in women.
D. Unlike breast cancer in women, endocrine manipulation plays no significant role in its management.
E. Gynecomastia is usually seen in association with male breast cancer.

Ref.: 1, 4

COMMENTS: Breast cancer in men accounts for approximately 1% of all cases of breast cancer in the United States. Its clinical presentation and natural history are similar to those in women. A mass in the male breast must be differentiated from gynecomastia (which is clearly the more common cause of breast enlargement in men); however, gynecomastia does not usually occur in association with male breast cancer. Because of the small amount of breast tissue present in men, pectoralis muscle involvement may be seen more frequently. As a consequence, it is frequently necessary to perform the classic Halsted radical mastectomy for proper local management. Stage for stage, the results of treatment are similar to those in women; however, men tend to present in later stages of the disease (due in part to the lack of awareness that breast cancer can occur in men), and so the overall prognosis for male breast cancer is poorer. Male breast cancer is similar to its female counterpart in that it may be affected by endocrine manipulation to a varying degree, and significant response rates in cases of advanced disease have been seen following orchiectomy and other hormonal manipulations.

ANSWER: A, B, C

26. With regard to mammography as a screening tool, which of the following is/are current American Cancer Society recommendations?

A. An initial screening mammogram should be obtained at age 35.
B. Following initial screening, mammograms should be obtained between ages 40 and 50 only if there is clinical suspicion of a lesion present.
C. Routine screening mammograms should be performed annually after the age of 50.
D. Routine screening mammograms should be performed every 3 years after the age of 50.

Ref.: 2, 4, 7

COMMENTS: The principal determinant of recommendations for routine mammography relate to the risk-benefit ratio of tumor induction by unnecessary radiation versus detecting cancers at an earlier and therefore more curable stage. Although unnecessary exposure to irradiation should always be avoided, especially in young persons, the benefits of appropriately prescribed and performed mammography probably outweigh the possible risks of oncogenesis. Weighing all of these factors, the American Cancer Society has recommended an initial screening mammogram at age 35. Annual mammography should be obtained after the age of 50. Between the time of the first screening mammogram and age 50, mammography should be performed at a variable interval ranging from every year to every 3 years, depending on the patient's risk factors, the findings on breast examination, and the results of the initial and subsequent mammograms. Recent Swedish data have shown the benefit of yearly mammography in women commencing at age 40. Swedish data indicate that tumor progression in the 40- to 49-year age group is faster than after age 50. Because of this increased progression, annual screening is needed if early detection is expected.

ANSWER: A, C

27. ER-positive and PR-positive tumors are associated with which of the following?

A. Better response to hormone manipulation.
B. Better response to chemotherapy.
C. Better prognosis following surgical therapy.
D. Better overall prognosis.
E. More well-differentiated tumors.

Ref.: 2, 4

COMMENTS: Although ER and PR analysis is performed to predict the response of breast cancers to endocrine manipulation, tumors that are receptor-positive appear to have a generally better response to all forms of therapy. Also, receptor-positive tumors tend to be well differentiated. Hormone receptor status is sufficiently reliable prognostically that receptor status is now an integral part of the evaluation of breast cancer and is a major factor in determining appropriate adjuvant therapy. Because of the importance of the results of hormone receptor analysis and the wide availability of this assay, it is considered inappropriate not to perform receptor analysis on operatively excised breast tissue. The only exception would be a tumor so small that all of the specimen is required for histologic examination, in which case receptor analysis should be done by immunohistochemical techniques.

ANSWER: A, B, C, D, E

28. If wide local excision (lumpectomy), axillary dissection, and radiotherapy are being considered as definitive treatment for a given breast carcinoma, which one or more of the following factors bear favorably on that choice?

A. T1 tumor.
B. Central (subareolar) location within the breast.
C. Extremely large breast.
D. Extremely small breast.
E. Synchronous second primary cancer within the breast.

Ref.: 1, 4

COMMENTS: The choice of wide local incision (lumpectomy), axillary dissection, and radiotherapy versus modified radical mastectomy for stage I and II breast cancers depends on both subjective and objective factors. Subjectively, one must pay heed to the patient's choice of operation after a fully informative preoperative consultation regarding the strengths and weaknesses of each operation. Objectively, certain features of the tumor and breast itself may play a role in the appropriateness of the therapeutic choice. Small lesions require a small resection and usually offer a better cosmetic result. The size of the breast tumor, however, must be considered in relation to the size of the breast. Extremely small breasts do not lend themselves particularly well to a wide local incision, as a significant portion of the breast must be removed to achieve clear margins. The large breast presents the radiotherapist with technical problems related to postoperative whole-breast radiotherapy, but technologic advances have diminished them. Large primary tumors, regardless of breast size, are a relative contraindication to wide local excision. A synchronous second primary cancer within the breast is considered a contraindication to breast preservation. Because the nipple–areolar area of the breast is rich in lymphatic channels, it is considered anatomically unsound to excise a tumor in the central portion of the breast without excising this lymphatic plexus. For these reasons, the usual choice for a subareolar carcinoma is mastectomy.

ANSWER: A

29. A 31-year-old woman underwent a modified radical mastectomy without reconstruction for a 3 cm, node-negative, ER-negative infiltrating duct carcinoma. Two years later she developed a 2 cm immobile nodule in her scar. Excisional biopsy showed infiltrating duct carcinoma. Chest film, bone scan, and liver function tests were normal. After adequate irradiation of the area with the local recurrence, what is her chance of being alive with no evidence of recurrence at age 50?

A. Less than 10%.
B. 20%.
C. 40%.
D. 60%.
E. More than 80%.

Ref.: 4

COMMENTS: Local recurrence of breast cancer following mastectomy occurs in approximately 10% of patients. Local excision plus irradiation is appropriate treatment. Whether systemic therapy should be used in this situation remains controversial. Local recurrence in this setting is almost always eventually accompanied by distant metastatic disease, even though evaluation may not detect it at the time. Long-term prognosis is poor.

ANSWER: A

30. A 10-week-pregnant 28-year-old woman is referred to you because her obstetrician felt a new breast mass. Mammography with proper shielding showed dense breast tissue with no evidence of malignancy, and an ultrasound examination failed to show a cyst. You can feel a 1.5-cm, firm, nontender, discrete mass just lateral to the areola. Which of the following treatments is appropriate?

A. Perform a biopsy if the mass is still present 1 month after delivery.
B. Locally excise the mass and, if cancer, proceed with treatment as soon as the patient delivers.
C. Locally excise the mass and, if cancer, recommend axillary dissection and irradiation.
D. Locally excise the mass and, if it is cancer, recommend mastectomy.
E. Locally excise the mass and, if it is cancer, recommend termination of the pregnancy and mastectomy.

Ref.: 4

COMMENTS: Stage for stage, the prognosis of breast cancer is the same in pregnant as in nonpregnant women. However, the overall prognosis for pregnant women is worse because they tend to present at a more advanced stage. Reluctance to evaluate breast masses on the part of both the patient and her physician are contributing factors. The evaluation and treatment of breast masses must not be delayed because of pregnancy. Diagnostic mammograms can be safely performed in pregnant women; however, radiation therapy, even with proper shielding, has a significant incidence of fetal injury and should be discouraged. Mastectomy is usually appropriate during early and middle pregnancy. During the third trimester, breast preservation may be considered if an early delivery would facilitate prompt commencement of whole-breast irradiation. There is no evidence that the pregnancy itself is detrimental; and for stage I or II disease termination is not warranted. The risk of chemotherapy during pregnancy is unclear, but it should be avoided during the first trimester.

ANSWER: D

31. Which of the following treatments is best for a 40-year-old woman with extensive microcalcifications involving the entire upper aspect of the right breast and biopsy results that show a comedo pattern of ductal carcinoma in situ (DCIS)?

A. Local excision alone.
B. Irradiation alone.
C. Local excision plus irradiation.
D. Right total mastectomy.
E. Bilateral total mastectomy.

Ref.: 4

COMMENTS: The pendulum has swung toward more conservative management of DCIS. For a small intraductal carcinoma of the solid, cribriform, or papillary variety, local excision with free margins with or without radiation is appropriate in many situations. The calcifications described in this patient are too extensive to allow complete excision with a good cosmetic result. In addition, a comedo pattern is more likely to be multifocal (i.e., two or more foci of disease separated by an apparently uninvolved portion of the duct system). DCIS spreads in a contiguous pattern from the peripheral locus centrally toward the nipple–areolar complex. Recent studies have shown that true multicentricity (i.e., foci of disease in separate quadrants or lobes of the breast) occurs in only 1–2% of cases studied. Both multifocality and multicentricity are associated with a higher rate of recurrence after conservative surgical treatment because wide excision (lumpectomy) is less likely to remove all of the tumor. Because the disease is noninvasive in this stage, axillary dissection is not necessary; however, many surgeons perform a conservative axillary dissection at the time of the mastectomy for the extensive process described in this question because of the possibility of invasive cancer being found in the mastectomy specimen. Postoperative irradiation offers no additional benefit, as total mastectomy has yielded essentially 100% survival.

ANSWER: D

32. A 44-year-old woman presents to your office with a movable, nontender, palpable mass in the 12 o'clock position of the left breast. She says it was not present on self-examination 5 weeks earlier. Mammogram shows a 2.5 cm well circumscribed density in the area of the palpable abnormality. There is no skin dimpling. Which of the following is the most appropriate first step in treatment?

A. Schedule her for excisional biopsy.
B. Perform a blind needle aspiration of the mass in the office.
C. Obtain an ultrasound scan of the breast.
D. Perform an ultrasound-guided needle aspiration of the mass in the office.
E. Recommend that she return in 1 month for follow-up.
F. Obtain magnification compression mammogram views.

Ref.: 4

COMMENTS: Fibrocystic disease is the most common cause of a mass in this age group, and the rapid onset in this patient suggests a cyst. The mammographic findings support this impression. Magnification compression views would add little information. In this patient, the most direct and certain way of establishing the diagnosis would be immediate needle aspiration guided by palpation or ultrasound. When performing an ultrasound-guided interventional procedure in lieu of a blind percutaneous aspiration, substantial advantages are realized. It allows precise placement of the needle within the lesion. By categorizing the ultrasound characteristics of the lesion, an appropriate interventional diagnostic technique can be utilized. Characteristics of benign solid lesions include sharp, smooth margins, a homogeneous (dark) interior, and posterior enhancement. In contradistinction, malignant characteristics include irregular and jagged margins, a nonhomogeneous (dark) interior, and posterior shadowing. Fine-needle aspiration (FNA) cytology or a core biopsy is the appropriate method of analysis for solid lesions. A benign cyst is characterized by a sharp, smooth contour, a homogeneous (black) interior, and strong posterior enhancement. Needle aspiration is easily performed and can be seen to achieve complete evacuation. If the fluid is not bloody and the mass completely disappears, cytologic evaluation rarely yields a diagnosis of carcinoma; it is not cost-effective but is often performed for medicolegal reasons. Follow-up examination within a month is often appropriate for ill-defined lobular areas of breast tissue, but a well defined mass such as this one would rarely disappear in 1 month.

ANSWER: B, D

33. A 53-year-old woman with no family history of breast cancer is discovered on routine examination to have a firm, movable, well defined, 2 cm mass in the upper outer quadrant of the right breast. Mammogram shows only bilateral dense breast tissue with no evidence of malignancy. No mass was seen on ultrasound examination. Which of the following evaluation steps is/are appropriate?

A. Follow-up mammogram in 3–4 months.
B. Fine-needle aspiration for cytology.
C. Needle localization and biopsy.
D. Excisional biopsy.
E. Reevaluation of the mass in 3 months.
F. Core biopsy.

Ref.: 4

COMMENTS: Because most patients with breast cancer do not have a family history of breast cancer, any palpable mass requires investigation regardless of history. A cyst would be seen on ultrasound examination. Needle aspiration of a solid mass for cytology is acceptable as an initial diagnostic step if an experienced cytopathologist is available. Positive cytology for carcinoma would allow definitive treatment in a one-step operation. Tissue obtained by core biopsy provides a histologic diagnosis. Excisional biopsy is also an appropriate diagnostic procedure. Dense breast tissue decreases the diagnostic sensitivity of mammography and can easily obscure a carcinoma. The absence of mammographic visualization in the presence of a palpable mass does not diminish the need for a tissue diagnosis. In fact, up to 10% of breast cancers are found in the presence of a "negative" mammogram. Needle localization prior to biopsy is unnecessary when the mass is palpable, and it is not possible when the lesion is not seen on mammography. Delaying evaluation of a well defined mass for 3 months is ill-advised, and a follow-up mammogram at 3–4 months is of little value because this lesion is not mammographically detectable.

ANSWER: B, D, F

34. A 33-year-old asymptomatic woman is referred to you with an abnormal mammogram. No masses are palpable in either breast. The mammogram shows a tight cluster of microcalcifications at the 2 o'clock position of the left breast. Magnification compression views show at least 20 tiny, irregular calcifications in a 2 cm area, varying in shape and density with no associated mass lesion. There are no other calcifications present in either breast. Which of the following is the most likely diagnosis?

A. Lobular carcinoma in situ.
B. Fibroadenoma.
C. Infiltrating duct carcinoma
D. DCIS (intraductal carcinoma).
E. Fibrocystic changes.

Ref.: 4, 8

COMMENTS: Mammographic calcifications are a hallmark of early breast cancer, particularly DCIS; but the etiology of common causes of calcifications identified on mammogram are varied. Specific patterns, however, have been identified that are often associated with and predictive of these pathologic processes. Parenchymal calcifications (i.e., those indicative of a pathologic breast process) occur in the lobar ductal system and in the terminal ductal lobular unit. Certain patterns of ductal calcification are almost pathognomonic of DCIS, as is a specific bilateral pattern seen with plasma cell mastitis. One mammographic feature common to both high-grade DCIS and plasma cell mastitis is the appearance of calcium in a linear branching pattern. Evenly scattered calcifications, more often than not bilateral, are indicative of a lobular process. This pattern is the one most commonly encountered and is indicative of either active or involutional fibrocystic change. Clustered calcifications, whether single or multiple, are a diagnostic dilemma because of the varied pathologic processes that give rise to this pattern. Close scrutiny of these areas by magnification views is required to delineate the finer characteristics of the calcifications. Coarse, granular-appearing calcifications are seen with partially calcified fibroadenomas and papillomas, fibrocystic change, and low- to intermediate-grade DCIS. Powdery calcifications are seen with sclerosing adenosis, with or without atypia, and low-grade DCIS. Large, coarse calcifications (popcorn-like) are classically associated with a degenerating fibroadenoma and are readily discernible on mammogram. Lobular carcinoma in situ and invasive lobular carcinoma are often mammographically featureless. The clustered geographic distribution and characteristics of the calcifications described above make a diagnosis of DCIS more likely than an invasive carcinoma.

ANSWER: D

35. A 47-year-old woman with a history of fibrocystic disease presents with a recent onset of bilateral green nipple discharge. She has generalized bilateral tenderness and no palpable mass on breast examination. The discharge is Hemoccult-negative. Mammogram shows diffuse fibroglandular tissue that is slightly more pronounced in the upper outer quadrants bilaterally but unchanged from a year earlier. Which of the following is the most appropriate first step in management?

A. Obtain an ultrasound scan.
B. Explore the ducts through a circumareolar incision.
C. Reassure the patient.
D. Obtain a galactogram.
E. Perform a blind biopsy in the upper outer quadrant of the more involved breast.

Ref.: 4

COMMENTS: Nipple discharge and breast tenderness are common complaints associated with mammary duct ectasia and fibrocystic change. If the drainage is bloody, serous, or watery, further diagnostic workup is indicated to reveal the etiology of the discharge. Although such discharges demand evaluation, the cause is often benign; it is commonly an intraductal papilloma or papillomatosis. Although some surgeons prefer a preoperative contrast radiograph of the involved duct (a galactogram) as a guide, the blood-distended duct is usually identifiable and can be removed through a circumareolar incision. If either preoperative or intraoperative ultrasonography is available, this modality can be used in real time to facilitate identification of the distended duct and to map precisely the area of operative excision. Blind biopsy is inappropriate. Reassurance is the appropriate management decision in this context particularly in light of the bilaterality and color of the nipple discharge.

ANSWER: C

36. A 35-year-old woman with no risk factors recently had her first mammogram. Mammographically, the breast tissue appeared fairly dense, but on the craniocaudad view a 1.5 cm well circumscribed, slightly lobulated, noncalcified density with smooth borders could be seen in the lateral aspect of the breast. The lesion was not seen on the mediolateral view. Ultrasound examination showed no evidence of a cyst. No masses were palpable. Which of the following management choices is/are appropriate?

A. Follow-up mammogram in 4–6 months.
B. Stereotactic localization for fine-needle cytology and core biopsy.
C. Stereotactic localization and excisional biopsy.
D. Reassure the patient that the lesion is benign.
E. Free-hand radiographic localization and excisional biopsy.

Ref.: 4

COMMENTS: The probability is high that the lesion described above is benign, most likely a fibroadenoma or a lymph node. If the patient is comfortable with accepting a small chance that the lesion represents a cancer, simple mammographic follow-up is acceptable. Stereotactic core biopsy is minimally invasive, is done on an outpatient basis, and provides a histologic diagnosis. Excisional biopsy is more invasive and more traumatic but avoids the small risk of sampling error inherent in needle biopsies. Localization of a lesion seen only on one view is best done stereotactically. However, if stereotaxis is unavailable, the lesion can be localized for excision by a free-hand method. Reassurance without follow-up is inappropriate.

ANSWER: A, B, C, E

37. With regard to tubular carcinoma, which of the following is/are true?

A. Lymph node involvement is seen in approximately 10% of cases.
B. It is a highly aggressive, frequently fatal carcinoma.
C. Lumpectomy with axillary dissection and irradiation is appropriate.
D. Modified radical mastectomy with reconstruction is appropriate.
E. Induction chemotherapy should usually be given preoperatively.

Ref.: 4

COMMENTS: Tubular carcinoma represents a somewhat uncommon, well-differentiated variety of infiltrating duct carcinoma that has a favorable prognosis. Lymph node metastasis is encountered in approximately 10% of patients. Either modified radical mastectomy or lumpectomy with axillary dissection and irradiation is an acceptable treatment option. The findings of a negative sentinel lymph node biopsy in pure tubular carcinoma reduces even further the need for axillary dissection in most patients. Preoperative induction chemotherapy is appropriate for inflammatory or other locally advanced breast cancers but not for a tubular carcinoma.

ANSWER: A, C, D

38. A 39-year-old woman with no family history of breast cancer underwent an excisional biopsy of a 2 cm breast mass. Histologic sections showed fibrosis, duct ectasia, atypical lobular hyperplasia, and several areas of lobular carcinoma in situ that involve the surgical margins. Which of the following statements is/are true?

A. At a minimum, she should undergo reexcision of the margins.
B. She has up to a ninefold increase in the chance of developing a subsequent breast cancer.
C. If she develops breast cancer, the area of the biopsy would be the most likely site.
D. If she develops breast cancer, it would most likely be lobular carcinoma.
E. Bilateral mastectomy is a reasonable option at this point.
F. Tamoxifen can be recommended to reduce her future risk of breast cancer.

Ref.: 4

COMMENTS: Lobular carcinoma in situ (LCIS) is a histologic finding that is usually seen in tissue from a biopsy of some other lesion. It represents a risk marker that predicts up to a ninefold increase in the chance of developing breast cancer. Atypical lobular hyperplasia alone increases the risk fourfold. In the face of a strong family history of breast cancer, atypical lobular hyperplasia also increases the risk ninefold. Acquisition of free margins does not decrease the incidence of a subsequent cancer. Either infiltrating lobular or infiltrating ductal carcinoma may develop, with the latter predominating. Both breasts are at equal risk; therefore if prophylaxis is chosen, bilateral total mastectomy should be performed. Alternatively, particularly over the past decade, less aggressive management of this particular lesion has developed; it consists of close follow-up with periodic physical examination and bilateral mammograms. A recently reported chemoprevention trial showed that in high risk individuals (including those with LCIS), tamoxifen resulted in a nearly 50% reduction in the risk of developing breast cancer. Treatment options should be fully discussed with the patient so it is clear that despite close, careful follow-up positive axillary nodes may develop prior to discovery of the invasive breast primary.

ANSWER: B, E, F

39. An otherwise healthy 42-year-old woman underwent excisional biopsy of a 2 cm mass in the upper outer quadrant of the right breast that showed a well-differentiated infiltrating duct carcinoma with a minimal intraductal component and free margins. She has a palpable firm but freely movable 2 cm right axillary node. Which of the following is/are considered appropriate local/regional therapy?

A. Right-modified radical mastectomy with immediate transverse rectus abdominis myocutaneous (TRAM) flap reconstruction.
B. Axillary dissection and breast irradiation.
C. Right modified radical mastectomy with delayed reconstruction.
D. Total mastectomy and axillary irradiation.
E. Radical mastectomy with immediate reconstruction.

Ref.: 4

COMMENTS: Because clinical examination of the axilla is notoriously unreliable (20–30% error rate), the presence of a palpable node should not automatically be considered a sign of metastatic involvement. Similarly, the absence of clinically palpable nodes does not ensure that they are microscopically free of cancer. The presence of positive axillary nodes, unless large and fixed, does not alter the local/regional management of breast cancer. If invasive cancer is present, an axillary dissection is indicated to determine overall prognosis and guide adjuvant therapy. Except in a small percentage of cases, the axillary dissection does not directly improve survival. The presence of axillary involvement does not preclude immediate reconstruction with either an implant or autologous tissue. In the face of a large, inflammatory, or fixed cancer, for which postoperative irradiation is likely, reconstruction is best deferred. Because postoperative irradiation increases the incidence of capsular contraction of implants and can cause fat necrosis in TRAM flaps, it may interfere with optimal cosmesis after reconstruction. Radical mastectomy offers no survival advantage over a modified radical mastectomy, is more difficult to reconstruct, and is associated with a poorer functional and cosmetic result. This patient would be best managed by a modified radical mastectomy, with or without reconstruction, or because the excisional biopsy has uninvolved margins axillary dissection and breast irradiation.

ANSWER: A, B, C

40. All the patients whose mammograms are shown below are in their early forties and asymptomatic. The calcifications shown are the only lesions present on the mammogram. On which of the patients would you perform a biopsy?

A. Patient 1.
B. Patient 2.
C. Patient 3.
D. None of the above.

Ref.: 4

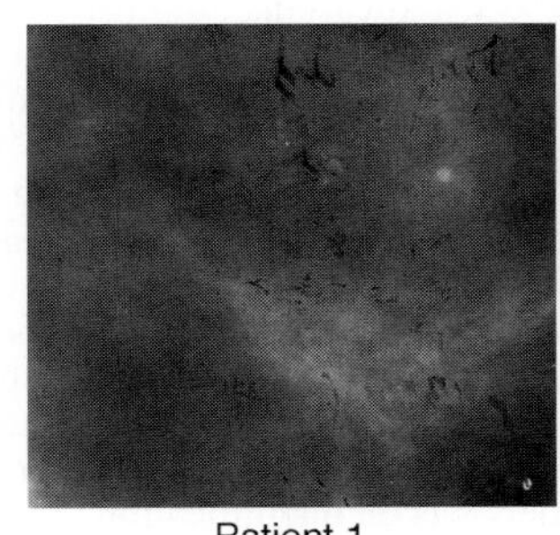

Patient 1 Patient 1

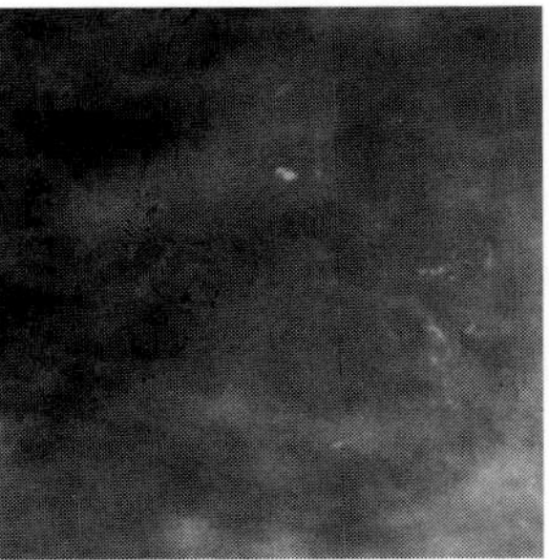

Patient 2

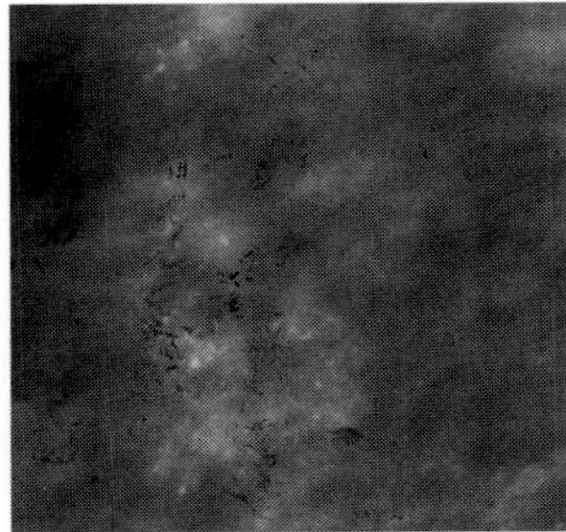

Patient 3

COMMENTS: See Question 41.

41. With regard to microcalcifications in the breast, which of the following statements is/are true?

A. More than 90% of the microcalcifications seen on mammography are not associated with a malignancy.
B. Clustered, round, smooth calcifications are highly suspicious for malignancy, and a biopsy should be performed.
C. Cup-and-saucer calcifications are highly suspicious for malignancy.

D. Casting calcifications are typical of ductal carcinomas.
E. Small, sharp, dense, tightly grouped calcifications are virtually always malignant.

Ref.: 4

COMMENTS: Calcium deposits in the breast are common; and a few small, round calcifications sparsely scattered throughout the breast or limited to a portion of the organ are seen in most patients. They have no clinical significance. Malignant calcifications tend to be multiple and close together, but size, configuration, and their relation to each other are equally important. Small, round, pearl-like calcifications in a rosette-like distribution often represent calcifications within a microcystic dilatation in a terminal duct lobular unit. Although this is technically a cluster, these calcifications are characteristic enough that, when properly studied in magnification views by an experienced observer, they can be confidently diagnosed as benign. Cup-and-saucer calcifications (patient 1, Question 40) correspond to "milk of calcium" sedimenting within microcysts and are the most characteristic of the benign or lobular-type calcifications. They appear as horizontal lines in 90-degree lateral projections, sometimes with a slightly concave upper border. In the craniocaudad projection, where the x-ray beam is perpendicular to the surface of the meniscus, they appear as ill-defined, low-density, rounded calcifications. Careful study of these calcium deposits on magnification views allows a definitive diagnosis, and a biopsy need not be performed. Thin, small, linear and branching calcifications are called "casting" (patient 2, Question 40). They represent calcified debris from necrotic tumor cells within the ducts. They are almost pathognomonic for malignant tumors, and a biopsy should always be performed. Small, sharp, dense, tightly grouped calcifications, often described as "crushed stones" (patient 3, Question 40), are another manifestation of necrotic debris within ducts invaded by a malignant growth. However, this type of calcification can be mimicked by some benign conditions, in particular blunt duct or sclerosing adenosis as well as lobular involution. The similarity between these conditions is such that even experienced observers working with optimal magnification views must describe them as "indeterminate"; a biopsy should be performed on each, but about half are benign.

ANSWER:
Question 40: B, C
Question 41: A, D

42. Mammography shows masses in two asymptomatic women in their midforties. There are no previous mammograms available. On which of the patients would an excisional biopsy be an appropriate next step?

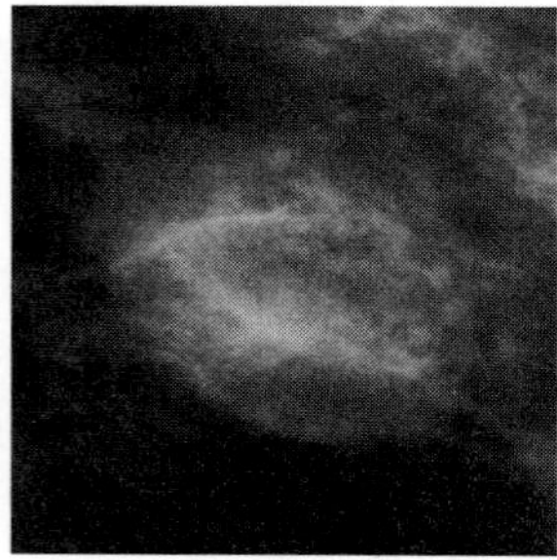

Patient 1

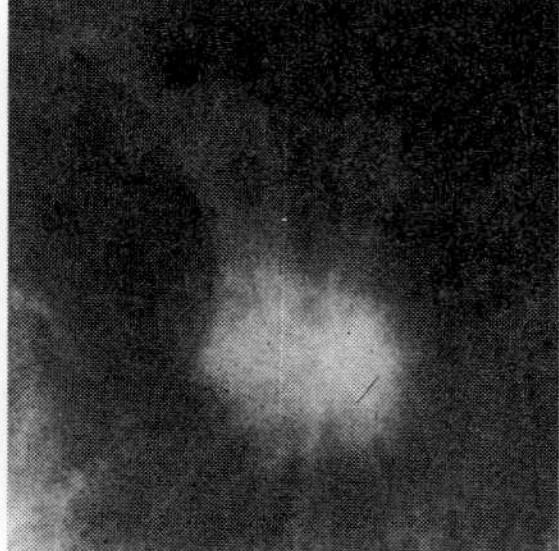

Patient 2

A. Patient 1.
B. Patient 2.
C. Neither of the above.

Ref.: 4

COMMENTS: See Question 43.

43. With regard to asymptomatic, mammographically found breast masses, which of the following statements is/are true?

A. As a first step, biopsy of a single, dominant mass more than 1 cm in diameter in women older than 40 years must be performed.
B. Masses with a small, well defined border and a "halo" sign around them are always benign.
C. The differential diagnosis of a small, dense stellate mass includes malignancy and postsurgical scar.
D. The presence of fat within a mass makes malignancy highly unlikely.

Ref.: 4

COMMENTS: Remember the ubiquitous cyst. Before performing an open biopsy for a smooth-bordered or even a lobulated mass within the breast, an ultrasound examination should be performed. Many such masses, even when they appear in postmenopausal women, are cysts (patient 1, Question 42), although solid focal lesions are also common. Smooth, rounded masses cannot be assumed to be benign even if prior mammograms demonstrate a stable appearance over a long period of time. Some malignant tumors, including mucinous and medullary carcinoma or cystosarcoma phylloides, can have a benign appearance on both ultrasonography and mammography. The stereotactic core biopsy and ultrasound-guided core biopsy offer good alternatives to open biopsy under these circumstances. Dense stellate masses (patient 2, Question 42) should always be considered malignant until proved otherwise. Although a surgical scar may give the same appearance as such a mass, the absence of a previous biopsy on history and physical examination excludes this possibility. Most masses that contain fat within them are benign. Typical examples are lymph nodes, with their fatty hilum, a posttraumatic oil cyst, and hamartomas or fibrolipoadenomas of the breast.

ANSWER:
Question 42: B
Question 43: C, D

44. Five 38-year-old women with otherwise normal physical, laboratory, and radiographic findings underwent biopsies for small, nonpalpable mammographic abnormalities. Photomicrographs of each are shown below. Assume that the disease extended right to the edge of resection in each case and that it is difficult to be certain that the margins of excision are totally free. For each patient, select the treatment options that is/are appropriate.

a. Modified radical mastectomy.
b. Routine follow-up with no further treatment.
c. Reexcision with free margins and close follow-up.
d. No further surgery; close follow-up.
e. Total mastectomy without axillary dissection.
f. Bilateral total mastectomy without axillary dissection.

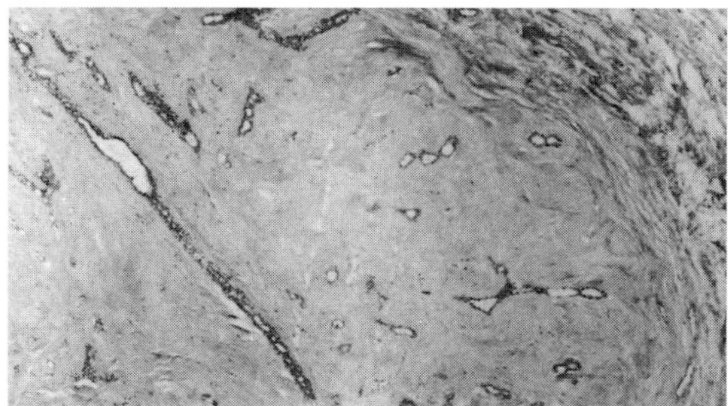
A

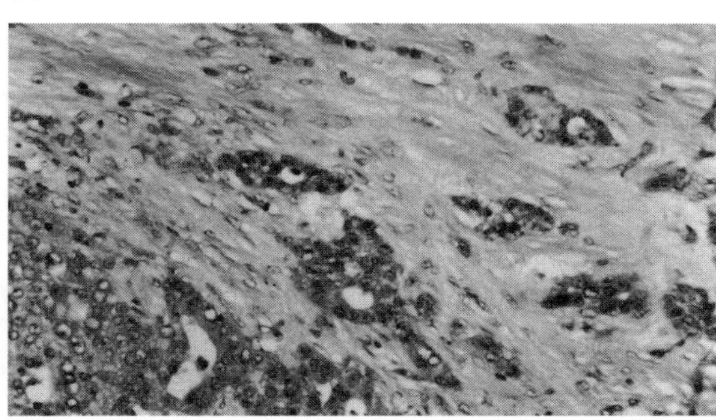
B

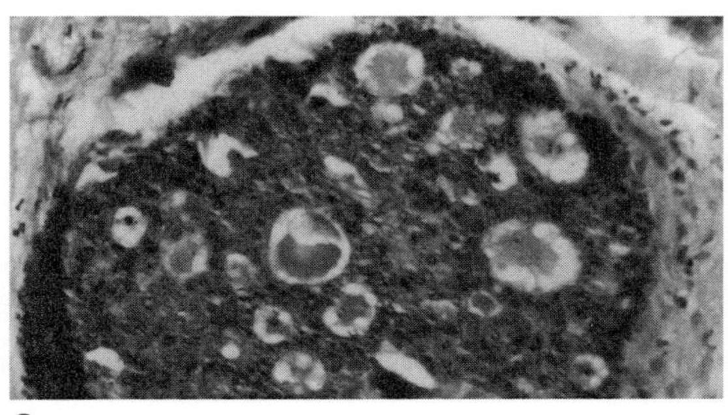
C

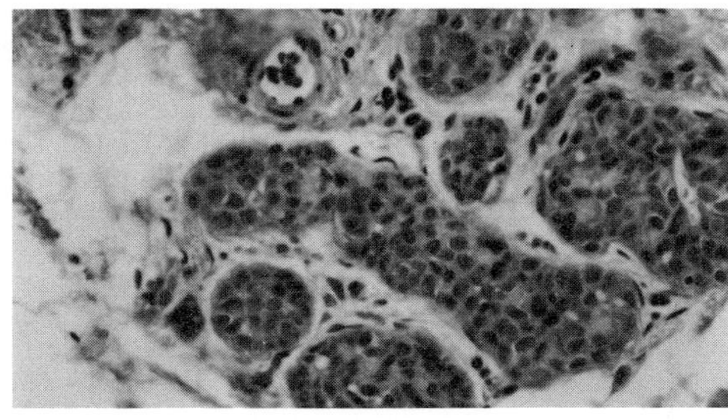
D

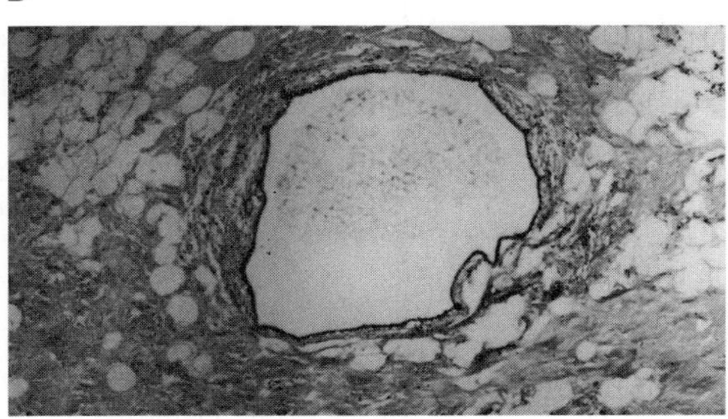
E

g. Reexcision with free margins, axillary dissection, and breast irradiation.
h. Reexcision with free margins and breast irradiation.

Ref.: 1, 2, 4

COMMENTS: *Photomicrograph A*: Prominent fibrous tissue compressing epithelial elements, as demonstrated here, is typical of a **fibroadenoma**. Involvement of margins is inconsequential, and reexcision is unwarranted. *B*: The nests of epithelial cells invading the stroma in random fashion with a suggestion of tubule formation, as shown, are typical of **infiltrating duct carcinoma**. Either modified radical mastectomy or wide local excision with axillary dissection and breast irradiation is appropriate. *C*: The hyperchromatic nuclei in a fairly uniform population of neoplastic-appearing cells filling and distending the ducts, along with sharply defined punched-out (Swiss cheese) spaces, are typical of a **cribriform intraductal carcinoma**. In contrast to a comedo pattern of intraductal carcinoma, this lesion can often be treated by excision to free margins and close follow-up. If free margins are not obtained, the rate of recurrence is high. Even if free margins are obtained, the lesion occasionally recurs in an invasive form. If the patient is unwilling to accept that small chance, total mastectomy or irradiation is appropriate, even though it may be overtreatment. Axillary dissection is unnecessary, and long-term survival following mastectomy is essentially 100%. *D*: The uniform population of cells filling, expanding, and distorting the lobules, as seen here, is typical of **lobular carcinoma in situ**. This is a risk marker that indicates a ninefold increase in the likelihood that the patient will eventually develop invasive breast cancer. There is no need to try to obtain free margins because it does not decrease the risk. Even though the margins are involved, the cancer that may subsequently develop and that may be ductal or lobular is no more likely to occur at the site of the biopsy than at any other location in either breast. For this reason, if one recommends a prophylactic operation, bilateral total mastectomy should be considered. This choice is rather aggressive when one considers that it would be unnecessary in two-thirds to three-fourths of patients (only 25–30% of women with the lesion develop invasive cancer). Many patients now choose close follow-up in place of bilateral mastectomy. *E*: The ectatic duct with a single or double (epithelial and myoepithelial) cell layer, as shown, is typical of **fibrocystic disease**. The condition is benign and requires only routine follow-up; there is no need to try to achieve free margins.

ANSWER: A-b; B-a,g; C-c,e,h; D-d,f; E-b

45. With regard to adjuvant tamoxifen therapy of invasive breast cancer, which of the following statements is/are true?

A. Significantly reduces recurrence among women with negative nodes.
B. Significantly reduces recurrence among women with positive nodes.
C. Significantly improves survival among women with negative nodes.
D. Significantly improves survival among women with positive nodes.
E. Is relatively more effective in postmenopausal than premenopausal women.
F. The longer the duration, the greater the effectiveness, up to 5 years.

G. Patients with ER-positive tumors derive greater benefit.

Ref.: 9

COMMENTS: See Question 46.

46. With regard to adjuvant chemotherapy of invasive breast cancer, which of the following statements is/are true?

A. Significantly reduces recurrence among women with negative nodes.
B. Significantly reduces recurrence among women with positive nodes.
C. Significantly improves survival among women with negative nodes.
D. Significantly improves survival among women with positive nodes.
E. Is relatively more effective in postmenopausal than premenopausal women.
F. Prolonged polychemotherapy is more effective than the same polychemotherapy for a shorter period of time.
G. Polychemotherapy is more effective than single-agent chemotherapy.

Ref.: 10

COMMENTS: Adjuvant systemic therapy (both cytotoxic chemotherapy and hormonal therapy) plays a significant and growing role in the primary management of locally and regionally confined breast cancer. In 1998 the Early Breast Cancer Trialists' Collaborative Group published updated results of their shared experiences with more than 130 randomized, prospective trials involving more than 75,000 women that investigated the role of adjuvant systemic therapy in breast cancer. This meta-analysis has provided a number of generally accepted conclusions about the effectiveness of this therapy. Both chemotherapy and tamoxifen resulted in a significantly reduced risk of both recurrence and death from breast cancer among women with negative nodes or positive nodes, regardless of age or menopausal status. Of note, however, was that tamoxifen resulted in greater risk reduction in postmenopausal women than in premenopausal women, and chemotherapy resulted in greater risk reduction in premenopausal women than in postmenopausal women. In terms of duration of treatment, tamoxifen seems to be more effective the longer it is used up to 5 years, with current recommendations being for a 5-year course. Multidrug chemotherapy, however, does not appear to gain in effectiveness if used longer than 6 months. Chemotherapy used up to 6 months, however, is more effective than a single pre- or perioperative treatment. Multiple-drug chemotherapy has been shown to be more effective than a single-drug regimen. Tamoxifen also appears to be more effective in patients with ER-positive tumors. Among all of these various groups and regimens, the reduction in "annual odds of death" or "annual odds of recurrence" ranged broadly from approximately 10% to 40%. Although one could draw the conclusion from these data that all patients should receive adjuvant systemic therapy, it must be remembered that for many populations of patients (e.g., a postmenopausal patient with a <1 cm, ER-positive, node-negative primary tumor) the likelihood of recurrence without adjuvant treatment may be only 5%. A 30% reduction in this risk would improve the overall recurrence rate to 3–4%. However, because the 5% of patients who experience recurrence cannot be identified at the outset, 98 of 100 or 99 of 100 would be receiving adjuvant therapy to benefit only one or two.

ANSWER:
Question 45: A, B, C, D, E, F, G
Question 46: A, B, C, D, G

47. Match the methodology of ER determination in the left column with one or more of its characteristics in the right column.

A. Dextran-coated charcoal assay (ER-DCC).	a. Quantitative
B. Enzyme immunoassay (ER-EIA)	b. Requires approximately 1 gm of tumor tissue
C. Immunocytochemical assay (ERICA)	c. Can be performed on formalin-fixed tissue
	d. Reveals heterogeneity of receptors in tumor

Ref.: 4

COMMENTS: The ER status of invasive breast cancer plays a critical decision-making role in terms of adjuvant therapy and determining therapy for subsequent distant metastatic disease. There are several methods for determining ER status. The standard for many years has been the **dextran-coated charcoal assay (ER-DCC)**, which is a "grind and bind" assay in which the tumor is ground and the amount of ER present is determined by a competitive binding technique. It is a labor-intensive assay that requires 2–3 days for results. Although a quantitative result is obtained (femtomoles of receptor per milligram of cytosol protein), a relatively large amount of tissue (approximately 1 gm) is required, and the tissue must be fresh. Therefore, small tumors or tumors that were found incidentally after formalin fixation cannot be assessed by this method. **Estrogen receptor enzyme immunoassay (ER-EIA)** is another "grind and bind" assay that involves binding of the tumor receptor with a monoclonal antibody, which can then react with O-phenylenediamine for spectrophotometric analysis. This assay also produces a quantitative result but requires only approximately 20% of the tissue needed for the ER-DCC assay. Non-cancer-containing tissues within the specimen can falsely lower the result; and as with ER-DCC, formalin-fixed tissue cannot be used. **Estrogen receptor by immunocytochemical analysis (ERICA)** is one of the newer and valuable methods for determining ER status. Many pathologists consider it to be the current "gold standard." This technique involves the binding of a monoclonal antibody to ER to tumor cells on a standard glass pathology slide. Although the result is given in terms of percent of cancer cells staining, it is considered a qualitative rather than a quantitative assay. It can be performed on minuscule amounts of tumor, it is relatively inexpensive, and results are usually available within 1 day. Moreover, this analysis can be performed on formalin-fixed tissue. One must note, however, that a negative result on formalin-fixed tissue may or may not be accurate, whereas a positive result is a true positive. Because the staining characteristics of individual tumor cells are viewed directly, the heterogeneity of the tumor's ER status can be assessed.

ANSWER: A-a,b; B-a; C-c,d

48. Which one or more of the following factors should influence the choice of systemic adjuvant therapy for invasive breast cancer?

A. Tumor size.
B. DNA ploidy.
C. HER-2/*neu*.
D. Axillary node status.
E. ER status.
F. Cathepsin D.
G. Age or menopausal status.

Ref.: 4

COMMENTS: Currently, the recommendation for adjuvant systemic therapy via cytotoxic chemotherapy or tamoxifen is based on consideration of tumor size, nodal status, ER status, and age or menopausal status. In general, tumors smaller than 1 cm and node-negative require no additional treatment. Recent evidence suggests that perhaps all node-positive patients should be treated with chemotherapy, regardless of menopausal status, adding tamoxifen in postmenopausal patients, but this recommendation has not yet been universally adopted. Many but not all oncologists recommend treating all node-negative tumors larger than 1 cm with adjuvant chemotherapy if they are ER-negative or with tamoxifen if they are ER-positive. Current studies are evaluating the more liberal combining of tamoxifen with chemotherapy for all of these categories. The other tumor characteristics mentioned above (DNA ploidy, HER-2/*neu* status, and cathepsin D status) have been variably reported to influence overall prognosis but are not yet considered to be factors that influence the choice of adjuvant therapy.

ANSWER: A, D, E, G

49. Germline mutations in which of the following genes is/are associated with a higher incidence of breast cancer.

A. *APC*.
B. *BRCA1*.
C. *BRCA2*.
D. *p53*.
E. *hPMS1*.

Ref.: 11

COMMENTS: A germline mutation is a mutation that exists in every cell of the body and therefore is capable of being passed to the offspring via the sperm or egg. The predominant genes responsible for hereditary breast cancer are *BRCA1* (BReast CAncer 1) and *BRCA2*. Women who carry a germline mutation in either of these genes have about an 85% likelihood of developing breast cancer by the age of 70, although most cancers occur before age 50. Women with these mutations also have an increased risk of developing ovarian cancer. Inherited mutations of the *p53* gene result in Li-Fraumeni syndrome, which is associated with the development of a number of malignancies including breast cancer, sarcomas, brain tumors, adrenocortical carcinomas, and leukemia. The *APC* gene is involved in cell growth regulation and when inherited in mutated form leads to **familial adenomatous polyposis** and an increased incidence of colon cancer. The *hPMS1* gene is responsible for repair of DNA strands that become mismatched during cell division. Mutations of this gene lead to **hereditary nonpolyposis colon cancer (HNPCC)**. The latter two genes do not increase the risk of breast cancer.

ANSWER: B, C, D

50. A germline mutation in either *BRCA1* or *BRCA2* is associated with which one or more of the following characteristics?

A. Autosomal dominant transmission.
B. High incidence of breast and ovarian cancer in women.
C. High incidence of breast cancer in men.
D. Equal likelihood of a woman inheriting the mutation from her father or mother.
E. Incomplete penetrance.
F. Late-onset breast cancer.

Ref.: 11

COMMENTS: Mutations in *BRCA1* or *BRCA2* result in a higher incidence of breast and ovarian cancer. The risk for breast cancer is about 85% among individuals who carry the mutation and have a family history of breast cancer in high risk families. The risk for ovarian cancer is about 40% for *BRCA1* mutations and 20% for *BRCA2* mutations. About 10% of males with *BRCA2* mutations develop breast cancer. This increased risk is not seen among males with *BRCA1* mutations. Because the gene resides on an autosome (and is therefore not sex-linked), men can pass the mutation to their daughters, although the man is usually unaffected. These genes are incompletely penetrant; that is, some mutation carriers can live to old age and not develop cancer. The mutation is autosomal dominant; that is, a mutation in only one of the pair of chromosomes usually produces the disease. Although women who carry germline mutations of these genes can develop postmenopausal breast cancer, most cancers arising in carriers occur premenopausally.

ANSWER: A, B, D, E

51. A 32-year-old woman presents with an invasive breast cancer. She has five sisters, two of whom have developed premenopausal breast cancer. Her mother died of ovarian cancer at age 45. You should:

A. Recommend that she be tested for a mutation in *BRCA1* or *BRCA2*.
B. Recommend bilateral mastectomy and prophylactic oophorectomy.
C. Begin tamoxifen.
D. Refer her for genetic counseling.
E. Recommend mammography every 6 months after she has been treated for her breast cancer.

Ref.: 11

COMMENTS: There is a significant likelihood that the patient described above has a *BRCA1* or *BRCA2* mutation. She could easily be tested for this with a simple but expensive blood test. If she tests positive for a mutation in either of these genes, she has an approximately 85% lifetime risk of developing breast cancer and a 20–40% lifetime risk of developing ovarian cancer. If such were the case, the patient might opt for aggressive prophylactic ablative surgery (mastectomy and oophorectomy). Alternatively, she could opt for conservative management with careful surveillance to include clinical breast and pelvic examination, mammography, ovarian ultrasonography, and ovarian tumor marker assessment at appropriate intervals. With regard to her breast cancer risk, she could opt for beginning tamoxifen, which has been shown in a recent chemoprevention trial to reduce the risk of developing breast cancer by close to 50% among patients considered to be at high risk. Choosing among these options requires a firm understanding by the patient of their respective risks and benefits. The patient should also understand that knowledge of one's status with regard to carrying a mutation of the *BRCA1* or

BRCA2 gene can result in discrimination by potential employers or insurance carriers unwilling to "take a chance" on such a high-risk individual. Finally, genetic testing has implications for the entire family, as one member being known to carry a mutation alters the likelihood of other family members also being carriers. For all these reasons, the current recommendation is for extremely high-risk individuals as described above to be referred for genetic counseling before actually undergoing testing for the presence of gene mutations.

ANSWER: D

52. A 45-year-old woman had her first child at age 40. She began menstruating at age 9. She had a breast biopsy a year ago that showed atypical hyperplasia. Her mother had postmenopausal breast cancer. Reasonable options for this woman include:

A. Bilateral prophylactic mastectomy.
B. Mammography every 6 months.
C. Tamoxifen for 5 years.
D. Raloxifene for 5 years.
E. Consuming a diet that is high in phytoestrogens.
F. Entering a clinical trial comparing tamoxifen with raloxifene.

Ref.: 11

COMMENTS: The Breast Cancer Prevention Trial (BCPT), conducted by the National Surgical Adjuvant Breast Cancer Project (NSABP) compared tamoxifen with placebo in 13,000 women at high risk for breast cancer. It showed that 5 years of tamoxifen reduced the short-term risk of breast cancer by 45%. Complications included blood clots (1%) and endometrial cancer (1%), which were largely limited to postmenopausal women. A randomized trial of postmenopausal women who received raloxifene versus placebo for osteoporosis resulted in a reduction in breast cancer, although breast cancer was not the primary endpoint of the trial. The NSABP will study 22,000 postmenopausal women at risk for breast cancer in the Study of Tamoxifen and Raloxifene (STAR) trial. Participants will be randomized to tamoxifen versus raloxifene for 5 years. Although there is tantalizing information from case-controlled and cohort studies that diets rich in phytoestrogens (e.g., soy, tofu) are associated with a reduced risk of breast cancer, there have as yet been no randomized trials addressing the issue. Although this patient is at increased risk for developing breast cancer, she is not at a level of risk for which prophylactic mastectomy would be strongly considered, nor would she require screening mammography more often than once annually unless there were specific mammographic changes that required more frequent imaging.

ANSWER: C, F

53. Human epidermal growth factor receptor-2 (*HER-2*) is a gene that:

A. Encodes a growth factor receptor.
B. Controls normal cell growth.
C. Is amplified in 25% of breast cancers.
D. Is a target for biologic therapy.
E. Is independently predictive of poor outcome in breast cancer.

Ref.: 11

COMMENTS: The *HER-2* gene is responsible for encoding a transmembrane tyrosine kinase, a protein with potent growth-stimulating activity. When the gene activity is amplified (i.e., the protein is present in abnormally increased amounts) in patients with breast cancer, more rapid growth and more aggressive behavior of the tumor can result. This amplification can be measured and is known to occur in 25–30% of human breast cancers. Such cancers are more likely to be associated with poor prognostic features such as being estrogen-receptor (ER)-negative, node-positive, and poorly differentiated. However, this overexpression of the gene is known to be an independent predictor of a worse prognosis regardless of the status of the other variables. The membrane receptor for the protein (not the gene itself) is a target for a new and promising monoclonal antibody therapy (Herceptin).

ANSWER: A, B, C, E

54. Select the *true* statement(s) regarding the use of tissue expanders for breast reconstruction.

A. Tissue expansion works by stretching and thinning the overlying tissues. Diminished epidermal mitoses and dermal collagen synthesis are seen in areas of tissue expansion.
B. Tissue expansion frequently produces wound disruption when it is employed for immediate reconstruction, so it is usually used for delayed reconstruction after mastectomy.
C. Tissue expansion is contraindicated in patients who are smokers. A pedicled TRAM flap is a safer method of reconstruction in these patients.
D. When a tissue expander is used for breast reconstruction, it is placed anterior to the pectoralis major muscle to produce an anatomically correct copy of the breast.
E. Breasts reconstructed with tissue expanders do not usually feel as natural as those reconstructed with TRAM flaps.

Ref.: 1, 2, 12

COMMENTS: Tissue expansion is the most commonly employed method of breast reconstruction in the United States. The device consists of a Silastic shell connected to an injection valve, through which saline solution can be added. Tissue expansion is well suited for immediate reconstruction after mastectomy, as the operative time and blood loss are considerably less than for other methods of reconstruction. The surgeon selects a tissue expander with a base dimension that matches the opposite breast and positions the device in the plane underneath the pectoralis major and serratus anterior muscles. This submuscular location is critical because it prevents wound disruption and provides sufficient soft tissue camouflage for a reasonably natural breast shape to be created. A small amount of saline solution is instilled at the time of reconstruction. Weekly expansion is usually begun approximately 3 weeks after surgery. The endpoint of tissue expansion is reached when sufficient saline solution has been added to produce a volumetric match of the opposite breast. This process takes 2–3 months for an average-sized breast. In most cases the tissue expander is removed at the completion of the expansion process and replaced with a softer saline- or silicone gel-filled reconstructive implant. Tissue expansion occurs by means of a combination of stretching overlying tissue, recruitment of adjacent tissue, and the production of new tissue. Increased epidermal mitosis and increased dermal collagen synthesis have been demonstrated in expanded tissue. The specific choice of reconstructive method is determined by a detailed analysis of the patient's medical history, goals, and personal preferences. In general, smoking is viewed as a contraindication to breast reconstruction with a pedicled TRAM flap because there is an unacceptably high incidence of flap necrosis in these patients. Although smoking increases the risk of complications for any surgical procedure, tissue expander reconstruction can usually be carried out in smokers with acceptable morbidity. One disadvantage of tissue expander and implant reconstruction is that the breast does not have as natural a feel as a breast reconstructed from the fat of the abdominal wall with a TRAM flap. This advantage must be balanced against the longer recovery and abdominal donor site scar of the TRAM flap.

ANSWER: E

55. Regarding breast reduction, which of the following statements is/are true?

A. The ability to lactate is frequently compromised by breast reduction surgery.
B. Back and neck pain are not considered acceptable medical indications for breast reduction surgery, as these symptoms are usually the result of obesity.
C. The superior pedicle technique is the safest method of breast reduction, because it preserves the most important blood supply to the breast, the branches of the thoracoacromial artery.
D. In patients with macromastia, breast reduction surgery has the additional advantage of making the breast easier to examine, both physically and mammographically.
E. For patients with extreme macromastia, in whom the nipple must be transposed a long distance, free nipple grafting may be the safest technique.

Ref.: 1, 2, 13

COMMENTS: The mechanical effects of massive breast enlargement are well documented. Patients with macromastia frequently suffer from back, neck, and shoulder pain directly caused by the abnormal size and position of the breasts. The effect of breast reduction surgery can often be dramatic in these patients, with reduction or elimination of symptoms within several days of the surgery. It is important to recognize that the mechanical effects of breast enlargement frequently make it difficult for patients to exercise. Patients who undergo breast reduction surgery often experience a beneficial weight reduction during the months following surgery because they are able to exercise comfortably for the first time in years. A variety of methods exist for breast reduction. The central mound technique maintains the greatest number of vascular attachments to the breast tissue. Significant contributions to the blood supply of the breast come from branches of the internal mammary, lateral thoracic, intercostal, and thoracoacromial vessels. In extreme cases of macromastia, it may be impossible to preserve sufficiently the vascular supply to the nipple, and free nipple grafting is indicated. With this technique, the nipple–areolar complex is detached from the breast parenchyma, reduced in circumference, thinned, and reattached as a skin graft to the reduced breast. Free nipple grafting has the disadvantage of sensory loss and depigmentation, which may be permanent. The volume reduction achieved often facilitates physical and mammographic evaluation, but this may be at the cost of lactation capability due to disruption of major ducts in the periareolar area.

ANSWER: A, D, E

56. Select the true statement(s) concerning breast reconstruction with autologous tissue.

A. When a breast is reconstructed with the latissimus dorsi myocutaneous flap, it is always necessary for the surgeon to position an implant behind the flap to produce adequate breast shape and volume.
B. The TRAM flap may be designed as a pedicled flap based on the inferior epigastric circulation or a free flap based on the superior epigastric circulation.
C. The most important perforators that maintain blood supply to the TRAM flap are in the periumbilical region.
D. Breasts reconstructed with the TRAM flap tend to be firmer and less pliable than breasts reconstructed with implants.
E. The TRAM flap should not be used as a method of breast reconstruction if there is a history of previous irradiation to the breast area or if irradiation is planned during the postoperative period.

Ref.: 1, 2, 12, 14

COMMENTS: The transverse rectus abdominis myocutaneous (TRAM) flap is comprised of the midabdominal fat and overlying skin. The flap derives its blood supply from the vascular arcade, which runs through the rectus muscle and is connected superiorly to the superior epigastric artery (a continuation of the internal mammary artery) and inferiorly to the inferior epigastric artery (a branch of the external iliac artery). With the pedicled version of the flap, the superior epigastric circulation is maintained, the inferior epigastric is divided, the rectus muscle is released from its sheath, and the flap is passed under the upper abdominal skin and into the mastectomy defect. With the free TRAM flap the muscle is divided superiorly, and the inferior epigastric vessels are transected and anastomosed to either the internal mammary vessels or the vessels of the lateral chest wall. With either flap design it is critical to preserve the periumbilical perforators, which travel up through the muscle and supply the skin and fat of the abdominal wall. The chief advantage of the TRAM flap is the natural consistency of the reconstructed breast, as it is comprised of abdominal fat. The chief disadvantages of the TRAM flap are the increased length and complexity of the operation and the need for the patient to recover from injury to the breast and abdominal wall areas. The TRAM flap is particularly suited to patients who are treated with radiation to the breast area, either pre- or postoperatively. Radiation often causes thickening of the capsule of scar tissue that forms around breast implants. This thickening, known as capsular contracture, can cause firmness, distortion, and discomfort in the reconstructed breast. The latissimus dorsi myocutaneous flap is another method of autologous tissue breast reconstruction. The latissimus dorsi muscle is rotated with an attached ellipse of skin into the mastectomy defect. An implant is usually positioned underneath the flap to provide a volumetric match to the opposite breast. In some patients it is possible to transfer sufficient fat from the back that an implant is not needed.

ANSWER: C

57. Select the true statement(s) concerning breast augmentation.

A. Both silicone gel- and saline-filled implants are currently used for breast augmentation in the United States.

B. Most scientific studies have demonstrated a reduced incidence of capsular contracture when implants are positioned in the subpectoral plane and when textured surface implants are used.
C. The incidence of breast cancer has been shown to be increased in patients with silicone gel breast implants when these patients are followed for 20 years.
D. Retrospective studies of large populations of patients with silicone gel implants have failed to demonstrate a statistically significant increase in collagen vascular disease compared to populations of patients without implants.
E. Breast implants in the subglandular plane allow easier mammographic evaluation compared to implants in the subpectoral plane.

Ref.: 1, 2, 15

COMMENTS: The U.S. Food and Drug Administration (FDA) allows the use of silicone gel breast implants in specific circumstances: breast reconstruction after mastectomy, replacement of existing gel implants, and correction of breast deformity. At the present time patients who desire breast augmentation are allowed to select only saline-filled implants. These implants have a less natural consistency than gel-filled implants, particularly in thin patients. Long-term studies have shown that patients with breast implants do not have an increased incidence of breast cancer. Breast cancer is not detected at a more advanced stage in patients with breast implants than in patients without breast implants. The mammographic technique must be altered in patients with breast implants to allow adequate visualization of the breast tissue. This includes additional views as well as technical maneuvers to lift the breast tissue away from the implant. Breast implants may be positioned subglandularly (underneath the breast tissue) or submuscularly (underneath the pectoralis major muscle). There are several advantages to the submuscular approach. Mammographic visualization of the breast tissue is more complete when an implant is submuscular. The superior aspects of the breast have a more natural configuration when the implant is submuscular. Several studies suggest a decreased incidence of capsular contracture (increased scar tissue around the implant) when the implant is positioned in the submuscular plane. Concerns have been raised regarding a possible association between silicone gel implants and collagen vascular disease. In response to this concern, several large-scale retrospective studies were carried out to study the incidence of collagen vascular disease in patients with breast implants. These studies document that there is not a statistically significant increase of any known collagen vascular disease in patients with breast implants.

ANSWER: B, D

58. For which one or more of the following situations would postmastectomy radiation therapy be indicated?

A. A primary breast tumor larger than 5 cm with positive axillary lymph nodes.
B. Four or more positive axillary lymph nodes.
C. A single positive axillary node with gross extracapsular extension.
D. Three of thirteen axillary nodes positive and matted together.
E. A node-negative 4 cm cancer involving the deep margin of the mastectomy specimen.
F. Inflammatory breast cancer.

Ref.: 5, 6, 16, 17

COMMENTS: In patients with T3 lesions (>5 cm) and positive axillary lymph nodes or in patients with four or more positive axillary lymph nodes (regardless of the primary tumor size), locoregional recurrence after mastectomy ranges from 25% to 30%. This figure can be reduced to approximately 10% with postmastectomy irradiation. Most commonly, the chest wall and regional nodal area (supraclavicular and axillary, with or without the internal mammary nodal regions) are treated to a dose of 50 Gy in 25–28 fractions. Additional fractions may be given for close or positive margins. Recently published trials from Denmark and British Columbia report that postmastectomy radiation therapy improves not only local control but also survival in node-positive patients. Postmastectomy radiation therapy in patients with T3N0 disease or patients with T1 and T2 tumors with one to three positive axillary lymph nodes is more controversial. Patients with T3N0 disease were included in the Danish study. Furthermore, patients with one to three positive nodes were included in both the Danish and British Columbia trials and represented more than 50% of the patients in these trials. Still, many argue that the risk of locoregional recurrence in these patients is less than 15%, and therefore postoperative radiation therapy may not be warranted. Other indications for postmastectomy irradiation include N2 to N3 disease, gross extracapsular tumor extension, positive surgical margins, inflammatory breast cancer, or involvement of the skin, pectoral fascia, or skeletal muscle.

ANSWER: A, B, C, D, E, F

59. Which of the following patients is considered an appropriate candidate for breast-preserving therapy with lumpectomy followed by radiation therapy?

A. A 40-year-old woman with a history of active scleroderma with a T1N0 infiltrating ductal carcinoma of the right breast.
B. A 45-year-old woman with a T1N1 infiltrating ductal carcinoma of the left breast status postlumpectomy with negative surgical margins and axillary lymph node dissection with 2 of 12 positive lymph nodes.
C. A 37-year-old woman with a T2N0 infiltrating ductal carcinoma of the right breast who has a history of Hodgkin's disease treated with 36 Gy to a mantle field 15 years ago.
D. All of the above.
E. None of the above.

Ref.: 18, 19

COMMENTS: The National Surgical Adjuvant Breast and Bowel Project (NSABP) B-06 trial demonstrated that lumpectomy followed by radiation therapy to the breast is appropriate treatment for patients with primary tumors 4 cm or less in diameter with either positive or negative axillary lymph nodes. Several other trials have confirmed these results for patients with stage I and II breast cancer. The 12-year results from the NSABP B-06 trial show equal overall survival and disease-free survival for all patients whether they were treated with breast preservation or mastectomy. However, the cohort of patients treated with lumpectomy alone without irradiation suffered a 35% recurrence rate in the ipsilateral breast. This recurrence rate is considered unacceptably high when compared to the 10% risk of ipsilateral breast recurrences in patients who received radiation to the breast followed lumpectomy. Several series have shown that patients with certain collagen vascular diseases may incur increased toxicity from radiation therapy. Though excessive complications have not been consistently shown with all types of collagen vascular disorders, severe fibrosis and soft tissue necrosis have been associated with scleroderma, suggesting that patients with scleroderma may be better served with a mastectomy. Patients with active systemic lupus erythematosus and rheumatoid arthritis may also be at increased risk for toxicity from radiation therapy. Mastectomy is recommended for patients who have had prior radiation therapy to the chest or to a mantle field (which includes the neck, axilla, mediastinum, and pulmonary hila) because radiation tolerance of the regional normal tissues may be exceeded, resulting in excessive toxicity.

ANSWER: B

60. What recommendation regarding mammography would you make to a woman whose mother was diagnosed with breast cancer at the age of 40 and her sister was diagnosed with breast cancer at the age of 45?

A. First mammogram at age 25 and annually starting at age 40.
B. First mammogram at age 30 and then annually thereafter.
C. First mammogram at age 35 and then annually thereafter.
D. First mammogram at age 40 and then annually thereafter.

Ref.: 7

COMMENTS: The current recommendation is for the patient to have a baseline mammogram 10 years before the youngest age at diagnosis of breast cancer among first-degree relatives in the family. This recommendation is often modified in cases where the first cancer is diagnosed earlier than age 35 because mammography in even high-risk women in their early twenties is rarely helpful.

ANSWER: B

61. A 40-year-old woman has undergone genetic testing recently and has been found to have a mutation of the *BRCA1* gene. There is a strong family history of breast cancer. Your recommendations would include which of the following?

A. Unilateral mastectomy.
B. Close follow-up with biannual clinical examination and an annual mammogram.
C. Bilateral mastectomy.
D. Prophylactic irradiation of both breasts.
E. Tamoxifen.

Ref.: 7, 20

COMMENTS: Women with a *BRCA1* gene mutation have an 85% lifetime risk of developing breast cancer. In these women bilateral mastectomy is a viable option for treatment. A unilateral mastectomy is not appropriate because there is no way to know which breast will develop cancer. These women should be followed closely with at least biannual clinical examinations and annual mammography starting 10 years before the youngest age at diagnosis of breast cancer in their family or at age 35. In a large recently completed chemoprevention trial, tamoxifen was shown to reduce the future risk of breast cancer by nearly 50% among women at high risk for developing breast cancer. The use of tamoxifen would therefore be a reasonable option for this patient. Because of the local tissue toxicity associated with irradiation and the fact that new cancers can develop in irradiated breasts, radiation as a means of breast cancer prophylaxis is not appropriate.

ANSWER: B, C, E

62. A 15-year-old girl is brought in by her mother because of asymmetric breast development. Your examination reveals normal breast development on the left, a hypoplastic breast on the right, with noted hypoplasia of the pectoralis major muscle also on the right. You would inform the mother that:

A. It is normal for the breast tissue to develop at different rates and be slightly asymmetric.
B. This is an example of Poland syndrome.
C. This is an example of Li-Fraumeni syndrome.
D. This is an example of amazia.

Ref.: 7

COMMENTS: This patient is demonstrating Poland syndrome, which is characterized by unilateral hypoplasia of the breast, pectoral muscles, and chest wall. Li-Fraumeni syndrome is one of the inherited breast cancer syndromes in which there is an increased incidence of breast cancer, soft tissue and osteosarcomas, brain tumors, adrenocortical cancer, and leukemias in the same family. Nearly 30% of the tumors in these families occur before the age of 15. Amazia refers to a condition in which the nipple is present but the breast mound is absent.

ANSWER: B

63. A 13-year-old girl is referred to you for a palpable breast mass. Her breast development is normal for her age and symmetric. Her mother was diagnosed with breast cancer at the age of 29. The appropriate management of this lesion would include which of the following?

A. Excision of the nodule.
B. Ultrasonography.
C. Mammography.
D. Fine-needle aspiration biopsy.
E. Clinical follow-up in 3 months.

Ref.: 7, 20

COMMENTS: Although there is a history of early-onset breast cancer in this girl's mother, the likelihood that this nodule is malignant is extremely low. In young patients, mammography is difficult to interpret because the breast tissue is so dense, and radiation to the early developing breast should be avoided. Ultrasonography would be the imaging technique of choice in this instance to delineate a solid lesion from a cystic lesion. Even if it is a solid lesion, it is most likely a fibroadenoma and could be followed with a repeat examination in 3 months or repeat ultrasound scanning. Excision of the nodule in a patient who is beginning breast development may result in abnormal breast development or amazia. A fine-needle aspiration biopsy could be performed to confirm the benign nature of the lesion.

ANSWER: B, D, E

64. Which of the following can mimic breast cancer on mammography or physical examination?

A. Radial scar.
B. Fibromatosis.
C. Granular cell tumor.
D. Fat necrosis.

Ref.: 7

COMMENTS: All of the above lesions can give an appearance similar to cancer on mammography or clinical examination. **Radial scars** appear as a soft-tissue density with irregular edges and spiculation on the mammogram. There is some controversy as to whether these lesions are premalignant. **Fibromatosis** is characterized by locally invasive, nonencapsulated, proliferation of well differentiated spindle cells. They present as a palpable mass and can have skin retraction or fixation to underlying muscle. They are indistinguishable from cancer on the mammogram. **Granular cell tumors** also simulate cancer on both clinical examination and mammography. These lesions present as palpable abnormalities with skin retraction and possible fixation to underlying structures. They resemble scirrhous carcinoma on the mammogram. **Fat necrosis** can appear similar to a cancer on mammography. It can present as a palpable mass with poorly defined borders and may cause skin retraction.

ANSWER: A, B, C, D

65. An initial mammogram of a 45-year-old woman reveals a cluster of indeterminate microcalcifications in the upper outer quadrant of the left breast. There is no family history of breast cancer, and the area in question is not palpable. Choose the most appropriate procedure.

A. Stereotactic-guided large core needle biopsy.
B. Ultrasound-guided large core needle biopsy.
C. Repeat mammogram of the involved breast in 6 months.
D. Excisional biopsy with wire localization and specimen radiography.

Ref.: 7

COMMENTS: See Question 68.

66. For which one or more of the following situations would additional intervention be warranted?

A. Stereotactic 14-gauge core biopsy for indeterminate microcalcifications revealing "sclerosing adenosis with calcification in benign ductules."
B. Stereotactic 14-gauge core biopsy for a well circumscribed mammographic density revealing "fibroadenoma."
C. Stereotactic 14-gauge core biopsy for a cluster of indeterminate microcalcifications revealing "atypical ductal hyperplasia."
D. Stereotactic 14-gauge core biopsy for a poorly defined 1 cm radiographic density revealing "apocrine metaplasia and fibrocystic changes."

Ref.: 7

COMMENTS: See Question 68.

67. A 38-year-old woman presents with a recently discovered 2 cm tender mass in the 10 o'clock position of the upper outer right breast. Ultrasonography reveals a 2 cm smooth-edged anechoic mass with bilateral edge shadowing and posterior acoustic enhancement as well as reverberation artifacts in the superficial portion of the mass. Which one or more of the following interventional procedures would be appropriate at this point?

A. Stereotactic-guided large-core needle biopsy.
B. Ultrasound-guided large-core needle biopsy.
C. Ultrasound-guided needle aspiration.
D. Excisional biopsy with wire localization and specimen radiography.
E. Fine-needle aspiration by palpation.

Ref.: 7

COMMENTS: See Question 68.

68. Routine screening mammography of a 57-year-old woman reveals a 1.5 cm spiculated centrally dense mass. An image-guided biopsy shows benign breast parenchyma. Which of the following is the most appropriate recommendation at this point?

A. Routine screening mammography in 1 year.
B. Additional imaging with contrast-enhanced magnetic resonance imaging (MRI).
C. Short-term follow-up with diagnostic mammography (in 4–6 months).
D. Excisional biopsy with wire localization and specimen radiography.

Ref.: 7

COMMENTS: One of the key advances in the diagnosis of breast pathology over the past 20 years has been the evolution of image-guided sampling of nonpalpable mammographically or sonographically detected lesions. Several principles of management that have emerged from our growing experience with these techniques are brought out in the preceding four questions. Indeterminate calcifications (Question 65) can be associated with a 10–30% chance of cancer accounting for the calcifications, and therefore some sort of tissue sampling would be indicated. Stereo-guided core biopsy permits sampling with a low false-negative rate and allows the 70–90% of persons whose pathology would be benign to avoid an open biopsy. Excisional biopsy with wire localization is not inappropriate but would be better utilized as the initial biopsy technique for calcifications that are highly suspicious rather than indeterminate. Although there is a small possibility of sampling error (falsely negative results), it is generally thought that in cases in which the mammographic target is not highly suspicious a clearly "benign" result without "atypia" would not require further intervention (Question 66). The presence of "atypical hyperplasia" (ductal or lobular) generally suggests the need for additional tissue sampling, most often a wire-localized excision. When the mammographic changes are highly suspicious, as described in Question 68, however, a negative core biopsy result must be viewed with caution, as the possibility of sampling error must always be considered. Definitive wide excision with wire localization in such circumstances would then be warranted. The reasons for the initial core biopsy in such suspicious cases are multiple and include the value of having a tissue diagnosis (rather than just a "suspicion") when discussing diagnosis and management options with the patient, and the ability to more accurately inject the radionuclide or blue dye into the area of the relatively undisturbed primary tumor when sentinel node biopsy is chosen as the method of axillary assessment. In Question 67 the ultrasound findings are those of a simple or slightly complex cyst. Such cysts carry essentially no risk of harboring cancer and therefore do not normally require any intervention unless they are symptomatic, as in this case. Aspiration is then appropriate and can be done either by palpation or with ultrasound guidance.

ANSWER:
Question 65: A
Question 66: C
Question 67: C, E
Question 68: D

69. In a patient who has undergone an axillary dissection for breast cancer, match the postoperative affliction on the left with the most likely cause on the right.

A. Hypesthesia of the upper inner aspect of the ipsilateral arm
B. Progressive atrophy of the pectoralis major muscle
C. Sudden painful early postoperative swelling of the involved arm
D. Painless, slow, progressive swelling of the involved arm beginning 18 months after surgery
E. Asymmetric protrusion of the ipsilateral scapula, especially during "pushing" maneuvers of the arm
F. Ischemic loss of the entire latissimus dorsi flap utilized for reconstruction

a. Lymphatic fibrosis
b. Medial pectoral pedicle injury
c. Thoracodorsal pedicle injury
d. Long thoracic nerve injury
e. Second intercostal brachiocutaneous nerve injury
f. Axillary vein thrombosis

Ref.: 7

COMMENTS: A number of neurovascular structures are identified and dissected during an axillary dissection and are at risk for injury. The axillary vein can be narrowed or ligated owing to surgical error during the procedure or can undergo acute spontaneous thrombosis during the immediate postoperative period. Because collateral channels have not had a chance to develop, the resulting swelling of the ipsilateral arm is usually acute and painful. The long thoracic nerve is the motor nerve to the serratus anterior muscle, which functions to stabilize the scapula against the posterior chest wall, especially during pushing maneuvers. Injury to this structure leads to "winging" of the scapula. The thoracodorsal pedicle contains the motor nerve and the principal artery and vein serving the latissimus dorsi muscle. Injury to the nerve leads to atrophy, but this is rarely clinically significant except in athletes. Loss of the vascular pedicle distal to its branch to the serratus muscle, however, would lead to ischemic loss of the latissimus dorsi myocutaneous rotation flap, one of the principal sources of autologous tissue for breast reconstruction and for closure of soft tissue deficits of the chest wall. The medial pectoral pedicle contains the principal motor nerve and partial blood supply to the pectoralis major muscle. Injury leads to atrophy but not ischemia, as the blood supply to this muscle is from many sources. The second intercostal brachiocutaneous nerve is sensory to the upper lateral chest wall and medial and posterior upper arm. It passes transversely across the axilla about 1–2 cm caudal to the axillary vein. In the past, it was routinely sectioned to allow cleaner "en bloc" removal of the axillary contents, but many surgeons now choose to preserve it in cases where it is not in close proximity to clinically suspicious lymph nodes. The axilla is rich in lymphatic vessels draining the ipsilateral arm. Some of these lymphatics are disrupted during axillary dissection; but continued fibrosis of the remaining lymphatics, especially in cases where the dissected axilla has been irradiated, may lead to progressive lymphedema of the arm, which can begin years after therapy. The possibility of developing occasionally unsightly and disabling lymphedema has led to a generally more conservative surgical approach toward axillary dissection for breast cancer in recent years.

ANSWER: A-e; B-b; C-f; D-a; E-d; F-c

70. A 48-year-old woman has undergone a lumpectomy for a 4 mm infiltrating ductal carcinoma of the lower outer quadrant of the right breast. The margins of resection are free of tumor. Which one or more of the following options for further local therapy would be appropriate?

A. Right modified radical mastectomy.
B. Right axillary sentinel lymph node biopsy followed by radiation therapy to the right breast.
C. Right axillary sentinel lymph node biopsy followed by radiation therapy only if the lymph node is positive for cancer.
D. A right level I axillary dissection followed by radiation therapy to the right breast.
E. A right level I axillary dissection followed by radiation therapy only if one or more of the axillary lymph nodes are positive for cancer.

COMMENTS: See Question 71.

Ref.: 21

71. Which of the following statements regarding axillary sentinel lymph node biopsy for breast cancer is/are true?

A. Axillary sentinel lymph nodes are successfully identified 75% of the time.
B. If there is concordance of identification of the sentinel lymph node by both radionuclide and blue dye techniques, the "false-negative" rate for diagnosing positive axillary lymph nodes is essentially zero.
C. The risk of arm swelling, sensory deficits, and shoulder stiffness is negligible following sentinel lymph node biopsy when compared with that which follows standard axillary dissection.
D. If the sentinel lymph node is positive for cancer, a more complete axillary dissection (level I or level I and II) should be performed.
E. Sentinel lymph node biopsy is especially well suited for primary tumors in close proximity to the axilla.
F. The accuracy of the sentinel lymph node biopsy is enhanced when the primary tumor is still present in the breast.

Ref.: 21

COMMENTS: All invasive breast cancers have the potential to metastasize to axillary lymph nodes. The accurate pathologic assessment of these nodes affects the prognosis and may affect the recommendation for adjuvant systemic therapy depending on features of the primary tumor. This is especially so for small cancers (<1 cm) for which systemic therapy would not generally be recommended if the nodes are negative. The increasing use of sentinel lymph node biopsy for axillary assessment for breast cancer has come from a desire to assess the axillary status accurately without the risks of lymphedema, numbness, and shoulder stiffness that are attendant to the more aggressive standard axillary dissection techniques. The sentinel lymph node biopsy procedure is especially well suited for small primary tumors where the likelihood of axillary metastasis is low (Question 70). In such cases, whether the axilla is assessed by sentinel lymph node biopsy or standard axillary dissection, radiation therapy is still indicated to reduce the incidence of in-breast tumor recurrence regardless of the nodal status. Mastectomy would not be required for such a patient, as the cure rate would not be improved. The sentinel lymph node biopsy technique is accomplished by injecting a small amount of radioactive material (technetium sulfur colloid) or blue dye (usually isosulfan blue dye), or both, into the area of the tumor. These materials are transported through the same lymph vessels to the same lymph node as cancer cells from the primary tumor would be if lymph node metastases were to have occurred. By scanning the axilla with a gamma probe for a "hot" area or by visually searching for a "blue" node, a much more limited incision and exploration of the axilla can be performed, reducing the risk of lymphedema, sensory deficits, and shoulder stiffness to negligible levels. One to three lymph nodes are usually identified and can be carefully assessed pathologically by both standard histologic and immunohistochemical staining techniques. Using one or both of these localizing techniques results in identifying at least one sentinel lymph node in approximately 95% of cases. Unfortunately, the sentinel lymph node technique is not 100% accurate. Among patients with histologically positive nodes, the sentinel lymph node technique failed to identify the positive node in approximately 10% of cases, even if the node was identified by both radioactive and blue dye techniques. When the sentinel lymph node is shown to contain tumor, it is generally thought that the axillary assessment should be completed with a level I or level I and II dissection to look for other nodal involvement, which could bear on the prognosis and postoperative therapy recommendations. This is somewhat controversial, however, because in most cases the recommendation for subsequent therapy is not changed. The overall accuracy of the sentinel node biopsy is likely enhanced when the primary tumor is still in place, as injection of the radionuclide or dye is more on target. After wide excision of the primary tumor, the localizing materials must be injected peripheral to the seroma cavity, which may be several centimeters remote from the primary tumor site, possibly leading to misidentification of the sentinel node. Identifying the sentinel lymph node is also more difficult when the primary tumor is located close to the axilla, especially with the radionuclide technique, because the "hot" area of the primary site overlaps the likely location of the "hot" sentinel node. Sentinel lymph node biopsy may become "standard of care" for small primary tumors within the next few years, pending the outcome of large multiinstitutional trials currently underway.

ANSWER:
Question 70: B, D
Question 71: C, D, F

REFERENCES

1. Sabiston DC Jr: *Textbook of Surgery*, 15th ed. WB Saunders, Philadelphia, 1997.
2. Schwartz SI, Shires GT, Spencer FC: *Principles of Surgery*, 7th ed. McGraw-Hill, New York, 1999.
3. American Joint Committee on Cancer: *Manual for Staging of Cancer*, 4th ed. JB Lippincott, Philadelphia, 1992.
4. Bland KI, Copeland EM: *The Breast: Comprehensive Management of Benign and Malignant Diseases.* WB Saunders, Philadelphia, 1991.
5. Overgaard M, Hanson P, Overgaard J, et al: Postoperative radiotherapy in high-risk premenopausal women with breast cancer who receive adjuvant chemotherapy. *N Engl J Med* 337:949–955, 1997.
6. Ragaz J, Jackson S, Le N, et al: Adjuvant radiotherapy and chemotherapy in node-positive premenopausal women with breast cancer. *N Engl J Med* 337:956–962, 1997.
7. Harris J, Lippman M, Morrow M, Helman S: *Diseases of the Breast.* Lippincott-Raven, Philadelphia, 1996.
8. *Tabar/Dean, Teaching Atlas of Mammography.* 2nd ed. Thieme, New York.
9. Early Breast Cancer Trialists' Collaborative Group: Tamoxifen for early breast cancer: an overview of the randomised trials. *Lancet* 351:1451–1467, 1998.
10. Early Breast Cancer Trialists' Collaborative Group: Polychemotherapy for early breast cancer: an overview of the randomised trials. *Lancet* 352:930–941, 1998.
11. Olopade O, Weber B: Breast cancer genetics: toward molecular characterization of individuals at increased risk for breast cancer. In: *PPO Updates: Principles & Practice of Oncology*, vol 12, Nos 10, 11, 1998.
12. Hartrampf C (ed): *Breast Reconstruction with Living Tissue.* Hammpton Press, Norfolk, 1991.
13. Goldwyn R (ed): *Reduction Mammoplasty.* Little, Brown, Boston, 1990.
14. Hunt KK, Baldwin BJ, Strom EA, et al: Feasibility of postmastectomy radiation therapy after TRAM flap breast reconstruction. *Ann Surg Oncol* 4:377–384, 1997.
15. Deapen DM, Bernsteri L, Brody GS: Are breast implants anticarcinogenic: a 14-year follow-up of the Los Angeles study. *Plast Reconstr Surg* 99:1346–1353, 1997.
16. Taylor ME: Breast: locally advanced (T3 and T4), inflammatory, and recurrent tumors. In: Perez CA, Brady LW (eds) *Principles and Practice of Radiation Oncology*, 3rd ed. Lippincott-Raven, Philadelphia, 1998.
17. Fowble B: Postmastectomy radiation: then and now. Oncology 11:213–239, 1997.
18. Fisher B, Anderson S, Redmond C, et al: Re-analysis and results after 12 years of follow-up in a randomized clinical trial comparing total mastectomy with lumpectomy with or without irradiation in the treatment of breast cancer. *N Engl J Med* 333:1456–1461, 1995.
19. Perez CA, Taylor ME: Breast: stage Tis, T1 and T2 tumors. In: Perez CA, Brady LW (eds) *Principles and Practice of Radiation Oncology*, 3rd ed. Lippincott-Raven, Philadelphia, 1998.
20. Cameron J: *Current Surgical Therapy.* Mosby, St. Louis, 1998.
21. Krag D, Weaver D, Ashikaga T, et al: The sentinel node in breast cancer: a multicenter validation study. *N Engl J Med* 339:941–946, 1998.

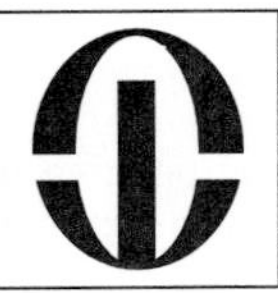

CHAPTER 20

Head and Neck

1. With regard to disorders of the external ear, which of the following statements is/are true?

A. The "cauliflower ear," as seen in wrestlers and boxers, is caused by repeated soft tissue infection of the pinna.
B. Full-thickness lacerations of the pinna should be managed with sutures placed on both cutaneous surfaces as well as through the perichondrium or disrupted cartilage.
C. Infections of the pinna superficial to the perichondrium should not be surgically drained, as this may be the cause of perichondritis.
D. A foreign body in the ear canal should be removed immediately.

Ref.: 1, 2, 3

COMMENTS: The presence of cartilage and its relation to the perichondrium are important anatomic considerations when determining management of disorders of the pinna. *Hematomas* usually occur between the perichondrium and underlying cartilage and should be drained by aspiration if possible or by incision. Suturing a bolster to the site of drainage avoids reaccumulation. Untreated hematomas can organize and calcify, resulting in a cauliflower ear.

For *full-thickness lacerations* of the pinna, sutures placed through cartilage help with alignment. Such full-thickness lacerations should be repaired by reapproximating cartilage and both skin surfaces.

Infections deep to the perichondrium should be promptly drained because, if untreated, they can lead to cartilage necrosis. Superficial furuncles may also need to be drained if they do not resolve with warm soaks and antibiotics.

A *foreign body* in the ear canal is a problem particularly common in children. A microscope is usually essential. A foreign body is never an emergency, and removal should not be attempted by one not trained to do so. The use of forceps may push a foreign body farther into the ear canal, injuring the tympanic membrane and ossicles. With an uncooperative child, general anesthesia may be warranted for removing foreign bodies from the ear canal. Animal or vegetable matter should not be irrigated in an attempt at removal, as they may swell and make removal more difficult. Removal of inanimate objects may be delayed if the canal is already irritated from previous attempts. Irregularly shaped objects may be removed with fine forceps under the operating microscope. Round objects such as beads can be removed only with strong suction or by passing a right-angle hook deep to them, turning them, and teasing them out. After removal, the canal should be inspected for a second foreign body and to assess the status of the canal wall and tympanic membrane.

ANSWER: B

2. With regard to neoplasms of the ear, which of the following statements is/are true?

A. Most carcinomas of the pinna are related to excessive exposure to ultraviolet irradiation.
B. Rhabdomyosarcoma is the most common childhood aural malignancy.
C. Squamous cell carcinoma of the ear may require neck dissection.
D. Squamous cell carcinoma of the ear may metastasize to parotid lymph nodes.

Ref.: 1, 4, 5

COMMENTS: Squamous cell carcinoma of the ear is relatively common, whereas both are related to exposure to ultraviolet light. Basal cell carcinoma is uncommon. Squamous cell carcinomas do metastasize (12–18% to parotid and cervical lymph nodes) and may require regional node resection when the nodes are palpable. The lymphatic drainage of the external ear passes through the parotid gland, and treatment for regional metastasis should include parotidectomy and neck dissection. Postoperative irradiation should be applied for positive margins or extensive disease. Rhabdomyosarcoma is the most common aural tumor of childhood. For limited disease surgery is indicated, with combination irradiation and chemotherapy required for more advanced tumors.

ANSWER: A, B, C, D

3. With regard to nasal trauma, which of the following statements is/are true?

A. Undisplaced nasal fractures require wire fixation to prevent subsequent displacement during the healing process.
B. Septal hematomas are clinically significant conditions that require surgical intervention.
C. Cerebrospinal fluid rhinorrhea requires urgent surgical intervention if one is to prevent meningitis.
D. Lacerations through the skin of the nose that penetrate to or through nasal bone or cartilage are open fractures that require immediate repair.

Ref.: 1, 2, 3, 4, 5, 6

COMMENTS: *Nasal fractures* are the most common fractures of the facial skeleton and are nearly always associated with tearing of the overlying mucosa, thereby making them open fractures. Clinical examination revealing displacement of nasal bones or crepitance on light palpation usually suggests the diagnosis. Nonetheless, facial radiographs should be obtained to confirm the fracture as well as to look for fractures of other facial bones. Undisplaced fractures, however, require no specific therapy except for external splinting for protection. Radiographs of the nasal bones show the bones in lateral view and can therefore detect only anteroposterior displacement. Lateral displacement can be assessed clinically and by CT scans.

Septal hematomas develop between the perichondrium and the underlying cartilage of the nasal septum. Such hematomas frequently become infected and may produce avascular necrosis of the underlying cartilage because of separation from the perichondrium, resulting in a "saddle nose" deformity. To prevent this problem, early diagnosis, incision and drainage, septal splinting, and antibiotics are indicated.

Severe nasal injury may be associated with *cerebrospinal fluid rhinorrhea*, which may be suspected if clear fluid drains from the nose after injury; it is strongly suggested if there is a high glucose content in the fluid; the presence of β_2-transferrin in the fluid confirms it as being cerebrospinal fluid (CSF). Thin-cut computed tomography (CT) scans should be used in all cases of traumatic CSF rhinorrhea to determine the site of the skull base injury. Usually a cribriform plate fracture is identifiable. Most traumatic leaks seal without treatment; the initial management is observation, head elevation, avoidance of nose blowing and straining, and possibly administration of antibiotics. If the leak persists for more than 4–6 weeks or meningitis develops, the leak should be repaired surgically. In most cases the leak can be repaired via an endoscopic or traditional extracranial approach, whereas a frontal craniotomy approach is best utilized for the more recalcitrant or cryptically located leaks. Repair of facial fractures should not be delayed during a trial of conservative management for a CSF fistula because realignment of the bony fragments helps speed healing of the dural tear. If leaking fluid cannot be collected, or if the site of the leak cannot be determined, radiologic contrast studies are indicated. As an adjunct to both surgical and conservative management, lumbar puncture and the use of a closed drainage system helps decrease the intracranial pressure (ICP), thus allowing the dura a better chance to heal.

ANSWER: B

4. With regard to epistaxis, which of the following statements is/are true?

A. In most cases, epistaxis occurs from the anteroinferior part of the nasal septum.
B. Properly applied anteroposterior packing controls bleeding in 95% of cases.
C. Hypoxemia is a potential complication of nasal packing.
D. Ligation of the internal maxillary artery is ineffective for controlling epistaxis and should be avoided.

Ref.: 1, 2, 3, 4, 5, 6

COMMENTS: Approximately 90% of cases of epistaxis arise from a plexus of vessels (Kiesselbach's plexus) in the anteroinferior part of the nasal septum. In most cases it is easily controlled with simple digital pressure. If this fails and if the bleeding site can be visualized, it can be cauterized chemically or electrically, although occasionally anterior nasal packing is required. Absorbable packing is recommended for patients with coagulopathies. In 10% of cases of epistaxis, the source is posterior, in the area of Woodruff's plexus. This situation poses a potentially serious problem, as posterior epistaxis frequently occurs in patients with arteriosclerosis and hypertension and may be difficult to control; it has significant associated morbidity, including hypoxia, sepsis, respiratory obstruction, cardiac arrhythmia or ischemia (or both), aspiration pneumonia, nasal necrosis, and sinusitis. The initial attempt at controlling the bleeding should be with readily available anterior or combined anterior and posterior packs and this will be successful in up to 95% of cases. When such packing is utilized, antibiotics should be given prophylactically in an effort to prevent sinusitis and otitis media. Air exchange is frequently hindered by the packing; and as many of these patients have associated systemic and cardiopulmonary disease, supplemental oxygen (28% O_2 or less) should be administered. Patients with cardiac or severe pulmonary disease should be placed on a monitor. Posterior epistaxis that cannot be controlled with packing may be treated by transantral or transnasal endoscopic ligation of the internal maxillary artery. The anterior ethmoid artery should be ligated if the bleeding site can be identified high in the lateral nasal walls. Alcoholics or patients with chronic obstructive pulmonary disease should be considered for early internal maxillary or ethmoid artery ligation (or both). This maneuver avoids nasal packing in this high risk group. Transfemoral carotid angiography and embolization with absorbable gel foam or polyvinyl alcohol particles is an option that may be utilized for recurrent epistaxis after unsuccessful surgical intervention in patients with nonoperable nasal tumors or who are poor anesthetic risks.

ANSWER: A, B, C

5. Endoscopic sinus surgery is the most common surgical procedure performed by head and neck surgeons. Postoperative care may require which of the following?

A. Immediate orbital decompression for orbital hematoma.
B. Immediate CT scan to look for intracerebral bleed or pneumocephalus to assess a postoperative mental status change.
C. Stat chest radiograph to rule out pneumomediastinum.
D. Collection of nasal drainage for β_2-transferrin to rule out CSF leak.

Ref.: 1, 6

COMMENTS: Although complications of endoscopic sinus surgery are rare, those that occur can be serious or even life-threatening. Bleeding, the most common complication, can usually be controlled by anterior and posterior nasal packing. Penetration of the lamina papyracea can result in orbital bleeding, which in turn can lead to orbital swelling, limitation of ocular movements, or blindness. Treatment involves immediate decompression with a lateral canthotomy and inferior cantholysis, which can be done at the bedside. These steps are followed by surgical decompression accomplished by removing the entire lamina papyracea and incising the periorbita. Penetration of the skull base can occur and can result in pneumocephalus, intracerebral bleeding, or CSF leak. Postoperative lethargy or alteration in mental status may be signs of intracerebral injury. A CT scan of the brain should be obtained immediately to rule out a hematoma, intracerebral bleed, or pneumoencephalic CSF leak, which also can result from skull base penetration. A leak should be identified and repaired. Undetected leaks may lead to meningitis. There is no risk of pneumomediastinum with these procedures.

ANSWER: A, B, D

6. With regard to pharyngeal foreign bodies, which of the following statements is/are true?

A. Round or oval foreign bodies tend to lodge in the conical piriform sinus.
B. Long, sharp objects tend to lodge in the tonsillar area.
C. Because of the protection afforded by the soft palate, foreign bodies reach the nasopharynx only via the nasal cavity.
D. Foreign bodies of the pharynx should be retrieved under general anesthesia.

Ref.: 1, 4

COMMENTS: Foreign bodies of the pharynx are most likely found in one of five locations: lingual tonsil, palatine tonsils, piriform sinuses, valleculae, or nasopharynx. Small, round, or oval objects (e.g., peanuts) are usually found in the valleculae because in other locations they would probably be easily swallowed. Long, sharp objects such as fish bones are likely to lodge in the palatine or lingual tonsils. Small, sharp, or irregularly shaped objects, including pills, are frequently found in the piriform sinuses of the hypopharynx. Foreign bodies located in the tonsillar fossa or base of the tongue can usually be removed by direct laryngoscopy with the patient under local anesthesia or light sedation. Occasionally, foreign bodies of any type are coughed into the nasopharynx. Entrapment of foreign bodies in this location or in the hypopharynx usually requires general anesthesia for removal.

ANSWER: B

7. With regard to neoplasms of the nasopharynx, which of the following statements is/are true?

A. Lymphoma is the most common nasopharyngeal neoplasm in children.
B. A viral association with lymphoepithelioma of the nasopharynx has been found.
C. There is an unusually high incidence of nasopharyngeal carcinoma among the Chinese.
D. Surgery is the treatment of choice for small, well localized nasopharyngeal carcinomas.

Ref.: 1, 2, 4, 5

COMMENTS: Malignant neoplasms of the nasopharynx include squamous carcinoma, adenocarcinoma (usually of minor salivary gland origin), sarcoma, lymphoma, and melanoma. Among children, lymphoma is the most common malignancy in the nasopharynx. In adults, squamous carcinoma and its variant lymphoepithelioma are the most common types. There is an unusually high incidence of nasopharyngeal carcinoma among the Chinese, and it appears at an earlier age than other squamous carcinomas of the upper aerodigestive tract. Elevated titers of anti-Epstein-Barr virus antibodies are seen in almost half of patients with nasopharyngeal carcinoma, suggesting a possible viral etiology. Clinical presentation may include bleeding or nasopharyngeal obstruction as well as the sequelae of invasion of the skull base, which includes cranial nerve involvement. Imaging with CT and magnetic resonance imaging (MRI) helps delineate disease in the nasopharynx and neck. Carcinoma of the nasopharynx is best treated with irradiation. Difficult access and the inability to obtain a wide surgical margin because of the proximity of the nasopharynx to the base of the skull and vertebral column make surgical excision of even the earliest lesions inappropriate. The tumor has a high propensity to metastasize to cervical lymph nodes. The overall 5-year survival rate for those with carcinoma of the nasopharynx is approximately 35%.

ANSWER: A, B, C

8. With regard to oropharyngeal abscesses, which of the following statements is/are true?

A. Peritonsillar, parapharyngeal, and retropharyngeal abscesses occur with approximately equal frequency among children younger than 10 years of age.
B. Parapharyngeal and retropharyngeal abscesses can progress rapidly to cause airway obstruction.
C. Drainage of peritonsillar, parapharyngeal, and retropharyngeal abscesses is best accomplished through the pharyngeal wall.
D. As with abscesses in other locations in the body, small drains should be placed into transpharyngeally drained abscesses to promote continued evacuation of the abscess cavity.

Ref.: 1, 3, 4

COMMENTS: Oropharyngeal abscesses have distinct characteristics regarding their epidemiology and management depending on their location. *Peritonsillar* abscesses are rare in children younger than age 10, even though they represent complications of acute tonsillitis. The patient may be quite ill and present with trismus and severe odynophagia. An initial trial of antibiotics and needle aspiration of the abscess are warranted; if there is no response within 24 hours, aspiration should be repeated or incision and drainage bed performed. Unlike a parapharyngeal or retropharyngeal abscess, which may progress rapidly and cause airway obstruction, the peritonsillar abscess is more limited and rarely causes airway obstruction. *Retropharyngeal* abscesses occur in infants, young children, and older adults; they are rare after the age of 10 years. In children these infections are due to the lymphadenitis associated with pharyngitis. In the elderly they are caused by foreign bodies or Pott's disease. The infant may present in opisthotonus, and the clinical picture is often confused with that of meningitis. The fever is often high, and the patient may drool secondary to odynophagia. Physical examination reveals a boggy, fluctuant texture to the retropharyngeal tissues and inability to palpate the normally palpable vertebral bodies. The swelling is unilateral because of the midline laryngeal raphe. Radiologic evaluation may show gas in the retropharyngeal soft tissue or widening of this space. Loss of the airway is a potential hazard. Antibiotics and surgical drainage through the posterior pharyngeal wall or the neck are the treatments of choice. With both peritonsillar and retropharyngeal abscesses, aspiration of pus into the tracheobronchial tree is a distinct hazard and can be prevented by careful endotracheal intubation and positioning the patient in the Trendelenburg position prior to drainage. Drains are not required, as these abscess cavities tend to empty themselves during each swallowing motion. *Parapharyngeal* abscesses occur in all age groups and may be secondary to dental infection, pharyngitis, or tonsillitis. Because these abscesses occur more laterally, drainage through the oropharynx is hazardous owing to the proximity to the internal carotid artery and jugular vein. Parapharyngeal abscesses should be drained through the lateral neck, with a drain left in place to permit continued evacuation of the cavity. An important concern is the ability of infection to spread from one space to another. The greatest morbidity associated with these abscesses is from internal jugular vein thrombosis, vascular erosion, or spread into the mediastinum or abdomen via the prevertebral or retropharyngeal spaces.

ANSWER: B

9. With regard to carcinoma of the tonsil, which of the following statements is/are true?

A. Because of the irritation from the passage of food, tonsillar carcinomas tend to present early.
B. Cervical lymph node metastases are rare because of the ability of the abundant peritonsillar lymphatic network to confine regional spread of the tumor.
C. The heavy use of tobacco and alcohol has been associated with tonsillar carcinoma.
D. Appropriate therapeutic options include surgery or irradiation, alone or in combination.

Ref.: 1, 2, 4, 5

COMMENTS: The most common malignant tumor of the tonsil is squamous carcinoma; and as with most squamous carcinomas of the upper aerodigestive tract, there is a distinct male predominance and an association with excessive use of tobacco and alcohol. Tonsillar carcinoma usually remains asymptomatic until it has reached considerable size, spreading along the pharyngeal wall. It can invade the base of the tongue, larynx, piriform sinus, and nasopharynx; or it can spread by direct lateral extension into the neck. This type of local growth, as well as the abundant lymphatics of the tonsillar fossa, are in part responsible for the relatively high frequency of cervical lymph node metastases (66–76% at presentation). Depending on the size of the primary lesion and the presence or absence of cervical lymph node metastases, initial curative therapy may involve surgical excision, or irradiation or both, with irradiation being the mainstay of treatment. Biopsy of a small tonsillar lesion is best accomplished by tonsillectomy.

ANSWER: C, D

10. With regard to laryngeal trauma, which of the following statements is/are true?

A. Trauma is the most common cause of laryngeal stenosis.
B. Iatrogenic laryngeal stenosis occurs most often in the supraglottic location as a result of traumatic intubation attempts.
C. Because the rigid component of the larynx is cartilage and not bone, fractures of the larynx do not occur.
D. Laryngeal trauma with associated difficulty breathing should be initially managed with urgent tracheostomy rather than endotracheal intubation.

Ref.: 1, 4

COMMENTS: Because of appropriate vaccination programs and improved antibiotic therapies, trauma has replaced infectious diseases as the most common cause of laryngeal stenosis. A significant proportion of laryngeal injuries are iatrogenic, relating primarily to subglottic injury caused by prolonged intubation with a cuffed endotracheal tube. However, the incidence of complications has been reduced significantly by the use of endotracheal tubes with soft, low-pressure cuffs. These posttraumatic stenoses may be managed by dilatation, laser therapy, or local excision with reconstruction of the stenotic segment.

Direct blows to the neck may result in fracture of the laryngeal cartilage or laryngotracheal disruption. When such an injury is suspected and the patient is having difficulty breathing, urgent tracheostomy should be performed, as attempts at endotracheal intubation may be unsuccessful, compound the injury, or result in loss of airway. If the patient is stable, the preliminary evaluation involves fiberoptic nasolaryngoscopy and CT scanning. When the patient's condition is stabilized, surgical reduction and repair of the fracture are carried out. Earlier repair leads to better results. Fractures may require approximation with miniplates; and mucosal lacerations require meticulous closure; stenting should be considered.

ANSWER: A, D

11. With regard to foreign bodies of the larynx and tracheobronchial tree, which of the following statements is/are true?

A. The ability to speak is an important differentiating sign for diagnosing the cause of cyanosis and respiratory difficulty that occurs while eating.
B. Complete occlusion of the larynx with a food bolus should be managed immediately by tracheostomy.
C. Radiographs may be of benefit for localizing the site of bronchial obstruction by radiolucent foreign bodies.
D. The cessation of coughing 30 minutes after inhalation of a foreign body indicates that the foreign body has been coughed out.
E. Infectious complications are the principal long-term sequelae of retained tracheobronchial foreign bodies.

Ref.: 1, 4

COMMENTS: The "café coronary," in which a patient becomes dyspneic and cyanotic while eating, may be due to myocardial infarction, arrhythmia, or airway obstruction from a food bolus. The inability to exchange air and to speak suggests aspiration as the cause of the difficulty. If the choking person is able to exchange adequate amounts of air, he or she should be left alone but observed closely. If there is complete obstruction to air exchange, initial treatment includes an attempt to dislodge the foreign body with the Heimlich (abdominal thrust) maneuver. Emergency tracheostomy is hazardous and should be employed only as a last-resort, life-saving measure. Inhalation of foreign bodies into the tracheobronchial tree where air exchange is still ongoing, usually produces severe coughing that lasts up to 30 minutes. By this time, however, the foreign body has settled into one specific location, and, because of sensory neural adaptation, the coughing may stop. This may be erroneously interpreted as a sign that the foreign body has been expelled. In most cases of retained foreign body, this relatively asymptomatic latent period is followed by a cough productive of purulent sputum. Infectious complications, including bronchiectasis, recurrent pneumonitis, lung abscess, and empyema, can follow. Even when radiolucent objects have been inhaled, standard chest radiographs may assist in localizing the site of bronchiolar obstruction, as in cases in which a ball-valve type of expiratory obstruction produces a localized pulmonary emphysema or air trapping with mediastinal shift.

The proper initial management of aspirated foreign bodies is retrieval via tracheobronchial endoscopy.

ANSWER: A, C, E

12. With regard to foreign bodies of the esophagus, which of the following statements is/are true?

A. Most esophageal foreign bodies are found just below the cricopharyngeus muscle.
B. Fever during the first 12 hours after esophagoscopy is usually a sign of atelectasis.
C. Dysphagia without pain is the clinical hallmark of the presence of a foreign body in the esophagus.
D. Retrieval of esophageal foreign bodies through a rigid esophagoscope with the patient under general anesthesia is the treatment of choice.

Ref.: 1, 4, 7

COMMENTS: Esophageal foreign bodies lodge at points of natural narrowing: below the cricopharyngeus muscle, near the arch of the aorta, behind the right main stem bronchus, and at the gastroesophageal junction. Approximately 95% of all esophageal foreign bodies are immediately below the cricopharyngeus muscle. Large foreign bodies in this area can produce partial airway obstruction as a result of extrinsic pressure on the membranous trachea. In most instances the clinical presentation is that of dysphagia and associated suprasternal pain. Perforation may occur immediately, or it may be delayed; the risk of perforation increases with the length of time the foreign body remains in the esophagus. Perforation is diagnosed by the presence of tachycardia, fever, pain radiating to the back, soft tissue crepitance or by radiographic demonstration of air in soft tissues. Documentation of the presence of a foreign body may be achieved by standard and contrast radiography. Appropriate treatment involves rigid endoscopic retrieval of the foreign body with the patient under general anesthesia. Fever or pain after esophagoscopy must be considered a sign of perforation until proved otherwise. Chest radiography to rule out air in the mediastinum and barium swallow should be performed immediately. Urgent drainage of the mediastinum is essential and minimizes the mortality associated with esophageal perforation.

ANSWER: A, D

13. Which one or more of the following are appropriate indications for tracheotomy?

A. Inability to handle upper respiratory secretions.
B. Inability to handle lower respiratory secretions.
C. Respiratory obstruction.
D. Endotracheal intubation longer than 5 days.

Ref.: 1, 2, 3, 4

COMMENTS: The principal indications for tracheotomy include respiratory obstruction that cannot be properly managed with endotracheal intubation and the inability to evacuate secretions from the upper or lower respiratory tree. Prolonged endotracheal intubation may lead to interarytenoid scarring or subglottic stenosis and necessitate tracheotomy; however, the currently available low-pressure soft cuffs allow safe endotracheal intubation for up to 14 days, depending on associated factors such as concomitant use of a nasogastric tube, patient movement, gastroesophageal reflux, and traumatic or multiple intubations. Although tracheobronchial toilet is more easily obtained through a tracheostomy tube, the presence of a tracheostomy tube is not without complications, such as an inability of the patient to cough (because of bypass of the glottic closure mechanism), bypassing of the normal warming and humidification of inspired air in the upper respiratory tract, and direct exposure of the lower respiratory tract to environmental pathogens. Nonetheless, the decrease in tracheobronchial deadspace and the accessibility of the upper airway to nursing personnel for pulmonary toilet, along with humidification via ventilators or a tracheal collar, are sufficient to correct these problems.

ANSWER: A, B, C

14. Match the lettered parts (A–F) of the illustrated pharynx and larynx with the anatomic structures listed below.

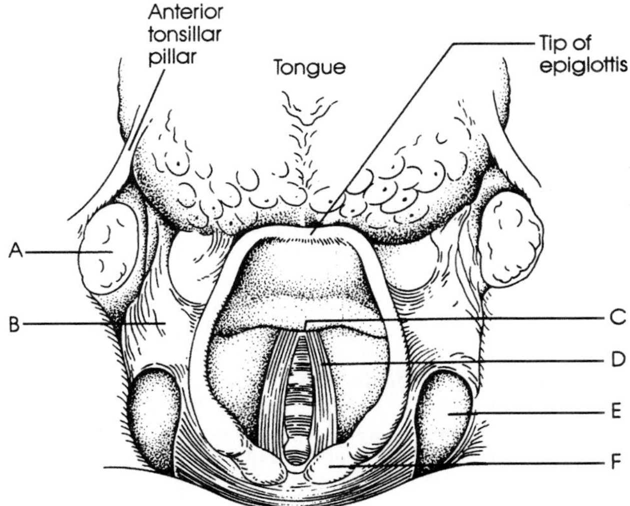

a. Arytenoid process
b. Vocal cord
c. Pharyngoepiglottic fold
d. Anterior commissure
e. Palatine tonsil
f. Piriform sinus

Ref.: 4

COMMENTS: Anatomically, the larynx may be divided into three regions: the glottic, supraglottic, and subglottic larynx. The **glottic larynx** consists of the true vocal cords only. The **supraglottic larynx** consists of structures superior to the true vocal cords and includes the laryngeal ventricle, false vocal cords, arytenoids, aryepiglottic folds, and epiglottis. The **subglottic larynx** extends from the undersurface of the true cords to the inferior border of the cricoid cartilage. The **hypopharynx** is made up of the piriform sinuses (including both medial and lateral walls), the postcricoid mucosa, and the posterior pharyngeal wall. Knowledge of these anatomic sites is required for proper staging of tumors in this area and for planning appropriate therapy.

ANSWER: A-e; B-c; C-d; D-b; E-f; F-a

15. Match each of the clinical characteristics of laryngeal/pharyngeal carcinoma in the left column with the appropriate anatomic site or sites of origin in the right column.

A. Symptoms occur early	a. Supraglottic larynx
B. Regional node metastases common	b. Glottic larynx
C. May be managed with voice preservation	c. Hypopharynx
D. Radiotherapy may be the treatment of choice even in symptomatic patients	

Ref.: 1, 2, 4

COMMENTS: Glottic carcinomas, in contradistinction to other laryngeal and hypopharyngeal tumors, produce symptoms early because of the relatively small degree of anatomic change required to produce hoarseness. Therefore glottic carcinomas tend to be diagnosed in their early stages. Additionally, because true glottic cancers have limited access to lymphatics, the likelihood of regional nodal metastases is low. For T1 and early T2 lesions, surgery and irradiation are of nearly equal effectiveness. The choice rests on patient preference, cost, and the surgeon's training. Lasers have added a new dimension to the treatment of glottic cancer, with high cure rates and low morbidity. Carcinomas of the supraglottic larynx and hypopharynx usually grow to a considerable size before producing symptoms (hoarseness, dysphagia, dyspnea). Because of this large tumor size and the greater access to the abundant lymphatics of the supraglottic and hypopharyngeal areas, regional lymph node metastases are relatively common (30–50%) at the time of initial clinical presentation. For these same reasons, symptomatic tumors in these areas can rarely be managed successfully by radiotherapy alone. Surgery, with or without irradiation, is the preferred treatment. Direct involvement of the glottic larynx or paralysis of the vocal cords by supraglottic or hypopharyngeal lesions may require total laryngectomy. In selected patients with the glottis free of tumor and fully mobile, resection can be carried out with preservation of voice function. Supraglottic and vertical hemilaryngectomies are surgical variations that allow preservation of the voice and swallowing in selected patients. Postlaryngectomy rehabilitation includes esophageal speech, use of the electrolarynx, and the surgically created tracheoesophageal fistula with one-way valve.

ANSWER: A-b; B-a,c; C-a,b,c; D-b

16. Acceptable alternatives to standard tracheotomy include which of the following?

A. Cricothyrotomy.
B. Percutaneous tracheotomy.
C. Prolonged intubation.
D. Permanent tracheostomy.

Ref.: 1, 6

COMMENTS: *Cricothyrotomy* is a procedure to establish an immediate airway when airway obstruction is imminent or present and endotracheal intubation is not possible. Packaged cricothyrotomy kits are easy to use, but any incision through the skin and directly through the cricothyroid membrane can establish an airway. An endotracheal tube should be pushed through the incision if possible. It should be converted to a standard tracheotomy within 5 days. • *Percutaneous tracheotomy* has been proven to be a safe and reasonable alternative to standard tracheotomy. Standard systems include a needle that pierces the soft tissue and trachea. A guidewire is then used to guide dilators through the perforation until a tracheotomy tube is placed. • *Prolonged intubation* is likely to be far more uncomfortable than tracheotomy. Patients with tracheotomy tubes can eat and speak, unlike patients with endotracheal tubes. Prolonged intubation can lead to permanent laryngeal tracheal scarring. Patients who require permanent tracheotomy for severe sleep apnea or laryngeal scarring not amenable to correction should have a tracheostomy instead of a tracheotomy.

Tracheostomy involves suturing skin flaps directly to the trachea so the stoma is epithelium-lined and remains open without a tube.

ANSWER: B, D

17. Match each of the clinical characteristics of cleft lip and palate in the left column with the appropriate anatomic defect in the right column.

A. Involves the lip, alveolus, or both	a. Cleft of primary palate
B. Involves hard and soft palates	b. Cleft of secondary palate
C. Should be closed within the first 3 months of life	
D. Should be closed between 1 and 2 years of age	

Ref.: 1, 4

COMMENTS: Vertical paramedian clefts of the lip and palate are considered in two principal categories: clefts of the primary palate (the lip and alveolar ridge) and clefts of the secondary palate (hard and soft palate). These clefts may occur alone or in association with each other, but the most common anomaly is a combined cleft lip and palate. The timing of surgical correction varies with the specific type of defect. Clefts of the lip are best repaired during the first 3 months of life, enabling the infant to achieve more normal patterns of feeding. Repair of a cleft palate is usually delayed until sometime between 1 and 2 years of age to facilitate the technical closure. Lip coaptation may be performed earlier to decrease the gap at the time of definitive surgery. Delay beyond the age of 2 years, when the child is beginning to develop skills of speech, may result in permanent speech disability. These closures are usually performed by means of local rotation flaps and are technically challenging.

ANSWER: A-a; B-b; C-a; D-b

18. Which one or more of the following statements accurately pertain to the management of full-thickness lacerations of the lip?

A. Layered closure is preferred.
B. A frequent cause of wound breakdown is ischemic necrosis secondary to the relatively poor labial blood supply.
C. The extent of soft tissue loss in labial lacerations is frequently underestimated.
D. Proper apposition of the vermilion border is the principal determinant of cosmetic outcome.

Ref.: 4

COMMENTS: The proper management of full-thickness labial lacerations involves débridement of devitalized tissue and a layered closure of the mucosa, labial musculature, and skin with fine absorbable and nonabsorbable sutures, paying particular attention to the accurate apposition of the vermilion border. Because of the circular and radial orientation of the labial musculature, labial lacerations frequently open widely, leading to the erroneous assumption that there has been significant soft tissue loss. The blood supply of the perioral area is excellent and is rarely of concern when repairing these wounds. Pathogenic oral anaerobes have occasionally been implicated as the cause of wound breakdown and local infection, and for this reason some clinicians recommend prophylactic antibiotic therapy.

ANSWER: A, D

19. Regarding obstructive sleep apnea (OSA), which of the following statements is/are true?

A. It is a rare disorder.
B. It is seen only in morbidly obese patients who are more than 100% over their expected body weight.
C. Treatment is uvulopalatopharyngoplasty.
D. It is associated with mycocardial cardiac arrhythmias, infarction, and death.

Ref.: 1, 6

COMMENTS: Obstructive sleep apnea is a common disorder that affects at least 10% of the population.

It is more common and more severe in morbidly obese patients but occurs in patients who are not obese. It is more common in patients with relative micrognathia or retrognathia. It is often associated with difficult anesthetic intubation. Symptoms include snoring and excessive daytime somnolence.

There are many surgical and nonsurgical treatments available to treat OSA. Nasal continuous positive airway pressure (CPAP) used by the patient during sleep is the mainstay of treatment. Surgical options include uvulopalatopharyngoplasty, hyoid suspension procedures, and permanent tracheostomy. Other surgical procedures that are more specific and less common include orthognathic surgery to correct retrognathia and procedures to reduce the volume of tissue at the tongue base.

Patients with OSA desaturate during periods of apnea. This is usually worse if a patient has been sedated or received narcotics. Desaturation may be a cause of arrhythmias, myocardial infarction, and death in the postoperative patient.

ANSWER: C, D

20. Which one or more of the following statements accurately describes carcinoma of the lip?

A. It is approximately equally distributed between the upper and the lower lip.
B. It has a strong relation to prior excessive exposure to the sun.
C. More than 90% are epidermoid carcinomas.
D. Regional nodal metastases usually first appear in the submental and submandibular triangles.

Ref.: 1, 2, 4

COMMENTS: Almost all (as many as 99%) of all lip cancers are epidermoid (squamous cell) carcinoma. These are found more frequently in patients with a fair complexion and in those who have a history of excessive exposure to the sun. Excessive use of tobacco (particularly pipes) and heavy consumption of alcohol are also considered to be risk factors. Sun exposure as a risk factor may explain why these carcinomas are usually found on the lower lip. Regional node metastases usually occur late in the course of the disease and tend to be found initially in the submental and submandibular triangles and later along the internal jugular chain. Commissure lesions are more aggressive with earlier metastases and a greater tendency to spread intraorally. Distant metastases are rare at initial presentation.

ANSWER: B, C, D

21. Which of the following anatomic sites are considered to be part of the oral cavity?

A. Floor of mouth.
B. Palatine tonsil.
C. Posterior upper gingiva.
D. Soft palate.
E. Posterior third of tongue.

Ref.: 1, 4

COMMENTS: When considering neoplasms of the upper aerodigestive tract, it is important to be specific in terms of the site of origin of the tumor, as it may have a bearing on management and prognosis. The **oral cavity** is bounded *anteriorly* by the lips and includes the vestibule of the mouth (including buccal mucosa and gingivobuccal sulcus); the buccal, alveolar, and lingual aspects of the gingiva; the floor of the mouth; the anterior two-thirds of the tongue; and the hard palate. *Posteriorly*, the oral cavity is bounded by the junction between the hard and soft palates and the junction between the anterior two-thirds and the posterior one-third of the tongue. The **lateral** borders are defined by the anterior tonsillar pillars. The **oropharynx**, which is not considered part of the oral cavity, is bounded by the palatine tonsils, soft palate, posterior third of the tongue, and posterior pharyngeal wall. The more posterior oropharyngeal tumors have a higher likelihood of regional lymph node metastases than those in a more anterior location because of the rich lymphatic network in the pharyngeal submucosa. Within the oral cavity are also general differences in the likelihood of regional nodal disease (e.g., tumors of the gingiva are less likely to have nodal metastases than are tumors of the floor of the mouth).

ANSWER: A, C

22. With regard to carcinoma of the oral cavity, which of the following statements is/are true?

A. Most cancers of the oral cavity are epidermoid carcinomas.
B. Male predominance and a history of excessive use of tobacco or alcohol (or both) characterize the epidemiology of most oral cavity carcinomas.
C. Minor salivary gland carcinomas are the second most common type of oral cavity cancer.
D. Radiotherapy should be avoided in the management of oral cavity cancers because of the debilitating side effects of xerostomia.

Ref.: 1, 2, 4

COMMENTS: As with all cancers of the upper aerodigestive tract, epidermoid carcinoma accounts for most cancers in the oral cavity. Most patients have a history of significant use of tobacco or alcohol (or both). Men have a greater incidence of cancer of the aerodigestive tract, but that difference is narrowing, apparently as a result of increased smoking by women. The second most common cancer in the oral cavity is of minor salivary gland origin. These tumors should be considered in the differential diagnosis of any submucosal lesion in the upper aerodigestive tract. Sarcomas, lymphomas, and melanomas of the oral cavity are rare. There is no general agreement on the proper therapy for cancers in the oral cavity. Early lesions may be treated by surgical excision or irradiation alone. To arrive at a treatment plan, one must weigh the relative risks of anesthesia and the cosmetic and functional deficits caused by surgery against the problems of xerostomia, dental disease, and poor healing caused by irradiation. Also, a specific area of oral mucosa that undergoes malignant degeneration may signify more generalized mucosal disease and a tendency to future carcinomas, a concept explained by the theory of "field cancerization." Radiation of an oral carcinoma in a young patient makes treatment of subsequent lesions more difficult. Advanced lesions of the oral cavity are frequently treated by surgery and radiotherapy in combination. The use of chemotherapy, alone and in combination with radiotherapy and surgery, is currently under investigation and has yielded excellent results in selected patients.

ANSWER: A, B, C

23. In which of the following ways do cancers of the oropharynx differ from those of the oral cavity?

A. Oropharyngeal cancers have an equal distribution between males and females.
B. Minor salivary gland tumors are the most common malignancies of the oropharynx.
C. Lymphoma is more common in the oropharynx than in the oral cavity.
D. The overall prognosis for cancer in the oropharynx is worse than that for cancer in the oral cavity.

Ref.: 1, 2, 4

COMMENTS: Similar to carcinoma of the oral cavity and other sites in the upper aerodigestive tract, oropharyngeal carcinoma has a male predominance, and most of the lesions are epidermoid carcinomas. In contrast to the oral cavity, however, there is much higher incidence of lymphoma (occurring primarily in the lymphoid-rich Waldeyer's ring). Overall, the prognosis of patients with oropharyngeal carcinoma is worse than that of patients with lesions in the oral cavity. This is due to a number of factors, including the greater likelihood of lymph node metastases being present at the time of clinical presentation and the larger size that the primary tumor usually achieves before it produces symptoms or is detected clinically.

ANSWER: C, D

24. With regard to reconstruction techniques in head and neck cancer surgery, which of the following statements is/are true?

A. The most significant advance in the rehabilitation of the head and neck cancer patient in recent years has been the development of the technique for esophageal speech following laryngectomy.
B. The use of myocutaneous flaps has significantly reduced the total hospital time required for reconstruction of defects after head and neck cancer operations.
C. Free microvascular composite grafts have contributed significantly to the reconstruction of complicated surgical defects, particularly those involving mandibulectomy.
D. The increasingly complicated extirpative procedures utilized during the last 10 years of head and neck surgery have resulted in a corresponding increase in the need for staged reconstruction techniques.

Ref.: 1, 2, 4

COMMENTS: Advances in the extirpative portion of the surgical management of head and neck cancer include the increased scope of anesthesia, the development of larynx-conservation techniques, and the introduction of lasers and microscopically controlled stepwise excision of neoplasms. Advances in head and neck reconstructive surgery have also occurred in recent years with the development of myocutaneous flaps and free microvascular flaps. As a consequence, decreased hospital stay and improved patient rehabilitation have become a reality. Prior to these developments, reconstruction frequently involved the delay and staged transfer of pedicle flaps. It is now common, even in complicated cases, for the entire reconstruction to be performed at the same time as the extirpative surgery. In addition to reducing the cost and time of the reconstruction, this has also allowed the patient to begin adjuvant radiation therapy or chemotherapy at an earlier time, if indicated. An important additional benefit has been the opportunity for these patients to avoid the prolonged disfigurement and social ostracism they might otherwise suffer. Although much has yet to be learned regarding the use of free composite grafts with microvascular anastomoses, their value in the reconstruction of the patient with head and neck cancer (particularly in cases involving mandibulectomy) appears to be well established.

ANSWER: B, C

25. Match each of the benign conditions involving the tongue in the left column with its appropriate characteristic in the right column.

A. Lingual thyroid	a. Failure of fusion
B. Thyroglossal duct cyst	b. Arises from perineural fibroblasts
C. Median rhomboid glossitis	c. Resection may necessitate lifelong medication
D. Granular cell myoblastoma	d. Surgical treatment involves resection of bone

Ref.: 4, 8

COMMENTS: The four entities listed above are among many benign conditions that may involve the tongue. **Lingual thyroid** results from failure of descent of the thyroid gland into the lower anterior neck. This results in the clinical appearance of a reddish brown mass emanating from the base of the tongue. Resection of a lingual thyroid may be necessary because of pharyngeal obstruction from the mass. One must be alert, however, to the possibility that this structure may represent the patient's only thyroid tissue. In such cases, resection would render the patient hypothyroid and necessitate thyroid replacement therapy. Thyroid scanning can establish the existence of other thyroid tissue. **Thyroglossal duct cysts**

also represent an anomaly of thyroid embryology in which there is failure of obliteration of the midline pharyngeal diverticulum during thyroid descent. Clinical presentation is that of a midline cystic mass, usually appearing during childhood or adolescence. Proper surgical treatment involves excision of the entire tract, including the midportion of the hyoid bone. **Median rhomboid glossitis** results from the failure of fusion of the lateral halves of the tongue. It is a clinically innocuous anomaly and requires no treatment. **Granular cell myoblastoma** is a benign proliferation of peripheral neurogenic elements of the Schwann cell that frequently occurs in the tongue. It may appear clinically similar to carcinoma of the tongue but has no malignant potential and is properly treated by local surgical excision.

ANSWER: A-c; B-d; C-a; D-b

26. With regard to carcinoma of the tongue, which of the following statements is/are true?

A. Most tongue carcinomas occur on the large dorsal surface.
B. Lymph node metastases are present in approximately half of all patients presenting with carcinoma of the tongue.
C. When tongue carcinomas are sufficiently large to involve the mandible, surgery is no longer an appropriate option, and the patient should be treated with radiation therapy.
D. Iron deficiency anemia may be associated with carcinoma of the tongue.

Ref.: 1, 2, 4, 8

COMMENTS: The epidemiology of carcinoma of the oral tongue is similar to that of other oral cavity tumors (male predominance, epidermoid carcinoma prevalence, history of tobacco and alcohol abuse). There is also an increased incidence of tongue carcinomas in patients with Plummer-Vinson syndrome (cervical dysphagia, iron deficiency anemia, atrophic oral mucosa, brittle spoon-shaped fingernails). Despite its larger surface area, the dorsum of the tongue is rarely the site of epidermoid carcinoma; most of these tumors occur on the lateral and ventral surfaces. Because 50% of patients with carcinoma of the tongue present with cervical lymph node metastases, combined treatment of the primary lesion with the ipsilateral cervical lymph nodes should be considered in most cases. Carcinoma of the tongue frequently presents with close approximation to, or invasion of, the inner table of the mandible. In such circumstances, resection must involve a partial mandibulectomy. Radiation therapy alone is unlikely to be successful with such large lesions, and most are currently treated with surgery in combination with radiation therapy or chemotherapy (or both).

ANSWER: B, D

27. With regard to mandibular trauma, which of the following statements is/are true?

A. Most fractures of the mandible are clinically undetectable, and radiographs are needed for diagnosis.
B. Most mandibular fractures are effectively treated with simple intermaxillary wiring or elastic band fixation.
C. Teeth lying within the fracture line of the mandible should be removed to prevent root abscesses.
D. For dislocations of the temporomandibular joint, open reduction and repair of the anterior capsule with the patient under general anesthesia are usually required.

Ref.: 4, 8

COMMENTS: The diagnosis of mandibular fracture is usually easily made on careful clinical examination; common signs to look for are point tenderness, malocclusion, intraoral mucosal ecchymosis and laceration, instability on bimanual manipulation, and numbness of the lower lip due to inferior alveolar nerve damage. Radiographs should be obtained to confirm the clinical impression and to search for associated occult facial bone fractures.

Most mandibular fractures are adequately treated by intermaxillary wiring or with arch bars and elastic band stabilization. Open reduction of mandibular fractures results in faster healing than after intermaxillary fixation and is gaining popularity.

It was formerly recommended that teeth lying within the fracture line be removed; more recently, however, it has been recognized that many of these teeth are salvageable if the fracture is managed conservatively.

Temporomandibular joint dislocations usually occur when the head of the mandibular condyle moves forward through a tear in the anterior joint capsule. This problem can usually be managed with injection of anesthetic into the joint capsule and downward traction on the posterior molar teeth. Cases of recurrent dislocation may require operative intervention.

ANSWER: B

28. Match each type of maxillary fracture in the left column with its appropriate anatomic description in the right column.

A. Le Fort I	a. Transverse maxillary fracture
B. Le Fort II	b. Craniofacial dissociation
C. Le Fort III	c. Pyramidal fractures

Ref.: 4, 8

COMMENTS: In 1900 Rene Le Fort classified midface fractures as described above. With Le Fort I fractures (transverse), fracture segments include the upper teeth, palate, lower portions of the pterygoid processes, and a portion of the wall of the maxillary sinus. Le Fort II fractures (pyramidal) also contain the nasal bones and frontal processes of the maxilla. Clinically, the malar eminences are usually not displaced, but there may be significant widening of the inner canthi of the eyes and bridge of the nose. Le Fort III fractures (craniofacial dissociation) involve separation of the maxillae, nasal bones, and zygomas from their usual cranial attachments. Treatment of these fractures is best carried out with direct operative exposure and miniplating of the fracture segments. The incidence of these injuries has decreased significantly with the increased use of air bags, shoulder–lap belts, padded dashboards, collapsible steering wheels, and the 55 mph speed limit. Multiple Le Fort fractures are common (e.g., a Le Fort I on one side with a Le Fort II on the other).

ANSWER: A-a; B-c; C-b

29. Match each of the tumors of the jaw in the left column with its appropriate characteristic in the right column.

A. Radicular cyst	a. Usually requires multimodality therapy
B. Ameloblastoma	b. Local excision or curettage is appropriate
C. Osteogenic sarcoma	c. Slow-growing malignancy with "soap-bubble" radiographic appearance
D. Carcinoma	d. May be metastatic from other primary site

Ref.: 4, 8

COMMENTS: Although the mandible and maxilla are most often involved in head and neck cancer by virtue of direct extension of contiguous epithelial tumors, a number of benign and malignant primary tumors of the jaws exist. **Radicular cysts** (dental cysts or root cysts) are usually easily diagnosed by their appropriate lucent appearance on radiographs. Local resection or enucleation with curettage of the cyst cavity is usually all that is required for treatment. **Ameloblastoma** (adamantinoma) is a slow-growing, low-grade malignancy that has the capability to metastasize to distant sites. The characteristic radiographic appearance is that of "soap bubbles." Wide excision with appropriate bone reconstruction is the treatment of choice. **Osteogenic sarcoma** may occur in either the mandible or maxilla and usually carries a grave prognosis. Wide surgical excision alone may be curative, but recent studies have shown improved results with multimodality therapy, including preoperative chemotherapy and possible adjuvant radiotherapy. **Carcinoma** from another site (most often breast, thyroid, or prostate) can metastasize to the mandible and present clinically as a primary tumor. Many other benign jaw cysts exist, and they require preoperative radiologic assessment and a histologic diagnosis before appropriate treatment can be instituted. These steps are necessary to avoid under- or overtreatment.

ANSWER: A-b; B-c; C-a; D-d

30. With regard to acute suppurative parotitis, which of the following statements is/are true?

A. Tends to occur in the elderly or debilitated patient.
B. Dehydration is a major contributing factor.
C. Immediate surgical drainage is mandatory.
D. *Staphylococcus aureus* is the organism most likely to be found.

Ref.: 1, 4, 8

COMMENTS: Acute suppurative parotitis is a severe, life-threatening infection most often seen in dehydrated elderly or debilitated patients. Its pathogenesis is thought to relate to stasis within the salivary ducts as a result of increased viscosity. *S. aureus* is the organism most often found in this severe infection. Initial treatment with appropriate intravenous hydration, heat, sialagogues, and antibiotics active against *Staphylococcus* may be successful. If improvement is not seen within 12 hours of initiating this treatment, surgical drainage is warranted.

ANSWER: A, B, D

31. With regard to nonneoplastic parotid disease, which of the following statements is/are true?

A. Lacerated Stensen's duct may be successfully reapproximated over a small-catheter stent.
B. Recurrent acute sialoadenitis is thought to be an ascending infection from the oral cavity.
C. Most calculi within the parotid duct are found near the duct orifice.
D. Parotidectomy, with its inherent risk of facial nerve injury, is considered too morbid a procedure for treatment of nonneoplastic conditions of the parotid gland.

Ref.: 1, 2, 4

COMMENTS: Transection of Stensen's duct should be repaired, if possible, with direct sutured approximation over a small-catheter stent. Ligation of the duct is sometimes required but may result in painful atrophy of the parotid gland, producing a contour deformity of the face.

Inflammatory conditions of the parotid gland include calculous disease and sialectasis, both of which may result in recurrent sialoadenitis. Infection is thought to result from ascending involvement of the parenchyma from the oral cavity by way of the major duct.

In the case of calculous disease, improper diet and abnormal salivary pH may predispose to the formation of stones in the major ducts. These stones are usually present near the duct orifice and may be successfully treated by incising the duct orifice and removing the stone transorally.

Occasionally, infections continue to occur despite stone extraction, alteration of diet and oral hygiene, stimulation of salivary secretions, adequate hydration, and antibiotics. In such circumstances, parotidectomy may be indicated. Observing the principles of facial nerve identification and dissection using the facial nerve monitor reduces the risk of the operation.

ANSWER: A, B, C

32. With regard to the anatomy of the salivary glands, which of the following statements is/are true?

A. The parotid gland is divided into two well defined lobes (superficial and deep) based on the neurovascular supply of the gland and embryologic lobar encapsulation.
B. The facial nerve and its branches course superficial to the external parotid fascia and therefore may be injured during parotid surgery.
C. Injury to one or more branches of the facial nerve may occur during operations on the submandibular salivary gland as well as on the parotid gland.
D. There are approximately 40–60 minor salivary glands scattered in the submucosal plane of the oral cavity of most individuals.

Ref.: 4, 8

COMMENTS: Were it not for the relation of the parotid gland to the facial nerve, parotid surgery would not be particularly challenging technically. The parotid gland is a unilobar structure embryologically and is considered clinically to be divided into a superficial and deep lobe as defined by the portions of the gland that lie, respectively, superficial and deep to the facial nerve, which ramifies through the gland.

Superficial lobe tumors necessitate identification of the trunk and branches of the facial nerve, with dissection of the tumor and superficial lobe off the underlying nerve. Deep lobe tumors are usually approached by an initial superficial lobectomy followed by removal of the deep lobe from between or underneath the branches of the facial nerve.

Injury to the marginal mandibular branch of the facial nerve may also occur during submandibular salivary gland surgery, as this nerve courses deep to the platysma over the external facial vessels, which are in close approximation to the lateral capsule of the gland. The lingual and hypoglossal nerves are also at risk during submandibular gland surgery and should be identified to avoid inadvertent injury.

Minor salivary glands, formerly and incorrectly considered to be ectopic salivary tissue, are scattered throughout the submucosal plane of the entire upper aerodigestive tract. They are particularly numerous in the oral cavity underneath the palatal, buccal, and labial mucosa. In normal individuals, the minor salivary glands probably number 700–1000.

ANSWER: C

33. Match each site of salivary gland tumor in the left column with its likelihood of being malignant in the right column.

A. Parotid gland	a. 75%
B. Submandibular gland	b. 50%
C. Minor salivary gland	c. 25%

Ref.: 1, 2, 4, 8

COMMENTS: The above likelihood of malignancy of the various salivary gland tumors is a rough approximation, with variation depending on the series cited. Although the likelihood of a given tumor being malignant is lowest in the parotid gland (approximately 25%), followed by the submandibular salivary gland (approximately 50%), and minor salivary glands (approximately 75%), one must remember that because approximately 70% of all salivary gland tumors occur in the parotid gland that gland accounts for most of the malignant salivary gland tumors. Although the sublingual gland is considered by many to be a major salivary gland, the likelihood of malignancy in sublingual glands is approximately that seen in minor salivary glands. The clinical approach to tumors of the sublingual gland is likewise similar to that for minor salivary gland tumors.

ANSWER: A-c; B-b; C-a

34. Match each histologic type of salivary gland tumor in the left column with its appropriate characteristic in the right column.

A. Pleomorphic adenoma	a. High likelihood of perineural involvement
B. Warthin's tumor	b. Most common salivary gland tumor
C. Mucoepidermoid carcinoma	c. Widest range of biologic aggressiveness
D. Adenoid cystic carcinoma	d. May represent malignant change in a previously benign tumor
E. Malignant mixed tumor	e. Marked male predominace

Ref.: 1, 2, 4, 8

COMMENTS: Tumors of the major and minor salivary glands represent a broad array of clinical presentations and biologic variability. Among the benign tumors, the **pleomorphic adenoma** (benign mixed tumor) is the most common overall. It is found most often in the parotid gland and is best managed by appropriate lobectomy with dissection of the facial nerve. Attempts to remove this tumor by a more limited "enucleation" have led to a 40–50% recurrence rate. The second most common benign tumor is **Warthin's tumor** (papillary cystadenoma lymphomatosum). These tumors are more common in males and may be bilateral (10%). One can sometimes detect a cystic component to this type of tumor on physical examination. **Mucoepidermoid carcinomas** as a group represent a wide range of biologic aggressiveness. Low-grade mucoepidermoid carcinomas carry a good prognosis, whereas high-grade mucoepidermoid carcinomas are rarely controlled by surgery alone and carry a poor prognosis. **Adenoid cystic carcinoma** (formerly cylindroma) is characterized by an indolent clinical course in which there may be long disease-free intervals followed by local or regional recurrence. A 5- or even 10-year disease-free status is no guarantee against eventual recurrence. These tumors have a propensity to invade and proliferate along nerves, which may account for their high likelihood of local recurrence. **Malignant mixed tumors** are considered by many clinicians to be a malignant transformation of a previously benign mixed tumor. This possibility has been suggested by finding malignant elements in tumors that otherwise appear to be pleomorphic adenomas, which supports the generally held surgical principle that major salivary gland tumors should be removed, even if they have been present and unchanged for many years.

ANSWER: A-b; B-e; C-c; D-a; E-d

35. With regard to the technical aspects of parotid surgery, which of the following statements is/are true?

A. The facial nerve is best identified by locating its trunk after it has exited the stylomastoid foramen near the posterior aspect of the parotid gland.
B. Complete postoperative paralysis of the muscles supplied by one or more divisions of the facial nerve suggests that there has been disruption of, or permanent injury to, that division during surgery.
C. The auriculotemporal nerve, although not specifically sought during parotid surgery, may be involved in postoperative morbidity.
D. Sectioning the facial nerve during parotid surgery results in permanent degeneration of the nerve distal to the cut, making attempts at nerve reconstruction futile.
E. The greater auricular nerve is rarely injured during parotid surgery, as it lies outside the usual anatomic borders of parotid dissection.

Ref.: 1, 2, 4

COMMENTS: Proper identification and preservation of the facial nerve and its branches are the keys to successful parotid surgery. Formerly, it was believed that most parotid malignancies should be treated by radical parotidectomy with deliberate sacrifice of the facial nerve. Currently, it is generally thought that deliberate sacrifice of the nerve or its branches may be required only in instances of direct nerve invasion by tumor. Nerve preservation and adjuvant postoperative radiation therapy have yielded local control rates equivalent to those seen with more radical surgery but without the inherent morbidity of facial nerve sacrifice. The facial nerve is best protected by identifying its trunk as it exits the stylomastoid foramen at the posterior aspect of the gland. Meticulous attention to technique, knowledge of surgical landmarks, and use of a facial nerve monitor make identification safer. When scarring or tumor prevents dissection in this area, the nerve may be found in a retrograde fashion by dissecting out its more peripheral branches first. Paresis or even complete paralysis of the muscles supplied by the facial nerve may occur in the absence of obvious nerve injury. This is almost always a temporary phenomenon, and function usually returns within several months. If the facial nerve or one of its major branches is deliberately or inadvertently cut during parotid surgery, immediate nerve repair or interposition nerve graft should be attempted, as there is at least some expectation of partial recovery in such circumstances. When this fails, there are numerous techniques of neuromusculofascial transfers that may be employed in an effort to restore facial symmetry and animation. Although the auriculotemporal nerve is not specifically sought during parotid surgery, its disruption and subsequent possible cross-reinnervation with branches of the sympathetic supply to the skin may result in postoperative gustatory sweating (Frey syndrome). The most frequently injured nerve during parotid surgery is not the facial nerve but the greater auricular nerve, which ramifies through the posteroinferior portion of the gland. Sectioning the nerve produces numbness of the lower portion of the auricle and periauricular skin.

ANSWER: A, C

36. During performance of a classic radical neck dissection, which of the following structures is/are routinely sacrificed?

A. Internal jugular vein.
B. Phrenic nerve.
C. Spinal accessory nerve.
D. Sternocleidomastoid muscle.
E. Levator scapulae muscle.
F. External carotid artery.

Ref.: 1, 2, 8

COMMENTS: The classic radical neck dissection is an operation designed to remove the lymph node-bearing tissue that accompanies the great vessels within the carotid sheath as well as that found in the submandibular and posterior cervical triangles. The dissection involves removal of the sternocleidomastoid muscle, internal jugular vein, spinal accessory nerve, and submandibular salivary gland and the associated lymph node-bearing fibrofatty tissue. Although branches of the external carotid artery may be sacrificed during this operation, the external, internal, and common carotid arteries are left intact. The cervical branch of the facial nerve is, of necessity, sacrificed, but the marginal branch is preserved. The sensory branches of the anterior roots of C-2, C-3, and C-4 are sacrificed during the procedure, accounting for the relatively low level of pain during the postoperative period. The lingual nerve, hypoglossal nerve, and phrenic nerve with its contributing cervical roots are preserved, as are the branches of the brachial plexus and the intrinsic deep musculature of the neck.

ANSWER: A, C, D

37. With regard to modifications of the standard approach to neck dissections, which of the following statements is/are true?

A. Bilateral simultaneous radical neck dissections are well tolerated and should be performed in cases of midline lesions that may have metastasized to either side of the neck.
B. The term "modified neck dissection" refers to the dissection of all but the posterior triangle portion of the classic radical neck dissection.
C. Modified neck dissection may be used for treatment of the clinically negative neck in which there is a significant risk of occult nodal metastases.
D. The dissection and preservation of the spinal accessory nerve significantly reduce the morbidity of neck dissection in most patients.

Ref.: 1, 2, 8

COMMENTS: Occasionally, clinical bilateral cervical nodal disease necessitates bilateral radical neck dissection. Such an operation significantly increases the morbidity associated with the surgery in terms of marked facial and pharyngeal edema, orbital edema, and occasionally changes in mental status due to increases in central nervous system venous pressures. Temporally staging the neck dissections (to allow some collaterals to develop) and preserving one of the internal jugular veins, if technically feasible, may reduce these postoperative risks. Prophylactic or elective bilateral simultaneous neck dissections should be avoided.

The terms used for neck dissection mean different things to different surgeons; in general, however, for the *modified neck dissection* the lymph node-bearing areas are dealt with as for the classic radical neck dissection but with preservation of one or more of the following: sternocleidomastoid muscle, internal jugular vein, or spinal accessory nerve. This technique has gained acceptance for dissection of the clinically negative neck that is being explored because of the possibility of occult nodal disease; in fact, it is recommended by many for the clinically node-negative neck with a more than 30% likelihood of harboring occult lymph node metastases. The modified neck dissection is also valuable for managing the clinically positive neck in patients with metastatic well differentiated thyroid cancer.

The shoulder droop, discomfort, and weakness that accompany loss of the spinal accessory nerve are major sources of morbidity following neck dissection. In patients who are candidates for modified neck dissection, preservation of this nerve significantly reduces the likelihood of this aspect of postoperative morbidity. Selective node dissection entails preservation of one or more lymph node groups. With these dissections the internal jugular vein, sternocleidomastoid muscle, and spinal accessory nerve are routinely spared.

ANSWER: C, D

38. With regard to the diagnosis and management of a solitary lump in the neck, which of the following statements is/are true?

A. A 1-month period of observation and antibiotic therapy should be carried out in all patients because of the possibility of the lump being an inflammatory lymph node.
B. The first step in management is an incisional or excisional biopsy to establish the diagnosis, avoiding other unnecessary testing.
C. One must consider primary tumors in the chest and abdomen to be potential sources of cervical lymph node metastases.
D. Radical neck dissection should not be performed for metastatic cervical disease if the primary tumor has not been found.

Ref.: 1, 2, 8

COMMENTS: Solitary lumps in the neck may represent congenital abnormalities, inflammatory lymph nodes, metastatic carcinoma from sites in the upper aerodigestive tract, metastases from sites other than the upper aerodigestive tract (e.g., lung, breast, gastrointestinal tract, kidney), lymphoma, or rare primary tumors (e.g., carotid body tumor). The age of the patient, clinical presentation, and physical characteristics of the mass frequently give some indication as to the nature of the pathology. The first step of management should be a thorough examination of the head and neck area, including indirect laryngoscopy and nasopharyngoscopy. If no primary pathology is found in the upper aerodigestive tract and the mass is thought clinically to be inflammatory in nature, it is reasonable to observe it over a brief period (2–4 weeks) with or without antibiotics. If the mass persists or enlarges during this time, one must consider the diagnosis of neoplasm. Any mass that is hard is neoplastic until proven otherwise. Fine-needle aspiration (FNA) for cytology and culture should be considered as an early diagnostic test insofar as it is safe, is accurate when positive, and has not been shown to result in implantation of tumor cells along the needle tract if a 21-gauge or smaller needle is used. One must not, however, accept a negative needle aspiration result if the clinical index of suspicion of malignancy is high. Further workup before biopsy includes CT neck scans, chest radiography, and, if indicated by the results of the FNA biopsy, a gastrointestinal workup. Incisional or excisional biopsy of the mass may be required to establish the diagnosis but should be preceded by panendoscopy (direct laryngopharyngoscopy, bronchoscopy, and esophagoscopy) to search for an occult upper aerodigestive tract primary tumor. Direct laryngoscopy under anesthesia should include multiple random biopsies of the likely sites of occult primary tumors (e.g., nasopharynx, tonsillar fossa, valleculae, base of tongue, and piriform sinus). When no primary tumor is found despite these efforts, open biopsy may be performed; but the patient and physician must be prepared for a neck dissection if metastatic squamous cell carcinoma is found. Neck dissection for an unknown primary tumor should be followed by irradiation to the pharynx and the neck. Approximately one-third of the patients so managed survive 5 years free of disease despite the fact that the primary tumor may never be found. A finding of adenocarcinoma suggests the gastrointestinal tract, breast, or lung as likely primary sites. One must remember, however, that salivary gland malignancies can metastasize to regional nodes.

ANSWER: C

39. With regard to the use of chemotherapy for regionally advanced head and neck cancer, which of the following statements is/are true?

A. Neoadjuvant chemotherapy has improved disease control and survival.
B. Combining chemotherapy with irradiation has improved disease control and survival.
C. Alternating cycles of chemotherapy with irradiation has improved disease control and survival.
D. Adjuvant chemotherapy, given after surgery and irradiation, has improved disease control and survival.

Ref.: 9

COMMENTS: Chemotherapy for management of head and neck cancer confined to local/regional sites may be utilized in one of three ways: neoadjuvant chemotherapy, giving a course of chemotherapy prior to surgery or irradiation; combined modality therapy, giving chemotherapy concomitantly with local/regional radiation therapy; and conventional adjuvant therapy, giving chemotherapy to a clinically disease-free patient following definitive local/regional therapy. **Neoadjuvant chemotherapy** with cisplatin and 5-fluorouracil (5-FU) infusion for three cycles prior to other local therapy has produced the highest complete response rate (25–55% of cases in most series) of the many induction chemotherapy regimens reported. However, this regimen and all other neoadjuvant regimens that have been tested in randomized trials have failed to improve disease control or survival over regional treatment alone. A singular exception to these negative findings exists with intraarterial methotrexate or intraarterial bleomycin and vincristine. Randomized studies of these drugs have shown improved control of early, predominantly intraoral cancers. Because regionally advanced cancers extend beyond any one arterial supply, however, intraarterial chemotherapy would not be expected to include the entire disease extent, thereby explaining the failure of this approach in such situations. In contrast, randomized studies of **combined-modality therapy,** adding just one drug to radiation therapy, have shown improved disease control with either 5-FU, methotrexate, bleomycin, mitomycin C, or cisplatin. Each of these drugs also improved survival over irradiation alone, but only the studies with 5-FU, methotrexate, and cisplatin showed a significant difference. Randomized studies with cisplatin, 5-FU infusion, and concomitant irradiation, with a split course of irradiation, have also improved disease control compared to cisplatin and 5-FU neoadjuvant chemotherapy followed by irradiation. These studies justify the addition of chemotherapy to irradiation in patients with inoperable head and neck cancer or to postoperative irradiation on patients with poor prognostic features (e.g., extracapsular spread in node-positive patients), as median survival with irradiation alone is 12 months or less. Alternating 1 week of cisplatin and 5-FU chemotherapy with 2 weeks of irradiation for three cycles has also shown disease control and survival benefit over conventional irradiation alone, with low toxicity in those with inoperable head and neck cancer. **Conventional adjuvant chemotherapy**, on the other hand, has been poorly accepted by patients, with up to 70% of patients not completing treatment. It may reduce the incidence of distant metastases, but regional disease control (the more frequent and more morbid problem) has not improved; therefore the survival benefit is limited. Thus, it appears that combined modality therapy offers the opportunity for disease control and long-term survival in patients with locally advanced head and neck cancer and may in fact be preferred in cases in which surgical therapy would be functionally or cosmetically disabling.

ANSWER: B, C

40. Which of the following statements regarding Kaposi's sarcoma (KS) are true?

A. Oral and pharyngeal mucosa are common sites for KS.
B. Severe odynophagia and dysphagia are often seen with oral KS.
C. The primary goal of treating KS is prevention of malignant degeneration.
D. The primary goal of treating KS is palliation of symptoms.
E. KS is the most common neoplasm associated with acquired human immunodeficiency syndrome (AIDS).

Ref.: 10

COMMENTS: Human immunodeficiency virus (HIV)-infected patients experience a variety of problems related to the head and neck. Kaposi's sarcoma, once rare, is now the most common neoplasm associated with AIDS. Interestingly, hemophiliacs with AIDS do not have KS, whereas 43% of homosexual or bisexual AIDS patients and 4% of intravenous drug abusers have the neoplasm. Symptoms are minor until the lesion undergoes ulceration or secondary infection; pharyngeal or laryngeal KS may cause airway obstruction. Treatment is primarily palliative. Although low dose radiotherapy is effective for cutaneous KS, mucosal lesions do not respond satisfactorily. Laser ablation, photodynamic therapy, and intralesional vinblastine have been tried with varying degrees of success. Ultimate survival is determined by the infectious complications of AIDS, not by the neoplasm.

ANSWER: A, B, D, E

REFERENCES

1. Cummings CW: Otolaryngology: *Head and Neck Surgery*, 2nd ed. CV Mosby, St. Louis, 1993.
2. Thawley S, Panje W: *Comprehensive Management of Head and Neck Tumors*. WB Saunders, Philadelphia, 1998.
3. Gates GA: *Current Therapy in Otolaryngology: Head and Neck Surgery*, 6th ed. Mosby, St. Louis, 1998.
4. Sabiston DC Jr: *Textbook of Surgery*, 15th ed. WB Saunders, Philadelphia, 1997.
5. Myers EN, Sven JY: *Cancer of the Head and Neck*, 3rd ed. WB Saunders, Philadelphia, 1996.
6. Bailey BJ: *Head and Neck Surgery: Otolaryngology*. JB Lippincott, Philadelphia, 1993.
7. Eisele DW: *Complications in Head and Neck Surgery*. CV Mosby, St. Louis, 1993.
8. Schwartz SI, Shires GT, Spencer FC: *Principles of Surgery*, 7th ed. McGraw-Hill, New York, 1999.
9. Economou SG, Witt TR, Deziel DJ, et al: *Adjuncts to Cancer Surgery*. Lea & Febiger, Philadelphia, 1991.
10. Tami TA, Lee KC: *AIDS and the Otolaryngologist*. A Self Instructional Package from the American Academy of Otolaryngology, Head and Neck Surgery Foundation, Inc. Rochester, New York, 1993.

CHAPTER 21

Thyroid

1. With regard to the vascular structures and their relations to the thyroid gland, which of the following is/are true?

   A. Thyroidea ima arteries can arise from the aorta.
   B. The superior thyroid artery originates from the external carotid, and the inferior thyroid originates from the subclavian artery.
   C. The inferior thyroid artery is in close proximity to the recurrent laryngeal nerve, which generally runs posterior to the artery.
   D. The superior thyroid artery supplies the parathyroid glands.
   E. Venous vessels parallel the arterial circulation.
   F. The superior laryngeal nerve can be injured when ligating the superior thyroid artery.

Ref.: 1, 2, 3

COMMENTS: The thyroid gland is a highly vascular organ that is second only to the carotid body in this respect. It is supplied by two superior and two inferior arteries. The superior thyroid arteries branch from the external carotid artery just above the carotid bifurcation. The inferior thyroid arteries arise from the thyrocervical trunk and course posterior to the carotid sheath then downward and medial to enter the middle of the thyroid gland. The inferior thyroid arteries also provide blood supply to the superior and inferior parathyroid glands. The relation with the recurrent laryngeal nerve has important surgical implications. In 1–4% of individuals, thyroidea ima arteries arise from either the innominate artery or aorta. They generally course along the trachea and then enter the lower surface of the isthmus. Venous drainage of the thyroid gland is comprised of three pairs of principal veins. The superior thyroid veins course along with the superior thyroid artery and then empty into the internal jugular vein. The middle thyroid vein, present in only 50% of individuals, drains directly into the internal jugular vein. This vein is ligated during thyroid surgery to provide adequate mobilization of the thyroid lobe. Inferior thyroid veins follow the course of the thyrothymic ligament prior to draining into the innominate or brachiocephalic veins.

ANSWER: A, C, F

2. With regard to the anatomic relation of the thyroid gland to nearby nerves, which of the following statements is/are true?

   A. Both superior and inferior thyroid arteries bear a fairly constant relation to the recurrent laryngeal nerves.
   B. The superior laryngeal nerves provide both sensory and motor function to the larynx.
   C. Injury to the external branch of the superior laryngeal nerve may go unnoticed in most individuals.
   D. The "recurrent" nature of the recurrent laryngeal nerves is one of the few anatomic relations for which anomalies or variations have not been reported.
   E. Unilateral recurrent laryngeal nerve injury results in airway compromise that may necessitate tracheostomy.

Ref.: 1, 2, 3, 4

COMMENTS: The thyroid gland is innervated via sympathetic fibers from the cervical ganglion and parasympathetic fibers from the vagus that reach the gland through the laryngeal nerves. Because of their proximity to the gland, the laryngeal nerves are at risk of injury during thyroidectomy.

The **superior laryngeal** nerve provides both sensory and motor function to the larynx. Its external branch provides motor innervation to the cricothyroid muscle and is at risk during thyroid surgery because of its close relation to the superior thyroid vessels. Injury to this nerve branch results in bowing of the vocal cord during phonation; this effect may go unnoticed except in individuals such as singers who find themselves unable to reach high-pitched notes or professional speakers who notice an increased fatigability of their voice.

The **recurrent laryngeal** nerve is so named because of its oblique course around the subclavian artery on the right and the aorta near the ductus arteriosus on the left. The nerve then ascends on either side in the tracheoesophageal sulcus to the thyroid gland. The relation of the recurrent nerve to the inferior thyroid artery is variable. In 75% of persons the nerve traverses posterior to the inferior thyroid artery, whereas in 25% it courses anterior to the artery and in as many as 10% it courses over the thyroid gland before entering the larynx.

In rare instances (<0.5% of persons) and almost exclusively on the right side, a **nonrecurrent** nerve exists, usually in association with vascular anomalies of the aortic arch. In such circumstances the nerve approaches the cricothyroid membrane obliquely from above, and during thyroid surgery it may be inadvertently divided if not recognized.

The recurrent laryngeal nerve provides motor function to most of the intrinsic laryngeal muscles, and its unilateral injury results in paralysis of the vocal cord, which changes the quality of the voice but rarely compromises the airway. Bilateral recurrent laryngeal nerve injury, in contrast, may severely compromise airflow, necessitating tracheostomy.

ANSWER: B, C

3. With regard to thyroid anatomy and associated structures, which of the following is/are true?

A. Delphian lymph nodes are located along the internal jugular vein.
B. The ligament of Berry is a posteromedial suspensory ligament that is in close relation to the recurrent laryngeal nerve.
C. The tubercle of Zuckerkandl is the most lateral posterior extension of thyroid tissue and is closely associated with the recurrent laryngeal nerve.
D. The tubercle of Zuckerkandl is removed during a subtotal thyroidectomy.
E. Injury to the loop of Galen is associated with ligation of the superior thyroid artery.

Ref.: 1, 2, 3

COMMENTS: The thyroid gland lies in the visceral compartment covered with a thin layer of connective tissue derived from pretracheal fascia. **Delphian lymph nodes** are closely associated with the pyramidal process and are enveloped by pretracheal fascia. Another name for the **ligament of Berry** is the posteromedial suspensory ligament. The location of this ligament is surgically important owing to its close proximity to the recurrent laryngeal nerve. In most patients the nerve lies lateral to the ligament of Berry, but in 25% of patients the ligament surrounds the nerve. The most lateral posterior extension of thyroid tissue is referred to as the **tubercle of Zuckerkandl**. To identify the location of the recurrent laryngeal nerve, this portion of thyroid tissue must be rotated medially. Because of the posterior location and close approximation to the recurrent laryngeal nerve, this portion of tissue is left behind during subtotal thyroidectomy. The superior laryngeal nerve branch of the vagus arises high in the neck and descends medial and deep to the internal carotid artery along the pharynx toward the superior cornu of the hyoid bone. It lies on the middle constrictor muscle and divides into internal and external branches. The **loop of Galen** is where the pharyngeal branches of the recurrent laryngeal nerve communicate with the branches of the superior laryngeal nerve. This structure may be injured when dissecting/ligating the superior thyroid artery.

ANSWER: B, C, E

4. With regard to anomalous variations in thyroid embryologic development, which of the following statements is/are true?

A. Lingual thyroid tissue should always be removed because it carries a high risk of malignancy.
B. Removal of a thyroglossal duct cyst generally requires resection of the midportion of the hyoid bone to prevent cyst recurrence.
C. In 70% of patients with lingual thyroid, it is the only thyroid tissue.
D. Most mediastinal thyroid glands result from an abnormally caudad embryologic descent.
E. So-called lateral aberrant thyroid rests may in fact be metastases of well-differentiated thyroid cancer.

Ref.: 1, 2, 3, 4, 5

COMMENTS: Embryologically, the thyroid gland is derived from the endoderm of the primitive foregut. It results from a median endodermal downgrowth from the first and second pharyngeal pouches in the area of the foramen cecum. These cells separate from the pharyngeal connections by the fifth gestational week and migrate caudally. During their descent, the follicular cells fuse with parafollicular cells, which are derived from the ultimobranchial bodies of the fourth and fifth branchial pouches. Abnormalities in descent of the thyroid tissue from the pharyngeal floor may result in a lingual thyroid or persistence of solid or cystic structures along the course of the midline descent, which results, respectively, in a persistent **pyramidal lobe** or a **thyroglossal duct cyst**.

In about 70% of patients with **lingual thyroids** it represents the only thyroid tissue. It is rarely symptomatic unless it enlarges and produces pharyngeal obstruction. It carries a 3% risk of becoming malignant. Treatment by radioiodine ablation or surgical excision is required only for symptoms or suspicion of malignancy.

A **thyroglossal duct cyst** may occur anywhere in the midline from the base of the tongue to the thyroid gland, but it is generally found just inferior to the hyoid bone. The cyst classically moves upward with swallowing. These lesions should be removed because they are susceptible to infections and in rare instances may be premalignant. Removal of the cyst generally requires resection of the midportion of the hyoid bone to prevent recurrence.

Although the initial embryologic descent of the thyroid may proceed into an abnormally caudad position, resulting in a mediastinal or substernal thyroid, most intrathoracic goiters represent inferior extensions of acquired pathologic processes in a normally located gland.

Most benign "**lateral aberrant thyroid rests**," in fact, represent metastases of well-differentiated thyroid cancers. This is certainly true when papillary features or severely atypical follicular features are found. However, failure of lateral thyroid elements to be incorporated into the thyroid capsule occasionally results in embryologic thyroid rests in the lateral neck.

ANSWER: B, C, E

5. With regard to thyroid hormone synthesis and physiology, which of the following statements is/are true?

A. The iodide used in thyroid hormone synthesis is derived primarily from dietary sources.
B. The amino acid threonine binds to iodine to form active thyroid hormone.
C. When the active thyroid hormones triiodothyronine (T_3) and thyroxine (T_4) are released into the plasma, they bind to thyroglobulin for transport.
D. In the periphery, T_3 is converted to the metabolically more active T_4.
E. Thyroid-stimulating hormone (TSH) regulates most aspects of iodine uptake and oxidation.

Ref.: 1, 3, 4, 5, 7

COMMENTS: Thyroid hormones play an active regulatory role in many aspects of energy substrate metabolism, including increased oxygen consumption and calorigenesis, stimulation of protein synthesis, regulation of most aspects of carbohydrate metabolism, and metabolism of cholesterol and phospholipids.

Thyroid hormone synthesis begins with the active transport of iodide (a process referred to as *iodide trapping*) from dietary sources into the thyroid gland, in which iodide is oxidized by thyroid peroxidase to iodine. Successive organic iodinization

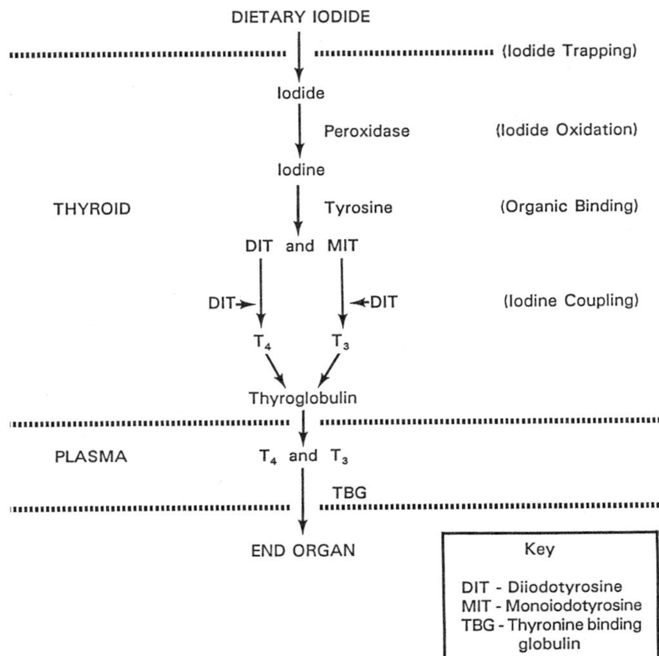

of tyrosine to monoiodotyrosine (MIT) and diiodotyrosine (DIT) results in the eventual production of triidothyronine (T_3) and tetraiodothyronine (T_4). Through a process of coupling, two molecules of DIT form T_4, and one of DIT and one of MIT form T_3. There is evidence that T_3 may be formed from T_4 within the thyroid and in the peripheral circulation. T_3 and T_4 are stored in the thyroid bound to the protein thyroglobulin. When cleaved from thyroglobulin, T_3 and T_4 are released into the plasma and become bound to thyronine-binding globulin (TBG) for transport. In plasma the T_4/T_3 ratio is between 10:1 and 20:1. Most T_4 is converted to T_3, which is several times more active than T_4 and accounts for approximately half the metabolic effect of the thyroid hormone. Most of the aspects of iodide uptake, oxidation, organic iodine binding, and thyroid hormone release are regulated by TSH, which is synthesized and released from the anterior pituitary gland. Thyrotropin-releasing hormone (TRH), which is produced in the hypothalamus, and both thyroid hormones modulate TSH secretion. Thyroid hormones inhibit TSH release, whereas TRH stimulates TSH production.

ANSWER: A, E

6. With regard to thyroid scanning, which of the following statements is/are true?

A. The dose of radiation delivered to the thyroid is the same regardless of whether iodine 131 (^{131}I), iodine 123 (^{123}I), or technetium 99m (^{99m}Tc) is used.
B. Thyroid scanning is useful for assessing the thyroid gland when it is normally located, but it does not evaluate ectopic thyroid tissue.
C. Thyroid scintigraphy is highly accurate even for detecting lesions as small as 1 cm in diameter.
D. Metastases from well-differentiated thyroid carcinoma are unlikely to be detected by ^{131}I imaging if substantial normal thyroid tissue is present.

Ref.: 1, 3, 4, 5, 6, 7

COMMENTS: See Question 7.

7. Match each thyroid test in the left column with one or more appropriate test characteristics in the right column.

A. ^{99m}Tc
B. ^{131}I
C. Ultrasonography
D. T_3 and T_4 assays
E. Fine-needle aspiration (FNA) biopsy
F. Thyroid autoantibodies

a. May be used in conjunction with TSH level to determine thyroid function and status of the thyroid/pituitary feedback mechanism
b. Useful for identifying metastatic deposits of differentiated thyroid cancer
c. May be used to treat cystic thyroid nodules and determine the need for operating on solid thyroid nodules
d. Low-radiation nuclide used to provide information about the function of a thyroid nodule
e. May provide information on thyroid anatomy and the solid or cystic nature of thyroid nodules
f. Useful for diagnosing Graves' disease and Hashimoto's thyroiditis

Ref.: 1, 3, 4, 6

COMMENTS: Thyroid scanning involves measuring the emitted radioactivity of a radionuclide that is taken up by the thyroid gland. The nuclides technetium 99m pertechnetate (^{99m}Tc) and iodine (both ^{123}I and ^{131}I) are used primarily to assess the function of nodules (generally those >1.5 cm in diameter) within the thyroid gland but also to identify ectopic thyroid tissue such as a lingual thyroid. ^{99m}Tc and ^{123}I are the standard agents used because the radiation exposure to the patient is relatively small (10 and 30 mrad, respectively). ^{131}I (500 mrad) remains useful for detecting distant metastases of differentiated thyroid cancer and for detecting retrosternal thyroid masses. The use of ^{131}I for detecting thyroid metastases is limited by the presence of normally functioning thyroid tissue, which preferentially takes up the iodine. The amount of radioactivity detected during the scan is a measure of the thyroid uptake of the nuclide and thus indirectly indicates the metabolic activity of the gland. **Ultrasonography** of the thyroid is useful for determining the number and distribution of thyroid nodules and whether they are cystic or solid; but it does not assess thyroid function. **Thyroid hormone** (T_3 or T_4) and **TSH** assays of peripheral blood are useful for determining the presence of hyper- or hypofunction of the gland and the status of the thyroid/pituitary feedback mechanism. The TSH level is more sensitive to subclinical hypothyroidism than are the thyroid hormone levels. **Fine-needle aspiration** biopsy is the prime method of evaluating thyroid nodules. Cystic lesions with a negative cytologic evaluation can be entirely treated by aspiration. If the lesion is solid, cytologic studies can be performed to estimate the likelihood of underlying malignancy and to determine reliably the need for resection. To decrease the already low rate of false-negative diagnoses, current recommendations are for repeat aspiration of cytologically benign nodules at a later time. Atypical, suspicious, or malignant cytologic findings mandate resection. High titers of **thyroid**

autoantibodies may be useful for identifying Graves' disease (hyperfunction) or Hashimoto's disease (hyper- or hypofunction).

ANSWER:
Question 6: D
Question 7: A-d; B-b; C-e; D-a; E-c; F-f

8. With regard to thyroid function tests, which of the following statements is/are true?

A. Estrogens increase the amount of TBG and therefore may falsely suggest hyperthyroidism.
B. Administration of exogenous thyroid may lead to an increase in the radioactive iodine uptake (RAIU).
C. Both barium enema and intravenous pyelography can affect the RAIU.
D. Failure of exogenous T_3 to suppress TSH secretion may be seen in Graves' disease and in toxic adenomas.

Ref.: 1, 4, 5, 6

COMMENTS: Most plasma T_4 assays measure total T_4, which reflects the amount bound to TBG as well as T_4. Estrogen administration or pregnancy usually results in elevated TBG values, which elevates the total T_4 level even though the patient has a normal free T_4 level and is not hyperthyroid. Androgens have the opposite effect. Administration of exogenous thyroid hormone or of dietary or intravenous iodine usually results in a reduction of RAIU even though the patient is clinically not hypothyroid. Contrast studies that do not involve iodine use do not affect the iodine uptake assay. Normally, plasma TSH levels should fall to 50% of control values when T_3 is administered for 7–10 days. In conditions exhibiting autonomous function of the thyroid (as may be seen in Graves' disease and toxic adenomas) TSH may already be suppressed, and further depression cannot be obtained by administration of exogenous thyroid hormone.

ANSWER: A, D

9. With regard to thyroid function tests, which of the following is/are true?

A. TSH levels are decreased in hyperthyroidism.
B. Suppression of iodine uptake in patients with increased T_3 and T_4 levels is pathognomonic for subacute thyroiditis.
C. Serum antibodies (antimicrosomal and antithyroglobulin) are present in both Graves' disease and Hashimoto's thyroiditis.
D. The TRH assay can evaluate the pituitary TSH-secreting mechanism.
E. The RAIU is elevated in patients receiving L-thyroxine or iodine.

Ref.: 1, 2, 3

COMMENTS: Many consider the measurement of **circulating TSH** concentrations to be the single best test of thyroid function in most patients. Normal levels are between 0.4 and 4.2 μU/ml. Hypothyroid patients have a TSH level of more than 4.0, whereas hyperthyroid patients have a level less than 0.5.

Serum T_4 assay is completed by measuring the total T_4 by radioimmunoassay (RIA). Both bound and free T_4 levels are measured. Total T_4 levels are elevated in most patients with hyperthyroidism but are also elevated in normal patients who have elevated TBG levels from estrogen use, pregnancy, and congenital TBG excess. Total T_4 levels are reduced in patients with hypothyroidism, with nephrotic syndrome, or who are taking anabolic steroids. The increase in serum T_3 and T_4 levels with thyroiditis and consequent hyperthyroidism result from leakage of colloid and thyroid hormone into the interstitial tissue and blood from disrupted follicles. Suppression of iodine uptake in patients with increased T_3 and T_4 levels is pathognomonic for subacute thyroiditis.

The **TRH** stimulation test determines the functional status of the pituitary TSH secretory mechanism. It has currently been replaced by the more sensitive serum TSH assay. Its use is confined to evaluating pituitary gland function. Serum thyroid antibodies such as anti-microsomal and anti-thyroglobulin may be present in autoimmune diseases such as Hashimoto's thyroiditis and Graves' disease. About 80% of patients with Hashimoto's thyroiditis have detectable autoantibodies.

RAIU is also an effective measure of thyroid function but is less frequently used. This study works on the premise that more iodine is trapped by the thyroid in those with hyperthyroidism, resulting in an elevated value. The opposite is true for hypothyroidism. Importantly, both L-thyroxine and iodine administration during radiologic studies such as angiography, computed tomography (CT), and cystography can give falsely low results.

ANSWER: A, B, C, D

10. Ultrasonography is beneficial for which of the following clinical applications in the neck?

A. Defining cystic versus solid thyroid nodules.
B. Facilitating fine-needle aspiration (FNA) in patients with difficult-to-palpate nodules.
C. Assess thyroid nodules and their response to therapy.
D. Demonstrate parathyroid and cervical lymph node pathology.

Ref.: 1, 2, 3, 4, 5

COMMENTS: Recent development of high-frequency, real-time ultrasound equipment has greatly improved the clinician's ability to image the thyroid and parathyroid glands. Ultrasonography of the neck has become extremely sensitive for detecting thyroid, parathyroid, and cervical lymph node pathology, even with lesions as small as 2–3 mm under appropriate conditions. Although the indications for routine use of ultrasonography remain poorly defined, it has increased the detection of asymptomatic nodules by 13–41%. A recognized use for ultrasonography is to aid in performing FNA of thyroid lesions. It also can be utilized to assess a thyroid nodule's response to thyroid hormone suppression. Surrounding anatomic structures in the neck can be identified, which may reveal parathyroid or cervical lymph node pathology. With the advantages of low cost, no radiation exposure, noninvasiveness, and brief examination time, further developments of this modality may benefit patients with thyroid pathology by improving accuracy of diagnosis.

ANSWER: A, B, C, D

11. Match the imaging modality on the left with the statement on the right.

A. MRI
B. Radioiodine
C. Gallium
D. Ultrasonography
E. Computed tomography

a. May be used for imaging as well as treatment
b. Most useful as an imaging agent for lymphoma or anaplastic cancer
c. Optimal for imaging the mediastinum
d. Assess adenopathy and assist in node biopsy
e. May be promising for differentiating follicular cancer from follicular adenoma

Ref.: 1, 3, 6

COMMENTS: No current imaging method is capable of reliably differentiating a benign nodule from a malignant one. **Radioactive iodine** is most specific and predicts the subsequent ability to treat with a larger iodine dose. It is useful only for well-differentiated thyroid cancer. Even so, some papillary tumors and approximately 50% of metastases from both papillary and follicular carcinomas cannot be detected. ^{123}I is the best isotope for diagnosis, and ^{131}I is best for treatment.

Gallium is most useful as an imaging agent for patients with anaplastic carcinoma or thyroid lymphoma. It frequently is positive in these iodine-negative tumors. Although a negative scan essentially excludes thyroid lymphoma, interpretation of a positive scan is complicated by the frequency of uptake in Hashimoto's thyroiditis, a common underlying disorder.

Positron emission tomography (PET), although not widely available, is useful for measuring nodule volume. Its combination with **fluorine-18-fluorodeoxyglucose (FDG) imaging** is intriguing and requires further study. Nonisotopic imaging is useful as an adjunct to the methods described previously.

Ultrasonography is useful for evaluating the neck for adenopathy or recurrence. It has the additional benefit of allowing directed biopsy of the nodule or area in question.

CT scanning may be optimal for imaging the mediastinum. Its use in thyroid cancer should be limited to noncontrast studies, if possible, to avoid interference with iodine imaging or treatment.

MRI, although more expensive than CT, introduces no radiation exposure, does not use iodinated contrast, and can produce images in three planes. It permits differentiation of fibrosis from residual/recurrent disease and identification of muscle invasion.

The recent demonstration of the use of proton magnetic imaging to distinguish between follicular cancer and follicular adenoma is encouraging.

ANSWER: A-e; B-a; C-b; D-d; E-c

12. With regard to the recurrent laryngeal nerve (RLN), which of the following statements is/are true?

A. Following a month without clinical improvement, unilateral injured vocal cords should be assessed and treated with injection of collagen or Teflon.
B. Bilateral injury may result in tracheostomy.
C. Anatomically, the most common location of the RLN is along the tracheoesophageal groove.
D. Reexploration is associated with an increased risk of injury.
E. If tumor has encompassed the RLN, the nerve should always be divided to obtain adequate margins.

Ref.: 1, 2, 3, 7

COMMENTS: The anatomic relations of greatest importance to the thyroid are those that relate to the recurrent laryngeal nerve (RLN). Injury to the RLN results in paralysis of the vocal cords on the ipsilateral side. The cord may remain in a paramedial position or be adducted, toward the midline. Clinically, patients present with hoarseness, a weakened voice, and occasionally shortness of breath. It is important to assess cord function preoperatively as well as postoperatively. The RLN generally courses in the tracheoesophageal groove posterior to the inferior thyroid artery, although in approximately 20% of patients it travels anterior to the inferior thyroid artery. Permanent RLN injuries occur during 1–2% of thyroid operations performed by experienced surgeons. Reexplorations increase the risk to 5%. Temporary RLN injuries occur more commonly. Therefore one should follow the patient for a period of 6–9 months to see if vocal cord function returns. If no function returns by then, injection of the paralyzed vocal cord with collagen or Teflon helps tighten it, thereby improving function. Bilateral injury is much more serious because both cords assume a median or paramedian position, resulting in airway obstruction. If this occurs the patient often requires an emergent tracheostomy. Sometimes the RLN must be sacrificed because of tumor involvement, although generally it can be preserved and dissected free from the tumor when it is functioning preoperatively. When it is encompassed by tumor, the nerve should be identified where it enters the tumor and then dissected free from the tumor. This is not possible is some patients.

ANSWER: B, C, D

13. Match each cause of hyperthyroidism in the left column with one or more appropriate descriptions in the right column.

A. Graves' disease
B. Toxic multinodular goiter
C. Toxic adenoma

a. Autonomous function independent of TSH, long-acting thyroid stimulator (LATS), and thyroid-stimulating immunoglobulins (TSI)
b. Diffuse gland involvement with increased vascularity and lymphoid aggregates
c. Extrathyroidal manifestations
d. Possible presence of cervical compression symptoms

Ref.: 1, 2, 4, 5

COMMENTS: Overactivity of the thyroid gland may manifest only as an elevation of the amount of circulating thyroid hormone, or it may be clinically evident from a number of signs and symptoms, many of which mimic catecholamine excess (e.g., hypertension, tachycardia, flushing, sweating). Overproduction of thyroid hormone may occur with diffuse involvement of the gland (diffuse toxic goiter or Graves' disease); alternatively, it may occur in the setting of a single "hot" nodule (toxic adenoma) or in a multinodular gland (Plummer's disease). Each of these causes of hyperthyroidism is several times more common in women than in men. Graves' disease occurs most commonly during the third and fourth decades, whereas toxic thyroid nodules are found most commonly in patients over 50 years of age. Other rare causes of hyperthyroidism include trophoblastic tumors and TSH-secreting pituitary tumors. With toxic adenoma or toxic multinodular goiter, the hyperfunctioning nodules are thought to represent adenomas that are functioning autonomously. In contradistinction, Graves' disease is thought to be an autoimmune phenomenon in which TSH receptors within the thyroid gland are stimulated by binding with immunoglobulins (LATS and TSI). Increased vascularity (a bruit) and lymphoid tissue may be present. Among the entities producing hyperthyroidism, Graves' disease is unique in its association with extrathyroidal manifestations (exophthalmos, pretibial myxedema), which may bear no relation to the presence or severity of thyroid overactivity. Enlargement of the thyroid gland associated with any of the aforementioned causes of thyrotoxicosis may produce tracheal or pharyngoesophageal compression symptoms.

ANSWER: A-b,c,d; B-a,d; C-a,d

14. With regard to the use of radioiodine to treat hyperthyroidism, which of the following statements is/are true?

A. Hypothyroidism occurs in essentially all cases.
B. There is a marked increased risk of future thyroid cancers after radioiodine therapy.
C. Radioiodine ablation is generally accomplished through the use of ^{123}I.
D. Radioiodine may pass through the placenta and lactating breasts to produce hypothyroidism in fetuses and infants.

Ref.: 1, 4, 5, 6

COMMENTS: See Question 15.

15. Match each clinical situation in the left column with the most appropriate treatment in the right column.

A. A 25-year-old with Graves' disease and a markedly enlarged gland with compressive symptoms	a. Surgery
B. An 8-year-old with Graves' disease and a small gland	b. Radioiodine
C. A 38-year-old with a toxic adenoma	c. Antithyroid drugs
D. A 35-year-old with a toxic, diffuse goiter and keloid formation	
E. A 40-year-old with Graves' disease and a nodule in one lobe	

Ref.: 1, 4, 5

COMMENTS: The treatment of Graves' disease is controversial and may be accomplished effectively with a subtotal or total thyroidectomy, radioiodine therapy, or antithyroid drugs; all of these forms of treatment have particular advantages and shortcomings. **Antithyroid drugs** exert their effect by interfering with the conversion of iodine to organic compounds (iodine-binding) and by preventing the coupling of iodotyrosine. Treatment with these drugs is long term—up to 2 years—and may be associated with drug fever, rash, and granulocytopenia. Agranulocytosis occurs in fewer than 0.4% of treated patients, but it can be fatal. Furthermore, recurrence of hyperthyroidism after cessation of the drugs occurs in as many as 60% of patients. **Radioiodine ablation** of the thyroid with ^{131}I may take several weeks to months to exert its effect and is associated with the almost certain occurrence of future hypothyroidism. Radioiodine may pass through the placenta and lactating breasts, thereby producing hypothyroidism in fetuses and infants. Radioiodine should be avoided in children. Although the carcinogenic effects of radioiodine are theoretically possible, clinical experience has not supported this concern. Such therapy is safe and effective and, in comparison with surgery, relatively inexpensive. **Thyroidectomy** confers the risk of anesthesia and trauma to the recurrent laryngeal nerves and parathyroids. Thyroidectomy has the advantage of an immediate response and the reversal of compression symptoms. Hypothyroidism after subtotal thyroidectomy also is common.

Each of these three forms of treatment may be appropriate for a particular patient with Graves' disease; specific circumstances occasionally influence the therapeutic choice. Antithyroid medications are used initially in most patients to render them euthyroid. Antithyroid medications are also used for young patients and for patients with relatively small goiters and only mild elevation of serum thyroid hormone levels. Patients with extremely large glands, particularly those causing compressive symptoms, are most readily treated by thyroidectomy. Surgery is indicated in patients with "cold" nodules within toxic glands because these nodules carry the same risk of malignancy as those found in a euthyroid gland. Toxic multinodular goiters probably are most effectively treated by surgical excision; radioiodine may be less effective for this condition than it is for Graves' disease because of the inhomogeneous uptake of the nuclide by the multinodular gland. Toxic adenomas are best treated by surgery involving lobectomy on the involved side, which provides an immediately effective treatment, frequently with preservation of enough thyroid tissue that there is no need for thyroid replacement therapy. Finally, pregnant patients whose condition is not readily controlled with antithyroid medications should undergo surgical resection of the thyroid.

ANSWER:
Question 14: A, D
Question 15: A-a,c; B-c; C-a,c; D-b,c; E-a,c

16. Which of the following is/are true about the treatment and management of Graves' disease?

A. Treatment of choice is subtotal thyroidectomy.
B. Subtotal thyroidectomy and irradiation have similar recurrence rates.
C. Radioactive iodine is the treatment of choice other than in children and women of childbearing age.
D. Recurrence rates for antithyroid drugs are comparable to that for subtotal thyroidectomy.
E. Subtotal thyroidectomy results in an improvement in exophthalmos.

Ref.: 1, 2, 3

COMMENTS: Graves' disease is an autoimmune disorder that targets the thyroid, extraocular muscles, and skin. Patients with this disorder complain of fatigue, palpitations, tremors, shortening of menstrual cycles, anxiety, weight loss, and heat intolerance. The diagnosis of thyrotoxicosis can be established by demonstrating elevation of the free thyroxine (T_4) index and suppression of the serum concentration of TSH. The diagnosis of Graves' disease is established by high thyroid radioactive iodine uptake (RAIU) in a thyrotoxic patient who has a diffuse goiter. Therapy may consist of treatment with ^{131}I, antithyroid drugs, and subtotal thyroidectomy. Radioactive iodine therapy is most commonly used, rendering 90% of patients euthyroid or hypothyroid. The relapse rate is 10–25%.

This form of therapy is contraindicated during pregnancy. Antithyroid drugs, propylthiouracil or methimazole, are used with the intent of inducing remission of Graves' disease. Remission rates approach 40% at 1 year and 65% at 2 years, but recurrence rates can be as high as 72%. Subtotal thyroidectomy removes most of the thyroid tissue, leaving behind a thyroid remnant of 2–7 gm, which may cause the patient to become euthyroid. The recurrence rates are equal to that of irradiation (up to 10%). Subtotal thyroidectomy can be associated with recurrent laryngeal nerve injury and transient or permanent hypocalcemia. It is imperative that the patient be made pharmacologically euthyroid preoperatively to avoid thyroid storm. Surgery does not reliably result in an alleviation of exophthalmos, but there are reports that total thyroidectomy may be beneficial.

ANSWER: B, C

17. With regard to thyroid storm, which of the following statements is/are true?

A. Thyroid storm is secondary to insufficient thyroid hormone release.
B. Thyroid storm is characterized by weakness, hypothermia, and bradyarrhythmias.
C. Trauma in a patient with untreated Graves' disease may precipitate thyroid storm.
D. Propranolol, hypothermia, and antithyroid medication such as propylthiouracil are some of the first-line treatments.
E. Radioiodine may be used to alleviate a refractory case of thyroid storm.

Ref.: 1, 4, 5

COMMENTS: Thyroid storm results when there is excessive release of thyroid hormone from a toxic gland. The clinical manifestations are hyperthermia, tachycardia, irritability, sweating, anxiety, and hypertension, which can eventually lead to prostration, hypotension, and death. Thyroid surgery in a patient with Graves' disease used to be the most common inciting event. Now it is more often precipitated in patients with untreated hyperthyroidism by trauma, infection, pregnancy, or other metabolic stresses such as diabetic acidosis. The fundamentals of treating thyroid storm center on treating the inciting factor, providing the substances needed to support the increased metabolic rate (oxygen, glucose, fluid), counteracting the peripheral adrenergic manifestations of the syndrome (with propranolol, hypothermia), and preventing iodine binding and release of thyroid hormone (propylthiouracil, potassium iodide). Radioiodine therapy does not have any value in the treatment of thyroid storm and may in fact precipitate thyroid storm.

ANSWER: C, D

18. A 50-year-old woman presents with a 2-year history of mild, diffuse, tender thyroid enlargement, a 10-pound weight gain, and fatigue. Of the following diagnoses, which is the most likely?

A. Riedel's thyroiditis.
B. Hashimoto's thyroiditis.
C. Subacute thyroiditis.
D. Acute suppurative thyroiditis.
E. Papillary thyroid carcinoma.

Ref.: 1, 2, 3, 4

COMMENTS: See Question 19.

19. Match each form of thyroiditis in the left column with the proper clinical description in the right column.

A. Acute suppurative thyroiditis	a. May be associated with retroperitoneal fibrosis
B. Subacute (de Quervain's) thyroiditis	b. Acute illness of bacterial origin
C. Hashimoto's disease	c. Most common form of thyroiditis
D. Riedel's thyroiditis	d. Probably of viral origin

Ref.: 1, 2, 4, 6

COMMENTS: Hashimoto's disease is the most common form of chronic thyroiditis. It most often occurs in middle-aged women, who present with complaints of fatigue and a diffusely enlarged thyroid that may be tender. Although hyperthyroidism may be present in patients with Hashimoto's disease, most are either euthyroid or hypothyroid. The disease is thought to be an autoimmune process, and one of the confirming diagnostic findings is the presence of antithyroid antibodies. Frequently, no treatment is needed; however, thyroid replacement therapy is used if the patient is hypothyroid. The incidence of papillary thyroid carcinoma among patients with Hashimoto's disease is not higher than that among the general population, so prophylactic thyroidectomy is not warranted. Operation generally is reserved for symptoms of compression or for removal of nodules within the diseased gland that are potentially malignant. **Acute suppurative thyroiditis** is rare. It manifests as a sudden onset of severe pain associated with fever, chills, and dysphagia. It almost always follows an acute upper respiratory infection and is of bacterial origin. Treatment is with antibiotics and occasionally drainage. **Subacute (de Quervain's) thyroiditis** also frequently follows an upper respiratory infection. Although association with a viral etiology is considered most likely, an autoimmune mechanism has been suggested because of the presence of thyroid antibodies. Although the onset is fairly abrupt, the clinical course is less fulminant than that of acute suppurative thyroiditis. It is characterized by moderate swelling and tenderness of the thyroid gland with repeated exacerbations and remissions over several months. Recovery is frequently spontaneous but may be facilitated by a course of salicylate or corticosteroid therapy. **Riedel's struma** is a rare, chronic inflammatory condition characterized by dense fibrosis throughout the thyroid and periglandular tissues. It frequently results in hypothyroidism and symptoms of tracheal and esophageal compression. It has been associated with other fibrotic reactions, including retroperitoneal fibrosis and sclerosing mediastinitis. When unilateral, it is difficult to distinguish from carcinoma. Treatment usually includes thyroid hormone therapy, and operation may be necessary for relief of tracheoesophageal obstruction.

ANSWER:
Question 18: B
Question 19: A-b; B-d; C-c; D-a

20. With regard to goiter, which of the following statements is/are correct?

A. The term *goiter* can refer to any abnormal enlargement of the thyroid gland.
B. The term *familial goiter* implies that a genetic defect may play a role in the etiology.
C. The most identifiable cause of endemic goiter is iodine deficiency.

D. Immediate operation is indicated for patients with extremely large iodine-deficiency goiters because of the increased risk of cancer in the larger glands.

Ref.: 1, 4, 6, 7

COMMENTS: The term *goiter* refers broadly to any abnormal enlargement of the thyroid gland, whether diffuse or nodular. Diffuse enlargement of the thyroid without evidence of a functional abnormality is usually the result of a colloid goiter (simple or nontoxic goiter). On occasion, there is a familial tendency toward diffuse thyroid enlargement (*familial goiter*), in some circumstances caused by an inherited enzymatic defect that results in impaired iodine metabolism. Affected patients are often hypothyroid. Diffuse thyroid enlargement is often caused by environmental effects, including the ingestion of goitrogenic foods or drugs (e.g., paraaminosalicylic acid), but the most common is dietary iodine deficiency. Many countries have so-called goiter belts (endemic goiter), the result of environmental iodine deficiencies that occur in specific geographic locations. In the United States this is primarily of historical interest today because the use of iodized table salt has become nearly routine. Diffuse goiters may cause problems by virtue of their cosmetic effect or compression symptoms. They can occasionally be made smaller with iodine or thyroid hormone administration, but operation may be required. The risk of cancer is not increased in these glands and is not an indication for operation.

ANSWER: A, B, C

21. Which of the following statements about a substernal goiter is/are true?

A. It may be associated with subclinical hypothyroidism.
B. CT scan is the best modality for its imaging.
C. Airway compression is an unusual presentation clinically.
D. It can involve the posterior mediastinum as well as the anterior mediastinum.
E. Primary substernal goiter vessels originate from the innominate artery, whereas secondary substernal goiter vessels originate from the superior and inferior thyroid arteries.
F. Treatment is total thyroidectomy.

Ref.: 1, 2, 3, 5

COMMENTS: Endemic goiter is primarily the result of dietary iodine deficiency. It results in primary hypothyroidism, which is associated with an elevated TSH level. A plain radiograph may demonstrate tracheal deviation, but CT scanning of the neck demonstrates continuity of the mediastinal mass with a cervical goiter and permits identification of tissue planes of intrathoracic goitrous components. Airway compression is the most common symptom of substernal goiter. Other symptoms include dysphagia, wheezing, vocal cord paralysis, and rarely superior vena cava (SVC) compression syndrome. Anatomically, substernal goiters are classified into two types: primary, in which the origin of the blood supply is intrathoracic; and secondary, in which the blood supply is cervical in origin. Both can be present in either the anterior or the posterior mediastinum. The surgical procedure of choice is total lobectomy on the side of the substernal goiter. If patients are kept on thyroid hormone substitution therapy, the recurrence rate is low (2.5%). Total thyroidectomy is not recommended as an approach to this benign disease unless both lobes are clearly involved.

ANSWER: A, B, D, E

22. Which of the following is/are associated with an increased risk for developing thyroid cancer.

A. Smoking.
B. Dental radiography.
C. Medical treatment with ^{131}I.
D. Child undergoing radiation therapy for a Wilms' tumor.
E. Individual who lived near Chernobyl.

Ref.: 1, 2, 3, 7

COMMENTS: A family history of thyroid neoplasms, benign or malignant, of follicular cell origin does not appear to increase the risk of thyroid cancer significantly. However, a family history of medullary carcinoma of the thyroid (parafollicular cell origin) does increase the risk of developing the same type of thyroid cancer. Risk is also increased in patients exposed to external radiation (e.g., those receiving upper mantle radiation therapy for Hodgkin's disease up to 5000 rad). Patients with Wilms' tumor and associated childhood tumors such as neuroblastoma and leukemias have an increased risk for developing thyroid cancer secondary to their radiation exposure. Therapeutic radioiodine administration, as used for treatment of hyperthyroidism, has not been associated with an increased subsequent risk of thyroid cancer; it is presumed that this is because of the nearly total destruction of the follicular cells. Smoking is not a risk factor for the development of thyroid carcinoma. Medical treatment with ^{131}I at low doses for diagnostic imaging or high doses for thyroid ablation does not appear to increase the incidence of thyroid cancer. On the other hand, the nuclear fallout present at Chernobyl released multiple short-lived isotopes ^{131}I, ^{133}I, and ^{135}I, and there has been an increase in the incidence of papillary carcinoma with a high incidence of lymph node metastases in patients living in the Chernobyl region. Papillary cancer is the most common thyroid cancer associated with radiation exposure. Patients with a history of radiation exposure and who have papillary cancer require total thyroidectomy. It is of note that patients are at increased risk for developing thyroid cancer for periods as long as 50 years after exposure. Dental radiographs are usually not associated with an increased risk.

ANSWER: D, E

23. Which of the following thyroid adenomas in rare instances behaves in a malignant manner?

A. Colloid adenoma.
B. Embryonal adenoma.
C. Fetal adenoma.
D. Hürthle cell adenoma.

Ref.: 1, 2, 5, 6

COMMENTS: The clinical significance of thyroid adenomas relates to the need to differentiate them from thyroid carcinoma. Such differentiation frequently requires thyroid lobectomy for tissue diagnosis; once the histologic diagnosis is known, no further treatment is necessary. Some clinicians believe that thyroid suppression should be used to reduce the risk of development of future adenomas. The **colloid**, **embryonal**, and **fetal** adenomas are all considered subcategories of follicular adenoma and are differentiated from each other by the relative amount of colloid present and the architectural arrangement of the epithelial cells. Cytologically, all these cells appear to be similar to the normal thyroid follicular cell. These follicular adenomas are entirely benign and do not increase the risk of carcinoma. **Hürthle cell adenoma** is characterized by Hürthle cells (variable enlargement, hyperchromatic nuclei, and granular cytoplasm) and is considered by some pathologists to be, in fact, a low-grade follicular carcinoma. Although it is rare for a benign-appearing Hürthle cell adenoma to behave in a malignant manner, the noncommittal term *Hürthle cell tumor* has been used to describe these neoplasms; the term *Hürthle cell carcinoma* is reserved for the clearly malignant variant. Some clinicians believe that a more aggressive surgical approach (total thyroidectomy) is indicated for routine management of Hürthle cell tumors because of their potentially (albeit rare) malignant behavior.

ANSWER: D

24. From each of the following pairs of features of thyroid nodules, select the one that is associated with the greater likelihood of malignancy.

A. Solid vs. cystic.
B. Solitary vs. multiple.
C. "Hot" vs. "cold."
D. Rapid enlargement overnight vs. slow enlargement over many months.
E. Hard vs. soft.
F. Male vs. female patient.
G. Child vs. adult patient.

Ref.: 1, 3, 4, 6

COMMENTS: The management of thyroid nodules, particularly the decision as to whether surgical intervention is required, depends on the clinical index of suspicion that the nodule is malignant. Numerous factors in the history, physical examination, and laboratory examination of the patient raise or lower one's index of suspicion. Epidemiologically, thyroid cancers are more common in adults than in children and in women than in men because thyroid nodules themselves are more common in those populations. The likelihood that a given nodule is malignant, however, is greater in males than in females and in children than in adults. Most thyroid cancers grow slowly and indolently. Extremely rapid growth (e.g., described as sudden enlargement overnight) usually is caused by hemorrhage into a previously undetected nodule. A history of recent voice change or difficulty swallowing, particularly when the lesion is small, should raise the index of suspicion of malignancy. On physical examination, soft or fleshy lesions suggest benign disease, whereas hardness is more often associated with malignancy. Indirect laryngoscopy should be performed to search for ipsilateral vocal cord paresis or paralysis, which suggests that the thyroid nodule may be invading or compressing the recurrent laryngeal nerve. Radionuclide scans can provide information about the metabolic activity of the nodule and the number of nodules present; ultrasonography can provide information about the number of nodules and their solid or cystic nature. A single nodule, decreased or absent function ("cold"), and solid consistency increase the likelihood of malignancy in comparison with multiple nodules, hyperfunction ("hot"), and cystic consistency. A solitary, solid, cold thyroid nodule carries a 10–20% risk of malignancy; whereas cystic structure, multinodularity, and normal or hyperfunctioning status carry risks in the range of 5% or less.

ANSWER: A-solid; B-solitary; C-cold; D-slow; E-hard; F-male; G-child

25. With regard to the technique of fine-needle aspiration (FNA) biopsy of the thyroid, which one of the following statements is/are true?

A. It is generally contraindicated because of the extremely vascular nature of the thyroid gland.
B. False-positive results are rare.
C. False-negative results occur less often than false-positive results.
D. There is a 3% risk that cancer cells will implant along the needle tract.
E. Benign versus malignant follicular neoplasms can be easily differentiated.

Ref.: 1, 4, 5, 7

COMMENTS: Fine-needle aspiration biopsy is a standard technique for evaluating thyroid nodules. **Core needle biopsy** was initially the technique employed but was associated with a risk of hematoma. This technique has been supplanted by **FNA cytology** (using 18- to 25-gauge needles). In the absence of coagulopathy, hemorrhagic complications are rare with this technique. The theoretic complication of cancer cell implantation along the needle tract has not been observed. Although false-negative results are rare (< 5%), when the clinical suspicion of malignancy is high a negative needle biopsy should not deter surgery. Because of the possibility of a false-negative result, patients should undergo repeated needle aspirations and follow-up observation. Changes in examination or cytologic findings to those of a more suspicious nature dictate surgical resection of the nodule. False-positive results are rare (< 1%) when the specimens are of good quality and examined by an experienced cytologist; therefore such nodules should be resected. The area of greatest difficulty during interpretation is with follicular neoplasms, for which differentiation of benign from malignant depends more on gross and histologic tumor architecture than on cytologic findings. Nodules whose cytologic features are reportedly atypical, suspicious, possibly malignant, or consistent with a follicular neoplasm should be resected because approximately 20% of them are carcinomas.

ANSWER: B

26. Match each type of thyroid cancer in the left column with the appropriate response on the right column.

A. Papillary	a. Worst prognosis
B. Follicular	b. Most commonly associated with radiation exposure
C. Medullary	c. Associated with hyperparathyroidism
D. Anaplastic	d. Hematogenous metastatic spread to bone
E. Lymphoma	e. Usually requires systemic chemo/radiation therapy

Ref.: 1, 2, 3

COMMENTS: Cancers of the thyroid encompass a wide range of biologic aggressiveness. At the least aggressive extreme is **papillary** carcinoma, which has a propensity for local or regional recurrence rather than systemic metastases. Papillary carcinoma is the most common thyroid malignancy associated with previous exposure to ionizing radiation. **Follic-**

ular carcinomas also carry a generally favorable prognosis but are characterized by a propensity for blood-borne/hematogenous metastases; fortunately, many of these tumors respond to radioiodine therapy. **Medullary** carcinomas occur sporadically or in a familial pattern, occasionally as part of the multiple endocrine neoplasia, type II (MEN-II) syndrome (medullary carcinoma of the thyroid, pheochromocytoma, parathyroid hyperplasia). These tumors carry an intermediate prognosis, depending on the stage of presentation. Medullary cancer spreads by nodal involvement and distant metastatic disease. **Lymphomas** of the thyroid gland also carry an intermediate prognosis, depending on the stage of presentation. In rare instances, patients with thyroid lymphoma are cured by surgery alone; in most cases, however, the disease is considered to be part of a more widespread process, and regional irradiation, systemic chemotherapy, or both are indicated. **Anaplastic** thyroid carcinoma is an extremely rapid-growing, almost uniformly fatal disease that manifests characteristically with massive involvement in the neck in association with tracheoesophageal obstruction. Palliative surgery, radiotherapy, or chemotherapy results in an occasional short-lived response.

ANSWER: A-b; B-d; C-c; D-a; E-e

27. With regard to papillary carcinoma, which of the following is/are true?

A. It is the most common thyroid malignancy.
B. It has the best prognosis.
C. Children are more likely to have lymph node metastases on presentation.
D. It often metastasizes to bone and lung.
E. It is the most common thyroid malignancy associated with previous radiation exposure.
F. Gardner syndrome is a risk factor for the development of papillary cancer.
G. Most tumors are unilateral.

Ref.: 1, 3, 6

COMMENTS: Papillary thyroid carcinoma is the most common form of thyroid cancer and carries the best prognosis. It manifests primarily as local and regional involvement; distant metastases are present in fewer than 1% of patients at initial presentation. It accounts for most thyroid cancers seen in patients with prior exposure to radiation. There is a high likelihood (up to 80%) of occult multicentric disease when the gland is examined pathologically with special care. These pathologic findings and autopsy data reveal a much higher incidence of occult disease than clinical disease indicates and raise the question as to the biologic importance of these occult papillary cancers. In contrast to most other epithelial cancers, the presence of regional lymph node metastases in patients does not appear to affect prognosis adversely so long as the disease is resectable. The incidence of local metastases is high with papillary carcinoma, ranging from 37% to 65% in adults; but the incidence is higher for children, ranging from 50% to 80%. Evaluations of large numbers of patients with papillary carcinoma in several series have failed to demonstrate any significant adverse mortality effects of local metastases of papillary carcinoma. The overall mortality rate from papillary thyroid cancer ranges from 1% to 10%, generally occurring only in older patients with large primary tumors. Death from papillary thyroid cancer is usually caused by aggressive local and regional behavior with tracheoesophageal and mediastinal involvement or by differentiation to a more anaplastic form. It is of note that familial adenomatous polyposis (Gardner syndrome) is associated with excessive rates of differentiated thyroid carcinoma: 89% papillary with a high 17:1 female/male ratio.

ANSWER: A, B, C, E, F

28. Fine-needle aspiration of a 3 cm thyroid nodule reveals papillary cancer. Which of the following is/are true?

A. Orphan Annie-eye nuclei can be present histologically.
B. The patient should undergo further radiologic evaluation of the neck with CT scans to assess lymph nodes and tumor extension due to the large size of the nodule.
C. Psammoma bodies can be present histologically.
D. Multiple histologic subtypes of papillary carcinoma exist.
E. The tall cell variant of papillary cancer carries a poor prognosis.

Ref.: 1, 3, 5, 6

COMMENTS: Fine-needle aspiration is considered the gold standard for evaluation of a thyroid nodule. The false-negative rate is less than 5% and the false-positive rate less than 1–2% when an experienced cytologist evaluates the specimen. Distinctive features of papillary carcinoma include large nuclei with a pale-staining, "ground glass appearance." These optically clear nuclei are referred to as *Orphan Annie-eye nuclei.* Also present are *psammoma bodies*, which represent degenerative changes in the papillae of papillary carcinoma that appear as laminated, basophilic structures. They appear in 40–50% of papillary carcinomas and are virtually pathognomonic. Further radiologic evaluation of the neck with CT does not change the treatment of this patient, which is total thyroidectomy. A more cost-effective means of identifying suspicious but not palpable lymph nodes is ultrasonography of the neck. There are multiple histologic subtypes of papillary carcinoma: encapsulated, follicular, tall cell, diffuse sclerosing, oxyphilic, and others including columnar cell, clear cell, insular, lipomatous, and trabecular. Tall cell carcinoma of the thyroid is a histologic variant that is more invasive, highly aggressive, and more common in elderly patients. Tall cell variants carry a poor prognosis. It is of note that according to the World Health Organization (WHO) classification, all carcinomas displaying any papillary features, either pure or in mixed form (with follicular elements), are classified as papillary carcinomas.

ANSWER: A, C, D, E

29. A 29-year-old man presents with a firm 2 cm mass in the right thyroid lobe and an ipsilateral lower deep jugular lymph node 1.5 cm in diameter. Both are examined cytologically by FNA biopsy and are found to contain papillary cancer. Which of the following therapies is/are most appropriate?

A. Thyroid lobectomy with external beam radiotherapy to the involved part of the neck.
B. Total thyroidectomy and ipsilateral radical neck dissection.
C. Total thyroidectomy with ipsilateral modified radical neck dissection.
D. Total thyroidectomy and bilateral modified radical neck dissection.
E. Excision of thyroid lobe and isthmus with ipsilateral modified radical neck dissection.

F. Enucleation of the primary tumor from the thyroid gland.
G. Excision of thyroid lobe and isthmus and paratracheal node dissection.

Ref.: 1, 2, 4

COMMENTS: Papillary thyroid cancer is primarily a surgically treated disease. External beam radiation therapy is indicated only for unresectable disease. Radioiodine ablation is appropriate in high risk patients (i.e., those who are older, have large primary tumors, and whose tumors have extrathyroidal extension or lateral cervical metastases). The extent of the surgical management of the primary tumor is also controversial.

Enucleation of the tumor without anatomic dissection of the involved lobe is not appropriate; it carries the risk of hemorrhage, injury to the nonvisualized recurrent laryngeal nerve, and implantation of the wound with cancer.

Excision of the involved thyroid lobe and isthmus is an acceptable approach for small (< 1.5 cm in diameter) papillary carcinomas that are contained within that lobe. Clinicians who prefer this approach do so because of the risk of hypoparathyroidism and nerve injury and the lack of evidence of a survival benefit when the clinically uninvolved contralateral lobe is resected.

Other clinicians believe that a near-total or total thyroidectomy is warranted. The rationale for this more aggressive approach is based on the recognized incidence of multicentric disease (albeit with an unclear clinical significance), facilitation of possible postoperative radioiodine therapy by surgical ablation of the remaining thyroid parenchyma, and a decreased incidence of recurrence in the contralateral lobe. Some authors have advocated subtotal resection of the contralateral lobe (particularly in high risk patients) to obtain the potential benefits of the more extensive resections without the added risks of nerve or parathyroid injury.

The management of cervical lymph node metastases has become more conservative. It is now generally accepted that a modified radical neck dissection (sparing the sternocleidomastoid muscle, internal jugular vein, and spinal accessory nerve) is appropriate management of clinically evident cervical node metastases.

Some clinicians believe that even less radical surgery that removes only the grossly positive nodes (the so-called berry-picking procedure) may also be appropriate.

Prophylactic dissection of the clinically uninvolved part of the neck for papillary thyroid carcinoma (ipsilateral or contralateral) has not been shown to be beneficial. For patients in whom the neck is clinically uninvolved with a proven papillary carcinoma, prophylactic paratracheal lymph node dissection may be appropriate because it can easily be performed without extending the incision and without functional or cosmetic compromise. Furthermore, it involves removal of the stage I lymph nodes that are most likely to be involved by papillary carcinoma.

ANSWER: C

30. In regard to follicular thyroid cancer, which of the following is/are true?

A. It is more common in geographic regions that are iodine-deficient.
B. It occurs predominantly in females, and estrogens have been recently found to be a risk factor.
C. The major histologic criterion for diagnosis is unequivocal capsular and vascular invasion.
D. Both minimally invasive and widely invasive follicular cancers are likely to have regional lymph node involvement on presentation.
E. Cytologically, it can be easily differentiated from a benign adenoma.

Ref.: 1, 3, 4, 6

COMMENTS: Follicular carcinoma comprises approximately 15% of all thyroid cancers. Patients with follicular thyroid cancer (FTC) tend to be older than those with papillary thyroid cancer. Due to the preponderance of FTC in female patients, it has been suggested that estrogens may be associated with thyroid cancer. Experiments have shown that thyrocytes express estrogen receptors, and estrogen stimulates the growth of thyrocytes. However, pregnancy has not been shown to increase the risk for thyroid cancer, and the role of estrogen in thyroid cancer currently remains unresolved. FTC is common in regions that are iodine-deficient, and rates of FTC have decreased in regions that have received iodine supplementation. Characteristics of both papillary and follicular tumors are frequently found within the same neoplasm, and these so-called mixed cancers tend to behave like a pure papillary thyroid cancer. Pure follicular carcinoma is difficult to diagnose on the basis of cytologic characteristics alone because its cells appear similar to those of its benign counterpart, the follicular adenoma. The diagnosis is more reliably obtained by the identification of vascular or capsular invasion of the tumor. Such invasive characteristics may be present, even though the capsule appears to be discrete and intact grossly. This is why one must do a thyroid lobectomy on a patient with an FNA diagnosis of a follicular neoplasm. These patients have a 20% risk of malignancy. If the thyroid lobectomy reveals follicular cancer, the patient undergoes total thyroidectomy. Unlike papillary carcinomas of the thyroid, follicular carcinomas usually spread hematogenously, and their metastatic potential is more likely distant than regional. Both minimally invasive and widely invasive follicular carcinomas involve the regional lymph nodes in only 10% of patients on presentation. The most common sites of distant metastases are lung and bone.

ANSWER: A, C

31. A 45-year-old woman with a firm 3 cm nodule in the left thyroid lobe undergoes left thyroid lobectomy; frozen section reveals a follicular carcinoma with capsular invasion. Which of the following additional therapeutic modalities are appropriate in this situation?

A. Near-total or total thyroidectomy.
B. Radical neck dissection on the involved side.
C. Exogenous thyroid administration to suppress TSH.
D. Radioiodine scan to detect pulmonary metastases with appropriate surgical resection if found.
E. Ablation of residual thyroid tissue and any demonstrated metastases with radioiodine.

Ref.: 1, 3, 4, 5, 6

COMMENTS: Near-total or total thyroidectomy is favored for follicular carcinoma because it allows detection of metastases by radioiodine postoperatively. Regional lymph node metastases from pure follicular thyroid carcinomas are relatively uncommon, and so prophylactic neck dissection is inappropriate. Involved cervical lymph nodes are best managed by a modified neck dissection with preservation of the sternocleidomastoid muscle, internal jugular vein, and spinal accessory nerve. Radioiodine scanning for the presence of metastases is useful for diagnosing follicular thyroid carcinoma, but its accuracy increases when the residual normal thyroid tissue has been ablated either by surgery or by a prior ablative dose of radioiodine. If metastases are subsequently found by radioiodine scanning, they are best treated by ablative doses of radioiodine. In rare instances, resection of isolated metastases is appropriate if they do not have an affinity for iodine. The growth of well-differentiated (papillary and follicular, nonmedullary) thyroid carcinomas may to some extent be under the influence of TSH, and many such cancers have cell surface TSH receptors. The recurrence and survival rates appear to be improved with thyroid hormone administration to obtain TSH suppression. In fact, regression of known metastatic follicular carcinoma with exogenous thyroid therapy alone has been reported.

ANSWER: A, C, E

32. With regard to thyroid cancer, which of the following are indications for the use of radioiodine therapy (^{131}I)?

A. Primary inoperable.
B. Postoperative residual disease in neck.
C. Distant metastases.
D. Invasion of thyroid capsule.
E. Cervical or mediastinal node metastases.
F. Recurrent thyroid cancer.

Ref.: 1, 3, 5, 6

COMMENTS: All of the above are indications of the use of ^{131}I for thyroid cancer. Patients who undergo near-total or total thyroidectomy improve the ability of ^{131}I to ablate the remaining gland and treat distant metastases. Patients with treated well-differentiated thyroid cancer are maintained on suppressive doses of thyroid hormone. Prior to body imaging with ^{131}I, thyroid hormone must be discontinued to allow the TSH level to rise. The TSH level usually reaches a maximum 4–6 weeks following total thyroidectomy. Elevated TSH is needed to optimize the ^{131}I scan. A suggested protocol is as follows: During the fourth to sixth week after discontinuing thyroid hormone, patients are given a diagnostic dose of 5 or 10 mCi ^{131}I and are scanned 3–4 days later. If there is any meaningful uptake, patients undergo radioiodine ablation or therapy. Patients undergo posttherapy scanning 3–7 days later to evaluate the responsiveness of the tumor. Side effects consist of sialadenitis, gastrointestinal symptoms, male and female infertility, bone marrow suppression, parathyroid dysfunction, and leukemia.

ANSWER: A, B, C, D, E, F

33. With regard to medullary thyroid carcinoma, which of the following statements is/are correct?

A. It is derived from a dedifferentiated variant of the same cell that produces papillary and follicular carcinomas.
B. Its pattern of metastatic spread is almost exclusively to distant sites.
C. The serum calcitonin level is useful for diagnosis and management.
D. The prognosis is approximately the same as that of papillary carcinoma.

Ref.: 1, 2, 4, 6

COMMENTS: Medullary carcinoma accounts for less than 10% of all thyroid carcinomas. Its cell of origin is the C-cell, or parafollicular cell, which originates in the neural crest. It bears no embryologic association with the epithelial cell origin of papillary and follicular tumors. This cell produces calcitonin, which is involved in calcium homeostasis. Elevations of serum calcitonin levels occur with C-cell hyperplasia (considered to be a premalignant condition) and frank medullary carcinoma; changes in the serum calcitonin level may be useful for monitoring the success of treatment and the presence of recurrent disease. Medullary thyroid carcinoma has the propensity to spread to both regional lymph nodes and distant metastatic sites, and its prognosis depends on the presence or absence of regional and distant metastases. The overall 5-year survival is approximately 50%, which is considerably less than that for papillary or follicular thyroid carcinoma.

ANSWER: C

34. Match the following characteristics of medullary thyroid carcinoma (MTC) in the left column to either its sporadic form, or its hereditary form, or both.

A. Contains parafollicular cells that secrete calcitonin	a. Sporadic MTC
B. Multifocal and bilateral	b. Hereditary MTC
C. Associated with MEN-IIA and MEN-IIB	c. Both
D. Worse prognosis	
E. Treatment consists of total thyroidectomy with central node dissection	

Ref.: 1, 2, 3, 5

COMMENTS: Medullary thyroid cancer (MTC), first described in 1959, is a tumor of the C-cells, or parafollicular cells. These cells secrete calcitonin, which is involved in calcium homeostasis. Calcitonin is used as a tumor marker to screen patients with multiple endocrine neoplasia types IIA and IIB (MEN-IIA, MEN-IIB) and is useful for following these patients for recurrence and response to treatment. Medullary cancer can occur in a sporadic form (75% of cases) and a familial form (25% of cases). In its sporadic form, the tumor is often single and unilateral and occurs without a pattern of familial predisposition. The tumor generally presents as a solitary thyroid nodule with lymph node metastases at the time of exploration. In the hereditary form, the tumor occurs as multifocal, bilateral disease with an autosomal dominant pattern of inheritance. These tumors also occur at an earlier age. The familial form can be associated with pheochromocytoma and parathyroid hyperplasia (MEN-IIA) or with pheochromocytoma, multiple mucosal neuromas, intestinal ganglioneuromas, and megacolon (MEN-IIB). MTC tends to be more aggressive in MEN-IIB. The overall 5-year survival is 50%, with a better prognosis for the sporadic than the hereditary or familial form.

ANSWER: A-c; B-b; C-b; D-b; E-c

35. With regard to the management of a patient with medullary thyroid carcinoma, which of the following statements is/are correct?

A. The patient should be screened for hyperparathyroidism and pheochromocytoma.
B. Total thyroidectomy is the procedure of choice.
C. If cervical lymph node metastases are present and no distant metastases are evident, neck dissection results in little benefit with regard to long-term survival.

D. If pheochromocytoma is found, adrenal surgery should precede the thyroid surgery.
E. If hyperparathyroidism is found, it may be surgically managed at the time of thyroidectomy by removing the two largest parathyroid glands.

Ref.: 1, 3, 5, 6

COMMENTS: The incidence of familial medullary thyroid carcinoma (MTC) is probably underestimated, inasmuch as the disease may go unrecognized (or unreported) in other family members. It is also possible that any patient with an MTC may be the index case for a familial type. It is reasonable therefore to screen for hyperparathyroidism (parathyroid hormone and calcium levels) and pheochromocytoma (urinary catecholamine, metanephrine, and vanillylmandelic acid levels) in all patients with MTC. The best current method of screening for familial MTC is genetic analysis for abnormality of the *ret* proto-oncogene or chromosome X.

If evidence of pheochromocytoma exists, this problem must be dealt with first because there is a significant risk of catastrophic blood pressure fluctuations during other (thyroid) surgery.

Hyperparathyroidism, if present, is almost always caused by four-gland hyperplasia and is best treated by excision of three and one-half glands (subtotal parathyroidectomy) or by a total parathyroidectomy with implantation of a small amount of parathyroid tissue in the forearm musculature. The parathyroid surgery should be carried out at the same time as the thyroid surgery.

Truly sporadic cases of MTC can be managed by excision of the involved thyroid lobe and isthmus alone because multicentricity is rare in the sporadic form. Total thyroidectomy, however, is considered to be the treatment of choice because the patient may have an unrecognized familial form in which multicentricity is common. MTC tends to spread first to the regional lymph nodes and then to distant sites; therefore thyroidectomy with neck dissection in the presence of clinically evident cervical lymph nodes is appropriate therapy and is associated with 10-year survival rates approaching 50%.

ANSWER: A, B, D

36. With regard to genetic analysis in patients with thyroid cancer, which of the following is/are true about the *ret* proto-oncogene?

A. Is associated with anaplastic thyroid cancer.
B. Is located on chromosome 10.
C. Is associated with familial medullary thyroid cancer (MTC).
D. Is associated with MEN-IIA and MEN-IIB.
E. Is associated with follicular cancer of the thyroid.

Ref.: 1, 8, 9

COMMENTS: The *ret* proto-oncogene was first cloned by Takahashi et al. in 1985. The gene was translocated and rearranged on the same chromosome 10 to an unknown 5′ sequence. A relation has been described between the *ret* proto-oncogene and papillary thyroid cancer. In Italy approximately 30% of patients with thyroid cancer had *ret* rearrangements. Recently, studies of the tyrosine kinase domain of the *ret* proto-oncogene revealed that specific germline mutations of *ret* led to MEN-IIA, MEN-IIB, and familial MTC. The oncogene was mapped on chromosome 10q11-12. In 1994 Lips et al. documented that patients who have the *ret* proto-oncogene mutation develop MTC and that *ret*-negative patients are not at risk. In fact, the presence of the *ret* proto-oncogene on chromosome 10 more accurately detected MTC than calcitonin. Continuing research in the field of genetics will provide further information about familial disease processes and help physicians manage these ailments clinically.

ANSWER: B, C, D

REFERENCES

1. Clark HO, Duh QY: *Textbook of Endocrine Surgery*. WB Saunders, Philadelphia, 1997.
2. Nyhus LM, Baker RJ, Fischer JE: *Mastery of Surgery*, 3rd ed. Little, Brown, Boston, 1997.
3. Sabiston DC Jr: *Textbook of Surgery*, 15th ed. WB Saunders, Philadelphia, 1997.
4. Greenfield LJ, Mulholland M, Oldham KT, et al: *Surgery: Scientific Principles and Practice*. Lippincott-Raven, Philadelphia, 1997.
5. Inabnet WB, Fisher SW, Staren ED: Thyroid and parathyroid ultrasound. *Probl Gen Surg* 14:54–65, 1997.
6. Schwartz SI, Shires GT, Spencer FC: *Principles of Surgery*, 7th ed. McGraw-Hill, New York, 1999.
7. Mack E: Management of patients with substernal goiters. *Surg Clin North Am* 75(3), 1995.
8. Takahashi M, Ritz J, Cooper GM: Activation of a novel human transforming gene, ret, by DNA arrangement. *Cell* 42:581, 1985.
9. Lips CJM, Landsvater RM, Hoppener JWM, et al: Clinical screening as compared with DNA analysis in families with multiple endocrine neoplasia type 2A. *N Engl J Med* 331:828–835, 1994.

CHAPTER 22

Parathyroid

1. With regard to the embryology of the inferior parathyroid glands, which of the following statements is/are correct?

A. They arise from the third branchial pouch.
B. They arise from the fourth branchial pouch.
C. They are embryologically associated with the thyroid gland.
D. They are embryologically associated with the thymus gland.

Ref.: 1, 2

COMMENTS: The superior parathyroid glands arise from the fourth branchial pouch in association with the lateral thyroid complex. Paradoxically, the inferior parathyroid glands arise from a higher branchial pouch (the third) in association with the thymus (hence the name *parathymus*). They achieve their characteristically lower position in adults because of the more caudal descent of the thymus gland into the mediastinum. Because of this long descent by elements of the third branchial pouch, the inferior parathyroids are found over a wider anatomic range (from the pharynx to the pericardium) than are the superior parathyroids, which bear a fairly constant relation to the posterolateral aspect of the thyroid gland.

ANSWER: A, D

2. With regard to parathyroid anatomy, which of the following statements is/are correct?

A. The superior parathyroids usually receive their blood supply from the superior thyroid artery.
B. The inferior parathyroids usually receive their blood supply from the inferior thyroid artery.
C. Either the superior or the inferior parathyroids may be located in the mediastinum.
D. Supernumerary glands are found in one-third of patients.

Ref.: 1, 2

COMMENTS: Normal parathyroid glands in adults are flat, ovoid structures measuring approximately 3 × 6 mm and weighing approximately 25–40 mg each. In most cases both the superior and inferior parathyroids derive their blood supply from the inferior thyroid artery. On occasion, the superior parathyroids are supplied by branches of the superior thyroid artery. The superior parathyroids are almost always located on the dorsal aspect of the thyroid at the level of the cricoid cartilage. The inferior parathyroids are more variable in their location; in 50% of patients they are found on the lateral surface of the lower pole, whereas in the remaining 50% they are associated with the thymus (mostly in the neck and occasionally in the superior mediastinum). About 90% of patients have four parathyroid glands; the other 10% have supernumerary glands (usually totaling five or six), which may be a result of fragmentation of the original four glands during embryologic descent. The presence of fewer than the usual four glands has been reported, but such reports must be viewed with caution because the inability to find a gland is not proof of its absence.

ANSWER: B

3. With regard to the physiology of parathyroid hormone (PTH), which of the following statements is/are correct?

A. Normally, PTH secretion is inversely related to the serum calcium level.
B. PTH secretion is under partial control of the pituitary via the parathyroid-stimulating hormone (PSH).
C. PTH has a direct action on bone, stimulating osteoclastic activity.
D. PTH has an indirect effect on the renal reabsorption of phosphate, which is controlled primarily by the action of vitamin D.
E. Assays specific for the N-terminal fragment are the most accurate for evaluating the serum PTH level.

Ref.: 1, 2

COMMENTS: PTH, the principal mediator of calcium homeostasis, is secreted from the parathyroid gland in response to fluctuations in the serum calcium concentration. This is a direct feedback system in which PTH secretion is inversely related to the serum level of ionized calcium. There is no pituitary control over PTH secretion. PTH has direct effects on the bone and kidneys and an indirect effect on the gut, all of which result in an increased serum calcium concentration. In bone, PTH stimulates calcium release by enhancing resorption of bone matrix by osteoclasts. In the kidneys, PTH increases tubular reabsorption of filtered calcium and decreases tubular reabsorption of filtered phosphate (phosphaturic effect). Increased intestinal absorption of dietary calcium occurs indirectly through PTH stimulation of renal vitamin D complex synthesis. The PTH molecule is made up of a fully active amino (N)-terminal fragment and a carboxy (C)-terminal fragment with no known biologic activity. PTH assays specific for the C-terminal fragment are more useful for evaluating the serum PTH level in the presence of hyperparathyroidism because of the long half-life of this fragment. A more recent innovation has been the ability to measure the intact PTH molecule, which is the most sensitive and specific of the three assays. The intact PTH level is elevated in 95% of patients with primary hyperparathyroidism.

ANSWER: A, C

4. With regard to vitamin D physiology, which of the following statements is/are correct?

   A. The major source of vitamin D is dietary.
   B. Hydroxylation of vitamin D_3 results in a loss of metabolic activity.
   C. Vitamin D increases intestinal absorption of dietary calcium.
   D. Vitamin D has a direct effect on bone, resulting in its ossification.
   E. Increased levels of serum phosphate stimulate the hydroxylation of 25-hydroxycholecalciferol in the kidneys.

Ref.: 1, 2

COMMENTS: Vitamin D (in the form of vitamin D_3 or cholecalciferol) is produced primarily by ultraviolet activation of 7-dehydrocholesterol in the skin. Vitamin D_3 undergoes initial hydroxylation in the liver to 25-hydroxycholecalciferol and a second hydroxylation in the kidneys to its most active form, 1,25-dihydroxycholecalciferol. This dihydroxy vitamin D_3 is the form that is primarily responsible for the physiologic functions: facilitation of intestinal absorption of dietary calcium and ossification of the bone. Low serum phosphate and increased serum PTH levels stimulate the conversion of 25-hydroxycholecalciferol to 1,25-dihydroxycholecalciferol.

ANSWER: C, D

5. Which of the following is/are true regarding calcitonin?

   A. It is secreted by thyroid parafollicular cells.
   B. It induces urinary excretion of both phosphate and calcium.
   C. It is an effective tumor marker.
   D. Its absence following total thyroidectomy causes hypercalcemia.
   E. Its abundance with medullary carcinoma of the thyroid causes hypocalcemia.

Ref.: 1, 2, 3, 4, 5

COMMENTS: Calcitonin is a hormone secreted by the *parafollicular cells* (C-cells) of the thyroid. Its physiologic effects relate to lowering of serum calcium levels by promoting urinary excretion of calcium and phosphate. In rats, calcitonin has also been demonstrated to inhibit bone resorbtion. As a matter of fact, the physiologic effects of calcitonin appear to be more important for calcium homeostasis in certain animals than in humans. Calcitonin does not play a central role in the control of serum calcium in humans, exemplified by the relatively normal serum calcium levels found in patients who have undergone total thyroidectomy and in those with medullary carcinoma of the thyroid. Synthetic salmon calcitonin in large doses (200–800 U/day) reduces the serum calcium level rapidly and is a useful adjunct to pamidronate, whose action has a delayed onset. Its most potent secretagogues are calcium and pentagastrin. Others include β-adrenergic catecholamines, glucagon, and cholecystokinin. PTH and calcitonin activity are mediated by cyclic adenosine monophosphate (cAMP) through a number of specific enzyme activations that occur in the kidney and bone. Calcitonin is a tumor marker for medullary thyroid carcinoma and provides a mechanism to diagnose and monitor patients for the presence and recurrence of disease.

ANSWER: A, B, C

6. Match the calcium-regulating hormone on the left with the proper location(s) of action and function(s) on the right.

A. Parathyroid hormone	a. Stimulates transport of calcium in bone
B. Vitamin D	b. Stimulates reabsorption of calcium in the kidney
C. Calcitonin	c. Inhibits reabsorption of calcium in the kidney
	d. Stimulates absorption of calcium in the intestine
	e. No direct effect on the intestine

Ref.: 1, 2, 3

COMMENTS: Parathyroid hormone is composed of 84 amino acids with a hormonally active N-terminal and an inactive C-terminal. In the skeleton, PTH inhibits osteoblasts and stimulates osteoclasts, resulting in a decrease in bone density. In the kidney, PTH causes a decrease in calcium clearance by stimulating the reabsorption of calcium and conversion of 25-hydroxy vitamin D_3 [25(OH)D_3] to 1,25(OH)2D_3. This metabolite then goes on to stimulate absorption of calcium and phosphate in the intestine. In contrast, PTH does not have a direct effect on calcium absorption in the intestine. Vitamin D_3 is derived from the ultraviolet activation of 7-dehydrocholesterol in the skin. Vitamin D is then hydroxylated in both the liver [25(OH)D_3] and the kidney [1,25(OH)2D_3]. Vitamin D increases the intestinal absorption of calcium and phosphate and the mobilization of calcium and phosphate from bone to blood. Calcitonin inhibits resorption of calcium and phosphate from bone and inhibits reabsorption of calcium and phosphate in the kidneys of some animals. Calcitonin does not have any direct effect on the intestine.

ANSWER: A-b,e; B-a,d; C-c,e

7. Match each laboratory or physiologic finding in the left column with the appropriate categorization of hyperparathyroidism in the right column.

A. High-normal to elevated serum calcium levels; high serum PTH levels	a. Primary hyperparathyroidism
B. Low-normal to low serum calcium levels; high serum PTH levels	b. Secondary hyperparathyroidism
C. Compensatory hyperfunction	c. Tertiary hyperparathyroidism
D. Autonomous hyperfunction	
E. When surgery is indicated, treatment is always by subtotal parathyroidectomy or total parathyroidectomy with autotransplantation	
F. Most patients do not require surgical intervention	

Ref.: 1, 2

COMMENTS: Hyperparathyroidism is the production of abnormally large amounts of PTH. This condition may be associated with high, normal, or low serum calcium levels, depending on the underlying mechanism. In **primary** hyperparathyroidism, one or more parathyroid glands are autonomously functioning without the normal negative feedback response to the serum calcium level, which usually results in elevations of serum calcium and PTH levels. **Secondary** hyperparathyroidism is considered a compensatory response by the parathyroid glands to hypocalcemia. Most often the hypocalcemia is secondary to underlying renal disease (causing hyperphosphatemia and a reduction of 1,25-dihydroxy vitamin D_3) or to intestinal malabsorption syndromes. In secondary hyperparathyroidism the PTH level is elevated; but because of abnormal calcium losses the serum calcium level rarely rises above the low-normal range. Most patients (approximately 90%) with secondary hyperparathyroidism from renal failure can be managed by diet, calcium, or vitamin D and phosphate-binding agents (or some combination); however, patients in whom severe renal osteodystrophy develops require subtotal parathyroidectomy or total parathyroidectomy with autotransplantation. **Tertiary** hyperparathyroidism generally refers to cases of secondary hyperparathyroidism in which long-standing stimulation of the parathyroid glands by hypocalcemia results in autonomous hyperfunction of those glands. In such cases, the parathyroid hormone level remains high and the serum calcium level becomes high-normal to elevated. Patients with tertiary hyperparathyroidism generally are asymptomatic. Surgery is required for only about 10% of those patients; indications are persistent hypercalcemia and elevated PTH with normal renal function. As with secondary hyperparathyroidism, surgery involves either subtotal parathyroidectomy or total parathyroidectomy with autotransplantation.

ANSWER: A-a,c; B-b; C-b; D-a,c; E-b,c; F-b,c

8. Which of the following is/are risk factor(s) for hyperparathyroidism?

A. Premenopausal female.
B. Previous exposure to ionizing radiation.
C. Family history of multiple endocrine neoplasia type I (MEN-I) syndrome.
D. Renal failure.

Ref.: 1, 2, 3, 4, 5

COMMENTS: The incidence of hyperparathyroidism is approximately 25 per 100,000 (0.025%) general population. The incidence of the disease markedly increases with age especially in postmenopausal women. In women older than 65, the incidence is 2.5%. Although the cause of primary hyperparathyroidism is unknown, some studies have identified associated risk factors. Exposure to low-dose ionizing radiation during childhood increases the risk for development of hyperparathyroidism, analogous to the increased incidence of well-differentiated thyroid cancer and salivary gland tumors in similarly exposed patients. Some reports suggest that exposure to radioactive iodine, as used for treatment of Graves' disease, may increase the risk of developing hyperparathyroidism. Members of a family with MEN-I or MEN-IIA syndrome are at risk for developing hyperparathyroidism. Genetic studies have identified a proto-oncogene, *PRAD1*, that has been associated with overexpression in parathyroid adenomas. Male gender and renal failure are not risk factors for primary hyperparathyroidism.

ANSWER: B, C

9. Most patients with primary hyperparathyroidism have elevations of all of the following *except*:

A. Total serum calcium.
B. Ionized serum calcium.
C. Serum alkaline phosphatase.
D. Urinary cAMP.
E. Urinary calcium.

Ref.: 1, 2, 3

COMMENTS: The diagnosis of hyperparathyroidism is usually based on the presence of elevated serum levels of calcium and intact PTH. Measurement of ionized calcium is superior to the total calcium level for evaluating patients with hyperparathyroidism. Only a few patients (10–40%) with hyperparathyroidism have an elevated alkaline phosphatase level, so this assay is not helpful for diagnosis. PTH interacts with cells lining the renal tubule, resulting in activation of cAMP. This results in cAMP leaking into tubular fluid, leading to an elevated urinary cAMP level. This finding has been demonstrated in up to 95% of patients with hyperparathyroidism. Hyperparathyroidism is associated with elevated urinary calcium levels, whereas benign familial hypocalciuric hypercalcemia (BFHH), which also causes hypercalcemia, is not. This distinction is critical because patients with BFHH do not benefit from an operation. Other typical biochemical features of primary hyperparathyroidism include elevated serum chloride and decreased serum phosphate levels. A chloride/phosphate ratio exceeding 33 is highly suggestive of the condition.

ANSWER: C

10. With regard to the pathologic features of primary hyperparathyroidism, which of the following statements is/are correct?

A. The presence of hyperplastic tissue surrounded by a rim of normal-appearing parathyroid tissue essentially confirms the diagnosis of adenoma.
B. Chief-cell hyperplasia is the most common form of parathyroid hyperplasia.
C. Clear-cell hyperplasia of the parathyroid gland is incapable of producing primary hyperparathyroidism.
D. When more than one gland is pathologically enlarged, the diagnosis of hyperplasia must be made.

Ref.: 1, 2

COMMENTS: The differentiation of **adenoma** from **hyperplasia** as the cause of primary hyperparathyroidism is difficult at times. The classic gross findings diagnostic of adenoma are a single enlarged gland with three normal or small remaining glands associated with the histologic finding of hyperplastic tissue surrounded by a rim of normal-appearing parathyroid tissue. This adenoma is the cause of primary hyperparathyroidism in approximately 80% of cases. When two glands are found to be enlarged and one or more glands are normal, the diagnosis is **multiple adenomas**, rather than hyperplasia. This condition is uncommon, accounting for fewer than 5% of cases. When three (or more) glands are abnormally enlarged, the likely diagnosis is hyperplasia. **Chief-cell hyperplasia** is the most common subtype of parathyroid hyperplasia. **Clear-cell hyperplasia** and **carcinoma** are rare causes of primary hyperparathyroidism. It often is difficult to differentiate hyperplasia from adenoma on the basis of frozen sections. Unless the characteristic rim of normal tissue is seen, the hyperplastic nature of adenomas is similar to that of true hyperplasia. Most commonly, the decision as to whether the entity is an adenoma or hyperplasia depends on the gross characteristics of the glands identified at exploration.

ANSWER: A, B

11. Which of the following may be associated with hyperparathyroidism?

A. Muscle weakness.
B. Myalgia, arthralgia.
C. Nephrolithiasis.
D. Pancreatitis.
E. Peptic ulcer disease.
F. Depression.

Ref.: 1, 2, 3

COMMENTS: Most patients with primary hyperparathyroidism are not overtly symptomatic, the condition being diagnosed most frequently after routine polychemistry serum testing. The most common complaints consist of myalgias, arthralgias, constipation, muscle weakness, and polyuria. These symptoms are nonspecific and often do not cause the examining physician to suspect hyperparathyroidism. Nephrolithiasis is present in approximately 10–25% of patients, whereas nephrocalcinosis (calcification within the parenchyma) is present in 5%. Renal function can be impaired with time, which may be a reason 70% of patients with hyperparathyroidism have hypertension. Patients with MEN-I syndrome and hyperparathyroidism have an increased risk for peptic ulcer disease. In these patients an elevated PTH augments the hypergastrinemia caused by gastrinoma, leading to further increased gastric acid secretion. Of 1000 patients with hyperparathyroidism at 26 hospitals in Great Britain, only 1% were found to have a history of pancreatitis. Although pancreatitis can occur with other disease processes associated with hypercalcemia, the relation between hyperparathyroidism and pancreatitis remains unconfirmed. Patients with hypercalcemia can develop neurologic or psychiatric disturbances ranging from depression or anxiety to psychosis or coma.

ANSWER: A, B, C, D, E, F

12. Which of the following is/are an indication(s) for operative treatment of *asymptomatic* patients with primary hyperparathyroidism?

A. Serum calcium of 13 mg/dl.
B. Reduced creatinine clearance.
C. Presence of kidney stones detected by abdominal radiography.
D. Markedly elevated 24-hour urinary calcium excretion.
E. Substantially reduced bone mass as determined by direct measurement.

Ref.: 1, 2, 3

COMMENTS: In 1990 the National Institute of Health Consensus Development Conference reviewed available data on the subject of managing patients with asymptomatic primary hyperparathyroidism. The panel agreed that a patient who is symptomatic requires operative therapy. The indications for operating on asymptomatic patients are as follows: history of an episode of life-threatening hypercalcemia, reduced creatinine clearance, presence of kidney stones detected by abdominal imaging, markedly elevated 24-hour urinary calcium excretion, and substantially reduced bone mass as determined by direct measurement. Patients who do not fall into one of the above categories may be followed with semiannual examinations. Operative treatment was recommended if one of the following developed: typical symptoms of the skeletal, renal, or gastrointestinal systems; sustained serum calcium of more than 1.0–1.6 mg/dl above normal; substantial decline in renal function; nephrolithiasis or worsening calciuria; substantial decline in bone mass; onset of neuromuscular or psychological symptoms; or inability or unwillingness of a patient to continue medical surveillance. Some studies have demonstrated an increased death rate from cardiovascular disease among patients with asymptomatic hyperparathyroidism followed nonoperatively.

ANSWER: A, B, C, D, E

13. Which of the following would *not* be elevated in patients with hypercalcemia due to malignancy?

A. Urinary cAMP.
B. Intact PTH.
C. C-Terminal PTH.
D. PTH-related peptide.

Ref.: 1, 2, 3

COMMENTS: In hospitalized patients, malignancy rather than hyperparathyroidism is the most common cause of hypercalcemia. Most patients with hypercalcemia and malignancy have suppressed PTH levels. Generally, hypercalcemia from malignancy can be divided into two groups: (1) those with hematologic malignancies; and (2) those with solid tumors. Hematologic diseases associated with hypercalcemia include multiple myeloma, lymphoma, and leukemia. These patients typically have lytic bone lesions radiographically and demonstrate increased osteoclast activity histologically. At the cellular level, the cause of hypercalcemia is stimulation of osteoclast activity by interleukin-1B and tumor necrosis factor-β. Unlike patients with hyperparathyroidism, these patients have low urine levels of cAMP. The solid tumors generally associated with hypercalcemia are in the breast, lung, and kidney and neuroendocrine tumors of the pancreas. These patients have a normal serum PTH, but urinary cAMP levels are elevated. The cause of hypercalcemia in these solid tumors has been linked to tumor production of a PTH-related peptide, which may be elevated in 85–90% of patients.

ANSWER: B, C

14. Of the following imaging studies, which is/are necessary prior to operating on a newly diagnosed patient with primary hyperparathyroidism?

A. Ultrasonography.
B. Computed tomography.
C. Sestamibi scan.
D. All of the above.
E. None of the above.

Ref.: 1, 2, 3, 4

COMMENTS: Preoperative localizing studies are not necessary for a patient undergoing a first-time neck exploration with a biochemically secure diagnosis of primary hyperparathyroidism. Nevertheless, most patients at many institutions still undergo such studies. In the hands of an experienced surgeon, operative management is successful 95–99% of the time, and the outcome is not improved by imaging studies. In fact, imaging studies are occasionally misleading and result in inappropriate treatment if both sides of the neck are not explored. These studies can certainly provide useful information, but they have a cost; and for a first-time exploration they do not generally alter the operative management. However, localizing studies are clearly important for patients with prior neck explorations.

ANSWER: E

15. A pregnant mother in her first trimester arrives at your office with the diagnosis of primary hyperparathyroidism. What is the correct management?

A. Parathyroidectomy during the first trimester.
B. Parathyroidectomy during the second trimester.
C. Cesarean section and parathyroidectomy at term.
D. Close observation and parathyroidectomy following delivery.

Ref.: 1, 2, 3

COMMENTS: Primary hyperparathyroidism during pregnancy, though rare, is associated with complications of fetal tetany, stillbirth, and abortion. The risk of fetal complications is higher if the hyperparathyroidism remains untreated. Therefore such a patient should undergo parathyroidectomy during the second trimester. The procedure is not done during the first trimester because of the risk of miscarriage and the teratogenic effects of anesthesia on the fetus. Operations during the third trimester have an increased risk of inducing labor. Overall, for operations that must be done during pregnancy, the second trimester offers the lowest morbidity and mortality for both mother and fetus.

ANSWER: B

16. In regard to secondary hyperparathyroidism, which of the following is/are true?

A. Bone pain is the most common indication for operation.
B. Intractable pruritus is alleviated in 85% of patients following parathyroidectomy.
C. Total parathyroidectomy with autotransplantation is superior to subtotal parathyroidectomy.
D. Transcervical thymectomy should be performed routinely in operated patients.

Ref.: 1, 2, 3, 5

COMMENTS: Only 5–10% of patients with secondary hyperparathyroidism require operative management. Most respond well to medical treatment with phosphate binders, supplemental calcium and vitamin D_3, and diet. Bone pain is the most common indication for operation, and the symptoms are relieved in 85% of patients following parathyroidectomy. Intractable pruritus is the second most frequent indication for parathyroidectomy and is also alleviated in 85% of patients. Malaise is another frequent symptom that diminishes in most patients undergoing parathyroidectomy. **Subtotal parathyroidectomy** was first introduced by Stanbury and colleagues in 1960. The procedure typically involves resection of three and a half of the four glands. **Total parathyroidectomy**, popularized by Wells in 1975, consists of removing all four enlarged parathyroidectomy glands and **autotransplanting** part of one parathyroid gland into the forearm. Roughly equivalent results have been obtained with the two procedures, and debate continues as to which is better. A **transcervical thymectomy** is performed routinely to remove supernumerary parathyroid glands or embryologic nests of parathyroid tissue. The most common cause of persistent hyperparathyroidism after subtotal or total parathyroidectomy plus autotransplantation is an undiscovered or supernumerary parathyroid gland in the neck or anterior mediastinum.

ANSWER: A, B, D

17. A patient with a previous diagnosis of primary hyperparathyroidism presents with rapidly developing muscular weakness, nausea, vomiting, and confusion. Initial management should include which of the following?

A. Vigorous hydration with intravenous saline.
B. Intravenous furosemide.
C. Intravenous mithramycin.
D. Intravenous calcitonin.
E. Immediate parathyroid exploration.

Ref.: 1, 2, 4

COMMENTS: For reasons that are unclear, patients with mild to moderate hypercalcemia from primary hyperparathyroidism may suddenly develop **hypercalcemic crisis** in which the serum calcium level rises to 14.5 mg/dl or higher. Symptoms may include weakness, nausea, vomiting, confusion, and even coma. Such a crisis is considered a medical emergency, and the initial management should be designed to lower the serum calcium level acutely. This is best accomplished by vigorous saline intravenous infusion to expand the intravascular volume, followed by administration of loop diuretics such as furosemide to increase urinary calcium excretion. Cardiac monitoring is required, particularly when the calcium level is higher than 16 mg/dl. When calcium levels remain elevated, other hypercalcemia agents are administered. **Calcitonin** given intravenously or subcutaneously has a rapid effect. Intravenous **mithramycin** (inhibits bone resorption) can effectively lower the serum calcium concentration within 24 hours of administration. Its potential hematologic, renal, and hepatic toxicity limits its use to (1) palliation of malignancy and (2) cases in which conventional therapy for hypercalcemia is ineffective or contraindicated. **Parathyroid exploration** with resection of the offending gland or glands represents the definitive treatment of this entity but should be delayed until the serum calcium level is reduced to a safer level.

ANSWER: A, B

18. A patient requires parathyroid exploration for primary hyperparathyroidism. During the exploration an abnormally large parathyroid gland is found posterior to the lower pole of the right thyroid lobe. Which of the following choices is/are appropriate at this point?

A. Excise the enlarged gland without identifying the other parathyroid glands.
B. Excise the enlarged gland and then identify the three remaining glands. If they appear normal, perform biopsies of all three to confirm normal histologic features.
C. Identify the remaining glands, and if they appear normal in size, excise the largest one only.
D. Identify the remaining glands and excise the largest one or two of the three remaining ones.

E. Identify the remaining glands; and if they appear normal in size, obtain a biopsy specimen from one of the remaining glands.

Ref.: 1, 2, 3, 4

COMMENTS: See Question 19.

19. On further exploration of the patient described in Question 18, the three remaining glands are encountered, and all appear to be abnormally enlarged, like the first gland found. Which one or more of the following options is/are appropriate at this point?

A. Resect all four glands.
B. Resect only the two largest glands.
C. Resect three glands and a portion of the fourth.
D. Resect all four glands and implant a portion of one in the forearm musculature.
E. Resect the largest gland and half of each of the three remaining glands.

Ref.: 1, 2, 3, 4

COMMENTS: The differentiation between an adenoma and four-gland hyperplasia as the cause of hyperparathyroidism frequently is most easily made by the gross findings at operation rather than by the histologic findings. When a large gland is found during exploration, the surgeon must identify at least one normal-sized gland to confirm the diagnosis of an adenoma. Nevertheless, because multiple adenomas are encountered in up to 5% of cases, the surgeon must attempt to identify the remaining three glands. Ideally, all three remaining glands are found; if they are normal in size, only the enlarged gland need be removed. A shave biopsy of one of the three normal-appearing glands may be useful for confirming its normal histologic features. A biopsy of all three remaining glands carries the risk of injuring or devascularizing all three and causing permanent hypoparathyroidism. If one large and one normal-sized gland are found but the other two glands are not easily identified, many surgeons would not pursue a more intense search for the remaining glands on the grounds that the risk of injuring those glands and causing hypoparathyroidism may outweight the small possibility of multiple adenomas. If more than one enlarged gland is found, four-gland hyperplasia must be suspected as the cause of the hyperparathyroidism; and in such cases it is even more important that all four glands be identified. If indeed all four are enlarged, the generally accepted options for management include either subtotal parathyroidectomy—resecting three glands and portion of the fourth (leaving approximately 40–60 mg of a single gland in place)—or a total parathyroidectomy—resecting all four glands and implanting a morcellated portion of one of the glands into a readily accessible muscle. Implantation into the forearm musculature permits reexploration of that area should hyperparathyroidism persist, without the inherent dangers of a cervical reexploration. The obvious goal of managing four-gland hyperplasia it to leave enough parathyroid tissue to prevent permanent hypoparathyroidism.

ANSWER:
Question 18: C, E
Question 19: C, D

20. During exploration for primary hyperparathyroidism, two normal-appearing glands on the left and one normal-appearing gland on the right are found after the paratracheal areas are explored bilaterally. The fourth gland is not found. Which of the following courses of action is/are the most appropriate?

A. Terminate the operation with no further dissection.
B. Extend the exploration through the existing cervical incision to include the central compartment of the neck between carotid arteries, posteriorly to the vertebral body, superiorly to the level of the pharynx and carotid bulb, and inferiorly into the mediastinum. Terminate the operation if the fourth gland is not found.
C. Resect the three glands found, leaving the fourth to maintain normal PTH levels.
D. Extend the incision into the right side of the neck laterally to explore the entire neck, including the posterior triangle.
E. Close the cervical incision and perform a median sternotomy to explore the mediastinum for an ectopic parathyroid.

Ref.: 1, 2, 4

COMMENTS: One of the more frustrating aspects of parathyroid surgery is the inability to find one of the parathyroid glands that is suspected to be the cause of hyperparathyroidism. In the clinical situation described, three normal-appearing glands are found, raising the likelihood that an adenoma of the fourth gland exists in an ectopic location. An understanding of the embryology of the parathyroids enables the surgeon to select the areas in which the gland is most likely to be found, which includes the central compartment of the neck between the carotid arteries, moving posteriorly to the vertebral body, superiorly to the level of the pharynx and carotid bulb, and inferiorly into the mediastinum. All of these areas, including the upper portion of the mediastinum, can be explored through the existing cervical collar incision, and this exploration should be conducted at the time of the initial operation. If the adenoma is not found after this extensive search, it is likely that the adenoma is in the mediastinum in an area not accessible through the collar incision. There is a small possibility that the adenoma is truly subcapsular within the ipsilateral thyroid lobe, and some surgeons would perform a thyroid lobectomy on the side of the missing gland. Extending the cervical exploration to include the posterior triangle would not be fruitful because the parathyroid gland would not be found in that location. Although sternotomy may be required to identify the missing gland, most surgeons delay this procedure until after the performance of sophisticated localization studies. Before closing, normal histologic features (i.e., nonhyperplastic tissue) should be confirmed by biopsy of one or two of the three normal-appearing glands that were found. Most surgeons mark the normal glands with surgical clips or nonabsorbable suture [the latter is preferred to avoid computed tomography (CT) scan interference] to facilitate their identification if reexploration becomes necessary. It is inappropriate to resect all three glands because hypoparathyroidism would result once the adenoma is found and resected.

ANSWER: B

21. Signs or symptoms of hypocalcemia include which of the following?

A. Electrocardiogram (ECG) with a shortened QT interval.
B. ECG with peaked T waves.
C. Bone pain due to "bone hunger."

D. Muscular paralysis.
E. Muscular tetany.

Ref.: 1, 2, 3

COMMENTS: Hypocalcemia can occur in as many as 30% of patients following parathyroidectomy, but only 1% develop permanent hypocalcemia. The major clinical manifestations result from reduced plasma ionized calcium and consequent neuromuscular excitability. The earliest manifestations are numbness and tingling in the circumoral area, fingers, and toes. Tetany may develop, characterized by carpopedal spasm. In severe cases, patients have mental status changes eventually leading to coma. On physical examination, contraction of the facial muscles is elicited by tapping on the facial nerve anterior to the ear (Chvostek's sign). Trousseau's sign (development of carpopedal spasm) can be elicited by occluding blood flow to the forearm for 3 minutes using a blood pressure cuff. The ECG may reveal a prolonged QT interval and peaked T waves. Mild symptoms can be treated with oral calcium; up to 6 gm of oral calcium may be given daily. One must be careful when giving intravenous calcium peripherally, as calcium can damage the skin and surrounding tissue, resulting in full-thickness skin burns and, in severe cases, loss of the distal extremity. If possible, intravenous calcium is administered centrally. Three causes of postoperative hypocalcemia are hungry bone syndrome, hypomagnesemia, and failure of the parathyroid remnant or autograft. In patients with long-standing hyperparathyroidism and bone disease, there may be substantial skeletal calcium deposition, so called bone hunger. Postoperatively, these patients have decreasing calcium levels for 2–3 days, which returns to normal over the next couple of days.

ANSWER: B, E

22. A 50-year-old woman presents to your office with a history of renal stones, peptic ulcer disease refractory to H_2-blockers, and nipple discharge. Which of the multiple endocrine neoplasia (MEN) syndromes does this suggest?

A. MEN-I.
B. MEN-IIA.
C. MEN-IIB.
D. Any of the above.

Ref.: 1, 2, 3, 4

COMMENTS: See Question 24.

23. For each MEN syndrome in the left column choose the appropriate biochemical screening test(s) from the right column:

A. MEN-I
B. MEN-IIA
C. MEN-IIB

a. Serum PTH
b. Serum somatomedin C
c. Serum gastrin
d. Serum calcitonin
e. Urinary catecholamines

Ref.: 1, 2, 3

COMMENTS: See Question 24.

24. Which of the following is/are appropriate treatment of the patient in Question 22?

A. Adrenalectomy.
B. Bromocriptine.
C. Unilateral parathyroidectomy.
D. Total parathyroidectomy.
E. Total thyroidectomy.

Ref.: 1, 2, 3

COMMENTS: Most cases of primary hyperparathyroidism occur in sporadic distribution in the general population. There is a small subset of patients, however, who manifest a familial tendency to develop hyperparathyroidism. It may occur alone as the only endocrine abnormality, or it may occur in association with other endocrine abnormalities (MEN syndromes). The **MEN-I syndrome** in its fully expressed state consists of pituitary adenomas (prolactin-secreting adenomas are the most common), parathyroid hyperplasia, and pancreatic islet cell neoplasia (e.g., gastrinoma, insulinoma). The **MEN-II syndrome** consists of medullary carcinoma of the thyroid variably associated with hyperparathyroidism and pheochromocytoma. The hyperparathyroidism may be due to hyperplasia or adenomas. In the fully expressed form of the subtype **MEN-IIA**, all three of these entities are present. **MEN-IIB syndrome** consists of medullary carcinoma of the thyroid and pheochromocytoma in association with ganglioneuromas, soft tissue nodules, and a marfanoid habitus but without hyperparathyroidism.

Screening for MEN-I consists of: (1) an intact serum PTH and an albumin-corrected total serum calcium level to detect hyperparathyroidism; (2) prolactin and somatomedin C assays to detect pituitary adenoma; and (3) fasting glucose and insulin, pancreatic polypeptide, and serum gastrin levels to detect pancreatic islet cell neoplasia. The calcitonin assay is used for diagnosing and following patients with medullary thyroid cancer, which can be present in MEN-IIA and MEN-IIB patients. A 24-hour urine collection for catecholamines and their metabolites is used as a screening test for pheochromocytoma, which can be present with MEN-IIA and MEN-IIB.

The **management** of patients with MEN-I depends on the severity of symptoms associated with the individual components. Resection of the pituitary adenoma, parathyroidectomy, and pharmacologic or surgical management of the pancreatic tumor may be appropriate and need not be performed in any set sequence. In MEN-I patients, hyperparathyroidism is associated with hyperplasia of all four glands rather than a single adenoma. Patients with evidence of hyperparathyroidism with an elevated gastrin level are advised strongly to undergo parathyroidectomy. Hypercalcemia is associated with increased gastrin levels, which may result in peptic ulcer disease. Peptic ulcer disease is the number one cause of death among families with MEN-I syndrome. Elevated gastrin in patients with MEN-I indicates the presence of gastrinoma resulting in Zollinger-Ellison syndrome. Identification and resection is the preferred treatment. Small duodenal gastrinomas must be directly searched for. Antisecretory drugs or parietal cell vagotomy may reduce medication requirements. Insulinoma is treated operatively; pharmacologic agents such as diazoxide and octreotide may be useful, as may streptozocin for patients with metastases. The prevalence of pituitary adenomas in patients with MEN-I varies from 10% to 65%. Prolactin-secreting adenomas are the most common followed by growth hormone-secreting adenomas. Surgery has been supplanted by medical treatment with dopamine analogues because of their ability to inhibit prolactin release. Approximately 70–90% of patients respond to the dopamine agonist bromocriptine. Somatostatin analogues and surgery are the preferred treatment for pituitary acromegaly. Patients with MEN-II and medullary thyroid cancer must be evaluated for pheochromocytoma. If present, the pheochromocytoma is resected first followed by staged neck exploration. Total parathyroidectomy with heterotopic transplantation is performed for patients with MEN-IIA and hyperparathyroidism and for those undergoing thyroidectomy even if normocalcemic.

ANSWER:
Question 22: A
Question 23: A-a,b,c; B-a,d,e; C-d,e
Question 24: B, D

25. With regard to parathyroid carcinoma, which of the following statements is/are correct?

A. It is a rare cause of hyperparathyroidism.
B. Only 5–10% of patients with parathyroid carcinoma manifest hypercalcemia.
C. The cytologic criteria differentiating parathyroid carcinoma from adenoma are well established.
D. A palpable neck mass suggests cancer.
E. Parathyroidectomy is usually curative.

Ref.: 1, 2, 5

COMMENTS: Parathyroid carcinoma is a rare cause of hyperparathyroidism, accounting for fewer than 1% of cases. Like many other neuroendocrine tumors, carcinoma of the parathyroid may not prevent the gland from carrying out its normal endocrine function (i.e., PTH production). However, regulation of PTH production is usually impaired, and as many as 85% of patients with parathyroid carcinoma present with hypercalcemia. It is of note that the hypercalcemia is usually severe, frequently manifesting serum calcium concentrations in excess of 14 mg/dl. Approximately 50% of patients with parathyroid cancer have a palpable tumor, in contrast to its rarity in patients with benign hyperparathyroidism. The cytologic criteria for malignancy are poorly defined, and it may be difficult to differentiate a parathyroid carcinoma from adenoma on histologic basis alone. Evidence of local invasion or regional or distant metastases may be needed to confirm the diagnosis of carcinoma. The surgeon must therefore be suspicious of carcinoma when the tumor is firmly attached to adjacent structures. The likelihood of cure is greatest when all known disease can be surgically resected, which involves en bloc resection of the parathyroid and ipsilateral thyroid lobe with adjacent muscle and fibrofatty tissue. Surgical debulking of known disease may be beneficial in reducing the PTH levels and thereby palliating the symptoms of severe hypercalcemia. The long-term prognosis is usually poor.

ANSWER: A, D

26. Which of the following is the most common cause of hypoparathyroidism?

A. Prior thyroid surgery.
B. Prior parathyroid surgery.
C. Prior viral infection involving the parathyroid glands.
D. Genetic disorder of PTH metabolism.

Ref.: 1, 2

COMMENTS: The most common cause of hypoparathyroidism is surgical trauma to the parathyroid glands during thyroid or parathyroid exploration. Because thyroid operations are much more common than parathyroid operations, prior thyroid surgery accounts for most cases of hypoparathyroidism. There is no known association between viral infections and the development of hypoparathyroidism. There is a rare genetic disorder (pseudohypoparathyroidism) in which the serum PTH level is normal to elevated but the end-organ response of the kidney to circulating PTH is abnormal, resulting in hyperphosphatemia and hypocalcemia. Most cases of postoperative hypocalcemia are temporary; and if viable parathyroid tissue does remain, the PTH and serum calcium levels return to normal. These patients may need to be supported temporarily with exogenous calcium and, on occasion, vitamin D. If the patient remains asymptomatic, it usually is wise to avoid calcium administration on the basis of a low serum calcium level alone because this low level serves as the stimulus for the compensatory growth and function of the remaining parathyroid tissue. If clinical signs of hypocalcemia develop (e.g., carpopedal spasm, tetany, Chvostek's sign, Trousseau's sign, ECG changes) or if the hypoparathyroidism appears to be permanent, treatment with exogenous calcium (up to 2 gm of elemental calcium/day) and vitamin D_3 (up to 100,000 units/day) is needed.

ANSWER: A

REFERENCES

1. Sabiston DC Jr: *Textbook of Surgery*, 15th ed. WB Saunders, Philadelphia, 1997.
2. Schwartz SI, Shires GT, Spencer FC: *Principles of Surgery*, 7th ed. McGraw-Hill, New York, 1999.
3. Greenfield LJ, Mulholland M, Oldham KT, et al: *Surgery: Scientific Principles and Practice*, 2nd ed. Lippincott-Raven, Philadelphia, 1997.
4. Clark OH, Duh QY: *Textbook of Endocrine Surgery*. WB Saunders, Philadelphia, 1997.
5. Clark OH, Duh QY, Siperstein AE: *Surg Clin North Am* 75(3), 1995.

CHAPTER 23

Pituitary

1. With regard to the anatomy of the pituitary gland, which of the following statements is/are true?

   A. As with other portions of the central nervous system (CNS), there is an anatomic and physiologic blood–brain barrier present within the neurohypophysis.
   B. The adenohypophysis does not have its own direct arterial blood supply.
   C. The neurohypophysis contains both neuronal cell bodies and axons.
   D. The adenohypophysis contains axons only.
   E. No nerves terminate within the adenohypophysis.

Ref.: 1, 2

COMMENTS: The special neuroendocrine function of the pituitary gland and its interrelation with the hypothalamus are facilitated by several distinct anatomic features. For example, the hormonal mediators released within the neurohypophysis gain access to the vascular system through fenestrated epithelium, and thus the neurohypophysis does not have a "blood–brain barrier" like the barrier that characterizes most of the rest of the CNS. The vascular anatomy of the adenohypophysis is unusual in that it does not derive its blood supply from a direct arterial source but, rather, from a system of portal vessels that first pass through the capillary bed of the neurohypophysis. Because no nerves directly terminate within the adenohypophysis, it is dependent on this portal capillary system for receiving the hormones that influence its function. The neurohypophysis, on the other hand, is regulated in part by hormonal influences from the periphery (and possibly feedback directly from the adenohypophysis) and by direct neural input from the hypothalamus. The latter is by means of axons, the cell bodies of which lie within the hypothalamus. The neurohypophysis itself contains no neuronal cell bodies. Such an anatomic arrangement allows complicated interplay of neural and endocrine factors between the hypothalamus, neurohypophysis, adenohypophysis, and peripheral endocrine function.

ANSWER: B, E

2. A 33-year-old woman develops a visual field loss, and computed tomography (CT) of the brain demonstrates a cystic sellar mass with calcification. Which of the following statements about this patient is/are true?

   A. The most common tumors involving the sellar and parasellar region include pituitary adenomas, hypothalamic/optic nerve gliomas, craniopharyngiomas, aneurysms, meningiomas, germinomas, and inflammatory lesions.
   B. Calcification is typical of pituitary adenomas.
   C. Craniopharyngiomas are usually cystic.
   D. Suprasellar extension of the tumor can lead to obstructive hydrocephalus.

Ref.: 2

COMMENTS: Certain lesions are commonly found in the sella and parasellar region. They include pituitary adenomas, gliomas of the optic nerve or chiasm and of the hypothalamus, craniopharyngiomas, aneurysms, meningiomas, germinomas, and inflammatory lesions such as a sarcoid. Although most of these abnormalities can cause visual symptoms, the presence of calcification in a cyst on a CT scan makes the most likely diagnosis of this lesion a craniopharyngioma. These tumors account for 2–4% of brain tumors and originate from remnants of Rathke's pouch. Pathologically, most craniopharyngiomas contain a solid and a cystic component containing calcifications; and they are composed of columnar epithelium with squamous cells forming the interior. These tumors can present with visual symptoms, headache, or hydrocephalus. Treatment consists of surgical resection followed by radiation therapy. As with any tumor of the sellar region, suprasellar extension of sellar tumors commonly leads to compression of the third ventricle and the foramen of Monro, with resultant obstructive hydrocephalus.

ANSWER: A, C, D

3. A patient undergoes removal of a pituitary microadenoma, and 24 hours after surgery the urine output increases to 300–500 ml/hr with a specific gravity of 1.000. Which of the following statements with regard to this patient is/are true?

   A. Electrolyte analysis would show hyponatremia.
   B. Vasopressin excess causes diabetes insipidus.
   C. The neurohypophysis is derived from an invagination of Rathke's pouch.
   D. Treatment of this disorder includes immediate administration of deamino-D-arginine-vasopressin (DDAVP).
   E. A rough estimate of serum osmolarity can be calculated if the blood urea nitrogen (BUN), glucose, and sodium levels are known.

Ref.: 1, 2

COMMENTS: This history of excessive dilute urine after pituitary surgery is highly suggestive of diabetes insipidus, which is the result of suppressed vasopressin release. Vasopressin is excreted into the portal circulation from the neurohypophysis. The adenohypophysis is generally believed to be derived from a diverticulum of the primitive foregut known as the stomodeum, whereas the neurohypophysis is directly related to the diencephalon, specifically the hypothalamus. Axons derived from the cells of the supraoptic nuclei and paraventricular nuclei in the hypothalamus terminate their neurons in the neurohypophysis and secrete vasopressin and oxytocin. Vasopressin, or antidiuretic hormone (ADH), binds to receptors on the distal renal tubules and collecting ducts, where it activates the generation of cyclic adenosine monophosphate (cAMP), which increases reabsorption of water from the nephron into the circulation. Osmolar receptors in the anterior hypothalamus are sensitive to increases in serum osmolarity and are the prime factors in the release of ADH. In other words a hyperosmolar state simulates the release of ADH. Diabetes insipidus results in an excessive volume of dilute urine, hypovolemia, and hypernatremia, with thirst usually a prominent clinical feature. Serum osmolarity can roughly be estimated by the following formula if one knows the serum electrolytes:

$$2 \times \text{serum sodium} + \text{blood glucose}/18 + \text{BUN}/3$$

When treating a patient who develops diabetes insipidus after pituitary surgery and who is alert and able to eat, fluid intake is usually dictated by the patient's normal thirst mechanism. Only in situations of inadequate oral intake is exogenous vasopressin necessary.

ANSWER: E

4. With regard to prolactin secretion and physiology, which of the following statements is/are true?

A. Prolactin is secreted from the neurohypophysis in response to suckling.
B. Males and nonpregnant females have similar blood levels of prolactin.
C. Prolactin has physiologic effects on the breast, ovary, and testis.
D. The principal hypothalamic effect on prolactin secretion is inhibitory.
E. Prolactin secretion may be stimulated by pregnancy, stress, exercise, and breast stimulation.

Ref.: 1, 2

COMMENTS: Prolactin is a peptide secreted from eosinophilic cells of the adenohypophysis in response to numerous peripheral factors, including pregnancy, stress, exercise, and direct breast stimulation. Hypothalamic control of prolactin secretion is primarily inhibitory via prolactin-inhibiting factor, which some evidence suggests may be dopamine. In the nonstimulated state, men and women have similar blood levels of prolactin. Its most significant physiologic effect is mammotropic, stimulating duct development and lactation. It also has gonadal effects and is thought to modulate to some degree ovarian progesterone synthesis and testicular testosterone synthesis.

ANSWER: B, C, D, E

5. With regard to adrenocorticotropic hormone (ACTH), which of the following statements is/are true?

A. ACTH release is presumed to be under partial hypothalamic control.
B. ACTH release may be affected by direct feedback inhibition of circulating cortisol levels on the adenohypophysis.
C. ACTH levels are fairly constant during any given 24-hour period but may rise abruptly in response to stress.
D. There is a circadian rhythm to ACTH release that cannot usually be overcome by peripheral stimulatory influences.

Ref.: 1, 2

COMMENTS: ACTH is secreted by the adenohypophysis under the influence of both hypothalamic control via corticotropin-releasing factor (CRF) and the negative feedback control of circulating cortisol levels. Although there are several surges of ACTH release during a given 24-hour period, the largest one occurs characteristically at night and during the early morning hours, accounting for the typical diurnal variation of blood cortisol levels. These central and negative feedback regulatory mechanisms are easily overridden during periods of stress, such as acute illness, fever, hypoglycemia, and emotional upset. An abrupt increase in ACTH secretion in response to these factors can lead to as much as a 10-fold increase in cortisol production within a short period of time.

ANSWER: A, B

6. Match each of the physiologic effects in the left column with its respective gonadotropic hormone in the right column.

A. Promotes spermatogenesis	a. Follicle-stimulating hormone (FSH)
B. Stimulates testicular testosterone production	b. Luteinizing hormone (LH)
C. Facilitates development of corpus luteum	c. Both FSH and LH
D. Promotes ovarian follicle maturation	d. Neither FSH nor LH
E. Production stimulated by gonadotropin-releasing hormone (GnRH)	

Ref.: 1, 2

COMMENTS: Sexual and reproductive physiology involves a complex interaction of hypothalamic, pituitary, gonadal, adrenal, and circulating hormonal factors. The role of the pituitary in this complex scheme involves the production of FSH and LH. These two hormones are produced by the same basophilic adenohypophyseal cell under the influence of a single GnRH from the hypothalamus. This hypothalamic–pituitary interaction is modulated by feedback from adrenal and gonadal hormone production.

ANSWER: A-a; B-b; C-d; D-a; E-c

7. With regard to thyroid-stimulating hormone (TSH), which of the following statements is/are true?

A. TSH release is under hypothalamic influence by means of thyrotropin-releasing hormone (TRH).
B. TSH release is directly influenced by circulating thyroid hormones.

C. As with other adenohypophyseal hormones, TSH has numerous effects in addition to its stimulatory effect on the thyroid gland.
D. TSH levels can be pharmacologically manipulated to affect the growth of thyroid neoplasms.

Ref.: 1, 2

COMMENTS: Unlike prolactin and growth hormone, which have numerous metabolic effects, TSH appears to exert influence only on the thyroid gland. It stimulates both growth of the gland and secretion of thyroid hormones. Circulating thyroid hormones exert a well defined feedback inhibition on TSH-producing cells in the adenohypophysis, directly and by inhibiting the effect of hypothalamically derived TRH. The growth of thyroid neoplasms, similar to the growth of the normal thyroid gland, may be stimulated by high TSH levels. For this reason, pharmacologic reduction of TSH levels through the administration of exogenous thyroid hormone may shrink both benign and malignant thyroid tumors.

ANSWER: A, B, D

8. Match each of the terms in the left column with its synonymous term in the right column.

A. Infundibular process	a. Median eminence
B. Pars distalis	b. Anterior pituitary
C. Infundibulum	c. Posterior pituitary
D. Infundibular stem	d. Pituitary stalk

Ref.: 1, 2

COMMENTS: To some degree there is a lack of standardization of the nomenclature pertaining to pituitary anatomy. The most widely accepted terminology is attributed to Wislocki. According to this terminology, the pituitary is composed of the neurohypophysis and the adenohypophysis. The **neurohypophysis** is composed of the infundibulum (median eminence), the infundibular stem (pituitary stalk), and the infundibular process (posterior lobe, posterior pituitary, or pars nervosa). The **adenohypophysis** consists of the pars tuberalis (wrapping around the infundibular stem) and the pars distalis (anterior lobe or anterior pituitary). The concept of the pituitary gland as two separate but closely related entities—the neurohypophysis, or posterior pituitary, and the adenohypophysis, or anterior pituitary—is important when considering the numerous aspects of clinical pituitary pathology.

ANSWER: A-c; B-b; C-a; D-d

9. Match each of the secretions in the left column with the portion of the pituitary from which it originates in the right column.

A. Growth hormone	a. Adenohypophysis
B. Oxytocin	b. Neurohypophysis
C. Thyrotropin-releasing factor	c. Both adenohypophysis and neurohypophysis
D. ACTH	d. Neither adenohypophysis nor neurohypophysis
E. Cortisol	
F. Vasopressin	
G. Prolactin	

Ref.: 1, 2

COMMENTS: Hormones secreted by the anterior pituitary (e.g., growth hormone, ACTH, TSH, LH, FSH, prolactin) are controlled in part by direct feedback inhibition from the periphery and by releasing factors from the hypothalamus and neurohypophysis (e.g., thyrotropin-, corticotropin-, gonadotropin-, or growth hormone inhibitory-releasing factors). In addition to these releasing factors, the neurohypophysis produces two hormones (oxytocin and vasopressin) that have their primary effect peripherally.

ANSWER: A-a; B-b; C-b; D-a; E-d; F-b; G-a

10. With regard to excess ACTH of pituitary origin, which one or more of the following statements is/are true?

A. Cushing syndrome and Cushing's disease are synonymous terms.
B. ACTH-producing pituitary adenomas are the most common cause of excess adrenal cortisol production.
C. Most hypothalamic/pituitary causes of excess ACTH production are due to pituitary microadenomas.
D. The sella is enlarged in most patients with ACTH-producing pituitary adenomas.
E. Bilateral adrenalectomy is preferable to hypophysectomy for the management of Cushing's disease.

Ref.: 1, 2

COMMENTS: Cushing syndrome refers to the clinical sequela of excess adrenal cortisol production. It may be due to an adrenal carcinoma, adrenal adenoma, nodular dysplasia of the adrenal, or diffuse adrenal hyperplasia in response to excess CRF production from the hypothalamus, ectopic ACTH production, or excess ACTH production from a pituitary adenoma. When Cushing syndrome is due to a pituitary adenoma, it is known as Cushing's disease. Of the hypothalamic/pituitary causes of **Cushing syndrome**, pathologic studies have demonstrated that up to 80% are due to a pituitary microadenoma that produces ACTH. In most of these cases, the adenoma is too small to cause any changes in the radiographic appearance of the sella. When appropriate studies have revealed that a pituitary adenoma is the cause of bilateral adrenal hyperplasia, the preferred method of treatment is transsphenoidal excision of the adenoma rather than bilateral adrenalectomy.

ANSWER: B, C

11. Which one or more of the following statements characterize pituitary endorphins?

A. They are opiate-like peptides.
B. They share a common amino acid sequence with other adenohypophyseal hormones.
C. They are also found in the brain and gut.
D. Despite their biochemical identification, physiologic or behavioral effects of these substances have not yet been demonstrated.

Ref.: 1, 2

COMMENTS: Pituitary endorphins are opiate-like peptides that represent fragments of a larger prohormone called pro-opiocortin. Melanocyte-stimulating hormone and ACTH possess amino acid sequences that are identical to portions of the pro-opiocortin and β-lipotropin structures. These endorphins, which are also found throughout the brain and gut, are capable of exerting potent analgesic effects and may be key factors in an individual's behavioral and physiologic response to pain.

ANSWER: A, B, C

12. Amenorrhea and progressive hypothyroidism occurring after recovery from shock due to placental hemorrhage may be known as which one or more of the following?

A. Sheehan syndrome.
B. Postpartum pituitary ischemia.
C. Thyrogenital syndrome.
D. A form of pituitary apoplexy.

Ref.: 1, 2

COMMENTS: During pregnancy the size of the pituitary may increase as much as 50%, with a proportionate increase in blood flow. If a state of hypoperfusion should occur during late pregnancy or delivery, the pituitary may become ischemic and subsequently necrotic, resulting in panhypopituitarism. The most obvious subsequent clinical manifestations of this condition are amenorrhea and hypothyroidism. Once the diagnosis is made, treatment involves appropriate hormone replacement therapy.

ANSWER: A, B, D

13. With regard to growth hormone hypersecretion, which of the following statements is/are true?

A. Acromegaly may occur in both adults and children.
B. Growth hormone secreting adenomas may be eosinophilic or chromophobic.
C. Growth hormone secreting tumors may produce symptoms that are not related to growth hormone excess.
D. Acromegalics frequently die of cardiac complications.
E. Surgery has been supplanted by radiation therapy as the treatment of choice for excessive growth hormone secretion.

Ref.: 1, 2

COMMENTS: Excessive production of growth hormone by pituitary adenomas (usually chromophobic but occasionally eosinophilic) leads to morphologic changes that differ according to the age and skeletal maturity of the patient. In children (before epiphyseal closure), there is generalized overgrowth of most of the somatic structures, resulting in gigantism. In adults (after epiphyseal closure), the somatic enlargement is most evident in the face, hands, and feet and is termed acromegaly. In patients with acromegaly, enlargement of the heart with subsequent valvular dysfunction and cardiomyopathy may also occur and is a common cause of death. Although the characteristic physical appearance of patients with growth hormone excess dominates the clinical presentation, the adenoma itself occasionally grows to such a size as to produce symptoms due to an expanding pituitary mass (e.g., visual disturbances, headaches, pituitary hypofunction). Surgical excision of the adenoma is the treatment in most circumstances, although radiation therapy is finding increasing applicability.

ANSWER: B, C, D

14. With regard to growth hormone, which of the following statements is/are true?

A. Growth hormone is a peptide that affects the growth of somatic structures such as bone and muscle but does not affect the growth of visceral organs or physiologic homeostasis.
B. Growth hormone secretion is stimulated by a hypothalamic-releasing factor, but as of the present no hypothalamic inhibitory factor has been identified.
C. Under normal circumstances, the largest surge of growth hormone in the peripheral blood occurs during the evening.
D. Growth hormone secretion may be stimulated by exercise, stress, or hypoglycemia.

Ref.: 1, 2

COMMENTS: Growth hormone is a large peptide secreted from the lateral aspect of the adenohypophysis. Its secretion is regulated by releasing factors and inhibitory factors (somatostatin) from the hypothalamus. Furthermore, its release is stimulated directly or indirectly by exercise, physiologic stress, and hypoglycemia. In addition to its positive effect on the growth of somatic structures, growth hormone also stimulates the growth of visceral organs. Additionally, it has numerous anabolic effects, including the elevation of blood glucose and free fatty acid levels and the incorporation of amino acids into protein. Growth hormone is released into the peripheral blood as a result of secretory surges occurring six to eight times daily, the largest one during the early morning hours. During adolescence the total amount of growth hormone secreted daily increases owing to an increase in the number of surges.

ANSWER: D

15. With regard to pituitary releasing factors, which of the following statements is/are true?

A. Releasing factors are formed in the hypothalamus and proceed directly to the adenohypophysis, bypassing the neurohypophysis.
B. Releasing factors are derivatives of steroids similar to those seen in the adrenal cortex.
C. Release of thyroid-stimulating hormone (TSH) is under partial control of thyroid-releasing hormone (TRH) and partial control of peripheral triiodothyronine (T_3) and thyroxine (T_4) levels.
D. The concept of feedback inhibition of pituitary function is outdated.

Ref.: 1, 2

COMMENTS: The concept of feedback inhibition is fundamental to the understanding of the hypothalamic-pituitary-peripheral endocrine axis. In its most simplified form, the hypothalamus, sensing and reacting to peripheral blood hormone levels, synthesizes releasing factors (small peptides), which are released as neurosecretory granules from the axons within the neurohypophysis. These are then transported through the portal vascular system to the adenohypophysis to influence adenohypophyseal hormone output. These hormones in turn influence endocrine function of the peripheral end organ that alters blood levels, completing the cycle. The adenohypophysis may be directly sensitive to blood levels of circulating hormones, as in the case of TSH production, which may be altered not only by TRH but also by peripheral T_3 and T_4 levels.

ANSWER: C

16. With regard to pituitary tumors, which one or more of the following statements is/are true?

A. The classification of pituitary tumors depends solely on their aniline dye affinity.
B. The most common pituitary tumor is endocrine-inactive.
C. Common parasellar symptoms include cerebrospinal fluid (CSF) obstruction.
D. Prolactin excess in males causes decreased potency and infertility.
E. Surgery and radiation therapy are the mainstays of treatment.

Ref.: 1, 2

COMMENTS: Pituitary tumors were formerly classified according to their affinity for aniline dyes (chromophobe, eosinophils, or basophilic adenomas). The more recent classification divides them into endocrine-active and endocrine-inactive tumors. The most common pituitary adenoma is the prolactin-producing adenoma, followed (in decreasing order of frequency) by endocrine-inactive tumors, growth hormone-producing tumors, ACTH-producing tumors, TSH-producing tumors, and finally LH/FSH-producing tumors. Tumors less than 1 cm in diameter are termed microadenomas, whereas those larger than 1 cm in diameter are called macroadenomas. Symptomatology depends on the type of hormone produced, the degree of compromise of the surrounding anterior pituitary (symptoms of hormone insufficiency), and the mass effect of the tumor itself producing parasellar neurologic deficits. In females prolactin excess causes menstrual irregularities, infertility, and galactorrhea. In males it leads to decreased potency and infertility. Growth hormone excess causes gigantism in young patients and acromegaly in patients whose epiphyses are closed. ACTH-producing adenomas cause Cushing's disease. TSH-producing adenomas are associated with hyperthyroidism, whereas LH/FSH-producing adenomas lead to gonadal insufficiency. Parasellar deficits include optic nerve dysfunction, extraocular motor loss, hypothalamic dysfunction, or frontal and medial temporal lobe signs and symptoms. The most effective therapies for symptomatic pituitary adenomas remain surgery and radiation therapy, although TSH-producing and FSH/LH-producing adenomas may shrink in response to bromocriptine therapy.

ANSWER: D, E

17. Match the sellar lesion with the common presenting symptom.

A. Macroadenoma	a. Gigantism in children, acromegaly in adults
B. Craniopharyngioma	b. Bitemporal hemianopsia
C. Growth hormone microadenoma	c. Galactorrhea, amenorrhea, impotence
D. ACTH microadenoma	d. Cushing's disease
E. Prolactin adenoma	e. Diabetes insipidus

Ref.: 1, 2

COMMENTS: The pituitary lies in the bony structure called the sella turcica at the base of the brain. It is connected to the hypothalamus via the infundibulum and the portal system. The pituitary gland acts as the master gland of the endocrine system. Its most common tumors are pituitary adenomas. Frequently, these adenomas are not hormonally active but, instead, cause symptoms by local mass effect. Because they present by pressing on local structures such as the optic chiasm or other cranial nerves, they are usually more than 1 cm in diameter and are referred to as macroadenomas. Microadenomas, pituitary tumors less than 1 cm in diameter, present because of the hormone releasing factors that they secrete. ACTH-secreting tumors cause Cushing's disease, which can be differentiated from adrenal tumors that produce cortisol and ectopic tumors that secrete ACTH by the dexamethasone suppression test. Growth hormone-secreting tumors cause gigantism in children and acromegaly in adults. These are best treated surgically if no contraindications exist. Prolactinomas cause amenorrhea, galactorrhea, impotence, and symptoms of mass effect. These symptoms can be controlled in some patients with bromocriptine, a dopamine agonist. Craniopharyngioma, an epithelium-lined tumor, usually involves the sella. It is more common during childhood and can present with mass effect or hypopituitary symptoms, such as diabetes insipidus.

ANSWER: A-b; B-e; C-a; D-d; E-c

REFERENCES

1. Schwartz SI, Shires GT, Spencer FC: *Principles of Surgery*, 7th ed. McGraw-Hill, New York, 1999.
2. Sabiston DC Jr: *Textbook of Surgery*, 15th ed. WB Saunders, Philadelphia, 1997.

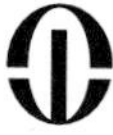

CHAPTER 24

Adrenal

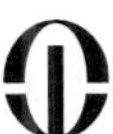

1. The arterial blood supply of *both* the right and left adrenal glands comes from which of the following?

A. Branch of the inferior phrenic artery.
B. Direct aortic branch.
C. Branch of the renal artery.
D. None of the above; each gland is supplied by a different pattern.

Ref.: 1, 2, 3

COMMENTS: The arterial blood supply to both the adrenal glands is somewhat similar and typically from three sources: The **superior adrenal artery** originates from a branch of the inferior phrenic artery, which comes off the aorta. The **middle adrenal artery** comes directly from the aorta. The **inferior adrenal artery** arises from the renal artery on each side. Recognition of these multiple arterial vessels is of obvious importance during adrenalectomy.

ANSWER: A, B, C

2. Which of the following statements correctly describe(s) the venous drainage of the adrenal glands?

A. Plexus of small veins drains each gland.
B. Primary central vein drains each gland.
C. Right gland typically drains into the renal vein.
D. Left gland typically drains into the renal vein.
E. Both glands typically drain directly into the inferior vena cava.

Ref.: 1, 2, 3, 4

COMMENTS: Each adrenal gland is usually drained by one main central vein. On the right side, the adrenal vein leaves the gland medially and goes directly into the inferior vena cava. This vein is typically short and wide and can be the source of hazardous bleeding if not handled correctly. On the left side, the adrenal vein leaves the gland anteriorly and joins the left renal vein. Because of this, selective catheterization of the adrenal vein for diagnostic sampling is simpler on the left. Occasionally, the left adrenal vein enters the inferior vena cava directly. Small accessory adrenal veins may also be present.

ANSWER: B, D

3. With regard to adrenal gland embryology, which of the following statements is/are true?

A. Adrenal cortex is derived from ectodermal tissue.
B. Adrenal medulla is derived from ectodermal tissue.
C. Extraadrenal medullary tissue is most commonly found adjacent to the gonads.
D. Extraadrenal cortical tissue is most commonly found along the sympathetic nerve chain.

Ref.: 1, 2, 3, 4

COMMENTS: The adrenal gland is composed of a cortex and a medulla, which have different embryologic origins and widely different physiologic functions. The cortex is derived from mesoderm between the dorsal mesentery and the primitive gonad located along the urogenital ridge. This development occurs between the fourth and sixth weeks of fetal life. The medulla is derived from ectodermal cells and the neural crest during the seventh week of fetal development. Migration of these ectodermal cells from the neural crest of the periaortic area is responsible for the eventual development of the sympathetic ganglia and the adrenal medulla. In lower vertebrates, the cortical and medullary tissues remain separate; in humans, the cortex envelops the medulla to form a single gland. This gland is larger than the kidney during the midportion of fetal development but gradually decreases in size through the end of the first postpartum year. During the course of fetal development, both adrenal cortical and adrenal medullary rests may persist along the paths of cellular migration. Extraadrenal medullary (chromaffin) tissue is found more commonly and over a much wider anatomic range than is extraadrenal cortical tissue, and it is responsible for the occurrence of extraadrenal pheochromocytoma. The most common extraadrenal site of medullary tissue is the organ of Zuckerkandl, located along the aorta adjacent to the origin of the inferior mesenteric artery.

ANSWER: B

4. Match each of the hormones in the left column with one or more of the parts of the adrenal gland where it is primarily manufactured in the right column.

A. Cortisol	a. Zona glomerulosa
B. Aldosterone	b. Zona fasciculata
C. Sex steroids	c. Zona reticularis
D. Epinephrine	d. Adrenal medulla
E. Norepinephrine	

Ref.: 1, 2

COMMENTS: See Question 5.

5. Match each of the enzymes in the left column with one or more of the anatomic zones of the adrenal cortex in which it is found in the right column.

A. 17-Hydroxylase	a. Zona glomerulosa
B. 11-Hydroxylase	b. Zona fasciculata
C. 21-Hydroxylase	c. Zona reticularis
D. Corticosterone methyloxidase	

Ref.: 1, 2

COMMENTS: Adrenal cortical hormones are manufactured as a result of hydroxylation and oxidation of certain sites on the cholesterol molecule. These processes occur in different areas of the adrenal cortex, depending on the presence or absence of specific enzymes. Anatomically, the adrenal cortex consists of three zones that are arranged concentrically from the capsule inward to the medulla: zona glomerulosa, zona fasciculata, and zona reticularis. Adrenal cortical hormones are synthesized from cholesterol, which is converted to 5-pregnenolone. In the presence of 17-hydroxylase (contained in the zona fasciculata and zona reticularis but *not* in the zona glomerulosa), 5-pregnenolone is converted to 17-hydroxypregnenolone, which is the precursor of both cortisol and the androgens. In the absence of 17-hydroxylase, 5-pregnenolone is converted to progesterone, which is the precursor of aldosterone. Each of the three zones in the adrenal cortex contains 11- and 21-hydroxylating enzymes. As a consequence of "anatomically specific" enzyme differences, aldosterone is produced exclusively by the zona glomerulosa because of the presence of corticosterone methyloxidase, whereas cortisol is produced in both the zona fasciculata and the zona reticularis. The sex steroids are thought to be produced primarily by the zona reticularis but may also be manufactured by cells within the zona fasciculata. The catecholamines are products of phenylalanine and tyrosine rather than being derived from cholesterol. The conversion of norepinephrine to epinephrine requires methylation by the enzyme phenylethanolamine-*N*-methyltransferase, which is present almost exclusively in the adrenal medulla and organ of Zuckerkandl. Therefore nearly all of the epinephrine is synthesized in the adrenal medulla.

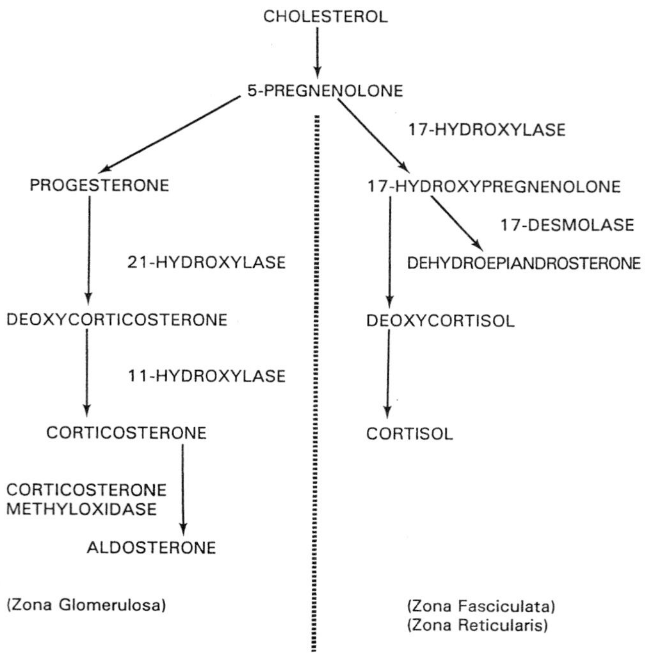

CHOLESTEROL
5-PREGNENOLONE
17-HYDROXYLASE
PROGESTERONE
17-HYDROXYPREGNENOLONE
17-DESMOLASE
21-HYDROXYLASE
DEHYDROEPIANDROSTERONE
DEOXYCORTICOSTERONE
DEOXYCORTISOL
11-HYDROXYLASE
CORTICOSTERONE
CORTISOL
CORTICOSTERONE METHYLOXIDASE
ALDOSTERONE
(Zona Glomerulosa)
(Zona Fasciculata)
(Zona Reticularis)

ANSWER:
Question 4: A-b,c; B-a; C-b,c; D-d; E-d
Question 5: A-b,c; B-a,b,c; C-a,b,c; D-a

6. Which of the following is/are a result of physiologic cortisol production?

A. Gluconeogenesis.
B. Protein catabolism.
C. Fat storage.
D. Decreasing excretion of urinary calcium.
E. Immunosuppression.

Ref.: 1, 2

COMMENTS: Cortisol is produced in the zona fasciculata and zona reticularis of the adrenal gland. After cortisol is excreted by the adrenal gland, it binds to a glucocorticoid receptor in a cell, promoting the transcription of target genes, which produce the metabolic effects of cortisol. Glucocorticoids are necessary to maintain hepatic glycogen stores (perform gluconeogenesis). Cortisol also stimulates protein catabolism and lipolysis and causes hyperinsulinemia. The pathway by which immunologic function is affected is unclear, but glucocorticoid excess suppresses immune and antiinflammatory responses. Physiologic levels of cortisol have not been demonstrated to affect either wound healing or the inflammatory process. Also, glucocorticoids can exhibit an effect on calcium homeostasis by decreasing intestinal calcium absorption and increasing excretion of urinary calcium.

ANSWER: A, B

7. Which of the following is the most common cause of endogenous hypercortisolism?

A. Adrenal adenoma.
B. Adrenal carcinoma.
C. Pituitary adenoma.
D. Ectopic ACTH production.

Ref.: 1, 2

COMMENTS: **Cushing syndrome** refers to the clinical manifestations of excess glucocorticoids. The overall most common cause is iatrogenic due to exogenous administration of corticosteroids. Endogenous overproduction of cortisol is most commonly due to a pituitary adenoma, which accounts for about 70% of all cases. Cortisol excess from a pituitary tumor is known as **Cushing's disease**, which is thus responsible for only a portion of patients with Cushing syndrome. Other **ACTH-dependent** causes of cortisol excess include ectopic ACTH produced by various tumors and, rarely, sources of corticotropin releasing hormone (CRH). About 10–20% of endogenous hypercortisolism is **ACTH-independent**. This includes the primary adrenal causes, which most frequently are an adrenal adenoma followed by adrenal carcinoma and the rare adrenocortical hyperplasia (nodular dysplasia).

ANSWER: C

8. Which type of adrenal pathology can occur in patients with ACTH-dependent hypercortisolism?

A. Bilateral adrenal hyperplasia.
B. Single adrenal adenoma.
C. Multiple adrenal adenomas.
D. All of the above.

Ref.: 1

COMMENTS: ACTH-dependent causes of excess cortisol production all result in bilateral adrenal hyperplasia. ACTH-independent hypercortisolism is due to primary adrenal pathology, which includes single or multiple adenomas, adrenal cancer, and adrenal hyperplasia.

ANSWER: A

9. Clinical features of Cushing syndrome include which of the following?

A. Hypertension.
B. Alopecia.
C. Truncal obesity.
D. Hypoglycemia.
E. Hyperkalemia.

Ref.: 1, 2, 4

COMMENTS: The clinical manifestations of excess glucocorticoid are similar regardless of the cause. Truncal obesity, hypertension, and glucose intolerance are typical. Abnormal patterns of fat deposition produce the characteristic "buffalo hump" and "moon facies." Females manifest hirsutism and menstrual disorders; sexual dysfunction is common in both sexes. Purple striae over the abdomen and extremities, proximal muscle atrophy, peripheral edema, acne, easy bruisability, and osteoporosis are seen. Other features may include back pain, poor wound healing, neurologic symptoms, and psychiatric disturbances. Hypokalemia can occur owing to the weak mineralocorticoid effect of cortisol.

ANSWER: A, C

10. An obese 45-year-old man complains of impotence. Examination demonstrates a blood pressure of 180/90, proximal muscle wasting, and purple abdominal striae. Which of the following is the most sensitive screening test for hypercortisolism?

A. Plasma cortisol level at 8 a.m.
B. Plasma cortisol level at 4 p.m.
C. Random plasma cortisol level.
D. 24-Hour urinary free cortisol level.
E. 24-Hour urinary 17-OH corticosteroid level.

Ref.: 1, 2, 3, 4

COMMENTS: The diagnostic strategy for evaluating a patient with suspected Cushing syndrome is to first confirm excess cortisol production and then to determine its cause or source. Cortisol is normally secreted intermittently with a diurnal variation such that evening levels are lower (by about one-half) than morning levels. Therefore a random sample is not useful. Likewise, even though patients with Cushing syndrome typically have elevated evening levels, there is sufficient overlap with normal levels to limit the accuracy of this approach. The most sensitive screening test is a 24-hour determination of urinary free cortisol. Normally, little free cortisol is excreted in the urine, but when excess cortisol is present the levels are elevated because cortisol-binding sites are saturated. Measurement of two or three consecutive urine samples should be obtained; and urinary creatinine should be measured concomitantly to ensure that the sample is adequate. Comparison of the urinary steroid/creatinine ratio may limit the false-positive results that might occur in obese patients because of increased body mass. 17-Hydroxy (OH) corticosteroids and 17-OH ketosteroids are metabolites of cortisol and androgens that can be measured in the urine, but this method is less accurate than the free cortisol assay.

ANSWER: D

11. The patient described in Question 10 is found to have mild elevation of urinary free cortisol. Which test would you next perform to confirm a diagnosis of Cushing syndrome?

A. Low-dose dexamethasone suppression.
B. High-dose dexamethasone suppression.
C. Plasma ACTH level.
D. Metyrapone stimulation.
E. Corticotropin-releasing hormone stimulation.

Ref.: 1, 2, 3, 4

COMMENTS: The low-dose dexamethasone suppression test can confirm hypercortisolism and in combination with urinary-free cortisol can increase the accuracy of the biochemical diagnosis. The other methods have been used to determine the cause of Cushing syndrome once a diagnosis has been made but are not used to establish the diagnosis. Dexamethasone is a synthetic corticoid that suppresses pituitary secretion of ACTH and consequent adrenal corticosteroid production. Plasma cortisol is sampled in the morning after oral administration of 1 mg dexamethasone the night before. Plasma cortisol levels are low (<3 mg/dl) in normal individuals but elevated in Cushing syndrome patients. False-positive tests may occur in patients who are obese, chronically ill, or alcoholic or in those taking certain medications (Dilantin, rifampin, estrogens, tamoxifen).

ANSWER: A

12. A patient with hypercortisolism (Cushing syndrome) is found to have an elevated serum ACTH level and a plasma cortisol level that suppresses to less than 50% of baseline following a single high dose of dexamethasone. The most likely diagnosis is which of the following?

A. Adrenal adenoma.
B. Adrenal hyperplasia.
C. Pituitary adenoma.
D. Ectopic ACTH production.

Ref.: 1, 2, 3, 4

COMMENTS: Once the diagnosis of excess cortisol production has been confirmed by urinary-free cortisol and low-dose dexamethasone suppression, a number of biochemical tests can be useful for identifying the cause. First, an attempt is made to differentiate primary adrenal pathology from excess pituitary or ectopic ACTH. Serum ACTH levels are low when the cortisol is from an adrenal problem, elevated (or normal) with a pituitary adenoma, and usually markedly elevated with ectopic ACTH. High-dose dexamethasone (a glucocorticoid) suppresses cortisol production due to a pituitary adenoma but does not diminish cortisol production from primary adrenal neoplasms or ectopic ACTH-producing tumors. There may be some overlap, however, so the accuracy of high-dose dexamethasone suppression is about 70–80%. Measurement of serum ACTH in response to administration of corticotropin-releasing hormone (CRH) can also aid in differentiating adrenal from nonadrenal causes. With pituitary adenomas (and in normal individuals) there is a rise in ACTH, but there is no response in patients whose hypercortisolism is due to excess ACTH from pituitary or ectopic sources.

ANSWER: C

13. Which of the following is/are true regarding the role of inferior petrosal sinus sampling in the evaluation of a patient with hypercortisolism (Cushing syndrome)?

A. Differentiates pituitary from nonpituitary ACTH-dependent Cushing syndrome.
B. Differentiates ACTH-independent from ACTH-dependent Cushing syndrome.
C. Can localize microadenomas within the pituitary.
D. Procedural complications limit its clinical usefulness.

Ref.: 1, 2, 4

COMMENTS: Bilateral simultaneous inferior petrosal sinus sampling is the most accurate method for distinguishing between ACTH excess from pituitary and ectopic sources. Comparisons are made between the ACTH levels in peripheral blood and blood from the inferior petrosal sinus draining the pituitary gland, both before and after stimulation with CRH. This test is appropriate when other biochemical and imaging studies have not succeeded in differentiating the source of ACTH-dependent Cushing syndrome. Comparison between the right and left sides may also be useful for lateralizing a pituitary adenoma. Inferior petrosal sinus sampling is an invasive test that requires skilled intervention to catheterize the sinuses via the internal jugular vein. In experienced hands, it has proved safe and reliable.

ANSWER: A, C

14. A 29-year-old man presents with truncal obesity, hypertension, and muscular weakness. He is found to have increased serum cortisol levels, an elevated plasma ACTH level, and suppression of urinary free cortisol after administration of high-dose, but not low-dose, dexamethasone. A CT brain scan reveals a small mass in the pituitary. Which of the following is the preferred treatment?

A. Pituitary irradiation.
B. Transsphenoidal resection of the microadenoma.
C. Bilateral adrenalectomy.
D. Aminoglutethimide administration.

Ref.: 1, 2, 3

COMMENTS: See Question 16.

15. A 35-year-old woman presents with clinical and laboratory evidence of Cushing syndrome and is found to have a depressed plasma ACTH level and a well defined 3 cm left adrenal mass. Which of the following is the preferred treatment?

A. Bilateral adrenalectomy.
B. Left adrenalectomy.
C. o,p′-DDD administration.
D. Left adrenal irradiation.

Ref.: 1, 2, 3

COMMENTS: See Question 16.

16. A 45-year-old man presents with Cushing syndrome and a 7 cm right adrenal mass invading the perinephric fat that is compatible with an adrenal carcinoma. After thorough evaluation, no disease can be found elsewhere. Which of the following is the preferred treatment?

A. External beam radiation therapy to the right adrenal area.
B. o,p′-DDD administration.
C. Right radical adrenalectomy.
D. Intraarterial doxorubicin (Adriamycin) via the right adrenal artery.

Ref.: 1, 2, 3

COMMENTS: The management of the patient with Cushing syndrome depends on the specific cause. For **Cushing's disease**, wherein the primary pathology relates to excess pituitary production of ACTH, the initial therapy should be directed toward the pituitary. Most patients have a small microadenoma; 50% can be imaged by CT scan. Transsphenoidal resection of the microadenoma is the preferred treatment, with 90–95% cure rates obtained by highly experienced neurosurgeons. Pharmacologic management of patients with Cushing's disease has been tried with drugs such as aminoglutethimide, which blocks the production and secretion of adrenocortical steroids. This treatment may be of value in patients who are poor surgical risks but certainly is not considered an appropriate initial treatment. Hypercortisolism due to **ectopic ACTH** production most commonly results from a neuroendocrine carcinoma of the lung, although this syndrome may also be associated with thymomas, bronchial adenomas, and islet cell tumors. Treatment is best approached by resecting the tumor producing the ACTH, if possible. If this cannot be achieved, bilateral adrenalectomy may be appropriate, depending on the overall status of the patient and the likelihood of long-term survival from the primary tumor. Cushing syndrome due to **adrenal adenomas** or **carcinoma** is best treated by total surgical resection of the involved gland. Approximately 50% of adrenocortical carcinomas are found to be hormonally functional, with glucocorticoid elevation leading to Cushing syndrome being the most common endocrinopathy. Adrenocortical carcinoma, in which there is no demonstrable distant disease, is best managed by aggressive surgical resection, even if it means en bloc inclusion of contiguous resectable tissues. Radiation therapy may be beneficial when the carcinoma cannot be totally excised or when the margins are close; however, information supporting the use of adjuvant postoperative radiation therapy is sparse. In cases of metastatic adrenocortical carcinoma producing Cushing syndrome, resection of metastases may provide palliation by reducing cortisol levels. The administration of o,p′-DDD (an adrenolytic agent related to the insecticide DDT) may produce regression of metastatic disease in up to 60% of patients.

ANSWER:
Question 14: B
Question 15: B
Question 16: C

17. Which one of the following findings is most consistent with the diagnosis of primary hyperaldosteronism?

A. Sodium 145 mEq/L, potassium 4.8 mEq/L, blood pressure 90/60, expanded blood volume.
B. Sodium 132 mEq/L, potassium 5.4 mEq/L, blood pressure 160/100, expanded blood volume.

C. Sodium 149 mEq/L, potassium 3.0 mEq/L, blood pressure 160/100, contracted blood volume.
D. Sodium 149 mEq/L, potassium 3.0 mEq/L, blood pressure 160/100, expanded blood volume.

Ref.: 1, 2, 3, 4

COMMENTS: The clinical and laboratory findings characteristic of primary hyperaldosteronism are hypokalemia, inappropriate kaliuresis, elevated plasma aldosterone, normal cortisol, expanded blood volume, and sustained hypertension. These are all attributable to aldosterone's physiologic effect on the distal convoluted tubule, causing sodium retention in exchange for potassium and hydrogen ion excretion. Alkalosis, polydipsia, nocturnal polyuria, and paresthesias also are common.

ANSWER: D

18. Match each of the anatomic locations in the left column with its physiologic function in the right column.

A. Liver
B. Juxtaglomerular cells
C. Zona glomerulosa
D. Macula densa
E. Lung

a. Sensitive to decreases in renal arterial blood pressure
b. Produces angiotensinogen
c. Synthesizes renin
d. Sensitive to decreases in serum sodium concentration
e. Converts angiotensin I to angiotensin II
f. Produces aldosterone

Ref.: 1, 2, 3, 4

COMMENTS: In humans, aldosterone is the only clinically important mineralocorticoid. It is secreted by the zona glomerulosa of the adrenal cortex under the influence of the renin-angiotensin system, serum potassium concentration, and plasma ACTH levels. Among these factors, stimulation by plasma ACTH appears to be the weakest, as it is seen only when pathologic states of ACTH excess are present or when pharmacologic doses of ACTH are given. Elevated serum potassium directly stimulates adrenal secretion of aldosterone. The major regulator of aldosterone secretion is the renin-angiotensin system, in which decreases in renal arterial blood pressure stimulate renin secretion from the juxtaglomerular cells of the kidney. Renin release precipitates a series of enzymatic reactions that convert hepatic angiotensinogen to the inactive angiotensin I. Angiotensin-converting enzyme in the lung converts angiotensin I to angiotensin II, which functions as both a potent vasoconstrictor and a stimulant of aldosterone secretion. Aldosterone acts primarily on the renal tubule, resulting in sodium and chloride retention in exchange for potassium and hydrogen. In pathologic states of hyperaldosteronism, this results in the classic findings of hypertension, hypokalemia, and metabolic alkalosis. Hyperaldosteronism may be a "primary" event, in which autonomous production of aldosterone (e.g., an aldosterone-producing adenoma) functions outside the influence of the normal negative feedback loop.

"Secondary" hyperaldosteronism is a normal physiologic compensatory mechanism in which elevated serum aldsoterone levels are found in response to increased renin secretion.

ANSWER: A-b; B-a; C-f; D-d; E-e

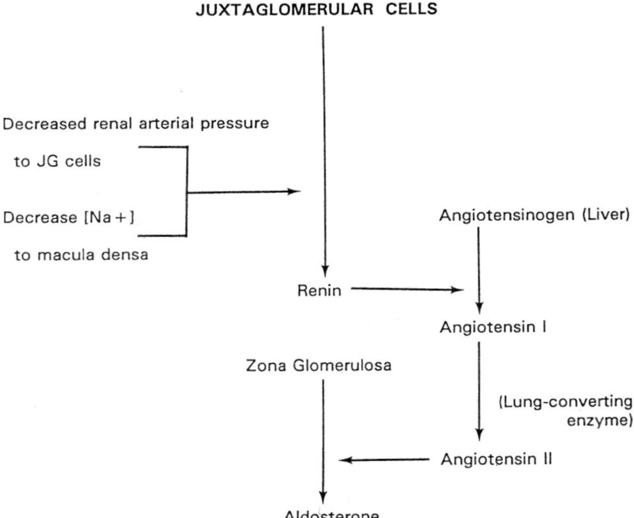

19. Which one of the following is the most common cause of primary hyperaldosteronism?

A. Bilateral adrenocortical hyperplasia.
B. Adrenocortical carcinoma.
C. Solitary adrenal adenoma.
D. Pituitary neoplasm.
E. Ovarian or testicular neoplasm.

Ref.: 1, 2, 3, 4

COMMENTS: Primary hyperaldosteronism is an uncommon disease, first described by Conn in 1955 and characterized by autonomous excess secretion of aldosterone from the adrenal cortex. **Secondary** hyperaldosteronism is a relatively common clinical condition in which a relative deficit of circulating volume or sodium content stimulates renin synthesis, leading to aldosterone production. Secondary hyperaldosteronism can occur in patients with renal artery stenosis, congestive heart failure, or hepatic cirrhosis and during pregnancy. In 60–70% of cases, primary hyperaldosteronism is due to a solitary adrenal adenoma. Most of the remaining cases are due to bilateral adrenocortical hyperplasia, the exact cause of which is unknown. Occasionally, adrenocortical carcinoma is associated with excess aldosterone secretion; there have been a few reports of ectopic production of aldosterone from ovarian neoplasms. Autosomal dominant glucocorticoid suppressible aldosteronism is another rare cause of primary hyperaldosteronism.

ANSWER: C

20. Primary hyperaldosteronism can be differentiated from secondary hyperaldosteronism based on which of the following?

A. Plasma aldosterone level.
B. Plasma renin activity.
C. Plasma cortisol level.
D. Computed tomography (CT) scan.
E. Adrenal vein sampling.

Ref.: 1, 2, 3, 4

COMMENTS: Primary hyperaldosteronism is characterized by elevated plasma aldosterone and suppressed plasma renin activity. In secondary hyperaldosteronism, plasma renin activity is not suppressed. Various tests that rely on the normal feedback control mechanisms have been used to confirm primary aldosterone overproduction by demonstrating persistent elevation of aldosterone under conditions that would normally decrease aldosterone secretion. These tests include saline loading to cause volume expansion and administration of captopril (which inhibits conversion of angiotensin I to angiotensin II) to produce the same result pharmacologically. The plasma aldosterone/plasma renin activity ratio may also be useful (>20 with primary hyperaldosteronism). Measurements of 24-hour urinary aldosterone may be more accurate than plasma levels. Antihypertensive medications such as spironolactone, ACE inhibitors, and diuretics affect renin-aldosterone regulation and should be discontinued prior to performing these studies.

ANSWER: B

21. Which of the following statements is/are true regarding the differentiation of hyperaldosteronism due to adrenal adenoma from that due to adrenal hyperplasia?

A. Preoperative distinction is critical because the primary treatment is unilateral adrenalectomy for adenoma and bilateral adrenalectomy for hyperplasia.
B. Initial distinction is not critical, as the primary treatment of either is medical, with potassium-sparing diuretics.
C. Operation can usually be performed based on biochemical determination of postural aldosterone and renin and measurement of 18-hydroxycorticosterone.
D. Iodocholesterol scan (NP-59) with dexamethasone suppression accurately identifies hyperfunctioning glands.

Ref.: 1, 2, 3

COMMENTS: Once primary hyperaldosteronism has been diagnosed, the distinction between a functioning adrenal adenoma and bilateral adrenal hyperplasia is critical. Adrenal adenoma is treated by unilateral adrenalectomy. The treatment of aldosterone excess caused by adrenal hyperplasia is pharmacologic, with spironolactone and calcium channel blockers. Biochemical tests can aid in distinguishing these entities but do not localize an adenoma. Postural measurements of aldosterone and renin in patients with adenomas show persistent elevation and suppression, respectively, with standing; variations are observed in patients with hyperplasia. The aldosterone precursor 18-hydroxycorticosterone is elevated with adenomas but not usually with hyperplasia. CT is the first localizing study of choice. Adrenal scintigraphy with iodocholesterol can identify hyperfunctioning cortical tissue with about 90% accuracy. If these noninvasive imaging attempts are equivocal, sampling of adrenal venous blood is still a useful technique for patients with primary hyperaldosteronism.

ANSWER: D

22. With regard to androgen and estrogen physiology, which of the following statements is/are true?

A. Adrenocortical production of androgens and estrogens exceeds gonadal production during most of childhood and early adult life.
B. Adrenal androgen secretion inhibits pituitary release of ACTH.
C. During fetal development, male physiognomy occurs by default unless estrogens are present in sufficient quantity to direct feminization.
D. Virilizing tumors in male adults are difficult to detect on clinical grounds alone.
E. Estrogen-producing tumors are clinically silent in female adults.

Ref.: 1, 2, 3, 4

COMMENTS: Both the adrenal cortex (primarily the zona reticularis) and the gonads are responsible for androgen and estrogen production, with the largest quantity of these steroids produced by the gonads under normal circumstances. Both androgen and cortisol release are stimulated by anterior pituitary production of ACTH; but unlike cortisol, androgens do not exert a negative feedback on further ACTH secretion. During fetal development the ''dominant'' sexual development pattern is female unless androgens are present in sufficient quantity to direct masculinization. Abnormally high androgen or estrogen production by the adrenal may occur during fetal development, childhood, or adulthood as a result of adrenocortical hyperplasia, adrenal enzymatic defects, or adrenal neoplasms. The clinical syndrome produced depends on the age of the patient and the degree of hormone excess. Probably the most difficult syndrome to detect clinically is virilization in a male adult. Estrogen-producing tumors in female adults also may be difficult to detect but frequently manifest as abnormal breast enlargement and menstrual irregularities. In prepubertal patients, estrogen excess produces precocious breast development and menstruation in females and gynecomastia in males, whereas androgen excess produces clitoral or phallic enlargement, increased muscle mass, and precocious development of axillary and pubic hair.

ANSWER: D

23. Which of the following enzymatic defects is/are associated with most cases of the adrenogenital syndrome (congenital adrenal hyperplasia)?

A. 3-Hydroxydehydrogenase deficiency.
B. 11-Hydroxylase deficiency.
C. 17-Hydroxylase deficiency.
D. 21-Hydroxylase deficiency.

Ref.: 1, 2, 3, 4

COMMENTS: Numerous enzymes are required for the appropriate conversion of cholesterol to the various adrenal corticosteroids required for normal physiology. Insufficient amounts of one or more of these enzymes may result in excess or deficient production of glucocorticoids, mineralocorticoids, or the sex steroids. This in turn leads to various combinations of electrolyte abnormalities, sexual maldevelopment, and hypertension. The most common enzymatic defect, accounting for approximately 95% of patients with the various adrenogenital syndromes, is 21-hydroxylase deficiency. Recall that 21-hydroxylase is an enzyme in the final metabolic pathway leading to both aldosterone and cortisol synthesis (see Question 5 and Figure above). Partial 21-hydroxylase deficiency occurs in two-thirds of the cases and results in block of normal cortisol and aldosterone synthesis. The block in cortisol synthesis results in a compensatory increase in ACTH release with increased production of androstenedione. The androstenedione is converted to testosterone, leading to virilization in females and precocious sexual development in males. When the enzyme deficiency is complete, these sexual changes are also associated with a severe salt-losing syndrome (secondary to no aldosterone). Other, less common enzymatic defects leading to the adrenogenital syndrome include deficiencies in 11-hydroxylase, 3-hydroxydehydrogenase, and 17-hydroxylase. Deficiency of 11-hydroxylase leads to an accumulation of adrenal androgens and the mineralocorticoid desoxycorticosterone, resulting in the clinical findings of virilization and hypertension. Deficiency of 3-hydroxydehydrogenase leads to a marked deficit of cortisol and aldosterone production, with a severe and usually fatal salt-losing syndrome associated with mild degrees of pseudohermaphroditism. Deficiency of 17-hydroxylase results in deficits of androgens, estrogens, and cortisol; this in turn leads to sexual infantilism and hypertension.

ANSWER: D

24. Which of the following is the most common cause of adrenal insufficiency?

A. Tuberculosis.
B. Autoimmune disease.
C. Adrenal hemorrhage.
D. Metastases to the adrenal gland.
E. Exogenous steroid administration.

Ref.: 1, 2, 4

COMMENTS: Exogenous steroid administration is overall the most common cause of adrenal insufficiency. Among the *primary* disorders that result in adrenal insufficiency, autoimmune disease is the most common, accounting for two-thirds or more of spontaneous cases. Tuberculosis remains an important cause as well, although it is less commonly so than in the past. Acquired immunodeficiency syndrome (AIDS)-related infections have been increasingly important. Adrenal hemorrhage may occur as a result of trauma, coagulopathy, or fulminant bacterial sepsis (Waterhouse-Friderichsen syndrome). Metastases to the adrenal glands are common in a number of malignancies (breast, lung, melanoma) and may also produce insidious adrenal insufficiency.

ANSWER: E

25. Typical characteristics of acute adrenal insufficiency include:

A. Fever, hypertension, high cardiac output, low systemic vascular resistance.
B. Hypothermia, hypotension, low cardiac output, high systemic vascular resistance.
C. Fever, hypotension, high cardiac output, low systemic vascular resistance.
D. Hyperkalemia, hyponatremia, hypoglycemia.
E. Hypokalemia, hypernatremia, hyperglycemia.

Ref.: 1, 2, 5

COMMENTS: See Question 26.

26. Treatment of acute adrenal insufficiency involves administration of which one or more of the following?

A. Normal saline and glucose.
B. Normal saline, potassium, and glucose.
C. Hypertonic saline and potassium.
D. Intravenous glucocorticoids.
E. Intravenous mineralocorticoids.

Ref.: 1, 2, 5

COMMENTS: Acute adrenal insufficiency or adrenal crisis results in cardiovascular collapse. Clinical features include fever, hypotension due to high-output circulatory failure and low systemic vascular resistance, nausea, vomiting, abdominal pain and distension, and mental lethargy or obtundation. This presentation obviously overlaps with a large number of other surgical and medical catastrophes, and diagnosis requires a high index of suspicion. Laboratory features of adrenal crisis include hyponatremia, hyperkalemia, hypoglycemia, and azotemia. Treatment must be prompt and intensive. Volume resuscitation is achieved with normal saline; glucose is administered; and intravenous glucocorticoids in the form of dexamethasone and hydrocortisone must be given. After the patient has been stabilized, the cause of the crisis and the underlying adrenal deficit is investigated. Mineralocorticoids are not necessary for the management of acute adrenal crisis, but fluorocortisone can be started later when saline infusion has been discontinued and mineralocorticoids are important for the maintenance of patients with chronic adrenal insufficiency.

ANSWER:
Question 25: C, D
Question 26: A, D

27. A 46-year-old woman who has been on long-term prednisone therapy for rheumatoid arthritis needs an abdominal hysterectomy for fibroid tumors. Which one or more of the following complications might be expected to occur in this patient with greater-than-average frequency?

A. Poor wound healing.
B. Pulmonary embolus.
C. Myocardial infarction.
D. Ileus.
E. Renal failure.

Ref.: 1, 2, 5

COMMENTS: See Question 28.

28. Appropriate perioperative steroid support for the patient described in Question 27 includes which one of the following?

A. Cortisone (10 mg) 8 hours before and after operation.
B. Prednisone (10 mg) 8 hours before and after operation.
C. Hydrocortisone (300 mg) in a single dose immediately after operation.
D. Cortisone (200 mg) in divided doses before operation; 100 mg hydrocortisone during the procedure; then in doses tapered over several days to baseline.
E. Cortisone (10 mg) 8 hours before operation and 1 gm methylprednisolone 8 hours after operation.

Ref.: 1, 2, 5

COMMENTS: Poor wound healing and increased frequency and severity of a variety of postoperative infections occur more commonly in patients on long-term steroid therapy. Poor wound healing is primarily due to the protein catabolic effect and inhibition of normal fibroblast function. The increased incidence of infection is related to the broad immunosuppressive activity of steroids. Although the association is somewhat controversial, chronic steroid therapy is also frequently linked to an increased incidence of several other complications including gastric and duodenal ulcers and pancreatitis. Pulmonary embolus, myocardial infarction, ileus, and renal failure do not occur with greater frequency in a patient on long-term steroids. **Adrenocortical insufficiency** may occur in patients on chronic corticosteroid therapy because of inhibition of the normal adrenal response to stress. Both pituitary ACTH and endogenous adrenal steroid production are suppressed by exogenous steroid administration and cannot, therefore, respond to physiologic or surgical stress in a normal manner. The adrenal cortex normally produces 10–30 mg cortisol per day; however, in times of stress, many times this amount may be required. To protect the patient against acute adrenal insufficiency, a "steroid prep" should be administered prior to surgery. One of the acceptable regimens includes administration of 100 mg hydrocortisone the evening before and the morning of a major operation, with 100 mg of hydrocortisone administered every 8 hours for the next 24 hours. Cortisone (or other corticosteroids in doses with comparable potency; see table, below) 300 mg/day perioperatively in divided doses, usually protects the patient even in cases of maximum stress. This dose is then tapered to the patient's baseline steroid requirements over a course of time, varying from several days to weeks, dictated by the preoperative steroid dose, the length of preoperative steroid treatment, and the degree of stress induced by the operative procedure and postoperative course. The dosage equivalents of corticoids are as follows.

Cortisone	25 mg
Cortisol (hydrocortisone)	20 mg
Prednisone (dehydrocortisone)	5 mg
Prednisolone (dehydrocortisol)	5 mg
Methylprednisolone	4 mg
Dexamethasone (fluoromethylprednisolone)	0.75 mg

ANSWER:
Question 27: A
Question 28: D

29. The rate-limiting step of catecholamine synthesis involves conversion of tyrosine to dihydroxyphenylalanine (DOPA) by which of the following?

A. Tyrosine hydroxylase.
B. Monoamine oxidase (MAO).
C. DOPA decarboxylase.
D. Catechol-*O*-methyltransferase (COMT).
E. Phenylethanolamine-*N*-methyltransferase (PNMT).

Ref.: 1, 2, 3, 4

COMMENTS: The corticosteroids of the adrenal cortex are derived from enzymatically mediated alterations in the cholesterol molecule. Catecholamine synthesis that occurs in the adrenal medulla begins with the amino acid tyrosine, derived from the diet or by endogenous conversion of phenylalanine. Tyrosine is hydroxylated by tyrosine hydroxylase to DOPA, which undergoes decarboxylation to form dopamine. Norepinephrine is then formed by hydroxylation of dopamine. Finally, norepinephrine may be converted to epinephrine by PNMT. Epinephrine is the major catecholamine in the adrenal medulla, accounting for approximately 80%. Catecholamines, particularly norepinephrine, exert a negative feedback inhibition of excess production by inhibiting the tyrosine hydroxylase enzyme necessary for conversion of tyrosine to DOPA. Inactivation of catecholamines may occur by uptake and retention in postganglionic neurons and sympathetic nerves and by metabolic degradation by the enzymes COMT or monoamine oxidase (MAO). The metabolites of catecholamine degradation include normetanephrine, metanephrine, and vanillylmandelic acid (VMA). These breakdown products are measurable in the urine and are of great use in the diagnosis

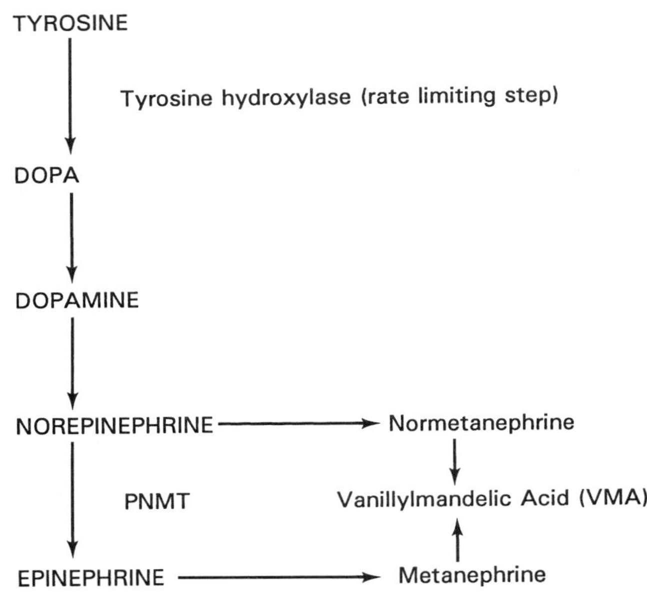

of states of catecholamine excess, as is seen in the case of pheochromocytoma.

ANSWER: A

30. A patient is diagnosed with pheochromocytoma. Which clinical symptom(s) is/are likely to be present?

A. Sweating.
B. Palpitations.
C. Headache.
D. Paroxysmal hypertension.
E. All of the above.

Ref.: 1, 2, 3, 5

COMMENTS: The clinical signs and symptoms seen in a patient with pheochromocytoma are due to excessive secretion of catecholamines. One would expect, therefore, to see the following typical physiologic response to catecholamine excess in these patients: hypertension, tachycardia, palpitations, excessive sweating, anxiety, tremulousness, and nausea and vomiting, among many others. Headache is quite common, occurring in approximately 80% of patients. The catecholamine secretion from these tumors may be episodic, in which case one sees paroxysmal hypertensive episodes, or it may be sustained secretion, wherein one sees persistent hypertension. Severe hypertension may be precipitated by induction of anesthesia in a patient with unsuspected pheochromocytoma. Indeed, about one-third of patients are diagnosed as a consequence of a hypertensive crisis or at autopsy.

ANSWER: E

31. Pheochromocytoma may be associated with which one or more of the following syndromes?

A. Multiple endocrine neoplasia type I (MEN-I).
B. MEN-IIA.
C. MEN-IIB.

D. von Recklinghausen's disease.
E. von Willebrand's disease.

Ref.: 1, 2, 3, 5

COMMENTS: Although most cases of pheochromocytoma occur in isolated form, one must be alert to the association of pheochromocytoma with several other neuroendocrine and neuroectodermal abnormalities. Pheochromocytoma is one of the tumors found in MEN-IIA or Sipple syndrome (pheochromocytoma, medullary carcinoma of the thyroid, and parathyroid hyperplasia) and in MEN-IIB (pheochromocytoma, medullary carcinoma of the thyroid, and multiple mucosal neuromas). It is also seen in several other neurocutaneous syndromes including von Recklinghausen's disease (neurofibromatosis), Bourneville's disease (tuberous sclerosis), and Sturge-Weber disease (meningofacial angiomatosis). It is generally believed that patients presenting with other manifestations of these syndromes should be screened for the presence of pheochromocytoma because of the danger of a catastrophic hypertensive crisis that can occur in a patient with undiagnosed pheochromocytoma.

ANSWER: B, C, D

32. With regard to pheochromocytoma, which one or more of the following statements is/are true?

A. Extraadrenal pheochromocytomas are rare.
B. Pheochromocytoma is found bilaterally in 50% of cases.
C. Malignant pheochromocytomas occur in approximately 50% of cases.
D. Approximately 10% of pheochromocytomas occur in patients younger than 20 years of age.

Ref.: 1, 2

COMMENTS: Pheochromocytomas may occur in locations other than the adrenal medulla; they may be bilateral, they may be malignant, and they may occur in patients younger than 20 years of age. When one considers all patients who have pheochromocytoma, each of the aforementioned clinical situations occurs in approximately 10–20% of cases. It is important to realize, therefore, that within subsets of patients with pheochromocytoma the likelihood increases that one or more of these clinical presentations will occur. For example, in cases of familial pheochromocytoma there is a significantly increased risk of bilateral tumors, extraadrenal tumors, and malignancy. Also, in familial cases the tumors tend to appear at an earlier age. With all cases of pheochromocytoma, one must be alert to the possibility of the tumor being present in an extraadrenal location. They may occur at any site where chromaffin tissue is located but most often are found in paraganglia of the periaortic area and specifically in vestigial structures located in the area of the inferior mesenteric artery and the aortic bifurcation (organ of Zuckerkandl). Pheochromocytomas have also been reported in the urinary bladder and outside the abdomen (carotid body and glomus jugulare). Adrenal pheochromocytomas have a right-sided predominance; the reason is not known.

ANSWER: D

33. All of the following may be useful for diagnosing pheochromocytoma *except*:

A. Plasma catecholamine levels.
B. 24-Hour urine metanephrine.
C. 24-Hour urine vanillylmandelic acid (VMA).
D. Clonidine suppression test.

Ref.: 1, 2, 3, 5

COMMENTS: See Question 34.

34. Each of the following imaging studies may be appropriate for localizing a pheochromocytoma *except*:

A. MRI scan.
B. CT scan.
C. Venography.
D. Iodocholesterol (NP-59) scan.
E. MIBG scan.

Ref.: 1, 2, 3, 5

COMMENTS: The biochemical diagnosis of pheochromocytoma depends on increased urinary catecholamines and metabolites. Plasma catecholamine levels are insufficient, as they are also elevated in essential hypertension. Biochemical testing for pheochromocytoma should be performed on patients with paroxysmal hypertension, pregnant patients with new hypertension, and those with a history of pheochromocytoma or associated conditions discussed previously. An incidental adrenal mass on CT or MRI should also be evaluated. Fewer than 2% of pheochromocytomas have been missed when the combination of 24-hour urine collection of metanephrines and VMA is done. Of note, iodine contrast media, labetolol, and the combination of α- and β-blockers can render these tests inaccurate. Another test that can be used is the clonidine suppression test. Failure to suppress catecholamine levels following administration of clonidine is considered a positive test. The CT scan reveals approximately 90% of adrenal tumors and is usually the first localization test performed. Patients should be scanned from the base of the diaphragm to at least below the level of the bifurcation of the aorta to prevent overlooking extraadrenal pheochromocytoma. MRI provides both anatomic and physiologic imaging. Pheochromocytomas can be demonstrated best on T2 weighted images. Both CT and MRI provide excellent images of the liver and periaortic lymph nodes, both possible sites of metastatic disease. Radionuclide scanning with ^{123}I monoiodobenzylguanidine (MIBG) may be helpful for identifying pheochromocytomas and may be particularly useful for extraadrenal tumors, in which the scan has an 80–90% sensitivity. Due to the possibility of inducing a lethal hypertensive crisis, venography is no longer performed. Iodocholesterol scintigraphy identifies adrenocortical tissue.

ANSWER:
Question 33: A
Question 34: C, D

35. Which of the following should be administered first in the preoperative preparation of a patient with pheochromocytoma?

A. α-Antagonist.
B. β-Antagonist.
C. β-Agonist.
D. Fluid, blood, or both.
E. Diuretic.

Ref.: 1, 2, 3

COMMENTS: The principal physiologic mechanism at work in cases of pheochromocytoma relates to excessive α- and (frequently) β-catecholamine stimulation. This leads to an increase in peripheral vascular resistance, hypertension, tachycardia, and a contracted blood volume. At the point in the operation when the pheochromocytoma is removed, there is abrupt cessation of this stimulation, which may lead to profound hypotension and hypovolemia. To protect against this eventuality, the patient should be prepared preoperatively with α- and often with β-blockade. α-Blockade may be achieved by administration of phenoxybenzamine, prazosin, or phentolamine for 1–3 weeks preoperatively. β-Blockade is indicated in patients with significant tachycardia (>110 or 120 bpm), arrhythmias, or tumors that secrete predominantly epinephrine. β-Blockade may be achieved by administration of propranolol or other agents. It is mandatory to achieve α-blockade prior to the administration of β-blockers because β-blockade alone in a patient with pheochromocytoma may precipitate heart failure due to cardiomyopathy and unrelieved afterload. Because vasodilation occurs as a result of effective α-adrenergic blockade, there is frequently the need to administer fluid or blood (or both) to achieve an effective circulating blood volume prior to operation. Of course, diuretics would be contraindicated in such a situation, as diuresis would lead to further contraction of the blood volume.

ANSWER: A

36. A 60-year-old man is found to have a 3 cm adrenal mass on CT scan. His history and physical are unrevealing. Which of the following is/are *correct*?

A. The adrenal mass should be resected.
B. Serum potassium, 24-hour levels of VMA, metanephrines, and catecholamines should be checked.
C. The patient should be observed with a repeat CT scan in 6 months.
D. Fine-needle aspiration should be done to rule out malignancy.

Ref.: 1, 2, 5

COMMENTS: Incidental adrenal masses are commonly seen owing to the greater frequency and use of abdominal CT scans. It is expected that as many as 2% of individuals undergoing abdominal CT scanning will be found to have adrenal masses. Important aspects about adrenal masses are that (1) benign, clinically inactive adrenocortical adenomas are common autopsy findings; (2) adrenocortical carcinomas are rare, with an annual incidence estimated from 0.06 to 0.17 per 100,000 population; and (3) the adrenal glands are a common site for metastasis. • The differential diagnosis consists of cortical adenoma, adrenocortical carcinoma, pheochromocytoma, ganglioneuroma, cyst, organized hemorrhage or fibrosis, myelolipoma, adenolipoma, or metastasis from a nonadrenal malignancy. Adrenocortical carcinoma is rare, and size is the most important predictor of malignancy. In a review of six series, 90% of adrenocortical carcinomas were larger than 6 cm. Age is also taken into account because the number of adrenal nodules increases in older patients. • Most surgeons advocate surgery on patients with nonfunctioning adrenal masses larger than 6 cm, and some perform adrenalectomy on masses larger than 4 cm. In younger patients, who have decreased operative risk, adrenalectomy has been recommended for adrenal masses larger than 3 cm. • In asymptomatic patients, one should rule out functional tumors as well as metastatic disease. A serum potassium should be ordered to rule out aldosteronoma; 24-hour VMA, metanephrines, and catecholamines to rule out pheochromocytoma; and 24-hour urine collection for 17-hydroxycorticosteroids and 17-ketosteroids to rule out Cushing syndrome. • Tumors that most commonly metastasize to the adrenals are melanoma, hypernephroma, and carcinoma of the lung, breast, and stomach. Therefore even patients without a history of malignancy should have a minimum of laboratory screening studies including stool for occult blood, chest radiograph, and in women a mammogram. Patients with a history of malignancy should undergo fine-needle aspiration of the adrenal mass. • Any adrenal mass of 3–6 cm with ominous CT characteristics should be resected. Observation is appropriate for patients 50 years of age and older who have masses between 3 and 6 cm and for all lesions <3 cm that are not hormonally active. Such observation consists of serial CT scans done at 3-month intervals for the first year and annually thereafter.

ANSWER: B

37. A 50-year-old woman presents with typical clinical features of Cushing syndrome. CT scan demonstrates an 8 cm right adrenal mass extending into the adjacent liver and kidney. Recommended treatment is:

A. Transsphenoidal hypophysectomy.
B. En bloc surgical resection.
C. Radiation therapy.
D. Mitotane.
E. Radiation therapy and mitotane followed by surgical resection.

Ref.: 1, 2, 5

COMMENTS: Adrenocortical carcinoma is a rare but deadly malignancy. Its peak incidence is during the first and fifth decades of life, and it is more common in women. About one-half of adult patients have clinically functional tumors due to excess production of cortisol, aldosterone, or sex steroids. A large adrenal mass (>6 cm) and masses with extraadrenal extension are virtually always malignant. Unfortunately, nearly 80% of patients have advanced disease (local invasion, positive nodes, metastases) at the time of diagnosis. En bloc resection of localized disease is the only chance for cure and may provide useful, albeit transient, palliation for most patients, even though they cannot be cured. Overall survival is probably about 20% at best. Mitotane is the only known chemotherapeutic agent that may be of benefit. It has been used as a postresectional adjunct but most often is used for patients with metastatic or unresectable disease. Radiation has not been effective.

ANSWER: B

38. Which of the following operative approaches is most appropriate for a unilateral 8 cm right adrenal mass?

A. Anterior transperitoneal.
B. Posterior retroperitoneal.
C. Thoracoabdominal.
D. Laparoscopic transperitoneal.
E. Laparoscopic retroperitoneal.

Ref.: 6, 7

COMMENTS: See Question 39.

39. Which of the following is/are a contraindication(s) to laparoscopic adrenalectomy?

A. Pheochromocytoma.
B. Adrenocortical cancer.
C. Bilateral adrenal lesions.
D. Prior abdominal surgery.
E. A 2 cm nonfunctioning incidentaloma.

Ref.: 6, 7

COMMENTS: The surgeon treating adrenal disease must be familiar with various operative approaches. Selection of the appropriate route in any given situation must consider the size and nature of the adrenal pathology, the patient's body habitus and general medical condition, and the experience of the surgeon. The **anterior transabdominal approach**, which permits exploration of the entire peritoneal cavity and both adrenal beds, is the indicated approach for treatment of adrenocortical cancers (which must be suspected for any mass >6 cm) because of the exposure necessary to assess fully the extent of disease and potentially resect adjacent structures. Many surgeons believe that pheochromocytomas should be approached anteriorly because of the possibility of multicentric, contralateral, or extraadrenal tumors. However, increasing accuracy in the preoperative localization of pheochromocytoma with CT, MRI, or MIBG scans has diminished the likelihood of encountering unsuspected tumors at exploration, allowing a direct **retroperitoneal approach** (posterior or flank) for unilateral tumors. Disadvantages of the transabdominal approach are postoperative pain, ileus, and respiratory complications. A **thoracoabdominal** incision is occasionally required for a large lesion but has the disadvantage of postoperative pain and morbidity. Posterior approaches are generally associated with a more rapid, less complicated recovery than the transabdominal approach and may be useful for patients with multiple prior abdominal operations. However, exposure is more limited and is inadequate for large tumors. Bilateral disease requires two incisions when approached from the back or flank, and abdominal exploration is precluded. The adrenal gland can be removed **laparoscopically** via the **transperitoneal** or **retroperitoneal** route. The patient is typically placed in the lateral position for transperitoneal laparoscopic access. Advantages of laparoscopic adrenalectomy include less postoperative pain and shorter hospital stays. In experienced hands, laparoscopic removal is emerging as the procedure of choice except for malignant or large tumors. Laparoscopic removal of adrenal cancers risks dissemination. The laparoscopic retroperitoneal approach can be difficult owing to limited space and anatomy, but it may be useful for patients with difficult abdominal situations (multiple operations, portal hypertension). Moreover, with the patient in the prone position, bilateral disease can be approached without repositioning the patient. As with any minimal access surgery, the availability of laparoscopic adrenalectomy is not a valid reason to extend the indications for an operation. Thus small, nonfunctioning, incidental adrenal masses are not operated on.

ANSWER:
Question 38: A
Question 39: B, E

REFERENCES

1. Sabiston DC Jr: *Textbook of Surgery*, 15th ed. WB Saunders, Philadelphia, 1997.
2. Schwartz SI, Shires GT, Spencer FC: *Principles of Surgery*, 7th ed. McGraw-Hill, New York, 1999.
3. Greenfield LJ, Mulholland M, Oldham KT, et al: *Surgery: Scientific Principles and Practice*, 2nd ed. Lippincott-Raven, Philadelphia, 1997.
4. O'Leary JP: *The Physiologic Basis of Surgery*, 2nd ed. Williams & Wilkins, Baltimore, 1996.
5. Clark HO, Duh QY: *Textbook of Endocrine Surgery*. WB Saunders, Philadelphia, 1997.
6. Staren ED, Prinz RA: Adrenalectomy in the era of laparoscopy. *Surgery* 120:706–711, 1996.
7. Gagner M, Pomp A, Heniford BT, et al: Laparoscopic adrenalectomy: lessons learned from 100 consecutive procedures. *Ann Surg* 226:238–247, 1997.

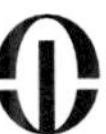

CHAPTER 25

Physiologic Basis of Gastrointestinal Symptoms

1. Which one or more of the following accurately describes the act of deglutition?

   A. The omohyoid muscle moves the food bolus from the back of the tongue into the pharynx.
   B. Elevation of the hard palate closes off the nasopharynx.
   C. The respiratory tract is normally completely sealed off by approximation of the vocal cords and anterior displacement of the epiglottis.
   D. Relaxation of the cricopharyngeus muscle permits the food bolus to enter the esophagus.

Ref.: 1

COMMENTS: Deglutition is a complicated orchestration of neuromuscular events classically considered in three stages. During the **oral** stage, the food bolus is moved into the pharynx by action of the oral tongue and mylohyoid muscle. During the **pharyngeal** stage, the bolus is transported through the pharynx by involuntary contractions of the pharyngeal muscles. Reflux into the nasopharynx is prevented by elevation of the soft palate; and aspiration into the trachea is prevented by apposition of the vocal cords, posterior displacement of the epiglottis, and reflex inhibition of respiration. The food bolus enters the cervical esophagus through the relaxed cricopharyngeus muscle, and the **esophageal** stage proceeds with esophageal peristalsis.

ANSWER: D

2. With regard to dysphagia, which of the following statements is/are true?

   A. Dysphagia can be caused by motility disorders or mechanical obstruction.
   B. The reason painful lesions of the mouth or tongue do not cause dysphagia is that they are not involved in the involuntary pharyngeal and esophageal stages of deglutition.
   C. Dysphagia may be a manifestation of neuromuscular disorders.
   D. In cases of mechanical esophageal obstruction causing dysphagia, the patient can usually pinpoint the site of obstruction.

Ref.: 1, 2

COMMENTS: The term dysphagia refers to *difficulty* swallowing, which may be due to a disturbance of muscular action or a physical obstruction. This is in contradistinction to odynophagia, which refers to *painful* swallowing. Because swallowing involves oral, pharyngeal, and esophageal stages, painful lesions or disorders affecting any of these stages may cause not only odynophagia but dysphagia. Abnormalities not necessarily intrinsic to the deglutition mechanism may also be responsible for dysphagia, including neuromuscular disturbances (e.g., poliomyelitis, myasthenia gravis), acute thyroiditis, and emotional disorders (e.g., anxiety states, conversion hysteria, anorexia nervosa). Esophageal dysphagia may be caused by both hypermotility and hypomotility states. In cases of obstruction due to tumor or stricture, the patient is frequently able to localize the site of obstruction.

ANSWER: A, C, D

3. With regard to hiccups, which of the following statements is/are true?

   A. The hiccup reflex arc is believed to include the phrenic and vagus nerves and the sympathetic chain arising from thoracic segments T2 to T6.
   B. Benign self-limiting hiccups can be caused by gastric distension, change in ambient temperature, alcohol ingestion, and tobacco use.
   C. Pharmacologic treatments of hiccups include chlorpromazine, haloperidol, phenytoin, and phenobarbital.
   D. Direct pharyngeal stimulation with a rubber catheter successfully treats hiccups approximately 90% of the time.

Ref.: 1

COMMENTS: The hiccup reflex arc is composed of afferent and efferent portions. The afferent portion consists of the phrenic and vagus nerves and the sympathetic chain arising from thoracic segments T6 to T12. Hiccups are divided into benign self-limited and persistent, or intractable, episodes. Benign self-limited hiccups are caused by gastric distension, sudden changes in ambient temperature, alcohol ingestion, and tobacco use. Intractable hiccups are organic, psychogenic, or idiopathic. Therapies for hiccups can be nonpharmacologic or pharmacologic. Pharmacologic treatments include positive-pressure ventilation, chlorpromazine, haloperidol, phenytoin, phenobarbital, carbamazine, and sodium valproate. An example of a nonpharmacologic treatment is direct pharyngeal stimulation with a rubber catheter. Nonpharmacologic treatments usually rely on some form of nasopharyngeal stimulation.

ANSWER: B, C, D

4. With regard to nausea and vomiting, which of the following statements is/are true?

A. Reversed peristalsis of the stomach plays a significant role in the mechanism of vomiting.
B. The chemoreceptor trigger zone is important in the mechanism of vomiting due to drugs, uremia, and radiation sickness.
C. Afferent pathways to the vomiting center emanate almost exclusively from the stomach and duodenum.
D. The act of vomiting involves contraction of the abdominal wall muscles, antral and pyloric contraction with coordinated gastric cardia elevation, and relaxation of the lower esophageal sphincter.

Ref.: 1

COMMENTS: The pathophysiology of nausea and vomiting is multifactorial and incompletely understood. There is general agreement that vomiting is controlled through two medullary centers: a sensory chemoreceptor trigger zone and an integrated center that coordinates the physical act of vomiting. The chemoreceptor trigger zone is important in initiating emesis associated with drugs, uremia, infections, and radiation sickness. Other afferent impulses causing vomiting may involve the autonomic nervous system and may emanate from many sites within the body, both gastrointestinal and nongastrointestinal. Mechanical obstruction, autonomic disorders of the alimentary tract, severe somatic and visceral pain, sepsis, shock, metabolic derangements, and emotional disturbances are among the many causes of nausea and vomiting. The physical act of vomiting is a complicated, coordinated motor function involving the respiratory, somatic, and gastrointestinal muscular systems. Appropriately timed contraction or relaxation of abdominal musculature, intrinsic gastric musculature, the diaphragm, and pharyngeal and laryngeal muscles results in the forceful expulsion of gastrointestinal contents through the mouth with protection of the airway. Reverse peristalsis in the stomach does not contribute significantly to the mechanism of vomiting.

ANSWER: B, D

5. Match each of the vomiting characteristics in the left column with one or more of its associated causes in the right column.

A. No antecedent nausea	a. Chronic gastric outlet obstruction
B. Projectile	b. Central nervous system (CNS) lesion
C. Immediately following eating	c. Hypertrophic pyloric stenosis
D. Large amounts of partially digested food at 12- to 48-hour intervals	d. Toxic etiology

Ref.: 1, 2

COMMENTS: Recognition of the pattern of vomiting can often assist in diagnosing the underlying cause. Although none of the associations listed above is present in every instance, taken together with other aspects of the patient's history and physical findings, they may be valuable in suggesting the cause of vomiting. Vomiting without antecedent nausea often suggests a primary lesion of the CNS as the cause. Projectile vomiting is likewise seen in cases of primary CNS pathology but is also associated with hypertrophic pyloric stenosis. Pyloric stenosis usually leads to vomiting immediately after eating, whereas more chronic or long-standing forms of gastric outlet obstruction (e.g., chronic scarring from peptic ulcer disease) is more characteristically associated with delayed vomiting of large volumes of partially digested food. Vomiting due to toxic etiologies is often repetitive and consequently produces only small volumes of emesis.

ANSWER: A-b; B-b,c; C-c; D-a

6. Which of the following accurately characterize(s) the metabolic consequences of protracted vomiting?

A. Hypovolemia.
B. Hypernatremia.
C. Hypochloremia.
D. Acidosis.
E. Paradoxical alkaline urine.

Ref.: 1, 2

COMMENTS: Protracted vomiting results in significant loss of fluid, hydrogen, chloride, and sodium in the vomitus, which results in a hypovolemic, hypokalemic, hypochloremic alkalosis. Volume depletion stimulates adrenocortical and renal mechanisms to conserve sodium at the expense of hydrogen and potassium, which results in worsening of the hypokalemia and excretion of a paradoxically acidic urine with subsequent worsening of the systemic alkalosis. The proper initial management to offset these changes includes intravenous administration of appropriate amounts of fluid, sodium, and chloride. With severe disturbances, administration of hydrochloric acid may be indicated.

ANSWER: A, C

7. Which of the following pathophysiologic mechanisms may result in diarrhea?

A. Excessive intestinal secretion.
B. Osmotic retention of intraluminal water.
C. Malabsorption of ions.
D. Disordered contact between chyme and the absorptive mucosal surface.

Ref.: 1, 2

COMMENTS: Diarrhea is usually produced by one or more of the four pathophysiologic mechanisms described above. The most important aspect of **secretory** diarrhea is excessive ion secretion by the small intestine, which may be a response to such underlying factors as bacterial toxins and gastrointestinal hormones. Secretory diarrhea is characterized by voluminous isotonic diarrhea, which usually persists even during fasting. **Osmotic** diarrhea results from the presence of poorly absorbable solutes within the intestine, possibly due to the type of food ingested or the inability of pancreatic or mucosal enzyme systems to properly digest the solutes present. Osmotic diarrhea usually abates when the patient fasts. **Malabsorption** of a normal ion is a rare cause of diarrhea. Congenital chloridorrhea, in which there is a defective transport mechanism for the absorption of chloride across the bowel mucosa, is an example.

Altered motility or disordered contact between chyme and the absorptive mucosal surface may be seen with conditions such as diabetic enteropathy, scleroderma, and radiation injury to the bowel.

ANSWER: A, B, C, D

8. With regard to the clinical manifestations of intestinal obstruction, which of the following statements is/are true?

A. Severe cramping pain occurs simultaneously with the hyperperistalsis of the intestine proximal to the obstruction.
B. Abdominal distension is not considered an early sign of obstruction.
C. With long-standing bowel obstruction, the vomitus frequently becomes dark and malodorous as a result of regurgitated feces.
D. Vomiting is a feature of all forms of bowel obstruction.

Ref.: 1, 2

COMMENTS: The cramping pain associated with bowel obstruction is a direct result of the hyperperistalsis proximal to the obstruction and therefore occurs simultaneously with it. Abdominal distension occurs as the bowel proximal to the obstruction distends with air and fluid. As this may take hours or days to develop, abdominal distension is not an early sign of obstruction. In instances of high intestinal obstruction, in which the contents of the obstructed gastrointestinal tract may be expelled by vomiting, abdominal distension may not be a feature at all. The vomitus from a patient who has been obstructed over a longer period of time may be dark and malodorous and even feculent. This is due to bacterial overgrowth within the stagnant intestinal contents and does not represent regurgitated feces. In cases of colonic obstruction with a competent ileocecal valve (the "closed-loop" syndrome), there can be massive distension and severe pain. Perforation of the colon can occur without vomiting being present.

ANSWER: A, B

9. Which of the following statements is/are true concerning the physical findings of a patient with a mechanical bowel obstruction?

A. Fever and tachycardia are usually not present within the first 12 hours of the obstruction.
B. Dehydration is usually present before vomiting develops.
C. Even in the absence of peritonitis, palpation during attacks of pain may reveal tenderness and cause guarding.
D. Except for instances in which blockage is incomplete, auscultatory findings are sufficiently nonspecific that they do not assist in the evaluation of the patient with a bowel obstruction.

Ref.: 1, 2

COMMENTS: Physical examination of a patient presumed to have a suspected bowel obstruction is of value not only for diagnosing the obstruction but also for determining the presence of complications of obstruction, such as strangulation. With a simple mechanical obstruction, there may be few if any physical findings within the first 24 hours. Fever and tachycardia would be rare in the absence of peritonitis or significant dehydration. Even before vomiting develops, however, large amounts of fluid can be sequestered within the lumen and wall of the bowel, resulting in significant intravascular volume depletion and subsequent oliguria. Although tenderness to palpation may be absent between episodes of pain, it may be severe during colicky episodes, sufficiently so even to falsely suggest the presence of peritonitis. The typical bursts or rushes of loud, high-pitched bowel sounds are characteristic of mechanical obstruction. Paralytic ileus is usually characterized by a fairly quiet abdomen, although a few bowel sounds may remain. Complete silence suggests the presence of gangrenous bowel. Evidence of systemic sepsis or toxemia is a grave sign, also suggesting the presence of gangrenous bowel.

ANSWER: A, B, C

10. With regard to the laboratory findings associated with intestinal obstruction, which of the following statements is/are true?

A. Significant electrolyte abnormalities are common during the early stages of intestinal obstruction.
B. The acid-base disturbances associated with intestinal obstruction vary according to the duration and location of the obstruction.
C. The white blood cell count is sufficiently variable as to be of minimal help in differentiating between the various types of obstruction.
D. The serum amylase level may be of benefit in suggesting the presence of an adynamic ileus rather than a bowel obstruction.

Ref.: 1, 2

COMMENTS: Although the diagnosis of bowel obstruction is generally a clinical and radiographic one, some laboratory findings may be of benefit in the evaluation of patients with bowel obstruction. Serum amylase levels may be elevated because of primary pancreatic pathology or abnormal renal amylase clearance; keep in mind, however, that their presence in cases of bowel obstruction may signal the possibility of ischemic bowel. Mild leukocytosis is commonly seen with uncomplicated mechanical obstruction; moderate elevations of the white blood cell count strongly suggest the presence of strangulation; marked leukocytosis suggests primary mesenteric vascular occlusion. Acid-base abnormalities may be severe with long-standing bowel obstruction, but there is no one characteristic picture. Metabolic acidosis may be seen as a result of dehydration, ketosis, and loss of alkaline secretions; metabolic alkalosis may be seen with high jejunal obstructions because of loss of the acidic gastric contents through vomiting. Even respiratory acidosis may be seen when the abdominal distension is so severe diaphragmatic excursion is hindered. Although significant dehydration does occur and may result in an associated rise in hematocrit, the plasma concentrations of sodium, potassium, and chloride are rarely affected.

ANSWER: B

11. Which one or more of the following statements accurately characterizes normal gastrointestinal transit of food?

A. Following a meal, the stomach usually empties within 3–4 hours.
B. Digested food reaching the cecum in less than 4 hours suggests abnormally increased small bowel motility.
C. Most of the large intestinal water absorption occurs in the right colon.

D. Defecation is primarily controlled by the autonomic nervous system.

Ref.: 1

COMMENTS: Although there is a relatively wide range of "normal" transit times through the gastrointestinal tract, ingested food usually leaves the stomach within 3–4 hours. It passes through the small intestine at an average rate of 1 inch per minute, with total passage of a meal into the cecum requiring 2–9 hours. The chyme entering the cecum and right colon is semiliquid, and it is within this segment of the colon that most of the water reabsorption occurs. Beyond the hepatic flexure, the primarily solid stool is propelled by mass peristaltic waves down to the rectum. Defecation is a complicated physiologic act that depends on afferent and efferent fibers of both the somatic and the autonomic nervous systems.

ANSWER: A, C

12. Match each of the terms in the left column with one or more associated types of abdominal pain in the right column.

A. Diffuse, poorly localized
B. Hollow viscus wall tension
C. Parietal peritoneum
D. Convergence-projection hypothesis
E. Associated sweating, nausea, tachycardia

a. Visceral pain
b. Somatic pain
c. Referred pain

Ref.: 1, 2

COMMENTS: Appreciation of the mechanisms of abdominal pain is important for understanding the pathophysiology of intraabdominal disease processes. **Visceral** or **splanchnic** pain is caused by stimulation of visceral afferent fibers, which are part of the autonomic nervous system. Visceral afferent nerve endings are located in the visceral peritoneum and walls of hollow viscera and in the capsule of solid viscera. They are sensitive to increased wall tension or stretching; and because of their relatively sparse numbers, they result in sensation of pain that is diffuse and poorly localized. **Somatic** pain arising from the abdomen is mediated by segmental spinal nerves whose endings are in the abdominal wall (including the parietal peritoneum), root of the mesentery, and diaphragm. Somatic pain tends to be more localized. **Referred** pain relates to the perception of pain in an area that is remote from the site of the pathology. It is explained according to the convergence-projection hypothesis, which suggests that pain fibers from multiple visceral and skin sites converge on a single tract for projection to the thalamus or brain cortex. The pain may be interpreted as having come from one of the converging afferent fibers that may not be involved in the pathologic process. Any type of pain, when severe enough, can cause associated autonomic responses, including sweating, nausea, vomiting, tachycardia, and hypotension.

ANSWER: A-a; B-a; C-b; D-c; E-a,b,c

13. Neurosurgical intervention is occasionally needed in the management of intractable abdominal pain. Match each of the statements in the left column with one or more associated forms of neurosurgical intervention in the right column.

A. Alleviates visceral pain
B. Alleviates somatic pain
C. Subsequent painful paresthesias
D. Altered reaction to pain

a. Splanchnicectomy and celiac ganglionectomy
b. Posterior rhizotomy
c. Anterolateral chordotomy
d. Prefrontal lobotomy

Ref.: 1, 2

COMMENTS: In cases of intractable pain, prolonged opiate use may become ineffective, necessitating neurosurgical intervention. Splanchnicectomy and celiac ganglionectomy are useful for controlling abdominal pain of visceral afferent origin but do not alleviate somatic pain. Posterior rhizotomy and interruption of the spinothalamic tract (anterolateral chordotomy) occur at a point at which the visceral and somatic afferent fibers have joined and therefore are effective in controlling both forms of pain. Unfortunately, pain and temperature sensation is also lost as a result of these procedures, which introduces the risk of subsequent injury to the anesthetized area. The anesthetic areas created by rhizotomy and chordotomy are frequently replaced (after approximately 1 year) by painful paresthesias. This point may be a consideration when choosing this form of neurosurgical intervention for patients with a long life expectancy. Prefrontal lobotomy does not alter the degree of pain but, rather, the patient's reaction to pain; it results in flattening affect globally.

ANSWER: A-a,b,c; B-b,c; C-b,c; D-d

14. With regard to some characteristics of pain, which of the following statements is/are true?

A. Sensitivity to pain varies throughout the life of an individual.
B. Repeated painful stimuli result in an accommodation to the stimuli and subsequent raising of the threshold of pain perception.
C. Underlying metabolic disorders can alter an individual's response to pain.
D. The autonomic response to pain is limited to sympathetic effects.

Ref.: 1

COMMENTS: The perception of pain is a subjective reaction to noxious stimuli that involves the highest levels of integration of the central nervous system. The perception of pain and the physical responses to it vary with a number of factors. Sensitivity to pain tends to increase from infancy to adult life and then gradually decreases in the elderly. This explains, in part, the somewhat atypical presentation of peritonitis that may occur in the very young and very old. Repeated painful stimuli result in a hypersensitivity (facilitated pain) in which the threshold for pain perception is lowered. The pain threshold may also be affected by underlying metabolic conditions such as hyperthyroidism and hyperadrenalism, which are associated with a lowered threshold, and by hypothyroidism, which is associated with a higher threshold. Pain frequently results in sympathetic nervous system responses. Severe, deep pain, however, may be accompanied by bradycardia and hypotension.

ANSWER: A, C

15. During the clinical evaluation of abdominal pain, which of the following characteristics of the pain is/are important to elicit?

A. Character.
B. Severity.
C. Location.
D. Duration.
E. Aggravating and alleviating factors.

Ref.: 1, 2

COMMENTS: In clinical practice, as we come to rely more and more on laboratory and radiographic investigation to diagnose the cause of abdominal pain, our ability to interpret its clinical features has tended to suffer. Obviously, all of the features listed above are important for determining the cause of abdominal pain. In teaching centers, where patients frequently must repeat their history to several observers, one must be alert to the possibility that some aspects of the patient's pain may have been "suggested" to the patient by earlier examiners. When possible, questioning a patient about abdominal pain is open-ended, and the terms used to describe the pain and its associated characteristics should be of the patient's choosing. Also, each physician should obtain the patient's history of abdominal pain and not rely on that offered to earlier examiners, as it is not uncommon for new and potentially helpful aspects of the pain to be elicited on repeated questioning. One should learn how the specific characteristics of abdominal pain, listed above, relate to specific underlying disease processes. As a general rule, however, abdominal pain persisting for more than 6 hours or associated with clinical signs of peritoneal irritation raises the possibility of an underlying surgically correctable cause. The decreased response to abdominal pain in the elderly makes evaluation of their pain more difficult.

ANSWER: A, B, C, D, E

16. With regard to anorexia, which of the following statements is/are true?

A. Anorexia is mediated through the hypothalamus.
B. Anorexia may be associated with extraabdominal endocrinopathies.
C. Anorexia is a potential side effect of many drugs.
D. The presence of anorexia is of significant help when differentiating between various forms of intraabdominal pathology.

Ref.: 1, 2

COMMENTS: Anorexia refers to the absence of the desire to eat. It is thought to be mediated through a satiety center in the hypothalamus. It is a nonspecific symptom that can be found in association with many forms of inflammatory and neoplastic abdominal pathology. It is similarly associated with many extraabdominal and systemic abnormalities, including endocrine disorders such as adrenal insufficiency and hyperparathyroidism. Most drugs are capable of causing anorexia through either toxic or idiosyncratic reactions. Anorexia is a sufficiently common complaint that it is not often helpful for making a specific diagnosis. Its absence, however, may be valuable for excluding certain pathologic processes. For example, appendicitis rarely occurs in the absence of some degree of anorexia.

ANSWER: A, B, C

17. Constipation may be associated with which one or more of the following?

A. Psychogenic factors.
B. High-fiber diet.
C. Pregnancy.
D. Multiple sclerosis.
E. Anal fissure.
F. Colorectal tumor.

Ref.: 1

COMMENTS: Constipation is considered to be abnormal retention of feces or delay in fecal discharge. There is a moderately broad range of what constitutes "normal" bowel movements. Most individuals have one bowel movement each day, whereas many have two, and still others have one only every other day. So "abnormal" refers considerably to the difference from what was the usual and ordinary for a particular patient. Constipation has numerous causes. Improper toilet training during childhood can cause psychogenic constipation. Diets consisting of highly refined foods and minimal fiber are also associated with constipation. Expulsion of fecal matter depends on involuntary bowel contraction as well as voluntary somatic contraction, principally of the abdominal and diaphragmatic muscles. Weakness of the abdominal muscles, as can be seen during pregnancy and with marked ascites, and atony of the intrinsic intestinal muscle, as seen with some electrolyte imbalances, can cause constipation. Neurogenic abnormalities (e.g., multiple sclerosis, spinal cord tumors) may affect the autonomic intestinal function, leading to constipation. Constipation can also be a side effect of numerous drugs. Painful anorectal conditions may be the cause of constipation; and they may be an unsuspected cause in children. Of course, new onset of constipation must always cause the clinician to consider mechanical obstruction to the gastrointestinal tract as, for example, by tumors, strictures, or impactions.

ANSWER: A, C, D, E, F

18. Which of the following are potential consequences of prolonged diarrhea?

A. Alkalosis.
B. Elevated hematocrit.
C. Hypokalemia.
D. Hyponatremia.

Ref.: 1, 2

COMMENTS: Diarrhea usually contains concentrations of sodium and chloride that are lower than those found in plasma, and concentrations of potassium and bicarbonate that are higher than those found in plasma. The relative losses of these electrolytes, together with the fluid loss and associated dehydration, lead to the predictable findings of acidosis, hypokalemia, and elevated hematocrit (as a result of dehydration) seen with prolonged diarrhea. Serum sodium concentrations are usually not significantly affected.

ANSWER: B, C

19. Match each of the clinical situations in the left column with the cause of intestinal obstruction *most likely* to be involved in the right column.

A. A 5-year-old boy with small bowel obstruction	a. Neoplasm
B. A 68-year-old man with colonic obstruction; no previous surgery	b. Adhesive bands
C. A 40-year-old woman with small bowel obstruction 3 years after abdominal hysterectomy for fibroids	c. Incarcerated hernia
D. A 35-year-old African man who recently migrated to the United States	d. Volvulus
	e. Diverticulitis

Ref.: 1, 2

COMMENTS: When all ages are grouped together, adhesive bands, followed by incarcerated hernia, followed in turn by neoplasm are the most common causes of intestinal obstruction. This order may vary, however, in specific age groups. For example, hernia is a much more common cause of obstruction during childhood, and colorectal carcinoma is a much more common cause in the elderly. In a given patient, the historical features and physical findings associated with the obstruction, together with the presence or absence of a history of previous abdominal surgery, assist greatly in determining the most likely cause of obstruction. Immigrants from countries yielding fiber and grain diets have a high incidence of sigmoid volvulus.

ANSWER: A-c; B-a; C-b; D-d

20. With regard to the abdominal distension seen with intestinal obstruction, which of the following statements is/are true?

A. The gaseous distension of the intestine is primarily due to swallowed air.
B. Intraluminal sequestration of fluid is the only significant way in which intraabdominal fluid contributes to distension.
C. Free peritoneal fluid implies perforation of the intestine and suggests the presence of severe concomitant peritonitis.
D. With distal small bowel obstruction, repetitive vomiting of large volumes of fluid does not prevent the development of significant abdominal distension.

Ref.: 1, 2

COMMENTS: The abdominal distension seen with intestinal obstruction is due to the accumulation of both gas and fluid. Although gas can be produced by intestinal bacteria, swallowed air accounts for the major portion of intraluminal gas seen in both normal and pathologic states. The fluid component of abdominal distension is primarily due to the sequestration of fluid within both the lumen and the wall of the bowel. The edematous bowel can exude fluid into the peritoneal cavity without perforation being present. Thus finding free peritoneal fluid in cases of intestinal obstruction does not necessarily imply that perforation or peritonitis is present. In the absence of other pathologic states (e.g., portal hypertension), the free peritoneal fluid seen with intestinal obstruction does not contribute significantly to the abdominal distension. Vomiting effectively empties the stomach, and even the duodenum, of its gaseous and fluid contents and is responsible for the occasional appearance of a nondistended abdomen in the setting of high intestinal obstruction. With low intestinal obstruction, the abdominal distension is primarily due to intraluminal fluid and gas that cannot be evacuated by vomiting.

ANSWER: A, D

21. Match each of the types of intestinal obstruction in the left column with one or more of its clinical characteristics in the right column.

A. Closed loop; small bowel	a. May lead to perforation
B. Simple mechanical; ileum	b. Most rapid clinical progression
C. Colon; competent ileocecal valve	c. Laplace's law predicts location of perforation
D. Colon; incompetent ileocecal valve	d. May have minimal distension

Ref.: 1, 2

COMMENTS: When an obstructed segment of bowel loses its blood supply, it is referred to as strangulation; it is the most hazardous consequence of intestinal obstruction. Strangulation may occur because of a twist of the mesentery, leading to obstruction of its vessels, or because of a pressure phenomenon within the lumen of the obstructed bowel, leading to occlusion of the venules, then the capillaries, and finally the arterioles. Untreated, strangulation eventually leads to perforation, which is a potential complication of any bowel obstruction. A closed-loop obstruction occurs when both the afferent and efferent limbs of the involved bowel are obstructed. This leads to rapid distension of the loop and a clinical progression to strangulation that is faster than in other forms of obstruction. Therefore strangulation and perforation can occur with closed-loop small bowel obstruction in the presence of minimal abdominal distension. Colonic obstruction may also be a form of closed-loop obstruction when the ileocecal valve is competent. In such cases there usually is massive colonic distension, which may lead to perforation. With colonic obstruction, the site of perforation is usually the cecum, as dictated by Laplace's law, which states that wall tension is directly related to intraluminal pressure and diameter. When the ileocecal valve is incompetent and the small bowel also can distend, the clinical course may be slower but with more abdominal distension. In such cases, colonic perforation is still possible but less likely.

ANSWER: A-a,b,d; B-a; C-a,c; D-a,c

22. Match each of the radiographic findings in the left column with one or more associated forms of bowel obstruction in the right column.

A. Moderate gaseous dilatation of the entire small and large bowel	a. Colonic obstruction with competent ileocecal valve
B. Gaseous distension of the small bowel with no gas in the colon	b. Ileus
C. Gaseous distension of the small bowel with small amount of gas in the colon	c. Complete small bowel obstruction
D. Distended colon from cecum to descending colon with no small bowel gas	d. Partial small bowel obstruction

Ref.: 1, 2

COMMENTS: The origin of the term *ileus* suggests that it should mean intestinal obstruction from any cause. By common usage, however, ileus has come to mean failure of progression of bowel contents due to disordered motility. The characteristic radiographic findings of ileus include moderate gaseous distension of both small and large bowel. If the large bowel is not distended all the way to the rectum, one must also consider a left-sided colonic obstruction with an incompetent ileocecal valve. Colonic obstruction with a competent ileocecal valve causes distension of the colon alone. An incomplete small bowel obstruction causes significant distension proximal to the obstruction but with some gas present distal to the obstruction because of its incomplete nature. When an incomplete obstruction goes on to completion, it takes some time for the gas beyond the obstruction to be expelled, and therefore early complete small bowel obstructions may be confused radiographically with partial small bowel obstructions. When fully established, however, the characteristic appearance of distended small bowel with absent colonic gas is seen.

ANSWER: A-b; B-c; C-c,d; D-a

23. Which of the following principles of management of intestinal obstruction is/are correct?

A. A closed-loop obstruction represents a surgical emergency.
B. With a partial small bowel obstruction, there is no advantage to delaying surgical intervention.
C. The use of long intestinal tubes is sufficiently cumbersome and time-consuming that it has no significant role in the modern management of intestinal obstruction.
D. Most strangulated obstructions progress sufficiently quickly that they are rarely associated with fluid and electrolyte abnormalities.

Ref.: 1, 2

COMMENTS: All forms of intestinal obstruction should be considered potential surgical problems, the urgency of which is dictated by the likelihood of associated strangulation. In cases of colonic obstruction (particularly with a competent ileocecal valve) or closed-loop obstruction of the small bowel, or when the diagnosis is bowel strangulation, the situation is considered a surgical emergency and the patient prepared as rapidly as possible for abdominal exploration. Dehydration and electrolyte abnormalities may be significant with all forms of obstruction, and the time one has to correct these abnormalities depends on the presence or absence of the factors listed above. In instances of partial small bowel obstruction without evidence of strangulation, it is appropriate first to correct fluid and electrolyte abnormalities before considering operation. In such instances, decompression of the proximal bowel with a long intestinal tube may result in relief of the obstruction and obviate the need for an operation. If not, this maneuver may be of benefit in reducing abdominal distension and relieving the intraluminal pressure, which may subsequently reduce the bowel wall edema. This may in turn lead to safer exploration, as there is less likelihood of spillage of intestinal contents and more secure anastomoses if they are required.

ANSWER: A

24. With regard to adynamic ileus, which of the following statements is/are true?

A. Ileus is due to muscular inhibition, muscular spasticity, or vascular occlusion.
B. Except for the stomach, all segments of the gastrointestinal tract recover from adynamic ileus at approximately the same rate.
C. Pseudoobstruction of the colon is easily differentiated from mechanical colonic obstruction with plain films of the abdomen.
D. In most instances, the management of ileus is nonoperative and is directed at the underlying predisposing abnormality.

Ref.: 1, 2

COMMENTS: The most common form of ileus seen in surgical practice is adynamic ileus, which is due to the inhibition of intestinal neuromuscular function, usually in response to manipulation at the time of operation or from localized inflammation or infection. In uncomplicated cases, the recovery of intestinal motility from adynamic ileus occurs at rates that are specific for the area of gastrointestinal tract involved (small bowel 8 hours, stomach 48 hours, colon 3–5 days). Spastic ileus refers to uncoordinated hyperactivity of the intestine and is seen in toxic and abnormal metabolic states. Specific therapy here is directed at the underlying pathology. Ileus of vascular occlusion results from the inability of ischemic muscle to contract properly. In chronic states, this problem may be alleviated by revascularization. A specific form of adynamic colonic ileus (Ogilvie's syndrome) is a form of colonic pseudoobstruction; on plain films it appears similar to a mechanical obstruction of the left colon, and a contrast study or colonoscopy may be needed to differentiate between the two. One must always consider underlying electrolyte abnormalities and drugs as contributing to adynamic ileus. In general, the therapy is expectant relative to cause but includes nasogastric and rectal decompression and correction of underlying fluid and electrolyte abnormalities.

ANSWER: A, D

25. With regard to gastrointestinal bleeding, which of the following statements is/are true?

A. The definition of hematemesis is limited to the vomiting of fresh blood from a source proximal to the pylorus.
B. Approximately 250 ml of gastrointestinal blood loss is required to produce melena.
C. The presence of occult blood in the stool may persist for up to 3 weeks following an acute episode of gastrointestinal bleeding.
D. The hematocrit level is a reliable measure of one's blood volume during the first 6 hours following an acute gastrointestinal bleed.
E. The degree of azotemia seen in gastrointestinal bleeding relates in part to the site of bleeding and the status of bacterial colonization of the gut.

Ref.: 1

COMMENTS: Hematemesis may occur as a result of any significant bleeding at a site from the pharynx to the ligament of Treitz. The blood vomited may be fresh and red, indicating fairly rapid or recent bleeding, or it may be dark and resemble "coffee grounds" owing to the acid effect on the blood that may occur at slower rates of bleeding. Melena refers to the passage of tarry stool and may be seen with as little as 50 ml of blood in the intestinal tract. Melena may persist for as long as 5 days after a significant gastrointestinal bleed, and occult blood may be detected for up to 3 weeks. Because it takes several hours for extracellular fluid shifts to occur in the setting of acute blood loss, the hematocrit is an unreliable indicator of the degree of hemorrhage early in the clinical course. Tachycardia and orthostatic blood pressure changes are more reliable indicators of significant blood loss. Azotemia may be seen with many forms of gastrointestinal hemorrhage, although it is most commonly seen during bleeding from esophageal varices because of the frequently associated liver disease. The production of urea from intraluminal blood requires bacterial action and therefore may vary with changes in the bacterial colonization of the gut (e.g., as occurs with the use of broad-spectrum antibiotics). Other factors, such as the site of bleeding within the gastrointestinal tract and coexisting renal impairment or hypotension, may also affect the degree of azotemia.

ANSWER: C, E

26. Match each of the techniques for assessing upper gastrointestinal hemorrhage in the left column with one or more of its characteristics in the right column.

A. Upper gastrointestinal contrast study	a. Most important assessment technique
B. Endoscopy	b. May hinder subsequent assessment
C. Arteriography	c. May be utilized for therapy as well as diagnosis
	d. Most hazardous

Ref.: 1, 2

COMMENTS: The three techniques listed above are the most common ones used for assessing upper gastrointestinal bleeding. Despite its relative safety, **upper gastrointestinal contrast study** should not be employed as an initial technique in cases of active bleeding. It fails to determine adequately the presence of erosive gastritis, for example. Also, the retained barium handicaps any subsequent arteriography. Instead, it is more appropriately utilized in patients suspected of having chronic bleeding when one is looking for a tumor or a discrete ulcer. **Endoscopy** has become the favored technique for initially evaluating these patients; it has the advantage of being able to visualize directly (and, when appropriate, to obtain a biopsy specimen) such causes as ulcers, erosive gastritis, esophageal varices, Mallory-Weiss tears, or tumors. Also, it can be used therapeutically to sclerose esophageal varices and to electrocoagulate or laser photocoagulate or inject sclerosants into bleeding sites. Its effectiveness is enhanced greatly by clearing the stomach of retained blood and clots prior to the procedure. **Arteriography**, although the most invasive and hazardous of these three techniques, can pinpoint the site of bleeding in selected patients (hemobilia); for this to be possible, bleeding must be at a rate of approximately 5 ml/min. After the diagnostic phase of the study, the arteriographic catheter may be left in place and used for therapeutic administration of vasopressin or embolic materials. Radionuclide imaging utilizing technetium-labeled erythrocytes is also a useful study, providing diagnostic information similar to that obtained by arteriography.

ANSWER: A-b; B-a,c; C-c,d

27. With regard to lower gastrointestinal tract bleeding, which of the following statements is/are true?

A. Bleeding from the proximal jejunum usually presents as hematemesis and melena.
B. Recognition of the right colon as the site of colonic bleeding has increased in recent years.
C. Diverticulosis and vascular ectasia are the most common causes of massive rectal bleeding in the adult.
D. The presence of inflamed hemorrhoids in the presence of rectal bleeding should preclude further investigation of the rectum and colon.

Ref.: 1

COMMENTS: Bleeding from sites distal to the ligament of Treitz usually manifests as the passage of bloody stools, which may vary from bright red to tarry depending on the site and rate of bleeding. Hematemesis is rarely associated with bleeding distal to the ligament of Treitz. Causes of bleeding from the distal small bowel include Meckel's diverticulum, intestinal duplication, inflammatory bowel disease, neoplasms, and vascular ectasia. In the colon the causes include diverticular disease, vascular ectasia, and neoplasm. Increasingly, vascular ectasia (particularly in the right colon) has been recognized as the cause of lower gastrointestinal bleeding; indeed, in some patient populations it is the most common cause. The rate of bleeding may give some clue as to its source; the bleeding episodes from vascular ectasia and diverticulosis are more likely to be moderate to massive; those from diverticulitis or colorectal cancer tend to be mild. Hemorrhoids and benign anorectal conditions that may present with bleeding are sufficiently common that their presence should not preclude evaluation of the remainder of the rectum and colon to search for other causes of rectal bleeding.

ANSWER: B, C

28. With regard to heartburn, which of the following statements is/are true?

A. Approximately 5% of Americans have daily symptoms for heartburn.
B. Gastroesophageal reflux is the leading cause of heartburn.
C. "Water brash" is defined as regurgitated gastric contents.
D. Most heartburn sufferers seek and are relieved by nonprescription medications.

Ref.: 1

COMMENTS: Heartburn is typically described as substernal burning associated with a bitter taste in the back of the mouth. Approximately 10% of Americans suffer from heartburn on a daily basis. Gastroesophageal reflux is the leading cause of heartburn. Approximately 10% of heartburn sufferers require prescription medication. "Water brash" is described as the sudden filling of the mouth with clear, slightly salty fluid; it is a salivary gland secretion response to acid irritation of the distal esophagus. This term is frequently misused and is definitely not regurgitated gastric contents.

ANSWER: B, D

29. Match each of the disease states that produce jaundice in the left column with its pathophysiology in the right column.

A. Gilbert's disease	a. Bilirubin production exceeds excretory capacity
B. Hemolysis	b. Extrahepatic biliary obstruction
C. Physiologic neonatal jaundice	c. Deficient hepatocyte secretion
D. Crigler-Najjar syndrome	d. Deficient hepatocyte uptake
E. Dubin-Johnson syndrome	e. Deficient conjugation
F. Suppurative cholangitis	

Ref.: 1

COMMENTS: It is useful to consider patients with jaundice in terms of possible pathophysiologic mechanisms: excess bilirubin production, deficient hepatocyte uptake, deficient conjugation, deficient hepatocyte secretion, and deficient bilirubin excretion. These mechanisms have been classically grouped as prehepatic, hepatic, and posthepatic causes. One of the first tests to be performed when evaluating the jaundiced patient is a fractionated bilirubin assessment to determine the relative proportion of conjugated and unconjugated bilirubin. A predominance of unconjugated bilirubin suggests prehepatic causes (**hemolysis**) or hepatic deficiencies of uptake or conjugation of bilirubin. Predominance of conjugated bilirubin suggests defects in hepatocyte secretion into the bile duct or biliary excretion into the gastrointestinal tract. Combined conjugated and unconjugated hyperbilirubinemia usually suggests complex pathophysiology in which there has been acquired liver damage or in which prehepatic or posthepatic causes have become associated with hepatocyte damage. **Gilbert's disease** is a relatively common abnormality of hepatic uptake of bilirubin and usually presents as a mild hyperbilirubinemia without other associated abnormalities. **Crigler-Najjar syndrome** represents an inability to conjugate bilirubin with the hepatocyte owing to a deficiency of glucuronyl transferase. The **physiologic jaundice** of the newborn also represents a deficiency in conjugation, but here it is due to a self-correcting immaturity of bilirubin glucuronide synthesis. **Dubin-Johnson syndrome** is caused by a deficiency in liver cell secretion and therefore presents as an intrahepatic form of obstructive jaundice. Clearly, the most significant category of jaundice as relates to surgical practice is that of extrahepatic biliary obstruction. It is usually caused by gallstones, stricture, or neoplasm. Clinically, the patient may present with a spectrum of findings ranging from asymptomatic jaundice to the sepsis and moribund state of the patient with acute **suppurative cholangitis**.

ANSWER: A-d; B-a; C-e; D-e; E-c; F-b

30. Match each of the diagnostic procedures utilized for evaluation of jaundice in the left column with one or more of its characteristics in the right column.

A. Computed tomography (CT)	a. Overall, the most cost-effective initial procedure
B. Percutaneous transhepatic cholangiography (PTC)	b. May be of help in obtaining a tissue diagnosis
C. Endoscopic retrograde cholangiopancreatography (ERCP)	c. Greater utility in assessing periampullary causes of obstruction
D. Upper gastrointestinal contrast study	d. May be utilized in biliary decompression
E. Ultrasonography	e. Helps determine resectability
	f. Rarely indicated

Ref.: 1

COMMENTS: Proper evaluation of a patient with obstructive jaundice involves assessment of the intra- and extrahepatic biliary tree and the periampullary area of the duodenum. All of the tests listed above may have a role to play in this assessment. Of these tests, the upper gastrointestinal contrast study is the least helpful and would be of benefit only in showing an intraduodenal mass or extrinsic involvement of the duodenum with a periduodenal tumor. Ultrasonography as the initial method of investigation is probably the most cost-effective in that it can confirm the presence of biliary dilatation and assess the pancreas, liver, and retroperitoneal nodal areas for the presence of mass lesions or involvement that may preclude curative resection. Furthermore, needle aspiration biopsy of mass lesions and percutaneous biliary decompression may be performed with ultrasound control. CT is also useful for demonstrating biliary dilatation and searching for mass lesions in the periampullary area and liver. It may further help assess resectability by defining the relation of the peripancreatic vessels (particularly the superior mesenteric vessels) to the tumor mass. As with ultrasonography, CT scans may also be utilized for directing percutaneous needle biopsies. PTC is useful for visualizing the site of biliary obstruction. During this procedure, transbiliary brush biopsies for cytology may be performed and drainage catheters placed to decompress the biliary tree. ERCP is useful for determining the site of obstruction; and when this site is suspected to be distal in the biliary tree, it offers the added advantage of visual inspection of the ampulla as the possible source of neoplastic obstruction. Biopsies for histology and cytology may be performed during ERCP, and therapeutic intervention in the form of catheter drainage or endoscopic papillotomy may be carried out. Magnetic resonance cholangiography (MRC) is an extremely promising method for imaging the bile duct that may soon become the imaging modality of choice for many situations. MRC is rapid and noninvasive and does not require any contrast administration. Computer hardware and software programs for MR imaging are advancing rapidly and are expanding its already impressive capabilities.

ANSWER: A-b,e; B-b,d,e; C-b,c,d; D-f; E-a,b,d,e

31. With regard to bacterial translocation, which of the following statements is/are true?

A. Enteral feedings in intensive care patients reduces bacterial translocation.
B. Promoters of bacterial translocation include injured tissue, hypotension, protein malnutrition, and altered gut flora.

C. Conditions associated with bacterial translocation include hemorrhagic shock, burns, malnutrition, sepsis, and jaundice.
D. Selective gut decontamination reduces bacterial translocation and its associated mortality.

Ref.: 1

COMMENTS: Bacterial translocation is defined as transmigration of living bacteria or their endotoxins from the lumen of the gut through the epithelium to distant sites such as the mesenteric lymph nodes, spleen, peritoneal cavity, and blood. Patients in the intensive care unit who are not receiving enteral nutrition have a permeable gastrointestinal tract, which leads to bacterial translocation. Promoters of bacterial translocation include injured tissue, hypotension, protein malnutrition, and altered gut flora. Conditions associated with bacterial translocation are hemorrhagic shock, burns, malnutrition, sepsis, and jaundice. Selective decontamination of enteric flora with nonabsorbable antibiotics has decreased nosocomial infections.

ANSWER: A, B, C

REFERENCES

1. Schwartz SI, Shires GT, Spencer FC: *Principles of Surgery*, 7th ed. McGraw-Hill, New York, 1999.
2. Sabiston DC Jr: *Textbook of Surgery*, 15th ed. WB Saunders, Philadelphia, 1997.

CHAPTER 26

Esophagus

1. With regard to the history of esophageal surgery, match the following:

A. Transmediastinal esophagectomy in cadaver	a. Turner 1933
B. Proper techniques of rigid endoscopy	b. Denk 1913
C. Stressed anatomic repair of hiatal hernia to correct reflux	c. Chevalier-Jackson
D. First successful transmediastinal esophagectomy for cancer with second-stage skin tube reconstruction	d. Allison
E. First successful transthoracic esophagectomy without reconstruction	e. Torek 1915

Ref.: 1

COMMENTS: The development of modern esophageal surgery is a fascinating subject and causes modern surgeons to appreciate those who came before them. Following are some of the sentinel events. The development of guidelines by Chevalier-Jackson for rigid endoscopy have held the test of time for the last 50 years. Because of the absence of anesthetic techniques, resection of the esophagus was limited to the cervical area. Billroth in 1871 and Czerny in 1877 successfully resected the cervical esophagus for carcinoma. Mikulicz in 1886 reconstructed the cervical esophagus using a skin tube. The first successful resection of the thoracic esophagus without reconstruction was accomplished in 1915 by Torek. Interestingly, blunt esophagectomy is not new, as Denk in 1913 performed transmediastinal esophagectomy in animals and cadavers using a vein stripper. Turner in 1933 performed the first successful transmediastinal esophagectomy for cancer with a second-stage skin-tube reconstruction, and the same year Oshawa performed the first distal transhiatal esophagectomy and esophagogastric anastomosis in the chest. Heller is credited for performing the first esophagomyotomy for achalasia in 1913. For reflux surgery, Allison in 1951 coined the phrase reflux esophagitis. He believed that reflux was caused by a hiatal hernia and emphasized repair of the anatomic defect rather than correction of the sphincter mechanism in the repair named after him. Successful repairs of hiatal hernia and correction of reflux were introduced by Nissen in 1961 and Skinner and Belsey in 1967.

ANSWER: A-b; B-c; C-d; D-a; E-e

2. With regard to the anatomy of the esophagus, which of the following statements is/are true?

A. The esophagus is 35 cm long.
B. The esophagus is divided into four segments.
C. There are five predictable areas of narrowing: (1) thyropharyngeus muscle; (2) thoracic inlet; (3) left subclavian artery; (4) left bronchus; (5) crossing of the thoracic duct.
D. The arterial blood is supplied by the splenic, right gastric, pulmonary, and innominate arteries.
E. The pharyngoesophageal segment of esophagus consists of three constrictors and the stylopharyngeus muscle.

Ref.: 1, 2

COMMENTS: See Question 3.

3. With regard to the anatomy of the esophagus, which of the following statements is/are true?

A. The outer muscular layer of the upper thoracic esophagus lies adjacent to the membranous portion of the trachea.
B. In patients with cirrhosis with portal hypertension, venous drainage flows through the azygous system.
C. The cervical and the lowest portion of the thoracic esophagus lie slightly to the left of the midline.
D. The left and right vagal plexi are intimately attached to the esophagus and emerge as two main anterior and posterior trunks just above the esophageal hiatus.
E. The thoracic duct travels from right to left at the upper third of the esophagus.

Ref.: 1, 2

COMMENTS: Proper surgical management of diseases of the esophagus requires thorough understanding of esophageal anatomy. The esophagus is a muscular tube 25 cm long with an inner circular layer and an outer longitudinal layer. The absence of a serosal covering, which has substantial strength, may contribute to the risk of anastomotic leakage after esophageal resection or repair of transmural esophageal defects. The esophagus is lined by squamous epithelium except for its distal 2 cm, which is lined by columnar epithelium. The absence of mucous glands renders it susceptible to acid peptic injury.

For convenience, the esophagus is divided into four segments: (1) The **pharyngoesophageal** segment is between the laryngopharynx and cervical esophagus and includes the superior, middle, and inferior constrictors and the stylopharyngeus muscle. The stylopharyngeus muscle is an inferior constrictor and courses obliquely upward. The cricopharyngeal muscle is believed by some to be part of the inferior constrictor, and its fibers course transversely. The cricopharyngeal muscle blends intimately with the upper fibers of the cervical esophagus and the lower fibers of the thyroglossus muscle. Because these fibers have divergent directions, it is believed that a weakness develops allowing for the development of a Zenker's diverticulum. The cricopharyngeal muscle serves as the upper sphincter of the esophagus and relaxes when the thyropharyngeus portion of the inferior constrictor contracts to propel a bolus of food. (2) The **cervical** esophagus is a segment 5–6 cm long. It begins at the cricopharyngeal muscle and ends at T1. (3) The **thoracic** esophageal segment begins at T1 and ends at the hiatus. (4) The **abdominal** esophageal segment varies in length from 1 to 5 cm. It begins at the hiatus and ends at the cardia.

In its course from the pharynx to the stomach, the esophagus is positioned to the left or the right of the midline at various levels, thereby influencing surgical accessibility. The cervical esophagus lies behind the trachea and slightly to its left; it then deviates to the right in the subcarinal area, gradually returning to the left behind the pericardial sac at the level of the 7th thoracic vertebra. As it lies behind the trachea adjacent to its membranous aspect, it is susceptible to involvement in tracheoesophageal fistulas.

The caliber of the normal esophagus is not uniform; rather, it has predictable areas of narrowing at the levels of the cricopharyngeal muscle, the aortic arch, and the diaphragm; of these, the cricopharyngeal muscle marks the narrowest point of the esophagus.

The **arterial blood supply** of the esophagus is segmental and arises from numerous and abundant terminal sources. The cervical esophagus receives branches from the superior thyroid and thyrocervical arteries; the thoracic esophagus is supplied by four to six branches—bronchial, inferior phrenic, left gastric, and inferior thyroid arteries—terminating in a fine capillary network before penetrating the musculature, allowing safe, blunt esophagectomy without the need for individual arterial ligation. The **submucosal venous plexus** of the thoracic esophagus drains into the azygos and hemizygous system and that of the abdominal portion into the left gastric vein; continuity is established by three submucosal vein plexi.

Lymphatic drainage may extend longitudinally in the wall of the esophagus before continuing on to regional lymph nodes; this point is important when determining proximal margins at the time of esophagectomy for malignant disease.

The **thoracic duct** courses from right to left behind the upper third of the esophagus and is thus exposed to possible surgical damage.

The **vagus nerves** lie on either side of the esophagus, forming a plexus on its musculature. Just above the hiatus, they form two major trunks: left anterior and right posterior.

The **esophagogastric junction** is a complex area, anatomically and physiologically. Supportive structures in this area include the diaphragmatic crura and the phrenoesophageal ligament, which is a continuation of the endoabdominal fascia and circumferentially attaches the esophagus to the muscular diaphragm. The anatomy of the phrenoesophageal membrane is an important factor in the pathophysiology of gastroesophageal reflux. It is important to know that it is a continuation of the transversalis fascia of the abdomen.

ANSWER:
Question 2: B, E
Question 3: A, B, C, D, E

4. With regard to normal esophageal motility, which of the following statements is/are true?

A. The pressure of the upper esophageal sphincter is higher than that of the lower esophageal sphincter.
B. Secondary waves are initiated when the entire bolus of food has not cleared the esophagus.
C. The most common method for measuring pressures employs micropressure transducers.
D. Normal postdeglutition contraction of both the upper and lower esophageal sphincters results in pressures greater than the predeglutition resting pressure.

Ref.: 1, 2

COMMENTS: Manometric studies have defined normal esophageal motility and characterized anomalies in various pathologic states. Studies are typically performed with the use of multiple perfused catheter systems and pull-through techniques. Recently, micropressure transducers have provided an accurate, simple measurement method without using a water-perfused system. These techniques are expensive, however, and difficult to maintain so they are not used widely. Two high-pressure zones can be identified within the esophagus: one corresponding to the upper esophageal sphincter (UES) at the level of the cricopharyngeal muscle and another representing the lower esophageal sphincter (LES) near the gastroesophageal junction.

The normal act of deglutition involves coordination of both voluntary and involuntary movements. After the act of swallowing, the UES allows a food bolus to enter the esophagus. A primary peristaltic wave progressively moves the food to the stomach, which is entered after coordinated relaxation of the LES. After relaxation, a postdeglutition contraction of the sphincters occurs before resumption of a resting pressure. If the esophagus is not cleared of material by the primary peristaltic wave, secondary peristaltic waves are initiated in the smooth muscle of the lower two-thirds of the esophagus. Tertiary waves are not peristaltic. Numerous hormonal, neural, pharmacologic, chemical, and mechanical factors can affect esophageal motility, although the precise mechanisms of control are incompletely defined.

Entry of air into the esophagus with inspiration or swallowing is prevented by the UES, which normally stays closed as a result of tonic contractions of the cricopharyngeal muscle.

ANSWER: A, B, D

5. Which of the following are the most important for maintaining competence of the gastroesophageal junction?

A. Small diameter of the esophagus at the hiatus.
B. Level of insertion of the phrenoesophageal ligament on the esophagus.
C. Angle of esophageal entry into the stomach.
D. Orientation of muscle fibers of the lower esophageal sphincter.
E. Intraabdominal segment of esophagus.

Ref.: 1, 2

COMMENTS: See Question 6.

6. Which of the following factor(s) play(s) a role in limiting esophageal exposure to acid?

A. Saliva.
B. Tertiary peristaltic waves.
C. Gastric emptying.
D. Secretin.
E. Gastrin.

Ref.: 1, 2, 3, 4

COMMENTS: The anatomic arrangement of the gastroesophageal (GE) junction and the physical means by which competence of the GE junction is maintained to limit esophageal exposure to acid have been studied extensively but are still not completely understood. In humans, unlike other animals, there is no distinct anatomic muscular sphincter. Pharmacologic studies in humans, however, have demonstrated variations in background basal tone in response to excitatory and inhibitory neurohumoral exposure, the knowledge of which is being applied clinically to the therapy of reflux. Among hormones, for example, gastrin, motilin, and bombesin increase the high pressure zone (HPZ) whereas secretin, cholecystokinin, glucagon, progesterone, estrogen, and prostaglandins E_1 and E_2 decrease it.

Several anatomic considerations affect the competence of the GE junction, but it is generally agreed that the presence of a segment of esophagus exposed to intraabdominal pressure is the most important. The laws of physics pertaining to wall tension and to pressure in hollow tubes of different diameters, as well as many years of clinical experience with various antireflux operations, support this concept. According to the law of Laplace, the pressure required to distend a pliable tube is inversely proportional to the diameter of the tube. With a sliding esophageal hiatal hernia, the phrenoesophageal membrane is stretched, thus exerting centrifugal tension on the distal esophagus and increasing its diameter; likewise, the rate of reflux varies inversely with the length of the abdominal segment of the esophagus. In patients with reflux, the attachment of the phrenoesophageal ligament is closer to the stomach, and the intraabdominal esophagus is shorter. The critical anatomic factor in maintaining a segment of the esophagus in the intraabdominal position appears to be insertion of the phrenoesophageal membrane to the esophagus at a point approximately 3–4 cm above the manometrically determined GE junction. The LES is better named the LES mechanism or distal esophageal HPZ, as no anatomic sphincter exists. There is no absolute value for the HPZ, but it is somewhere between 10 and 20 mm Hg. Patients with no reflux may have low values, and others with massive reflux have high values. This discrepancy results from variations in the anatomic characteristics just mentioned and the recently discussed evidence that there is uneven and eccentric pressures around the circumference of the HPZ. Two other important mechanisms when limiting exposure of the distal esophagus to acid are (1) esophageal clearing through primary and secondary peristaltic activity, salivation, and gravity and (2) proper gastric function, such as timely emptying and peptic acid activity. Patients with these problems may require modification of the antireflux procedure or additional operations on the stomach, such as emptying procedures or parietal cell vagotomy. Patients with symptoms and endoscopic evidence of esophagitis but normal manometric findings and pH should be evaluated for other causes of this condition, such as drug-induced esophagitis, alkaline reflux, and gastric disease.

ANSWER:
Question 5: A, B, E
Question 6: A, C, E

7. With regard to GE reflux, which of the following statements is/are true?

A. Reflux occurs less than 7% of the day in all patients regardless of the presence or absence of hiatal hernia.
B. Symptomatic GE reflux does not occur without a hiatal hernia.
C. Patients with columnar epithelium-lined esophagus have reflux 26% of the day.
D. Most patients with symptomatic GE reflux have hiatal hernia.

Ref.: 1, 2

COMMENTS: See Question 11.

8. Which of the following tests is the most sensitive for the detection of GE reflux?

A. Barium swallow.
B. Manometry.
C. 24-Hour pH monitoring.
D. Acid perfusion (Bernstein) test.
E. Standard antireflux test (SART).

Ref.: 1, 2, 5

COMMENTS: See Question 11.

9. A 50-year-old woman complains of pyrosis, nightly cough, and a sour taste in her mouth. Which of the following are helpful when deciding for antireflux surgery?

A. Failure of medical therapy to control symptoms.
B. Defect of lower esophageal sphincter.
C. Increase of esophageal exposure to gastric juice.
D. Positive histology.
E. Positive Bernstein test.

Ref.: 1, 2

COMMENTS: See Question 11.

10. A 45-year-old woman has a history of a prior vagotomy and antrectomy for recurrent duodenal peptic ulceration. She now has severe heartburn, nausea, and emesis. Endoscopy reveals severe esophagitis. Which of the following are important before antireflux surgery?

A. 24-Hour pH monitoring.
B. Fiberoptic bile probe.
C. Acid perfusion (Bernstein) test.
D. One week of metronidazole (Flagyl) therapy.
E. Barium swallow.

Ref.: 1, 2

COMMENTS: See Question 11.

11. The patient described in Question 10 is found to have normal esophageal motility, a normal barium swallow, and 24-hour pH in the basic-to-neutral range. Which of the following are helpful?

A. Angelchik prosthesis.
B. Conversion of a Billroth II anastomosis to a Roux-en-Y anastomosis.
C. Bile-chelating agents.
D. Allison procedure.

Ref.: 1, 2

COMMENTS: Limited acid reflux into the esophagus is a normal physiologic event. Reflux and its attendant complications are clinically significant when the HPZ at the lower end of the esophagus is of inadequate degree or length. This is not necessarily related to the presence of a sliding hiatal hernia, in which the stomach and transversalis (endoabdominal) fascia protrude through the esophageal hiatus. Most patients with significant reflux, however, can be demonstrated to have a sliding hernia. The cause of the reflux is not the hernia per se; in fact, most patients with sliding hiatal hernias do not have significant or symptomatic reflux. The overlap between the symptoms of GE reflux and those of other upper abdominal or mediastinal problems necessitates accurate documentation of pathologic reflux before definitive therapy is undertaken. **Contrast studies** that include the pharynx, esophagus, and stomach can reveal anatomic problems such as diverticula, various types of hiatal hernia, and gastric abnormalities, which help the endoscopist perform safer, more complete endoscopy. In addition, well done videofluoroscopic contrast studies detect abnormal peristaltic activity and spontaneous reflux. Reflux during the Valsalva maneuver can be demonstrated as a matter of course and is not pathologic. Numerous other tests have been used to identify abnormal reflux. **Twenty-four hour pH monitoring** is now the gold standard and the most precise measurement of acid reflux. An electrode probe placed 5 cm above the LES records the frequency and exposure time of pH dips. A log is kept by the patient to document symptoms and type of activity, which are then correlated to the pH recording. Bile reflux can be measured by a fiberoptic probe that recognizes bilirubin. It is important to note that both pH and bile probes measure concentration, not the amount of acid or bile present. Normal acid exposure time in 24 hours is considered to be 4–7%, 12% for mild esophagitis and 26% in those with Barrett's epithelium. Other tests using the pH probe may be performed in special circumstances.

The **standard acid reflux test** (SART) is a test in which 300 ml of 0.1 N hydrochloric acid is instilled in the stomach, and the pH is measured while performing various maneuvers.

The **Bernstein test**, in which 0.1 N hydrochloric acid is instilled into the esophagus in an attempt to reproduce symptoms, and acid-clearing tests in which there is measurement of the ability of the esophagus to remove instilled acid are less accurate.

Endoscopy is useful for assessing anatomic damage produced by reflux such as esophagitis, ulceration, or stricture and is critical to rule out cancer.

Manometry of the esophagus should be performed when a motility disorder is suspected from symptoms of dysphagia or reflux. Manometry before antireflux procedures may disclose primary esophageal disease, which could alter plans for the type of procedure employed. For instance, in a patient with poor peristaltic waves a partial wrap may be required, whereas a patient with simultaneous contractions or failure of relaxation of the distal esophagus may require an entirely different procedure altogether. Before embarking on a surgical procedure, the results of endoscopy, histology, pH monitoring, and manometry are tabulated, and the patient is given a score. Patients whose tests are negative or give equivocal results are given the score 0 and 1, respectively, and are not candidates for surgery. Patients with a score of 2 have positive tests but no mucosal damage. Patients given a score of 3 have all positive tests, and those with a score of 4 have severe disease. These last three categories are candidates for surgical therapy.

Medical therapy, of course, should be attempted for a period of 8–12 weeks in most patients prior to surgery.

Ref.: 1, 2, 3, 4, 5

ANSWER:
Question 7: A, C
Question 8: C
Question 9: A, B, C, D
Question 10: A, B, E
Question 11: B, C

12. For each factor in the left column, select the appropriate effect on the distal lower esophageal sphincter (LES) pressure from the right column.

A. Atropine	a. Increased LES pressure
B. Coffee	b. Decreased LES pressure
C. Metoclopramide	c. No significant effect
D. Cigarettes	
E. Gastric acidification	
F. Alcohol	
G. Tobacco	
H. Bacon and eggs	
I. Protein meal	

Ref.: 1, 2

COMMENTS: The control of the distal HPZ in the esophagus, which acts as a physiologic sphincter, is complex and is affected primarily by mechanical factors and secondarily by neural, hormonal, and chemical factors. Therapeutic administration of agents that increase sphincter pressure and avoidance of factors that reduce sphincter pressure are important to the medical management of patients with symptomatic reflux. Cholinergic agents (e.g., bethanechol), anticholinesterases, and α-adrenergic agents (e.g., metoclopramide) increase sphincter tone, whereas anticholinergic agents (e.g., atropine), α-adrenergic antagonists, and β-adrenergic agonists decrease sphincter pressure. Nicotine, alcohol, chocolate, and fatty meals have detrimental effects on sphincter tone, whereas a high protein meal increases sphincter tone. Hormonal influences include the stimulatory effects of gastrin and the inhibitory influences of secretin and cholecystokinin; it is not clear, however, what effect these hormones have in physiologic doses. Gastric alkalinization and distension tend to increase LES pressure, whereas gastric acidification decreases sphincter tone.

ANSWER: A-b; B-b; C-a; D-b; E-b; F-b; G-b; H-b; I-a

13. Recognized complications of GE reflux include which one or more of the following?

A. Ulcer.
B. Aspiration.
C. Columnar epithelium-lined esophagus.
D. Motility disturbance.
E. Zenker's diverticulum.
F. Stricture.
G. Laryngeal inflammation.

Ref.: 1, 2, 4, 5

COMMENTS: See Question 14.

14. Which of the following is/are related to the nonsurgical therapy of reflux?

A. Alginic acid.
B. Prokinetic agents.
C. Living at a higher altitude.
D. Low fat meals.
E. Proton pump inhibitors.

Ref.: 1, 2, 4, 5

COMMENTS: Significant reflux of acid gastric contents into the esophagus can produce mucosal inflammation, ulceration, chronic blood loss, and eventual stricture or shortening from scar contracture. Pulmonary aspiration of refluxed material can lead to laryngeal edema, bronchospasm, recurrent pneumonia, bronchiectasis, and lung abscess. The chronic destructive influences of reflux can produce metaplasia of the normal squamous esophageal epithelium, resulting in lining of the esophagus by columnar epithelium; this condition is known as Barrett's esophagus. Abnormal motility disorders, including spasm and disordered peristalsis, can result from chronic reflux or stenosis.

In general, the indications for operative intervention include symptoms or complications intractable to medical management or the desire to escape the need for continual drug treatment. Medical management consists of mechanical measures, such as avoidance of positions or activities that cause reflux, for example, total recumbency by keeping the head of the bed elevated (particularly after meals), weight loss, and avoidance of constricting garments, as well as pharmacologic measures that might include simple antacids, alginic acid, H_2-blockers, proton pump inhibitors (omeprazole), and prokinetic agents (metoclopramide). Fortunately, medical management is sufficient for most patients with symptomatic gastroesophageal reflux disease (GERD). Even the complication of esophageal stenosis can often be effectively treated by esophageal dilatation, but an antireflux procedure should accompany the dilatation to prevent recurrence and irreversible stricture. Surgery has been demonstrated to be superior to medical management for patients with complications of GERD.

ANSWER:
Question 13: A, B, C, D, F, G
Question 14: A, B, D, E

15. With regard to Barrett's esophagus, which of the following statements is/are true?

A. It is congenital in origin.
B. The columnar lining may be discontinuous with the gastric epithelium.
C. It is associated with an increased risk of epidermoid cancer of the esophagus.
D. Surgical indications are those for reflux.
E. Esophageal resection is indicated when severe dysplasia is present.

Ref.: 1, 2, 6

COMMENTS: See Question 17.

16. Which one or more of the following are effects of antireflux operations on Barrett's esophagus?

A. Regression of esophagitis.
B. Prevention of further columnar metaplasia.
C. Regression of columnar esophageal lining.
D. Prevention of malignancy.

Ref.: 1, 2, 6

COMMENTS: See Question 17.

17. Match each condition in the left column with the appropriate therapy in the right column.

A. Asymptomatic Barrett's esophagus	a. Nissen
B. Barrett's esophagus with severe dysplasia on repeated biopsy	b. Nonsurgical management
C. Barrett's esophagus with ulceration unresponsive to H_2-blockers	c. Esophagectomy
D. Metastatic cancer from Barrett's in patients who can eat	d. Periodic endoscopy and biopsy

Ref.: 1, 2, 6

COMMENTS: Barrett's esophagus is a condition of columnar metaplasia of the normal squamous epithelial lining of the esophagus found in 7–10% of patients with long-standing reflux. It is not to be mistaken for the embryologically inherited heterotopic gastric mucosa in the proximal esophagus. Patients with Barrett's esophagus have been demonstrated to have had longer periods of acid exposure of the esophagus than those without it. Both continuous and discontinuous patterns of involvement of the esophageal mucosa occur. Complications include esophageal stenosis, ulceration in the columnar epithelium (Barrett's ulcer), and an increased risk of dysplasia and subsequent development of adenocarcinoma of the esophagus. The exact risk of malignant transformation is not known, but it is believed to be 40 times that of the normal population. The indications for antireflux operations for Barrett's esophagus not complicated by malignancy are no different from the indications in any patient with GE reflux. Antireflux operations effectively relieve esophagitis and prevent further metaplastic epithelial change, but they do not reliably cause the columnar lining already present to regress, nor have they been shown clearly to eliminate the risk of cancer. Any patient with Barrett's esophagus, regardless of whether symptomatic, requires careful follow-up with serial endoscopic examination and biopsy. If severe dysplasia is demonstrated, esophageal resection is indicated. Various methods of endoscopic ablation (photochemical, laser) are being actively investigated for treatment of Barrett's esophagus both with and without dysplasia. These treatments are not without complications and their efficacy has not been established, as metaplastic epithelium can persist underneath reepithelialized areas.

ANSWER:
Question 15: B, D, E
Question 16: A, B
Question 17: A-b,d; B-c; C-a,d; D-b

18. Which one or more of the following principles are common to the Belsey, Nissen, and Hill and laparoscopic Nissen antireflux operations?

A. Effective antireflux procedure.
B. Gastric plication around the distal esophagus.
C. Restoration of normal GE anatomy.
D. Restoration of an intraabdominal segment of esophagus.
E. Pyloroplasty.

Ref.: 1, 2, 3, 4, 5

COMMENTS: See Question 20.

19. Match each operative characteristic in the left column with one or more appropriate operations in the right column.

A. Thoracic approach
B. Abdominal approach
C. Median arcuate ligament
D. Prosthetic device
E. Anatomic repair
F. Short esophagus
G. Partial wrap

a. Belsey
b. Nissen
c. Hill
d. Allison
e. Angelchik
f. Collis gastroplasty

Ref.: 1, 2, 3, 4, 5

COMMENTS: See Question 20.

20. Which is/are true of laparoscopic Nissen fundoplication?

A. Contraindicated in the presence of short esophagus.
B. Is rarely performed.
C. No medical therapy indicated prior to the procedure.
D. Only history is required prior to procedure.

COMMENTS: Simple reconstitution of normal GE anatomy, as with the transabdominal **Allison** repair, is not an effective antireflux operation because of the high rate of recurrence of GE reflux. Several well conceived, standardized operations have now been devised as effective antireflux procedures. These operations include the Nissen fundoplication, the Belsey Mark IV operation, and the Hill posterior gastropexy with calibration of the cardia. Common to all of these procedures are restoration of an intraabdominal segment of esophagus, a variable degree of gastric plication around the distal esophagus, and reconstitution of the esophageal hiatus. Certain principles must be adhered to when an antireflux operation is performed. The procedure should permanently establish an adequate length of esophagus in the abdomen and restore the sphincteric pressure to twice that of the gastric pressure; the cardia must not be constricted and must be allowed to relax. Also, it must not impede the bolus of food from progression when the propulsive force of the esophagus is diminished. The factors to be considered before the reflux operation is performed are the propulsive force of the esophagus, the presence or absence of concomitant esophageal disorders, gastric reflux that mimics esophageal reflux symptoms, and the presence of gastroduodenal disorders that may necessitate additional procedures. The referenced surgical texts should be referred to for simple anatomic understanding of the operations.

The **Belsey** operation is difficult to learn. It is performed only through the chest and involves two layers of plicating sutures placed between the gastric fundus and the lower esophagus with subsequent creation of approximately a 280-degree anterior gastric wrap and posterior approximation of the crura.

With the **Nissen** fundoplication, which can be performed via an abdominal or a thoracic approach, a 360-degree circumferential wrap of the gastric fundus around the distal esophagus is created. Whereas Nissen originally had recommended a 4 cm wrap, the frequent occurrence of the gas bloat syndrome has led surgeons to use a 2 cm "floppy" wrap to achieve better results.

With the **Hill** operation, performed only through the abdomen, posterior approximation of the crura is followed by anchoring both the anterior and posterior aspects of the GE junction to the median arcuate ligament adjacent to the aorta, thereby creating a gastric wrap of approximately 180 degrees. Calibration of the plication by intraoperative manometric measurements is considered critical for success of the Hill procedure. All of these operations can effectively prevent GE reflux; whether one operation is clearly superior to another is controversial, but most surgeons prefer the Nissen fundoplication for uncomplicated reflux. When there is insufficient esophageal motility, a partial fundoplication such as the Belsey Mark IV may be preferred.

In the presence of a short esophagus, a **Collis** gastroplasty combined with the Belsey Mark IV or Nissen is suggested. With this procedure, performed through the chest, the esophagus is lengthened by dividing the stomach parallel to the lesser curvature starting at the angle of His and then constructing the fundoplication from around the esophagus. Each procedure has a place in the management of GE reflux, depending on the characteristics of the individual patient, technical considerations, and the surgeon's experience.

The **Angelchik** device is a horseshoe-shaped Silastic device placed around the distal esophagus, thus keeping this segment in the abdomen. Its simplicity invites use through the abdominal approach. Its disadvantages are erosion of the device into the esophagus or stomach and migration. Its use is not recommended.

Laparoscopic Nissen fundoplication now performed widely is a safe and effective procedure that has been tested for several years. The indications are the same as for the open procedure; but, most important, the presence of a short esophagus must be excluded lest the wrap be placed around the cardia of the stomach, which would lead to complications. Skilled laparoscopic surgeons have developed techniques of laparoscopic Collis procedures in conjunction with fundoplication but experience is relatively limited.

ANSWER:
Question 18: A, B, D
Question 19: A-a,b,f; B-b,c,d,e; C-c; D-e; E-d; F-f; G-a,c
Question 20: A

21. With regard to paraesophageal hiatal hernia, which of the following is/are characteristic?

A. Symptomatic GE reflux is the most common complication.
B. Often there is an associated sliding hiatal hernia.
C. Large asymptomatic hernias necessitate repair.
D. Dissection may destroy HPZ integrity.
E. Hematemesis.
F. Infarction.
G. Colon is never part of contents.

Ref.: 1, 2, 3, 4

COMMENTS: There are two main types of anatomically defined esophageal hiatal hernias: type I (sliding) hernia and type II (paraesophageal) hernia. Other types of hernia that have anatomic features and complications of both are described also. With **type I** (*sliding*) hiatal hernia (H1) the cardia enters the chest through a widened hiatus and a stretched, but intact, phrenoesophageal ligament. Because the phrenoesophageal ligament is intact, abdominal pressure is still applied to the distal esophagus, so in most patients reflux does not develop. However, most patients with reflux do have a sliding hiatal hernia. The point of insertion of the phrenoesophageal ligament on the esophagus and lateral tension on the esophagus are factors that may contribute to reflux. With **type II** (*paraesophageal*) hiatal hernia (H2) the anatomic problem involves a defect in the phrenoesophageal membrane with herniation of the stomach into a peritoneum-lined pouch adjacent to the esophagus. With other hernias, such as **type III** paraesophageal hernia (H3), the esophagogastric junction is in the mediastinum; and with **type IV** paraesophageal hernia (H4), the entire stomach and other viscera are in the mediastinum.

Occult gastrointestinal bleeding from gastritis, ulceration in the herniated portion of the stomach, and gastric volvulus are the most common complications of paraesophageal hernia.

Acute gastric volvulus is a surgical emergency; it may manifest with a classic triad of pain, nausea with inability to vomit, and inability to accept passage of a nasogastric tube. There is a significant risk of serious complications and high mortality with paraesophageal hernias, even when asymptomatic; for this reason, repair is generally indicated when the condition is diagnosed. Although a pure paraesophageal hernia is not associated with GE reflux and theoretically should not require an antireflux procedure for its correction, a significant incidence of postoperative reflux has been observed after simple hernial reduction. This has been attributed to attentuation of tissues and the consequences of the dissection required for the reduction of large paraesophageal hernias. An antireflux procedure therefore is performed by many surgeons when the paraesophageal hernia is reduced, even if there is not an associated sliding component.

ANSWER: B, C, D, F

22. A 45-year-old man complains of dysphagia and regurgitation. The esophagram shows a narrow distal esophagus. Manometric studies demonstrate an absence of peristaltic waves and a lower esophageal sphincter (LES) that does not relax with swallowing. Which one or more of the following descriptions apply?

A. Bilateral vagal injury.
B. Weight loss.
C. Midbrain lesion.
D. LES relaxes with deglutition.
E. "Bird's beak."

Ref.: 1, 2, 4

COMMENTS: See Question 25.

23. Appropriate treatment for the patient described in Question 22 may include which one or more of the following?

A. Botulin neurotoxin.
B. Balloon dilatation.
C. Cervical esophagomyotomy.
D. Distal esophagomyotomy.
E. Esophagectomy.

Ref.: 1, 2, 4, 5

COMMENTS: See Question 25.

24. A 40-year-old woman complains of chest pain and dysphagia. An esophagram is normal. Manometric studies demonstrate simultaneous moderately high amplitude contractions with normal relaxation of the lower esophageal sphincter (LES). Which of the following applies?

A. Nutcracker esophagus.
B. Diffuse esophageal spasm.
C. "Vigorous" achalasia.
D. Scleroderma.
E. Coronary angiography.

Ref.: 1, 2, 3, 4, 5

COMMENTS: See Question 25.

25. What is the appropriate treatment for the patient described in Question 24 if medical measures fail?

A. Antispasmodics.
B. Balloon dilatation.
C. Cervical esophagomyotomy.
D. Thoracic esophagomyotomy.
E. Forceful dilatation.

Ref.: 1, 2, 3, 4, 5

COMMENTS: Esophageal motility disorders may be primary, or they may occur secondarily as the result of mechanical obstruction or various neuromuscular disorders. Ruling out mechanical problems such as tumor or stricture and accurate characterization of the type of motility disorder are mandatory before definitive therapy. Motility disorders often can be differentiated on the basis of the findings of esophagoscopy, esophagography, manometry, and 24-hour pH measurement.

In **achalasia**, the LES fails to relax, the inner circular muscle is greatly hypertrophied with interstitial fibrosis, and there is absence or degeneration of ganglia in Auerbach's plexus. Manometrically there is absence of peristaltic waves late in the disease and simultaneous contractions earlier. The HPZ shows normal pressure but no relaxation. The cause of achalasia is not known, but a similar condition is found in Chagas' disease and can be produced experimentally by causing midbrain lesions in cats and vagal nerve dysfunction in dogs. An esophagram may demonstrate esophageal dilatation and a typical "bird's beak" narrowing of the distal esophagus. Clinically, patients experience dysphagia, regurgitation, and weight loss. Although the problem may occur at any age, it is most commonly diagnosed in patients between 30 and 50 years of age and is somewhat more common in men. Diagnostic tests should exclude cardiac disease, but angiography is seldom indicated. Therapy is focused on destruction of the muscular apparatus of the hypertonic and hypertrophic lower esophageal segment. This can be effectively accomplished in about 60% of patients by *forceful dilatation* with hydrostatic or pneumatic balloons and in 90% of patients with surgical *myotomy* of the lower thoracic esophagus. Operative treatment is essentially more effective and carries a lower risk of perforation. The extent to which the myotomy should be carried down onto the stomach and the need for concomitant performance of an antireflux procedure are controversial features about the surgical management of achalasia, but most surgeons perform complete myotomy with a loose or partial (Dor, Toupet) wrap. Recently, minimal access myotomy is performed through the transabdominal or transthoracic approach with good results. *Botulin neurotoxin* injected into the LES through flexible endoscopy inhibits neural release of acetylcholine and has a favorable effect in patients with achalasia, but effects are usually temporary and injection may make operative dissection more difficult.

Diffuse esophageal spasm (DES) manifests with chest pain and dysphagia. The etiology is unclear, although in many patients it is associated with emotional factors and functional gastrointestinal disorders. Manometric studies demonstrate repetitive simultaneous high-amplitude contractions, although peristalsis may be observed in the upper, striated portion of the esophagus. In contrast to achalasia, the LES usually has a normal relaxation response; manometric findings may be intermittent, obscuring the diagnosis. The esophagram frequently is normal, although the classic "corkscrew" esophagus is occasionally demonstrated. Surgical treatment for diffuse esophageal spasm is less satisfactory than that for achalasia. For this reason, medical management with antispasmodics, dietary modulation, and psychiatric counseling constitute the initial therapeutic management. When surgical therapy is necessary, an extended thoracic esophagomyotomy is indicated.

Nutcracker esophagus is a motor abnormality characterized by chest pain and extremely high amplitude peristaltic waves up to 400 mm Hg. Twenty-four hour manometry is important for identifying a subgroup with a manometric pattern of DES. These patients, similar to those with DES and dysphagia, can obtain relief from a long myotomy. Esophagectomy is occasionally indicated for patients with advanced esophageal dilatation because of motility disorders of any type.

Variants of achalasia and diffuse esophageal spasm may be seen, and precise diagnosis is sometimes difficult. One example is so-called **vigorous achalasia**, in which the patient may present with symptoms of dysphagia, regurgitation, and chest pain. Manometric findings are suggestive of diffuse spasm and abnormal relaxation of the LES.

A note of caution: in any patient with a suspected esophageal motility disorder, organic obstruction and particularly carcinoma must be carefully ruled out.

Scleroderma is a collagen vascular disease resulting in fibrous replacement of the esophageal smooth muscle with secondary lack of peristalsis of the distal esophagus. There is also a loss of the HPZ leading to reflux, ulceration, and shortening of the esophagus. If standard medical therapy fails, an antireflux operation with a partial wrap is performed. If there is a short esophagus, a Collis gastroplasty with a partial wrap is undertaken.

ANSWER:
Question 22: A, B, C, E
Question 23: A, B, D
Question 24: B
Question 25: D

26. Which of the following are prerequisites for a successful result after cricopharyngeal myotomy?

A. Adequate function of cranial nerves 5, 7, 10, 11, 12, and 1st, 2nd, and 3rd cervical roots.
B. Occlusion of the nasopharynx by the soft palate.
C. Adequate HPZ.
D. Absence of Zenker's diverticulum.
E. Presence of upper esophageal web.

Ref.: 1, 2, 5

COMMENTS: See Question 28.

27. With regard to Zenker's diverticulum, which of the following statements is/are true?

A. Severity of symptoms is not determined primarily by the size of the diverticulum.
B. Diagnosis is best established endoscopically.
C. Cricopharyngeal myotomy alone without diverticulectomy is adequate treatment for small diverticula.
D. Diverticulopexy is adequate in poor risk patients with large diverticuli.
E. Endoscopic excision is the preferred method.

Ref.: 1, 2, 5

COMMENTS: See Question 28.

28. Cricopharyngeal myotomy may be an appropriate treatment for which one or more of the following conditions?

A. Plummer-Vinson syndrome.
B. Incomplete relaxation of the cricopharyngeal muscle.
C. Cerebrovascular accident (CVA) with involvement of nerves 5, 7, 10, and 11.
D. Decreased compliance of hypopharyngeal muscle.

Ref.: 1, 2, 5

COMMENTS: The transfer of food and liquid from the mouth into the upper esophagus is a complicated process and requires proper function of the tongue, pharynx, larynx, epiglottis, and soft palate. For instance, occlusion of the nasopharynx by the soft palate prevents nasal regurgitation of oral contents. The upper esophageal sphincter in turn must relax properly to allow food to be transferred into the esophagus. The function of the cricopharyngeal muscle is believed to prevent air from entering the esophagus during breathing and swallowing.

Symptoms of cervical dysphagia may be manifestations of neurologic, muscular, or mechanical disorders affecting the pharyngoesophageal region. Proper evaluation of swallowing begins with a thorough neurologic evaluation, and pharyngoesophagography and cervical manometry may be required. The presence of a Zenker's diverticulum is best established radiographically. Cranial nerves 5, 7, 10, 11, 12, and 1st, 2nd, and 3rd cervical roots must be intact. If there is a question of gastrointestinal reflux, 24-hour pH monitoring is required; and if reflux is found, cricopharyngotomy is not advised. Endoscopy and biopsy may be indicated when mucosal damage is suspected.

Cricopharyngeal myotomy has been used widely with variable success, often because of inadequate evaluation and improper diagnosis. A good result can be expected in the surgical therapy of cervical dysphagia when performed for the following conditions: (1) presence of Zenker's diverticulum; (2) incomplete relaxation or discoordinated cricopharyngeal relaxation; (3) poor pharyngeal contraction resulting from a CVA that reduces the ability to transverse the bolus against the cricopharyngeal pressure; and (4) manometrically recorded hypopharyngeal "shoulder pressure" with normal relaxation resulting from decreased compliance because of restrictive myopathy.

The cause of **Zenker's** diverticulum is not clear. Manometric findings often are normal but may demonstrate incoordination, failure of relaxation, or restrictive myopathy. The severity of symptoms is not determined primarily by the size of the diverticulum, except in patients whose diverticulum is completely dependent and obstructs the esophagus. Cricopharyngeal myotomy alone abolishes symptoms in most patients with Zenker's diverticulum (except in those with a large diverticulum), and so removal of the diverticulum is not necessary in most patients. If the diverticulum persists, excision is recommended in stable patients; in poor risk patients, a diverticulopexy in an upside-down position on the prevertebral fascia can be performed. Cricopharyngeal myotomy is easily performed even with the use of local anesthesia.

Cervical dysphagia also occurs in patients with **sideropenic dysphagia** (Plummer-Vinson or Paterson-Kelly syndrome) in which the mechanism is usually an upper esophageal web related to a nutritional deficiency. The treatment consists of esophageal dilatation and nutritional supplementation.

Esophageal motility problems can occur with **scleroderma** and other collagen vascular diseases, which may present as cervical dysphagia. The primary disturbance, however, is not specific to the cricopharyngeal region and generally involves motility disturbances of the distal esophagus and incompetence of the gastroesophageal sphincter.

ANSWER:
Question 26: A, B, C
Question 27: A, C, D
Question 28: B, D

29. Match each characteristic in the left column with the appropriate type or types of esophageal diverticula in the right column.

A. Acquired
B. Muscular wall
C. Esophagobronchial fistula
D. Treatment usually nonoperative
E. Killian's triangle
F. Tuberculosis

a. Zenker's
b. Traction
c. Epiphrenic
d. None of the above

Ref.: 1, 2

COMMENTS: Diverticula can occur at any level of the alimentary tract. They can be considered *true* diverticula when they contain a complete wall of mucosa, submucosa, and muscle. They can also be considered *false* diverticula, which lack a muscular layer.

Diverticula can further be categorized as *acquired* or *congenital*. In the esophagus, most herniations are acquired defects.

The pharyngoesophageal (**Zenker's**) and **epiphrenic** outpouchings lack a muscular layer, referred to as *false* diverticula. They result from functional or mechanical obstruction. The pharyngoesophageal diverticulum lies posteriorly, and all other diverticula usually lie laterally. Zenker's diverticula form in Killian's triangle, a point posteriorly where there is a divergence of direction of the thyropharyngeus and cricopharyngeal muscles. **Traction** diverticula generally are located in the midesophagus and represent a small area of distortion that involves the entire muscular wall of the esophagus. Referred to as *true* diverticula, they are caused by inflammation in adjacent mediastinal lymph nodes and are usually a result of granulomatous disease or tuberculosis. Traction and epiphrenic diverticula usually are inconsequential; operation is occasionally necessary for a large epiphrenic diverticulum or for a traction diverticulum complicated by perforation or an esophagorespiratory fistula.

ANSWER: A-a,b,c; B-b; C-b; D-b,c; E-a; F-b

30. A 50-year-old healthy conventioneer is brought to the emergency room with retching followed by hematemesis.

A. Treatment is by balloon tamponade.
B. Bleeding often stops spontaneously.
C. It is caused by forceful vomiting.
D. There is air in the mediastinum.
E. Diagnosis is made by endoscopy.

Ref.: 1, 2

COMMENTS: In 1929 Mallory and Weiss described four cases of gastric bleeding that followed repeated emesis and in which there were linear tears in the esophagogastric mucosa. The mechanism is similar to that of the Boerhaave syndrome (postemetic esophageal rupture) in which there is associated perforation and vomiting against a closed cardia. It is diagnosed by endoscopy, and the bleeding usually stops spontaneously. Because the bleeding is arterial, a pressure tamponade does not help and may in fact lead to esophageal disruption. If bleeding does not stop, gastrotomy and oversewing of the bleeding point is the proper therapy, although various nonsurgical alternatives, such as endoscopic injection of epinephrine and cautery, have been attempted.

ANSWER: B, C, E

31. A smooth filling defect, 3 cm in its greatest dimension, is found in the middle third of the esophagus. Which of the following procedures is/are correct?

A. Perform endoscopy and obtain a biopsy specimen of the lesion.
B. Usually presents with hematemesis.
C. Excise lesion by enucleation.
D. Composed of spindle cells.

Ref.: 1, 2, 4

COMMENTS: Benign esophageal tumors are far less common than malignant neoplasms. Often they are completely asymptomatic but may cause dysphagia and pain. **Leiomyomas** are the most common benign esophageal lesions and are usually found in the lower two-thirds of the esophagus composed of smooth muscle; they are extramucosal lesions that produce a characteristic smooth defect with intact mucosa on radiographic studies. In contrast to those located in the stomach, they rarely bleed. Treatment consists of simple enucleation. Endoscopy is indicated, but biopsy should not be performed because the secondary scarring hinders proper enucleation of the leiomyoma.

ANSWER: C, D

32. With regard to epidermoid cancer of the esophagus, which of the following statements is/are true?

A. Increased incidence among African-American men.
B. Increased incidence in American women.
C. Domestic chickens in Linxian, China, have exhibited the same increased incidence of epidermoid cell cancer as their owners.
D. Tylosis is associated with a decrease in epidermoid cell cancer.
E. Increased incidence in nitrosoamine exposure.

Ref.: 1, 2, 4

COMMENTS: See Question 33.

33. Which of the following factors is/are associated with adenocarcinoma of the esophagus?

A. Achalasia.
B. Barrett's esophagus.
C. Corrosive stricture.
D. Ectopic gastric mucosa.
E. Upper esophageal web.

Ref.: 1, 2, 4, 7

COMMENTS: The incidence of **epidermoid cell cancer** of the esophagus varies widely throughout the world, and for men varies from 6/100,000 to more than 140/100,000 in some areas of Asia, South Africa, and the former USSR. In the United States the highest incidence is among African-American men at approximately 12/100,000. In Western countries a high risk area is the wine district of southern France (e.g., Bordeaux). Risk factors have been found to vary from region to region. In the United States and western Europe, tobacco and alcohol each have been found to be independent risk factors, and together they have a synergistic effect. In South Africa, tobacco is a more significant risk factor because the tobacco is chewed after it is smoked in pipes. In Linxian, China, domestic chickens sharing food and water with their owners have a cancer incidence of 175/100,000, whereas among humans the incidence is 142/100,000. Other risk factors are nitrosamines in Kenya and Asia, resulting from pickled vegetables and cured meats. There is an increased incidence of epidermoid cancer in individuals with achalasia, corrosive esophageal stricture, sideropenic dysphagia, tylosis, or celiac disease. Most malignant esophageal neoplasms are epidermoid carcinomas.

Adenocarcinoma may occur in the distal esophagus at the columnar–epithelial junction or in other columnar-lined areas of the esophagus, as observed with Barrett's esophagus or ectopic gastric mucosa. Adenocarcinoma in the distal esophagus may also be seen as an extension of a primary gastric neoplasm. The incidence of adenocarcinoma of the esophagus and gastric cardia has been increasing from 1976, in contrast to the steady incidence of epidermoid cancer. The increase among men ranges from 4% to 10% per year—more of an increase than for any other type of cancer. This phenomenon occurs disproportionately among white men and rarely among women. Risk factors have not been discovered, and the subject has not been studied well, but Barrett's esophagus is a possible risk factor.

ANSWER:
Question 32: A, C, E
Question 33: B, D

34. Select one or more of the following *true* statements about epidermoid esophageal cancer.

A. Presents with dysphagia and weight loss.
B. Diagnosis confirmed with barium esophagogram and endoscopic biopsy.
C. Lymph nodes usually not involved.
D. There is no submucosal spread.
E. Exploration is best determinant of resectability.

Ref.: 1, 2, 4

COMMENTS: See Question 37.

35. With regard to the use of the colon as an esophageal substitute after complete esophageal resection, which of the following statements is/are true?

A. Three anastomoses are required.
B. The colon resists peptic stricture.
C. The colon is the organ of choice in young patients with benign disease.
D. It functions best when placed substernally.
E. The blood supply and venous drainage depend on the marginal vessels.

Ref.: 1, 2, 4, 6

COMMENTS: See Question 37.

36. With regard to the use of the stomach as an esophageal substitute after total esophagectomy, which of the following statements is/are true?

A. The blood supply is derived from the fundal branch of the splenic artery.
B. It can usually be made to reach the cervical esophagus.
C. A narrow gastric tube is preferred.
D. A drainage procedure is always required.

Ref.: 1, 2, 4, 6

COMMENTS: See Question 37.

37. Select one or more of the following *true* statements. Esophagectomy for esophageal cancer is:

A. Contraindicated in the presence of liver metastasis.
B. Indicated for palliation only if endoscopic intubation is unsuccessful.
C. Seen to have improved results when preceded by chemotherapy and irradiation.
D. Potentially curative in about 20% of patients.

Ref.: 1, 2, 4

COMMENTS: Esophageal cancer is a disease with a dismal outlook. The most frequent symptoms of esophageal cancer are dysphagia and weight loss. Both of these symptoms occur late owing to the ability of the esophagus to accommodate. Any patient with dysphagia should undergo barium esophagography followed by upper endoscopy and biopsy. It is important to stage these patients because those with distal metastases (i.e., lung, liver, adrenals) are not usually considered candidates for esophagectomy, as their survival is less than 12 months. Local lymphadenopathy does not preclude resection. Transesophageal ultrasonography is extremely accurate for detecting depth of invasion and lymphadenopathy, but the computed tomography (CT) scan is the most often used test. Even though many cases have been judged unresectable on CT scan, at exploration the cancer was found to be resectable. Therefore exploration is the best method to judge resectability in patients with questionable CT findings. Bronchoscopy is mandatory in upper- and middle-third lesions to rule out tracheobronchial invasion. The extensive submucosal lymphatic network of the esophagus predisposes a patient to early involvement of mediastinal, supraclavicular, and abdominal lymph nodes. Hematogenous spread to lung and liver also occurs but less frequently. Furthermore, these tumors tend to be locally invasive, with involvement of adjacent mediastinal structures such as the tracheobronchial tree, recurrent laryngeal nerve, aorta, pericardium, and diaphragm. Submucosal extension proximally is common, which is an important point to remember when proximal surgical margins are obtained. Although operation for esophageal cancer is most often noncurative, many clinicians consider esophagectomy the best method of providing palliation. Reconstruction generally is performed by either pulling up the stomach or using a colon interposition.

There are a number of disadvantages associated with using the colon as an esophageal substitute: (1) the colon has the tenuous marginal vessels for blood supply and venous drainage; (2) bacteria are present; (3) three anastomoses are required; and (4) the operation is long. It is now believed that for advanced malignant disease the stomach is the substitute of choice and the colon should be used only when the stomach is not available. The colon, however, is the preferred substitute when resection is for benign disease of the esophagus (e.g., advanced achalasia and long-standing corrosive or peptic strictures) and for diseases with a favorable outlook (e.g., early cancer, benign tumors, and premalignant conditions). Many of these conditions are seen among young patients who are healthy and have a long life expectancy. It is advantageous in these patients to preserve gastric function. The colon is resistant to peptic stricture; and when it is anastomosed posteriorly in the stomach and with a partial wrap, reflux is avoided. The subcutaneous approach has the poorest functional result.

The stomach is considered the safest esophageal substitute because only one anastomosis is required. Its blood supply and drainage is abundant, because of the right gastroepiploic vessels, which send anastomotic branches to the lesser curvature through an abundant submucosal network. The vascular supply and venous drainage of the fundus especially depend on the plexus of the subcardial region. This information has changed the approach to preparing the fundus for cervical and pharyngeal anastomosis. It is best to preserve the subcardial plexus in this instance and not try to transect the stomach longitudinally to shape it as a tube (i.e., tubulation) as was formerly done on the assumption that it would improve vascularity. The best vascularity is maintained when the whole stomach is used, especially for pharyngogastric anastomosis. However, partial tubulation of the stomach may be necessary for cervical anastomosis to reduce the bulk of the stomach or to resect the cardia and lesser curvature to ensure margins and nodal removal in malignant disease. The requirement for an emptying procedure is controversial. Pyloric obstruction and postoperative gastric dilatation have been reported when an emptying procedure has not been performed. Pyloroplasty leads to shortening of the gastric tube; and the possible increased tension of the suture line may increase the risk of anastomotic disruption. For these reasons, pyloromyotomy may be performed, but conversion to pyloroplasty may be necessary when the duodenal mucosa is perforated. The trend is toward intraoperative finger dilatation or endoscopic postoperative balloon dilatation when delayed gastric emptying occurs. The mortality rate after esophagectomy is 2–5%.

Endoscopic intubation of unresectable obstructing esophageal cancers appears to be an attractive technique but has not been uniformly acceptable because of the complications of tube obstruction or dislodgement and because of esophageal perforation. Placing an esophageal tube, however, may be the preferred method of palliation for the difficult problem of malignant tracheoesophageal fistula. Use of the stomach or colon for retrosternal bypass of the obstructed esophagus is associated with a high morbidity rate and has not been proved superior to esophagectomy for palliation. For many patients unsuitable for surgery, irradiation provides palliation, as epidermoid cancer is radiosensitive. The University of Michigan group used chemotherapy and radiation prior to blunt esophagectomy with results better than those seen with surgery alone. Skinner and associates have demonstrated a similar experience.

ANSWER:
Question 34: A, B, E
Question 35: A, B, C, D, E
Question 36: B
Question 37: A, C, D

38. Match each surgical approach in the left column with one or more appropriate comments in the right column.

A. Ivor Lewis
B. Left thoraco-abdominal

a. Two separate incisions
b. Transect diaphragm
c. Inadvertent injury to azygos vein
d. Increased incidence of pulmonary complications
e. Poor exposure of upper esophagus
f. One incision

Ref.: 4, 6, 8

COMMENTS: See Question 39.

39. Complications of esophagectomy performed without thoracotomy for esophageal cancer include which one or more of the following?

A. Chylothorax.
B. Increased mortality from anastomotic leakage.
C. Increased incidence of GE reflux.
D. Increased blood loss.
E. Pneumothorax.

Ref.: 1, 2, 4, 9

COMMENTS: Standard approaches to the thoracic esophagus include a left thoracoabdominal incision, a combined abdominal incision and separate right thoracotomy, and most recently an esophagectomy without thoracotomy but with the use of abdominal and cervical incisions.

The **abdominal and right thoracic incision**, known as the Ivor Lewis procedure, was described by Ivor Lewis in 1946 in his Hunterian Lecture. It was intended primarily for middle esophageal lesions. The advantages of the Ivor Lewis approach are (1) excellent exposure of the entire esophagus with an improved opportunity to obtain clear margins; (2) ready accessibility to the azygos vein; and (3) the fact that the aortic arch is out of the way and protects the left pleural cavity. The **left thoracoabdominal approach** gained popularity because it afforded excellent exposure of the distal esophagus but poor exposure for the upper esophagus. This approach is associated with high morbidity and mortality as a result of transection of the costal margin and diaphragm, greater risk of injury to the azygos vein during the mobilization (because it is not seen clearly), and poor visualization of the upper esophagus.

The approach more recently popularized involves a **transhiatal blunt** resection of the thoracic esophagus from the abdomen with subsequent pullup of the stomach and an esophagogastric anastomosis in the neck. The "blunt," or transhiatal, approach for esophagectomy was conceived by Denk in 1913 (see Comments, Question 1) and popularized by M.B. Orringer in 1980. Such an approach violates the dictum of traditional cancer surgery that calls for a **radical en bloc resection** of the affected organ and regional lymph nodes in planes away from the tumor. Nonetheless, proponents of blunt esophagectomy argue that the avoidance of thoracotomy minimizes morbidity from the operation, leakage from the cervical anastomosis is far less catastrophic than an intrathoracic leakage, postoperative GE reflux is less common than with an intrathoracic anastomosis, the technique has not detrimentally affected survival, and finally much of the distal esophagectomy is performed under direct vision. Blunt esophagectomy, however, is not without complications: Pneumothorax is common; and serious injury to the trachea, recurrent laryngeal nerve, aorta, or thoracic duct can occur. Randomized prospective clinical trials comparing the blunt technique with standard radical esophagectomy have not been reported.

ANSWER:
Question 38: A-a; B-b,c,d,e,f
Question 39: A, E

40. A 4-year-old child is brought to the emergency room 15 minutes after ingesting drain cleaner. The child is hoarse and stridorous. Which of the following apply?

A. Laryngeal ulceration.
B. Instillation of vinegar in stomach.
C. Immediate fiberoptic endoscopy.
D. Tracheostomy.

Ref.: 1, 2, 4

COMMENTS: See Question 42.

41. With regard to the role of endoscopy in the acute therapy of a patient who has ingested a corrosive substance, which of the following statements is/are true?

A. It should be performed after 24 hours if the patient is stable.

B. It is contraindicated before esophagography because of the risk of perforation.
C. It is contraindicated if obvious oropharyngeal burns are present.
D. It is used to remove a button-type alkaline battery from the esophagus.
E. The full extent of the injury must be visualized to determine appropriate therapy.

Ref.: 1, 2, 4

COMMENTS: See Question 42.

42. Which of the following is/are indications for emergency surgical intervention for corrosive ingestion?

A. Cervical subcutaneous crepitance.
B. Presence of alkaline gastric contents.
C. Extensive damage to esophagus and stomach.
D. Scattered exudate in the esophagus, found on endoscopy.

Ref.: 1, 2, 4

COMMENTS: When caustic alkaline burns of the esophagus are suspected, the ingested agent should promptly be identified and the extent of injury assessed early. Superficial burns usually heal without complication, whereas deeper injury must be aggressively but judiciously treated to avoid late formation of stricture and yet not cause iatrogenic perforations. Early endoscopy is important for verifying the presence or absence of esophageal injury and for assessing its severity. It is critical that the endoscope not be advanced any farther than the proximal extent of injury to avoid perforation, and it is contraindicated when perforation is suspected. The distal extent of injury can be assessed radiographically at a later date when the patient is stable. Esophagoscopy is contraindicated in patients with evidence of perforation or potential airway obstruction.

Aggressive attempts to neutralize or dilute the corrosive agent are not helpful because the injury is instantaneous, and as little as 1 ml of lye has been known to cause extensive esophageal injury. Likewise, induced emesis and lavage also are contraindicated because they may aggravate the injury. Patients who swallow disk-shaped alkaline batteries should have them removed endoscopically if they are lodged in the esophagus.

The child described in Question 40 exhibits laryngeal or epiglottic edema, and preservation of the airway must be the priority of treatment. Endoscopy is therefore deferred, and tracheostomy may be required. When an esophageal burn is confirmed or when the presence of absence of an esophageal injury cannot be verified because of airway considerations, treatment consisting of the administration of antibiotics and steroids has been advocated, although there is no statistical evidence that steroids lessen early complications or late stricture formation. Early esophageal dilatation has been advocated by some clinicians, but this too has not been demonstrated to prevent later stricture formation; indeed, it may lead to iatrogenic injury. Silastic stents have been beneficial for avoiding strictures when left in 2–3 weeks. Steroids may be better avoided in patients with suspected perforation or acid ingestion; in such patients, the site of injury is more frequently the stomach, rather than the esophagus; and the addition of steroid therapy may increase the risk of hemorrhage or peptic ulceration.

In most cases, oral intake is allowed after several days when the edema of the initial injury has subsided and the patient can swallow effectively. Oral intake, in fact, provides a natural method of esophageal dilatation and may help prevent stricture formation. Radiographic studies at this time disclose the full extent of the injury. Swallowing usually is possible for 2–3 weeks, at which time stricturing may begin. At this time, radiographic studies are repeated to confirm the full anatomy, and dilatation is begun.

The presence or absence of oropharyngeal burns in a patient with suspected corrosive injection is not a reliable indicator of esophageal injury. In general, acids such as sulfuric acid and nitric acid cause coagulation injuries, whereas alkali substances cause liquefaction injury.

Emergency surgery after ingestion of corrosive substances may necessitate thoracotomy, laparotomy, or both. Indications for emergency *thoracotomy* are signs and symptoms of mediastinitis or perforation of the esophagus: severe chest pain, tachycardia, cervical subcutaneous crepitance, wide mediastinum, pneumomediastinum, pneumothorax, and pleural effusion. The only indication for radiopaque contrast studies of the esophagus or stomach at this time is a suspicion of perforation secondary to the burn or to instrumentation. Indications for *laparotomy* are signs of perforation, free abdominal air, interstitial air in the wall of the stomach, and radiologic confirmation of perforation. Laparotomy is also indicated if nasogastric intubation was erroneously performed, when there is advanced injury to the esophagus or stomach seen on endoscopy, or when nasogastric alkali contents from the stomach have been aspirated because once alkali contents have reached the stomach, direct visualization of the stomach is necessary to rule out full thickness liquifaction necrosis.

ANSWER:
Question 40: A, D
Question 41: D
Question 42: A, B, C

43. With regard to the late sequelae of ingestion of corrosive substances, which of the following statements is/are true?

A. Stricture is best treated by botulin neurotoxin injection.
B. Acid ingestion is complicated more commonly by gastric outlet obstruction than by esophageal stricture.
C. Tracheoesophageal fistula is best treated by leaving an excluded segment of esophagus attached.
D. Cancer that develops after corrosive injury carries a better prognosis than does esophageal cancer in general.

Ref.: 1, 2, 4

COMMENTS: Late complications of corrosive burns of the esophagus include stricture, GE reflux, malignancy, and rarely tracheoesophageal fistula. Strictures often are multiple and involve the cervical esophagus, the region of the aortic arch, and the cardia. Spasm of the cricopharyngeal muscle may entrap the corrosive agent in the pharynx, resulting in pharyngeal obstruction and often severe laryngeal injury, necessitating permanent tracheostomy. The standard treatment for stricture is esophageal dilatation, often performed in a retrograde manner through a gastrostomy. There is limited experience with treatment of localized strictures by direct injection of steroids. Refractory strictures may necessitate esophagectomy or a bypass operation. Direct approach to the repair of tracheoesophageal fistula should be avoided. It is best to leave a small segment of excluded esophagus attached to the fistula. For patients in whom severe GE reflux develops as the result of scarring and shortening of the esophagus and hiatus hernia, dilatation of the stricture may necessitate an associated antireflux operation.

Malignant degeneration is a well recognized complication of corrosive esophageal stricture and should be suspected in any patient with long-standing stricture who exhibits a change in symptoms. The prognosis of these cancers, however, has been more favorable than that of patients without this predisposing injury or with sporadic epidermoid cancer, and resection may provide cure. In contradistinction to alkaline ingestion, acid ingestion more commonly produces gastric injury. This is because the squamous epithelium of the esophagus is somewhat resistant to acid injury and because the pylorospasm that accompanies acid ingestion prolongs contact time with the stomach.

ANSWER: B, C, D

44. After diagnostic esophagoscopy, a patient complains of odynophagia and chest pain, but results of a water-soluble contrast swallow are negative. Which of the following apply?

A. Discharge if the electrocardiogram is normal.
B. Barium in the chest is devastating.
C. Esophageal manometry should be performed immediately.
D. Repeated swallow with barium.

Ref.: 1, 2, 4

COMMENTS: Chest pain, fever, tachycardia, subcutaneous emphysema, dysphagia, and dyspnea are typical of esophageal perforation. Perforation may result from iatrogenic operations (periesophageal endoscopy), external trauma, primary esophageal disease, or postemetic ("spontaneous") esophageal hypertension. The incidence of mortality from esophageal perforation is clearly related to the time interval between perforation and definitive treatment. Whenever perforation is suspected, a contrast study should be performed with water-soluble contrast material; but if this study does not demonstrate the perforation, it should be repeated with barium. Although barium is contraindicated in the presence of colonic injuries because of the harmful effects of feces and barium, it does not cause a problem in the chest. Barium is more accurate for delineating esophageal leakage. Contrast studies are important not only for verifying esophageal rupture but also for documenting the level of injury, which has important implications for treatment. Although endoscopy can be used in cases of suspected esophageal perforation and may enable retrieval of a foreign body, it is usually not required and is associated with the potential hazard of extending the perforation.

ANSWER: D

45. For each clinical situation described in the left column, choose the most appropriate treatment in the right column.

A. Septic patient with 48-hour-old perforation of the thoracic esophagus and pneumohydrothorax
B. Stable patient with fever, subcutaneous emphysema, and cervical perforation 2 hours after endoscopy
C. Patient with epidermolysis bullosa, minimal chest pain, and low-grade fever 2 days after endoscopy; esophagram shows thoracic perforation with limited mediastinal involvement
D. Patient with 6-hour-old stab wound, temperature of 102°F, left pleural effusion, and thoracic esophageal perforation
E. A 65-year-old patient with cancer of the esophagus, chest pain, and pneumohydrothorax 6 hours after endoscopy

a. Antibiotics, nothing orally, parenteral nutrition
b. Emergency esophagectomy
c. Pleural drainage, esophageal exclusion, gastrostomy, cervical esophagostomy
d. Primary transthoracic racic esophageal repair
e. Transcervical esophageal repair and drainage
f. Emergency esophagectomy and colon interposition

Ref.: 1, 2, 4

COMMENTS: Treatment of esophageal perforation depends on the site and extent of injury, the etiology, the presence or absence of underlying esophageal disease, the patient's general status, and importantly the time interval between perforation and diagnosis.

Cervical perforations usually can be managed with transcervical drainage; repair is desirable if technically possible.

Recognized early perforations of the *thoracic* esophagus can be managed successfully by primary esophageal repair, the principles of which include layered closure of the esophagus, buttressing of the repair, and thoracic drainage. The gastric fundus or pleural or pericardial flaps can be useful for buttressing the sutured closure and are important for decreasing postoperative leakage.

Among *septic patients with late perforations*, the mortality rate is high. These patients require aggressive control of the septic focus; attempts at primary repair are doomed to failure. Techniques of esophageal exclusion may be useful in this setting; some surgeons also favor esophagectomy. In patients with esophageal perforations and underlying esophageal disease, such as obstructing distal lesions, surgical management of the perforation includes definitive treatment of the underlying pathologic process. It may necessitate esophagectomy, for example, in patients with perforation and concomitant esophageal cancer.

There is a subset of patients who may be managed conservatively without operation. They include stable patients with perforations that are recognized late, patients with epidermolysis bullosa who often demonstrate asymptomatic limited perforations, those who are clinically stable and improving, those in whom perforation is radiographically limited without pleural extension, and those preferably with evidence of spontaneous drainage of the periesophageal cavity back into the esophagus.

ANSWER: A-c; B-e; C-a; D-d; E-b

REFERENCES

1. Sabiston DC Jr: *Textbook of Surgery*, 15th ed. WB Saunders, Philadelphia, 1997.
2. Schwartz SI, Shires GT, Spencer FC: *Principles of Surgery*, 7th ed. McGraw-Hill, New York, 1999.
3. Skinner DB: Pathophysiology of gastroesophageal reflux. *Ann Surg* 202:546–556, 1985.
4. Skinner DB, Belsey RHH: *Management of Esophageal Disease*. WB Saunders, Philadelphia, 1988.
5. Stein HJ, DeMeester TR, Hinder RA: Outpatient physiologic testing and surgical management of foregut motility disorders. *Curr Probl Surg* 24:413–555, 1992.
6. Rüedi TP: *State of the Art of Surgery 1991/92* [summaries of the Luncheon Panels, held at the 34th World Congress of Surgery of the International Society of Surgery, organized as International Surgical Week in Stockholm, 1991]. Schwabe, Basel, 1992.
7. Blot WJ, Devesa SS, Kneller RW, Fraumeni JF Jr: Rising incidence of adenocarcinoma of the esophagus and gastric cardia. *JAMA* 265: 1287–1289, 1991.
8. Weiss GD, Read RC: The Ivor Lewis procedure. *Surg Rounds* 7: 41–48, 1984.
9. Orringer MB: Transhiatal esophagectomy without thoracotomy for carcinoma of the thoracic esophagus. *Ann Surg* 200:282–288, 1984.

CHAPTER 27

Stomach and Duodenum

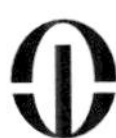

1. With regard to the blood supply of the stomach, which of the following statements is/are true?

A. The right gastric artery arises from the common hepatic artery and constitutes the major vascular supply to the antrum.
B. The left gastric artery often originates anomalously from the superior mesenteric artery.
C. The gastroepiploic arcade arises from both the gastroduodenal and splenic arteries.
D. Ligation of the splenic artery results in necrosis of the greater curvature of the stomach.

Ref.: 1, 2, 3

COMMENTS: The arterial blood supply of the stomach is derived primarily from the celiac trunk, which gives off the hepatic, left gastric, and splenic arteries. The **left gastric artery** usually arises directly from the celiac trunk and is found at the proximal lesser curvature, where it divides into ascending and descending branches. An anatomic variation of surgical significance is origination of a left hepatic artery from the left gastric artery. The **right gastric artery** typically originates from the common hepatic artery distal to the gastroduodenal artery. This vessel contributes to the pyloroduodenal blood supply and does not generally anastomose widely with the left gastric artery, as is sometimes pictured. The **right gastroepiploic artery** usually comes from the gastroduodenal artery (occasionally from the superior mesenteric artery), whereas the left gastroepiploic artery arises from the splenic artery. The extent of connection between the right and left gastroepiploic vessels is variable. The **vasa brevia**, or **short gastric arteries**, arise from the branches of the splenic or left gastroepiploic artery. Because of the abundant collateral blood supply present the stomach is well protected from ischemia and can survive with ligation of all but one of its major vessels. The splenic artery may also contribute a branch to the posterior fundus, referred to as the **posterior gastric artery**.

ANSWER: C

2. When the stomach is mobilized for esophageal replacement, the arterial supply is primarily based on which of the following vessels?

A. Left gastric artery.
B. Right gastric artery.
C. Left gastroepiploic artery.
D. Right gastroepiploic artery.
E. Superior mesenteric artery.

Ref.: 1, 2, 3

COMMENTS: The left gastric artery arising from the celiac trunk and the short gastric vessels arising from branches of the splenic artery are routinely divided when the stomach is mobilized for esophageal replacement. The main blood supply of the gastric interposition is derived from the right gastroepiploic artery. The gastroduodenal artery from which the right gastroepiploic vessel originates must therefore be preserved during dissection. Under usual circumstances, the right gastric artery and the superior mesenteric artery contribute a less significant proportion of the blood supply to the mobilized stomach.

ANSWER: D

3. Match each item in the left column with the appropriate vagal innervation-related item in the right column.

A. Right thoracic vagus	a. Anterior abdominal vagus
B. Left thoracic vagus	b. Posterior abdominal vagus
C. Sympathetic innervation	c. Both
D. Hepatic vagal branch	d. Neither
E. Celiac vagal branch	
F. Nerve of Latarget	
G. "Crow's foot"	
H. Criminal nerve of Grassi	

Ref.: 1, 2, 3, 4

COMMENTS: Parasympathetic innervation of the foregut and midgut is supplied by the vagus nerves (sacral parasympathetic nerves supply the hindgut). Sympathetic innervation of the stomach travels via the splanchnic nerves (preganglionic) and fibers along branches of the celiac artery (postganglionic). In the thorax, vagal trunks are right and left of the esophagus. As the result of embryonic gastric rotation, the vagal trunks assume anterior (left vagus) and posterior (right vagus) positions at the level of the cardia. The anterior vagus divides into anterior gastric (anterior nerve of Latarget) and hepatic branches. A separate pyloric nerve (nerve of McCrea) may arise from the anterior vagus or its hepatic branch. The posterior vagus divides into posterior gastric (posterior nerve of Latarget) and celiac branches. The "crow's foot" refers to the distal branches of the gastric vagal divisions in the pyloroantral region where the nerves of Latarget terminate. The term was first used in reference to the distal branches of the descending left gastric artery. The vagal branches to the proximal fundus do not originate from a constant level, and if they are missed incomplete vagotomy can result. Indeed, a simple anterior vagus nerve is present in only 60% of patients and a simple posterior one in 40%. One of those proximal branches, originating from the posterior vagal innervation, is known as the criminal nerve of Grassi. Selective vagotomy divides the nerves of Latarget below the hepatic and celiac branches; highly selective vagotomy divides individual branches of the nerve of Latarget, preserving the "crow's foot."

ANSWER: A-b; B-a; C-d; D-a; E-b; F-c; G-c; H-b

4. Match each cell type in the left column with the appropriate secretory product or products in the right column.

A. Parietal cell
B. Chief cell
C. G-cell
D. Brunner's gland
E. Neck cells

a. Intrinsic factor
b. Gastrin
c. Pepsinogen
d. Hydrochloric acid
e. Mucus

Ref.: 1, 2, 3, 5

COMMENTS: See Question 5.

5. Match the cell types with their primary anatomic location.

A. Parietal cell
B. Chief cell
C. G-cell
D. Brunner's gland
E. Delta cell

a. Gastric cardia
b. Gastric corpus and fundus
c. Gastric antrum
d. Duodenum

Ref.: 1, 2, 3, 5

COMMENTS: The gastric mucosa consists of surface columnar epithelial cells and glands containing various cell types. The mucosal cells have different specific secretory functions and anatomic distributions. These relations constitute the physiologic foundation on which surgical management of peptic ulcer disease is based. **Parietal cells** (which produce hydrochloric acid and intrinsic factor) and **chief cells** (which produce pepsinogens) are located predominantly in the fundus and corpus. The **G-cells** of the antrum are the primary source of gastrin. The duodenum in humans contains 10–20% as much gastrin as does the antrum, and it appears to be physiologically active. Mucus, for lubrication, is secreted by gastric surface epithelial cells, neck cells of the gastric glands, and **Brunner's glands**. Brunner's glands are found in the submucosa of the proximal duodenum and are also a source of pepsinogens. Somatostatin presumably is synthesized and stored by the **delta (antral) cells**. Other mediators, such as serotonin and prostaglandins, are also produced in the stomach. Subtotal gastrectomy removes a large portion of the acid-secreting parietal cell mass. Antrectomy removes the main source of acid-stimulating gastrin. The effectiveness of highly selective vagotomy is based on denervation of the parietal cell mass. After resections of the corpus and fundus, periodic injections of vitamin B_{12} are required to prevent a deficiency caused by lack of intrinsic factor.

ANSWER:
Question 4: A-a,d; B-c; C-b; D-c,e; E-e
Question 5: A-b; B-b; C-c,d; D-d; E-c

6. The oxyntic portion of the stomach consists of which anatomic area(s)?

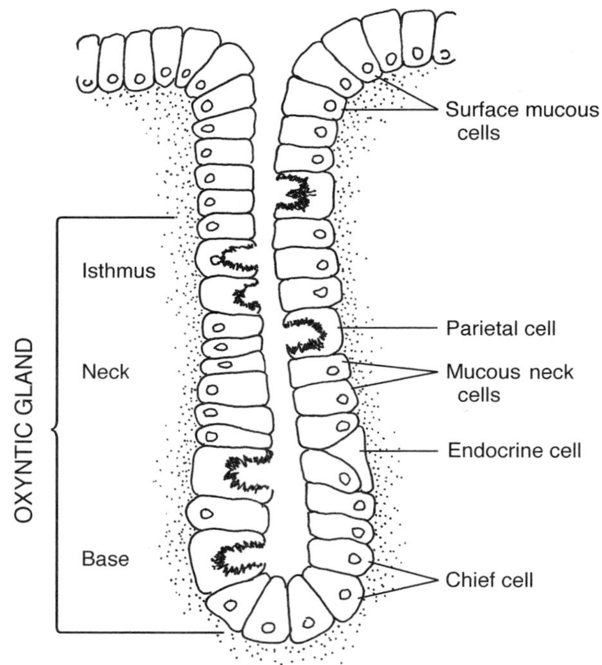

A. Cardia.
B. Fundus.
C. Corpus.
D. Antrum.
E. Pylorus.

Ref.: 3, 5

COMMENTS: The oxyntic portion of the stomach contains the oxyntic, or parietal, glands, which are the acid-producing glands. The oxyntic glands, as illustrated, have a characteristic histologic arrangement and contain surface mucous cells and mucous neck cells near the top, scattered parietal cells and enteroendocrine cells, and chief cells at the bottom. The oxyntic glands occupy the gastric fundus and corpus. The gastric cardia is the area just distal to the gastroesophageal (GE) junction, and the fundus is above and to the left of the GE junction. The border between the corpus and more distal antrum is more distinct histologically than grossly. The pylorus can readily be identified by its thick muscular ring.

ANSWER: B, C

7. What parietal cell receptors stimulate acid secretion?

A. Histamine.
B. Gastrin.
C. Acetylcholine.
D. Prostaglandin E_2.
E. Somatostatin.

Ref.: 1, 3, 5

COMMENTS: See Question 8.

8. The final common pathway of acid secretion by parietal cells involves which one of the following?

A. Adenylate cyclase.
B. H^+-K^+-ATPase.
C. Increased intracellular Ca^{2+}.
D. Protein kinase.

E. Phosphorylase kinase.

Ref.: 1, 3, 5

COMMENTS: Understanding the cellular basis for parietal cell acid secretion is important to appreciate the pharmacologic control of acid in clinical practice. The parietal cell has three specific plasma membrane receptors that stimulate acid: histamine, acetylcholine, and gastrin receptors. These three receptors eventually activate a common proton pump, H^+-K^+-ATPase, resulting in an exchange of hydrogen ions for potassium. The mechanisms and second messenger systems by which this occurs are different for different secretogues. Histamine activates adenylate cyclase and subsequently a protein kinase that leads to protein phosphorylation and H^+-K^+-ATPase activation. Gastrin- and acetylcholine-stimulated secretion depends on specific membrane phospholipases plus increases in intracellular calcium with subsequent phosphorylase kinase-induced protein phosphorylation and H^+-K^+-ATPase activity. Parietal cells also have somatostatin and prostaglandin receptors that inhibit acid secretion. Pharmacologic agents act at different sites during this process.

ANSWER:
Question 7: A, B, C
Question 8: B

9. Gastric acid secretion is stimulated by all of the following *except*?

A. Acetylcholine.
B. Duodenal gastrin.
C. Intraluminal protein.
D. Secretin.
E. Gastric distension.

Ref.: 1, 2, 3, 5

COMMENTS: There are cephalic, gastric, and intestinal phases of gastric acid secretion. As previously mentioned, the parietal cell has receptors for acetylcholine, gastrin, and histamine that stimulate acid secretion. The **cephalic phase** is primarily mediated by the vagus nerve but also by neuropeptides. Vagal cholinergic stimulation directly releases acid from parietal cells in addition to releasing gastrin from the antrum. The **gastric phase** is mediated by gastrin released in response to gastric distension, peptides, and amino acids. Although the antrum is the predominant source of gastrin, secretion from the duodenal mucosa also occurs, accounting for part of the **intestinal phase** of gastric acid secretion. An intestinal hormone, enterooxyntin, has also been implicated as a stimulant of gastric acid secretion during the intestinal phase, but this entity has not been specifically characterized. Duodenal acidification releases secretin, which blocks gastrin receptors on the parietal cell without affecting histamine or acetylcholine sites. Antral acidification releases somatostatin, which inhibits acid and gastrin release. Cholecystokinin and enterogastrones also inhibit acid secretion.

ANSWER: D

10. Match the intestinal peptide hormone in the left column to its function in the right column.

A. Cholecystokinin
B. Gastric inhibitory peptide
C. Motilin
D. Somatostatin
E. Bombesin
F. Vasoactive intestinal peptide

a. Stimulates gastric acid secretion
b. Stimulates intestinal secretion and motility
c. Inhibits release of gastrin
d. Regulates phase III interdigestive migrating motor complex
e. Inhibits gastric acid secretion and potentiates insulin secretion
f. Stimulates pancreatic exocrine secretion

Ref.: 1, 2, 3

COMMENTS: The gastrointestinal (GI) mucosa is rich in endocrine cells that produce single-chained polypeptides to act as hormones and neurotransmitters. These peptides act in a complex interplay to control GI tract secretion, motility, and absorption and gut growth. **Cholecystokinin** is produced in the I-cells of the duodenum and upper jejunum. Amino acids and fatty acids in the upper intestine stimulate its release. The main actions in the GI tract are the stimulation of pancreatic exocrine secretion and gallbladder contraction. It has two known receptors. **Gastric inhibitory peptide (GIP)** is found in K-cells of the duodenum and jejunum and is released in response to ingested nutrients. Inhibition of gastric acid secretion and potentiation of glucose-induced insulin release are its two main actions. Motilin is secreted by M-cells in the duodenum, jejunum, and upper ileum. It regulates the activity front (phase III) of the interdigestive migrating motor complex. **Somatostatin** is found in greatest concentration in the GI tract in pancreatic islet D-cells and in the gastric antrum. It has a wide range of inhibitory actions on the release of insulin, glucagon, gastrin, secretin, GIP, motilin, neurotensin, and enteroglucagon. The result of somatostatin release is inhibition of gastric emptying, pancreatic endocrine and exocrine secretion, and gallbladder contraction. **Bombesin**, or gastric releasing peptide, is found throughout the enteric and central nervous systems. It has stimulating effects on intestinal motor activity, pancreatic enzyme secretion, and gastric acid secretion. **Vasoactive intestinal peptide (VIP)** is mainly a neurotransmitter in the enteric nervous system. It is a strong stimulus for intestinal secretion and motility.

ANSWER: A-f; B-e; C-d; D-c; E-a, f; F-b

11. With regard to normal gastric emptying, which of the following statements is/are true?

A. Emptying of solids is dependent on fundal tone.
B. The rate of emptying of solids is linear.
C. Emptying of liquids is dependent on antral propulsion.
D. Rate of emptying of liquids is exponential.
E. Patterns of emptying of solids and liquids are similar.

Ref.: 1, 3, 5

COMMENTS: Gastric emptying, regulated by changes in gastric motor activity, is a complicated process influenced by meal composition and by neural and hormonal factors. Emptying of solids is different from emptying of liquids. Emptying of solids depends on mechanical action of the pyloroantral region; propulsive and retropulsive activity breaks solids into small particles that become mixed with the liquid gastric contents. The pattern of emptying of solids is linear after an initial lag period. Gastric emptying of liquids depends primarily on the pressure gradient between the proximal stomach and the pylorus and is largely determined by fundal tone. The pattern of emptying of liquids is exponential, and the rate is determined by the volume of gastric contents.

ANSWER: B, D

12. Which of the following clinical conditions is/are associated with rapid gastric emptying?

A. Hyperglycemia.
B. Hypokalemia.
C. Scleroderma.
D. Gastric resection.
E. Zollinger-Ellison syndrome.

Ref.: 1, 3, 5

COMMENTS: Abnormalities in gastric emptying can produce significant and disabling clinical situations. Most clinically significant problems of gastric motility are related to delayed gastric emptying. Other than mechanical obstruction, important causes of delayed gastric emptying include drugs (opiates, anticholinergics), electrolyte imbalances (hypokalemia, hypocalcemia), metabolic derangements (myxedema, hyperglycemia), and systemic diseases (diabetes mellitus, scleroderma). Disorders of rapid gastric emptying are encountered less frequently and are most commonly a consequence of previous gastric surgery, such as resection. Other situations associated with rapid gastric emptying include Zollinger-Ellison syndrome, caused by hypergastrinemia and lack of inhibition by duodenal acidification, and conditions producing steatorrhea caused by loss of inhibition of gastric emptying from impaired fat absorption (pancreatic insufficiency, short bowel syndrome, gluten enteropathy). Duodenal ulcer may be associated with normal or rapid gastric emptying.

ANSWER: D, E

13. Gastric emptying of solids is best assessed by which one of the following tests?

A. Saline load test.
B. Serial intubation and aspiration of test meal.
C. Technetium 99m pertechnetate (^{99m}Tc)-labeling radionuclide scintigraphy.
D. Indium 111 (^{111}In)-labeling radionuclide scintigraphy.
E. Barium burger upper gastrointestinal series.

Ref.: 1, 3, 5

COMMENTS: Gastric emptying of solids is most accurately assessed by radionuclide scans after ingestion of ^{99m}Tc-labeled chicken liver or egg white. The isotope remains bound to the solid phase, and computer quantification of emptying is possible by analysis of appropriately selected windows through use of the geometric mean of the anterior and posterior counts. The radioisotope ^{111}In remains in the liquid phase of gastric contents and is thus a marker for assessment of liquid emptying. Traditional radiographic contrast studies provide only a rough qualitative assessment of gastric emptying; barium may empty with the liquid phase, and labeling of ingested solids is not an accurate method for determining solid emptying. The saline load test (whereby 750 ml of saline is instilled into the stomach and the residual volume is aspirated 30 minutes later) and other intubation tests involving nonabsorbable markers are inconvenient, less sensitive, and limited to assessment of liquid emptying.

ANSWER: C

14. With regard to postoperative effects on gastric emptying, which of the following statements is/are true?

A. Truncal vagotomy delays emptying of liquids.
B. Truncal vagotomy accelerates emptying of solids.
C. Parietal cell vagotomy does not affect gastric emptying.
D. Pyloroplasty accelerates emptying of solids.
E. Roux-en-Y gastrojejunostomy delays gastric emptying.

Ref.: 1, 3, 5

COMMENTS: Changes in gastric emptying result from operative procedures on the stomach. These changes occasionally produce clinically significant problems, ranging from delayed emptying to the dumping syndrome. Resective procedures with Billroth I or Billroth II reconstruction are usually accompanied by more rapid emptying. Reconstruction by Roux-en-Y gastrojejunostomy, on the other hand, can result in impaired emptying of the gastric remnant and the Roux limb of the jejunum, perhaps in relation to interruption of neural impulses from the duodenal pacemaker. Vagal denervation of the proximal stomach accelerates emptying of liquids as a result of the loss of receptive relaxation and accommodation. Parietal cell vagotomy is therefore associated with increased emptying of liquids but normal emptying of solids. Complete gastric vagotomy, in the form of truncal vagotomy or selective vagotomy, also delays emptying of solids. The addition of a pyloroplasty initially increases the rate of emptying of solids; later, emptying may be delayed or remain rapid. The pattern of emptying of solids after various types of vagal denervation often normalizes over time.

ANSWER: D, E

15. Gastric infection with *Helicobacter pylori* has been associated with all of the following conditions *except*?

A. Duodenal ulcer.
B. Gastric ulcer.
C. Chronic gastritis.
D. Gastric cancer.
E. Eosinophilic gastroenteritis.

Ref.: 1, 3

COMMENTS: *Helicobacter pylori* (formerly *Campylobacter pylori*) is a gram-negative microaerophilic spiral bacterium that chronically infects the gastroduodenal mucosa in a high percentage of patients with gastroduodenal disorders. Investigators have demonstrated *H. pylori* infection in most patients with antral gastritis, duodenal ulcer, and gastric ulcer. Infection may play an etiologic role in these conditions, inasmuch as treatment of *H. pylori* has resulted in healing of gastritis, more rapid healing of duodenal ulcers, and significantly lower recurrence rates for both duodenal and gastric ulcers. In addition, *H. pylori* has been associated with chronic atrophic gastritis, which in turn is associated with gastric cancer. *H. pylori* infection may be a cofactor in gastric carcinogenesis. Colloidal bismuth subcitrate in combination with one or two antibiotics has proved effective in eradicating *H. pylori* infection. Gastric cancers below the cardia are approximately three times more common in patients with *H. pylori* infection than in noninfected controls. Eosinophilic gastroenteritis is an unusual infiltrative disorder typically affecting the gastric antrum; its etiology is unknown.

ANSWER: E

16. Which of the following tests is/are *not* appropriate for the detection of *H. pylori* in dyspeptic patients?

A. Urea breath test.
B. Rapid urease test of mucosal biopsy.
C. Culture and sensitivity of mucosal biopsy.
D. Histologic evaluation of mucosal biopsy.
E. Serologic assay for *H. pylori* antibodies.

Ref.: 6

COMMENTS: Because of the important role *H. pylori* has assumed in the etiology of peptic ulcer disease, it is important to document the presence or absence of the organism to optimally treat dyspeptic patients. Several methods have been developed to detect host colonization with *H. pylori*, but there continues to be debate on the optimal detection strategy. The rapid urease test (RUT) on mucosal biopsies utilizes a change in pH resulting from the breakdown of urea in culture media caused by a urease enzyme in the bacteria. It is probably the test of choice because of its accuracy, low cost, simplicity, and rapid availability of results. Histology is the gold standard and should always be performed when endoscopic biopsy specimens are obtained to confirm RUT results and assess the integrity of the gastric mucosa. Cultures with sensitivities should also be obtained from the biopsy specimen at the same procedure. Urea breath tests are reported to be 90–100% sensitive and are indicated when endoscopy is not performed. Serologic tests for the presence of antibodies to the organism have been questioned for all but epidemiologic purposes. Polymerase chain reaction methods to detect the organism in biopsy specimens are also available and highly accurate but expensive. At present the optimal strategy to detect *H. pylori* in dyspeptic patients should employ at least two of the above methods utilizing random biopsies from the antrum and corpus of the stomach.

ANSWER: E

17. Gastric secretion tests in an unoperated patient demonstrate a basal acid output (BAO) of 2 mmol/hr and a peak acid output (PAO) of 25 mmol/hr. These findings are most consistent with which of the following conditions?

A. Duodenal ulcer.
B. Zollinger-Ellison syndrome.
C. Normal acid secretion.
D. Pernicious anemia.
E. Antral G-cell hyperplasia.

Ref.: 4

COMMENTS: Normal mean BAO is about 2 mmol/hr (range 0 to >5 mmol/hr); and the normal mean PAO is 20–35 mmol/hr (range <1 to 60 mmol/hr). Patients with duodenal ulcer commonly have increased gastric acid output, whereas patients with gastric ulcer typically have outputs in the normal range. Adults with pernicious anemia are achlorhydric. Patients with gastric cancer may also be achlorhydric or have subnormal acid outputs. In contrast, Zollinger-Ellison syndrome and antral G-cell hyperplasia are conditions associated with hypergastrinemia and high gastric acid output. Gastric secretory studies in gastrinoma patients may demonstrate a BAO of more than 15 mmol/hr and a BAO/maximal acid output ratio that exceeds 60%, although acid secretory studies alone are not reliable for establishing the diagnosis.

ANSWER: C

18. Elevated serum gastrin levels during fasting are typical in each of the following conditions *except*:

A. Pernicious anemia.
B. Chronic gastritis.
C. Duodenal ulcer.
D. Postvagotomy state.
E. Gastric outlet obstruction.

Ref.: 2, 4

COMMENTS: Hypergastrinemia has a broad differential diagnosis that can be narrowed considerably by consideration of several clinical factors. Conditions associated with elevated serum gastrin *and* increased acid secretion include Zollinger-Ellison syndrome, antral G-cell hyperplasia, retained antrum, renal failure, gastric outlet obstruction, and short bowel syndrome. In contradistinction, hypergastrinemia is associated with normal or diminished acid production in pernicious anemia, chronic gastritis, gastric cancer, and postvagotomy states and in patients receiving pharmacologic agents for acid suppression. Serum gastrin levels during fasting are normal in patients with uncomplicated duodenal ulcer but may be excessively elevated postprandially. The absolute level of an abnormally elevated serum gastrin is not necessarily indicative of the cause. Although marked elevations (>1000 pg/ml) are often associated with Zollinger-Ellison syndrome, the elevations are not always as pronounced and may overlap considerably with those seen in other conditions. Pernicious anemia can also be associated with high gastrin levels.

ANSWER: C

19. Match each finding in the left column with the appropriate condition or conditions in the right column.

A. Serum gastrin level is elevated	a. Zollinger-Ellison syndrome
B. Gastric acid output is elevated	b. Antral G cell hyperplasia
C. Secretin stimulation markedly increases gastrin level	c. Both
D. Protein meal markedly increases gastrin levels	d. Neither
E. Bombesin stimulation markedly increases gastrin level	

Ref.: 4

COMMENTS: Zollinger-Ellison syndrome, antral G-cell hyperplasia, and retained antrum are conditions causing peptic ulcer that are associated with hypergastrinemia as a cause of elevated gastric acid secretion. Although these conditions are unusual, they must be differentiated to determine proper therapy; they can be differentiated on the basis of the serum gastrin response to several provocative tests. A pronounced increase in serum gastrin level after intravenous infusion of secretin is typical of Zollinger-Ellison syndrome; elevations can be seen with other conditions, but they are not as dramatic. In contradistinction, more marked increases in gastrin levels occur after stimulation by a protein meal in patients with G-cell hyperplasia or retained antrum than in patients with Zollinger-Ellison syndrome. Bombesin stimulates release of gastrin from the antrum but not from gastrinomas and may also aid the differentiation of these entities.

ANSWER: A-c; B-c; C-a; D-b; E-b

20. With regard to the medical treatment of duodenal ulcer, which of the following statements is/are true?

A. Antacids alone provide symptomatic relief but have not been demonstrated to promote healing.
B. Diets have not been demonstrated to promote healing.
C. Minimal relapse has been observed after an adequate 6-week course of H_2-blockers.
D. Omeprazole binds to necrotic tissue at the ulcer base to prevent back-diffusion of hydrogen ion.
E. *Helicobacter pylori* infection is usually controlled by antibiotics alone.

Ref.: 1, 2, 3

COMMENTS: Much of the traditional medical therapy for duodenal ulcer is unfounded. Controlled clinical studies have not demonstrated any type of diet or feeding schedule to affect ulcer healing or recurrence, although aspirin, nonsteroidal antiinflammatory drugs (NSAIDs), and cigarettes should be avoided. Antacids and H_2-receptor antagonists are equally effective; and both have been demonstrated to promote ulcer healing, in comparison with placebo. Traditionally, there has been a high rate of relapse after cessation of any medical therapy, and medical treatment has not altered the natural history of the disease. More recently, however, the combination of antisecretory therapy with antibiotics for eradication of *H. pylori* infection has been shown to reduce dramatically the recurrence of both duodenal and gastric ulcers. Treatment of *H. pylori* introduces the potential risks of antibiotic side effects and development of resistant organisms. For these reasons, routine treatment is controversial for first-time ulcer patients, who may respond to antisecretory therapy alone. However, combination therapy is appropriate when *H. pylori* infection is demonstrated in patients with recurrent peptic ulcer disease.

ANSWER: B

21. A 45-year-old man requires surgery for intractable duodenal ulcer. Which operation best prevents ulcer recurrence?

A. Subtotal gastrectomy.
B. Truncal vagotomy and pyloroplasty.
C. Truncal vagotomy and antrectomy.
D. Selective vagotomy.
E. Highly selective (parietal cell) vagotomy.

Ref.: 1, 2 , 3, 4

COMMENTS: See Question 22.

22. Which operation for duodenal ulcer is least likely to produce undesirable postoperative symptoms?

A. Subtotal gastrectomy.
B. Truncal vagotomy and pyloroplasty.
C. Truncal vagotomy and antrectomy.
D. Selective vagotomy.
E. Highly selective (parietal cell) vagotomy.

Ref.: 1, 2, 3, 4

COMMENTS: The goal of surgical therapy for duodenal ulcer is to reduce acid in a manner that is safe and has the fewest possible side effects. Acid can be reduced by eliminating vagal stimulation, removing the antral source of gastrin, and removing the parietal cell mass. Traditionally, subtotal two-thirds gastrectomy has carried the highest mortality rate. Truncal vagotomy with antrectomy has the lowest recurrence rate. Highly selective vagotomy, also known as parietal cell vagotomy or proximal gastric vagotomy, aims to denervate the parietal cell-bearing portion of the stomach but preserve innervation to the pyloroantral region and thus maintain more normal gastric emptying. This operation carries the lowest mortality rate, the lowest incidence of side effects, but the highest recurrence rate, particularly in patients with prepyloric and pyloric ulcers. Procedures that involve gastric resection, pyloroplasty, or truncal vagotomy may be complicated by diarrhea, postprandial dumping, or bile reflux. Selective vagotomy, which preserves the hepatic and celiac vagal branches, has been associated with a lower rate of diarrhea than truncal vagotomy.

ANSWER:
Question 21: C
Question 22: E

23. A 75-year-old man on NSAIDs for arthritis presents with an acute abdomen and pneumoperitoneum. His symptoms are 6 hours old, and his vital signs are stable after infusion of 1 liter of normal saline. His management should next include:

A. Operation.
B. Esophagogastroduodenoscopy.
C. Upper GI contrast study.
D. Antisecretory drugs, antibiotics for gram-negative organisms, and operation if he fails to improve in 6 hours.
E. Antisecretory drugs, antibiotics for *H. pylori*, and operation if he fails to improve in 6 hours.

Ref.: 1, 2, 3, 4

COMMENTS: See Question 24.

24. The patient in Question 23 is found to have a perforated duodenal ulcer. Which of the following *best* describes the required operation?

A. Suture closure of perforation.
B. Omental patch of perforation.
C. Repair of perforation and highly selective vagotomy.
D. Repair of perforation and truncal vagotomy.
E. Repair of perforation and gastric resection.

Ref.: 1, 2, 3, 4

COMMENTS: The preferred treatment for perforated duodenal ulcer is resuscitation and prompt operation. Nonoperative management is reserved for old contained or forme fruste-type perforations or for terminally ill patients who otherwise cannot undergo surgery. The diagnosis is a presumptive one based on clinical grounds and should not be excluded if pneumoperitoneum cannot be demonstrated, as about 20% of patients with perforations do not have this typical radiographic feature. Operative management requires closure of the perforation, which is generally best accomplished by an omental

(Graham) patch. Following simple repair alone, the traditional natural history has been that about one-third of patients have no further ulcer problems, one-third have ulcer recurrence amenable to medical management, and one-third require a subsequent operation for ulcer disease. How precisely this concept applies to patients whose ulcer may be due to drugs or *H. pylori* infection is not clear. It has been suggested that chronicity of symptoms before perforation or operative findings of chronicity increase the advisability of performing a more definitive antiulcer operation at the time a perforation is repaired. Definitive operations should be performed only in stable patients. A highly selective vagotomy is an excellent choice. Truncal vagotomy may be more rapid but has a greater incidence of side effects. Resective procedures are generally avoided in the setting of perforation owing to higher morbidity. Following surgery, ulcerogenic drugs should be withheld, and any concomitant *H. pylori* infection should be treated if present.

ANSWER:
Question 23: A
Question 24: B

25. With regard to hemorrhage complicating duodenal ulcer, which of the following statements is/are true?

A. It is a more common complication of duodenal ulcer than perforation.
B. Endoscopic treatment prior to operation decreases mortality.
C. Endoscopic treatment decreases the need for operation.
D. Operative management is indicated only if endoscopic treatment fails.
E. Operative management should include an acid-reducing procedure.

Ref.: 1, 2, 3, 4

COMMENTS: Hemorrhage is the most common complication of duodenal ulcer. It usually presents with melena or hematemesis; there may be massive bleeding from an eroded gastroduodenal artery or one of its tributaries. Endoscopy is critical for diagnosing the site of upper gastrointestinal hemorrhage. Endoscopic techniques can be useful for controlling hemorrhage, but whether they decrease mortality rates or the need for subsequent operation has not been universally established. The most important endoscopic predictor of persistent or recurrent bleeding is active bleeding (arterial spurting) at the time of endoscopy. The presence of a "visible vessel" implies a high risk of recurrent bleeding even if the vessel is not bleeding at the time of endoscopy. When operation is necessary, bleeding is controlled by suture-ligation with attention to proper suture placement for control of the posterior complex of gastroduodenal vessels. A definitive antiulcer operation should then be performed because of the high risk of recurrent hemorrhage. Selection of the appropriate definitive procedure is highly dependent on the physiologic status of the patient. If the patient has been in shock or is otherwise ill, truncal vagotomy and pyloroplasty is advisable. For fit patients, parietal cell vagotomy or truncal vagotomy and antrectomy are considered.

ANSWER: A, E

26. Advanced gastric outlet obstruction is characterized by which one or more of the following metabolic abnormalities?

A. Hypochloremia and increased urinary chloride.
B. Hypokalemia due to urinary potassium loss.
C. Metabolic alkalosis with alkaline urine.
D. Metabolic alkalosis with acid urine.
E. Increased serum ionized calcium.

Ref.: 1, 2, 3

COMMENTS: The classic metabolic abnormality resulting from gastric outlet obstruction and prolonged vomiting is a hypochloremic, hypokalemic metabolic alkalosis. Initial loss of hydrochloric acid causes hypochloremia and a mild alkalosis compensated for by renal excretion of bicarbonate, so in the early stages the urine is alkaline. Continued vomiting produces a severe extracellular fluid deficit and sodium deficit from both renal and gastric losses. The kidneys begin to conserve sodium and, in exchange, excrete hydrogen and potassium as the cation to accompany bicarbonate. The kidneys are the predominant site of potassium loss, and the urine is paradoxically acidic. Urine chloride content is reduced throughout and eventually absent. Serum ionized calcium is decreased because it is mildly alkaline and shifts to its nonionized form to reduce alkalosis. Treatment of this metabolic situation is accomplished primarily by administration of isotonic saline, which replenishes the deficits of volume, sodium, and chloride. Potassium is replaced when renal function has been optimized.

ANSWER: B, D

27. Concerning the treatment of patients with Zollinger-Ellison syndrome, which of the following statements is/are true?

A. Operative treatment of associated hyperparathyroidism takes precedence over abdominal operation.
B. Pancreatic tumors can be removed by enucleation.
C. Duodenal tumors usually require pancreaticoduodenectomy.
D. Total gastrectomy is indicated if the tumor cannot be localized.
E. Resection of liver metastases is not indicated.

Ref.: 1, 2, 3, 4

COMMENTS: The treatment of Zollinger-Ellison syndrome is two-pronged and is aimed at both resecting tumor when possible and protecting the gastric end-organ. Therapy must be individualized. Patients with known endocrine tumors should undergo careful evaluation for other potential endocrine tumors. In the patient with gastrinoma and hyperparathyroidism, parathyroidectomy should first be performed to eliminate hypercalcemia; abdominal operation is not urgent with current antisecretory medications. Although gastrinomas are often multiple and are usually metastatic, long-term survival is possible. Aggressive attempts to localize and resect tumors can provide cure in 5–20% of patients and can diminish gastrin secretion in others. Both pancreatic and duodenal gastrinomas can be resected by enucleation when appropriately located. Blind pancreatic resections are not generally indicated. When complete tumor removal is not possible, a gastric operation may be appropriate. Proximal gastric vagotomy may be useful, but total gastrectomy still provides the best long-term quality of life for some patients. Lifelong pharmacologic treatment with antisecretory agents may control the ulcer diathesis in some patients, but problems with high doses, compliance, and side effects may occur. Resection or ablation of metastatic disease, although not curative, can provide important palliation and decrease the need for drug therapy.

ANSWER: A, B

28. Concerning "stress" bleeding from acute erosive gastritis, which of the following statements is/are true?

A. Polyphylactic treatment with H_2-blockers or antacids is equally effective.
B. The incidence of such bleeding has been decreasing.
C. The site of hemorrhage is most often in the antrum.
D. There is minimal recurrent bleeding after treatment by oversewing of bleeding sites, vagotomy, and pyloroplasty.
E. Effective surgical treatment necessitates total gastrectomy.

Ref.: 1, 2, 3

COMMENTS: Stress bleeding in critically ill patients is best prevented by the use of antacids whose dosage is monitored by titration of the gastric pH. H_2-receptor antagonists alone are not as effective as antacids alone, but use of the two conjointly may decrease the volume of buffer required. Sucralfate is effective as an acute cytoprotective topical agent, and it works in an acidic environment. It may decrease oropharyngeal colonization by enteric bacteria and the subsequent rate of pneumonia. For reasons that are not known the incidence of major bleeding from acute mucosal erosions has decreased greatly; however, the lesions should be anticipated in malnourished patients with septic syndrome or septic shock. Bleeding often begins insidiously, but major bleeding may develop rapidly. Gastroscopy usually demonstrates acute, superficial lesions that appear first in the proximal stomach (fundus) and then spread distally. If an operation is indicated for protracted bleeding, gastroscopic findings should dictate the procedure needed. Total gastrectomy is warranted if the bleeding sites cannot be controlled by means of a lesser operation (vagotomy and pyloroplasty).

ANSWER: B

29. The pathogenesis of benign type I gastric ulcers is predominantly which one of the following?

A. Hypersecretion of acid as a result of increased parietal cell mass.
B. Hypergastrinemia as a result of gastric stasis.
C. Defective gastric mucus barrier.
D. Defective gastric mucosal barrier.
E. Hyperpepsinogenemia.

Ref.: 1, 2, 3, 5

COMMENTS: Type I gastric ulcers occur along the lesser curvature, typically on the antral side of the junction between the acid-secreting and non–acid-secreting mucosa. Type II gastric ulcers are those combined with duodenal ulcers; type III ulcers are prepyloric. Type II and III gastric ulcers are similar to duodenal ulcers in terms of acid-secretory behavior and types of therapy to which they are amenable. Isolated benign gastric ulcers are thought to result from a defect in the mucosal barrier to hydrogen ion diffusion in the presence of acid. A variety of factors, such as duodenogastric reflux of bile, mucosa-damaging drugs (aspirin, nonsteroidal antiinflammatory drugs), and ethanol, may be involved in the mucosal injury. The gastric mucous layer primarily acts as a lubricant and is not particularly important in protection from acid. Dragstedt's theory of antral stasis as the primary cause of gastric ulcer is no longer accepted; most patients with gastric ulcer have normal gastric emptying.

ANSWER: D

30. Match each clinical feature in the left column with the appropriate ulcer type in the right column.

A. Most frequent peptic ulcer	a. Gastric ulcer (type I)
B. More common after 50 years of age	b. Duodenal ulcer
C. Slower healing with medical therapy	c. Both
D. Hemorrhage associated with higher mortality rate	d. Neither
E. Malignant transformation common.	

Ref.: 1, 2, 3, 4

COMMENTS: In the United States isolated gastric ulcers are about four times less common than duodenal ulcers, whereas in Japan gastric ulcers are more common. Gastric ulcers occur more commonly in older patients; and when they are complicated by bleeding, perforation, or obstruction the corresponding prognosis is generally worse than it is for patients with duodenal ulcer. Antisecretory therapy promotes healing of gastric ulcers, but healing is in general slower and therapy is not as effective as for duodenal ulcer. *Helicobacter pylori* infection must be treated. All gastric ulcers should be examined by biopsy (and repeated biopsy as necessary) to rule out malignancy. Approximately 5% of benign-appearing gastric ulcers are malignant. In uncommon cases, cancer develops in the mucosa peripheral to a chronic ulcer.

ANSWER: A-b; B-a; C-a; D-a; E-d

31. With regard to surgical therapy of gastric ulcer, which of the following statements is/are true?

A. A type I ulcer at the incisura is effectively treated by distal gastrectomy without vagotomy.
B. A type I ulcer at the incisura is preferably treated by vagotomy and pyloroplasty.
C. A type III prepyloric ulcer without obstruction is best treated by parietal cell vagotomy.
D. Type II (combined duodenal and gastric) ulcers are best treated by subtotal (70–80%) gastrectomy without vagotomy.
E. A type I ulcer on the lesser curve near the gastroesophageal junction is best treated by total gastrectomy.

Ref.: 1, 2, 3, 4

COMMENTS: Surgical therapy of benign gastric ulcer depends on the type of ulcer and associated acid secretion. Isolated type I ulcers are usually well treated by antrectomy or hemigastrectomy (including removal of the ulcer) without vagotomy. Although the addition of vagotomy to distal resection for type I ulcers has not improved outcome, vagotomy is sometimes used because of the possibility of associated duodenal ulcer or when the distinction between a type I ulcer and a type III ulcer is not clear. Vagotomy with pyloroplasty for type I ulcers has been associated with a higher recurrence rate than has resection and has conferred no advantages. Limited experience with parietal cell vagotomy for type I ulcers has yielded reasonable clinical results. Type I ulcers near the gastroesophageal junction can be treated by modifications of distal gastrectomy that include ulcer excision. Type II and III ulcers are treated as duodenal ulcers with vagotomy and resection or drainage. Parietal cell vagotomy is generally not indicated for prepyloric ulcers because of high recurrence rates, although there are data demonstrating that parietal cell vagotomy in combination with a pyloric drainage procedure may be effective therapy in this situation.

ANSWER: A

32. Malignant gastric ulcers can preoperatively be distinguished from benign gastric ulcers based on which of the following?

A. Size larger than 2 cm.
B. Location on the greater curvature.
C. Acid secretory studies demonstrating achlorhydria.
D. Multiple biopsies.
E. Failure to heal by 8 weeks.

Ref.: 1, 2, 3

COMMENTS: Although certain characteristics suggest that an ulcer is malignant (size, location, achlorhydria), the only accurate method of distinction is adequate histologic sampling. Even the visual endoscopic appearance of a malignant lesion can be misinterpreted as that of a benign ulcer. Multiple (four or more) biopsies at different quadrants increase the accuracy of histologic diagnosis. Benign gastric ulcers can be slow to heal, especially if large; and malignant gastric ulcers also can show partial healing. Repeated biopsy is advised for ulcers that have not healed after 8–12 weeks of medical therapy.

ANSWER: D

33. With regard to the epidemiology of gastric cancer, which of the following statements is/are true?

A. The highest incidence is in Japan.
B. Predominance among males or females varies geographically.
C. Both incidence and death rates in the United States have decreased.
D. There is a higher incidence among patients with blood group O.
E. There is a higher incidence among patients who have undergone gastric resection for duodenal ulcer.

Ref.: 1, 2, 3, 4

COMMENTS: The significant geographic variations in the incidence of gastric cancer are likely related to environmental and dietary differences that result in exposure to *N*-nitrosocompounds, polycyclic hydrocarbons, and other potential carcinogens. The highest incidence is in Japan, where the death rate is about eight times higher than that in the United States. Gastric cancer occurs more frequently in males in all areas of the world. Parallel dramatic declines in the incidence and death rates of gastric cancer in the United States have been observed since the early 1940s, although a slight increase may now be occurring, the reasons for which are unknown. Although most risk factors for gastric cancer are probably exogenous, genetic factors may also be involved, as exemplified by patients with pernicious anemia and by the slightly increased risk among patients with blood group A. There appears also to be an increased risk 10–15 years after gastric resection for benign disease, perhaps indicating the role of chronic bile reflux.

ANSWER: A, C, E

34. Which one or more of the following conditions are associated with gastric cancer?

A. Adenomatous gastric polyps.
B. Autoimmune chronic gastritis.
C. Hypersecretory chronic gastritis.
D. Environmental chronic gastritis.
E. Ménétrier's disease.

Ref.: 4

COMMENTS: Certain gastric lesions have a significant association with gastric cancer and can be considered precursors to malignancy. Adenomatous polyps in the stomach have a malignant potential, as do adenomatous polyps of the colon. Chronic atrophic gastritis, of which several forms are recognized, underlies most gastric cancers; epithelial changes of intestinal metaplasia and dysplasia are premalignant. Autoimmune chronic gastritis (type A gastritis) involves the body and fundus of the stomach; it is associated with pernicious anemia, parietal cell antibodies, achlorhydria, very high gastrin levels, and a high risk of cancer. Hypersecretory chronic gastritis (type B gastritis) involves the gastric antrum and is associated with peptic ulcer disease but *not* malignancy. Environmental chronic gastritis is multifocal, involving the body and antrum, and occurs in geographic areas with a high incidence of gastric cancer. Ménétrier's disease, one of the hyperplastic gastropathies and characterized by enlarged rugae, is no longer considered premalignant. Earlier descriptions of cancer in Ménétrier's disease referred to patients with gastric polyposis.

ANSWER: A, B, D

35. With regard to the prognosis of gastric adenocarcinoma, which of the following statements is/are true?

A. The polypoid gross type carries a better prognosis than does the diffusely infiltrating type.
B. The intestinal histologic type carries a better prognosis than does the diffuse type.
C. The overall 5-year survival rate in the United States is approximately 50% after resection.
D. Cure rates of 80–90% are obtained for lesions confined to the mucosa.
E. Length of survival is improved by chemotherapy and radiation therapy after curative resection.

Ref.: 1, 2, 3, 4

COMMENTS: Gastric cancers can be classified according to gross and histologic appearances with some correlation between the two. On gross examination, polypoid, ulcerating, superficial spreading, and diffusely infiltrating (linitis plastica) types are recognized. The polypoid and superficial spreading types carry a better prognosis, whereas the prognosis of patients with linitis plastica is dismal. Histologically, Lauren distinguished intestinal and diffuse types. The intestinal variety, which is decreasing in incidence in the United States, is better differentiated and is associated with longer survival stage for stage than is the diffuse type. The intestinal pattern predominates in polypoid and superficial spreading tumors. Resection of stage I tumors, confined to the mucosa, yields excellent survival rates. However, these lesions are unusual in the United States in comparison with Japan, where they constitute 20–40% of tumors. In the United States the overall 5-year survival rate after treatment is only about 10% because most of the patients have more advanced disease. Survival rates of 40–50% are found in node-negative patients and even in node-positive patients with intestinal histologic findings. Adjuvant therapy after potentially curative resection has yielded no clear benefit.

ANSWER: A, B, D

36. With regard to the surgical treatment of gastric adenocarcinoma, which of the following statements is/are true?

A. Total gastrectomy for antral lesions results in longer survival than does partial gastrectomy.
B. Routine splenectomy does not improve survival rates.
C. Extended lymph node dissection improves survival rates for patients with stage I and II lesions.
D. Total gastrectomy for palliation is contraindicated.
E. Linitis plastica should be resected to histologically negative margins.

Ref.: 1, 2, 3, 4

COMMENTS: Gastric adenocarcinoma is preferably treated by resection, although resection usually proves to be palliative. The general strategy for curative resection is to remove as much stomach as necessary to obtain free margins and to perform limited node dissection. Although data from Japan support the benefit of extended nodal dissections (celiac, mesenteric, hepatic, paraaortic), studies in the United States have not generally confirmed this benefit. Furthermore, these extended dissections can be associated with substantial morbidity. Most resections entail distal subtotal gastrectomy. Total gastrectomy is appropriate for locally extensive tumors, proximal tumors (to avoid esophageal anastomosis to distal stomach remnant), and even palliation if necessary. Extending clear margins on a distal tumor by total rather than subtotal gastrectomy is of no benefit. Resections for linitis plastica are palliative, usually necessitate total gastrectomy, and are carried out to grossly negative margins only. Splenectomy is performed according to the location of gastric resection, but its routine performance does not improve the survival rate.

ANSWER: B

37. An upper gastrointestinal series demonstrates enlarged rugae in the corpus and fundus of the stomach. Which of the following is *not* included in the differential diagnosis?

A. Ménétrier's disease.
B. Lymphoma.
C. Pseudolymphoma.
D. Eosinophilic gastroenteritis.
E. Adenocarcinoma.

Ref.: 2, 4

COMMENTS: A number of disorders are associated with grossly enlarged gastric folds. In Ménétrier's disease, mucosal folds of the fundus and corpus may be markedly enlarged as a result of mucous cell hyperplasia. The condition may be associated with protein-losing enteropathy and typically spares the antrum. Eosinophilic gastroenteritis, in contrast, is a process characterized by polypoid or diffuse eosinophilic infiltration that occurs in the antrum. Gastric malignancy, adenocarcinoma or lymphoma, can manifest with thickened folds. These radiographic characteristics may also be demonstrated in pseudolymphoma, which represents lymphoid hyperplasia.

ANSWER: D

38. With regard to primary gastric lymphoma, which of the following statements is/are true?

A. Gastrointestinal bleeding is the most common symptom.
B. Mucosal biopsy can establish the diagnosis in nearly all cases.
C. Primary therapy is surgical resection.
D. Primary therapy is irradiation.
E. The long-term survival rate is equivalent to that for adenocarcinoma.

Ref.: 1, 2, 3, 4

COMMENTS: Gastric lymphoma is not common, but the stomach is the most common site of extranodal non-Hodgkin's lymphoma. Patients usually present with abdominal pain and weight loss. Endoscopic visualization and biopsy may not establish the diagnosis because the lesion begins as a submucosal process. Even when ulceration is present, biopsy specimens may yield only nondiagnostic necrotic material. The primary treatment is surgical resection, for both cure and palliation. The 5-year survival rate with curative resection is 75%. Radiation therapy has been used as primary therapy, as an adjunct to resection, and for unresectable tumors. Although the value of adjuvant radiation has not been fully established, it is often employed, particularly if there is nodal or serosal involvement. Chemotherapy is also used for patients with unresectable lesions or systemic disease and might be considered for resected tumors with poor prognostic factors, such as nodal disease or transmural involvement.

ANSWER: C

39. Concerning the Mallory-Weiss syndrome, which of the following statements is/are true?

A. It is a complication of gastroesophageal reflux.
B. It involves esophageal rupture near the gastroesophageal junction.
C. Profuse hemorrhage is the most common manifestation.
D. Bleeding can generally be managed medically.
E. Vagotomy is indicated for patients requiring surgical treatment.

Ref.: 1, 2

COMMENTS: Mallory-Weiss syndrome refers to a tear of the mucosa and submucosa near the gastroesophageal junction that occurs as a result of retching. The tear is usually on the gastric side and on its lesser curvature. The bleeding can often be managed medically; there is profuse hemorrhage in about 10% of cases. Should operation be necessary, bleeding can be controlled simply by oversewing the site of the tear, an acid-reducing operation is not required.

ANSWER: D

40. With regard to gastric volvulus, which of the following statements is/are true?

A. Symptoms consist of severe nausea with inability to vomit.
B. It is associated with congenital anomalies of gastric fixation.
C. It frequently is relieved simply by passage of a nasogastric tube.
D. It constitutes a surgical emergency.
E. It is associated with an increased incidence of sigmoid volvulus.

Ref.: 2

COMMENTS: Gastric volvulus is a serious complication of paraesophageal hernia. Two types of gastric volvulus may occur, depending on the axis of rotation. *Organoaxial* volvulus, the more common type, involves rotation around the axis of a line connecting the cardia and pylorus. With *mesenterioaxial volvulus*, the axis is approximately at a right angle to the cardiopyloric line. Combined types have also been described. Patients generally have severe pain and nausea but are unable to vomit, and a nasogastric tube cannot be passed. Strangulation can follow; hence gastric volvulus requires prompt reduction. Because of the risk of volvulus, patients with paraesophageal hiatal hernia should undergo repair.

ANSWER: A, D

41. Which of the following is the preferred treatment for a symptomatic duodenal diverticulum?

A. Antibiotics for suppression of bacterial overgrowth.
B. H_2-blockers.
C. Surgical excision.
D. Gastrojejunostomy.
E. Pancreaticoduodenectomy.

Ref.: 4

COMMENTS: A duodenal diverticulum is usually an asymptomatic, incidental finding that does not necessitate specific therapy. In a patient with gastrointestinal symptoms, other pathologic processes should be carefully sought. Duodenal diverticula occasionally cause abdominal pain, obstruction, bleeding, bacterial overgrowth, perforation, or pancreaticobiliary problems. The diverticulum is most commonly located on the medial wall of the second portion of the duodenum near the papilla of Vater. When treatment is required, surgical excision is recommended. In general, this can be accomplished after a Kocher maneuver, although transduodenal excision is occasionally necessary. Care must be taken to identify the bile duct and pancreatic duct.

ANSWER: C

42. Which of the following conditions is/are associated with an increased risk of duodenal adenocarcinoma?

A. Heterotopic pancreas.
B. Adenoma of Brunner's glands.
C. Nodular hyperplasia of Brunner's glands.
D. Familial polyposis coli.
E. Gardner syndrome.

Ref.: 4

COMMENTS: A variety of benign and malignant duodenal neoplasms can occur, and surgeons should be familiar with them. Adenocarcinoma, the most common malignant duodenal neoplasm, has been associated with a number of conditions, including adenomatous polyps, villous adenomas, familial polyposis coli, Gardner syndrome, and von Recklinghausen's disease. Heterotopic pancreas is not neoplastic, but it can manifest as a submucosal duodenal nodule. Adenomas of Brunner's glands are probably hamartomas; they are benign but enter into the differential diagnosis of duodenal tumors. Nodular hyperplasia of Brunner's glands is a diffuse benign process that can be seen in patients on hemodialysis or after renal transplantation.

ANSWER: D, E

43. An 18-year-old woman presents with abdominal pain and weight loss. Examination reveals a soft, moveable epigastric mass. Endoscopy demonstrates a large mass of black hair in the stomach. Which of the following is the most appropriate therapy?

A. Endoscopic extraction.
B. Oral administration of papain.
C. Psychiatric consultation.
D. Gastrotomy and removal.
E. Gastrojejunostomy.

Ref.: 4

COMMENTS: Gastric bezoars caused by ingested hair are termed *trichobezoars*; they most typically occur in young women. The hair is not digestible, and endoscopic removal is generally inadequate. Additional bezoars may be present in the small intestine. For these reasons, laparotomy, gastrotomy, and operative removal are indicated. *Phytobezoars* are made up of vegetable or fruit fiber. These are more common in older patients and may occur in association with diabetes, prior gastric surgery, or other causes of delayed gastric emptying. A unique type of phytobezoar resulting from persimmon fruit (*diopyrobezoar*) may necessitate operation. Otherwise, most phytobezoars can be treated with liquid diets, enzymatic digestion, and endoscopic manipulation.

ANSWER: D

44. A spot film from an upper gastrointestinal study was obtained on a patient who had vague abdominal pain. From the radiographic findings, which of the following is the most likely diagnosis?

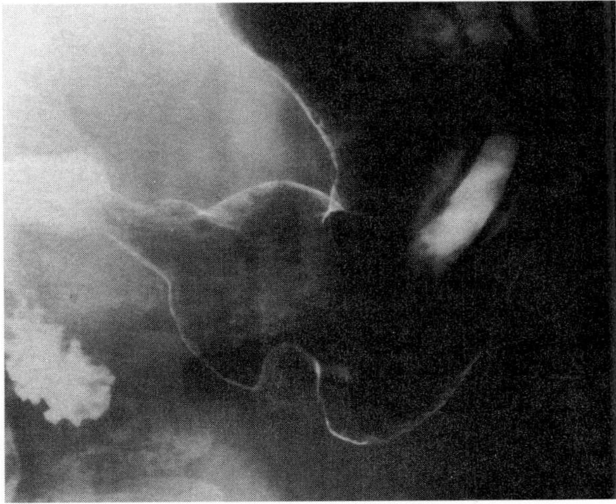

A. Mucosal polyp.
B. Gastric ulcer.
C. Ectopic pancreas.
D. Adenocarcinoma.

Ref.: 4

COMMENTS: Note that there is a mass along the greater curvature portion of the antrum with radiographically smooth mucosa. The mass makes 90-degree angles with the gastric lumen, which places the mass in the *submucosal* location. Radiographically, *mucosal* masses produce angles with the lumen that are acute. Adjacent masses that push on the stomach to create the image of a mass have angles greater than 180 degrees. • A **mucosal polyp**, either hyperplastic or an adenoma, is unlikely because of the suspected submucosal origin. Hyperplastic polyps are usually multiple and are found in the fundus and proximal stomach. Adenomas usually are single, are found in the antrum, and carry the same ominous implications as do adenomas in the colon. **Leiomyomas** are the most common submucosal masses found in the gastrointestinal tract, and the radiologic findings in the patient in Question 44 are compatible with a submucosal mass. On occasion, if the mass is large, the mucosa ulcerates. The differential diagnosis between benign leiomyoma and leiomyosarcoma cannot be made on radiographic grounds alone. Other submucosal masses include neuromas, neurofibromas, hemangiomas, lipomas, and lymphoma. **Ectopic pancreas** is a rest of pancreatic tissues in an unusual location. Usually these rests are found in the gastric antrum or duodenum. They are submucosal in location, as in this patient. On occasion, as in this case, there is an aborted pancreatic duct that fills with contrast material (it appears as a white dot in the center of the mass). The definitive diagnosis is established by excision. **Gastric carcinoma** destroys the mucosa, which is reflected by an ulceration within the mucosal pattern radiographically. Early gastric cancer may be found as a small polypoid lesion that resembles a gastric polyp. Other appearances of early gastric cancer include a plaque-like area of ulceration that can mimic the appearance of a benign ulcer. **Lymphoma** is another lesion that can occur submucosally and should be ruled out each time a submucosal mass is discovered. Ruling out malignancy in submucosal masses is difficult because endoscopic evaluation with biopsy often reaches only the mucosa. The endoscopist must therefore be aware of the submucosal nature of the mass; repeated biopsies in the same area or surgical excision may be needed to establish the diagnosis.

ANSWER: C

REFERENCES

1. Sabiston DC Jr, Lyerly HK (eds): *Textbook of Surgery: The Biological Basis of Modern Surgical Practice*, 15th ed. WB Saunders, Philadelphia, 1997.
2. Schwartz SI, Shires GT, Spencer FC, et al (eds): *Principles of Surgery*, 7th ed. McGraw-Hill, New York, 1999.
3. Greenfield LJ, Mulholland M, Oldham KT, et al: *Surgery: Scientific Principles and Practice*, 2nd ed. Lippincott-Raven, Philadelphia, 1997.
4. Wastell C, Nyhus LM, Donahue PE (eds): *Surgery of the Stomach and Duodenum*, 5th ed. Little, Brown, Boston, 1995.
5. O'Leary JP: *The Physiologic Basis of Surgery*, 2nd ed. Williams & Wilkins, Baltimore, 1996.
6. Burette A: How (who?) and when to test for *Helicobacter pylori*. *Acta Gastroenterol Belg* 61:336–343, 1998.

CHAPTER 28

Small Intestine

1. During an operation for presumed appendicitis, the appendix is found to be normal. The terminal ileum, however, is markedly thickened and feels rubbery to firm; its serosa is erythematous and inflamed; and several loops of apparently normal small intestine are adherent to it. The terminal ileum mesentery is thickened, with fat growing about the bowel circumference. Which of the following is the most likely diagnosis?

   A. Crohn's disease of the terminal ileum.
   B. Perforated Meckel's diverticulum.
   C. Ulcerative colitis.
   D. Ileocecal tuberculosis.
   E. Acute ileitis.

Ref.: 1, 2

COMMENTS: Crohn's disease can present acutely and, when it involves the terminal ileum, can closely resemble appendicitis clinically. Segments of bowel in a patient with Crohn's disease have a characteristic gross appearance: In addition to the features described previously, the mesenteric fat "creeps" over the serosa. The mesentery is thickened, dull, and rubbery; and it may contain lymph nodes as large as 4 cm in diameter. Not infrequently, partial obstruction of the involved segment can produce dilatation of the proximal bowel. Enteric fistulas may also be seen. **Acute ileitis** may clinically mimic appendicitis and grossly appear as inflammation of the terminal ileum; the operative findings, however, do not resemble those of advanced Crohn's disease. **Meckel's diverticulitis** can mimic appendicitis, but it presents as an inflammatory phlegmon process located approximately 50 cm proximal to the ileocecal valve and does not have the bowel wall or mesenteric changes seen with Crohn's disease. **Tuberculosis of the terminal ileum**—rare in the United States—can produce scarring and stenosis of the distal ileum and enlargement of the mesenteric lymph nodes. Demonstration of caseation and acid-fast bacilli on biopsy of a mesenteric lymph node confirms the diagnosis. **Ulcerative colitis** is confined to the large bowel, and any associated pain can usually be distinguished from that of appendicitis.

ANSWER: A

2. During exploratory surgery for presumed appendicitis, the cecum and appendix are found to be normal. The terminal 50 cm of ileum, however, is inflamed, beefy red, and slightly edematous. It is soft, and there is no proximal ileal distension. Which of the following is the most appropriate operative choice?

   A. Appendectomy.
   B. Resection of involved ileum and appendix.
   C. Placement of irrigation catheters and appendectomy.
   D. Closure without appendectomy or ileal resection.
   E. Bypass ileo-ascending colostomy.

Ref.: 1, 2

COMMENTS: When **acute regional enteritis** of the terminal ileum is encountered during exploration for presumed appendicitis, the appropriateness of appendectomy is somewhat controversial. The incidence of enterocutaneous fistula after operation in patients with Crohn's disease is high, but the fistulas usually arise from the diseased ileum, not the appendiceal stump. Also, 90% of patients in whom acute regional enteritis is found at operation do not progress to chronic Crohn's disease; symptoms resolve without sequelae. Therefore if the stump of the appendix is not involved, most surgeons favor performance of an appendectomy. This step ameliorates the dilemma of the differential diagnosis if right lower abdominal pain should develop at a later date. When acute regional enteritis is encountered, as in this clinical setting (i.e., without evidence of obstruction or fistula formation), the ileum should not be resected.

ANSWER: A

3. With regard to Crohn's disease, which of the following statements is/are correct?

   A. It is the most common primary disease of the small intestine that requires operation.
   B. Black males and males of Mediterranean descent are most commonly affected.
   C. The disease involves both the terminal ileum and the right colon in 90% of cases.
   D. The disease may involve any portion of the gastrointestinal (GI) tract from the mouth to the anus.

Ref.: 2

COMMENTS: Although uncommon in comparison with other GI diseases, Crohn's disease is the most common primary disease of the small intestine that requires operation. The incidence is highest in the United States, England, and Scandinavia. Crohn's disease is three times more common in Jews than in non-Jews, more common in whites than in nonwhites, and slightly more common in males than in females. It occurs in all age groups but is most frequently diagnosed in young adults. The distribution of involvement is such that 30% of patients have disease limited to the small intestine and 20% to the colon; about 50% have both small and large intestine involvement. Diseased segments may be separated by normal bowel (i.e., skip areas). Isolated involvement of the esophagus, stomach, or duodenum does occur but is rare.

ANSWER: A, D

4. As to the microscopic appearance of Crohn's disease, which of the following statements is/are true?

A. The disease is confined to the mucosa.
B. The disease is confined to the mucosa and submucosa.
C. Granulomas demonstrating caseation without acid-fast bacilli confirm the diagnosis.
D. Submucosal fibrosis occurs secondary to bacterial invasion.
E. Marked lymphangiectasia is a prominent microscopic feature.

Ref.: 1, 2

COMMENTS: Several microscopic features characterize, but are nonspecific for, Crohn's disease. These features progress from an early to a late phase of involvement and can be described as a granulomatous fibrotic inflammation progressing through all layers of the bowel wall. **Early phase**: Edema of the entire bowel wall is seen accompanied by lymphangiectasia and hyperemia, associated with an increased proportion of goblet cells in an otherwise normal mucosa. **Intermediate phase**: Thickening is caused by fibrosis of the submucosal and subserosal areas of the bowel. Focal mucosal ulcers become numerous; and in 60% of patients sarcoid-like granulomas appear, particularly in the submucosa, subserosa, and regional lymph nodes. These granulomas contain epithelioid giant cells, do not caseate, and do not contain acid-fast bacilli. The absence of granulomas does not exclude the diagnosis of Crohn's disease. Lymphangiectasia remains visible throughout the intermediate and late phases. **Late phase**: Dense fibrosis exceeds that expected from the simple healing of an inflammatory insult, producing a fixed stenosis and partial obstruction of the lumen. The mucosa is denuded over wide areas with occasional islands of intact mucosal cells (pseudopolyps). Glands deep in the mucosa resemble those of the pyloric region and are termed "aberrant pyloric glands" or Brunner's gland metaplasia. The ulcers can be deep, and progression through the bowel wall may occur, sometimes resulting in fistula formation.

ANSWER: E

5. With regard to the etiology of Crohn's disease, which of the following statements is/are true?

A. The primary pathologic mechanism is a progressive, obstructive lymphangitis.
B. Crohn's disease is a form of sarcoidosis limited to the gastrointestinal tract.
C. A mouse-footpad virus has been identified as the etiologic agent.
D. The disease is the result of a local hypersensitivity reaction.
E. The disease is primarily a psychosomatic illness.
F. The etiology is unknown.

Ref.: 1, 2

COMMENTS: Despite extensive investigation, the etiology of Crohn's disease is unknown. The possibility of a transmissible agent has emerged as a result of work demonstrating the development of granulomatous lesions in the mouse footpad following injection of intestinal homogenates obtained from patients with Crohn's disease. These results, however, have been difficult to reproduce, and their precise meaning requires further investigation. Although the granulomas of sarcoidosis and Crohn's disease are similar, the Kveim test, positive in 80% of patients with active sarcoidosis, is almost always negative in those with Crohn's disease. It is generally thought that the immunologic alterations and psychosomatic manifestations seen in patients with Crohn's disease reflect responses to the disease rather than indicate its cause.

ANSWER: F

6. Regarding the clinical manifestations of Crohn's disease, which of the following statements is/are true?

A. Most patients present acutely with pain, nausea, and diarrhea.
B. Bloody diarrhea is an infrequent symptom.
C. Bloody diarrhea almost always produces anemia.
D. There is steatorrhea as a result of pancreatic involvement.
E. Fever and signs of systemic toxicity are common.

Ref.: 1, 2

COMMENTS: Although 10% of patients with Crohn's disease present acutely and with symptoms similar to those of appendicitis, in most instances the onset is insidious, with intermittent **pain** or discomfort being the most frequent and sometimes the only symptom. The pain often is precipitated by a dietary indiscretion. With advanced disease, the pain may become associated with signs and symptoms of partial obstruction. Constant, localized pain, especially if associated with a palpable mass, suggests the presence of an abscess or bowel fistula. **Diarrhea** is the next most frequent symptom; and unlike the diarrhea of chronic ulcerative colitis, it rarely contains mucus, pus, or blood. Diarrhea is the result of several factors: The involved segment of small bowel has a decreased capacity to absorb intestinal contents. Also, the **obstruction** produced by this involved segment alters the absorptive capacity of the proximal bowel. **Decreased absorption** of bile salts in the terminal ileum leads to bile salt-induced damage of the absorptive cells of the colonic mucosa. One-third of patients present with **fever** and one-half with **weight loss, weakness**, and **easy fatigability**. Persistent occult loss of blood frequently produces **anemia**, which may be aggravated by a vitamin B_{12} deficiency. **Hypoproteinemia** occurs because of increased loss of protein from the inflamed bowel mucosa. **Vitamin and mineral deficiencies** are the result of decreased ingestion, altered metabolism, and decreased absorption.

ANSWER: B

7. With regard to the complications of Crohn's disease, which of the following statements is/are true?

A. When obstruction is present, it usually is partial rather than complete.
B. Perforation of the bowel wall occurs in 15–20% of patients.
C. Free perforations into the peritoneal cavity are as common as confined perforations.

D. Fistulization rarely occurs in patients who have not had an operation.
E. Perianal disease rarely occurs in patients with Crohn's disease confined to the small bowel.
F. Crohn's disease of the small bowel is not associated with an increased risk of malignancy.

Ref.: 1, 2

COMMENTS: *Complete* obstruction is uncommon in Crohn's disease. *Partial* obstruction is common; and when it is high grade, an elective operation may be necessary. *Perforation* occurs in 15–20% of patients, usually resulting in formation of an abscess or an internal fistula to the bowel, bladder, or vagina. • *Enterocutaneous fistulas* rarely occur in patients not previously operated upon, but they are common after operation. *Free* perforations into the peritoneal cavity are rare. When they do occur, they usually are on the antimesenteric border of the distal ileum, proximal to a stenotic lesion. • Up to 30% of patients with Crohn's disease of the small bowel develop *perirectal abscesses* or *fistulas*, usually without evidence of communication with the diseased small bowel. • Frank *hemorrhage* is rare, but it can occur if an ulcer erodes into a large blood vessel. • There is an increased risk of developing *cancer* in patients with Crohn's disease in comparison with the general population; but with regard to the colon, it does not approach the level seen in patients with chronic ulcerative colitis. This difference may be related to the shorter period between diagnosis and colectomy for Crohn's disease compared with ulcerative colitis. The risk, however, is not considered high enough to warrant prophylactic resection. Most cases of small bowel cancer associated with Crohn's disease have occurred in patients with long-standing disease and have appeared in a previously bypassed segment of bowel.

ANSWER: A, B

8. Regarding the radiographic findings of Crohn's disease of the small intestine, which of the following statements is/are true?

A. Barium enema with reflux into the terminal ileum is adequate for defining the extent of disease.
B. The string sign of Kantor is produced by luminal narrowing.
C. When present, fistulas are almost always seen on small bowel follow-through studies.
D. Studies with barium should be avoided because they can convert partial-thickness bowel wall involvement to a full-thickness lesion.
E. Increased space between bowel loops or deviation of the bowel wall may be due to thickening of the bowel wall and mesentery or to abscess formation.

Ref.: 1, 2

COMMENTS: An upper GI series of x-ray films with small bowel follow-through studies, as well as a barium enema with reflux into the terminal ileum, should be obtained when evaluating patients suspected of having Crohn's disease. Luminal narrowing of the terminal ileum as a result of acute edema or chronic fibrosis produces the string sign of Kantor seen on barium examination. Thickening of the bowel wall and mesentery increases the space between adjacent loops of bowel and may give the impression of extraluminal abscess formation. Fistulas may be seen, but they often are obscured by adjacent loops of bowel. The mucosal pattern may be markedly distorted, but it is more difficult to evaluate than the mucosal changes seen with Crohn's colitis. Skip areas of diseased bowel with intervening normal bowel segments may also be detected and help to differentiate Crohn's disease from ulcerative colitis.

ANSWER: B, E

9. With regard to the medical management of Crohn's disease, which of the following statements is/are true?

A. Nonabsorbable antibiotics (e.g., sulfasalazine) may alleviate symptoms.
B. Steroids relieve symptoms and can induce remission but do not alter the natural course of Crohn's disease.
C. Azathioprine is no more effective than a placebo in relief of symptoms or induction of remission.
D. 6-Mercaptopurine is more effective than a placebo in decreasing symptoms, healing fistulas, and allowing steroid dosage to be reduced.
E. Elemental diets and total parenteral nutrition do not affect the natural course of Crohn's disease.
F. Prednisone is most effective for small bowel involvement, while sulfasalazine is most effective for colonic involvement.

Ref.: 1, 2

COMMENTS: There is no curative therapy for Crohn's disease. Although certain therapeutic agents can effectively control symptoms, none has been shown to influence the natural course of the disease. The goal of medical management therefore is to control symptoms and to provide nutritional support. Failure of medical therapy that necessitates operation usually results from progression of the disease at the established site rather than from longitudinal extension along uninvolved bowel. Most patients with Crohn's disease ultimately require an operation; but because the rate of recurrence after operation is high, medical management is preferred until a complication makes an operation mandatory. Occasionally, a patient with an incomplete obstruction or with an internal fistula responds to aggressive nonoperative management; these complications therefore should not be considered as absolute indications for operation.

ANSWER: A, B, C, D, E, F

10. As to an operation for Crohn's disease, which of the following statements is/are true?

A. Operation is curative.
B. Perirectal disease may respond to resection of diseased small bowel.
C. The most common indication for operation is obstruction.
D. The recurrence rate after operation is 15%.

Ref.: 1, 2

COMMENTS: Up to 90% of all patients with Crohn's disease ultimately need an operation. Because Crohn's disease is panintestinal and typically recurrent, surgery is not curative (all tissue at risk for Crohn's disease cannot be removed). Therefore surgery is reserved for treating the complications of Crohn's disease, not to cure the disease. The most common indications for operation, in decreasing order of frequency, are obstruction, persistent symptomatic abdominal mass, abscess, fistula, perirectal disease that fails to respond to local therapy, and intractability of symptoms despite adequate medical management. Less common indications are free perforation, hemorrhage, and the blind-loop syndrome. Whichever operation the surgeon chooses to perform, the foremost goal is preservation of intestinal length whenever possible. As a consequence, most surgeons practice conservative resection of grossly diseased bowel. Neither the use of frozen-section microscopic examination to assess the margins of resection nor resection of involved mesenteric lymph nodes improves the long-term course of the disease. Simple bypass and bypass with exclusion are no longer used routinely. The bypassed segment often continues to be a source of active disease, prone to the development of bacterial overgrowth, obstruction, perforation, and possibly malignant transformation. A bypass procedure is reserved for use in elderly, poor-risk patients; in patients with obstructive gastroduodenal disease, which is treated with gastrojejunostomy; and in patients who have undergone previous extensive small bowel resection. Multiple fibrotic strictures in a patient who has had previous resections can be treated with strictureplasty in an attempt to conserve bowel length. Recurrence of symptoms after operation occurs in up to 50% of patients, and the yearly rate for reoperation remains constant at approximately 15%.

ANSWER: B, C

11. With regard to tuberculous enteritis, which of the following statements is/are true?

A. Primary infection usually results from ingestion of milk contaminated with the bovine strain of *Mycobacterium tuberculosis.*
B. Secondary infection results from the ingestion of bacilli contained in contaminated sputum.
C. The ileocecal region is the site of involvement in 85% of cases.
D. Primary infection frequently mimics the chronic form of Crohn's disease.
E. Secondary infection frequently produces radiographic findings indistinguishable from carcinoma of the colon.

Ref.: 1, 2

COMMENTS: Primary tuberculosis is rare in the United States but is still common in underdeveloped countries. Usually it produces minimal symptoms, but occasionally it causes a hypertrophic reaction in the ileocecal area that produces stricture and stenosis of the distal ileum and cecum. Radiographic findings are frequently indistinguishable from those of carcinoma of the colon. In some instances exploration and biopsy are advisable. Although it may be necessary to resect bowel because of high-grade obstruction, it is not appropriate to do so simply to *certify* the diagnosis. Treatment with isoniazid, paraaminosalicylic acid, and streptomycin usually suffices. **Ulcerative tuberculosis** is a form that develops **secondary** to pulmonary disease. Symptoms are variable, but when present they most often consist of pain and diarrhea. (**Primary** tuberculosis, not secondary tuberculosis mimics colon cancer.) The diagnosis is made by barium enema examination; confirmation is obtained by documenting the patient's response to antitubercular therapy. Antitubercular chemotherapy effectively allows healing of the lesion, and operation is contraindicated except for the complications of perforation, obstruction, or hemorrhage.

ANSWER: A, B, C

12. Regarding typhoid enteritis, which of the following statements is/are true?

A. The diagnosis can be made by culturing *Salmonella typhi* from the blood or stool.
B. Chloramphenicol is the preferred drug for treatment.
C. Bleeding requiring operative intervention occurs in 10–20% of patients.
D. Steroids should be used in patients who are toxic and who fail to respond after several days of antibiotic therapy.

Ref.: 2

COMMENTS: Typhoid enteritis, a systemic infection caused by *S. typhi*, is accompanied by fever, headache, cough, maculopapular rash, abdominal pain, and leukopenia. There is hyperplasia and ulceration of Peyer's patches, mesenteric lymphadenopathy, and splenomegaly. Chloramphenicol no longer is the drug of choice because of the emergence of resistant strains of bacteria and the risk of marrow toxicity. Currently, trimethoprim and sulfamethoxazole are preferred. Patients who remain toxic after 1 week of therapy often benefit from a short course of prednisone. Bleeding occurs in 10–20% of patients and usually is treated with transfusion. Perforation through ulcerated Peyer's patches occurs in 2% of patients and is most often free, solitary, and located in the terminal ileum. Operative closure and appropriate peritoneal toilet is required; occasionally, the perforations are multiple, necessitating intestinal resection with primary anastomosis.

ANSWER: A, D

13. With regard to benign tumors of the small intestine, which of the following statements is/are true?

A. Most are found in the ileum.
B. Often they produce no symptoms and are difficult to diagnose by either clinical or radiologic examination.
C. The most common clinical manifestations are bleeding and obstruction.
D. They obstruct the bowel by encroachment on the lumen or by causing intussusception.

Ref.: 1, 2

COMMENTS: The types and relative frequency of benign neoplasms of the small intestine vary among series, but common lesions include leiomyoma, lipoma, adenoma, and hemangioma. About 15% occur in the duodenum, 25% in the jejunum, and 60% in the ileum, usually the distal third. Often benign neoplasms are asymptomatic; when symptoms are present, they are vague and nonspecific. Bleeding and obstruction are the two most common symptoms; the bleeding usually is occult and intermittent and may even lead to iron-deficiency anemia. Leiomyoma and hemangioma are the lesions that most often bleed. The differential diagnosis of small bowel bleeding should include hereditary hemorrhagic telangiectasis (Osler-Rendu-Weber syndrome). Intussusception in adults usually has an organic cause; 50% of cases are caused by benign small bowel neoplasms. When small bowel neoplasms are suspected, barium small bowel follow-through is indicated and usually is diagnostic. When identified, small bowel tumors should be excised because of the risk of complications and the possibility that they are malignant.

ANSWER: A, B, C, D

14. A 26-year-old man presents in the emergency room with the complaint of recurrent, colicky, midabdominal pain. Physical examination reveals a palpable abdominal mass and several areas of increased pigmentation on his lips, palms, and soles. He states that his father had a colon polyp removed several years ago. Which of the following is the most likely diagnosis?

A. Familial polyposis with malignant degeneration.
B. Gardner syndrome with intussusception.
C. Peutz-Jeghers syndrome with intussusception.
D. Symptomatic Crohn's disease.

Ref.: 1, 2

COMMENTS: Peutz-Jeghers syndrome is an autosomal dominant familial disease characterized by intestinal polyposis and mucocutaneous hyperpigmentation. The polyps are hamartomas that most frequently are located in the jejunum and ileum, but they also can be found in the stomach, duodenum, colon, and rectum. It is generally believed that their malignant potential is extremely low. Peutz-Jeghers syndrome can produce abdominal symptoms caused by intussusception or hemorrhage; up to one third of patients present with abdominal pain and a palpable mass. An operation is indicated for obstruction or bleeding; it should be limited to conservative resection of the involved portion of the bowel rather than be an attempt to resect all polyps detected during exploration.

ANSWER: C

15. With regard to malignant small bowel tumors, which of the following statements is/are true?

A. They account for 2% of all GI malignancies.
B. Carcinoid is the most common malignancy of the small intestine.
C. The 5-year survival rate is highest with adenocarcinoma, followed by lymphoma and leiomyosarcoma.
D. Wide resection with regional lymphadenectomy is the correct operation.

Ref.: 2

COMMENTS: Malignant tumors of the small bowel account for 2% of all GI malignancies. The most frequent type is adenocarcinoma, followed in decreasing frequency by carcinoid, lymphoma, and sarcoma, principally leiomyosarcoma. Although adenocarcinoma occurs with equal frequency in the duodenum, jejunum, and ileum, the other types tend to occur most often in the ileum. Their clinical manifestations may include any combination of diarrhea, obstruction, or chronic blood loss with anemia. The preferred therapy is wide resection with regional lymphadenectomy. For each entity, survival is dependent on a number of factors and is variable, but in general leiomyosarcomas and lymphomas are associated with the highest 5-year survival rates (about 40%) and adenocarcinoma with the lowest (about 20%). Postoperative chemotherapy and radiation therapy can be useful for treating a patient with lymphoma but are not useful adjuncts for adenocarcinoma or sarcoma. Histiocytic lymphoma may develop in patients with long-standing celiac sprue and has a worse prognosis than conventional small bowel lymphomas. The Mediterranean-type lymphoma, a lymphoma variant associated with monoclonal alpha heavy chains and a dense plasma cell tumor infiltration, also carries a bad prognosis.

ANSWER: A, D

16. Which of the following statements regarding carcinoid tumors is/are true?

A. The cell of origin is the Kupffer cell.
B. The rectum is the most common site of origin.
C. There is a tendency toward multicentricity.
D. Prognosis is related to tumor size, location, and histologic pattern.

Ref.: 1, 2, 3

COMMENTS: The origin of carcinoid tumors is the Kulchitsky cell, which is thought to arise from the neural crest. Carcinoids can occur anywhere in the GI tract; the most frequent site is the appendix, followed by the ileum and the rectum. Extraintestinal sites include the bronchus and ovary. Small bowel carcinoid tumors tend to be multiple in 30% of cases, and a second GI tumor of another histologic type can be found in 30%. The prognosis is a function of the size of the tumor and its site of origin. Ileal carcinoids tend to metastasize more commonly than those that originate in the appendix. Ileal tumors less than 1 cm in diameter have a 20–30% incidence of nodal metastasis (metastasis not seen in appendiceal carcinoid <1 cm). Ileal tumors 1–2 cm in diameter have a 60–80% incidence of nodal metastases (0–11% for appendix), and tumors larger than 2 cm have a more than 80% incidence of nodal metastases (30–60% for appendix). Recent information suggests that the histologic pattern also may affect prognosis: Patients with well-differentiated lesions fare better than those with small-cell, anaplastic lesions.

ANSWER: C, D

17. With regard to carcinoid tumors and their surgical management, which of the following statements is/are true?

A. They produce a characteristic luminal deformity seen on barium examination.
B. They are usually easily palpable on external physical examination of the bowel.
C. Often their metastases are much larger than the primary tumor.
D. Resection is not indicated when there is metastatic disease.

Ref.: 1, 2, 3

COMMENTS: The usual submucosal location of carcinoid tumors often makes them difficult to find on radiographic examination or with cursory palpation during an exploratory laparotomy. The tumors are sometimes associated with a surrounding fibrosis that can produce luminal narrowing. Mesenteric lymph node metastases can be large, and they may be accompanied by an extensive desmoplastic reaction that results in fixation and kinking of the bowel. Tumors less than 1 cm in diameter and without demonstrable metastases can be treated by excision or segmental resection. Those larger than 1 cm or with regional metastases should be excised widely; this excision should include right hemicolectomy for lesions of the distal ileum and appendix. In patients with metastases and in whom the carcinoid syndrome is present, removal of as much of the tumor mass as is resectable can provide significant palliation.

ANSWER: C

18. Concerning the clinical manifestations of the carcinoid syndrome, which of the following statements is/are true?

A. Episodic manifestations include cutaneous flushing, hyperperistalsis, diarrhea, and asthma.
B. Cardiac manifestations occur early and primarily affect the mitral and aortic valves.
C. Cutaneous phenomena are the most characteristic and frequently recognized manifestations.
D. Diarrhea is a significant complaint in fewer than 30% of patients.
E. Asthmatic attacks occur in most patients.

Ref.: 1, 2, 3

COMMENTS: Episodic manifestations of the carcinoid syndrome include flushing, diarrhea, and asthma. The cutaneous manifestations are the most common and consist of episodes of flushing of the face, neck, arms, and upper trunk, occasionally accompanied by vasomotor collapse. Diarrhea is significant in more than 80% of patients and usually is sudden in onset, watery, and accompanied by cramping pain and borborygmi. Asthmatic attacks occur in 25% of patients. Manifestations of long-standing involvement include the development of facial hyperemia with telangiectasias of the cheeks, nose, and forehead; development of the cutaneous lesions of pellagra; and valvular heart disease. The valves most commonly involved are the tricuspid and pulmonic, although the mitral and aortic valves are sometimes affected. Peripheral edema is present in about 70% of patients and can occur in the absence of valvular disease.

ANSWER: A, C

19. With regard to carcinoid syndrome, which of the following statements is/are true?

A. Carcinoid tumors, which produce serotonin, consume up to 60% of dietary tryptophan.
B. The most useful diagnostic test for suspected carcinoid syndrome is the determination of serum serotonin levels.
C. Patients with normal serotonin levels do not develop carcinoid syndrome.
D. 5-Hyroxyindoleacetic acid (5-HIAA) is the active form of serotonin.

Ref.: 1, 2, 3

COMMENTS: Functioning carcinoid tumors divert up to 60% of dietary tryptophan in the production of serotonin, thereby contributing to the development of pellagra and protein deficiency. Serotonin is metabolized in the liver to 5-HIAA, which then is excreted into the urine. For this reason, the most useful diagnostic test in patients suspected of having a carcinoid tumor is the determination of 5-HIAA in a 24-hour collection of urine. Serotonin, produced by tumors located in organs that are drained by the portal system, is converted to inactive 5-HIAA, which, because it is inactive, does not cause carcinoid syndrome. A tumor therefore may produce large amounts of serotonin without causing the syndrome, because the liver metabolizes serotonin to an inactive substrate. The carcinoid syndrome is produced by release of serotonin into the systemic circulation by liver metastases or by tumors outside the portal distribution. Whereas it is generally believed that patients with carcinoid syndrome have tumors that produce serotonin, the role of serotonin in the mediation of the syndrome is not clear. Not all patients with elevated production of serotonin have the syndrome; some patients with the syndrome have normal levels of 5-HIAA in the urine, and injection of pure serotonin does not create all of the manifestations of the disease. It is likely that carcinoid tumors have the capacity to produce a number of biologically active peptides, which accounts for the variability of the syndrome and discrepancies between a patient's serotonin levels and the clinical presentation. Other substances produced by carcinoid tumors include histamine, dopamine, kallikrein, substance P, prostaglandins, and neuropeptide K.

ANSWER: A

20. Regarding the treatment of carcinoid syndrome, which of the following statements is/are true?

A. Exploration is indicated in nearly all patients with malignant carcinoid syndrome.
B. The antiserotonin agents methysergide, cyproheptadine, and *p*-chlorophenylalanine may be helpful for controlling bowel symptoms.
C. Phenothiazines and α-adrenergic blockers may ameliorate flushing attacks.
D. Occasionally, corticosteroid therapy can decrease the symptoms of carcinoid syndrome.
E. In some patients with carcinoid syndrome and unresectable tumor, a combination of streptozotocin and 5-fluorouracil (5-FU) can provide palliation through their antineoplastic effect.

Ref.: 2

COMMENTS: As previously stated, exploration may be worthwhile in patients with carcinoid syndrome and noncurable metastasis because in many patients even subtotal tumor excision can provide relief of symptoms for prolonged periods. A number of pharmacologic agents can be used to ameliorate the symptoms; a combination of streptozotocin and 5-FU has provided palliation of the syndrome in some patients.

ANSWER: A, B, C, D, E

21. Somatostatin has emerged as a safe and effective agent with a broad range of applications. These applications include which of the following for patients with carcinoid tumors?

A. Somatostatin may be used as a provocative agent prior to measuring 5-HIAA levels.
B. Somatostatin receptor scintigraphy is more efficacious at localizing primary and metastatic carcinoid tumors than computed tomography (CT) or magnetic resonance imaging (MRI).
C. Somatostatin is ineffective for management of carcinoid crisis.
D. Somatostatin therapy improves survival in patients with carcinoid syndrome.
E. Somatostatin therapy response may be predicted by the results of somatostatin receptor scintigraphy.

Ref.: 1, 3

COMMENTS: Somatostatin was first identified in 1973. Since then, a great deal of interest has been directed at characterizing and identifying the physiologic effects and the clinical utility of somatostatin and its analogues. Somatostatin is a 14-amino-acid protein with several analogues of shorter length that maintain clinical effectiveness. The general effects of somatostatin are those of an inhibitory hormone. • Several provocative agents may be used prior to conducting tests for neuroendocrine tumors, including pentagastrin, secretin, and calcium infusion. Somatostatin is not effective as a provocative agent. • Somatostatin receptor scintigraphy is a new modality using indium[111] pentreotide and a gamma camera. This study has several advantages over conventional imaging with CT or MRI. The sensitivity of this study is higher (80–90%) than that for CT scan (60–70%) when defining metastatic disease. Furthermore, somatostatin receptor scintigraphy is more effective for identifying the primary tumor site and visualizing the entire body to detect metastases in clinically occult sites. Carcinoid tumors visible by somatostatin receptor scintigraphy suggest that these particular tumors manifest somatostatin receptors and are therefore subject to the inhibitory effects of somatostatin. • Carcinoid crisis is a life-threatening attack that may occur during episodes of flushing, anesthesia, or surgery. Severe hypotension and bronchospasm may result during carcinoid crisis, and they may be refractory to the usual supportive care. The reported incidence of such crises is variable, between 2% and 50%. Somatostatin may be administered preoperatively as a prophylactic agent or during a carcinoid crisis as a therapeutic agent. It is usually successful in reversing the condition. • Somatostatin has also been found to be highly effective for relieving symptoms of carcinoid syndrome. It has even been suggested that chronic octreotide therapy results in longer survival for patients with carcinoid syndrome compared with survival for patients treated with chemotherapy, but this hypothesis remains to be proved by randomized, controlled trials.

ANSWER: B, E

22. With regard to Meckel's diverticulum, which of the following statements is/are true?

A. They are found in various anatomic forms and clinical presentations in 50% of the population.
B. They are true diverticula.
C. Some can be visualized on technetium 99m pertechnetate (^{99m}Tc) scans.
D. Most complications occur in the elderly.
E. Diverticulitis is the most common complication.

Ref.: 1, 2

COMMENTS: Meckel's diverticulum is the most frequently encountered diverticulum of the small intestine; it occurs in 2–4% of the general population. It is a true diverticulum, arising from the antimesenteric border of the ileum, 50–75 cm from the ileocecal valve. Often there is a persistent band of tissue extending from the tip of the diverticulum to the umbilicus. • Sometimes the diverticulum contains ectopic gastric mucosa capable of producing peptic ulceration and bleeding in adjacent ileal mucosa. This ectopic gastric mucosa can be visualized using ^{99m}Tc scans. • Clinical problems most often present in the pediatric population. The most frequent complications are bleeding, intussusception, and obstruction; the latter usually is caused by volvulus or kinking around the persistent band. The least common manifestation is diverticulitis, which presents clinically as lower abdominal pain and usually is diagnosed as appendicitis. • Therapy consists of diverticulectomy for uncomplicated diverticulitis and segmental ileal resection for bleeding or for complicated diverticulitis. Prophylactic diverticulectomy generally is not performed when a diverticulum is found incidentally unless there is evidence of ectopic gastric mucosa or the neck of the diverticulum is narrow.

ANSWER: B, C

23. Concerning duodenal, jejunal, and ileal diverticula, which of the following statements is/are true?

A. Duodenal diverticula are true diverticula.
B. Duodenal diverticula often are multiple, whereas jejunal diverticula are often solitary.
C. Asymptomatic duodenal diverticula should be resected to avoid potentially serious complications.
D. Asymptomatic jejunal diverticula do not require therapy.

Ref.: 2

COMMENTS: Diverticula of the duodenum, jejunum, and ileum are false (pulsion) diverticula containing only mucosa, submucosa, and serosa. Duodenal diverticula usually are solitary and project medially toward the head of the pancreas. Although most are asymptomatic, 10% of patients present with nonspecific epigastric symptoms such as bleeding and perforation. In instances of perforation the local site should be drained; gastrojejunostomy is the operation most often applicable, although occasionally biliary decompression is necessary. In instances of bleeding without inflammation, diverticulectomy is indicated, either from a dorsal approach utilizing the Kocher maneuver or via a duodenotomy. • Jejunal and ileal diverticula are often multiple and project from the mesenteric border of the bowel into the leaves of the mesentery. This type of diverticulum is more common in the jejunum than in the ileum. The usual treatment for symptomatic diverticula in these areas is segmental resection. Asymptomatic diverticula of the duodenum, jejunum, or ileum do not require therapy.

ANSWER: D

24. A 56-year-old woman has a history of pelvic radiation therapy 5 years ago for cervical cancer. Now, 5 days after she underwent a right hemicolectomy for a villous adenoma of the cecum, her surgical wound is red and tender. You open her wound, and the initial drainage is obviously purulent; she becomes afebrile. The drainage persists as a continuous brown, liquid discharge. Which of the following is the most likely diagnosis?

A. Simple wound infection.
B. Clostridial infection.
C. Anastomotic leakage with enterocutaneous fistula.
D. Dehiscence.

Ref.: 2

COMMENTS: Most fistulas are iatrogenic and result from anastomotic leakage, inadvertent injury to the bowel during the operation, laceration of the bowel during abdominal closure, or retained foreign bodies. Fewer than 2% of fistulas are the result of diseased bowel; when they are, the most common contributing factors are preoperative radiation therapy, intestinal obstruction, and inflammatory bowel disease. Although small bowel fistulas occasionally lead to generalized peritonitis, they most commonly produce a walled-off abscess that presents as an infection of the operative incision. The initial drainage may be purulent; however, if the infection is caused by anastomotic leakage of the small bowel, the drainage becomes enteric within 1–2 days.

ANSWER: C

25. For the patient described in Question 24, which of the following might be included in appropriate initial management?

A. Packing of the subcutaneous tissue with wet-to-dry dressings.
B. Packing of the subcutaneous tissue with dry, absorbent dressings.
C. Placing a rubber sump catheter attached to suction.
D. Protecting the skin around the fistula with Stomahesive karaya powder, aluminum paste, or zinc oxide and collecting the draining fluid in an attached plastic bag.
E. Inserting a nasogastric tube and administering appropriate intravenous fluids.

***Ref.*:** 2

COMMENTS: The initial management of a small bowel fistula includes the administration of appropriate intravenous fluids, proximal decompression with nasogastric suction, control and quantification of the fistula output, and protection of the surrounding skin. Fistulas are classified according to their location and to the volume of their output. Proximal fistulas tend to have a higher output and lead to more severe electrolyte and fluid imbalance. Nasogastric suction can be helpful in diminishing the output of proximal intestinal fistulas, but the output of those more distal in the gut may not be influenced by this maneuver. Sump catheters can provide a means of controlling and quantifying high-output fistulas, especially early in their formation. Once the fistula tract is established, suction catheters should be replaced with a stoma appliance fixed to the edges of the fistula. Enteric contents are highly corrosive, and the skin surrounding the fistula opening should be carefully protected. Gauze dressings are generally ineffective at absorbing all the drainage and protecting the skin. Therefore, their use is generally avoided. Most well established fistulas do not produce sepsis, but in patients with persistent fever, systemic administration of antibiotics and a careful search for an undrained abdominal abscess are indicated.

ANSWER: C, D, E

26. After the first several days, a diagnostic workup of the patient described in Question 24 should be performed to localize the fistula. Which of the following procedures should be included in the workup?

A. Upper GI series with small bowel follow-through.
B. Fluoroscopic examination of the colon with contrast material.
C. Instillation of contrast material via a catheter into the fistula.
D. CT scan of the abdomen.

***Ref.*:** 2

COMMENTS: Localizing the position of the fistula can be achieved with a combination of the tests listed above. In addition, instillation of contrast material through the fistula opening helps define the extent of the associated abscess cavity if one is present.

ANSWER: A, B, C, D

27. Diagnostic workup of the woman described in Question 24 reveals that she has a distal ileal fistula in communication with an associated small cavity. Which of the following is/are appropriate therapy?

A. Prompt exploration and interruption of the fistula tract.
B. Prompt exploration and bypass of the fistula.
C. Prompt exploration, with resection of the portion of ileum involved in the fistula and primary reanastomosis.
D. A 4- to 6-week trial of intravenous hyperalimentation.
E. A 4- to 6-week trial of low-residue or elemental enteral alimentation.

***Ref.*:** 2

COMMENTS: Knowing the location of the fistula is of important prognostic and therapeutic value. The overall mortality rate for small bowel fistulas is 20%; the rate is higher for jejunal fistulas and lower for those of the ileum. With proper supportive care, such as intravenous or enteral alimentation, and in the absence of distal obstruction, up to 40% of small bowel fistulas close spontaneously. Enteral alimentation has the advantage of avoiding the possible hepatic and septic complications of prolonged total parenteral nutrition. Even if there is a slight increase in fistula output after the start of enteral nutrition, the fistula still may close. Fistulas of the proximal jejunum may require transnasal insertion of a long tube through the stomach and duodenum and just beyond the fistula before starting enteral alimentation. The preferred operation for correcting a persistent fistula is resection of the fistula in continuity with the segment of involved bowel, followed by a primary anastomosis. Alternative therapies include complete or partial exclusion with primary anastomosis. After resolution of the inflammation, the isolated loop of bowel is excised. Simple bypass of the fistula without exclusion is avoided.

ANSWER: D, E

28. With regard to the blind-loop syndrome, which of the following statements is/are correct?

A. It manifests as abdominal pain, diarrhea, malabsorption, and vitamin deficiencies.
B. Bacteria successfully compete for vitamin B_{12}, which may lead to megaloblastic anemia.
C. Bacterial deconjugation of the bile salts can lead to steatorrhea.
D. Addition of intrinsic factor in the Schilling test causes urinary vitamin B_{12} excretion to return to normal.
E. The addition of tetracycline in the Schilling test causes urinary vitamin B_{12} excretion to return to normal.

***Ref.*:** 1, 2

COMMENTS: The blind-loop syndrome is caused by stasis of intestinal contents with subsequent bacterial overgrowth. This stasis can be caused by a number of abnormalities, including stricture, stenosis, fistula, diverticula, or the formation of a blind pouch. The syndrome presents with steatorrhea, diarrhea, anemia, weight loss, abdominal pain, multiple vitamin deficiencies, joint pains, and occasionally neurologic disorders. The steatorrhea is the result of bile salt deconjugation that takes place in the stagnant fluid in the blind loop of bowel. Megaloblastic anemia probably is a result of successful competition by the bacteria for vitamin B_{12}. The Schilling test reveals a type of urinary excretion of vitamin B_{12} similar to that seen with pernicious anemia, except it is not corrected by addition of intrinsic factor but is corrected with the use of oral tetracycline. Although the administration of tetracycline and parenteral vitamin B_{12} can correct megaloblastic anemia, surgical correction of the cause of the bowel stasis is curative.

ANSWER: A, B, C, E

29. Select the correct statement(s) in regard to the short-bowel syndrome.

A. Serious nutritional deficits are produced with resection of the entire jejunum.
B. Abnormal absorption of fat, vitamin B_{12}, electrolytes, and water constitutes the four major nutritional derangements.
C. Resection of up to 70% of the bowel can be tolerated if the terminal ileum and ileocecal valve are preserved.
D. Relative gastric hyposecretion with increased intestinal pH in conjunction with interruption of the enterohepatic bile salt circulation is the cause of steatorrhea.

Ref.: 2

COMMENTS: The entire jejunum can be resected without adverse nutritional sequelae. The entire ileum can be resected without harm so long as vitamin B_{12} is replaced postoperatively. Up to 70% of the small bowel can be safely resected if the terminal ileum and ileocecal valve are left intact; if they are resected, however, loss of 50–60% of the small bowel can lead to severely compromised nutrition. The deficiencies created by extensive resection of the small bowel are vitamin B_{12} malabsorption, altered fat absorption, and fluid and electrolyte problems. Vitamin B_{12} malabsorption leads to vitamin B_{12} deficiency and megaloblastic anemia. Altered fat absorption produces steatorrhea as a result of several factors: (1) Massive small bowel resection leads to gastric hypersecretion; decreased bowel pH stimulates the intestine, thereby shortening transit time and interfering with absorption of ingested fat. (2) Interruption of bile salt resorption interferes with micelle formation. (3) The unabsorbed fats are irritating to the colonic mucosa, thereby increasing the diarrhea and steatorrhea associated with the syndrome. Fluid and electrolyte problems are a function of the shortened transit time and the diarrhea that results from loss of small bowel absorptive area.

ANSWER: B, C

30. With regard to short-bowel syndrome, which of the following statements is/are true?

A. Initial therapy consists of control of diarrhea, restriction of oral intake, and intravenous administration of nutrients, fluid, and electrolytes.
B. Diarrhea is best controlled by administration of medium-chain triglycerides.
C. The administration of oral bile salts is of central importance in controlling steatorrhea.
D. Vagotomy/pyloroplasty and reversal of a segment of bowel are the two most important operations for early management of short-bowel syndrome.

Ref.: 1, 2

COMMENTS: Treatment of short-bowel syndrome centers on control of diarrhea and parenteral maintenance of nutrition. With time (2–3 years), the mucosa of as little as 30–45 cm of small bowel may undergo enough hypertrophy to allow withdrawal of intravenous alimentation and the start of carefully modified oral feedings. Treatment with growth hormone, glutamine and fiber has had some promising results in terms of gut regeneration. Diarrhea can be controlled with agents such as Lomotil or codeine, which slow intestinal motility. Oral calcium carbonate is also useful and acts by neutralizing hydrochloric acid and free fatty acids. When oral intake is resumed, dietary fat is restricted to 30–50 gm daily. Some patients benefit from the use of medium-chain triglycerides. Oral bile salts are tolerated and aid in the formation of micelles in some patients, whereas in others they cause increased diarrhea. Cholestyramine, an agent that sequesters bile acids, is useful in patients who have had less than 100 cm of small bowel resected. There is no standard approach to the resumption of oral intake, and the treatment must be highly individualized. Whereas some patients ultimately do well with a modified oral diet, others remain dependent on permanent parenteral nutrition. There are no operative procedures that reliably correct this problem, therefore operative treatment should be considered only in patients who cannot maintain their body weight to within 30% of normal without intravenous supplementation. Operations that may be useful are reversal of a segment of intestine, creation of a recirculating loop of small bowel, creation of an artificial sphincter, vagotomy and pyloroplasty, correction of bowel obstruction, and placing all bowel in continuity. Vagotomy and pyloroplasty is rarely performed for short-bowel syndrome since the introduction of H_2 blockers and protein pump inhibitors. Allotransplantation of small bowel in humans has been successfully performed but has a high failure rate and remains experimental.

ANSWER: A

31. The following medications may be used in the medical management of inflammatory bowel diseases. Match each medication in the left column with the associated possible complication in the right column.

A. Prednisone	a. Neutropenia
B. 5-Acetylsalicylic acid (5-ASA)	b. Peripheral neuropathy
C. Metronidazole	c. Diabetes mellitus
D. Cyclosporine	d. Renal failure
E. 6-Mercaptopurine and azathioprine	e. Watery diarrhea

Ref.: 4

COMMENTS: Systemic corticosteroids are used for management of Crohn's disease and severe ulcerative colitis. The initial dose of oral prednisone may vary from 40 to 60 mg per day. The onset of diabetes mellitus may complicate steroid therapy, and some patients require insulin therapy while on high doses of prednisone. The other common side effects are fluid retention, hypertension, mood swings, acne, and with long-term use osteoporosis, aseptic necrosis, and cataracts. • 5-ASA products are now used to treat Crohn's colitis and ulcerative colitis. The oral forms are replacing sulfasalazine to avoid side effects attributed to the sulfa moiety. One disturbing side effect seen with 5-ASA has been watery diarrhea, which occurs in 15–30% of patients. • Metronidazole is used for treatment of Crohn's disease, particularly when perianal disease and fistulas are present. It has been used also for treatment of pouchitis after ileoanal anastomosis. At high doses (>1.5 g/day) metronidazole has been associated with GI upset and peripheral neuropathy. Use of metronidazole (Flagyl) should be avoided during pregnancy because of its teratogenic effects. Alcohol should be avoided while using metronidazole, as a disulfiram-like reaction may develop. • Cyclosporine is an experimental medication that has been used in cases of severe refractory ulcerative colitis and rarely for Crohn's disease. Renal function deterioration and hypertension can be seen at the recommended doses, which limits its use. • 6-Mercaptopurine and azathioprine are immunosuppressive medications that can be used to allow a decrease in corticosteroid dose (i.e., steroid-sparing effect). In particular, 6-mercaptopurine can be used in Crohn's disease patients with fistula. The use of these agents to maintain Crohn's remission is controversial. Neutropenia and bone marrow depression is seen in 2% of patients and pancreatitis has been described. Secondary malignancies are rare.

ANSWER: A-c; B-e; C-b; D-d; E-a

32. The rational use of corticosteroids for medical management of idiopathic inflammatory bowel disease is based on which of the following statements?

A. Corticosteroids are safe to use in pregnant patients with an acute flare-up of Crohn's disease.
B. Corticosteroids effectively maintain remission of Crohn's colitis and ulcerative colitis.
C. Corticosteroids used in enema (topical) form are not absorbed into the systemic circulation and therefore have no systemic side effects.
D. Every-other-day therapy is effective in these patients.
E. Intravenous corticosteroids and adrenocorticotropic hormone (ACTH) are equally effective in patients with acute severe ulcerative colitis that is refractory to oral treatment.
F. Corticosteroid therapy can be used to control flare-ups, depending on their severity, for 4–8 weeks; the dose is then tapered for another 4–8 weeks, with the goal of discontinuation.

Ref.: 4

COMMENTS: The use of steroids in patients with an acute flare-up of Crohn's colitis or ulcerative colitis during pregnancy has been shown to be not only effective but also safe for the mother and fetus. The same statements apply to sulfasalazine. • Corticosteroids have never been shown to maintain remission of Crohn's colitis or ulcerative colitis. Sulfasalazine and the newer 5-ASA products olsalazine and coated 5-ASA are effective in maintaining remission only of ulcerative colitis. • Topical steroids in foam or enema preparations might be absorbed in small amounts (10–20%). Alternate-day dosing has not been effective in most patients with inflammatory bowel disease. • Intravenous ACTH is preferred to intravenous hydrocortisone by some, but controversy still exists regarding whether ACTH is more effective even for previously untreated ulcerative colitis. An ACTH dose of 40–60 units over 8 hours appears to be as effective as 300–400 mg of hydrocortisone per day. • The duration of steroid therapy varies depending on the severity of the disease, but it should always be tapered on an individual basis with the goal of discontinuation. Many patients (10–15%) are kept on a low maintenance dose when complete elimination leads to flare-up. This situation should not be confused with the incorrect practice of continuing a maintenance dose in patients who have achieved complete remission. Some consider failure to achieve remission after 2 months of administering more than 15 mg of prednisone an indication for surgery.

ANSWER: A, E, F

33. In patients with inflammatory bowel disease *refractory to medical treatment*, nutritional support may influence the course of disease. Which of the following statements is/are true?

A. Bowel rest and parenteral nutrition comprise the primary therapy for Crohn's colitis.
B. Parenteral nutrition helps prevent the need for total colectomy in patients with ulcerative colitis.
C. In patients with Crohn's ileitis, total parenteral nutrition (TPN) helps maintain lean body mass.
D. In those with Crohn's disease with high output fistula, TPN promotes fistula closing.
E. Elemental diet is the primary therapy for exacerbation of Crohn's disease.

Ref.: 5

COMMENTS: TPN has no role as primary therapy for ulcerative colitis, but it may help maintain a satisfactory nutritional state during bowel rest. TPN does not help prevent the need for colectomy in cases refractory to medical treatment. The role of TPN in patients with Crohn's colitis is not well established, but in those with Crohn's colitis and small bowel involvement TPN may induce remission and promote fistula closure. Elemental diets have been shown by some to be effective in inducing remission of active Crohn's disease. Patient tolerance may be poor, however, and results are not superior to those obtained with corticosteroids and sulfasalazine. Peripheral intravenous alimentation rarely provides adequate caloric replacement and may induce vein sclerosis and phlebitis.

ANSWER: C, D

34. A 30-year-old woman has a bowel obstruction secondary to Crohn's disease. She has had multiple previous small bowel resections. At laparotomy multiple strictures throughout the bowel are noted. Which of the following statements is/are true?

A. Strictureplasty should be considered only for cases in which there is an isolated stricture.
B. Strictureplasty is preferred to bowel resection at the initial laparotomy.
C. Anastomotic leak and fistula following strictureplasty has been seen in 50% of cases.
D. Restricture of the strictureplasty site has been seen in fewer than 5% of cases.
E. Because residual disease is left behind, reoperation for Crohn's disease is more likely with strictureplasty than for bowel resection.

Ref.: 6

COMMENTS: Strictureplasty for Crohn's disease was first performed in 1961; experience since then has shown it to be a safe alternative to resection in properly selected patients. Strictureplasty should be considered in any patient who has had extensive prior resections of diseased bowel and in whom further resection might create short-bowel syndrome. Multiple strictures can be safely treated at a single laparotomy; the entire small bowel must be inspected to avoid overlooking strictures that are not obvious. This can be accomplished by passing, via a proximal enterostomy, a long intestinal tube with the balloon inflated to 2 cm through the entire length of small bowel. Ideally, fibrotic rather than acute edematous strictures are treated. A longitudinal incision is made over the stricture and extended for 2 cm proximally and distally beyond the stricture. The enterotomy is then closed transversely. • If a stricture is encountered at a patient's first surgery, resection rather than strictureplasty is preferable, as it eliminates diseased bowel. However, in a small series patients treated by strictureplasty were compared with patients treated by resection. The need for reoperation for Crohn's disease at the original site was similar in the two groups. • Postoperative complications are low; at the Cleveland Clinic anastomotic leakage, abscess, or fistula has occurred in 9% of patients treated by strictureplasty; restricture of the strictureplasty site occurred in only 2%.

ANSWER: D

35. With regard to ileostomy physiology, which of the following statements is/are true?

A. Daily output from an established ileostomy is approximately 1500 ml/day.
B. Ileostomy output can increase by 50% at times of dietary indiscretion.
C. With dehydration, the concentration of the ileostomy sodium output rises.
D. Compared to normal ileal fluid, ileostomy effluent contains a 100-fold increase in number of aerobes and a 2500-fold increase in coliforms.

Ref.: 6

COMMENTS: The daily output from an established ileostomy is 500–800 ml/day. Although there is a great deal of variation in daily output among individuals, the output in a given patient varies only about 20% with changes in diet or with episodes of gastroenteritis. The usual ileostomy sodium concentration is 115 mEq/L, although the concentration rises and falls with changes in total body sodium. With dehydration, the sodium concentration falls and the potassium level rises, reflecting the ability of the terminal ileum to conserve sodium in times of salt depletion. Normally, the sodium/potassium ratio is about 12:1. • The microbiologic flora of ileostomy output is markedly different than that of normal ileal fluid. The total number of bacteria is 80 times greater; and there is a 100-fold increase in the number of aerobes, a 2500-fold increase in coliforms, and an increase in total anaerobes.

ANSWER: D

36. Which of the following statements about small bowel motility is/are true?

A. Oral feeding stimulates production of migrating motor complexes (MMCs).
B. If motility is impaired, absorption of nutrients is similarly affected.
C. The frequency of MMCs returns to normal within 6–24 hours after laparotomy.
D. Vagotomy-induced diarrhea is due to increased secretion secondary to denervation.
E. Segmental bowel resection causes a temporary interruption of the MMCs; the clinical results are usually insignificant.

Ref.: 3

COMMENTS: MMCs are propagated aboral peristaltic contractions occurring at 90-minute intervals. Activity fronts of MMCs usually originate high in the stomach, propagate distally, and end in the ileum, usually at the midileal level. • Oral feeding inhibits MMCs, resulting in irregular, nonpropagating contractions throughout most of the small intestine. This postprandial inhibition may persist 3–4 hours after a meal and is most pronounced with lipids. Although this motility pattern is disorganized, there is a distal progression of chyme. • Absorption is not affected by intestinal motility. Enteral feedings can therefore be safely and efficiently used in postoperative patients in which motility may be altered. • Both gastric and small bowel motility can be affected by exogenous conditions. The small bowel is less sensitive than the stomach to general anesthesia and laparotomy, each of which decreases the frequency of MMCs. The frequency of MMCs returns to normal within 6–24 hours in the absence of peritonitis or abscess formation. The tone of the stomach is affected more than that of the small bowel by general anesthesia and laparotomy, at times taking longer than 24 hours to normalize. This may explain the occurrence of postoperative nausea and emesis. Vagotomy-induced diarrhea is a result of persistence of the sustained, organized wave of MMCs during the postprandial state. • Segmental small bowel resection or denervation temporarily reduces the frequency of MMCs with a resultant temporary impairment of motility. Resection or denervation does not, however, produce long-term sequelae, provided intestinal length is not sacrificed.

ANSWER: C, E

37. A 60-year-old alcoholic man presents with a 24-hour history of nausea and vomiting, abdominal pain and distension, and decreased passage of stool and flatus. He had an abdominoperineal resection of the rectum for cancer 18 months ago with postoperative irradiation and chemotherapy. Examination reveals a distended, diffusely tender, tympanitic abdomen. Which of the following is the *least* likely diagnosis?

A. Pancreatitis with ileus.
B. Adhesive bowel obstruction.
C. Bowel obstruction due to extrinsic compression.
D. Bowel obstruction due to radiation injury.
E. Alcoholic hepatitis with ascites.

Ref.: 1, 2

COMMENTS: The classic presentation of bowel obstruction is the triad of nausea/vomiting, crampy abdominal pain, and decreased passage of stool and flatus. However, nonobstructive conditions may have a similar presentation. • **Ileus** is temporary paralysis of the bowel due to metabolic or neurofactors. *Electrolyte disorders* (especially hypokalemia) may cause paralytic ileus by disrupting the normal electrical activity of intestinal nerves and muscles. *Neuro reflexes*, which inhibit intestinal motor activity, may be caused by distension of a hollow viscus (ureter), retroperitoneal processes (hemorrhage, pancreatitis, spinal fracture), or peritonitis. • **Mechanical bowel obstruction** may be caused by a process extrinsic to the bowel wall, intrinsic to the bowel wall, or within the lumen of the bowel. *Extrinsic lesions* cause obstruction by kinking or compression of the lumen of the bowel. Intraabdominal adhesions form in up to 90% of patients after abdominal surgery and may also follow intraabdominal inflammatory conditions (diverticulitis, abscess). *Adhesions* may cause a fixed bend in the bowel or a tight band crossing a segment of bowel, or they can act as a focus for the bowel to twist upon itself (volvulus). Adhesions are the most common cause of small bowel obstruction in adults. The other two major categories of extrinsic bowel obstruction are hernias and masses. *Hernias* may be external (inguinal, femoral, ventral, perineal) or internal (due to congenital or surgical defects in the mesentery). Obstructing *masses* may be neoplastic (primary malignancy, carcinomatosis, desmoid tumor) or inflammatory (phlegmon, abscess). *Intrinsic lesions* may be congenital (atresia, duplication), anastomotic or inflammatory strictures (Crohn's disease, radiation injury, recovered ischemic bowel), or neoplastic (adenocarcinoma, melanoma, lymphoma, sarcoma). *Intraluminal lesions* that may cause bowel obstruction include intussusception and mass-like intraluminal contents (large gallstone, bezoar, inspissated barium, or stool). • Although abdominal distension may be due to ascites, its onset is much more gradual than 24 hours, and it is usually painless.

ANSWER: E

38. Which of the following statements is true regarding the radiographic appearance of small bowel obstruction?

A. Gas within the small bowel is distinguished from gas within the colon by luminal lines perpendicular to the bowel wall; the small bowel lines partially cross the lumen, whereas the colonic lines completely cross the lumen.
B. Ileus may be difficult to distinguish from small bowel obstruction, as both of these conditions can produce gas distension of the bowel with air-fluid levels.
C. The "string of pearls" sign refers to a series of radiolucent images in the small bowel representing the gallstones of gallstone ileus.
D. The gasless abdomen on plain films rules out a small bowel obstruction.
E. The distinction between complete and partial small bowel obstruction may be difficult during the early stages of presentation.

Ref.: 1, 2

COMMENTS: Plain radiographs of the abdomen are useful for evaluating patients with a possible diagnosis of small bowel obstruction. Gas-filled loops of small bowel are typically seen in the central portion of the abdomen. The presence of both dilated (>4 cm) and normal diameter (<2 cm) small bowel is typical of small bowel obstruction. Small bowel loops are recognized by the valvulae conniventes (plicae circulares), which are visible as lines that completely cross the lumen. Colonic loops are usually located peripherally and have lines within them that only partially cross the lumen (plicae semilunaris, haustra). • Air-fluid levels are seen with both small bowel obstruction and ileus. They are seen only on upright or decubitus views, which allow gravity to be directed perpendicular to the x-ray beam with pooling of intestinal fluid in the dependent portion of the bowel. • The "string of pearls" sign is a series of small radiolucent circles seen when a small amount of air at the top of an air-fluid level is broken up by several valvulae conniventes in a row. • A gasless abdomen may be seen in the presence of small bowel obstruction. It may be the result of decompression of the obstructed proximal bowel by emesis or nasogastric suctioning, or there may be a completely fluid-filled bowel with no visible air. • The distinction between partial and complete bowel obstruction is important. A partial obstruction is present when the patient is able to pass some gas and liquid stool beyond the obstruction. Radiographically, this condition is recognized by gas seen in decompressed bowel distal to the transition point. In contrast, complete small bowel obstruction manifests as an absence of flatus and stool (obstipation), and no gas is seen distal to the dilated proximal bowel. Early, complete bowel obstruction may be confused with partial obstruction, as distal gas and stool, present before the obstruction developed, have not yet been evacuated.

ANSWER: B, E

39. Initial treatment of the patient with acute, complete small bowel obstruction includes which of the following?

A. Immediate operation is warranted as soon as the diagnosis is made.
B. Nasogastric decompression for 24 hours allows spontaneous resolution of complete bowel obstruction in most patients.
C. The presence of fever, tachycardia, localized pain, or leukocytosis suggests strangulation and warrants prompt operation.
D. All patients with complete small bowel obstruction require blood and plasma for resuscitation.
E. If small bowel resection must be performed, a stoma and mucous fistula is necessary as anastomosis is unsafe.

Ref.: 1, 2

COMMENTS: Timing an operation for small bowel obstruction requires significant judgment. It is a balance between the need for resuscitation and for prevention of gangrene by prompt intervention. Severe intravascular volume depletion can occur owing to fluid sequestration (as much as 6 liters) in the lumen of the bowel and peritoneal cavity. Sodium, chloride, and potassium depletion frequently accompany bowel obstruction. Blood loss is unusual unless strangulation is present. Therefore prior to general anesthesia and operation, fluid and electrolyte replacement should be instituted with isotonic saline solution to normalize the heart rate, blood pressure, and urine output. Potassium repletion should begin once adequate urine output is established. Operation is delayed until the patient is stabilized and ready for general anesthesia. • Nasogastric decompression is an important component of supportive therapy of small bowel obstruction. Nausea and vomiting are controlled by this measure, and the risk of aspiration is reduced. Swallowed air is evacuated, limiting further intestinal distension. In cases of adhesive partial bowel obstruction without signs of strangulation (fever, tachycardia, localized abdominal pain, or leukocytosis) a 24- to 48-hour period of bowel rest and nasogastric decompression is warranted. The likelihood of strangulation is limited. In most patients the obstruction resolves spontaneously. Delay in surgical intervention for complete small bowel obstruction is not recommended, as the possibility of strangulation is much higher than with partial bowel obstruction. • There is no increase in the anastomotic leakage rate of small bowel anastomoses in urgent versus elective small bowel resections, providing the bowel used in the anastomosis is healthy. Therefore a proximal stoma and mucous fistula is seldom necessary following small bowel resection for obstruction.

ANSWER: C

REFERENCES

1. Sabiston DC Jr: *Textbook of Surgery*, 15th ed. WB Saunders, Philadelphia, 1997.
2. Schwartz SI, Shires GT, Spencer FC: *Principles of Surgery*, 7th ed. McGraw-Hill, New York, 1999.
3. Memon MA, Nelson H: Gastrointestinal carcinoid tumors: current management strategies. *Dis Colon Rectum* 40:1101–1118, 1997.
4. Sleisenger MH, Fordtran JS: *Gastrointestinal Disease: Pathophysiology, Diagnosis, Management*, 4th ed. WB Saunders, Philadelphia, 1989.
5. Wilson JD, Braunwald E, Isselbacher KJ, et al: *Harrison's Principles of Internal Medicine*, 12th ed. McGraw-Hill, New York, 1991.
6. Gordon PH, Nivatvongs, SH: *Principles and Practice of Surgery for the Colon, Rectum, Anus.* Quality Medical Publishing, St. Louis, 1992.

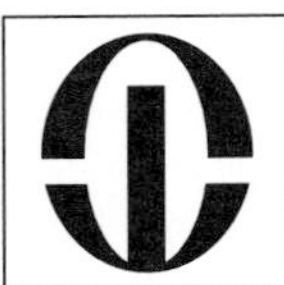

CHAPTER 29

Appendix

1. With regard to the function of the appendix, which of the following statements is/are true?

A. It is a vestigial organ with no known function.
B. It is a component of the secretory immune system.
C. Its immunologic function protects against the development of colon cancer.
D. The infantile appendix is the sole source of maturation for thymus-independent lymphocytes.

Ref.: 1, 2, 3, 4

COMMENTS: Although the appendix is dispensable, it functions as an immunologic organ, being part of the gut-associated lymphoid tissues (GALT) that secrete immunoglobulins. Lymphoid tissue appears in the appendix during infancy and involutes during adulthood. A few submucosal lymphoid follicles, present at birth, increase in number to a peak of 200 follicles at age 20; after age 60 they involute and may totally disappear. Concurrent with lymphoid atrophy is fibrosis, which obliterates the lumen in many older patients. Although there has been an increased incidence of colon cancer during the last several decades, there is no evidence that appendectomy predisposes to its development. • It has been postulated that the appendix, the tonsils, and Peyer's patches of the small intestine are sites where the processing of thymus-independent lymphocytes occurs in humans.

ANSWER: B

2. With regard to the appendix, which of the following statements is/are true?

A. In adults, its base is located at the apex of the cecum below the ileocecal valve.
B. The position of the tip in acute appendicitis may influence the presenting symptomatology.
C. The taeniae coli form its outer longitudinal muscle layer.
D. The lumen of the appendix is lined by colonic columnar epithelium.
E. The prodromal symptoms of appendicitis are unchanged in patients with malrotation of the cecum.

Ref.: 1, 2

COMMENTS: The relation of the base of the appendix to the cecum is relatively constant, but the position of the tip is variable. A low retrocecal position is found in 65% of patients; in about 30% the tip of the appendix is at the pelvis, and in the remaining 5% it lies in an extraperitoneal position, behind the cecum or the ascending colon. Malrotation of the cecum is associated with locations of the appendix anywhere between the right iliac fossae and the left upper quadrant and determines the location of the physical finding produced by the inflamed appendix against the parietal peritoneum. Because the embryologic origin of the colon and appendix remain unchanged, any prodromal symptoms are the same (i.e., anorexia, nausea, and vomiting). • Because the outer longitudinal muscular coat of the appendix is formed by the convergence of the taeniae coli, the anterior one in particular may be used as a landmark to find the appendix at operation. • The lumen of the appendix is lined by colonic columnar epithelium.

ANSWER: B, C, D, E

3. With regard to the pathogenesis of acute appendicitis, which of the following statements is/are true?

A. Fecaliths are identified in 90% of patients with uncomplicated appendicitis.
B. The amount of lymphoid tissue in the appendix is directly related to the incidence of acute appendicitis.
C. Luminal obstruction is the most important factor in the development of appendicitis.
D. The secretory capacity of the appendiceal mucosa is diminished in the elderly.
E. Gangrene of the appendix usually occurs at its base.

Ref.: 1, 2

COMMENTS: Appendicitis is initiated by obstruction of the lumen, which is commonly caused by a fecalith in adults and by lymphoid hyperplasia in children. Less commonly, inspissated barium, vegetable or fruit seeds, or parasites are the cause. Fecaliths have been identified in approximately 40% of patients with acute appendicitis, compared with 90% of patients with gangrenous appendicitis with rupture. • The amount of lymphoid tissue parallels the incidence of acute appendicitis, the peak for both occurring during the teenage years. • Following obstruction of the appendiceal lumen, bacterial infection ensues. The content of the lumen, degree of obstruction, mucosal secretory capacity, and degree of serosal fibrosis influence the resulting pathologic findings. Active secretion of mucus occurs after obstruction and may lead to a maximum intraluminal pressure of up to 126 cm H_2O after 14 hours of obstruction, leading to gangrene and perforation. • With appendiceal fibrosis, commonly seen in the elderly, there is diminished secretory capacity, which may account for the decreased incidence of appendicitis in this age group. • The area of the appendix with the poorest blood supply is the midportion of the antimesenteric border; hence this area most frequently shows evidence of gangrene and perforation.

ANSWER: B, C, D

4. With regard to the natural history of acute appendicitis, which of the following statements is/are true?

A. Rupture occurs most frequently in adolescent girls because of the difficulty establishing the diagnosis and the consequent delay in operation.
B. Perforation rates correlate with the severity of the initial illness.
C. Acute appendicitis does not resolve spontaneously.
D. Early antibiotic treatment decreases the incidence of perforation.
E. None of the above.

Ref.: 1, 2

COMMENTS: Although some episodes of acute appendicitis apparently resolve spontaneously and recurrent appendicitis is a recognized entity, the natural history of acute appendicitis is generally one of persistent obstruction leading to gangrene and perforation. Perforation occurs more commonly in patients at either end of the age spectrum, but clinical manifestations of the disease do not otherwise correlate with the risk of appendiceal rupture. Prompt appendectomy therefore is indicated when the diagnosis is made because it is the only certain way of preventing perforation and its attendant morbidity. Antibiotics are indicated for prophylaxis of infectious complications; nevertheless, antibiotics do not alter the natural history of the disease. Antibiotics should be directed against aerobic and anaerobic enteric bacteria, as they are most commonly involved in bacterial invasion of the appendix.

ANSWER: E

5. With regard to acute appendicitis, which of the following statements is/are true?

A. Anorexia is usually present.
B. Vomiting usually precedes pain.
C. Pain often begins in the periumbilical area.
D. Obstipation or diarrhea may occur.
E. All of the above.

Ref.: 1, 2

COMMENTS: Classically, abdominal pain, which begins in the periumbilical region and subsequently localizes to the right lower quadrant, is the hallmark of acute appendicitis. Distension of the appendix stimulates visceral afferent pain fibers, producing vague periumbilical pain of midgut origin; the inflammatory process eventually involves the serosa and the parietal peritoneum, producing the characteristic shift in pain to the right lower quadrant. Variations in the location of the appendix account for variations from the classic localization of somatic pain at McBurney's point (e.g., retrocecal appendix may cause flank or back pain). Atypical abdominal pain occurs in 45% of patients with proved appendicitis and is frequently found in the elderly and in patients receiving steroids or on chronic antibiotic therapy. Anorexia is a fairly constant symptom, and the diagnosis should be questioned if it is not present. Vomiting occurs in 75% of patients and typically follows the onset of pain. This sequence has diagnostic significance because in 95% of patients anorexia precedes the onset of pain and is followed by vomiting. Although many patients have vomiting, they have only one or two episodes. This is in contrast to the profuse and frequent vomiting seen in patients with gastroenteritis. • Variable patterns of bowel function may be seen and are usually not of diagnostic significance, although repeated diarrhea accompanied by vomiting is more suggestive of gastroenteritis than of appendicitis.

ANSWER: A, C, D

6. Which of the following is the most reliable physical finding associated with acute appendicitis?

A. Localized right lower quadrant tenderness.
B. Psoas sign.
C. Cutaneous hyperesthesia.
D. Tenderness on rectal examination.
E. All of the above are equally reliable.

Ref.: 1, 2

COMMENTS: Physical findings are determined by the anatomic location of the appendix and whether the appendix has already ruptured. With typical acute appendicitis, tenderness is maximal near McBurney's point, which is located one-third of the way from the anterior spinous process of the ilium to the umbilicus; however, the precise location of maximal tenderness varies with the position of the appendix, being more lateral or posterior with a retrocecal or retroperitoneal appendix and more medial or suprapubic with a pelvic location. Muscular resistance to palpation of the abdominal wall parallels the severity of the inflammatory process; as peritoneal irritation progresses, true reflex rigidity (in contrast to voluntary guarding) ensues. Following rupture of the appendix, physical findings are more defined; if the rupture is contained, a fullness in the lower quadrant is usually felt. Should the rupture fail to localize, tenderness becomes diffuse, and signs of spreading peritonitis occur. Fever higher than 38°C is unusual with simple appendicitis, and the temperature may even be normal; when ruptured appendicitis is present, the temperature is often above 38°C. • *Rovsing's* sign (pain in the right lower quadrant when pressure is exerted on the left lower quadrant), the *psoas* sign (pain on extension of the thigh), and the *obturator* sign (pain on flexion and internal rotation of the thigh) are indications of local peritoneal or retroperitoneal irritation. • Cutaneous hyperesthesia in the area supplied by the spinal nerves on the right at T-10, T-11, and T-12 is an inconstant finding but sometimes a helpful early sign. • A pelvic examination is essential in every female patient suspected of having appendicitis. Its primary purpose is to help exclude pelvic lesions such as ovarian cysts or tuboovarian processes. A rectal examination is most useful when an abscess or a phlegmon is present.

ANSWER: A

7. With regard to acute appendicitis, which of the following statements is/are true?

A. A normal total and differential white blood cell (WBC) count rules out the diagnosis of appendicitis.
B. The presence of white and red blood cells in the urine is compatible with the diagnosis of appendicitis.
C. The degree of abnormality in the total and differential WBC count correlates with the degree of appendiceal abnormality.

D. Symptoms of appendicitis and the finding of anemia should raise suspicion of a concomitant cecal neoplasm.
E. All of the above.

Ref.: 1, 2

COMMENTS: Moderate leukocytosis, ranging from 10,000 to 18,000/mm^3 with a moderate polymorphonuclear predominance, is typical for acute uncomplicated appendicitis. However, up to one-third of patients have a normal WBC count. The degree of abnormality in the serum WBC count does not correlate with the degree of pathologic findings with uncomplicated appendicitis, although counts higher than 18,000/mm^3 are frequently found with ruptured appendicitis. • Minimal albuminuria, some white blood cells, and even occasional red blood cells can be found in the urine of patients with appendicitis, particularly when the appendix is retrocecal. Nevertheless, patients with more than 30 red blood cells per field in a specimen of voided urine should be suspected of having urinary tract disease. The presence of bacteria in the urine does not exclude the diagnosis of appendicitis. • Anemia, particularly in the elderly, should raise suspicion for a carcinoma of the cecum. In cases of suspected appendicitis in which the laboratory findings are at variance with the clinical findings, the latter take precedence in terms of diagnostic value.

ANSWER: B, D

8. Which one or more of the following radiographic findings can be associated with the presence of acute appendicitis?

A. Distended loop of small bowel in the right lower quadrant.
B. Partial filling of the appendix with barium from a barium enema.
C. Gas-filled appendix.
D. Fecalith in the right lower quadrant.
E. Mass effect on the cecum with barium enema.

Ref.: 1, 2

COMMENTS: The diagnosis of acute appendicitis is usually based on the history and clinical findings, particularly when substantiated by laboratory findings of leukocytosis and normal urinalysis. Radiologic studies are useful in terms of the differential diagnosis and to demonstrate complications of appendicitis. Plain films may show cecal ileus. A radiopaque fecalith, the presence of gas in the lumen of the appendix, or the presence of a mass extrinsic to the cecum usually indicates a gangrenous, often perforated appendix. With complicated appendicitis, radiographs may reveal scoliosis toward the right as a result of spasm of the inflamed right paraspinal muscles, the absence of the right psoas shadow as a result of associated edema, the absence of small bowel gas in the right lower quadrant, or edema of the abdominal wall. • Barium enema examination may be helpful in selected patients, particularly in children or young women with abdominal pain in whom the diagnosis is obscure after observation. Complete filling of the appendix and absence of the mucosal changes in the region of the appendix can reliably exclude the diagnosis of appendicitis. This is especially true in children, whose appendix has a wider base than that in adults, in whom nonfilling of the appendix may represent fibrotic obliteration of the lumen. The false-negative rate of barium enema in selected cases is 10%. Pathognomonic findings of appendicitis on barium enema include nonfilling or partial filling of the appendix (the latter may be difficult to assess because of the variable length of the appendix) and a mass effect on the medial wall of the cecum (*reverse 3* sign).

ANSWER: A, B, C, D, E

9. Which of the following imaging techniques has been found to be useful for diagnosing acute appendicitis?

A. Ultrasonography.
B. Magnetic resonance imaging (MRI).
C. Gallium scan.
D. Computed tomography (CT) scan.
E. Positron emission tomography (PET) scan.

Ref.: 5, 6

COMMENTS: The diagnosis of appendicitis is largely based on a well performed, thorough history and physical examination. However, there remain many patients in whom the diagnosis is uncertain (young children, women of childbearing age, middle-aged and older patients). • The use of graded compression ultrasonography has been successfully applied to the diagnosis of appendicitis in equivocal cases of right lower quadrant pain. The appendix is visualized, and pain is then assessed as gradually increasing pressure is placed on the area of the appendix with the ultrasound probe. An abnormal appendix is defined as a tubular, immobile, noncompressible image; on transverse imaging it is seen as a target with an outer diameter at least 6 mm, a wall thickness at least 2 mm, or hyperechoic submucosa. Using these criteria, graded compression ultrasonography has high sensitivity (82%) and specificity (96%), with an overall accuracy of 88%. False-negative results are frequently associated with nonvisualization of the appendix. The advantages of this technique include wide accessibility, ability to identify other pathology responsible for pain, lack of ionizing radiation (for women of childbearing potential), and limited expense. Disadvantages include examiner variability and patient factors limiting the study (obesity, bowel gas, patient discomfort). • Focused appendix CT scanning has emerged as a useful diagnostic tool in cases of equivocal appendicitis. It involves administration of a limited amount of oral barium (up to 750 ml as tolerated 30 minutes before imaging) and Gastrografin via a rectal tube. Helical scanning with 5 mm images is then performed, limited to a 12- to 15-cm region centered 3 cm above the tip of the cecum. Diagnostic criteria for acute appendicitis include an enlarged appendix (at least 6 mm outside diameter), with periappendiceal inflammatory changes, an appendicolith, or an abnormal cecal contour. The exclusion of appendicitis requires visualization of a normal appendix. This technique has repeatedly shown high sensitivity and specificity (both 98%) and overall accuracy (98%). The advantages of focused appendix CT scanning include a high degree of accuracy, reproducible imaging, and less variability in examiner technique. Disadvantages include expense, availability (based on CT resources), and administration of oral contrast prior to possible general anesthesia.

ANSWER: A, D

10. With regard to appendicitis in young preschool children, which of the following statements is/are true?

A. It is more uncommon than in adults because of the relatively larger diameter of the appendiceal lumen.
B. It is often associated with higher fever and more vomiting than in adults.

C. There is a high rate of rupture because of commonly delayed diagnosis and more rapid progression of disease.
D. When rupture occurs, a localized periappendiceal abscess results more often than in adults.
E. All of the above.

Ref.: 1, 2

COMMENTS: Diagnostic accuracy of acute appendicitis in infants and young children is lower than in adults. First, the patient is unable to give a precise history; second, nonspecific abdominal pain is common in this age group; and third, appendicitis is infrequent in infants (probably because of the larger lumen of the appendix at its base than at the tip before differential growth of the cecum occurs); therefore it is less often considered a cause of abdominal pain. Vomiting, fever, and diarrhea are likely early complaints. On physical examination, abdominal distension is common. Leukocyte counts are not reliable. The presence of a fecalith on a plain film of the abdomen in a child with suspicious symptoms should be enough to establish the diagnosis. • Gangrene and rupture occur more commonly than in adults because of delay in diagnosis, more rapid progression of the disease, and atypical presentation. The rupture rate varies from 15% to 50%. In preschool children it is higher, ranging from 50% to 85%. • Rupture of gangrenous appendicitis in children is frequently followed by diffuse peritonitis and multiple intraabdominal abscesses. The walling-off process is less efficient than in adults, partly because of the incompletely developed greater omentum. The mortality rate has traditionally been reported to be as high as 5%. Recently, low mortality and low morbidity rates have been reported in pediatric centers, perhaps because of the acute awareness of the disease and earlier operation, thorough irrigation of the peritoneal cavity, and the use of antibiotics directed against aerobic and anaerobic organisms.

ANSWER: B, C

11. With regard to acute appendicitis in the elderly, which of the following is/are true?

A. Symptoms and physical findings are characteristic.
B. It is associated with a high rate of perforation.
C. Perforation is associated with a 50% mortality rate.
D. It may mimic bowel obstruction.
E. It may necessitate right hemicolectomy.

Ref.: 1, 2

COMMENTS: As in infants, acute appendicitis in the elderly may not present with typical signs and symptoms. Symptoms and clinical findings may be minimal or absent; leukocytosis may not be present. • A 60–90% rate of rupture has been described because of the delay in diagnosis; and when rupture occurs, the mortality rate is about 15%. As in infants, who have an incompletely developed (short) omentum, the atrophic omentum in the elderly is less capable of walling off the inflammatory process. Consequently, rupture may result in diffuse peritonitis or distant intraabdominal abscess. • Physical examination is characterized by a paucity of findings; abdominal distension is prominent, and symptoms and signs mimicking bowel obstruction are not uncommon. An occasional patient presents with a painless palpable mass in the right lower quadrant but due to a black, gangrenous appendix (pseudotumor appendix). • In addition, whenever a patient older than 60 years of age develops right lower quadrant peritonitis, the surgeon should be alert to the possibility that a phlegmonous mass of the cecum may be a cancer. Indeed, an inflammatory mass affecting the cecum may necessitate a right hemicolectomy, particularly if the diagnosis is in doubt.

ANSWER: B, D, E

12. With regard to ruptured appendicitis, which one or more of the following is/are appropriate management choices?

A. Drainage and prompt appendectomy for periappendiceal abscess.
B. Drainage and interval appendectomy for periappendiceal abscess if the appendix cannot be removed safely.
C. Antibiotics and nonoperative therapy.
D. Appendectomy, peritoneal lavage, and drainage for diffuse peritonitis.
E. All of the above.

Ref.: 1, 2

COMMENTS: A ruptured appendix may produce a localized periappendiceal abscess, diffuse peritonitis, or abscesses at other abdominal sites, notably in the pelvis, in the right subhepatic region, or between loops of bowel. Unrelenting obstruction of the appendix leads to gangrene and rupture of the organ, which occurs more commonly in the pediatric and geriatric groups. The diagnosis of perforation is usually not difficult. Because the patient is ill, the abdominal pain is more severe and diffuse, and evidence of sepsis is apparent. Physical signs are more obvious after rupture, depending on the position of the appendix. With a periappendiceal abscess or phlegmon, a mass is usually felt, and its nature can be further clarified by ultrasound examination. • Drainage of the abscess through a transverse or a gridiron incision is indicated; the appendix should be removed if easily identified, especially in patients younger than 40 years of age; otherwise, about one-third have recurrence of the appendicitis. • Selected patients presenting with a well localized abscess identified by ultrasound examination or CT scan may be treated by nonoperative therapy should the symptoms be of several days' duration and subsiding. An elective appendectomy within 6–8 weeks is advisable. The presence of a fecalith or retained barium in the appendix following nonoperative treatment of simple or ruptured acute appendicitis predisposes to recurrent attacks within 2–3 years. • Patients with ruptured appendicitis producing a spreading peritonitis should be promptly explored. Drainage of diffuse peritonitis is not warranted and, in truth, is not physically possible. In most such cases, the subcutaneous tissues and skin should be left open; whenever drains are used, they should be exteriorized through counterincisions to minimize wound dehiscence. Use of antibiotic irrigating solution is not universally accepted; nevertheless, preoperative antibiotics against aerobic and anaerobic bacteria should be continued until the patient has no evidence of wound infection or abscess. Complications occur in as many as 47% of patients, mainly due to abscess formation and wound infection. The overall mortality in patients with ruptured appendicitis is 3% and in the elderly about 15%.

ANSWER: A, B

13. With regard to appendicitis during pregnancy, which of the following statements is/are true?

A. Acute appendicitis is the most common cause of an acute abdomen in women after the first trimester of pregnancy.
B. It may present with right upper quadrant or right flank pain.
C. It should initially be treated with antibiotics in an attempt to avoid an operation.
D. It is more common than in nonpregnant women.
E. A perforated appendix is associated with a fetal mortality rate of 80% and a maternal mortality rate of 10%.
F. All of the above.

Ref.: 1, 2

COMMENTS: Appendicitis is the most common cause of an acute abdomen in pregnant women past the first trimester. Because during the third trimester the gravid uterus pushes the appendix (and cecum) to a more lateral and cephalad position, the typical location of somatic pain is altered; nevertheless, during the first 6 months of pregnancy, symptoms of appendicitis do not differ much from those in the nonpregnant patient. Acute pyelitis and torsion of an ovarian cyst can be difficult to distinguish from appendicitis. The common occurrence of abdominal pain, nausea, and leukocytosis during the normal course of pregnancy may also make the diagnosis more difficult. • When the diagnosis is strongly suggested, prompt operation is indicated. • The incidence of appendicitis is not increased by pregnancy. Most cases occur during the second trimester. • Appendicitis during the third trimester is associated with a higher incidence of rupture because of delay in diagnosis. Furthermore, the omentum cannot wall off the inflamed appendix. Premature labor occurs in 50% of women who develop appendicitis during the third trimester. The fetal mortality rate is approximately 2.0–8.5% overall and rises to 35% with rupture; the prognosis of the fetus is related to the birth weight and the effects of sepsis. The maternal mortality rate is less than 0.5%.

ANSWER: A, B

14. For which one or more of the following patients would nonoperative therapy of appendicitis be appropriate?

A. A pregnant woman during the third trimester.
B. A 35-year-old patient with subsiding symptoms and a right lower quadrant mass.
C. An elderly patient with concomitant cardiac disease.
D. A 20-year-old woman with Crohn's disease.
E. None of the above.

Ref.: 1, 2

COMMENTS: When the diagnosis of appendicitis is a strong consideration but not certain, in most instances operation should be undertaken because delay involves the risk of rupture with its accompanying increased morbidity and mortality. Operation should not be delayed during pregnancy because doing so increases the risk to both mother and fetus; nor should it be delayed in elderly patients because they carry an increased risk of appendiceal rupture and death. • Although the optimal timing of operation for ruptured appendicitis with established periappendiceal abscess has been controversial, most surgeons now favor prompt operation rather than nonoperative treatment and delayed appendectomy. However, initial nonoperative therapy followed by interval appendectomy in 6–8 weeks may be considered in selected patients whose symptoms are clearly subsiding and in whom a discrete right lower quadrant mass is palpable; such expectant treatment consists of intravenous fluids, nasogastric suction, and appropriate antibiotics. Vital signs, WBC count, and size of the mass are followed closely. With these measures, most abscesses resolve, yet prolonged hospitalization and antibiotic therapy are needed. Should progression occur, the abscess is drained. • The manifestations of acute regional enteritis often mimic appendicitis. Acute ileitis should be distinguished from Crohn's disease because progression of the former to the latter occurs in only 10% of cases. If exploration reveals an acutely inflamed ileum and a normal appendix, an appendectomy may be performed, but only if the cecum is normal. To do otherwise—that is, to perform an appendectomy in the face of cecal inflammation—risks the formation of a fecal fistula.

ANSWER: B

15. A 20-year-old woman is operated on through a McBurney incision for presumed appendicitis, but the appendix is normal. At this point, which of the following would be appropriate treatment?

A. Exploration and treatment of any associated pathology, as indicated, without appendectomy.
B. Exploration and, if no pathology is found, closure without appendectomy.
C. Exploration and diverticulectomy if Meckel's diverticulum is present and normal by inspection and palpation.
D. Exploration and ileal resection if the terminal ileum appears acutely inflamed.
E. None of the above.

Ref.: 1, 2

COMMENTS: If appendicitis is not found at the time of operation, a careful exploration for other pathology must be carried out. The accuracy of the preoperative diagnosis should be 85%. In general, appendectomy is performed except in some cases of Crohn's disease with extensive involvement of the ileum and cecum. The pelvic organs, gallbladder, colon, and gastroduodenal areas should be inspected to the extent possible. A laparoscopic approach may allow better evaluation of other areas than can be accomplished through a limited right lower quadrant incision. • Mesenteric lymph nodes are assessed; if they are enlarged, a biopsy is performed. The lymph nodes are examined histologically for granulomas (Crohn's disease), and tissue cultures are performed for mycobacteria and *Yersinia*. Infection with *Yersinia* causes mesenteric adenitis, ileitis, colitis, and acute appendicitis. • The small intestine is inspected in a retrograde manner for evidence of inflammatory bowel disease or an inflamed Meckel's diverticulum. The incidence of perforation or peritonitis with Meckel's diverticulitis is about 50%. Resection of Meckel's diverticulum is indicated if diverticulitis is present; an asymptomatic Meckel's diverticulum found incidentally during a laparotomy in adults should not necessarily be removed. If acute regional enteritis is discovered, appendectomy alone is indicated, provided the cecum is not involved.

ANSWER: E

16. During evaluation of a male patient with right lower quadrant pain, which of the following should be included in the differential diagnosis?

A. Acute mesenteric adenitis.
B. Gastroenteritis.
C. Diverticulitis.
D. Epiploic appendagitis.
E. Intussusception.

Ref.: 1, 2

COMMENTS: The differential diagnosis of appendicitis is basically that of the acute abdomen. Often it is impossible to differentiate the entities listed above and other inflammatory processes from acute appendicitis. An extensive diagnostic workup is usually not warranted. The surgeon must be prepared to treat other pathologic entities should they be found on exploration for appendicitis. • **Acute mesenteric adenitis** is most often confused with appendicitis in children. Often an upper respiratory tract infection precedes or is present at the onset of a more diffuse abdominal pain. Tenderness is not localized and may change as the patient assumes different positions. Generalized lymphadenopathy or relative lymphocytosis, when present, can be of help. If after observation the differentiation is in doubt, an operation is warranted. • Acute **gastroenteritis** is characterized by cramping pain followed by watery stools, nausea, and vomiting. Laboratory studies are usually normal. Diagnosis of a specific bacterial infection (*Salmonella*, typhoid fever) is made by stool culture. • **Diverticulitis** of the cecum or a perforated carcinoma of the cecum may be impossible to distinguish from acute appendicitis. Both often present as a right lower quadrant mass with evidence of infection and peritonitis. Frequently, a right hemicolectomy is needed because the diagnosis may be difficult to establish at operation. Sigmoid diverticulitis may also mimic appendicitis if a mobile, inflamed sigmoid colon is located in the right lower quadrant. • **Epiploic appendagitis** results from infarction of the appendage due to torsion. The pain shift is unusual, and the patient does not appear ill. Tenderness, rebound tenderness, and absence of rigidity over the site are common. • In contrast to the previously mentioned entities, it is important to differentiate **intussusception** from appendicitis. The patient's age, the type of pain, a palpable mass in the lower quadrant, and the passage of currant-jelly stool may help the diagnosis. A barium enema offers a diagnostic and therapeutic option for intussusception.

ANSWER: A, B, C, D, E

17. A 26-year-old woman presents to the emergency room at the midpoint of her menstrual cycle with right lower quadrant abdominal pain and tenderness, fever to 39°C, mild diarrhea, and two episodes of vomiting. The white blood cell (WBC) count is 12,500/mm^3. Which of the following is the most likely diagnosis?

A. Acute appendicitis.
B. Ruptured graafian follicle.
C. Acute gastroenteritis.
D. Pelvic inflammatory disease.
E. Crohn's disease.

Ref.: 1, 2

COMMENTS: See Question 18.

18. With regard to the patient in Question 17, which of the following is an appropriate course of action?

A. Laparotomy through a midline incision.
B. Laparoscopy.
C. Appendectomy via McBurney incision.
D. Observation and antibiotics.
E. Ultrasound examination.

Ref.: 1, 2

COMMENTS: The etiology of right lower quadrant abdominal pain includes numerous gastrointestinal, genitourinary, and infectious causes, which are best differentiated on the basis of the history, clinical examination, and laboratory findings. Occasionally, plain abdominal films, radiographic contrast studies of the colon, and ultrasonography are of use; to make a correct diagnosis, a laparotomy is sometimes needed. A false-positive rate of 15% is commonly considered acceptable. A policy of active surgical intervention on the basis of clinical suspicion reduces both morbidity and mortality of appendicitis. Removal of a normal appendix in appropriate circumstances can never be construed as an unnecessary appendectomy. Other causes of such symptoms most commonly include acute mesenteric lymphadenitis, acute pelvic inflammatory disease, torsion of an ovarian cyst, ruptured graafian follicle, acute gastroenteritis, and even no organic pathology. • A negative exploration rate for appendicitis of 32–45% has been reported in women of childbearing age and is compounded by a higher incidence of appendicitis during the latter half of the menstrual cycle than during the first half. • Careful observation is indicated if the pain is atypical, there is no guarding on the right lower quadrant, and fever and leukocytosis are absent. • Salpingitis offers the greatest diagnostic difficulty: the pain is usually bilateral and low in the abdomen, and pelvic examination may elicit extreme pelvic tenderness (*chandelier* sign). Intracellular diplococci may be demonstrable on a smear of purulent vaginal discharge. • Although laparotomy through a midline incision has been advocated in women presenting with equivocal findings, laparoscopy is being used increasingly to ascertain the cause of the process and to perform therapeutic operations. It allows rapid inspection of the abdominal cavity and assessment of possible intraabdominal pathology; it also directs the surgeon toward the most appropriate incision, if needed. • Many surgeons prefer a McBurney or a transverse (Rockey-Davis) incision in patients with suspected appendicitis. The transverse approach allows extension of the incision if it becomes necessary to address pelvic pathology and avoidance of a second incision.

ANSWER:
Question 17: A
Question 18: B, C, E

19. With regard to carcinoids of the appendix, which of the following statements is/are true?

A. The appendix is the most common location of gastrointestinal carcinoids.
B. Nearly one-third are multiple.
C. Carcinoids may present as acute appendicitis because they most often occur at the base of the appendix.
D. Appendiceal carcinoids are malignant and often produce carcinoid syndrome.
E. All of the above.

Ref.: 1, 2

COMMENTS: In order of decreasing frequency, the appendix, ileum, and rectum are the most common locations for gastrointestinal carcinoids. • Carcinoids of the small bowel are multiple in 30% of cases, whereas appendiceal carcinoids are usually solitary. With classic carcinoid syndrome, seen in patients with liver metastases, the primary lesion is most commonly in the ileum and rarely in the appendix. About 75% of appendiceal carcinoids occur at the distal tip; fewer than 10% occur at the base. They are usually an incidental finding and only rarely cause appendicitis. • Even though carcinoids are considered malignant, the behavior of appendiceal carcinoids is biologically benign. Metastasis occurs in only 3%. Malignant carcinoid syndrome due to an appendiceal carcinoid is rare.

ANSWER: A

20. If an incidental appendiceal carcinoid is recognized during simple appendectomy, which of the following statements is/are true?

A. If the tumor is 2 cm in size, the mesoappendiceal lymph nodes are negative, and the resection margins are clear, no further surgical treatment is necessary.
B. Right hemicolectomy is routinely indicated regardless of nodal status.
C. Right hemicolectomy is indicated if tumor is present at the surgical margins or if nodal involvement is present.
D. If mesoappendiceal lymph nodal metastases are present, surgical cure is unlikely and chemotherapy should be initiated.
E. None of the above.

Ref.: 1, 2

COMMENTS: A carcinoid of the appendix is usually found incidentally and is recognized by the presence of a small, firm, circumscribed, yellowish tumor. The malignant potential is related to the site of origin (foregut, midgut, hindgut) and the size of the tumor. Only 3% of appendiceal tumors metastasize, in contrast to 35% of those arising in the ileum. Tumors less than 1 cm in size rarely metastasize to regional lymph nodes and distant organs; tumors having diameters of 1–2 cm metastasize in 50% of cases; 80–90% of tumors larger than 2 cm metastasize. The microscopic growth pattern seems to correlate with long-term survival as well; the median survival time for a patient with mixed insular/glandular pattern is 4.4 years, whereas that for a patient with an undifferentiated tumor is 6 months. Simple appendectomy and resection of the mesoappendix are considered adequate treatment for carcinoids of the appendix that are small (<1 cm) and that do not have regional nodal metastases and that have been completely resected by appendectomy. • If nodes are involved or the tumor is larger than 2 cm, right hemicolectomy should be performed. For patients with tumors 1–2 cm in size, the decision to perform a right hemicolectomy must be individualized, as these patients have a substantial risk (50%) of metastasis. When extensive metastatic disease precludes cure, extensive debulking surgery for palliation is indicated; chemotherapy with a combination of 5-fluorouracil and streptozocin has provided some palliation of the carcinoid syndrome in patients with unresectable metastatic disease. Various antiserotonin agents have also been employed for controlling symptoms in patients with the carcinoid syndrome. Somatostatin can be used for controlling symptoms and as an antineoplastic agent. Up to 25% of patients who undergo palliative resections survive 5 years.

ANSWER: C

21. When a mucocele of the appendix is found at the time of surgery, which of the following is/are appropriate initial therapy?

A. Incisional biopsy with subsequent appendectomy if malignancy is confirmed by frozen section.
B. Routine right hemicolectomy with lymph node dissection.
C. Needle aspiration of cystic fluid for cytologic examination.
D. Appendectomy.
E. None of the above.

Ref.: 1, 2

COMMENTS: Appendectomy is adequate treatment for mucocele, but care must be taken to avoid rupture, as pseudomyxoma peritonei has been reported following rupture and peritoneal dissemination of the appendiceal contents. Histologically, mucocele can be categorized as a benign type, which is the result of an occlusion of the proximal lumen of the appendix, and a malignant type, which is a variant of a mucous papillary adenocarcinoma. Treatment of an appendiceal adenocarcinoma is right hemicolectomy.

ANSWER: D

22. Which of the following statements regarding laparoscopic and open appendectomy is true?

A. Laparoscopic appendectomy is associated with a shorter hospital stay by approximately 24 hours.
B. Laparoscopic appendectomy is associated with decreased postoperative pain.
C. There is no difference in the time to return to regular activity.
D. No differences in infection rates exist between the two techniques.
E. Laparoscopic appendectomy is the procedure of choice for appendicitis in almost all situations.

Ref.: 7

COMMENTS: A recent meta-analysis of 16 prospective randomized studies on laparoscopic versus open appendectomy has been performed. This evaluation demonstrated several advantages of laparoscopic appendectomy over open appendectomy. Specifically, patients have less postoperative pain, better cosmesis, and a faster return to normal activities. The operating room time is longer, and it is unclear whether there is a shorter length of hospital stay for patients having laparoscopic appendectomy. Some studies indicate a shorter length of stay for laparoscopic appendectomy, although it rarely reaches a difference of 24 hours. Differences in infection rates do exist. The wound infection rate for laparoscopic appendectomy is less than one-half the rate of open appendectomy. This is thought to be related to withdrawal of the inflamed appendix through a cannula rather than through the open wound. There is a trend toward a higher intraabdominal abscess rate in patients with appendicitis undergoing laparoscopic appendectomy, particularly for those who have advanced appendicitis at presentation. The overall comparison suggests that there is little advantage to laparoscopic appendectomy over open appendectomy on a routine basis. However, laparoscopic appendectomy is particularly well suited for the patient with equivocal appendicitis, particularly the female of childbearing age.

ANSWER: B

REFERENCES

1. Sabiston DC Jr: *Textbook of Surgery*, 15th ed. WB Saunders, Philadelphia, 1997.
2. Schwartz SI, Shires GT, Spencer FC: *Principles of Surgery*, 7th ed. McGraw-Hill, New York, 1999.
3. Stites DP, Stobo JD, Fudenberg HH, Wells JV: Gastrointestinal and liver diseases. In: *Basic and Clinical Immunology*, 5th ed. Lounge Medical Publications, Los Altos, CA, 1984.
4. Roitt I, Brostoff J, Male D: The lymphoid system. In: *Immunology*. CV Mosby, St. Louis, 1986.
5. Galindo Gallego M, Fadrique B, Nieto MA, et al: Evaluation of ultrasonography and clinical diagnostic scoring in suspected appendicitis. *Br J Surg* 85:37–40, 1998.
6. Rao PM, Rhea JT, Novelline RA, et al: Effect of computed tomography of the appendix on treatment of patients and use of hospital resources. *N Engl J Med* 338:141–146, 1998.
7. Golub R, Siddiqui F, Pohl D: Laparoscopic versus open appendectomy: a metaanalysis. *J Am Coll Surg* 186(5), 1998.

CHAPTER 30

Colon and Rectum

1. With regard to the anatomy of the colon and rectum, which of the following statements is/are true?

A. The colon has a complete outer longitudinal and an incomplete inner circular muscle layer.
B. The haustra are separated by plicae circulares.
C. The ascending and descending colon are normally fixed to the retroperitoneum.
D. The anatomic rectum is partially intraperitoneal and partially extraperitoneal.

Ref.: 1, 2, 3

COMMENTS: A thorough understanding of anatomy is integral to the surgical management of problems of the colon and rectum. • The colon has two muscle layers: an outer longitudinal layer and an inner circular layer. The **inner** layer completely encircles the colon; the **outer** layer, unlike in the small intestine, is in the form of three grossly recognizable longitudinal strips, **taeniae coli**, that do not cover the full circumference of the bowel. At the rectosigmoid junction, the three taeniae coli become broad and fuse together, and the rectum is totally invested with two complete muscle layers. • The **plicae semilunares** are spaced, transverse, crescentic folds that separate the tissue between the taeniae coli, forming haustra. They produce a characteristic, intermittently bulging pattern that radiologically permits differentiation of the colon from the small intestine, which has circular mucosal folds known as **plicae circulares** or **valvulae conniventes**. In contrast to the plicae semilunaris, the plicae circulares traverse the full diameter of the bowel lumen, facilitating radiographic distinction. • Normally, the ascending and descending portions of the colon are fused to the retroperitoneum, whereas the transverse and sigmoid portions are free. Developmental anomalies of fixation, as seen with malrotation and in some cases of volvulus, are not uncommon. Cecal volvulus, for example, could not occur unless incomplete fixation to the retroperitoneum made it possible for a mobile cecum to rotate around a narrow mesenteric pedicle. • Surgeons traditionally have placed the upper border of the rectum at the peritoneal reflection; an alternative definition is that point where the taeniae have completely merged. The distal rectum is void of any peritoneal covering; the middle rectum is covered by peritoneum ventrally; and the upper rectum is completely covered by peritoneum, except for a thin strip dorsally where the short mesorectum suspends the rectum to the presacral tissue.

ANSWER: C, D

2. With regard to the arterial system of the colon and rectum, which of the following statements is/are true?

A. The ileocolic, right colic, and middle colic arteries originate from the superior mesenteric artery.
B. The superior and middle rectal arteries originate from the inferior mesenteric artery.
C. Approximately 80% of intestinal blood flow circulates to the mucosa and submucosa; the remaining 20% passes to the muscularis.
D. The colon and small bowel are equally vulnerable to ischemic injury produced by acute reductions in blood flow.
E. An increase in the functional motor activity of the colon is accompanied by a corresponding increase in blood flow.

Ref.: 4, 5

COMMENTS: The total blood flow to the gastrointestinal tract is approximately 25 ml/kg/min, or 20% of the cardiac output. During a meal the blood flow to the intestine rises to 50% above normal without a corresponding rise in cardiac output. Physical exercise, in contrast, doubles cardiac output, with a 20% decrease in superior mesenteric artery flow. • The right and transverse colons are derived from the foregut and receive their blood supply from the superior mesenteric artery via its ileocolic, right colic, and middle colic branches. The left colon and sigmoid, derived from the hindgut, are supplied by the left colic and sigmoid branches originating from the inferior mesenteric artery. In general, there are well developed collaterals between the mesenteric arteries through a marginal arcade adjacent to the colon. The rectum, a hindgut structure, is supplied by the superior hemorrhoidal artery originating from the inferior mesenteric artery and by the middle and inferior hemorrhoidal arteries originating from the internal iliac artery or its internal pudendal branch. The venous and lymphatic drainage systems of the colon and rectum generally parallel the arterial supply, with the exception of the inferior mesenteric vein, which courses directly cephalad to empty into the splenic vein. • Approximately 80% of the blood flow to the colon wall reaches the mucosa and submucosa; the remaining 20% supplies the muscularis. Despite the extensive collateral vessels to the colon, it receives only about 50% of the blood flow that the small intestine receives; the colon therefore is more sensitive to ischemic injury during acute reductions in blood flow. • In contrast to other areas of the body, an increase in functional motor activity of the colon does not result in a parallel increase in absolute colonic blood flow.

ANSWER: A, C

3. Which of the following is/are the most effective method(s) of reducing the risk of wound infection in colorectal operations?

A. Systemic antibiotics alone.
B. Mechanical bowel cleansing alone.
C. Mechanical cleansing plus systemic antibiotics.
D. Mechanical cleansing plus nonabsorbable oral antibiotics.
E. Mechanical cleansing plus nonabsorbable oral antibiotics plus systemic antibiotics.

Ref.: 1, 2, 6

COMMENTS: The colon contains a higher concentration of bacteria, both aerobic and anaerobic, than any other area of the body; and infectious complications constitute the major morbidity of colorectal operations. The ability of intestinal antisepsis to lessen these complications has been well established in numerous laboratory and clinical studies, although there are conflicting data as to the best method of providing antisepsis. Mechanical cleansing of the colon can be achieved by administration of a cathartic in combination with enemas or by peroral lavage with a relatively large volume of solution. The lavage being used most frequently is a nonabsorbable polyethylene glycol-electrolyte solution administered during the afternoon before surgery. Metoclopramide, given orally or intramuscularly before the lavage begins, may reduce the relatively commonly associated nausea; no cathartics are necessary when using a lavage solution. Such mechanical cleansing clearly is important, but if used alone it does not significantly alter the concentration of bacterial flora nor does it decrease the incidence of postoperative septic complications. Wound infections still occur in approximately 50% of cases. A combination of mechanical preparation with the administration of nonabsorbable oral antibiotics effective against both aerobic and anaerobic colonic flora provides the most effective protection against infections. Systemic antibiotics are often combined with lavage and oral antibiotics, but such a combination has not been conclusively demonstrated to confer an advantage over the use of lavage and oral antibiotics alone. The use of systemic antibiotics in place of oral antibiotics is a less effective method of prophylaxis and may result in a higher rate of infection.

ANSWER: D, E

4. In the United States, what is the most common cause of mechanical obstruction of the colon?

A. Adhesions.
B. Diverticulitis.
C. Cancer.
D. Volvulus.
E. Inguinal hernia.

Ref.: 1, 2

COMMENTS: Whenever a patient presents with signs and symptoms of intestinal obstruction, one first attempts to define the level of obstruction (i.e., small bowel or large bowel). Colonic obstruction is often suggested by the gas pattern on plain abdominal radiographs and can be confirmed radiographically by a carefully performed enema with a water-soluble contrast medium. Barium used in this situation has potential hazards; one concern is causing peritonitis in the presence of a perforating lesion; another concern is inspissation proximal to a partially obstructing cancer or diverticulitis, effectively converting a partial obstruction to a complete one. In the United States, **colorectal cancer** is by far the leading cause of large bowel obstruction; **diverticulitis** is the next most common cause. In some parts of the world (e.g., Iran, Iraq, Pakistan) where there is a high fiber content in the diet resulting in large volumes of stool and an elongated colon, **volvulus** is the leading cause. In the United States sigmoid volvulus is rare and is usually seen in elderly, institutionalized patients. **Intussusception** is a common cause of colonic obstruction in infants and children but is unusual in adults unless a neoplasm has precipitated an intussusception. It is highly unusual to have large bowel obstruction secondary to **adhesions** or **incarceration** within an inguinal hernia; this is in contradistinction to an obstruction of the small intestine. Other causes of large bowel obstruction include **fecal impaction**, especially in the elderly and infirm, and **benign strictures** secondary to ischemia or inflammatory bowel disease. A neglected obstruction (from any mechanism) can be fatal. Colon obstruction in the presence of a competent ileocecal valve creates a closed-loop phenomenon; progressive distension of the colon between the point of obstruction and the ileocecal valve may lead to necrosis and perforation of the gut wall. Volvulus can behave in the same manner and have the same consequence.

ANSWER: C

5. Which of the following are the most common causes of massive colonic bleeding?

A. Cancer.
B. Ulcerative colitis.
C. Diverticulosis.
D. Diverticulitis.
E. Angiodysplasia.

Ref.: 2, 7, 8

COMMENTS: Massive colonic bleeding classically has been attributed to diverticulosis, but recent evidence suggests that **angiodysplasia**, also known as vascular ectasia, is as common. These two entities frequently coexist, and exact identification of the bleeding source may require a combination of endoscopic, radiographic, and histologic methods. Before the advent of angiography, angiodysplasia was not recognized as a source of colonic hemorrhage. Its cause is not known but may be related to degenerative changes associated with aging and to intramural muscular hypertrophy that obstructs the submucosal veins, leading to their dilatation and propensity to bleed. **Diverticulosis** can also cause **massive** bleeding, attributed to ruptured vasa recta at the apex or neck of a diverticulum. **Diverticulitis** also can cause bleeding as a result of superficial mucosal ulceration, but usually it is mild. **Ulcerative colitis** is more likely to cause mild to moderate bleeding and frequently is associated with diarrhea and systemic signs of a chronic illness, such as weight loss and failure to thrive. **Cancer** of the colon usually causes occult rather than massive gastrointestinal bleeding.

ANSWER: C, E

6. With regard to lower gastrointestinal hemorrhage, match each statement in the left column with the appropriate disease in the right column.

A. At least 50% of cases have bleeding originating in the right colon
B. The bleeding is arterial and severe
C. After the first episode, the rate of recurrent bleeding is 85%
D. Extravasation of dye during angiography can be seen in most cases
E. Total colectomy is the procedure of choice

a. Diverticulosis
b. Angiodysplasia
c. Both
d. Neither

Ref.: 3

COMMENTS: Diverticulosis and angiodysplasia account for 90% of cases of **massive lower gastrointestinal bleeding** in patients older than 50 years of age. Since the advent of angiography for evaluating colonic hemorrhage, angiodysplasia is being recognized as the cause with increasing frequency. • Although 80% of diverticular disease is concentrated in the sigmoid colon, 50% of diverticular bleeding originates from the right colon. Almost all colonic angiodysplasias are located in the cecum and right colon. • The bleeding associated with diverticulosis is secondary to a ruptured vasa recta at the neck or apex of a diverticulum and is arterial and usually severe. In contrast, bleeding from angiodysplasia is venous and is not as severe. After the initial episode, diverticular bleeding may recur in 25% of cases; rebleeding after the second episode occurs in 50%. Angiodysplastic bleeding may recur up to 85% of the time after the initial episode. • In most cases of diverticular hemorrhage, angiography reveals the source by demonstrating extravasation of radiopaque contrast material into the intestinal lumen. In contrast, only 8–10% of bleeding secondary to angiodysplasia exhibits angiographic extravasation. Other, more common angiographic findings associated with angiodysplasia include a dense, slowly emptying mesenteric vein (92%), a vascular tuft (68%), and an early filling mesenteric vein (56%). • If preoperative concise demonstration of a bleeding site is possible, a limited resection is preferred. This holds true for bleeding from cecal angiodysplasia, even though asymptomatic sigmoid diverticula are incidentally discovered. Total colectomy is reserved for cases in which the degree of bleeding warrants surgery but preoperative localizing studies are unsuccessful in pinpointing the site of bleeding.

ANSWER: A-c; B-a; C-b; D-a; E-d

7. A 68-year-old man is admitted to the hospital having passed three large maroon-colored stools. On arrival at the hospital, he passes more bloody stools as well as clots. He is pale, orthostatic, and tachycardic. Nasogastric aspirates are bilious. After resuscitation is begun, which of the following is the most appropriate initial test?

A. Angiography.
B. Nuclear medicine red blood cell scan.
C. Rigid proctoscopy.
D. Colonoscopy.
E. Barium enema.

Ref.: 3

COMMENTS: Although all of the aforementioned tests may play a role in evaluating a patient with massive loss of blood through the rectum, proctoscopy is the most appropriate initial test. Proctoscopy may reveal an anorectal source of the bleeding and a diffuse mucosal process such as ulcerative proctitis. • Proceeding directly to a barium enema examination is ill-advised, as the barium obscures details if angiography is subsequently needed. Furthermore, finding sigmoid diverticula does not prove that they were the source of the bleeding. • Mesenteric angiography is performed if the hemorrhage is brisk and persistent; a bleeding rate of approximately 1–5 ml/min is necessary to visualize the responsible vessel. The superior mesenteric artery should be injected first because most bleeding originates in the right colon; if no abnormalities are found, this step is followed by injecting the inferior mesenteric artery and *finally the celiac axis*. If a source of the bleeding is found, embolization may be performed using Gelfoam strips or autologous blood clots. Embolization, however, may occlude more than the single bleeding vessel and lead to ischemia and even colon infarction. Therefore embolization should be reserved for the patient who cannot tolerate surgery or vasopressin. Vasopressin may be selectively infused into the mesenteric vessel; although it stops the bleeding in many patients, it may also cause cardiac arrhythmias, heart failure, and hypertension. Cessation of the vasopressin may precipitate further bleeding. The use of vasopressin permits the physician time to complete resuscitation and to address coexisting medical disorders. • Technetium sulfur colloid nuclear scanning has also been used to address lower intestinal bleeding. Unfortunately, the isotope is cleared rapidly by the reticuloendothelial system. Alternatively, red blood cells may be tagged with technetium. This technique detects bleeding at a rate as low as 0.1 ml/min. Because this isotope is not cleared from the vascular system as rapidly, repeated scanning may be possible over an extended period. Sensitivity, specificity, and accuracy rates have varied widely among reported series, and the exact role of red blood cell scanning is controversial. • Colonoscopy has emerged as a valuable diagnostic and therapeutic tool for the stable patient who is not bleeding briskly. No bowel cleansing is needed, but the examination must be done by an experienced endoscopist. Angiodysplastic lesions can be treated successfully with colonoscopic fulguration.

ANSWER: C

8. A definite increased risk of developing colon cancer is associated with which one or more of the following?

A. Diet high in fiber.
B. Diet low in animal fat and protein.
C. Ulcerative colitis.
D. Familial polyposis.
E. Prior cholecystectomy.
F. Strong family history of colon cancer in several preceding generations.

Ref.: 1, 3

COMMENTS: In the United States colorectal cancer is second only to lung cancer as the leading cause of death from cancer. Environmental factors, particularly dietary habits, may explain the wide variation in geographic distribution of colon cancer. • Diets low in fiber and high in animal fats and protein are associated with an increased risk of colon cancer. The mechanisms may include alterations in intestinal transit time and an increase in the formation of carcinogenic compounds as a result of bacterial metabolism of dietary components. Gallstone disease appears to be more common in areas where colon cancer is prevalent. Some studies have suggested that cholecystectomy is associated with a higher incidence of subsequent colon cancer, particularly involving the right colon. A proposed mechanism relates to the carcinogenic potential of secondary bile acids to which the intestinal mucosa is increasingly exposed after cholecystectomy as a result of increased enterohepatic cycling. Evidence supporting this association is conflicting, however, and any association that might exist is minimal. • Genetic factors play a definite role in carcinogenesis, and mutational abnormalities have been identified in familial polyposis and hereditary nonpolyposis colorectal cancer syndromes (HNPCC). Almost 100% of patients with familial polyposis develop cancer, usually by age 40, if the colon is left untreated. The aforementioned notwithstanding, familial polyposis, the HNPCC syndrome, and ulcerative colitis account for only a small percentage of the total cases of colorectal cancer. • Risk factors for the development of cancer in patients with ulcerative colitis include disease of long duration (the incidence increases 1–2% per year after 10 years) and total colonic involvement. An increased risk of cancer has also been seen with Crohn's disease, of both the small and large intestine, especially in bypassed segments.

ANSWER: C, D, F

9. With regard to screening/surveillance for colorectal cancer, which of the following is/are true?

A. Barium enema alone is a cost-effective means of screening asymptomatic patients.
B. Population-based screening programs using guaiac tests for fecal occult blood have been able to detect a higher than expected number of early, superficial cancers.
C. The positive-predictive value of a positive fecal occult blood test (FOBT) is approximately 10% for cancer and 30% for adenomas.
D. When combined with flexible sigmoidoscopy, FOBT reduces mortality from colorectal cancer.
E. For patients with familial polyposis or hereditary nonpolyposis colorectal cancer, screening is best achieved with FOBT performed alone every 6 months.

Ref.: 6

COMMENTS: Screening asymptomatic, low-risk patients for colorectal cancer must be accomplished with a cost-effective means that encourages patient compliance. The test that best accomplishes these goals is annual examination of the stool for occult blood. This test utilizes the peroxidate-like activity of hemoglobin. Stools are collected on three separate occasions and smeared on filter paper impregnated with guaiac solution. Hydrogen peroxide is added, and if hemoglobin is present to catalyze the reaction the colorless guaiac is oxidized to a blue-colored quinone. Prolonged storage of the test slides may interfere with proper performance of the test. Normal blood loss in stool is 2 mg of hemoglobin per gram of stool; FOBT requires a fecal blood loss of 10 mg of hemoglobin per gram of stool to obtain a positive result. • Mass screening programs yield positive results in 1–8% of patients; the positive predictive value of a positive test is 10% for cancer and 30% for adenoma. These programs diagnose a higher percentage of Duke's A cancers than might be expected otherwise, a fact that lends support to performing FOBT as a matter of routine. The FOBT is not a perfect test; for example, small adenomas and cancers not actively bleeding may not yield a positive result. In fact, in patients with a known cancer, the sensitivity of FOBT is 50–85%. Furthermore, it is not clear whether the mortality from colorectal cancer is reduced by FOBT alone. When annual FOBT is combined with periodic flexible sigmoidoscopy, there is evidence to suggest that cancer mortality is reduced. When used as a screening tool barium enema is combined with sigmoidoscopy and is performed every 5 years. Alternatively, colonoscopy may be performed every 10 years. • Current screening practices for the asymptomatic patient endorsed by the American Cancer Society consist of the following: annual digital rectal examination with FOBT beginning at age 40 and flexible sigmoidoscopy at age 50 and 51. If these tests are normal they are then performed every 3–5 years. • Periodic barium enema and colonoscopy, although they examine the entire colon and eliminate speculation that pathology is present, are not approved screening tools for the asymptomatic, low-risk patient. • "Screening" is not a term that applies to high risk conditions such as familial polyposis and hereditary nonpolyposis colorectal cancer (HNPCC). For these conditions, the high likelihood of finding neoplastic lesions combined with their lethal nature should tumors be missed mandates tests additional to FOBT. Beginning at puberty, patients at risk for familial polyposis should be examined at yearly intervals with flexible sigmoidoscopy; if the disease does not become apparent by age 40, the patient likely does not have it. Patients at risk for HNPCC should undergo colonoscopy beginning at age 25.

ANSWER: B, C, D

10. Select the most common mode of spread of colon cancer.

A. Hematogenous.
B. Lymphatic.
C. Direct extension.
D. Implantation.

Ref.: 1, 2

COMMENTS: Of the various mechanisms by which colon cancer may spread, the **lymphatic** route to regional mesenteric lymph nodes is the most common. This fact has surgical importance because it dictates the extent of resection necessary when operating with curative intent. **Hematogenous** spread from colon cancer is primarily via the portal circulation to the liver. Cells that escape this effective filter can reach the lung and occasionally the brain. Rectal cancers can metastasize to the spine via Batson's plexus. Because the rectum has dual venous drainage—through the portal vein and the hemorrhoidal veins into iliac veins—malignant cells may reach the liver or the lungs. Distal rectal cancers may spread to the lungs without entering the portal circulation. **Direct extension** to adjacent structures can occur with or without distant metastases; with the latter, en bloc resection of portions of these organs may be necessary. If the colon cancer has broken through the serosal surface, **implantation** on the peritoneal surface, locally or widely, can result, accounting for metastatic deposits in the rectovesical pouch (Blumer's shelf), to the peritoneum under the umbilicus (Sister Joseph's nodule), and to the ovary (Krukenberg's tumor, originally described for metastases from the stomach to the ovary).

ANSWER: B

11. Which of the following is the most important prognostic determinant of survival after treatment for colorectal cancer?

A. Lymph node involvement.
B. Transmural extension.
C. Tumor size.
D. Histologic differentiation.
E. DNA content.

Ref.: 1, 2, 3

COMMENTS: Of the many variables that have an impact on the cure of patients with colon cancer, the status of the **lymph nodes** remains the most important. Long-term survival for node-positive patients is approximately half that of node-negative patients. The extent of nodal disease also has an impact on the prognosis, patients with three or more positive lymph nodes having a lower 5-year survival rate than patients with fewer than three positive nodes. **Transmural** extension also has an impact on prognosis, as demonstrated by the decline in 5-year survival rates from Dukes' A to Dukes' B lesions (80% versus 60%, respectively). The difference, however, is not as pronounced as with the effect of lymph node metastases (35% survival in patients with positive lymph nodes). **Tumor size** in and of itself has no bearing on metastatic potential or prognosis. The **DNA** content of colorectal tumors has been studied extensively, and aneuploidy seems to correlate well with histologic differentiation, transmural penetration, and the presence of nodal metastases. DNA content, however, has not been shown conclusively to be an important independent prognostic indicator.

ANSWER: A

12. Examine the following illustration of a colon cancer and select the appropriate stage or stages.

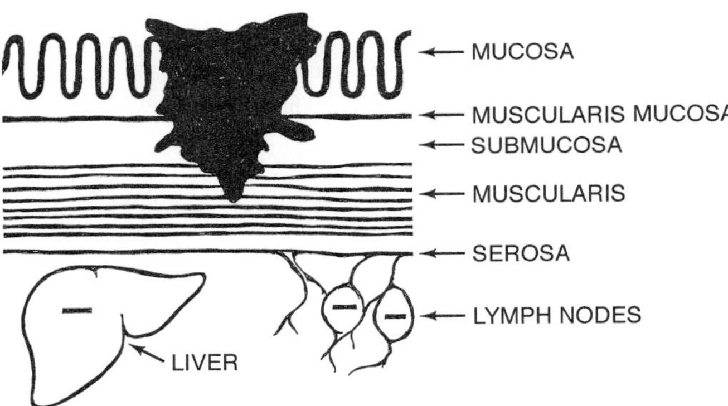

A. Dukes' A.
B. Astler-Coller A.
C. T2N0M0.
D. T1N0M0.
E. Dukes' B.
F. Astler-Coller B_2.
G. Astler-Coller B_1.

Ref.: 1, 2

COMMENTS: Dukes' classification was the original standardized method of staging colorectal cancer. In recent years, however, confusion has arisen because of numerous subsequent modifications. According to the original scheme proposed in 1932 by Cuthbert Dukes, an A lesion was confined to the bowel wall, a B lesion extended through the bowel wall but did not involve lymph nodes, and a C lesion indicated regional node involvement. It is not uncommon to hear someone refer to a colon cancer with distant metastases as a Dukes D lesion even though it was not, in fact, part of the original classification. In 1949 J.W. Kirklin and associates modified Dukes' classification, designating an A lesion as one confined to mucosa and submucosa; a B_1 lesion as one extending into, but not through, the muscularis propria; and a B_2 lesion as one extending through the muscularis propria into the pericolonic fat. In 1954, V.B. Astler and F.A. Coller modified the Kirklin classification (which itself, remember, was a modification of Dukes' classification) by designating a C_1 lesion as one limited to the bowel wall but with positive lymph nodes and a C_2 lesion as one invading all layers of the bowel wall with positive lymph nodes. In 1978 the staging classification was modified even further: An A lesion is confined to the mucosa and submucosa; B_1 is involvement of the muscularis; B_2 is involvement of the serosa; and B_3 is involvement of an adjacent organ. The C lesions are the same with respect to local involvement but with positive lymph nodes. D lesions are any of the aforementioned but includes distant metastases as well. The American Joint Committee on Cancer has proposed a TNM classification that also stages a tumor according to the extent of bowel wall involvement and the presence or absence of lymph node involvement (N1 or N0). A T1 tumor penetrates only into the submucosa, whereas a T2 tumor demonstrates partial invasion of the muscularis. Transmural penetration imparts a T3 designation. The designations M0 and M1 indicate the absence and presence, respectively, of metastases.

ANSWER: A, C, G

13. Which of the following is the appropriate operation for a sigmoid cancer that has not metastasized distantly?

A. Segmental resection of the sigmoid.
B. Resection of sigmoid and distal descending colon, sparing the main left colic artery.
C. Resection of the sigmoid and the descending colon, including the inferior mesenteric artery at its origin.
D. Resection of the entire colon proximal to the lesion with ileorectostomy.
E. Concomitant oophorectomy in women.

Ref.: 2, 3

COMMENTS: The respective draining mesenteric lymph nodes and the vascular supply to an area of the colon determine the amount of resection necessary when one is operating with intent to cure. For a sigmoid cancer without evidence of distal spread, the resection should include, at a minimum, the sigmoid and distal descending colon and the accompanying mesentery to include the sigmoidal and superior hemorrhoidal vessels but sparing the left colic artery. A more extensive mesenteric resection with ligation of the inferior mesenteric artery at its origin is advocated by some, although there is no conclusive evidence that it improves the survival rate. Resection of the entire intraabdominal colon can be considered for an obstructing cancer because resection of a dilated stool-laden colon may safely permit an ileorectostomy rather than colostomy. Other indications for total colectomy include synchronous cancers in separate segments of the colon or in high risk (younger) patients who require lifelong surveillance. Oophorectomy may be considered in postmenopausal women, because approximately 6% of these patients have simultaneous drop metastases to the ovaries. It has not been established that routine prophylactic oophorectomy improves survival; furthermore, only 1.4% of women with colorectal cancer subsequently require an operation for a recurrence in the ovary.

ANSWER: B

14. Which one or more of the following constitute appropriate operative management of a left colon cancer that is causing a high-grade obstruction?

A. Resection and primary anastomosis.
B. Resection and intraoperative colonic irrigation followed by primary anastomosis.
C. Initial decompressing colostomy followed by resection within 7–10 days.
D. Primary left colectomy and either a Hartmann procedure or a mucous fistula.
E. Primary subtotal colectomy and ileocolic anastomosis.

Ref.: 1, 2, 3

COMMENTS: Cancer is the leading cause of colon obstruction, and left-sided tumors in particular are susceptible to obstruction. **Right and transverse colon**: Most right and transverse colon cancers presenting with obstruction can be treated safely by primary resection and reanastomosis as a one-stage procedure. **Left colon**: For left-sided tumors producing obstruction, the traditional surgical approach has been an initial decompressing transverse colostomy, followed at a second stage by resection within 7–10 days and possibly a third-stage operation for colostomy closure. Initial treatment by decompressing colostomy only is still appropriate, particularly for poor-risk patients; but resection of the obstructing pathology is more commonly performed today. A primary colocolostomy remains hazardous in the patient with both an unprepared and distended bowel. Therefore for many patients with obstructing left-sided tumors, the preferred operation is primary resection accompanied by a Hartmann procedure or creation of a mucous fistula; the reanastomosis is performed at a second stage. Some advocate primary subtotal colectomy with an ileocolic anastomosis as a one-stage procedure. • In the absence of peritonitis or perforation, an alternative approach consists of resection followed by intraoperative colonic irrigation and then primary anastomosis. The irrigation is accomplished with several liters of saline solution administered through a cecostomy or an appendicostomy. The effluent is then discharged through large-caliber tubing inserted into the open end of the left colon. This operative approach carries with it a clinical leakage rate of 5–7%.

ANSWER: B, C, D, E

15. In which of the following situations should a combined abdominoperineal resection be performed?

A. A circumferential villous adenoma beginning at the dentate line and extending proximally 8 cm.
B. A rectal cancer in which a 5-cm distal margin cannot be obtained.
C. A rectal cancer that produces pain and tenesmus.
D. Anastomotic recurrence after low anterior resection.
E. Palliation of obstructing rectal cancer just above the dentate line with minimal liver metastases.

Ref.: 1, 2

COMMENTS: The Miles abdominoperineal resection is the most widely used operation for most cancers of the distal rectum. It means, however, a permanent colostomy and the potential serious morbidity of impotence and bladder dysfunction; therefore it is indicated for malignant rather than benign lesions. Large and even circumferential rectal adenomas can be removed with a variety of transanal techniques that preserve the sphincter muscle and fecal continence. Curative resection of cancers whose distal edge is 7–8 cm above the anal verge can be performed by low anterior resection and colorectostomy or by coloanal anastomosis without the need for permanent colostomy, depending on the exact extent of the lesion, the size of the patient's pelvis, and the skill of the surgeon. The end-to-end surgical stapling devices introduced through the rectum have greatly facilitated anastomoses deep in the pelvis. The traditional attempt to obtain a distal margin of 5 cm may not be necessary, especially if doing so sacrifices the sphincter; resections with distal margins of 2 cm have demonstrated equivalent survival and recurrence rates. Because stapling devices have increased our capability of performing deep pelvic anastomoses, there is concern that local recurrence rates will be higher as a result of compromising the distal margin. In fact, distal margins are not compromised, and the ability to obtain an even greater margin is enhanced. Recurrence rates comparing stapled versus hand-sewn anastomoses are the same. • Abdominoperineal resection is usually performed with curative intent, although it is justified for the symptomatic patient with minimal metastatic disease who is expected to survive 6 months or longer.

ANSWER: C, D, E

16. With regard to adjuvant chemotherapy, radiation therapy, or both for locally advanced rectal cancer, which of the following statements is/are true?

A. Postoperative radiation therapy alone decreases local recurrence rates of rectal cancer.
B. Postoperative radiation therapy alone increases survival rates of patients with rectal cancer.
C. Postoperative combined chemotherapy and radiation therapy yield improved local control and survival rates in comparison with irradiation alone.
D. Side effects of combined postoperative chemotherapy and radiation therapy are few; 95% of patients are able to complete treatment.
E. Preoperative chemotherapy and radiation down-stages the tumor and improves resectability.

Ref.: 6, 9, 10

COMMENTS: Adjuvant chemotherapy and radiation therapy have been studied in an attempt to determine their impact on survival and recurrence rates for rectal cancer. The Gastrointestinal Tumor Study Group (GITSG) and the National Surgical Adjuvant Breast and Bowel Protocol R-01 (NSABP) have shown that **postoperative** radiation therapy reduces regional recurrence rates, but its impact on survival was not significant. Recently, a randomized Swedish trial showed that a short course of 2550 cGy in five fractions administered **preoperatively** reduced locoregional failure and improved 5-year survival compared with surgery alone. Another Swedish study compared this preoperative regimen with 6000 cGy in 30 fractions administered postoperatively and showed significantly better locoregional control with the preoperative treatment. No chemotherapy was administered. • The GITSG and the North Central Cancer Treatment Group (NCCTG) have investigated the **combined** use of 5-fluorouracil and methyl chloroethylcyclohexyl nitrourea (methyl-CCNU) and **postoperative** irradiation for Duke's B and C cancers of the rectum and found a reduction in the recurrence rates and an improvement in 5-year survival rates. This combined therapy, however, is accompanied by significant toxicity; only approximately 65% of patients are able to complete treatment. Side effects include diarrhea, leukopenia, and enteritis. Nevertheless, combined postoperative treatment is the accepted regimen for Dukes' B and C cancers. • An encouraging trend in the management of rectal cancer is the use of **preoperative combined** chemotherapy and radiation therapy for T3 tumors or any tumor that has evidence of nodal metastases seen by rectal ultrasonography. This regimen acts to down-stage tumors and improve resectability. The advocates of this protocol claim that sphincter preservation is likely to be enhanced, but this advantage remains to be seen. It is of note that up to 30% of patients have a complete response to treatment; that is, no residual tumor is found in the resected specimen. It also remains to be seen whether locoregional control and survival rates are improved; and cooperative studies are underway to answer this question. • ***Summary comments***: (1) **postoperative radiation therapy alone** reduces locoregional recurrence rates but has not shown an effect on survival; (2) **postoperative radiation therapy combined with chemotherapy** reduces recurrence rates and improves survival and is indicated for Dukes' B and C tumors; (3) **preoperative radiation therapy alone** reduces recurrence rates and in a Swedish study also improved survival; (4) **preoperative radiation therapy combined with chemotherapy** down-stages tumors, improves resectability, and induces a complete response in some patients, but it remains to be seen whether it enhances sphincter preservation and improves local control and survival.

ANSWER: A, C, E

17. Hamartomas are found in which of the following situations?

A. Juvenile polyps.
B. Peutz-Jeghers syndrome.
C. Familial polyposis.
D. Gardner syndrome.
E. Chronic ulcerative colitis.

Ref.: 1, 2, 3

18. Match each characteristic in the left column with one or more syndromes in which it appears in the right column.

A. Malignant potential	a. Peutz-Jeghers syndrome
B. Extraintestinal manifestations	b. Familial polyposis
C. Small bowel polyps	c. Gardner syndrome
D. Mendelian dominant gene	d. Turcot syndrome
	e. Cronkhite-Canada syndrome

Ref.: 1, 2, 11, 12

COMMENTS: Hamartomas are lesions in which normal tissue is found in an abnormal structural configuration. Because the tissue itself is not neoplastic, there is no malignant potential. **Peutz-Jeghers syndrome** is transmitted as an autosomal dominant trait. The polyps are hamartomas and are found primarily in the jejunum and ileum, with involvement of the colon and rectum in one-third and the stomach in one-fourth of the cases. The polyps may cause obstruction, intussusception, or bleeding. It is now generally accepted that there is an increased incidence of gastrointestinal cancers associated with Peutz-Jeghers, and polypectomy is advised, especially if the patient has recurrent colicky pain or anemia. Colonic lesions are usually treated by polypectomy; colectomy is generally not needed. In addition to intestinal polyps, the syndrome is characterized by melanin spots of the oral mucosa, lips, palms of the hands, and soles of the feet. **Juvenile polyps** are solitary 70% of the time, and in 60% of cases these polyps are located within 10 cm of the anal verge. Occasionally, a patient is found to have a syndrome of juvenile polyposis, characterized by anemia, anergy, hypoproteinemia, and failure to thrive. Some authors have found a strong association between gastrointestinal malignancy and juvenile polyposis. In **Cronkhite-Canada syndrome** the polyps, which are hamartomas, are dispersed throughout the gastrointestinal tract. This entity is characterized by hyperpigmentation of the skin, alopecia, and atrophy of the fingernails and toenails. **Familial adenomatous polyposis** by itself lacks extraintestinal manifestations; Turcot and Gardner syndromes are the names used to describe familial polyposis in association with certain noncolonic manifestations. **Turcot syndrome** has the additional characteristic of central nervous system tumors. **Gardner syndrome**, in addition to the polyps, is typified by the presence of osteomas, exostoses, and desmoid tumors. The polypoid lesions observed with chronic ulcerative colitis are inflammatory "pseudopolyps," and the malignant potential of ulcerative colitis is not related to the presence of these lesions. **Summary statements:** Of the conditions listed, Cronkhite-Canada syndrome is not inherited and does not have malignant potential. • Familial polyposis, Gardner syndrome, and Turcot syndrome may represent different expressions of the same disease. • Patients with familial polyposis, Gardner syndrome, or Turcot syndrome must undergo surveillance upper endoscopy at 3- to 5-year intervals. In the Cleveland Clinic Polyposis Registry, duodenal polyps were found in 33% of patients and gastric polyps in 28%; and although most gastric polyps were of the fundic gland type, all duodenal polyps were adenomas. Following colorectal cancer, the most common cause of death in these patients was cancer of the periampullary region. • Small bowel polyposis is seen in all of the syndromes listed, with the exception of Turcot syndrome. • An autosomal dominant gene has been proposed for Peutz-Jeghers syndrome, familial polyposis, and Gardner syndrome, whereas it is believed that Turcot syndrome is due to an autosomal recessive gene or an autosomal dominant tract with incomplete penetrance.

ANSWER:
Question 17: A, B
Question 18: A-a,b,c,d; B-a,c,d,e; C-a,b,c,e; D-a,b,c,d

19. With regard to colorectal polyps, which of the following is/are considered precancerous?

A. Hyperplastic polyp.
B. Tubular adenoma.
C. Tubulovillous adenoma.
D. Villous adenoma.

Ref.: 1, 2

20. Match each statement in the left column with the appropriate pathologic entity in the right column.

A. Most common type of intestinal polyp	a. Tubular adenoma
B. Children and adolescents	b. Hyperplastic polyp
C. Mitoses at the depths of crypts	c. Both
D. Mitoses at the surface of crypts	d. Neither
E. Differentiation into mature goblet cells	

Ref.: 1, 2

21. Match each statement in the left column with the appropriate response in the right column.

A. Pedunculated	a. Tubular adenoma
B. Size usually less than 1 cm	b. Villous adenoma
C. Rectosigmoid the most common location	c. Both
D. Malignant potential related to size	d. Neither
E. Malignant potential related to location	

Ref.: 1, 2

COMMENTS: Polypoid colorectal lesions can be classified as being neoplastic or nonneoplastic. The **nonneoplastic polyps** include hyperplastic polyps, pseudopolyps, and hamartomas. The **neoplastic polyps** include tubular adenomas, tubulovillous adenomas, and villous adenomas. **Hyperplastic polyps** are the most common type of all polyps. They result from an imbalance between cell division and cell exfoliation. They are small, multiple, and sessile; and they occur most frequently in the rectosigmoid. Although hyperplastic polyps are nonneoplastic and have no malignant potential, they are nonetheless removed to differentiate them from neoplastic polyps (adenomas), which have varying malignant potential depending on their size, histologic pattern, and degree of cellular atypia. **Histology**: The distinction between hyperplastic polyps and adenomatous polyps (tubular, tubulovillous, villous) can be readily made on the basis of cellular differentiation and the location of cell division. In normal colonic mucosa and hyperplastic polyps, cell division is limited to the depths of the crypts of Lieberkühn, and differentiation into mature cells occurs as the cells migrate up the crypt to the surface. In adenomatous polyps, cell division occurs at all levels of the crypt, including the surface; and the differentiation is incomplete. **Neoplastic polyps** may be classified by histology (tubular versus villous) and morphology (sessile versus pedunculated). **Tubular adenoma** is the most common type of neoplastic polyp, constituting approximately 75% of this group. Generally, they are asymptomatic, pedunculated, less than 1 cm in size, and (as with all colon polyps) are found most commonly in the rectosigmoid region. The likelihood of a neoplastic polyp containing cancer is directly related to its size and configuration. Tubular adenomas less than 1 cm in diameter rarely harbor malignancy; this figure increases to 10% for those 1–2 cm and exceeds 30% for larger lesions. Sessile adenomas, of all the histologic types, are more likely to harbor an occult cancer than are pedunculated ones. **Villous adenomas** account for approximately 10% of neoplastic colon polyps. They generally are sessile, and when compared with tubular adenomas are larger, more likely to present with symptoms such as rectal bleeding, mucous discharge, or diarrhea. They also have a significantly higher risk of malignancy. Overall, approximately 40–50% of villous adenomas contain cancer, and one-half of these are invasive. **Mixed histologic pattern**: Approximately 15% of neoplastic colon adenomas contain both tubular and villous elements and are referred to as tubulovillous adenomas. The risk of malignancy in tubulovillous adenomas is 22%, greater than that seen with tubular adenomas but less than that reported with villous adenomas. **Nonneoplastic polyps** also may have a sessile or pedunculated morphology, so this characteristic has limited value in predicting the histologic nature of the polyp.

ANSWER:
Question 19: B, C, D
Question 20: A-b; B-d; C-c; D-a; E-b
Question 21: A-a; B-a; C-c; D-c; E-d

22. A pedunculated 1.5 cm tubular adenoma is removed endoscopically from the sigmoid colon and is found to contain well differentiated adenocarcinoma extending to, but not beyond, the muscularis mucosa. The margin of resection is free of tumor. Select the best therapeutic option.

A. Observation and repeat the endoscopic examination in 3 months.
B. Endoscopic fulguration of the polypectomy site.
C. Operative colotomy and excision of the polypectomy site.
D. Sigmoid colectomy.

Ref.: 1, 2, 13

COMMENTS: By definition, this lesion is classified as carcinoma in situ and is treated adequately by endoscopic polypectomy. A lymphatic plexus exists just below the muscularis mucosae, so lymphatic dissemination is possible only when invasion beyond this structure has occurred. The muscularis mucosa of the colon wall may extend for a variable distance into the stalk of the polyp and may not even reach the head. There are four anatomic levels of pedunculated polyps: Level 1 is the head itself; level 2 is the interface between the head and the stalk; level 3 is the stalk; and level 4 is the junction between the stalk and the colonic wall. Endoscopic polypectomy should be considered adequate treatment of a polyp containing invasive cancer at level 1, 2, or 3 if the carcinoma is well differentiated, does not exhibit invasion of the veins or lymphatics, and the resection margins are free of cancer. For example, endoscopic polypectomy would be sufficient for a tubular adenoma with a well differentiated cancer extending to level 3 so long as there was no evidence of venous or lymphatic invasion and the margin of resection was free of disease. A poorly differentiated cancer extending to level 2, however, would require a formal segmental resection; similarly, any polyp with cancer extending to level 4 requires segmental resection regardless of differentiation or vascular invasion.

ANSWER: A

23. Biopsy of a villous lesion of the rectum beginning 4 cm from the anal verge and extending proximally for 5 cm shows cellular atypia. Which of the following steps is the most appropriate for management?

A. Repeated biopsy.
B. Fulguration.
C. Transanal excision.
D. Abdominoperineal resection.
E. Intracavitary radiotherapy.

Ref.: 1, 2

COMMENTS: A villous adenoma, by these dimensions alone, has a 30–50% chance of harboring cancer. The sigmoidoscopic biopsy represents a limited sample size and is not adequate proof of the lesion's precise histology. In this instance, the finding of atypia suggests a high probability of cancer elsewhere in the adenoma. Complete full-thickness transanal excision of the lesion should be performed so that if a carcinoma is present its depth of penetration can be accurately assessed. If there is no invasive cancer, the patient is followed by interval endoscopic examinations because the risk of recurrence is approximately 20%, even though the initial lesion was benign. If invasive cancer is found, the need for further treatment is determined based on the depth of penetration. A T1 cancer is adequately treated with transanal excision provided the tumor is well differentiated and lacks vascular or lymphatic invasion. A T2 cancer should be treated with radical resection; alternatively, irradiation with or without chemotherapy may be appropriate, but long-term studies are needed to determine the efficacy of this treatment. Fulguration of the lesion can be performed in the elderly or poor risk patient in whom precise histologic staging is not essential. If there is a local recurrence after transanal excision, abdominoperineal resection may be considered, provided there are no metastases and the patient is an acceptable operative risk. Intracavitary radiotherapy can be considered for accessible, well differentiated cancers that are small and have minimal invasion of the rectal wall. However, because the cancer is irradiated rather than excised, no histologic verification of depth or degree of differentiation is available.

ANSWER: C

24. With regard to ulcerative colitis, which one or more of the following statements is/are true?

A. In at least half of the cases the entire colon is involved in a continuous pattern without skip areas.
B. The characteristic histologic finding of crypt abscesses is the sine qua non of ulcerative colitis and is not seen with other inflammatory conditions of the bowel.
C. The disease is most commonly a chronic relapsing one; an acute and fulminant course is seen in only 10–15% of patients.
D. Cancers arising in ulcerative colitis tend to be more evenly distributed throughout the involved colon, are more frequently multicentric, and usually are more aggressive than are similar lesions arising from colons without ulcerative colitis.

***Ref.*:** 1, 2

COMMENTS: Ulcerative colitis is a disease usually limited to the mucosal and submucosal layers of the bowel. The rectum is almost always involved, with continuous proximal spread to varying lengths of colon. The entire colon is involved in at least half of the cases. The characteristic crypt abscesses containing an infiltration of neutrophils and eosinophils extend down into the bases of the crypts of Lieberkühn and the lamina propria. Although crypt abscesses may be seen with other inflammatory conditions of the colon, they are always present with ulcerative colitis and usually in greater numbers. In contrast to Crohn's disease, in which the supply of goblet cells is preserved, the microscopic appearance of ulcerative colitis characteristically reveals goblet cell depletion. Ulcerative colitis is most commonly chronic and relapsing in character, although in 10–15% of the cases the disease runs an acute and fulminant course. • Cancers arising in colons with past or present ulcerative colitis are usually diagnosed later in their course, because the signs and symptoms may be confused initially with an inflammatory relapse; it is for this reason that these cancers are associated with a poorer prognosis. Studies have shown that, contrary to what has been believed, colitic cancers do not behave more aggressively than their noncolitic counterparts when similar stages are compared. Cancers arising within a colitic colon (compared to noncolitic cases) are more evenly distributed throughout the colon, have a higher incidence of proximal involvement, and are frequently multiple.

ANSWER: A, C

25. A 25-year-old woman presents with a history of repeated episodes of bloody diarrhea, general abdominal cramping with lower abdominal pain, and weight loss. The presumed diagnosis is ulcerative colitis. Which of the following is/are correct management?

A. A barium enema radiographic examination is done early to assess the extent and severity of her disease.
B. Hydrocortisone has been shown to induce remissions; but such steroid-induced remissions are more likely to be followed by a relapse than are spontaneous remissions.
C. Total parenteral nutrition, if administered early as part of the treatment, may delay or even prevent the need for colectomy.
D. Maintenance, low-dose steroids are effective in preventing relapses.
E. If medical therapy fails and an abdominal colectomy with ileorectal anastomosis is performed, there is a 15–20% chance that carcinoma will develop in the rectal remnant during the next 20 years.

***Ref.*:** 2

COMMENTS: **Endoscopy with biopsy** is the most widely used method for diagnosing ulcerative colitis; **barium enema** examinations can be performed but should be done with caution and avoided altogether during acute attacks because of the risk of perforation or of precipitating the development of toxic megacolon. **Prednisone** or **hydrocortisone** are highly effective for treating acute phases of the illness. Both drugs have sufficiently adverse side effects, however, that the dose is tapered early when possible. Administration of low-dose steroids on a maintenance basis has not been shown to prevent relapses. The risk of relapse is the same whether it follows a steroid-induced remission or a spontaneous remission. The optimal role of **total parenteral nutrition** for treatment of these patients has not been well defined, but it does not appear to delay the need for surgical intervention, nor should it be used as primary treatment. **Cancer risk**: Approximately 5–6% of patients with ulcerative colitis develop cancer; patients with pancolitis or disease of long-standing duration are at highest risk. When an ileorectal anastomosis is performed, lifetime proctoscopic surveillance for dysplasia or neoplasia is mandatory because of the risk of subsequent cancer, which is approximately 2% at 15 years and 15% at 30 years. Other than the cancer risk, proctitis symptomatic enough to require proctectomy is another concern following ileorectostomy for ulcerative colitis. Approximately 50% of patients undergoing this operation therefore require proctectomy because of cancer, dysplastic changes, or refractory proctitis.

ANSWER: E

26. Match the clinical comment on the left with the disease process on the right.

A. Anal involvement in 50%	a. Crohn's disease
B. Rectal involvement in nearly all	b. Ulcerative colitis
C. Small bowel involvement common	c. Both
D. Chronic diarrhea, cramps, fever	d. Neither
E. Curative surgery available	
F. Toxic megacolon	

Ref.: 2

COMMENTS: In ulcerative colitis, the anus is spared; in Crohn's disease, however, anal or perianal disease is the first manifestation in 25% of cases. Ultimately, 50–70% of patients with Crohn's colitis develop anal disease. Rectal involvement can be seen with both of these inflammatory diseases of the colon but is more common in ulcerative colitis (95% versus 50%). The small bowel is extensively involved in approximately 50% of patients with Crohn's disease, whereas "backwash ileitis," a nonspecific dilatation of the terminal ileum, occurs in perhaps only 10% of patients with ulcerative colitis and has no prognostic or physiologic implications. The clinical presentations of these two entities are similar: chronic diarrhea, cramping, abdominal pain, and fever. Bloody stools, common with ulcerative colitis, are less common with Crohn's disease. Total proctocolectomy or colectomy, rectal mucosectomy, and ileal pouch–anal anastomosis eliminate the disease process of ulcerative colitis, whereas there is no curative operation for Crohn's disease. Indeed, even after total proctocolectomy for pancolonic involvement with Crohn's disease, its recurrence rate may be as high as 50%; one-third of patients require additional surgery for such recurrence. • A toxic megacolon can be an emergent, life-threatening complication of either ulcerative colitis or Crohn's disease, although it occurs less frequently with the latter.

ANSWER: A-a; B-c; C-a; D-c; E-b; F-c

27. Match each clinical presentation in the left column with the appropriate clinical condition in the right column.

A. The principal mechanism is twisting of a segment of bowel on a narrow mesentery.	a. Sigmoid volvulus.
B. Most common in elderly debilitated persons with psychiatric or neurologic diseases.	b. Cecal volvulus.
C. Nonoperative reduction is successful in approximately 70% of patients.	c. Both.
D. Abdominal distension, pain, and radiographic signs of a small bowel obstruction.	d. Neither.
E. Mortality rates are not altered whether operating urgently for peritonitis or electively after successful nonoperative reduction.	

Ref.: 1, 2, 11

COMMENTS: The prerequisite for developing a sigmoid or a cecal volvulus is a mobile segment of bowel that can rotate around a mesentery whose points of fixation are in close proximity. Otherwise, there are surprisingly few similarities between a sigmoid and a cecal volvulus. **Frequency**: Volvulus of the cecum is found most frequently in persons 25–35 years of age, whereas it is unusual for sigmoid volvulus to occur in an active, otherwise healthy individual. Usually it is seen in elderly, debilitated persons or in those with psychiatric or neurologic disorders in which immobility, medications that impair bowel motility, and loss of accessory defecatory muscles may lead to constipation and elongation of the colon. **Signs and symptoms**: Both types of volvulus typically cause abdominal distension and pain. With cecal volvulus there may be radiographic evidence of small bowel obstruction; with sigmoid volvulus the distended twisted loop has a fairly characteristic appearance of a bent inner tube. **Therapy**: For **sigmoid volvulus** nonoperative detorsion by careful insufflation of air endoscopically and a rectal tube to evacuate the voluminous fecal contents is the preferred initial therapeutic approach but should be attempted only if the mucosa does not appear gangrenous. Although nonoperative detorsion is successful approximately 70% of the time, a recurrence rate of 33–60% mandates elective resection of the elongated colon if the patient is believed to be an acceptable operative risk. Physical findings of peritoneal inflammation or irritation mitigate against nonoperative reduction, and these patients must undergo laparotomy. For **cecal volvulus** nonoperative colonoscopic reduction of a cecal volvulus is successful in only 25% of cases and should not be attempted in the presence of peritoneal inflammation. If colonoscopy is unsuccessful or contraindicated (e.g., tenderness), an operation is indicated as soon as the patient can be prepared. If gangrenous, the cecum must be resected; in the absence of vascular compromise, a cecopexy with or without cecostomy is sufficient. The most important determinant of patient outcome is whether bowel gangrene is present, mortality being highest if surgery is performed for intestinal infarction or perforation. Mortality is also higher if operating for recurrent volvulus.

ANSWER: A-c; B-a; C-a; D-b; E-d

28. With regard to diverticular fistulas, which of the following statements is/are true?

A. Colocutaneous fistulas frequently occur spontaneously.
B. Colovesical fistulas normally present with urinary tract infections that may be accompanied by pneumaturia and fecaluria, and the diagnosis is best confirmed with barium enema.
C. Coloenteric fistulas may be totally asymptomatic.
D. Surgical correction should be in staged operations because of the hazards of primary anastomosis in the presence of extensive local prior inflammation.

Ref.: 1, 2

COMMENTS: Fistula formation occurs in 5% of complicated cases of colonic diverticulitis. Fistulas are usually adjacent to viscera: the bladder, uterus, vagina, or small bowel. **Colocutaneous fistulas** rarely form spontaneously; they are most commonly seen as a postoperative complication, draining through operative incisions or drain tracts. **Colovesical fistulas** are most commonly the result of diverticular disease, followed in frequency by cancer, Crohn's disease, radiation colitis, and foreign bodies. Their first symptoms (e.g., fecaluria and pneumaturia) are referable to the urinary tract. The patient may relate a history of abdominal pain and fever prior to the development of the fistula. Although a barium enema may give information regarding the site and extent of involvement of the colon with diverticulosis, the fistula is demonstrated in only half of the cases. Cystoscopy is more likely to demonstrate the fistula; findings may include bullous (edematous) edema of the dome of the bladder. Computed tomography may reveal a constellation of findings including air in the bladder, a thickened loop of bowel laying adherent to the bladder and enteric contrast in the bladder (before intravenous contrast has been administered). **Coloenteric fistulas** may cause no symptoms or may present with diarrhea. • The fistula can be corrected by a one-stage operation in most patients and thus is the preferred treatment. If the bowel preparation is inadequate or if there is extensive local inflammation or abscess formation, staged procedures may be preferable.

ANSWER: C

29. Match the characteristic features in the left column with the locations of diverticula in the right column.

A. Frequently are true diverticula and therefore are considered congenital in origin.
B. When inflamed, may be clinically and radiographically indistinguishable from cancer.
C. Resection and primary anastomosis may be hazardous in the presence of perforation with frank peritonitis.
D. Asymptomatic diverticula found incidentally on a barium enema should be treated operatively because of the high incidence of complications.

a. Sigmoid.
b. Cecal.
c. Both.
d. Neither.

Ref.: 2

COMMENTS: Sigmoid diverticula lack a muscular component and so are not considered true diverticula. Right-sided diverticula may occur as part of diffuse colonic diverticulosis and as such are pseudodiverticular and acquired. Occasionally, isolated, solitary, right-sided diverticula are found and possess all layers of the bowel wall; they are probably congenital in origin. Cecal diverticulitis is uncommon, and the correct preoperative diagnosis is rarely made because it is confused with acute appendicitis in 80% and with cancer in approximately 5% of cases. In rare cases of repeated attacks, the cecal inflammation with subsequent scarring and fibrosis can produce a radiographic picture and operative findings that may be indistinguishable from those of cancer. Similarly, an inflammatory mass of the sigmoid colon may resemble a cancer at laparotomy. The surgical options depend on the extent of inflammation: If inflammation is minimal and is limited to the diverticulum, resection of a solitary cecal diverticulum may be all that is necessary; if there has been perforation with frank peritonitis, most surgeons hesitate to perform a primary anastomosis and instead resect the involved segment and divert the stool proximally. For both types of diverticula, surgical therapy is not required if the diverticulum is discovered incidentally and the patient is asymptomatic.

ANSWER: A-b; B-c; C-c; D-d

30. With regard to radiation enterocolitis, which of the following statements is/are true?

A. Histologically, subintimal foam cells are pathognomonic; additional changes include a progressive vasculitis of the submucosal arteries.
B. The rectum is the most common site of injury.
C. Rectovaginal fistulas secondary to irradiation can be treated only by fecal diversion.
D. Long segments of strictured bowel are best treated with resection.
E. Prior pelvic irradiation predisposes to rectosigmoid cancer.

Ref.: 2

COMMENTS: The incidence of radiation injury to the bowel is dose-dependent. Substantial bowel injury is uncommon at external doses of less than 4000 rad. In addition to the radiation dose, other factors that may predispose to injury include advanced age, hypertension, arteriosclerosis, diabetes, and adhesions that fix the bowel to a constant location. After cessation of radiation therapy, the denuded intestinal epithelium regenerates. The vessels, however, develop a progressive vasculitis that may lead to thickening of the vessel wall with progressive diminution of the vessel lumen with occlusion or thrombosis (or both). • The rectum is the most common site of injury because of its proximity to the most frequently targeted organs (e.g., cervix, uterus, prostate) and its fixed location within the pelvis. When rectal ulcers occur, they are on the anterior wall about 4–6 cm from the dentate line; rectal strictures usually occur at the 8- to 12-cm level. • When faced with a rectovaginal fistula, every attempt should be made to rule out a recurrence of the cancer as the cause of the fistula; if present, fecal diversion usually palliates symptoms. In the absence of recurrent cancer and in selected patients, an attempt can be made to correct the fistula. Operative correction must interpose nonirradiated tissue between the rectum and the vagina after the fistulous openings have been closed. When possible, anterior resection or coloanal pull-through employing nonirradiated intestine for the proximal anastomotic limb is preferred. The aforementioned precautions to ensure primary healing notwithstanding, there should be proximal temporary fecal diversion in the form of a colostomy. • Prior pelvic irradiation does predispose to rectosigmoid cancer after a latent period of several years. For this reason, flexible sigmoidoscopy is advised on a periodic basis. • In summary, when treating radiation enterocolitis, certain principles should be observed: Avoid an operation unless no other option exists; resect short segments, but bypass long segments, of diseased bowel; avoid extensive adhesiolysis; safeguard anastomotic leak with a temporary proximal colostomy.

ANSWER: A, B, E

31. With regard to pseudomembranous colitis, which of the following statements is/are true?

A. Diarrhea that begins 1 week after antibiotics have been discontinued rules out pseudomembranous colitis.
B. Pseudomembranous colitis does not occur in the absence of antibiotic therapy.
C. Administration of vancomycin or metronidazole is appropriate treatment.
D. There is a relapse rate of 50% after treatment.

Ref.: 1, 2

COMMENTS: Pseudomembranous enterocolitis, which was first described by Billroth in 1867, has been seen with increased frequency and is associated with the use of many antibiotics. The disease has not been described with the use of vancomycin or with antimicrobials used to treat mycobacteria, fungi, or parasites. There is evidence that antibiotics change the intracolonic flora, allowing overgrowth of *Clostridium difficile*, which then produces enterocolitis. There is also evidence, however, that pseudomembranous colitis is infectious and is spread by patient-to-patient or staff-to-patient contact. • Pseudomembranous colitis should be suspected in any patient who develops diarrhea during or up to 3 weeks after the cessation of antibiotic therapy. • The diagnosis is established endoscopically by visualizing the characteristic raised mucosal plaques or by a cytotoxic assay for *C. difficile* exotoxin, which usually has a positive result in cases of pseudomembranous colitis. • Therapy should begin with prompt cessation of the offending antibiotic. Vancomycin (500 mg q.i.d. for 10 days) or metronidazole (500 mg q.i.d. for 10 days) has been used to treat this condition successfully; the relapse rate, however, is 20% for vancomycin and 23% for metronidazole. • Surgery is rarely necessary except in cases of toxic colitis or perforation.

ANSWER: C

32. With regard to carcinoid tumors of the colon and rectum, which of the following statements is/are true?

A. They occur with equal frequency at these two sites.
B. The incidence of invasive malignancy and metastases correlates with carcinoid size.
C. They frequently cause the carcinoid syndrome.
D. Superficial, small rectal lesions should be excised transanally.
E. Invasive rectal lesions larger than 2 cm are best treated by abdominoperineal resection.

Ref.: 6

COMMENTS: Carcinoid (neuroendocrine) tumors of the colon and rectum represent a wide and diverse group of neoplasms that range from completely benign lesions to poorly differentiated cancers with an extremely dismal prognosis. These lesions share the capability of storing large amounts of an amine precursor (5-hydroxytryptophan); and through the amine precursor uptake and decarboxylation system [APUD: amine precursor uptake (and) decarboxylation] these lesions produce several biologically active amines. The gastrointestinal tract is the most common site for carcinoid formation; and in decreasing order of frequency, the most common locations are the appendix, ileum, rectum, stomach, and colon. Colon carcinoids account for only 2.5% of all gastrointestinal carcinoids; rectal carcinoids account for 12–15%. The incidence of invasive malignancy and metastases to regional lymph nodes correlates well with the size of the carcinoid, for both colonic and rectal lesions. For example, when rectal carcinoids are larger than 2 cm only 5–10% are benign, whereas a lesion less than 2 cm is malignant only approximately 5% of the time. Because rectal carcinoids less than 2 cm rarely demonstrate invasion of the muscularis or lymph node metastases, they may be excised transanally. Lesions larger than 2 cm and located in the rectum are best treated by abdominoperineal resection or low anterior resection, if possible. If malignant, colon carcinoids should be treated by a formal segmental resection with the accompanying lymph node-bearing tissue. Up to two-thirds of patients with carcinoids of the colon have either local spread or systemic metastases at the time of diagnosis. If there is disseminated disease, resection of the primary lesion is still recommended to alleviate symptoms and avoid the potential for bleeding and obstruction. Carcinoids of the colon and rectum infrequently produce the carcinoid syndrome unless systemic metastases have occurred.

ANSWER: B, D, E

33. With regard to amebiasis, which of the following statements is/are true?

A. Approximately 10% of the people in the United States are asymptomatic carriers.
B. *Entamoeba histolytica* antibodies are detectable in the serum of more than 90% of those with active amebiasis.
C. Acute amebic dysentery closely resembles fulminant ulcerative colitis and should be treated aggressively with steroids.
D. Amebic abscess of the spleen is the most common complication of amebic colitis.
E. Colon perforation with peritonitis occurs in approximately half of the patients with an acute presentation.

Ref.: 1, 2

COMMENTS: Amebic colitis is caused by the protozoan *Entamoeba histolytica*, which infests primarily the colon and rectum and, secondarily, other organs such as the liver. It has been estimated that 10% of the American population are asymptomatic carriers. Transmission of the disease is through food or water contaminated with feces containing *Entamoeba* cysts. The disease can assume an acute and a chronic form. **Acute amebic dysentery** is seen with contamination of the water supply and has a presentation similar to that of acute ulcerative colitis (i.e., fever, cramps, and bloody diarrhea). The distinction between these two entities is important; steroids are given routinely on a short-term basis to treat ulcerative colitis but are contraindicated in the therapy of amebic dysentery; the desired effect of steroids of muting the inflammatory response would mask the clinicopathologic progression of amebic colitis. In a typical case, proctosigmoidoscopy should reveal extensive ulceration of the intestinal epithelium, and warm saline preparation of the stool usually demonstrates numerous trophozoites containing ingested erythrocytes. The diagnosis is strengthened by a serologic test for *E. histolytica* antibodies, which is positive in 90% of patients with active amebiasis. Treatment is with metronidazole 750 mg t.i.d. for 10 days. • Perforation of the colon during the acute form of the disease is rare. • Amebic abscess of the liver is the most common complication of amebic colitis, which may in turn rupture into the pleura, pericardium, or peritoneum. **Chronic amebic dysentery** is more common than the acute form and is characterized by three to four foul-smelling bowel movements per day along with abdominal cramping and fever. The diagnosis of chronic amebic dysentery is more difficult to establish because cysts or trophozoites are not always demonstrable in stool preparations and sigmoidoscopy is normal in up to 30% of such individuals. ***E. histolytica*** antibodies, however, should be detectable. The treatment is diiodohydroxyquin 650 mg t.i.d. for 20 days and metronidazole, or diloxamide furoate, 500 mg t.i.d. for 10 days.

ANSWER: A, B

34. Match each disease in the left column with the appropriate drug or drugs that may be used for their treatment in the right column.

A. Actinomycosis	a. Hydrocortisone
B. Lymphogranuloma venereum	b. Metronidazole
C. Tuberculous enteritis	c. Penicillin
D. *Yersinia* infection	d. Tetracycline
	e. Streptomycin

Ref.: 1, 2, 3

COMMENTS: Actinomycosis is a suppurative, granulomatous disease caused by *Actinomyces israelii*, an anaerobic, gram-positive bacterium that produces chronic inflammatory induration and sinus formation. Although the causative organism is part of the normal oral flora, infections may occur in the cervicofacial area, thorax, or abdomen. The cecal region is the most frequent site of abdominal infection, producing a pericecal mass, abscesses, and sinus. Rectal strictures have been reported as well. Treatment consists of surgical drainage and penicillin or tetracycline. • **Lymphogranuloma venereum** is a sexually transmissible disease due to *Chlamydia trachomatis*. It is seen most frequently in the homosexual population, in which it starts as proctitis and produces tenesmus, discharge, and bleeding. Perianal and rectovaginal fistulas may develop, as may rectal strictures. The diagnosis is made by the Frei intracutaneous test when the test is available. Otherwise, the diagnosis may be confirmed by a complement fixation test. Tetracycline is curative, and steroids have been recommended. • **Tuberculous enteritis** is seen most commonly in the ileocecal region and occasionally leads to stenosis of the distal ileum, cecum, and ascending colon, producing endoscopic and radiographic features that may be indistinguishable from those of Crohn's disease. Surgery is reserved for patients with obstruction. Triple-drug therapy of isoniazid, paraaminosalicylic acid, and streptomycin usually heals the intestinal lesions. • ***Yersinia*** infections are caused by a gram-negative rod that is transmitted through food contaminated by feces or urine; it produces a clinical picture frequently indistinguishable from that of acute appendicitis. *Yersinia* may also cause acute gastroenteritis, which affects primarily the ileocecal region. *Yersinia* responds to treatment with tetracycline, streptomycin, ampicillin, or kanamycin.

ANSWER: A-c,d; B-a,d; C-e; D-d,e

35. With regard to ischemic colitis, which of the following statements is/are true?

A. The most common symptoms are lower abdominal pain and bright red rectal bleeding.
B. Occlusion of the major mesenteric vessels is responsible for producing the ischemia in most cases.
C. The splenic flexure and descending colon are the most vulnerable areas, although any segment of colon may be involved.
D. Nonoperative management is not justified because in a significant percentage of such cases perforation and peritonitis eventually develop.

Ref.: 1, 2, 3, 11

COMMENTS: Ischemic colitis should be considered in the differential diagnosis of any elderly patient who presents with left lower quadrant pain. It can also be found in individuals of any age in association with periarteritis nodosa, systemic lupus erythematosus, rheumatoid arthritis, polycythemia vera, and scleroderma. • Ischemic colitis may present as three distinct clinical syndromes depending on (1) the extent and duration of vascular occlusion, (2) the adequacy of collateral circulation, and (3) the extent of septic complications. Mild or transient ischemia is compensated for by collateral blood flow; there may be a partial, reversible mucosal slough that heals in 2–3 days. Transmural ischemia may predispose to a stricture if healing takes place without perforation. If these ischemic changes progress to full-thickness gangrene, perforation and peritonitis will ensue. • Ischemic colitis appears to be a disease of the small arterioles. Occlusion of the major mesenteric vessels does not adequately explain the cause of this disease. For example, patients with frank ischemic colitis may have angiographic evidence of patent major arteries. Moreover, ligation of these vessels (e.g., when ligating the inferior mesenteric artery during aortic aneurysmectomy) may not cause ischemic colitis. Although this disease can occur in any segment of the large bowel, it is seen most commonly in the splenic flexure or distal sigmoid colon, a plausible explanation being the suboptimal blood flow in areas positioned between two vascular systems ("watershed areas"), which rely on an intact but meandering artery for their blood supply. **Sudeck's** point is the area between the blood supply from the last sigmoid artery and the superior rectal artery. The clinical significance of Sudek's point is questionable because of retrograde flow from the middle and inferior rectal arteries. **Griffith's** point is the vulnerable area at the splenic flexure that is positioned between areas perfused by the left branch of the middle colic artery and the ascending branch of the left colic artery. • The diagnosis is made by endoscopy, which reveals cyanotic, edematous mucosa that may be covered by exudative membranes, or by barium enema, which may show the typical "thumbprinting" of the bowel wall. If gangrenous colitis is suspected on the basis of ominous physical findings, these studies are contraindicated and prompt laparotomy is mandatory. • Transient ischemic colitis usually responds to nonoperative management. Ischemic strictures may be electively resected with primary anastomosis after the initial ischemic episode has subsided. If surgery is needed for peritonitis and gangrenous colitis, resection with end-colostomy is the preferred operation.

ANSWER: A, C

36. With regard to the operation that includes colectomy, mucosal proctectomy, and ileoanal anastomosis, which of the following statements is/are true?

A. It is indicated for either ulcerative colitis or Crohn's disease, provided the rectum is minimally involved.
B. Bladder and sexual function are preserved postoperatively.
C. The need for a permanent ileostomy is avoided.
D. Construction of an ileal pouch proximal to the anastomosis increases intestinal storage capacity and decreases stool frequency.

Ref.: 1, 2

COMMENTS: Patients who require total proctocolectomy and permanent ileostomy for ulcerative colitis may be eligible for a sphincter-preserving procedure. Colectomy, mucosal proctectomy, and ileoanal anastomosis offer advantages over proctocolectomy and permanent ileostomy because not only is the diseased mucosa eliminated but so is the need for a permanent abdominal stoma. The operative technique was described by Ravich and Sabiston in 1947 and has undergone certain modifications—most notably, construction of an ileal pouch proximal to the ileoanal anastomosis. The pouch may be S-shaped or J-shaped, increasing intestinal storage capacity and decreasing stool frequency. A temporary diverting ileostomy is usually required for 2–3 months while the pouch heals. The procedure is presently recommended for selected patients with ulcerative colitis and those with familial polyposis. It is not indicated for Crohn's disease because of the risk of recurrence within the pouch, which may lead to complex fistulas and septic complications. Although advanced age is not an absolute contraindication, the elderly patient with multiple comorbidities may be better served with a permanent ileostomy. Similarly, patients with preexisting fecal incontinence from anorectal surgery or obstetric injuries should probably avoid an ileoanal anastomosis. For appropriately selected patients, functional results are good, with preservation of the parasympathetic innervation to the bladder and genitalia; fecal sensation and continence are retained in most of these patients.

ANSWER: B, C, D

37. With regard to megacolon, which of the following statements is/are true?

A. The common denominator for congenital megacolon (Hirschsprung's disease) and acquired megacolon is chronic partial distal obstruction.
B. Hirschsprung's disease is due to the congenital absence of ganglion cells in the myenteric plexus.
C. There is a transition zone from the dilated nondiseased colon to normal-caliber aganglionic bowel.
D. Acquired megacolon may be seen in patients whose colon is infested with *Trypanosoma cruzi* and in patients with neurologic disorders, such as paraplegia and poliomyelitis.
E. The surgical importance of megacolon is in its formation of chronic bowel dilatation, elongation, and a propensity to volvulus formation.

Ref.: 1, 2

COMMENTS: **Megacolon** may be congenital or acquired; both forms have the common denominator of dilatation, elongation, and hypertrophy of the colon proximal to a segment of nonperistaltic collapsed bowel causing obstruction. Both have an increased risk of volvulus. **Hirschsprung's disease** is caused by the congenital absence of ganglion cells in the myenteric plexus of the bowel, resulting in loss of peristaltic activity in that segment of intestine. The rectosigmoid region is most frequently involved, with variable extension of the disease proximally. There is a transition zone from the normal bowel (that is dilated) to the abnormal bowel that is aganglionic, aperistaltic, and of normal or decreased caliber. Although primarily a disease of infants and children, occasionally Hirschsprung's disease does not manifest until later in life if an ultra-short segment of distal rectum is involved. In these cases patients relate a history of constipation dating back to infancy. The diagnosis is apparent during the first 24 hours of life if the infant fails to pass meconium. A rectal biopsy is diagnostic. In adolescents and young adults, Hirschsprung's disease can be diagnosed using anal manometry. If the disease is present, the normal relaxation of the internal sphincter, which is the expected response to rectal distension, is lost. The treatment of Hirschsprung's disease is primarily surgical, utilizing a coloanal anastomosis. **Acquired megacolon** may be seen in protozoal colon infections with *Trypanosoma cruzi*, which is endemic in South and Central America. *T. cruzi* causes widespread destruction of the intramural nervous system. Acquired megacolon is seen also in patients with colonic dilatation as a result of chronic constipation due to the loss of voluntary defecatory muscles (paraplegia), extreme inactivity (poliomyelitis), or voluntary inhibition of defecation (psychotic disorders). Resection of the excessive redundant colon is occasionally justified in the latter group of patients.

ANSWER: A, B, C, D, E

38. With regard to the polyposis coli syndromes, which of the following statements is/are true?

A. Screening family members at risk should begin at puberty and consists of an annual complete colonoscopy.
B. Death from colon cancer that develops in these patients occurs at a significantly earlier age than in nonpolyposis patients with colon cancer.
C. The risk of colon cancer developing is approximately 100%.
D. Abdominal colectomy and ileoproctostomy eliminate the risk of carcinoma.
E. Periampullary tumors are an important cause of death.

Ref.: 1, 2, 11, 12

COMMENTS: Most reports of polyposis syndromes reflect experience in American and European populations, but these diseases have been identified in Africans and Asians as well. There probably is no race or geographic area that is exempt. The polyposis syndromes occur in approximately 1 of every 12,000 births; thus 300 new patients are diagnosed each year in the United States. The disease is transmitted as an autosomal dominant trait; therefore approximately 50% of the offspring of an afflicted individual have the disease. About 30–40% of patients do not have a positive family history for polyposis, and these cases represent spontaneous mutations at the polyposis locus. • The polyps are not present at birth but first appear usually at puberty and gradually increase in number so that by age 21 the colon and rectum are carpeted by thousands of polyps. If the polyps are left untreated, the risk of developing cancer of the colon is approximately 100%, with death from colon cancer occurring at an average age of 41.5 years. • Subtotal colectomy with ileoproctostomy has been advocated by some authors; if done, close surveillance of the rectal remnant is mandatory and is accomplished with proctoscopy performed at 6-month intervals. The incidence of rectal cancer after ileorectostomy varies widely among reported series, with one being as high as 59% at 23 years. Other reports estimate the risk to be 5–15% and the chance of dying from rectal cancer extremely low. In fact, patients are less likely to die of rectal cancer than from periampullary tumors or desmoids. Nevertheless, the importance of surveillance proctoscopy cannot be overemphasized. Extensive carpeting of the rectum with polyps should dissuade one from recommending ileorectostomy. • Mucosal proctectomy with ileoanal anastomosis removes all neoplastic mucosa while avoiding the need for permanent ileostomy. • Screening asymptomatic family members at risk should begin at puberty. Because colon polyps rarely if ever develop in the absence of rectal polyps, sigmoidoscopy is adequate for screening. If polyps are found, a biopsy is recommended to verify the presence of adenomatous tissue. Upper endoscopy should be done at the time of diagnosis to document the involvement of the stomach and duodenum.

ANSWER: B, C, E

39. With regard to colonic fluid and electrolyte absorption, which of the following statements is/are correct?

A. The colon protects against hyponatremia by actively absorbing sodium against both concentration and electrical gradients.
B. Under normal conditions, absorption of sodium and water in the right colon is the same as in the rectum.
C. Chloride and bicarbonate ions participate in an exchange mechanism; chloride is actively absorbed from the colonic lumen.
D. The colon is not involved in urea metabolism.
E. The maximal absorptive capacity of the colon is 5–6 liters per day.

Ref.: 14

COMMENTS: In healthy subjects, the colon normally absorbs 1–2 liters of water and up to 200 mEq of sodium and chloride per day. This absorptive capacity can increase up to 5–6 liters per day, thereby protecting the person against severe diarrhea. Lack of a colon may lead to enteric losses of sodium and chloride. • Absorption of sodium is an active process and continues even when luminal concentrations are as low as 15–25 mM. Sodium absorption also takes place against a potential (electrical) gradient of 35–50 mV (mucosa negative). • Colonic absorption varies regionally: The cecum and right colon absorb sodium and water the most rapidly; the rectum is impermeable to sodium and water. • Chloride ions are actively absorbed at the expense of bicarbonate, which is secreted in exchange. Absence of luminal chloride inhibits bicarbonate secretion. When the sigmoid colon is used as a urinary conduit, urinary chloride is actively absorbed. As a consequence, bicarbonate is secreted, leading to the common and predictable complication of chronic acidosis. The ileal mucosa, in contrast, absorbs chloride less avidly, making it more suitable as a urinary conduit. • The daily urea production exceeds urinary excretion by 25%; the excess is metabolized by the colon. Through the mesenteric vessels, circulating urea reaches the mucosa, where bacterial ureases convert urea to ammonia, which is then reabsorbed.

ANSWER: A, C, E

40. Match each physician in the left column with the contribution to the management of colorectal cancer in the right column.

A. John B. Murphy
B. Nicholas Senn
C. Arthur Dean Bevan
D. Claude E. Dixon
E. W. Ernest Miles

a. Posterior approach to the rectum with division of the sphincter muscle
b. Instrumental in the suturing of anastomoses with a continuous inverting suture
c. Internal stent for constructing intestinal anastomoses
d. Low anterior resection
e. Abdominoperineal resection

Ref.: 3

COMMENTS: Prior to the advances in critical care and blood bank technology, the most frequently performed operations for rectal cancer were through transperineal or transsacral approaches. **Paul Kraske** (1851–1930) removed the coccyx and a portion of the sacrum (while preserving the sphincter) prior to resecting accessible rectal cancers. If intestinal continuity could not be restored, a sacral anus was created. Extension of the paracoccygeal incision down to and through the sphincter was first advocated by **Arthur Dean Bevan** (1861–1943). Bevan, who was a graduate of Rush Medical College in 1883 and subsequently appointed Chairman of Surgery at the same institution in 1909, used this approach "for small carcinomas of the rectum without any radical involvement." Because proximal lymphatic spread was not addressed by this method, **W. Ernest Miles** (1869–1947) concluded that the approaches used by Kraske and Bevan were inadequate operations for rectal cancer. Miles contended that all areas of potential lymphatic spread must be removed along with the anus, rectum, and a portion of the sigmoid. The abdominoperineal resection was reported by Miles in 1908; his operation lasted approximately 30 minutes. An alternative approach to the Miles operation is low anterior resection and primary anastomosis for properly selected patients. Fear of anastomotic leak and sepsis prompted **John B. Murphy** (1857–1916), a professor of surgery at Rush Medical College, to create in 1892 his "button," which by acting as an internal stent helped to coapt ends of intestinal tissue without the need of suturing. Primary anastomosis of the intestine was perfected by several surgical researchers including Halsted, Lembert, and Senn. **Nicholas Senn** (1844–1908) was one of the first surgeons in the Western Hemisphere to appreciate the importance of the animal laboratory for refining surgical technique. Senn, a professor of surgical pathology at Rush Medical College, worked with Connell in perfecting the continuous inverting suture for intestinal anastomoses. **Claude E. Dixon** (1893–1968), head of the Section of General Surgery at The Mayo Graduate School from 1928 to 1957, was one of the first advocates of low anterior resection and primary anastomosis without colostomy.

ANSWER: A-c; B-b; C-a; D-d; E-e

41. Colonoscopy is indicated in which of the following conditions?

A. Determining the extent of ulcerative colitis in a patient admitted to the hospital for an acute exacerbation.
B. Screening family members at risk for familial adenomatous polyposis.
C. Evaluation of an equivocal finding on barium enema.
D. If an adenomatous polyp is found in the upper rectum on screening sigmoidoscopy.
E. Evaluating gastrointestinal symptoms such as bleeding or pain when radiographic studies fail to reveal the cause.

Ref.: 3

COMMENTS: Colonoscopy is contraindicated in cases of acute peritoneal inflammation, such as acute diverticulitis, peritonitis, or perforation. Also, colonoscopy should not be performed during acute presentations of inflammatory bowel disease because of the potential for colonic perforation. Colonoscopy is also contraindicated in patients immediately after an acute myocardial infarction (because of the possibly adverse sequela associated with a vasovagal reflex), in patients with marked splenomegaly (traction on the splenic flexure may precipitate splenic bleeding), and during pregnancy (if fluoroscopy is to be used). • Because colonic polyps in patients with familial polyposis rarely develop in the absence of rectal polyps, screening family members at risk for polyposis is best accomplished with proctosigmoidoscopy. • Colonoscopy may confirm or refute suspected or equivocal radiographic findings during a barium enema examination. If the barium enema fails to reveal the cause of a patient's anemia, pain, or bleeding, colonoscopy is indicated. • If an adenomatous polyp or cancer is discovered during screening sigmoidoscopy, colonoscopy is indicated to exclude the possibility of primary synchronous polyps (30%) or cancers (4–8%). • Colonoscopy is indicated for sigmoid volvulus and pseudoobstruction of the colon, provided there are no signs of peritoneal inflammation. Decompression of the distended colon can be achieved successfully with minimal patient preparation.

ANSWER: C, D, E

42. For medical management of toxic megacolon, which of the following is/are true?

A. Nasoenteric decompression should be employed early.
B. Endoscopy is necessary for the correct diagnosis.
C. The patient should be rolled into a prone position on a flattened bed several times daily.
D. Intravenous steroids have no role in this condition.

Ref.: 11, 15

COMMENTS: Toxic megacolon is seen in patients with ulcerative colitis (1–13%) and less frequently in Crohn's colitis. Rapid fluid resuscitation and blood product transfusion are essential. A nasogastric tube should be inserted. Some authors insist on passage of a long small bowel tube. Whichever method is chosen, nasoenteric suction helps minimize the accumulation of swallowed air in the colon. • Air accumulates usually in the transverse colon, and such accumulation is promoted in patients lying supine. Therefore it is suggested to have patients roll into the prone position for 10–15 minutes every 2 hours. • There is little need to confirm the diagnosis with endoscopy; in fact, intubation of the colon above the peritoneal reflection may cause perforation. In patients with a fulminant presentation and no previous history of inflammatory bowel disease, a proctoscope, if inserted, should be advanced carefully to 10–15 cm and with little insufflation. It helps confirm suspected inflammatory bowel disease and rules out anorectal causes of blood per rectum, such as hemorrhoids. The diagnosis of toxic megacolon is based on clinical findings of fever, tachycardia, and abdominal bloating, combined with radiographs of the abdomen showing colonic distension. Response to medical management is assessed with serial abdominal radiographs. Prompt administration of steroids is an important factor when inducing a response. Broad-spectrum antibiotics are also used. Even if medical therapy is successful, most patients do not have a satisfactory long-term outcome; ongoing symptoms and even recurrent toxic colitis continue to be concerns. • Worsening colonic distension, fever, and leukocytosis are indications for surgery. In these instances the operative choice is abdominal colectomy without proctectomy. This procedure allows sphincter-preserving surgery to take place once health has been restored.

ANSWER: A, C

43. Match each colitic process in the left column to the appropriate statement in the right column.

A. Backwash ileitis	a. Responds to short-chain fatty acid instillation
B. Diversion colitis	b. Metronidazole used to treat this condition
C. Microscopic (lymphocytic) colitis	c. Seen in some cases of ulcerative colitis
D. Acute ileitis	d. Good response to sulfasalazine
E. Pseudomembranous colitis	e. *Yersinia* infection

Ref.: 15

COMMENTS: Backwash ileitis comprises nonspecific inflammation and dilatation of the ileum in patients with ulcerative colitis involving the entire colon. There is no thickening or narrowing as seen in Crohn's disease. Its presence does not imply a pre-Crohn's disease condition, nor does it imply a poor outcome following the ileal pouch/anal anastomosis procedure. • **Diversion colitis** is found in segments of defunctionalized bowel. The instillation of short-chain fatty acids ameliorates the condition, supporting the concept that these substances (being primary nutrients for the colonic mucosal cells) are deficient in this condition, leading to chronic inflammation. There have been preliminary trials in idiopathic ulcerative proctocolitis that show a response to short-chain fatty acid enemas. • **Microscopic colitis** (also known as **lymphocytic colitis**) is characterized by a history of watery diarrhea and microscopic inflammation of colonic mucosa. The colitis often responds favorably to sulfasalazine. **Collagenous colitis** (a collagenous band is seen on microscopy under the surface epithelium of the colon) may be a variant of this condition because patients present with similar symptoms and respond to sulfasalazine. Spontaneous remission of these two conditions is common. Most of these patients have been incorrectly labeled for years as having irritable bowel syndrome; colonoscopy with biopsy may yield the correct diagnosis. • **Acute inflammatory ileitis** presents with right lower quadrant pain and is commonly confused with appendicitis or Crohn's disease. Acute ileitis, often due to *Yersinia enterocolitica* infection, is capable of producing a self-limited acute ileitis and colitis, sometimes with a granulomatous reaction. • Antibiotic-induced colitis (also known as **pseudomembranous colitis**) presents with watery diarrhea, which is rarely bloody and is due to *Clostridium difficile* proliferation. The diagnosis is best made by detecting the *C. difficile* toxin in the stool. Either oral vancomycin or metronidazole is used to treat this condition; the latter is less expensive and is therefore used more often.

ANSWER: A-c; B-a; C-d; D-e; E-b

44. Colonoscopy is strongly indicated in which one or more of the following groups of patients?

A. In patients with Crohn's colitis to monitor the efficacy of treatment.
B. In patients with an 8- to 10-year history of ulcerative colitis.
C. In patients with recurrent anal fistula and fissures.
D. In patients with suspected colovaginal or colovesical fistulas.
E. Patients with colorectal cancer in first degree relative(s).

Ref.: 11, 15

COMMENTS: Endoscopy is not indicated simply for the purpose of monitoring the response of Crohn's disease to medical therapy. It can be done on a clinical basis alone. • Patients with a history of ulcerative colitis for more than 8–10 years are at higher risk to have adenocarcinoma of the colon and should undergo a surveillance colonoscopy with multiple-site biopsies for the determination of dysplasia. This procedure should be done even if the disease is in remission. Thereafter, if results are negative, surveillance should probably be done on at least an annual basis. Patients with pancolitis appear to be at higher risk for cancer than patients with limited left-sided disease, but the latter group should also undergo surveillance. In patients with Crohn's disease, there is no guideline for cancer surveillance. • Patients with recurrent or multiple anal fistulas and fissures should undergo colonoscopy to exclude Crohn's disease. If the ileum is not intubated, a small-bowel radiograph should be obtained. • The presence of a colovaginal or colovesicle fistula is difficult to demonstrate endoscopically or radiographically. With either fistula, the colon must be assessed; and even if a fistula is not demonstrated, indirect evidence with regard to its cause can be obtained. For example, diverticular disease, cancer, or inflammatory bowel disease can be responsible for fistula formation and should be seen. A barium enema is probably preferable to colonoscopy for workup of a colovesicle or colovaginal fistula because of its lower risk and cost and the enhanced total image of the colon and its flexures. • At-risk patients in families with hereditary nonpolyposis colorectal cancer must undergo colonoscopy beginning at age 25. First-degree relatives of patients with sporadic colorectal cancer have a two- to threefold increased risk of developing cancer, especially if the family member was younger than age 55 at the time of cancer diagnosis. The age at which to begin screening first degree relatives with colonoscopy is controversial, but it has been suggested that screening begin at an age 10 years younger than the age of the relative when cancer was diagnosed.

ANSWER: B, C, E

45. Match each type of radiation therapy used for treatment of rectal cancer in the left column with the appropriate feature or features in the right column.

A. Preoperative
B. Intraoperative
C. Postoperative

a. Minimizes or avoids radiation damage to the small intestine
b. Capable of improving local control by treating tumor cell spillage during surgery
c. When combined with chemotherapy has demonstrated definite benefit in local control and survival
d. Capable of down-staging the tumor

Ref.: 6

COMMENTS: All of the forms of radiation therapy listed are capable of improving local control and lowering recurrence rates by treating potential tumor cell spillage. Although **preoperative irradiation** has not consistently shown a survival benefit, resectability rates may be improved and tumors may be down-staged by ablating metastatic lymph nodes. When preoperative radiation is combined with chemotherapy, complete response rates of 20–30% have been noted for cancers in the distal rectum. Although this is encouraging, there are no randomized studies of a large number of patients yet available. Because the rectum fills the pelvis, the small bowel can be potentially spared owing to its mobility and lack of fixation within the pelvis. The radiation dose has varied widely in reported series. The dose most frequently used is 40–45 Gy over 4–6 weeks, with a 6-week hiatus before surgery. • **Intraoperative irradiation** is used to treat tumors or tumor beds where gross residual or microscopic disease remains. This technique allows some radiosensitive structures such as the small bowel to be shielded from the radiation beam, thereby minimizing damage to normal tissue. A single dose of 10–20 Gy is given, and patients are also usually treated with postoperative external beam radiation therapy as well. Results have not shown an improvement in survival, and a significant portion of patients develop ureteral obstruction and sacral neuritis. • **Postoperative irradiation** is usually administered for tumors at high risk for local recurrence, such as those demonstrating transmural penetration or lymph node metastases. When combined with chemotherapy, improved local control and survival have been noted. The main advantage of administering radiation postoperatively is that the exact stage of the cancer is known; patients with early lesions or those whose tumor has spread beyond the confines of the pelvis are spared treatment.

ANSWER: A-a,b,d; B-a,b; C-b,c

46. Pouchitis can frequently complicate the ileal pouch/anal anastomosis procedure. With regard to this condition, which of the following is/are true?

A. It occurs with equal frequency in patients with familial polyposis and ulcerative colitis.
B. It is found more frequently in patients with capacious S-shaped pouches than in those with J-shaped pouches.
C. Most patients can be treated successfully with oral metronidazole.
D. The responsible pathogen is usually *Bacteroides*.
E. Recurrent persistent pouchitis invariably necessitates pouch excision.

Ref.: 6

COMMENTS: Pouchitis is a nonspecific inflammation of the ileal reservoir following the ileal pouch/anal anastomosis procedure. It occurs in 5–40% of patients. The exact cause is not known, but pouchitis is seen more frequently in patients with ulcerative colitis than in those with familial polyposis. Pouchitis is not related to pouch design, stasis within the pouch, or a specific aerobic or anaerobic bacterial pathogen. Pouchitis manifests clinically as increased stool output and frequency, malaise, cramps, and arthralgias. Most cases respond to oral metronidazole, and hospitalization or pouch excision is rarely required.

ANSWER: C

47. Match each type of rectal cancer in the left column with one or more appropriate operations in the right column.

A. Fixed, circumferential adenocarcinoma just above the dentate line
B. Ulcerating adenocarcinoma whose lower edge is 7 cm from the dentate line
C. A 2 cm mobile adenocarcinoma arising in a villous adenoma 3 cm from the dentate line; ultrasonography shows an intact second hypoechoic band
D. Circumferential adenocarcinoma 12 cm from the anal verge
E. A 3.5 cm carcinoid at 4 cm

a. Abdominoperineal resection
b. Low anterior resection with descending colorectostomy
c. Low anterior resection with coloanal anastomosis
d. Local excision

Ref.: 6

COMMENTS: The most important determinant of which operation to perform for a rectal cancer is the location of the lesion within the rectum. Tumors located 0–5 cm from the anal verge, especially those that involve the sphincter muscle, producing pain, are best treated by abdominoperineal resection. Approximately 10–15% of tumors within this region, however, can be considered for local excision if they satisfy strict selection criteria. They should be no larger than 3–4 cm, have minimal penetration of the rectal wall on rectal ultrasonography, and should be well differentiated. • Lesions in the upper rectum (10–15 cm) are amenable to anterior resection with restoration of intestinal continuity by descending colorectostomy. • Lesions located in the midrectum (5–10 cm) are treated by a variety of operations, depending on the skill of the surgeon and the patient's body habitus. Most cancers in this region can be treated by low anterior resection with colorectostomy (which has been facilitated by use of surgical staplers) or coloanal anastomosis. In the latter case, a proximal temporary colostomy is constructed to divert stool away from the anastomosis. Impaired fecal continence has been noted in 10–35% of patients after coloanal anastomosis. The decision with regard to the appropriateness of sphincter preservation must be individualized, and safety is a primary concern. If the patient is obese or the pelvis is narrow and a satisfactory anastomosis cannot be done, abdominoperineal resection or low anterior resection with coloanal anastomosis is an option for midrectal cancers. Also, if the patient preoperatively has sphincter impairment due to age or previous surgery, avoiding a low anastomosis should be considered. • Abdominoperineal resection is indicated for low rectal carcinoids larger than 2 cm.

ANSWER: A-a; B-a,b,c; C-d; D-b; E-a

48. Regarding hereditary nonpolyposis colorectal carcinoma (Lynch syndrome), which of the following is/are true?

A. It is inherited as an autosomal-dominant trait.
B. Most cancers are in the right colon.
C. There is a greater likelihood of multiple, synchronous lesions.
D. Most patients are under 50 years of age.
E. Up to 40% of patients develop metachronous colorectal cancers within 10 years.
F. There is a high frequency of endometrial, ovarian, breast, and gastric cancers.

Ref.: 6, 16

COMMENTS: Hereditary nonpolyposis colorectal carcinoma (HNPCC) syndrome occurs in two varieties: (1) site-specific colorectal cancer (**Lynch syndrome I**) and (2) colorectal cancer associated with other forms of cancer (endometrial, ovarian, breast, gastric) (**Lynch syndrome II**). Accounting for approximately 5–6% of all colorectal cancers, HNPCC is due to mutations in mismatch repair genes that normally repair errors in DNA replication. It is inherited as an autosomal dominant trait and may affect multiple generations in succession. Afflicted individuals show a predominance of right-sided cancers (72.3%), are likely to have multiple carcinomas (18.1%), are usually young (mean 44.6 years), and often develop metachronous colorectal cancers (40% risk over 10 years). Interestingly, these individuals may have an improved survival compared to those with sporadic cancers. • Family members at risk should undergo biannual colonoscopy beginning at age 25; women should have an annual pelvic examination with endometrial biopsy every 3 years. Mammograms should be obtained earlier than what is usually advised. • If a new cancer is found in an HNPCC family, consideration should be given to subtotal colectomy because of the risk of metachronous tumors. If a woman has completed childbearing, one may also consider hysterectomy and bilateral salpingo-oophorectomy.

ANSWER: A, B, C, D, E, F

49. Match the gene on the left with its correct statement on the right.

A. Adenoma polyposis coli (*APC*)	a. Tumor-suppressor gene located on chromosome 17
B. *p53*	b. Late occurring alteration resulting in loss of cell-to-cell contact, thereby enhancing metastases
C. *hMSH2*	c. Located on chromosome 5
D. *DCC*	d. Most common mutation found in hereditary nonpolyposis colorectal cancer
E. K-*ras*	e. Oncogene that, when mutated, codes for a protein that cannot regulate cell growth and differentiation

Ref.: 16

COMMENTS: The **adenoma polyposis coli** (***APC***) gene is located on chromosome 5, is large (consisting of approximately 15 exons), and encodes for a cytoplasmic protein of 2843 amino acids. *APC* mutations occur in both sporadic colorectal cancers and familial polyposis, are frequent, are comparable in incidence between adenomas and carcinomas, and occur early in the development of cancer. The APC protein is normally involved in maintaining cellular adhesions and suppressing neoplastic growth, but the mutant protein may not be capable of serving this function. The *APC* gene thereby acts as a tumor-suppressor gene. Approximately 35% of sporadic cancers and up to 75% of polyposis cancers have *APC* mutations that can occur at variable points within the gene. This may explain the different phenotypes associated with the polyposis syndromes. • The ***p53* gene** is a tumor-suppressor gene located on chromosome 17. Mutations of this gene are the most common genetic abnormality found in various human cancers. The gene encodes for a nuclear phosphoprotein that regulates transcription and negatively influences cellular proliferation by binding at specific DNA sites. For example, cells damaged by ultraviolet light or radiation are kept from replicating by the wild-type (natural) P53 protein. Mutant P53 binds to wild-type P53, preventing specific binding to DNA; tumor growth is thereby permitted. • **Mismatch repair genes** correct errors of DNA replication. Alterations in these genes have been implicated in the pathogenesis of hereditary nonpolyposis colorectal cancer. The identified genetic sequences are (1) ***hMSH2*** on chromosome 2; mutation of this gene may account for up to 40% of the genetic alterations seen in HNPCC families; (2) ***hMLH1*** on chromosome 3, which may act as a tumor-suppressor gene; (3) ***hPMS1*** on chromosome 2; and (4) ***hPMS2*** on chromosome 7. Mutations of the latter two genes account for only 10% of the mutations seen in HNPCC families. Germ-line mutations of *hMSH2* and *hMLH1* genes, by themselves, are not enough to produce the HNPCC phenotype; a somatic mutation of the remaining wild-type allele is also necessary. • The ***DCC* gene** is located on chromosome 18 and encodes for a protein involved in cell-to-cell contact. Deletions of this gene have been found in 73% of colorectal cancers but only 11% of adenomas, suggesting that gene loss occurred late during tumorigenesis. Cancers with a loss of the *DCC* gene are more likely to present with advanced disease (compared to tumors maintaining this gene), and patient survival is consequently compromised. • The **K-*ras* gene**, an oncogene found on chromosome 12, encodes for a plasma membrane-based protein involved in transduction of growth and differentiation signals. Approximately 50% of colorectal cancers have *ras* mutations; large adenomas and adenomas with small areas of invasive cancer have nearly the same incidence of *ras* mutations, suggesting that genetic alterations in the *ras* gene occurs early (but not as early as *APC* mutations) during tumorigenesis. It has yet to be proved if *ras* mutations have any prognostic significance.

ANSWER: A-c; B-a; C-d; D-b; E-e

50. Which of the following are accepted applications of endorectal ultrasonography?

A. Assessing sphincter integrity in patients complaining of fecal incontinence.
B. Determining if a rectal cancer is suitable for local excision.
C. Ruling out recurrent cancer.
D. Evaluating anal fistulas.

Ref.: 17

COMMENTS: Endorectal ultrasonography has had significant impact on the diagnosis and management of a variety of anorectal diseases. The initial use of ultrasound instrumentation was for staging **rectal cancers**, whereby the depth of penetration and presence of abnormal lymph nodes was used to determine the stage of the cancer and its suitability for transanal, local excision. Generally, tumors that demonstrate deep penetration of the rectal wall are associated with lymph node enlargement and are not suitable candidates for transanal excision because of the unacceptably high recurrence rates associated with local excision of these advanced neoplasms. Recently, ths use of ultrasonography for staging rectal cancers has been expanded to determine whether a lesion is advanced enough to warrant preoperative therapy or chemotherapy. This application of ultrasonography and the use of preoperative therapy is not widely practiced, although preliminary data are encouraging that recurrence rates and potentially even survival can be enhanced by treating rectal cancers preoperatively. Certainly, ultrasonography can be used to assess the rectal wall and the extraluminal tissue for any sign of recurrent cancer following surgery. In this respect, it has distinct advantages over other imaging modalities, such as computed tomography (CT), in that the probe is placed in direct contact with the area of maximal interest, namely the operative site. Resolution capabilities are much better with ultrasonography than with CT scanning.

Regarding **benign diseases** of the anus and rectum, the endorectal ultrasound device can also be used to image the sphincter mechanism in patients complaining of fecal incontinence. In fact, before any patient is given a diagnosis of idiopathic or neurogenic incontinence, an ultrasound scan must be done to inspect the integrity of the sphincter. Although most anorectal abscesses and fistulas can be managed without elaborate imaging studies, ultrasonography has proved useful for determining the extent laterally and in a cephalad direction of abscess collections. Furthermore, the tract of the fistula in relation to the sphincter muscle can be assessed using ultrasonography whereby the internal opening can be identified as a hypoechoic disruption of the internal sphincter muscle. In some instances, hydrogen peroxide has been injected into the fistula tract during ultrasound scanning to further delineate the fistula tract.

ANSWER: A, B, C, D

51. Which of the following is/are true regarding anorectal ultrasonography?

A. Sedation is required.
B. The bowel must be prepared as if for colonoscopy or colectomy.
C. Scanning is best performed with a 3.0 MHz crystal.
D. Imaging lesions more than 10 cm from the anus is not possible.
E. Image-guided needle biopsy of extraluminal nodules is safe.

Ref.: 17

COMMENTS: Anorectal ultrasonography is generally performed as an office procedure without the need for sedation or a formal bowel preparation. Frequently, a single enema is given 1–2 hours before the examination to remove any stool from the rectal vault. Because minimal penetration of the rectal wall and perirectal tissues is required, a high-frequency ultrasound crystal is used (i.e., 7 or 10 MHz). High resolution of the superficial structures is thus obtained. With lower frequencies there would be better penetration of the deeper structures, but the information obtained from assessing the deep structures of the pelvic cavity have little bearing on the clinical management of anorectal diseases. It is possible to image lesions in the mid and upper rectum; but to be certain that the ultrasound probe is in contact with neoplasms at this level, it is necessary to insert the probe under direct vision through a commercially available 2 cm wide proctoscope. The proctoscope is advanced under direct vision to the desired level, and once the lesion is identified the ultrasound probe is inserted through the shaft of the proctoscope directly to the area of interest. Image-guided needle biopsy of extraluminal nodules is a safe procedure and can be performed with the ultrasound probe used by the urologist for imaging the prostate. Suspicious perirectal nodules can be biopsied in this fashion, although one must be careful with the interpretation of these biopsy data. If adipose tissue or skeletal muscle is obtained, one cannot assume that the nodule in question does not contain cancer. Only if the nodule contains benign lymphoid tissue can it be assumed that the nodule in question is truly free of cancer.

ANSWER: E

REFERENCES

1. Sabiston DC Jr: *Textbook of Surgery*, 15th ed. WB Saunders, Philadelphia, 1997.
2. Schwartz SI, Shires GT, Spencer FC: *Principles of Surgery*, 7th ed. McGraw-Hill, New York, 1999.
3. Corman ML: *Colon and Rectal Surgery*, 2nd ed. JB Lippincott, Philadelphia, 1989.
4. Kaleya RN, Boley SJ: Colonic ischemia. *Perspect Colon Rectal Surg* 3(1):62–81, 1990.
5. Taylor I: Intestinal blood flow. *Perspect Colon Rectal Surg* 1(2): 49–57, 1988.

6. Gordon PM, Nivatvongs S: *Principles and Practice of Surgery for the Colon, Rectum and Anus*. Quality Medical Publishing, St. Louis, 1992.
7. Boley SJ, Brandt LJ, Frank MS: Severe lower intestinal bleeding: diagnosis and treatment. *Clin Gastroenterol* 10:65–91, 1981.
8. Browder W, Cerise EJ, Litwin MS: Impact of emergency angiography in massive lower gastrointestinal bleeding. *Ann Surg* 204:530–536, 1986.
9. Diaz-Canton EA, Pazdur R: Adjuvant therapy for colorectal cancer. *Surg Clin North Am* 77:211–228, 1997.
10. Fleshman JW, Myerson RJ: Adjuvant radiation therapy for adenocarcinoma of the rectum. *Surg Clin North Am* 77:15–26.
11. Mazier WP, Levien DH, Luchtefeld MA, Senagore AJ: *Surgery of the Colon, Rectum and Anus*. WB Saunders, Philadelphia, 1995.
12. Fazio VW (ed): *Current Therapy in Colon and Rectal Surgery*. BC Decker, St. Louis, 1990.
13. Gordon MS, Cohen AM: Management of invasive carcinoma in pedunculated colorectal polyps. *Oncology* 3:99–105, 1989.
14. Pemberton JH, Phillips SF: Colonic absorption. *Perspect Colon Rectal Surg* 1(1), 1988.
15. Sleisenger MH, Fordtran JS: *Gastrointestinal Disease: Pathophysiology, Diagnosis and Management*, 4th ed. WB Saunders, Philadelphia, 1989.
16. Howe JR, Guillem JG: The genetics of colorectal cancer. *Surg Clin North Am* 77:175–196, 1997.
17. Staren ED: *Ultrasound for the Surgeon*. Lippincott-Raven, Philadelphia, pp 65–84.

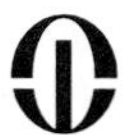

CHAPTER 31

Anus and Perianal Disease

1. Match each of the anatomic structures/landmarks listed below with its proper location in the coronal view of the anorectal area (only one side shown).

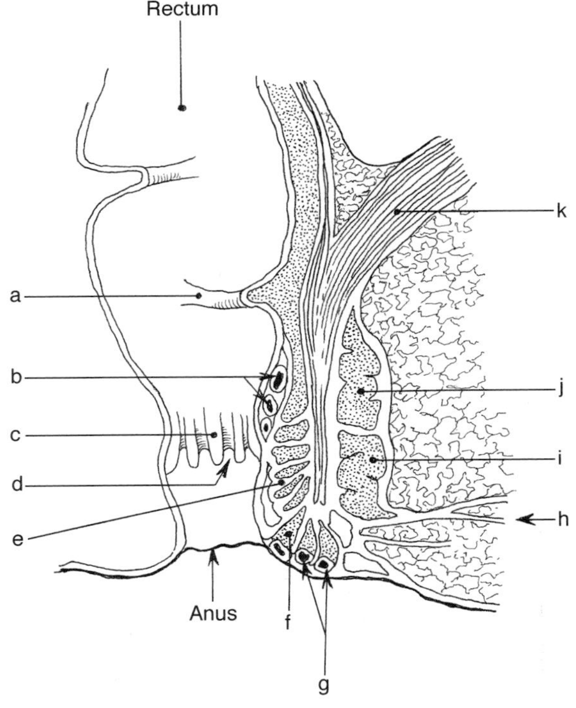

A. Levator ani.
B. Valve of Houston.
C. Subcutaneous external sphincter.
D. Transverse septum of ischiorectal fossa.
E. Deep external sphincter and puborectalis.
F. Internal rectal (hemorrhoidal) plexus.
G. Internal sphincter.
H. Superficial external sphincter.
I. Columns of Morgagni.
J. External rectal (hemorrhoidal) plexus.
K. Dentate line.

Ref.: 1, 2

COMMENTS: See Questions 2 and 3.

2. With regard to the anal sphincteric mechanism, which of the following statements is/are true?

A. The teniae of the colon thicken to form the internal sphincter.
B. The internal sphincter is made up of smooth muscle and surrounds the distal two-thirds of the anal canal.
C. The external sphincter is made up of striated muscle and is voluntary.
D. The puborectalis is a part of the levator muscle.
E. The anorectal ring is composed entirely of the palpable deep portion of external sphincter.

Ref.: 1, 2

COMMENTS: The teniae of the colon fuse at the upper border of the rectum to invest the rectum totally with longitudinal muscle. In the anal canal this muscle forms the **conjoined longitudinal muscle**, which descends in the plane between the internal and external sphincter. The circular muscle of the rectum thickens to form the involuntary **internal sphincter**, which surrounds the distal two-thirds of the anal canal. The lowest edge of the internal sphincter is 1.0–1.5 cm below the dentate line and is just above the lowest portion of the external sphincter. The **external sphincter** is formed of three parts—subcutaneous, superficial, and deep—which are striated muscles and under voluntary control. The **puborectalis muscle** is fused with the deep portion of the external sphincter and is not part of the levator muscle. The puborectalis originates from the posterior surface of the symphysis pubis and runs in a posterior direction to form a U-shaped loop around the rectum. Contraction of the puborectalis muscle pulls the rectum forward, thereby establishing a resting anorectal angle of 90–110 degrees. Unhindered defecation must involve relaxation of the puborectalis; inappropriate contraction during straining renders the anorectal angle more acute, thereby impairing defecation. The puborectalis muscle and the deep portion of the external sphincter along with the upper portion of the internal sphincter form the palpable anorectal ring. (See Question 3.)

3. With regard to the anatomy of the anal canal, which of the following statements is/are true?

A. The dentate line lies above the columns of Morgagni.
B. Anal gland ducts open into the anal crypts.
C. Anal glands rarely extend into the ischiorectal space.
D. The columns of Morgagni overlie the internal hemorrhoidal plexus.
E. The epithelium above the dentate line is innervated by the autonomic nervous system.

Ref.: 1, 2

COMMENTS: The dentate line is at the level of the anal crypts; above it are the vertical mucosal folds (columns of Morgagni), which overlie the internal hemorrhoidal plexus. The anal mucosa proximal to the dentate line is supplied by the autonomic nervous system and is insensitive to most painful stimuli; the anoderm distal to this is supplied by somatic nerves and is sensitive to painful stimuli. Anal glands, 6–10 in number, lie in the intersphincteric space, and their ducts open into the anal crypts.

ANSWER:
Question 1: A-k; B-a; C-f; D-h; E-j; F-b; G-e; H-i; I-c; J-g; K-d
Question 2: B, C
Question 3: B, D, E

4. With regard to perirectal spaces, which of the following statements is/are true?

A. The supralevator space is situated above the levator muscle and is connected with the contralateral side anteriorly.
B. The retrorectal space lies between the rectum and the sacrum above the rectosacral fascia.
C. The deep postanal space lies between the levator ani and the superficial external sphincter posteriorly.
D. The perianal space and the superficial postanal space lie deep to the superficial anal sphincter.
E. The intersphincteric space lies within the conjoined longitudinal muscle.

Ref.: 2

COMMENTS: The **supralevator space** is located above the levator ani on both sides and communicates with the contralateral side posteriorly. This space is bounded superiorly by the peritoneum, laterally by the pelvic wall, medially by the rectum, and inferiorly by the levator ani. Infection in this space can arise from a pelvic source (e.g., diverticulitis, pelvic inflammatory disease) or as an upward extension from an anorectal source. The **retrorectal space** lies above the rectosacral fascia between the upper two-thirds of the rectum and sacrum. The fascia runs downward and forward from the sacrum to the anorectal junction. The retrorectal space contains loose connective tissue and is a site for the formation of tumors arising from embryologic remnants (dermoids, teratomas, chordomas). The retrorectal space is bounded anteriorly by the rectum, posteriorly by the presacral fascia, laterally by the pelvic side wall, superiorly by the peritoneal reflection, and inferiorly by the rectosacral fascia, below which is the supralevator space. The **ischiorectal space** lies below the levator muscle, above the transverse septum of the ischiorectal fossa, and between the external sphincter and lateral pelvic wall. This space communicates posteriorly through the **deep postanal space** that lies between the levator ani and the superficial external sphincter. The lower border of the deep postanal space is the anococcygeal ligament which originates from the superficial portion of the external sphincter in the posterior midline. This communication allows a deep postanal space abscess to extend to both ischiorectal spaces (horseshoe abscess). The **perianal space** (the most common space involved in abscesses) lies superficial to the superficial external anal sphincter; and the **intersphincteric space** lies within the conjoined longitudinal muscle, where the anal glands also are located. The perianal, ischiorectal, and supralevator spaces may each connect posteriorly with its counterpart on the contralateral side, forming a horseshoe connection in any of these spaces.

ANSWER: B, C, E

5. With regard to hemorrhoids, which of the following statements is/are true?

A. Internal hemorrhoids are vascular cushions above the dentate line and are covered by anoderm.
B. Prolapsing hemorrhoids are external hemorrhoids covered by anoderm.
C. Bleeding internal hemorrhoids are best managed by surgical excision.
D. Thrombosed hemorrhoids are best treated by hemorrhoidectomy with the patient under general anesthesia.
E. Recurrence is uncommon after surgical hemorrhoidectomy.

Ref.: 1, 2

COMMENTS: **Internal** hemorrhoids are exaggerated submucosal vascular cushions normally located above the dentate line and therefore are covered by the mucous membrane of the anal canal and not by anoderm. **External** hemorrhoids are the dilated veins of the inferior hemorrhoidal plexus located below the dentate line and are covered by anoderm. **Prolapsing** hemorrhoids are internal hemorrhoids that prolapse beyond the dentate line. **Bleeding** is the main manifestation of internal hemorrhoids and is managed initially by injection sclerotherapy or rubber banding. Surgery is reserved for internal hemorrhoids that do not respond to conservative management. Surgery is the best initial therapy for prolapsing internal hemorrhoids that require manual reduction or for those that are incarcerated. **Thrombosed** hemorrhoids are best treated by incising the overlying anoderm with evacuation of the thrombus. **Recurrence** should be rare after surgical hemorrhoidectomy; when it occurs, it is related to inadequate removal of the rectal mucosa and hemorrhoidal tissue.

ANSWER: E

6. With regard to anal fissure, which of the following statements is/are true?

A. It is located above the dentate line.
B. It is located on the posterior midline in more than 90% of patients.
C. The operation of choice for a midline fissure is excision of the fissure and posterior internal sphincterotomy.
D. Lateral partial subcutaneous sphincterotomy is the operation of choice for nonmidline fissures.
E. Treatment should consist of fissurectomy and lateral partial subcutaneous external sphincterotomy.

Ref.: 1, 2

COMMENTS: Anal fissure, a tear of the skin-lined part of the anal canal, is located at or below the dentate line; gentle spreading of the buttocks is frequently all that is needed to reveal the fissure. About 90% of fissures (acute or chronic) are located at the posterior midline, an area where the anoderm is least supported by the sphincter. Fissures located laterally should arouse suspicion of Crohn's disease, ulcerative colitis, syphilis, tuberculosis, leukemia, or other causes; and therapy is directed toward the underlying disease. The initial treatment of a midline fissure is conservative, involving lubricants and bulk laxatives. If conservative management fails, operative treatment is a lateral subcutaneous partial internal sphincterotomy to relax the internal sphincter, with the sphincterotomy carried up to the dentate line. A major cause of nonhealing is inadequate sphincterotomy. Posterior fissurectomy and sphincterotomy can lead to a keyhole defect and constant soiling; it can be avoided by performing the sphincterotomy in the lateral location.

ANSWER: B

7. With regard to perirectal suppuration, which of the following statements is/are true?

A. The pathophysiology of perirectal abscess is related to infection of the perianal skin.
B. A horseshoe abscess begins as a posterior midline infection.
C. An intersphincteric abscess causes pain deep in the rectum without external manifestations.
D. Most perianal abscesses can be drained with the use of local anesthesia and without concern for subsequent formation of fistula in ano.
E. Ischiorectal abscesses should be drained with the patient under general anesthesia and the fistula identified and treated.

Ref.: 1, 2

COMMENTS: A **perirectal abscess** starts in the anal glands lying in the intersphincteric space. **Horseshoe abscesses** are bilateral ischiorectal, supralevator, or perianal abscesses communicating posteriorly. For example, a horseshoe ischiorectal abscess starts in the deep postanal space and extends in a U-shaped manner into each ischiorectal space. Horseshoe abscesses usually start from infection of the posterior midline anal glands. The patient is treated in the operating room under regional or general anesthesia and by incising the skin from the external sphincter to the coccyx. This step exposes the superficial external sphincter, which is split longitudinally but not transected; the incision provides access to the deep postanal space. A probe is inserted into the posterior midline crypt and then into the deep postanal space. A rubber seton is placed in this space and is wrapped around the internal sphincter and superficial external sphincter. Small counterincisions are made laterally along the extensions of the abscess. Sequential tightening of the seton should result in minimal if any sphincter impairment. An **intersphincteric abscess** usually presents with pain and bulging inside the rectum but with no external swelling. Treatment consists of transanally laying open the internal sphincter, beginning at its lower edge and extending cephalad to the top of the abscess cavity. Most **perianal abscesses** can be drained with the use of local anesthesia without serious concern about subsequent fistula formation.

ANSWER: B, C, D

8. With regard to the management of patients with fistula in ano, which of the following statements is/are true?

A. All internal openings of fistulas are located posteriorly according to Goodsall's rule.
B. The most common type of fistula is intersphincteric.
C. Excision of the entire fistulous tract is necessary for cure.
D. High fistulas are managed by means of a seton suture.
E. A horseshoe fistula can be treated by posterior midline internal sphincterotomy combined with opening the deep postanal space.

Ref.: 1, 2

COMMENTS: Anal fistulas are classified as intersphincteric (most common), transsphincteric, suprasphincteric, and extrasphincteric. **Goodsall's rule** states that if the external opening is anterior to an imaginary line drawn between the ischial tuberosities, the fistula usually runs directly into the anal canal; and if the external opening is posterior, the tract curves to the posterior midline. Anal fistulotomy and establishment of adequate drainage constitute sufficient therapy; excision of the tract is unnecessary and prolongs healing. High transsphincteric fistulas are best managed by means of a seton suture. A horseshoe fistula, which starts with infection at the posterior midline anal glands, is best treated by opening the deep postanal space and identifying and curetting the lateral extensions. Laying open the fistula extensions could be done but would result in large, gaping wounds that may require a long time to heal. The external opening in the posterior midline can be managed by placement of a Seton drain, or posterior midline internal sphincterotomy. The latter has a potentially higher recurrence rate.

ANSWER: B, D, E

9. Anal incontinence associated with rectal prolapse is caused primarily by which one of the following?

A. Levator diastasis.
B. Loss of the rectal angle.
C. Stretching of the anal sphincter.
D. Stretching of the pudendal nerve.
E. Loose endopelvic fascia.

Ref.: 1, 2

COMMENTS: Anal and urinary incontinence in advanced cases of prolapse is due to entrapment and stretching of the pudendal nerve, resulting in neuromuscular dysfunction. It is important, therefore, to repair rectal prolapse before incontinence develops. Chronic stretching of the sphincter by the prolapse itself may lead to sphincter impairment as well. Repair of the prolapse improves continence in approximately 50% of patients. The other defects listed above are associated with the prolapse but are not the cause of incontinence. Their correction therefore does not cure the problem of incontinence.

ANSWER: C, D

10. Match each of the anal conditions in the left column with the most appropriate initial therapy in the right column.

A. Bowen's disease	a. Local excision
B. Paget's disease	b. Local excision and postoperative radiotherapy
C. Basal cell carcinoma	c. Abdominoperineal resection
	d. External beam radiotherapy
	e. Chemotherapy and radiotherapy

Ref.: 1, 2

COMMENTS: **Bowen's disease** is an intraepidermal squamous cell carcinoma. It rarely metastasizes but can be locally recurrent. Local excision with clear margins is adequate. **Paget's disease** of the perianal skin is a malignant neoplasm of the intraepidermal portion of the apocrine glands. It usually appears as an eczematoid perianal lesion in women and is intensely pruritic. Paget cells stain with periodic acid-Schiff stain, which differentiates them from bowenoid cells. Invasion occurs late, and metastases are rare. Wide local excision with adequate margins is the procedure of choice. Both Bowen's and Paget's diseases are associated with other cutaneous or visceral malignancies. **Basal cell carcinoma** is usually noninvasive and nonmetastasizing. Local excision with adequate margins virtually ensures a cure.

ANSWER: A-a; B-a; C-a

11. In comparison with squamous cell cancers of the anal margin, which of the following statements is/are generally true of squamous cell cancers of the anal canal?

A. They are more common in women.
B. They are more often associated with benign anal conditions.
C. They are more advanced when diagnosed.
D. They are more frequently associated with basaloid histology.
E. They are associated with a better prognosis.

Ref.: 1, 2

COMMENTS: The **anal canal** is generally considered to be the region from above the dentate line to the top of the anorectal ring. The **anal margin** is distal to the dentate line. Squamous cell cancers of the anal canal are more common in women. Because they are often mistaken for benign anal disorders, they are usually advanced at the time of diagnosis and therefore have a worse prognosis. Basaloid and cloacogenic carcinomas are a histologic variant of squamous cell cancer of the anal canal. Conversely, perianal (anal margin) squamous cell carcinoma is four times more common in men and is usually slow-growing and late to metastasize. Basaloid features are uncommon. Wide local excision with a 2 cm margin may be adequate therapy for superficial squamous cell cancers of the anal margin, whereas squamous cell cancers of the anal canal generally necessitate multimodality therapy, involving irradiation and chemotherapy.

ANSWER: A, C, D

12. There is general agreement that survival after treatment for squamous cancer of the anus is related to which one or more of the following?

A. Tumor size.
B. Depth of invasion.
C. Basaloid versus squamous histology.
D. Lymph node involvement.

Ref.: 1, 2

COMMENTS: The poor prognosis of squamous cell carcinoma of the anal canal is related to delay in diagnosis. Poor prognostic factors include large tumor size, deeply invasive lesions, and lymph node metastases. In basaloid cancers, there is good correlation between histologic differentiation and the 5-year survival rate (90% for well-differentiated, 50% for moderately differentiated, and 0% for anaplastic lesions). Basaloid histology versus squamous histology alone, however, has not been conclusively shown to affect prognosis.

ANSWER: A, B, D

13. With regard to the management of inguinal lymph nodes in patients with squamous cell cancer of the anus, which of the following statements is/are true?

A. Prophylactic groin dissection is indicated when abdominoperineal resection is performed.
B. Groin dissection, whether for synchronously or metachronously appearing nodes, yields equivalent survival rates.
C. Metachronously appearing lymph nodes should be treated by radiation therapy because their surgical excision improves salvage only minimally.
D. Combined irradiation and chemotherapy may be applied to clinically normal inguinal lymph nodes with benefit.

Ref.: 2, 3

COMMENTS: Prophylactic inguinal lymph node dissection in every case yields positive nodes in only 10–30%; therefore the morbidity of this operation does not justify its performance on a routine basis. Synchronous inguinal lymph node metastasis is an ominous sign; in contrast, metachronous nodal disease carries a better prognosis (up to 75% of patients survive 5 years). Lymph node dissection is recommended in both clinical settings. When a combination of chemotherapy and irradiation is used as the initial treatment for the anal disease, prophylactic irradiation to clinically negative inguinal nodes reduces the incidence of lymph node involvement to less than 5% from a rate of 15–25% without such treatment.

ANSWER: D

14. Which of the following may be appropriate initial therapy for a 3 cm cancer of the anal canal with invasion of the internal sphincter and no inguinal adenopathy?

A. Local excision.
B. Abdominoperineal resection.
C. Combined external beam and interstitial radiotherapy.
D. Combined chemotherapy and radiotherapy.

Ref.: 1, 2

COMMENTS: The optimal management of a small (<5 cm) squamous cell cancer of the anal canal without palpable groin lymph nodes is multimodal, involving radiation therapy and chemotherapy. As the effect of chemotherapy is believed to be radiopotentiating, recent protocols that include external beam radiation and interstitial therapy have been tried with equal success. No randomized trial is available comparing these two protocols. The cure rate without abdominoperineal resection approaches 80–85%. Local excision of anal neoplasms is reserved for anal margin cancers that do not approach the dentate line or involve the sphincter. Similarly, local excision of anal canal cancers is indicated only for well-differentiated lesions that have not invaded the sphincter.

ANSWER: C, D

15. With regard to the results of initial combined radiation therapy with 5-fluorouracil (5-FU) and mitomycin C for squamous cell cancer of the anus, which of the following statements is/are true?

A. Complete regression of gross tumor has been observed in most patients.
B. Patients may be followed without abdominoperineal resection if posttreatment biopsies reveal no tumor.
C. Anal sphincter function may be preserved in at least one-half of patients.

D. Randomized prospective trials demonstrate improved survival compared with abdominoperineal resection alone.

Ref.: 1, 2

COMMENTS: A combination of radiation therapy and chemotherapy with 5-FU and mitomycin C results in regression of gross tumor in all cases and microscopic disappearance of tumor cells in more than 80% of patients. It is estimated that the anal sphincter can be saved in 85% of patients. Abdominoperineal resection therefore is reserved for patients with gross or microscopic persistent tumor or for those with treatment failure, recurrent disease, or anal complications of treatment. Based on the excellent results of multimodal therapy, randomization with abdominoperineal resection alone is not justified.

ANSWER: A, B, C

16. With regard to anal infection with condyloma acuminatum, which of the following statements is/are true?

A. The causative agent appears to be human papillomavirus.
B. Podophyllin, administered in a 25% solution, causes resolution of warts in 80% of patients; recurrence rates are less than 10%.
C. Immunotherapy with autologous condyloma is used as initial treatment for small condyloma.
D. Carcinoma frequently develops in untreated condyloma.

Ref.: 3

COMMENTS: Anal infection with papillomavirus is responsible for condyloma acuminatum, which appears as a group of cauliflower-like masses on the perianal skin. The disease is transmitted by close contact and is seen in both heterosexuals and homosexuals. It is especially prevalent in anal-receptive homosexual men, and in this population it is seen more often than genital warts. An explanation for this phenomenon is that the anus is a warm, moist traumatized area. Podophyllin, a cytotoxic agent available in 10% and 25% solutions, must be applied by a physician. Results have been disappointing; clearance of the warts has been noted in 22–77% of patients, with recurrence rates as high as 65%. Podophyllin may cause skin burns and cannot be used within the anal canal; multiple treatments may be necessary. Failure to treat intraanal lesions may cause higher recurrence rates. • Autologous vaccine prepared from the condyloma is injected weekly for 6 weeks. No adverse reactions have been seen, and resolution of the lesions has been noted in up to 95% of cases. At present, such therapy is considered for extensive, persistent, or recurrent cases of condyloma. Although malignant transformation can occur, few cases have been reported to date.

ANSWER: A

17. With regard to anal and perianal Crohn's disease, which of the following statements is/are true?

A. It is the first sign of the disease in 30% of patients.
B. Anal involvement is more common in patients with small bowel rather than colonic disease.
C. Multiple fistulas are the most common anal manifestation.
D. One-third of low fistulas may demonstrate spontaneous healing.
E. Healing after fistulectomy correlates with the presence of rectal disease and Crohn's activity elsewhere in the gastrointestinal tract.

Ref.: 3

COMMENTS: Anal or perianal disease is the first sign of Crohn's disease in approximately 10% of patients; ultimately, up to 30% of Crohn's disease patients manifest anal disease. The anus is more likely to be involved with distal gastrointestinal involvement; approximately 50% of patients with Crohn's colitis have anal involvement compared to 25% of patients with Crohn's disease of the small intestine. The most common anal manifestation is edematous, thickened skin tags 1–2 cm in size. They can cause pain and thus difficulty achieving satisfactory local hygiene. • Fistula in ano is the second most common anal manifestation. Most fistulas are low and simple; approximately one-third demonstrate spontaneous healing. If symptomatic and persistent, fistulotomy can be performed, but healing might not result. Preoperatively, every attempt should be made to control proximal disease within the gastrointestinal tract. Failure to do so results in a higher incidence of nonhealing perineal involvement. The absence of rectal disease correlates well with successful healing after fistulectomy. • Surgery for perianal Crohn's disease should be directed at relieving symptoms, such as draining of abscesses, gentle dilatation of strictures, and promotion of drainage of fistula tracts with curettage or placement of seton sutures.

ANSWER: D, E

18. With regard to rectovaginal fistulas, which of the following is/are true?

A. Repaired obstetric tears of the rectum and vagina dehisce in 10% of cases; 30–60% of fistulas due to obstetric trauma heal spontaneously.
B. Low rectovaginal fistulas may be treated with fistulectomy.
C. High rectovaginal fistulas are best treated through a transabdominal approach.
D. Rectovaginal fistulas associated with Crohn's disease usually necessitate proctectomy.
E. Radiation-induced fistulas generally necessitate a colostomy.

Ref.: 3

COMMENTS: Rectovaginal fistulas are classified according to location and etiology; both influence the type of corrective surgery required. *High* fistulas require an abdominal approach, whereas *low* or *mid* fistulas can be repaired through a transvaginal, transperineal, or transrectal approach. The causes of these fistulas include obstetric injuries, irradiation for pelvic cancers, inflammatory bowel disease, violent trauma, or infection (tuberculosis, lymphogranuloma venereum). • Episiotomy with a third- or fourth-degree rectal tear occurs in about 5% of deliveries; approximately 10% of the repairs disrupt, leading to impaired fecal control and, potentially, a rectovaginal fistula. Approximately 30–60% of fistulas heal spontaneously. Therefore if the patient's symptoms are not disabling, a 3- to 6-month wait is recommended. This waiting period also allows tissue inflammation and edema to subside prior to any surgical intervention. Repair of a fistula secondary to an obstetric injury can be accomplished with a local procedure that usually involves excision of the fistula tract with a layered closure. A diverting colostomy is not required unless multiple previous surgical attempts have failed. An *anovaginal* fistula may be treated with fistulotomy; but rectovaginal fistulas, even distal ones, should not be treated by this method. Partial or total incontinence may result if the fistula tract is divided. • *High rectovaginal* fistulas are best treated through a transabdominal approach so coexisting pathology such as diverticulitis, cancer, or inflammatory bowel disease can be addressed. If local tissues are normal, the rectovaginal septum is mobilized, the fistula is divided, the rectum and vagina are closed separately, and normal tissue such as omentum is interposed. If tissue is not normal as a result of inflammation or irradiation, bowel resection is usually necessary. • Fistulas secondary to *Crohn's disease* do not necessitate a proctectomy if symptoms are minimal, the rectum is relatively healthy, and continence is normal. In such cases an advancement flap can result in healing. On the other hand, refractory rectal Crohn's disease or incontinence usually necessitates proctectomy. Radiation-induced fistulas usually necessitate a colostomy as sole therapy in a poor-risk patient or in a patient with recurrent cancer or to divert stool from an anastomosis after resection of diseased bowel.

ANSWER: A, C, E

19. For patients with rectal cancer, radiation therapy is recommended in which of the following settings?

A. Preoperatively, in patients whose primary tumors are located close enough to the dentate line that sphincter preservation may not be possible.
B. Postoperatively, with chemotherapy for patients with T3-4 cancers and lymph node metastases.
C. Postoperatively, after low anterior resection for T2N0 adenocarcinoma of the rectum with negative margins.
D. All of the above.
E. None of the above.

Ref.: 4, 5, 6, 7, 8

COMMENTS: Preoperative radiation therapy may downstage and shrink a tumor, thereby permitting sphincter preservation in some patients who otherwise would have required abdominoperineal resection. The response rate is variable; and although the benefit of preserving the sphincter is undeniable, patients should be counseled that the chief advantage is a lower recurrence rate. A dose of 45–50 Gy is delivered to the pelvis with or without chemotherapy. The reported local failure rate with this treatment is low, ranging from 1% to 17%; and sphincter function is good to excellent in most patients. At least 80–90% of patients with stage I rectal carcinoma have 5-year survival with surgery alone, so adjuvant treatment is not recommended. Patients with stage II or III disease remain at high risk for disease recurrence. Randomized trials, including those from the Gastrointestinal Study Group (GITSG) and the North Central Cancer Treatment Group (NCCTG) have shown improved survival and freedom from local recurrence in patients with T3-4 cancers, lymph node metastases, or both who undergo postoperative irradiation with concurrent chemotherapy. In the GITSG study, local recurrence was decreased from 24% with surgery alone to 11% with adjuvant chemotherapy and radiation therapy. Overall recurrence rates with an 80-month median follow-up were 55% in the surgery alone arm versus 33% in the adjuvant chemoradiation arm.

ANSWER: A, B

20. The theoretic advantages of preoperative radiation therapy include which one or more of the following?

A. Radiation treatment to the tumor bed, the regional lymphatics, or both may be initiated without delay.
B. Elimination of viable cells potentially capable of metastatic dissemination at the time of surgery.
C. Improved wound healing over that seen with postoperative irradiation.
D. Improved ease of tumor resectability.

Ref.: 9

COMMENTS: The rationale for preoperative radiation therapy includes elimination of microscopic disease beyond the margins of surgical resection and improving the ease of tumor resectability (e.g., distal rectal cancers or large sarcomas). Another advantage is the elimination of viable cells that could at the time of surgery disseminate into the bloodstream to produce metastatic disease. Moreover, treatment may begin immediately without delay for postoperative recovery during which time remaining tumor cells may be multiplying. A potential disadvantage is that surgical staging information is not available prior to initiation of treatment, and so some patients are treated unnecessarily. Also, some studies have demonstrated increased wound healing complications with preoperative irradiation, though with proper technique and doses of 45–50 Gy the effect should be minimal.

ANSWER: A, B, D

21. The theoretic advantages of postoperative radiation therapy include which one or more of the following?

A. Higher doses of radiation may be given postoperatively than those given preoperatively.
B. The volume treated postoperatively is typically smaller than the volume treated preoperatively.
C. The altered vascularity of the postoperative tumor bed leads to greater radiosensitivity of any remaining cancer cells.

Ref.: 9

COMMENTS: Postoperative irradiation is used to eliminate any residual locoregional disease. One advantage of postoperative treatment is that higher doses may be used than those allowed for with preoperative irradiation, potentially offering a better chance of local control. However, the altered vascularity of the surgical bed may render tumor cells more hypoxic and as a result more resistant to radiation. The postoperative radiation volume is often larger than the preoperative volume because not only must the tumor volume be covered but also the entire operative bed where cells may have been implanted at the time of surgery.

ANSWER: A

REFERENCES

1. Schwartz SI, Shires GT, Spencer FC: *Principles of Surgery*, 7th ed. McGraw-Hill, New York, 1999.
2. Sabiston Jr DC: *Textbook of Surgery*, 15th ed. WB Saunders, Philadelphia, 1997.
3. Gordon PH, Nivatvongs S: *Principles and Practice of Surgery for the Colon, Rectum and Anus*. Quality Medical Publishing, St. Louis, 1992.
4. Minsky BD: Preoperative radiation therapy followed by low an-

terior resection with coloanal anastomosis. *Semin Radiat Oncol* 8: 30–35, 1998.
5. Martensen JA, Gunderson LL: Colon and rectum, In: Perez CA, Brady LW (eds) *Principles and Practice of Radiation Oncology*, 3rd ed. Lippincott-Raven, Philadelphia, 1998.
6. Gastrointestinal Tumor Study Group: Prolongation of the disease-free interval in surgically treated rectal carcinoma. *N Engl J Med* 312:1465–1472, 1985.
7. Krook JE, et al: Effective surgical adjuvant therapy for high-risk rectal carcinoma. *N Engl J Med* 324:709–715, 1991.
8. NIH Consensus Conference: Adjuvant therapy for patients with colon and rectal cancer. *JAMA* 264:1444–1450, 1990.
9. Perez CA, Brady LW, Roti Roti JL: Overview. In: Perez CA, Brady LW (eds) *Principles and Practice of Radiation Oncology*, 3rd ed. Lippincott-Raven, Philadelphia, 1998.

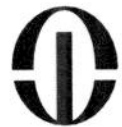

CHAPTER 32

Liver

1. Which of the following statements about the anatomy of the liver is/are true?

   A. The right lobe extends to the left of the umbilical fissure.
   B. The left lobe extends to the right of the falciform ligament.
   C. The quadrate lobe is a portion of the medial segment of the left lobe.
   D. The caudate lobe is a portion of the right lobe.

Ref.: 1, 2, 3

COMMENTS: See Question 2.

2. The anterior sector of the right lobe of the liver consists of which anatomic segment(s)?

   A. Segments II and III.
   B. Segment IV.
   C. Segments V and VI.
   D. Segments V and VIII.
   E. Segments VI and VII.

Ref.: 1, 2, 3

COMMENTS: The surgical anatomy of the liver is based on the distribution of the hepatic veins and portal structures. The liver is divided into right and left lobes by a vertically angled plane that extends from the gallbladder to the left of the inferior vena cava. This is known as the main interlobar fissure or the middle portal scissura, and it contains the middle hepatic vein. The liver is divided into sectors by the planes of the right, middle, and left hepatic veins and is further divided into segments by the branching of the portal structures. The right lobe is divided into anteromedial (segments V and VIII) and posterolateral (segments VI and VII) sectors by a vertical plane containing the right hepatic vein. The left lobe is divided into medial and lateral segments by a longitudinal plane extending through the umbilical fissure and falciform ligament. According to the segmental nomenclature introduced by the French anatomists Soupault and Couinaud, the left lobe is divided into posterosuperior (segment II) and inferoanterior sectors (segments III and IV) by the plane of the left hepatic vein (see reference 2). The anatomy of the left lobe is not always so described or so pictured, which leads to confusion. Sometimes the left hepatic vein is depicted as the superior division between the medial and lateral segments of the left lobe, with the plane of the umbilical fissure forming the inferior border (see reference 3). When drawn like this, the left hepatic vein appears to separate segments II and III from segment IV. The medial segment of the left lobe is segment IV and the lateral segment of the left lobe is segments II and III. The caudate lobe (segment I) is best considered anatomically independent from the right and left lobes, as it receives separate portal and arterial branches from both sides and as hepatic venous drainage is by way of separate veins directly into the inferior vena cava. The quadrate lobe is a topographic description of the area between the gallbladder fossa, umbilical fissure, and portal triad; thus it is within the medial aspect of the left lobe (segment IV).

ANSWER:
Question 1: B, C
Question 2: D

3. Which of the following statements is/are true about the hepatic arterial supply?

   A. It provides 75% of blood flow to the liver.
   B. "Normal" arterial anatomy is present in only 50% of persons.
   C. It parallels the portal venous system intrahepatically.
   D. The most common variant is origin of the right hepatic artery from the gastroduodenal artery.

Ref.: 1, 2, 3

COMMENTS: The hepatic arterial supply normally is derived from the celiac axis by way of the proper hepatic artery, which becomes the common hepatic artery after giving off the gastroduodenal branch and subsequently bifurcates into right and left hepatic branches. There is, however, significant variability in hepatic arterial anatomy. In approximately 15–20% of individuals the right hepatic artery arises from the superior mesenteric artery and is found at the posterolateral aspect of the hepatoduodenal ligament. In 15% of individuals the left hepatic artery originates from the left gastric artery and is located in the gastrohepatic ligament. These commonly encountered variants can have important surgical implications during upper abdominal operations. The arterial blood supply accounts for only 25% of hepatic blood flow, with the remainder supplied by the portal vein.

ANSWER: B, C

4. Which of the following statement(s) about the anatomy of the hepatic veins is/are true?

A. The left hepatic vein drains the entire left lobe.
B. Veins from the caudate lobe enter the inferior vena cava directly.
C. The middle hepatic vein usually drains into the right hepatic vein.
D. The hepatic veins parallel the hepatic arterial system intrahepatically.

Ref.: 1, 2, 3

COMMENTS: The hepatic veins begin in the liver lobules as the central veins and coalesce to form the right, left, and middle hepatic veins, which drain into the inferior vena cava and are of considerable surgical importance because they define the three vertical scissura of the liver. The **right vein**, which is generally the largest, drains most of the right lobe. The **left vein** drains the lateral segment of the left lobe and a portion of the medial segment as well. The **middle vein** drains the inferoanterior portion of the right lobe and the inferomedial segment of the left lobe; this vein joins the left hepatic vein in 80% of individuals and enters the inferior vena cava directly in the remainder. There are also smaller veins, particularly those draining the caudate lobe posteriorly, which enter directly into the inferior vena cava.

ANSWER: B

5. Which of the following statements is/are true about the anatomy of the portal vein?

A. It contains the valves of Mirizzi.
B. It is formed by the junction of the inferior mesenteric vein and splenic vein.
C. It is the most posterior structure in the hepatoduodenal ligament.
D. The right portal vein typically branches sooner than the left portal vein.

Ref.: 1, 2, 3

COMMENTS: The portal vein is usually formed dorsal to the neck of the pancreas by the junction of the superior mesenteric vein and splenic veins. It ascends dorsal to the common bile duct and hepatic artery in the hepatoduodenal ligament. There are no valves in the portal venous system. (Mirizzi described valves in the common hepatic duct that do not exist.) The portal vein bifurcates just outside the liver. The right portal vein has anterior and posterior branches that typically come off only a short distance from the bifurcation. The left hepatic vein has a longer transverse portion (*pars transversus*) and then angulates anteriorly in the umbilical fissure (*pars umbilicus*), where it gives off medial branches to segment IV and lateral branches to segments II and III.

ANSWER: C, D

6. Which of the following hepatic resection(s) involve(s) dissection in the plane of the umbilical fissure?

A. Right lobectomy.
B. Right trisegmentectomy.
C. Left lateral segmentectomy.
D. Left lobectomy.
E. None of the above.

Ref.: 1, 2, 3

COMMENTS: The umbilical fissure is the segmental plane between the medial and lateral segments of the left lobe of the liver. A portion of the left branch of the portal vein, known as the pars umbilicus, runs in the inferior portion of the umbilical fissure. Dissection is therefore never carried out directly in the segmental fissure. During left lateral segmentectomy the plane of the parenchymal dissection is to the left of the fissure; whereas with right trisegmentectomy the parenchyma is divided to the right of the fissure. Both right and left lobectomies involve dissection well to the right of this plane.

ANSWER: E

7. Which of the following ultrasound characteristics is/are typical of the hepatic portal vein branches?

A. Hyperechoic vessel walls.
B. Hepatofugal blood flow.
C. Diastolic reversal of blood flow.
D. Location between hepatic segments.

Ref.: 4

COMMENTS: The portal veins and hepatic veins can be readily differentiated from each other based on their distinctive sonographic features. The portal vein and its branches have prominent hyperechoic-appearing walls. This appearance has been attributed to the accompanying intrahepatic branches of the hepatic artery and bile duct, which generally are not individually seen by external ultrasonography. The hepatic veins, on the other hand, appear to be essentially "wall-less." They are anechoic or hypoechoic tubular structures that are vertically oriented and increase in caliber as they course toward the inferior vena cava. The portal veins are more transversely oriented and of larger caliber centrally. The portal vein branches are located within the anatomic liver segments, and the hepatic veins are found between the segments. Doppler ultrasonography permits characterization of flow patterns in the hepatic vessels. Under normal circumstances, portal vein flow is toward the liver (hepatopedal). Flow in the portal vein is usually of fairly low velocity with minor undulations and continued forward flow during diastole. Flow in the hepatic veins is hepatofugal and varies according to the cardiorespiratory cycle.

ANSWER: A

8. Ultrasonography demonstrates a hyperechoic liver with a geographic hypoechoic area adjacent to the gallbladder. This picture likely represents:

A. Duplication of the gallbladder.
B. Reverberation artifact.
C. Focal fatty sparing.
D. Hepatic abscess.
E. Bowel gas.

Ref.: 4

COMMENTS: Fatty infiltration of the liver is a common finding that produces a hyperechoic parenchymal pattern on ultrasound scans. It is not unusual to have focal areas of fatty sparing within an otherwise steatotic liver. These areas typically appear as zonal hypoechoic regions and are usually found adjacent to the gallbladder or anterior to the porta hepatis. Duplication of the gallbladder is a rare occurrence. Reverberation artifacts are echoes within cystic structures. The sonographic appearance of hepatic abscesses is variable depending on etiology and duration. Pyogenic abscesses are usually complex with cystic characteristics and internal echoes due to debris or septations. Bowel gas is highly reflective and impedes ultrasound imaging.

ANSWER: C

9. The hepatocytes most susceptible to hypoxic injury are located in which one or more of the following areas?

A. Central lobular region.
B. Central acinar region.
C. Acinar zone I.
D. Acinar zone III.

Ref.: 1, 3

COMMENTS: The functional histologic unit of the liver is the acinus. At the center of the acinus is a terminal branch of the portal vein along with an hepatic arteriole and bile ductule. Blood from the terminal portal venule goes into hepatic sinusoids around which the hepatocytes are located. Eventually the blood returns to the terminal hepatic venules at the periphery of the acinar unit. The hepatic venules are at the center of the histologic hepatic lobule. The hepatocytes of the acinus are divided into three zones, with zone I being closest to the afferent portal venule and zone III being nearest the efferent hepatic venule. Within the acinus there is a gradient of solute concentration and oxygen tension that is greatest near the portal venules at the center of the acinus. The hepatocytes in zone I are therefore exposed to more oxygen and are less subject to hypoxia than the hepatocytes near the periphery of the acinus. This explains the histologic pattern of centrilobular necrosis that occurs following ischemia.

ANSWER: A, D

10. Alkaline phosphatase is primarily located in which portion of the hepatocyte plasma membrane?

A. Sinusoidal membrane.
B. Basolateral membrane.
C. Canalicular membrane.
D. All of the above.

Ref.: 3

COMMENTS: The plasma membrane of the hepatocyte has different regions with ultrastructures designed for different functions. The sinusoidal membrane that borders the perisinusoidal space of Disse is covered with microvilli that project into the perisinusoidal space. Proteins, solutes, and other substances are actively transported across this border of the hepatocyte; and various transport proteins are located there. The flat basolateral membrane connects the hepatocyte to adjacent cells and is important for cellular interactions. The canalicular membrane is a specialized section of the hepatocyte membrane that is involved in bile formation and in the transport of various substances into bile. The canalicular regions comprise about 15% of the hepatocyte membrane and are separated from the pericellular space by tight junctions. The canalicular membrane also has a microvillous structure, and enzymes such as alkaline phosphatase and 5′-nucleotidase are found there.

ANSWER: C

11. During fasting, the liver provides energy substrates by all of the following mechanisms *except*:

A. Glycogenolysis.
B. Glycolysis.
C. Gluconeogenesis from alanine.
D. Gluconeogenesis from lactate.
E. Formation of ketone bodies from fatty acids.

Ref.: 1, 3, 5

COMMENTS: The liver plays a pivotal role in energy metabolism. In the fed state, glucose is converted to glycogen for storage. The liver itself primarily obtains its energy from ketoacids rather than glucose, although it can use glycolysis during periods of glucose excess (fed state). During fasting the liver provides glucose by breakdown of the stored glycogen (glycogenolysis); glucose is a critical energy source for red blood cells, central nervous system, and kidney. Glycogen stores are depleted after about 48 hours, however, so the liver generates glucose from other sources. Alanine, other amino acids, lactate, and glycerol can serve as carbon sources for gluconeogenesis. Lipolysis occurs during prolonged fasting, and the fatty acids released from adipose stores are oxidized in the hepatocytes to form ketone bodies. Ketone bodies are an important alternative fuel source for brain and muscle.

ANSWER: B

12. The reticuloendothelial function of the liver is primarily dependent on which of the following cells?

A. Hepatocytes.
B. Sinusoidal endothelial cells.
C. Kupffer's cells.
D. Ito cells.

Ref.: 1, 5

COMMENTS: The reticuloendothelial system (RES) functions to clear the circulation of particulate matter and microbes. The RES is comprised of fixed phagocytic cells, primarily located in the liver, spleen, and lung. Kupffer's cells are primarily responsible for the reticuloendothelial function of the liver. At their location, lining the hepatic sinusoids (along with the sinusoidal endothelial cells), they are uniquely positioned to phagocytize and process gut antigens from the splanchnic circulation. Kupffer's cells have been recognized to have an important role in the production and control of various cytokines and inflammatory regulators. Ito cells are perisinusoidal cells involved in collagen and vitamin A metabolism.

ANSWER: C

13. Which of the following proteins is/are *not* primarily synthesized in the liver?

A. Albumin.
B. Fibrinogen.
C. Factor VII.
D. Factor V.
E. Transferrin.

Ref.: 1, 3, 5

COMMENTS: The liver is the primary or sole source of numerous plasma proteins including albumin, α-globulins and an array of other transport proteins such as transferrin, hepatoglobulin, ferritin, and ceruloplasmin. Most urea is synthesized in the liver. About a dozen proteins involved in hemostasis are synthesized in the liver including fibrinogen, the vitamin K-dependent factors (II, VII, IX, X), and all of the procoagulation factors except for von Willebrand factor. Factor V is synthesized by vascular endothelial cells, so a determination of factor V activity may be useful when ascertaining whether a clinical coagulation disorder is primarily related to liver dysfunction or to other factors.

ANSWER: D

14. The cytochrome P-450 system transforms compounds by which of the following mechanisms?

A. Oxidative reactions.
B. Incorporation into the urea cycle.
C. Conjugation.
D. Formation of hydrophilic compounds.

Ref.: 1, 3, 5

COMMENTS: The liver is responsible for biotransformation of many endogenous and exogenous substances. For the most part, this process detoxifies potentially injurious substances and facilitates their elimination. In some instances, however, hepatic biotransformation produces more toxic metabolites. There are two general mechanisms by which the liver accomplishes biotransformation. The cytochrome P-450 enzyme system catalyzes phase I reactions, which are primarily oxidation, reduction, and hydrolysis. The second mechanism involves an array of enzymes that conjugate substances with other endogenous molecules; these are referred to as the phase II reactions. The purpose of phase II reactions is to convert hydrophobic compounds to hydrophilic ones that are water-soluble and can thus be eliminated in bile or urine. The liver is also the principal site of conversion of ammonia to urea via the urea cycle, which is a separate process.

ANSWER: A

15. The liver is integral to which one or more of the following steps in vitamin D metabolism?

A. Intestinal absorption.
B. 25-Hydroxylation.
C. 1-Hydroxylation.
D. All of the above.

Ref.: 1, 3

COMMENTS: The absorption, metabolism, and storage of vitamins is dependent on hepatic events. Intestinal absorption of the fat-soluble vitamins A, D, E, and K requires bile salts synthesized in the liver. Vitamin D undergoes 25-hydroxylation in the liver and subsequent 1-hydroxylation in the kidney to arrive at the metabolically active form. The liver is an important storage site for fat-soluble vitamins and is the only site of storage of vitamin A. Excessive vitamin A is hepatotoxic. The liver also produces a number of transport proteins required for vitamin metabolism.

ANSWER: A, B

16. During typical obstructive jaundice, marked elevations might be expected in:

A. Aspartate aminotransferase (AST).
B. Alanine aminotransferase (ALT).
C. γ-Glutamyltransferase (GGT).
D. 5′-Nucleotidase.
E. Leucine aminopeptidase.

Ref.: 1

COMMENTS: AST (serum glutamic oxaloacetic transaminase, SGOT), ALT (serum glutamate pyruvate transaminase, SGPT), and lactate dehydrogenase (LDH) are indicators of the integrity of the cell membrane and increases reflect hepatocyte injury with leakage. These enzymes usually are only mildly or moderately elevated in pure obstructive jaundice. On the other hand, enzymes including alkaline phosphatase, 5′-nucleotidase, leucine aminopeptidase, and GGT reflect the excretory capacity of the liver. These enzymes are typically elevated in the presence of extrahepatic bile duct obstruction or intrahepatic cholestasis. Elevations are also seen in hepatic parenchymal disease or liver tumors.

ANSWER: C, D, E

17. Eight weeks after open heart surgery with transfusions, a 56-year-old man notes dark urine, fatigue, and anorexia. An examination discloses only mild, tender hepatomegaly. Laboratory investigations reveal bilirubin 2 mg/dl, SGOT 540 IU/L, SGPT 620 IU/L, alkaline phosphatase 1120 IU/L, and negative hepatitis B surface antigen (HBsAg), hepatitis B core antibody (anti-HBc), immunoglobulin M anti-hepatitis A virus antibody (IgM anti-HAV), and anti-hepatitis C virus antibody (anti-HCV) assays. Which of the following is the most likely explanation for the patient's clinical condition?

A. Acute viral hepatitis A.
B. Acute viral hepatitis B.
C. Acute viral hepatitis C.
D. Acute viral hepatitis D.
E. Acute viral hepatitis E.

Ref.: 1, 3

COMMENTS: Posttransfusion non-A, non-B hepatitis is mostly the result of hepatitis C infection. The incubation period is usually 5–10 weeks, and the mean peak aminotransferase levels are 500–1000 IU/L. Anti-HCV antibody is commonly not detectable until 18 weeks after illness onset. Approximately 70% of patients with acute hepatitis C progress to chronic hepatitis and potentially cirrhosis. The negative serologic studies described above exclude acute infection with hepatitis A and B. Hepatitis D (delta) virus (HDV) is capable of infecting only patients who also have HBsAg, because HDV is an incomplete RNA virus. Hepatitis E (epidemic) virus is rare, except in association with water-borne epidemics in India, the Middle East, and South America.

ANSWER: C

18. Which of the following clinical conditions does the presence of antibodies in the serum against hepatitis-B surface antigen (anti-HBs) and hepatitis-B core antigen (anti-HBc) in the absence of hepatitis-B surface antigen (HBsAg) indicate?

A. Active, acute infection with the hepatitis B virus.
B. Normal response to vaccination with the hepatitis B vaccine.
C. Chronic active hepatitis due to the hepatitis B virus.

D. Recovery with subsequent immunity following acute hepatitis B.
E. Asymptomatic chronic carrier of the hepatitis B virus.

Ref.: 1, 3

COMMENTS: The pattern of negative HBsAg, positive anti-HBs, and positive anti-HBc assays is seen during the recovery phase following acute hepatitis B and clearance of HBsAg from the liver. This antibody pattern may persist for years and is not associated with liver disease or infectivity. Vaccination with the hepatitis B vaccine (genetically manufactured HBsAg particles *without* HBcAg or HBV-DNA) is associated with the development of anti-HBs antibody alone. Active, ongoing infection with the hepatitis B virus, whether acute hepatitis, chronic active hepatitis, or asymptomatic chronic carrier state, is manifested by the presence of HBsAg and anti-HBc in the serum.

ANSWER: D

19. Which of the following is/are appropriate for management of hepatic trauma?

A. Observation of subcapsular hematoma.
B. Simple suture closure of a nonbleeding laceration.
C. Ligation of the hepatic artery for a bleeding bilobar stellate laceration in a hypotensive patient.
D. Anatomic lobectomy for a deep stab wound of the right lobe.
E. Right thoracotomy and placement of an atriocaval shunt for retrohepatic vena cava injury.

Ref.: 1, 2, 3

COMMENTS: The liver is the intraabdominal organ most frequently injured by penetrating trauma and is the second most frequently injured organ by blunt trauma. Subcapsular hematomas may be observed if stable or evacuated if large. Many simple lacerations are not bleeding at the time of exploration; these lacerations should not be closed because of the risk of liver abscess. Drainage of nonbleeding lacerations may not be necessary, although it is advisable for deeper injuries because of the potential for bile leakage. Simple bleeding lacerations can generally be controlled by direct suture-ligation or by the use of topical hemostatic agents. The preferred method for controlling bleeding from deeper wounds is hepatotomy and direct vascular ligation. Compression of the portal vein and hepatic arterial inflow in the hepatoduodenal ligament (Pringle maneuver) may be useful for controlling bleeding from these deeper injuries. More extensive parenchymal injuries require resectional débridement to remove all necrotic or devitalized tissue; resection rarely follows precise anatomic lines. Perihepatic packing has been a useful method to control hemorrhage temporarily in patients with hemodynamic instability, extensive parenchymal injuries, or coagulopathy. These patients are reexplored after resuscitation, usually 24–72 hours later. At that time, the packing is removed, bleeding sites are controlled, and necrotic tissue is débrided. Extensive hemorrhage following inflow occlusion suggests hepatic venous or retrohepatic caval injury; it requires control of the vena cava above and below the liver and possible placement of an atriocaval shunt, which is accomplished via sternotomy. Selective ligation of the right or left hepatic artery for control of hemorrhage is rarely necessary but might be helpful for penetrating deep wounds involving one lobe when exposure of the wound would require extensive hepatotomy. Hepatic arterial ligation, particularly in the presence of hypotension, may produce hepatic necrosis; hence ligation of the proper hepatic artery should not be performed. Techniques of mesh hepatorrhaphy that involve wrapping the injured liver in absorbable mesh, similar to mesh splenorrhaphy, have been introduced.

ANSWER: A

20. Which of the following statements is/are true regarding the management of patients undergoing major hepatic resection?

A. Preoperative prothrombin time and serum albumin determinations accurately predict the functional adequacy of the remaining liver.
B. Postoperative hyperglycemia results from intraoperative release of glycogen stores and is best managed by continuous insulin infusion.
C. Postoperative coagulopathy reflects vitamin K deficiency and is best treated by parenteral vitamin K.
D. Transient postoperative elevations of serum ammonia levels are expected and are treated by lactulose and administration of branched-chain amino acids.
E. Local problems, such as bleeding or bile leak, are the most frequent postoperative complications.

Ref.: 1, 2, 3

COMMENTS: Operations that involve removal of one or more anatomic segments of the liver can be considered major resections. The elective operative mortality of major hepatic resection is now 5% or less, reflecting refinements in surgical technique and advances in preoperative preparation and postoperative support. Preoperative preparation involves correction of reversible defects, such as anemia, malnutrition, and vitamin K deficiency. Unfortunately, there are no single tests of liver function that accurately predict the adequacy of the remaining liver. Generalized abnormalities of hepatic function suggested by increased bilirubin and depressed synthetic parameters suggest that great care must be taken before performing major resection. Local complications such as bleeding, bile leak, and abscess are the most frequent postoperative problems after major resection, followed by metabolic and respiratory problems. Metabolic complications include liver and renal failure, hypoglycemia (treated by infusion of 10% dextrose), hypoalbuminemia (treated with exogenous albumin), and coagulopathy (treated by administration of fresh whole blood or platelets and fresh-frozen plasma). Transient elevations of alkaline phosphatase, bilirubin, or transaminases are not uncommon; but even with extensive hepatic resection, blood ammonia levels usually remain normal.

ANSWER: E

21. Which of the following techniques is/are appropriate to limit blood loss during major hepatic resection?

A. Portal triad clamping.
B. Normal thermic total hepatic vascular isolation.
C. Total hepatic vascular isolation with venovenous bypass.
D. Low central venous pressure anesthesia.

Ref.: 6

COMMENTS: Hemorrhage is one of the major hazards during liver resection. Troublesome bleeding is most likely to occur during division of the hepatic parenchyma, and life-threatening hemorrhage is most commonly from the hepatic veins and their branches. A variety of intraoperative techniques have been employed in efforts to avoid this problem. The downside of any vascular occlusion, however, is the potential for ischemic injury to the liver, particularly in patients with underlying hepatocellular disease. Occlusion of the portal triad (Pringle maneuver) can be useful for limiting bleeding from the hepatic artery and portal vein branches. It has generally been suggested that periods of occlusion not exceed 20 minutes and perhaps should be shorter. Total hepatic vascular isolation requires occlusion of the inferior vena cava above and below the liver in addition to the Pringle maneuver. Such management can be complex and is not well tolerated by some patients. Venovenous bypass, which has commonly been used during hepatic transplantation, has also been applied to major hepatic resections at some centers. Attempts to protect the liver during vascular occlusion using local hepatic hypothermia or systemic steroids have not been uniformly practiced or successful. Low central venous pressure anesthesia minimizes hepatic venous bleeding by fluid restriction, head-down positioning, and the vasodilatory effects of standard anesthetics. This technique has been successful in nearly 500 patients at Memorial Sloan-Kettering Cancer Center in New York. Low central venous pressure anesthesia during major hepatic resection has avoided perioperative blood transfusion in two-thirds of patients and has a reported mortality of 4% and only a 3% rate of clinically important postoperative increases in serum creatinine.

ANSWER: A, B, C, D

22. A 50-year-old woman is found to have a 4 cm hepatic cyst with no internal echoes on ultrasonography. Which of the following would be the most appropriate management?

A. Observation if asymptomatic.
B. Tamoxifen to prevent enlargement.
C. Resection because it is premalignant.
D. Percutaneous aspiration for cytology.

Ref.: 1, 3, 5

COMMENTS: Simple, nonparasitic hepatic cysts are presumed to be congenital. They may be single or multiple, are more common in women, and are usually asymptomatic. The absence of internal echoes is diagnostic of a simple cyst, rather than a complex cyst, a cystic neoplasm, or a solid lesion. No further intervention is indicated for asymptomatic liver cysts when the diagnosis is secure. Complications such as hemorrhage or infection are rare, and these lesions are not premalignant. Exogenous hormones are not recognized to be harmful, nor is antihormonal therapy indicated. Occasionally, large cysts are symptomatic, primarily due to local pressure and discomfort. Treatment of symptomatic cysts is by operative resection or unroofing, which is often accomplished laparoscopically depending on cyst location. Percutaneous drainage or injection of alcohol or other sclerosing agents does not suffice and is not recommended. If the cyst is found to communicate with the bile ducts, either closure of the communication or cyst jejunostomy may be necessary.

ANSWER: A

23. Polycystic liver disease in adults is associated with which one or more of the following?

A. Polycystic kidney disease.
B. Hepatic fibrosis and portal hypertension.
C. Increased risk of hepatoma.
D. Intracranial aneurysms.

Ref.: 1, 3, 5

COMMENTS: Adult polycystic disease is an autosomal dominant disorder. About one-half of patients with liver cysts also have cystic involvement of the kidneys or other organs such as the pancreas or spleen. Intracranial arterial aneurysms occur in up to 30% of patients. Symptoms or complications of the liver cysts per se are infrequent, so specific therapy may not be necessary. When symptomatic, pain is the predominant problem. Operations to unroof or excise superficial cysts and fenestrate deeper cysts may provide the best symptomatic relief, although the benefit may be temporary. These procedures can be accomplished laparoscopically. Cyst aspiration or sclerosis is ineffective because of recurrence. Infantile polycystic kidney disease often results in death from renal failure; congenital hepatic fibrosis may be present. Hepatic fibrosis also occurs in association with multiple dilatations of the intrahepatic biliary tree (Caroli's disease). Polycystic liver disease is not a premalignant condition, but Caroli's disease is associated with malignancy.

ANSWER: A, D

24. Select the type of hepatic abscess in the right-hand column that is best described by each statement on the left.

A. Organisms most commonly reach liver by portal vein
B. Predominantly involves the right lobe
C. Cultures of percutaneous aspirate usually sterile
D. Primary treatment is pharmacologic
E. Primary treatment is drainage

a. Amebic liver abscess
b. Pyogenic liver abscess
c. Both
d. Neither

Ref.: 1, 2, 3

COMMENTS: Although the clinical signs and symptoms of pyogenic and amebic liver abscesses may be similar, predominantly consisting of fever and pain, it is important to differentiate between the two for therapeutic purposes. *Escherichia coli* or other gram-negative bacteria are the most commonly isolated organisms from pyogenic abscesses; *Streptococcus* species and anaerobes such as *Bacteroides* are also common. Today, the most frequent source of pyogenic abscess is contiguous infection in the biliary tract. Other sources include infectious foci within the portal venous drainage system, direct extension from perihepatic sites, and hematogenous spread. Approximately 20% of pyogenic abscesses are cryptogenic. The right lobe is most commonly involved with any hepatic abscesses, which has been attributed to a streaming effect in the portal vein. Diagnosis is based on the clinical presentation and hepatic imaging and may be confirmed by fine-needle aspiration. Treatment of pyogenic abscess requires eradication of both the abscess and the source. Treatment of the abscess usually requires drainage by operative or percutaneous approaches. Antibiotic therapy alone may suffice for treatment of multiple small abscess. Amebic abscesses are caused by the protozoan *Entamoeba histolytica*; diagnosis requires hepatic imaging and serologic testing. The organisms reach the liver from the intestine via the portal vein and produce a liquefaction necrosis responsible for the classic "anchovy paste" appearance. Protozoa are not usually isolated from the abscess, as they are located in the peripheral rim of tissue. Hepatic amebiasis is treated primarily by the administration of amebicidal drugs, with metronidazole as the drug of choice. Percutaneous aspiration may be indicated if the patient does not respond to medical management; and percutaneous or operative drainage is indicated in the presence of secondary bacterial infection, which occurs in about 10% of amebic abscesses.

ANSWER: A-a; B-c; C-a; D-a; E-b

25. What is the preferred treatment in the case of a patient with a 6 cm calcified cystic lesion containing daughter cysts in the right lobe of the liver?

A. Metronidazole.
B. Percutaneous catheter drainage.
C. Transperitoneal surgical drainage.
D. Pericystectomy.
E. Hepatic lobectomy.

Ref.: 1, 2, 3

COMMENTS: The helminth *Echinococcus granulosus* is responsible for most hydatid disease of the liver. It is usually a unilocular process involving the right lobe, although it may present as multiple cysts. Complications include intrabiliary, intraperitoneal, or intrapleural rupture; secondary infection; anaphylaxis; and mass replacement of the liver. These lesions often have a calcified wall and can be diagnosed serologically by indirect hemagglutination tests, complement fixation tests, serum immunoelectrophoresis, and formerly by the Casoni skin test. CT and ultrasound imaging may demonstrate characteristic daughter cysts or hydatid sand within the cyst. Treatment is primarily surgical; percutaneous aspiration or drainage is contraindicated because of the risk of intraperitoneal dissemination. The principles of surgical therapy are to avoid spillage and to remove the entire germinal layer. The cyst consists of an inner germinal layer (endocyst) and an outer fibrous reaction (exocyst). Resection is usually accomplished by pericystectomy; anatomic hepatic resection is not generally required. Because 20% of echinococcal cysts have biliary communication, assessment by preoperative endoscopic retrograde cholangiopancreatography or intraoperative cholangiography is important in any patient with jaundice, cholangitis, elevated liver enzymes, or bile noted during resection. Scolicidal agents should be used with caution because of the risk of sclerosing the bile ducts in the event the agent finds its way into the ductal system.

ANSWER: D

26. Match the following characteristics on the left with the correct hepatic neoplasm on the right.

A. Clearly associated with oral contraceptive use	a. Hepatic adenoma
B. High-risk hemorrhage	b. Focal nodular hyperplasia
C. Malignant potential	c. Both
D. Glycogen storage disease	d. Neither
E. Contains Kupffer cells	

Ref.: 1, 2, 3, 5

COMMENTS: Hepatic adenoma (HA) and focal nodular hyperplasia (FNH) are benign neoplasms with important differentiating clinical and histologic features and therapeutic implications. Both occur most commonly in women of childbearing age. Hepatic adenoma is associated with use of oral contraceptives and anabolic steroids and is also seen in certain glycogen storage diseases. The relation of FNH with steroid use is questionable and not completely settled. Hepatic adenoma is usually symptomatic (80%) and is associated with rupture and bleeding in a substantial proportion of patients. Malignant transformation of HA is recognized. The risk of malignancy in FNH is unlikely but uncertain. Histologically, HA consists of hepatocysts without bile ducts or Kupffer cells. A central stellate scar is characteristic of larger FNH lesions but is not always present.

ANSWER: A-a; B-a; C-a; D-a; E-b

27. A 25-year-old woman on oral contraceptives develops right upper quadrant abdominal pain. A CT scan demonstrates a hypodense 6 cm mass in the right lobe of the liver. A technetium 99m (^{99m}Tc) scan reveals a defect in the area of the mass. Angiography shows a hypervascular tumor with a peripheral blood supply. Which of the following is the appropriate management?

A. Discontinuation of oral contraceptives and observation with serial CT scans.
B. Percutaneous needle biopsy.
C. Hepatic resection.
D. Arterial embolization.
E. Radiation therapy.

Ref.: 1, 2, 3, 5

COMMENTS: The imaging characteristics described are typical of hepatic adenoma (HA). Because HA does not contain Kupffer cells, it does not take up radioisotope. This point may be useful for differentiating HA from FNH but not necessarily from other mass lesions of the liver. Percutaneous biopsy of suspected HA is not advisable because of the risk of hemorrhage. HAs associated with oral contraceptives tend to be larger and have a higher risk of bleeding than do those not associated with steroid use. Regression does not reliably occur with cessation of oral contraceptives. Resection is indicated for most suspected hepatic adenomas and especially for symptomatic lesions, for patients not on oral contraceptives, and if the diagnosis is uncertain. Embolization might be useful for treating hemorrhage in a patient whose HA is inoperable. Irradiation has no role in the management of HA.

ANSWER: C

28. An asymptomatic 60-year-old man is found to have an 8 cm liver mass. A CT scan demonstrates an initial hypodense lesion with peripheral to central enhancement by contrast. Magnetic resonance imaging (MRI) shows a dense T2-weighted phase. Which of the following is the appropriate management?

A. Arteriography.
B. Percutaneous needle biopsy.
C. Resection.
D. Radiation therapy.
E. Observation.

Ref.: 1, 2, 3, 5

COMMENTS: Cavernous hemangiomas are hamartomatous transformations of blood vessels that can be diagnosed by their characteristic appearance on noninvasive imaging studies. Contrast CT reveals a typical pattern of enhancement; a dense T2-weighted image on MRI is a sensitive (although not specific) finding; radiolabeled red blood cell scans can also diagnose hemangiomas. Angiography would be diagnostic as well but is not necessary. These lesions are usually asymptomatic and simply can be observed. They do not have a high risk of spontaneous rupture. Percutaneous biopsy is contraindicated because of the risk of bleeding. Resection by enucleation is appropriate for symptomatic lesions, for enlarging lesions, or if the diagnosis if uncertain. There is no established role for treatment such as arterial ligation, embolization, or irradiation.

ANSWER: E

29. Hepatocellular carcinoma is epidemiologically associated with one or more of the following?

A. Hepatitis A infection.
B. Hepatitis B infection.
C. Hepatitis C infection.
D. Hepatic cirrhosis independent of hepatitis infection.
E. Primary biliary cirrhosis.

Ref.: 1, 3

COMMENTS: Primary hepatocellular cancer, although less common in North America, is the most common malignant neoplasm worldwide. Endemic areas include sub-Saharan Africa, Southeast Asia, and Japan. The primary risk factors are chronic liver disease with cirrhosis (from essentially any cause), chronic infection with hepatitis B or C virus, and various hepatotoxins. Hepatocellular carcinoma can develop in patients with liver disease related to alcohol abuse, hemochromatosis, α_1-antitrypsin deficiency, hepatic adenomas, and other conditions. Exogenous risk factors include dietary aflatoxins (found in grain, dairy products, and peanuts), oral contraceptives, anabolic steroids, vinyl chloride, and certain pesticides. Hepatitis A virus and primary biliary cirrhosis are not associated with hepatocellular cancer, nor apparently is Wilson's disease.

ANSWER: B, C, D

30. Marked elevations of α-fetoprotein (AFP) (>400 μg/L) may be found with which one or more of the following?

A. Hepatocellular carcinoma.
B. Normal 6-week-old infant.
C. Colon cancer.
D. Acute viral hepatitis.
E. Teratocarcinoma.

Ref.: 1, 3

COMMENTS: α-Fetoprotein (AFP) is an oncofetoprotein that is useful diagnostically in regard to hepatocellular carcinoma. It is abundant during fetal development but decreases rapidly after birth. Approximately 75% of patients with hepatocellular cancer and cirrhosis have levels above 400 μg/L, whereas AFP is elevated in only about one-third of patients with hepatocellular cancer and a noncirrhotic liver. Other conditions that may be associated with pronounced elevations of serum AFP levels include teratocarcinomas, yolk sac tumors, and occasionally metastatic pancreatic or gastric carcinoma. Milder elevations may be found in patients with chronic liver disease, acute viral hepatitis, and metastatic cancer. Interval measurements of AFP (every 3 months) in combination with ultrasonography has been effective in screening high risk patients for the development of hepatocellular cancer.

ANSWER: A, E

31. Which of the following best approximates the 5-year survival after complete resection of an hepatocellular cancer?

A. 5%.
B. 25%.
C. 50%.
D. 75%.

Ref.: 1, 3

COMMENTS: Resection is the only potentially curative treatment for hepatocellular cancer. Unfortunately, most lesions are not resectable due to tumor spread or underlying cirrhosis. Prognostic factors that influence long-term survival following resection include tumor size, tumor multiplicity, encapsulation, completeness of resection, portal or hepatic vein invasion, and histologic differentiation. The 5-year survival after resection approximates 25%. Survival rates of 50–70% have been reported for small tumors. Liver transplantation for hepatocellular cancer in cirrhotic patients that cannot undergo partial hepatic resection yields similar survival rates. Tumor recurrence most frequently is in the liver following either resection or transplantation.

ANSWER: B

32. Match the clinical characteristics in the left-hand column with the appropriate type of hepatocellular tumor in the right-hand column.

A. Better survival with resection	a. Standard hepatocellular cancer
B. More common in males	b. Fibrolamellar cancer
C. AFP usually elevated	c. Both
D. Associated with hepatitis B	d. Neither

Ref.: 1, 3

COMMENTS: The fibrolamellar variant of hepatocellular cancer is relatively uncommon but has clinical and pathologic features that distinguish it from standard hepatocellular cancer. Histologically, it consists of sheets of well differentiated hepatocytes separated by fibrous tissue. It tends to be well localized and occurs in younger patients, often in the 20–30 year range. Standard hepatocellular cancers have a distinct male predominance but fibrolamellar tumors are as common or perhaps even more common in females. Unlike typical hepatocellular cancer, the fibrolamellar variant is not commonly associated with hepatitis B infection, cirrhosis, or elevated AFP levels (all ≤10%). These tumors are more often resectable and the prognosis following resection is considerably better with five-year survivals of 50–60%.

ANSWER: A-b; B-a; C-a; D-a

33. Which of the following statements is/are true regarding intrahepatic cholangiocarcinoma?

A. Survival following resection is generally lower than for distal bile duct cancer.

B. Resection is contraindicated unless histologically negative margins can be obtained.
C. Best survival is obtained with liver transplantation.
D. Adjuvant chemotherapy improves survival following resection.

Ref.: 1, 7

COMMENTS: Cholangiocarcinoma arises from the bile duct epithelium and can occur anywhere along the biliary tract. Tumors arising from the extrahepatic bile ducts differ from those located intrahepatically in terms of their presentation, therapy, and prognosis. Tumors of the extrahepatic bile ducts typically present with biliary obstruction. Intrahepatic tumors present as a liver mass with absent or vague symptoms, such as pain, weight loss, nausea, and anorexia. The prognosis is best for tumors of the distal bile ducts that can be resected by pancreaticoduodenectomy with a 5-year survival of 30–40%. Tumors involving the bifurcation of the bile duct (Klatskin tumor) are less often resectable, although resection (usually with hepatectomy) can yield 5-year survivals of 20–25%. Intrahepatic cholangiocarcinoma accounts for about 10% of primary hepatic malignancies and is second in frequency to hepatocellular carcinoma. Resection is associated with 5-year survivals of 20–40%. Tumor size and the presence of satellite nodules correlate with outcome. Histologically negative margins are always desirable, but prolonged survival can be attained even with microscopically involved margins. The results of liver transplantation for cholangiocarcinoma have been troubled with frequent recurrence and have not generally been encouraging. Adjuvant chemotherapy has not typically been useful for bile duct cancer.

ANSWER: A

34. In which of the following situations would resection of an isolated hepatic segment for malignancy be contraindicated?

A. Primary hepatocellular cancer.
B. Metastatic colorectal cancer.
C. Malignant tumor in a noncirrhotic liver.
D. Malignant tumor in a patient with extrahepatic metastases.

Ref.: 8

COMMENTS: The surgical anatomy of the liver, based on the branching of the portal structures, permits anatomic resections of single or multiple hepatic segments. These resections allow conservation of hepatic parenchyma and may be appropriate for patients with cirrhosis, those undergoing multiple or bilobar resections, or those undergoing repeat liver resection. The segmental vascular pedicle is isolated and divided prior to parenchymal division. In appropriate patients the rate of margin positivity does not exceed that of nonanatomic wedge resections and may be lower. Disease recurrence is usually elsewhere in the liver and not at the resection margin. It must be emphasized that safe performance of these resections requires an experienced hepatic surgeon who is thoroughly familiar with hepatic anatomy and dissection techniques. Metastatic extrahepatic disease is a general contraindication to any type of hepatic resection.

ANSWER: D

35. Resection of hepatic metastases has most clearly benefitted patients with which of the following cancers?

A. Colon.
B. Breast.
C. Stomach.
D. Pancreas.
E. Lung.

Ref.: 1, 2, 3

COMMENTS: Resection of hepatic metastases from colorectal cancer provides a clear survival advantage compared to any other treatment and should be performed whenever possible. The 5-year survival is approximately 25% and is as high as 40% in favorable subgroups. Resection of metastatic neuroendocrine tumors (carcinoid, insulinoma, gastrinoma) can be valuable for controlling symptoms of excessive endocrine secretion. Experience with hepatic resection for metastases from other portal sites (stomach, pancreas, biliary) or nonportal sites (lung, breast, melanoma, gynecologic, head and neck, renal) has been more limited, and results have not generally been as encouraging. Occasionally, a patient with a noncolorectal primary is cured when he or she undergoes resection of the isolated hepatic metastasis. However, the natural history of noncolorectal primary malignancies is such that patients rarely develop metastases isolated to the liver. Hepatic resection for direct, contiguous growth of the primary tumor (stomach, biliary) into the liver sometimes produces long-term survivors.

ANSWER: A

36. Which of the following is/are contraindications for resection of colorectal hepatic metastases?

A. Extrahepatic metastases.
B. Synchronous metastases.
C. Bilobar metastases.
D. Multiple metastases.
E. Size >5 cm.

Ref.: 1, 3

COMMENTS: See Question 37.

37. Disease-free survival following resection of colorectal hepatic metastases is influenced by which one or more of the following?

A. Time interval between resection of primary lesion and hepatic metastases.
B. Resection margin >1 cm.
C. Resection margin >3 cm.
D. Adjuvant hepatic arterial chemotherapy.
E. Adjuvant radiation therapy.

Ref.: 1, 3, 9

COMMENTS: Resection is currently the preferred treatment for liver metastases from colorectal cancer provided the patient has adequate liver reserve and does not have extrahepatic metastases. The goal is to resect all hepatic disease; survival is adversely affected by margins that are positive or are less than 1 cm. So long as the resection margin is adequate, the specific type of liver resection (anatomic versus "wedge") does not influence survival. Many parameters have been evaluated for their prognostic importance following resection of colorectal metastases. Although long-term survival is not as good for patients with four or more tumors, resection, when possible, still provides some longevity. Factors that have not consistently been found to influence survival include synchronous versus metachronous lesions, tumor size, tumor distribution (unilobar versus bilobar), and stage of the primary tumor (although patients with positive mesenteric nodes are more likely to develop extrahepatic metastases). Most patients undergoing hepatic resection for colorectal metastases eventually have a recurrence at some site. Hepatic arterial infusion of chemotherapeutic agents has a higher response rate than does systemic administration, although adjuvant chemotherapy has not prolonged survival following hepatic resection in randomized studies. Irradiation is not useful for hepatic metastases. The role of ablative therapy such as cryosurgery or hyperthermia (radiofrequency, laser) for hepatic metastases is under evaluation. These approaches appear useful for patients who cannot undergo resection, but they cannot yet be considered appropriate alternative treatment for otherwise resectable tumors.

ANSWER:
Question 36: A
Question 37: B

38. Which of the following is the most accurate method for identifying hepatic metastases?

A. CT scan.
B. Laparoscopy.
C. Transabdominal ultrasonography.
D. Intraoperative ultrasonography.
E. Intraoperative palpation.

Ref.: 4

COMMENTS: Transabdominal ultrasonography is as accurate as CT scans for detecting liver tumors that are 2 cm in size or larger. For somewhat smaller lesions, CT is more accurate, although it can miss the smallest lesions (<1 cm). Laparoscopy is useful for identifying small metastases on the liver or peritoneal surfaces that escape discovery by noninvasive preoperative imaging modalities. Laparoscopy has been incorporated in the staging workup of a variety of intraabdominal malignancies including liver. However, one of its limitations is in its ability to assess the interior structure of solid organs. It is now well recognized that intraoperative ultrasonography (US) is the most accurate method for detecting and assessing hepatic tumors. Not only does intraoperative US discover more lesions than any other modality (including palpation), it also clearly demonstrates the anatomic relation of tumors to important vascular structures, which is a critical determinant of resectability or of the extent of resection necessary. Intraoperative US scans can be obtained with hand-held or laparoscopic transducers. Experience with intraoperative US during surgery for liver tumors has shown that the sonographic findings affect the surgical management of one-third to one-half of patients. Intraoperative US has become an indispensable component of hepatic surgery.

ANSWER: D

39. Which of the following studies may be important in determining treatment for a patient with hepatic encephalopathy?

A. Serum ammonia level.
B. Serum amino acid pattern.
C. Electroencephalography (EEG).
D. Paracentesis.
E. Angiography.

Ref.: 1, 2, 3

COMMENTS: Although the etiology of hepatic encephalopathy is not fully understood, current understanding focuses on toxic effects of ammonia, mercaptans, short-chain fatty acids, methane thiols, and false neurotransmitters. The mechanism involves hepatic dysfunction or portosystemic shunting, but usually a combination of the two. A number of situations can precipitate hepatic encephalopathy and should be sought during the initial evaluation of patients. These causes include gastrointestinal bleeding, infection, constipation, electrolyte or metabolic abnormalities, and diuretic and other drug therapy (particularly sedatives or hypnotic drugs). When evaluating patients for potential infection, it is important to recognize the possibility of spontaneous primary bacterial peritonitis in those with ascites and to perform paracentesis to clarify this point. Some cases of hepatic encephalopathy have no identifiable precipitating cause other than the patient's inability to metabolize protein adequately or the presence of portosystemic shunting. In cases of refractory encephalopathy, angiographic assessment and therapeutic occlusion of a prior surgical shunt or of major collaterals may bring about improvement in the patient's condition. Although serum ammonia levels are usually elevated with encephalopathy and amino acid patterns are altered, these findings do not indicate a specific therapeutic approach. EEG may provide confirmatory diagnostic information.

ANSWER: D, E

40. Which of the following should be used for initial treatment of a patient in hepatic coma?

A. Lactulose.
B. Nutritional supplementation with standard amino acid formulas.
C. Nutritional supplementation with branched-chain amino acids.
D. Systemic antibiotics.
E. Ileostomy.

Ref.: 1, 2, 3

COMMENTS: The treatment of hepatic encephalopathy and coma is aimed at limiting the nitrogen that the liver must metabolize by eliminating nitrogen materials from the gastrointestinal tract and by inhibiting their absorption. At the same time, precipitating causes are sought and treated. Lactulose acts as a cathartic and also inhibits absorption of ammonia by acidifying the colon. Intraluminal neomycin reduces the colonic flora and the production of ammonia. Although alterations in the balance of aromatic amino acids and branched-chain amino acid have been demonstrated in patients with hepatic disease and encephalopathy, there is no evidence that administration of branched-chain amino acids significantly alleviates encephalopathy. Nutritional support is important and can be initiated with standard amino acids and restriction of dietary protein. Branched-chain amino acids can be reserved for patients with intractable encephalopathy despite these initial measures. Systemic antibiotics may be useful for treating specific infections that precipitate encephalopathy but are not indicated empirically. Because the colon is the major site of ammonia absorption, colonic resection or exclusion has been used to improve encephalopathy but is not a widely employed therapeutic measure.

ANSWER: A, B

41. The initial management of ascites associated with cirrhosis should include which of the following?

A. Fluid restriction.
B. Sodium restriction.

C. Diuretic administration.
D. Diagnostic paracentesis.
E. Therapeutic large-volume paracentesis.

Ref.: 10

COMMENTS: Ascites is the most common major complication of hepatic cirrhosis. It is associated with a 2-year survival of 50%, and its onset in a cirrhotic patient should prompt an evaluation for liver transplantation. The treatment of ascites depends on its cause, so diagnostic paracentesis is required after a history and physical examination. Abdominal ultrasonography can confirm the presence of ascites if it is not certain by examination. The serum–ascites albumin gradient is useful diagnostically. A high gradient (≥1.1 gm/dl) indicates portal hypertension and suggests that the patient will be responsive to medical management consisting of sodium restriction (2000 mg/day) and oral diuretics. Usually, both spironolactone and furosemide are administered to produce fluid loss and natriuresis. Spironolactone alone may cause hyperkalemia, and furosemide alone is less effective. Fluid restriction is not necessary unless the patient has pronounced hyponatremia (<120 mmol/L). Medical therapy controls ascites in about 90% of patients. When the ascites is refractory, serial therapeutic paracenteses (with or without administration of albumin or other plasma volume expanders) is indicated. Liver transplantation is the ultimate treatment. A peritoneovenous shunt is an option for patients with refractory ascites who are not transplant candidates or who cannot undergo repeated paracenteses. These shunts are fraught with potential complications, however, and do not prolong survival compared to medical management. Transjugular intrahepatic portosystemic shunts (TIPS) or operative side-to-side type portosystemic shunts may control ascites in selected patients.

ANSWER: B, C, D

42. Which of the following is/are relative contraindication(s) to peritoneovenous shunting for intractable ascites?

A. History of variceal bleeding.
B. Oliguria.
C. Bacterial peritonitis.
D. Uncorrectable coagulopathy.
E. Malignant intraabdominal disease.

Ref.: 1, 3

COMMENTS: Patients with significant ascites due to cirrhosis or malignancy who do not respond to medical management may be candidates for peritoneovenous shunting. These shunts decrease ascites and increase cardiac output and renal blood flow. Some degree of coagulopathy, usually transient, occurs in nearly all patients with cirrhotic ascites; uncorrectable coagulopathy is considered a contraindication to shunting. Patients with portal hypertension and previous variceal bleeding may rebleed following shunting because of the increase in circulating blood volume. Other contraindications to shunting in patients with cirrhotic ascites include bacterial peritonitis, liver failure, and cardiac failure. Patients undergoing peritoneovenous shunts for malignancy have a higher incidence of shunt occlusion; relative contraindications include the presence of bloody ascitic fluid or fluid with high protein content.

ANSWER: A, C, D

43. Which of the following statements is/are true regarding spontaneous bacterial peritonitis (SBP)?

A. Diagnosis can be made clinically without paracentesis.
B. Infection is most commonly monomicrobial with an enteric organism.
C. Antibiotic therapy is reserved for patients with positive ascitic fluid cultures.
D. It can be differentiated from secondary bacterial peritonitis based on the clinical response to therapy.

Ref.: 3, 10

COMMENTS: Spontaneous bacterial peritonitis is a potentially lethal complication of ascites that affects about 10% of patients with cirrhotic ascites. Fever and abdominal pain are common manifestations, but the presentation may be subtle. Diagnosis requires paracentesis with demonstration of an elevated ascitic fluid polymorphonuclear neutrophil (PMN) count (≥250 cells/mm^3) or eventual positive cultures. Antibiotic therapy should be instituted promptly based on an elevated ascitic fluid PMN count or on symptoms even if the PMN count is lower. Infection is usually monomicrobial, the most common organisms are *Escherichia coli*, *Klebsiella*, and pneumococci. A third-generation cephalosporin is typically the preferred antibiotic. Differentiation from secondary bacterial peritonitis due to a surgical condition is critical. Patients with SBP typically respond to appropriate antibiotics within 48 hours, and ascitic PMN counts decrease. Failure to improve, the presence of polymicrobial infection, or ascitic fluid with a total protein level greater than 1 gm/dl, LDH greater than serum, or glucose less than 50 mg/dl suggests secondary peritonitis. Risk factors for SBP include prior SBP, variceal hemorrhage, and low protein ascites (<1.0 gm/dl). Short or long-term prophylactic antibiotics may be appropriate for high-risk patients.

ANSWER: B, D

44. With regard to hernias in patients with ascites:

A. The recurrence rate following repair of inguinal hernias is similar to that following repair of umbilical hernias.
B. Patients with asymptomatic groin hernias should be treated expectantly.
C. Incarceration occurs frequently in patients with ascites.
D. Ascites leak following a surgical procedure should be treated expectantly.

Ref.: 11

COMMENTS: Umbilical, and less frequently inguinal, hernias occur in patients with ascites. The recurrence rate following inguinal hernias is approximately 10% and approximately 40% following repair of umbilical hernias. Because of the high complication rate following hernia repair, it should not be entertained for the asymptomatic hernia. Incarceration is a rare event in patients with ascites. Ascites leak following a surgical procedure should be treated aggressively, and early wound exploration and repair of fascial dehiscence is necessary. Diuretic therapy alone is ineffective in this situation.

ANSWER: B

REFERENCES

1. Sabiston DC: *Textbook of Surgery: The Biological Basis of Modern Surgical Practice*, 15th ed. WB Saunders, Philadelphia, 1997.
2. Schwartz SI, Shires GT, Spencer FC: *Principles of Surgery*, 7th ed. McGraw-Hill, New York, 1999.

3. Greenfield LJ, Mulholland M, Oldham T, et al: *Surgery: Scientific Principles and Practice*, 2nd ed. Lippincott-Raven, Philadelphia, 1996.
4. Deziel DJ: Hepatobiliary ultrasound. *Probl Gen Surg* 14:13–24, 1997.
5. O'Leary JP: *The Physiologic Basis of Surgery*, 2nd ed. Williams & Wilkins, Baltimore, 1996.
6. Melendez JA, Arslan V, Fischer ME, et al: Perioperative outcomes of major hepatic resections under low central venous pressure anesthesia: blood loss, blood transfusion and the risk of postoperative renal dysfunction. *J Am Coll Surg* 187:620–625, 1998.
7. Roayaie S, Guarrera JV, Ye MQ, et al: Aggressive surgical treatment of intrahepatic cholangiocarcinoma: predictors or outcome. *J Am Coll Surg* 187:365–372, 1998.
8. Billingsley KG, Jarnagin WR, Fong Y, Blumgart LM: Segment-oriented hepatic resection in the management of malignant neoplasms of the liver. *J Am Coll Surg* 187:471–481, 1998.
9. Lorenz M, Müller HH, Schramm H, et al: Randomized trial of surgery versus surgery followed by adjuvant hepatic arterial infusion with 5-fluorouracil and folinic acid for liver metastases of colorectal cancer. *Ann Surg* 228:756–762, 1998.
10. Runyon BA: Management of adult patients with ascites caused by cirrhosis. *Hepatology* 27:264–272, 1998.
11. Rosemurgy AS, Statman RC, Murphy CG, et al: Postoperative ascitic leaks: the ongoing challenge [see comments]. *Surgery* 111: 623–625, 1992.

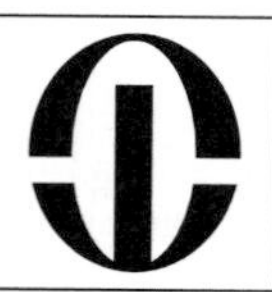

CHAPTER 33

Portal Venous System

1. A 51-year-old man is admitted to the hospital after hematemesis and upper gastrointestinal bleeding necessitating transfusion of 6 units of blood. The only positive finding in the workup is seen on the radiograph shown below. Which of the following is the preferred treatment option to prevent rebleeding?

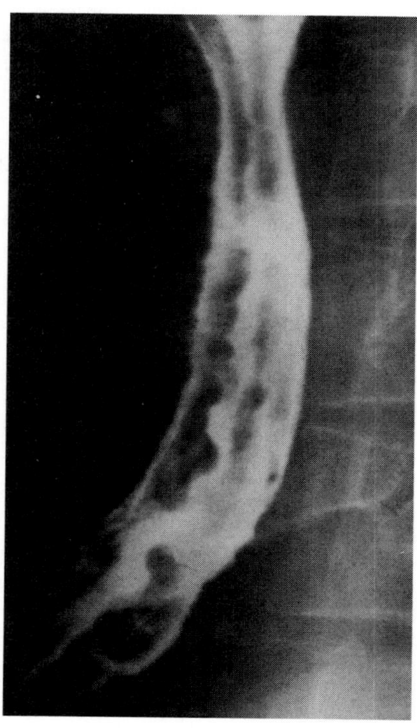

A. Observation.
B. Propranolol.
C. Vasopressin.
D. Balloon tamponade.
E. Sclerotherapy.
F. Portacaval shunt.
G. Transjugular intrahepatic portosystemic shunt (TIPS) procedure.
H. Liver transplant.

Ref.: 1

COMMENTS: This radiograph demonstrates esophageal varices and is likely a manifestation of portal hypertension. Varices are present in 50–60% of patients with cirrhosis. Bleeding ceases spontaneously in 20–30% of patients, but each episode is associated with 25–40% mortality. The risk of rebleeding is high. The immediate gcal is to stabilize hemodynamics. Once variceal hemorrhage is established endoscopically, therapy should address portal pressure (i.e., vasopressin and local control). Balloon tamponade is used for control of the acute bleed where other therapies fail or cannot be performed. After the acute hemorrhage is controlled, therapy should be directed at preventing recurrence. Oral β-blockers are the most commonly used agents for preventing variceal hemorrhage recurrence. The dose should be adjusted to heart rates around 55–60 bpm. Endoscopic sclerotherapy reduces the risk of rebleeding and mortality but when long-term sclerotherapy was compared to the use of β-blockers, no differences were reported. Variceal ligation is a good option, but clinical trials are still pending. Shunt surgery is usually indicated when the above methods of controlling bleeding have failed in patients who are good surgical candidates. TIPS is recommended in patients who have rebled on pharmacologic therapy but who are not good surgical candidates.

ANSWER: B

2. With regard to the portal vein, which of the following statements is/are true?

A. It is valveless.
B. It is formed by the junction of the inferior mesenteric vein and the splenic vein.
C. It commonly has various patterns of branching within the liver.
D. It can develop multiple portosystemic collaterals.

Ref.: 2, 3

COMMENTS: The portal vein is formed by the junction of the superior mesenteric vein and the splenic vein, provides 75% of hepatic blood flow, and has a relatively constant pattern of branching within the liver. Portal hypertension is a common sequela of hepatic diseases that produce portal venous obstruction; prominent clinical manifestations are often due to increased blood flow through the many portosystemic collateral pathways that are available. The portal venous system has no valves, which permits measurement of portal venous pressure from any point in the system.

ANSWER: A, D

3. For management of portal vein injury, which of the following is/are appropriate?

A. Direct venorrhaphy.
B. Portal vein ligation.
C. End-to-end anastomosis.
D. Graft interposition.
E. Portal vein ligation with portosystemic shunt.

Ref.: 2, 3

COMMENTS: Portal vein injuries generally result from penetrating trauma and have a high fatality rate. The preferred method of management is some form of repair, by lateral venorrhaphy when possible or by reanastomosis or graft interposition. If repair is not possible, the portal vein may be ligated. Portosystemic shunting is not advocated; it is more dangerous than ligation alone and poses a risk of hepatic encephalopathy.

ANSWER: A, B, C, D

4. In which of the following disorders does the pathophysiology of portal hypertension involve presinusoidal intrahepatic obstruction?

A. Budd-Chiari syndrome.
B. Cavernomatous transformation of the portal vein.
C. Hemochromatosis.
D. Alcoholic cirrhosis.
E. Schistosomiasis.

Ref.: 2, 3

COMMENTS: Portal hypertension may result from increased portal blood flow or increased resistance to flow. By far the most common cause is increased resistance due to some form of obstruction. The site of obstruction is most frequently intrahepatic but may be extrahepatic, as seen in the Budd-Chiari syndrome or portal vein thrombosis. It is useful to consider the site of obstruction as either presinusoidal or postsinusoidal because patients with presinusoidal obstruction may have normal hepatocyte function, whereas patients with postsinusoidal obstruction usually have hepatocellular damage. By far the most common intrahepatic cause of obstruction is cirrhosis, which produces postsinusoidal obstruction. Presinusoidal obstruction involving fibrosis of the terminal radicles of the portal vein is produced by schistosomiasis and congenital hepatic fibrosis.

ANSWER: E

5. With regard to the angiographic evaluation of patients with portal hypertension, which of the following statements is/are true?

A. Both venous anatomy and portal pressure can be determined by transhepatic portography, umbilical vein catheterization, or splenoportography.
B. Indirect portography is inadequate for assessment of the portal vein.
C. Wedged hepatic vein pressure is elevated with presinusoidal obstruction.
D. The degree of portal hypertension measured during angiography correlates with the risk of variceal bleeding.

Ref.: 2

COMMENTS: Angiographic evaluation of patients with portal hypertension permits both visualization of the venous anatomy and measurement of portal pressures. The first approach to visualization of the portal venous anatomy is usually indirect portography performed by percutaneous injection into the splenic and superior mesenteric arteries. Direct portography via transhepatic or transsplenic routes is usually reserved for cases that cannot be visualized by indirect methods. A number of approaches allow direct measurement of portal venous pressures. Wedged hepatic vein pressure reflects sinusoidal pressure and is usually normal with presinusoidal obstruction. Although manometric studies are of interest in patients with portal hypertension, the degree of pressure elevation has not been found to correlate with the subsequent risk of variceal hemorrhage or ascites.

ANSWER: A

6. Following resuscitation of a patient with acute hemorrhage from esophageal varices, which of the following is/are appropriate next therapeutic measures?

A. Intraarterial vasopressin.
B. Intravenous vasopressin.
C. Endoscopic sclerotherapy.
D. Portacaval shunt.
E. Gastroesophageal devascularization.
F. Terlipressin.
G. Octreotide.

Ref.: 2, 3, 4

COMMENTS: The approach to acute upper gastrointestinal hemorrhage in a patient with portal hypertension must focus on resuscitation followed by confirmation of the bleeding site and therapeutic measures directed at hemostasis. In general, the least invasive therapies are initiated first. Vasopressin can be administered via a peripheral vein as a bolus of 20 U over 20 minutes, followed by a continuous infusion of up to 0.4 U/min. This controls hemorrhage in 50–70% of patients. There is no particular advantage to intraarterial administration of vasopressin. Terlipressin is a synthetic derivative of vasopressin that has a longer duration of action and can be administered as a bolus injection. Octreotide reduces portal pressure by decreasing portal blood flow. It has been shown to be more effective than vasopressin for controlling the acute variceal hemorrhage with minimal side effects. If these agents do not control bleeding, endoscopic sclerosis of acute variceal hemorrhage can effectively achieve initial control in 80–90% of cases and results in a lower mortality rate than that achieved in patients managed medically without sclerosis. Balloon tamponade is no longer the preferred initial treatment for acute variceal hemorrhage, but it may be useful as a temporizing measure in patients who continue to bleed. For patients who continue to rebleed, either an emergency shunt or the TIPS procedure is recommended.

ANSWER: B, F, G

7. Which of the following is/are effect(s) of vasopressin?

A. Esophageal variceal vasoconstriction.
B. Splanchnic arteriolar vasoconstriction.
C. Coronary arterial vasoconstriction.
D. Cramping abdominal pain.
E. Dilutional hyponatremia.

Ref.: 2, 3

COMMENTS: Vasopressin produces generalized vasoconstriction. It is effective in reducing variceal hemorrhage because its constricts splanchnic arteriolar beds with a secondary fall in portal pressure. It does not directly affect the bleeding varices, which do not have smooth muscle. Vasopressin may also cause coronary vasoconstriction, contraindicating its use in patients with ischemic heart disease. Raynaud's phenomenon is also sometimes observed. Contraction of intestinal smooth muscle may produce cramping pain and diarrhea. Dilutional hyponatremia may occur as a result of the antidiuretic effect of vasopressin.

ANSWER: B, C, D, E

8. Which one or more of the following treatments may decrease recurrence of variceal bleeding?

A. Total portosystemic shunt.
B. Selective variceal shunt.
C. Gastric devascularization and portal-azygous disconnection.
D. Endoscopic variceal sclerosis.
E. Propranolol.
F. TIPS (transjugular intrahepatic portosystemic shunt).

Ref.: 2

COMMENTS: The natural history of variceal hemorrhage in cirrhotic patients indicates that 60% rebleed within 1 year of their initial hemorrhage, associated with significant mortality. Several therapeutic options are available and have been shown to decrease the incidence of recurrent variceal hemorrhage, although the criteria by which patients are selected for one treatment or another are not unequivocally defined. Both total and selective portosystemic shunts effectively prevent recurrent hemorrhage. Some surgeons favor selective shunts on the basis that they preserve hepatic blood flow and prevent hepatic failure and encephalopathy. Portal-azygous disconnection usually involves esophageal transection, splenectomy, and gastric devascularization; this approach may be useful in patients with compromised hepatic function or in those in whom shunting procedures cannot be performed for technical reasons (i.e., absence of portal, splenic, or superior mesenteric vein). Repeated endoscopic sclerotherapy has been shown to decrease rebleeding. Long-term survival following sclerotherapy has not yet been demonstrated to be superior to that after shunting procedures. Pharmacologic measures to decrease portal pressure, such as treatment with the β-adrenergic blocker propranolol, have been shown to decrease rebleeding. TIPS can be used in poor risk patients as a bridge to orthotopic liver transplantation.

ANSWER: A, B, C, D, E, F

9. With regard to prophylactic shunts in patients with cirrhosis and varices, which of the following is/are true?

A. They decrease risk of hemorrhage compared with medical therapy.
B. They improve survival compared with medical therapy.
C. They decrease risk of encephalopathy compared with medical therapy.
D. They decrease risk of hepatic coma compared with medical therapy.

Ref.: 2

COMMENTS: Clinical trials of portosystemic shunts performed prophylactically in patients with cirrhosis and documented varices (and who have not yet bled) have not demonstrated any overall advantage compared with standard medical therapy. Although the risk of bleeding is decreased, these patients are at risk for both encephalopathy and hepatic failure; and survival has not been improved. Consequently, prophylaxis is currently not considered an indication for portosystemic shunting. In this regard, it should be noted that Sugiura's experience with portal-azygous disconnection and Inokuchi's experience with coronary-caval shunts, both of whom report superior results, have included a significant proportion of patients for whom the procedures were performed prophylactically.

ANSWER: A

10. Which of the following is/are true with regard to cirrhotic ascites?

A. Ascites is commonly found in patients with prehepatic portal hypertension.
B. A serum–ascites albumin gradient of more than 1.1 is high and reflects portal hypertension.
C. The most rational diuretic treatment of cirrhotic ascites includes treatment with spironolactone and furosemide.
D. TIPS would be an appropriate first line therapy for patients with cirrhotic ascites.

Ref.: 5, 6

COMMENTS: Ascites is a common manifestation of cirrhosis of the liver. It occurs when the amount of peritoneal fluid is increased to more than 150 ml. Ascites is unusual in patients with prehepatic portal hypertension but is commonly found in those with hepatic and posthepatic causes of portal hypertension. It is usually first treated with salt restriction of less than 2 gm/day and diuretics. Second-line therapy includes large-volume paracentesis. Peritoneovenous shunt or TIPS is reserved for patients with refractory ascites.

ANSWER: B, C

11. Which of the following is/are considered to be total physiologic portosystemic shunts?

A. End-to-side portacaval.
B. Side-to-side portacaval.
C. Central splenorenal.
D. Distal splenorenal.
E. Coronary-caval.

Ref.: 2, 3

COMMENTS: Physiologically, portosystemic shunts eventually function either as total shunts, which deprive the liver of blood flow, or as selective shunts, which are performed with the goal of maintaining portal perfusion of the liver. End-to-side portacaval shunts function as Eck's fistulas, with complete diversion of portal hepatic blood flow. However, even shunts that maintain portal-hepatic continuity, such as the side-to-side, mesorenal, central splenorenal, and mesocaval shunts, effectively produce a total physiologic shunt, because the portal vein acts as an outflow tract from the high-pressure system. The distal splenorenal shunt and coronary-caval shunt, however, are examples of selective shunts, which decompress the gastroesophageal region while maintaining portal hepatic flow. Adequate division of collateral pathways during creation of a selective shunt may be important to prevent its eventual function as a total shunt.

ANSWER: A, B, C

12. Total portosystemic shunts effectively achieve which of the following?

A. Control of acute variceal bleeding.
B. Prevention of recurrent variceal bleeding.
C. Improvement in patient survival compared with medical management.
D. Prevention of hepatic encephalopathy.

Ref.: 2

COMMENTS: There is no question that total portosystemic shunts effectively control acute variceal hemorrhage and prevent recurrence of bleeding. The price, however, is the risk of encephalopathy and hepatic failure due to diversion of hepatic blood flow. Neither prophylactic nor therapeutic total shunts have been shown to improve overall survival significantly compared with nonshunt therapy.

ANSWER: A, B

13. In patients with alcoholic cirrhosis, the advantages of distal splenorenal shunts, compared with portacaval shunts, have been which of the following?

A. Improved survival.
B. More effective prevention of hemorrhage.
C. Reduced risk of encephalopathy.
D. Technically easier to perform.

Ref.: 2, 3

COMMENTS: Randomized prospective trials comparing the selective splenorenal shunt with total portosystemic shunts for treatment of portal hypertension due to alcoholic cirrhosis have demonstrated equivalent effectiveness for both types in terms of controlling hemorrhage and allowing long-term survival. In most studies, encephalopathy has been less common after selective shunts. Technically, an end-to-side portacaval shunt is easier to perform.

ANSWER: C

14. Which of the following is/are incorporated in the modified Child-Pugh classification of hepatic dysfunction?

A. Bilirubin determination.
B. Serum glutamic oxalic transaminase (SGOT; aspartate aminotransferase, AST) determination.
C. Prothrombin time.
D. Serum albumin determination.
E. Assessment of ascites.

Ref.: 2, 3, 7

COMMENTS: Child's classification incorporates a combination of clinical and laboratory parameters that correlate with the early mortality rates of shunting operations. These prognostic factors include clinical assessment of ascites, encephalopathy, and nutritional status and laboratory determinations of serum bilirubin and albumin. Patients are designated class A, B, or C, with their respective operative mortality rates for shunting procedures approximately less than 2%, 10%, and 50%. Prolongation of prothrombin time to more than 4 seconds above control (after vitamin K has been replaced) also suggests significant hepatic dysfunction. SGOT elevations suggest hepatitis and warrant delay of operation until this diagnosis can be excluded.

ANSWER: A, C, D, E

15. Which of the following veins is/are not ligated during distal splenorenal shunt?

A. Left adrenal vein.
B. Inferior mesenteric vein.
C. Superior mesenteric vein.
D. Coronary vein.
E. Pancreatic branches of splenic vein.

Ref.: 2

COMMENTS: The selective distal splenorenal shunt is performed by end-to-side anastomosis of the distal end of the divided splenic vein to the left renal vein, thereby decompressing gastroesophageal collaterals through the short gastric vessels. The left adrenal vein and inferior mesenteric vein are ligated during dissection of the renal vein and splenic vein respectively. It has additionally been recognized that pancreatic branches of the splenic vein should be divided to prevent the late development of peripancreatic collaterals, which would divert hepatic portal blood flow and negate the selectivity of the shunt. For this same reason, the left gastric vein (coronary vein) and right gastroepiploic vein are disconnected from the portal system.

ANSWER: C

16. Which one or more of the following technical considerations might preclude construction of a portacaval shunt?

A. Portal vein thrombosis.
B. Large caudate lobe of liver.
C. Previous splenectomy.
D. Previous operations for biliary stricture.

Ref.: 2

COMMENTS: Selection of the appropriate type of shunting operation for a particular patient must consider the cause of the portal hypertension, the clinical manifestations, the status of the liver, and the technical demands of each operation. Portacaval shunts cannot be performed when there are extensive adhesions from previous right upper quadrant operations. The presence of a large caudate lobe may prevent direct approximation of the portal vein and inferior vena cava; this can sometimes be circumvented by placing an interposition graft or resecting the caudate lobe. Previous splenectomy has no bearing on technical construction of a portacaval shunt but would preclude performance of a selective distal splenorenal shunt.

ANSWER: A, B, D

17. With regard to portal hypertension in children, which of the following is/are true?

A. Congenital hepatic fibrosis is the most common cause.
B. Variceal bleeding is the most common cause of massive hematemesis.
C. Acute variceal hemorrhage usually requires operation.
D. Portosystemic shunts are contraindicated because of the long-term risk of encephalopathy.

Ref.: 2, 3, 8

COMMENTS: Unlike portal hypertension in adults, most portal hypertension in children is caused by extrahepatic obstruction of the portal vein, usually the result of portal vein thrombosis. Although bleeding from esophageal varices accounts for less than 15% of upper gastrointestinal bleeding in adults, it constitutes the most common cause of massive upper gastrointestinal bleeding in children and is often the first manifestation of portal hypertension. Most episodes of acute variceal hemorrhage in children stop without invasive therapeutic measures. Survival following shunting procedures in children with extrahepatic portal vein obstruction is better than in adults with hepatic compromise. This has influenced some to suggest an aggressive approach to shunting procedures in children with recurrent hemorrhage. Because bleeding episodes are generally well tolerated, however, others advocate a conservative attitude and note that shunting procedures in children carry the risk of thrombosis and encephalopathy or of hepatic dysfunction. Total shunts, such as the mesocaval or central splenorenal type, have been performed in children with portal vein thrombosis. If the splenic vein is of sufficient size to avoid thrombosis, a selective distal splenorenal shunt may be preferable. Endoscopic sclerotherapy for variceal hemorrhage may be successful. Patients may eventually demonstrate spontaneous regression of varices as they grow and collaterals develop.

ANSWER: B

18. Which one or more of the following shunts may be appropriate for the treatment of Budd-Chiari syndrome?

A. End-to-side portacaval.
B. Side-to-side portacaval.
C. Mesocaval.
D. Mesoatrial.
E. Distal splenorenal.

Ref.: 9

COMMENTS: Budd-Chiari syndrome is characterized by obstruction of the hepatic veins, which produces hepatomegaly, ascites, and pain, progressing to hepatocyte necrosis with liver failure. Because the hepatic outflow tract is occluded, surgical decompression can be achieved only by some form of side-to-side shunt. The evaluation of patients with Budd-Chiari syndrome should include radiographic and manometric assessment of the inferior vena cava because obstruction or thrombosis of the inferior vena cava may also be present. This situation precludes a simple portacaval shunt and necessitates some form of portal-atrial or caval-portal-atrial shunt. A number of shunts have been proposed for this particular situation; mesoatrial interposition grafts have been successful but have a significant incidence of thrombosis. These cases are unusual, and experience treating them has been limited.

ANSWER: B, C, D

19. With regard to hepatic encephalopathy:

A. In patients with previous hepatic encephalopathy, oral protein intake should be less than 40 gm/day.
B. Lactulose is a nondigestable disaccharide; dosage should range from 45 to 90 gm and should be titrated to two to three soft stools per day.
C. Antibiotics such as neomycin are contraindicated for treatment of hepatic encephalopathy.
D. Branched-chain amino acids always help the patient with encephalopathy.

Ref.: 10

COMMENTS: Protein intake should never exceed 70 gm/day, although intake of less than 70 gm/day is rarely necessary. If it is less than 40 gm/day there may be a negative nitrogen balance. Lactulose is catabolized by colonic bacteria to form acids that may inhibit the growth of ammonia-forming bacteria; it works by a cathartic effect due to a hyperosmolar load. Neomycin is a nonabsorbable antibiotic with a usual dosage of 2–8 gm four times a day. A small percentage of this nephrotoxic drug is absorbed and if given for prolonged periods may result in increased side effects. It has been hypothesized that an imbalance in branched chain to aromatic amino acids leads to hepatic encephalopathy. Unfortunately, no benefit from administration of branched-chain amino acids is seen in protein-tolerant patients.

ANSWER: B

20. The risk of bleeding from esophageal varices is associated with which of the following?

A. Size of the varix viewed endoscopically.
B. Presence of red spot and red wale marking.
C. Absolute portal pressure.
D. Spleen size.
E. Pressure of ascites.
F. Child's classification.

Ref.: 11, 12

COMMENTS: Esophageal varices bleed by rupture rather than erosion. Although varices are rarely found if the corrected portal pressure is less than 12 mm Hg, there is a poor correlation between higher pressures and the risk of bleeding. The best assessment of bleeding risk (when studied prospectively) is the size of the varices when viewed endoscopically. The larger the varix the greater is the wall tension and hence the risk of rupturing. Additional endoscopic features associated with bleeding include varix-on-a-varix and red wale marking. Patients with Child's class C are more likely to have a first bleed.

ANSWER: A, B, F

21. With regard to the advantage of intrahepatic, in contrast to surgical extrahepatic, portacaval shunts, which of the following statements is/are true?

A. They involve less invasiveness, which makes their use possible in patients who are otherwise not operative candidates.
B. They allow preservation of antegrade flow in the portal vein, allowing possible conventional surgical shunt or transplantation.
C. They allow the possibility of tailoring the shunt diameter to the desired portosystemic pressure gradient.
D. They allow the possibility of occluding the shunt in case of intractable hepatic encephalopathy.
E. They allow immediate transcatheter embolization of collateral vessels connected to actively bleeding esophageal varices to be performed in the same session.

Ref.: 13

COMMENTS: Percutaneous transjugular portosystemic shunts were created in animals in 1969, and the technique was first applied to humans in 1988. Subsequent modifications have taken place, and the current technique involves the use of a transjugular-only approach with shunt patency maintained by balloon-expandable metallic stents. Because of the limited invasiveness of this technique, coagulopathy need not be corrected before the procedure. This procedure is most effective in patients with portal hypertension and end-stage liver disease who may be candidates for liver transplantation. Because of concern over long-term patency of TIPS, surgical shunts may be more appropriate in patients with preserved liver function. Preliminary color Doppler ultrasound examination should be performed to ensure patency of the portal venous system. The radiographs shown below are of a transjugular intrahepatic portosystemic shunt that has been created with a balloon-expandable metallic stent (long arrow). In this patient, persistent bleeding of esophageal varices prompted embolization of a large coronary vein (short arrow).

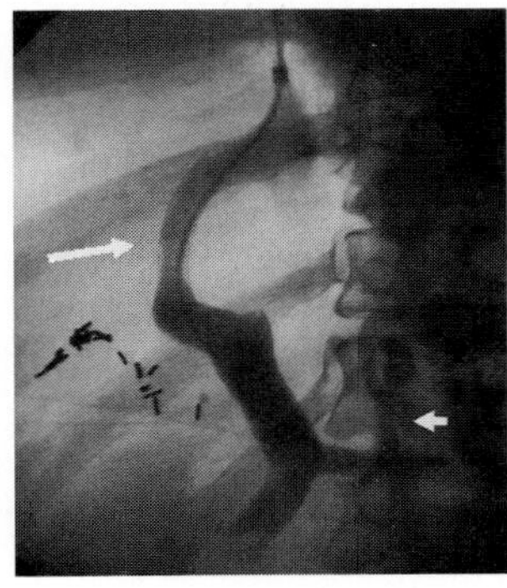

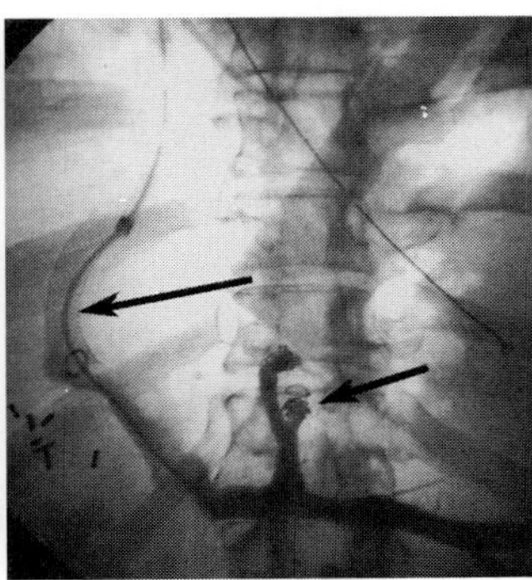

ANSWER: A, B, C, D, E

22. Technical complications following TIPS include which of the following?

A. Dislocation of the stent.
B. Perforation of the liver capsule.
C. Puncture of biliary ducts.
D. Encephalopathy.

Ref.: 14

COMMENTS: Although mortality following the TIPS procedure is fairly low (<5%), several technical complications can occur, including all of the above. Because the TIPS procedure reroutes blood away from the liver, encephalopathy may become problematic. The incidence of encephalopathy is approximately 20%, and it is usually treated with dietary modulation. Care during placement of TIPS is important in patients considered for liver transplantation. Placement into the extrahepatic portal or hepatic veins can result in major technical challenges, increasing the morbidity during the liver transplant procedure.

ANSWER: A, B, C, D

REFERENCES

1. Navarro VJ, Garcia-Tsao G: Variceal hemorrhage [review]. *Crit Care Clin* 11:391–414, 1995.
2. Sabiston DC Jr: *Textbook of Surgery*, 15th ed. WB Saunders, Philadelphia, 1997.
3. Schwartz SI, Shires GT, Spencer FC: *Principles of Surgery*, 7th ed. McGraw-Hill, New York, 1999.
4. Roberts LR, Kamath PS: Pathophysiology and treatment of variceal hemorrhage [review]. *Mayo Clin Proc* 71:973–983, 1996.
5. Martinet JP, Fenyves D, Legault L, et al: Treatment of refractory ascites using transjugular intrahepatic portosystemic shunt (TIPS): a caution. *Dig Dis Sci* 42:161–166, 1997.
6. Garcia-Tsao G: Cirrhotic ascites: pathogenesis and management [review]. *Gastroenterologist* 3:41–54, 1995.
7. Pugh RN, Murray-Lyon IM, Dawson JL, et al: Transection of the oesophagus for bleeding oesophageal varices. *Br J Surg* 60:646–649, 1973.
8. Hassall E: Nonsurgical treatments for portal hypertension in children [review]. *Gastrointest Endosc Clin North Am* 4:223–258, 1994.
9. Hemming AW, Langer B, Grieg P, et al: Treatment of Budd-Chiari syndrome with portosystemic shunt or liver transplantation. *Am J Surg* 171:249–254, 1996.
10. Ferenci P, Herneth A, Steindl P: Newer approaches to therapy of hepatic encephalopathy. *Semin Liver Dis* 16:330–337, 1996.
11. D'Amico G, Pagliaro L, Bosch J: The treatment of portal hypertension: a meta-analytic review. *Hepatology* 22:332–354, 1995.
12. Sherlock S: Esophageal varices. *Am J Surg* 160:9–13, 1990.
13. Ritcher GM, Noeldge G, Palmaz JC, et al: Transjugular intrahepatic portacaval stent shunt: preliminary clinical results. *Radiology* 174:1027–1030, 1990.
14. Catchpole RM: Transjugular intrahepatic portasystemic shunts. *JAMA* 273:1825–1827, 1995.

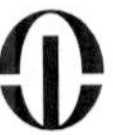

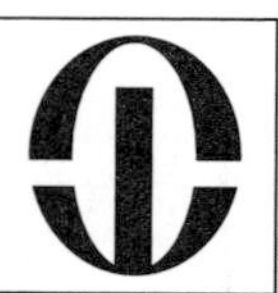

CHAPTER 34

Biliary System

1. Match the numbered layers (1–3) of the gallbladder wall with the following.

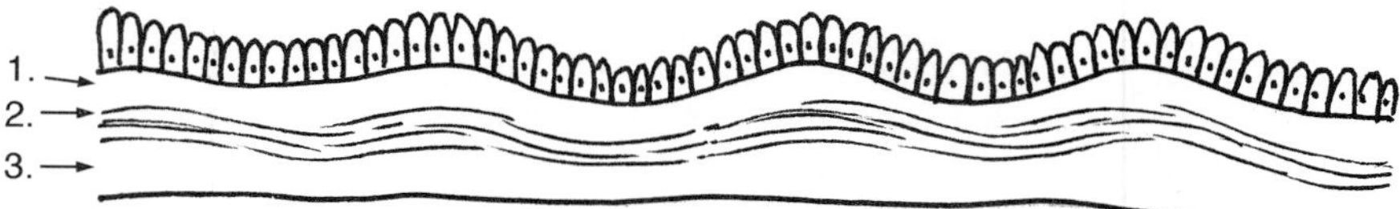

A. Lamina propria.
B. Smooth muscle.
C. Muscularis mucosa.
D. Submucosa.
E. Subserosa.

Ref.: 1

COMMENTS: The histologic structure of the gallbladder consists of five layers: (1) epithelium; (2) lamina propria; (3) smooth muscle; (4) subserosal connective tissue; and (5) serosa. Unlike the bowel, there is no submucosa or muscularis mucosa. The epithelium is composed of columnar cells. The lamina propria has nerves, vessels, lymphocytes, and supportive connective tissue. The smooth muscle is thin, loosely arranged, and not well defined.

ANSWER: 1-A; 2-B; 3-E

2. Which of the following statements best describes the anatomy of the bile duct shown in this cholangiogram?

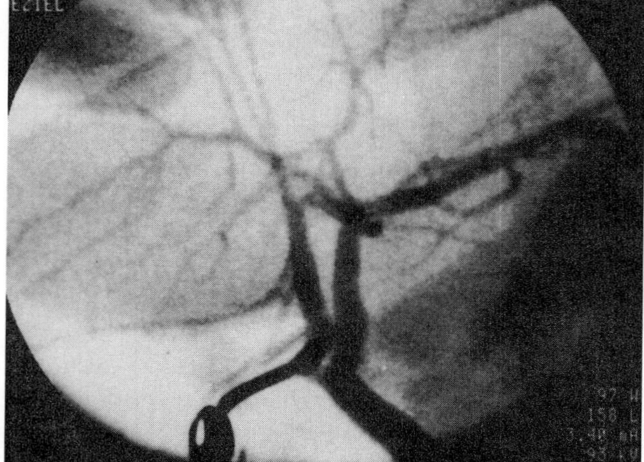

A. Normal "textbook" pattern.
B. Accessory right hepatic duct.
C. Separately inserting right sectoral duct.
D. "Crossover" right hepatic duct.

Ref.: 2, 3, 4

COMMENTS: Variations in the anatomy of the extrahepatic bile ducts occur commonly. The surgeon must be cognizant of this point and learn to recognize and identify these variations to prevent inadvertent injury of the bile ducts during cholecystectomy. Approximately two-thirds of individuals have the "textbook" anatomy with the anterior (segments V and VIII) and posterior (segments VI and VII) sectoral ducts from the right joining to form a main right hepatic duct, which then joins the main left hepatic duct to form the common hepatic duct. In 15–25% of individuals the anterior or posterior duct from the right inserts separately into the common hepatic duct. When the posterior duct inserts separately it is usually at a greater distance caudally from the junction of the left duct and the other right duct compared to when the anterior duct inserts separately. This duct is therefore at risk of injury during cholecystectomy if the anatomy is not recognized. Also, one of the most common variations in cystic duct anatomy is direct insertion into one of these separately inserting right hepatic ducts as the pictured cholangiogram demonstrates. The terms "crossover duct" and "accessory duct" are misnomers for describing this arrangement. True accessory ducts are rare and occur when there is embryologic duplication of the bud that forms the bile ducts and liver. True accessory ducts may enter the gallbladder or the bile ducts but are small and can be ligated. Use of the term "aberrant" ducts should be discouraged, as these are common normal anatomic variations.

ANSWER: C

3. During palpation of the hepatoduodenal ligament a pulsation is felt behind and slightly to the right of the common bile duct. It most likely represents:

A. Normal common hepatic artery.
B. Normal right hepatic artery.
C. Replaced right hepatic artery.
D. Gastroduodenal artery.

Ref.: 1, 2

COMMENTS: The most common variation in hepatic arterial anatomy is the origination of the right hepatic artery from the superior mesenteric artery. This is a replaced hepatic artery and not simply an accessory vessel that can be sacrificed with impunity. When an operation is performed in the right upper abdomen, the pulsations encountered in the porta hepatis and gastrohepatic ligaments should be assessed. If the hepatic artery is absent or small, the surgeon must be alert to the possibility of a replaced hepatic vessel. When the right hepatic artery originates from the superior mesenteric artery, it courses posterior to the head of the pancreas and the portal vein and is usually identified posterolateral to the common bile duct. Only rarely does a replaced right hepatic artery course through the pancreas. A replaced left hepatic artery originates from the left gastric artery and is located in the gastrohepatic ligament, where it is frequently encountered during operations on the stomach and gastroesophageal junction.

ANSWER: C

4. With regard to the blood supply to the common hepatic and common bile ducts, which of the following statements is/are true?

A. Blood supply to the supraduodenal bile duct has a primarily longitudinal pattern.
B. Blood supply to the bifurcation of the common hepatic duct is the least constant, which explains the high frequency of hilar strictures.
C. Blood supply to the common bile duct is derived primarily from the common hepatic artery.
D. The segmental, end-artery arrangement of the blood supply contributes to the occurrence of bile duct stricture.

Ref.: 1, 2, 3

COMMENTS: Ischemia is an important contributing factor in the development of postoperative bile duct stricture. The blood supply to the area of the bile duct bifurcation and the distal retropancreatic duct is primarily lateral in arrangement, whereas the blood supply to the supraduodenal portion of the bile duct has a primarily axial or longitudinal pattern. The so-called 3 and 9 o'clock arteries and other small vessels arise from the right hepatic artery and the retroduodenal artery, which is a branch of the gastroduodenal artery, and form the skeleton of a pericholedochal plexus of vessels. An additional source of blood supply to the common bile duct can be the retroportal artery. This vessel arises from the celiac axis or the superior mesenteric artery and generally joins the retroduodenal artery; but in approximately one-third of individuals it ascends the back of the common bile duct to the right hepatic artery. The portion of the bile duct supplied by the longitudinal vessels receives most of its arterial blood supply from below, rendering the proximal portion of the duct subject to ischemia after injury or transection.

ANSWER: A

5. Match the following structures with their location (A–D) in this *longitudinal* laparoscopic ultrasound scan of the hepatoduodenal ligament.

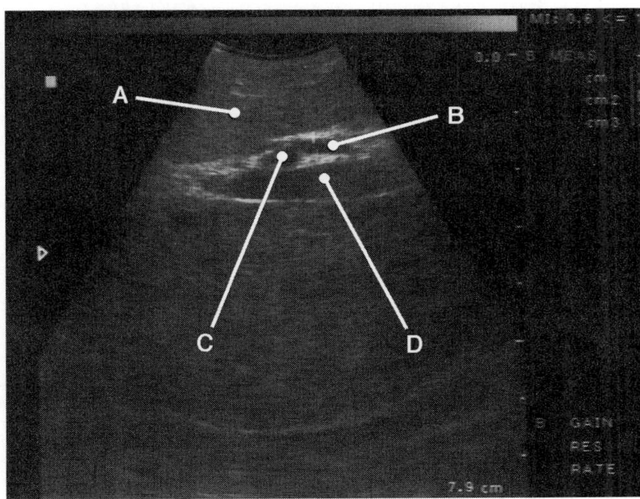

a. Liver.
b. Portal vein.
c. Right hepatic artery.
d. Common bile duct.

Ref.: 5

COMMENTS: See Question 6.

6. Match the following structures with their location (A–C) in this *transverse* laparoscopic ultrasound scan of the hepatoduodenal ligament.

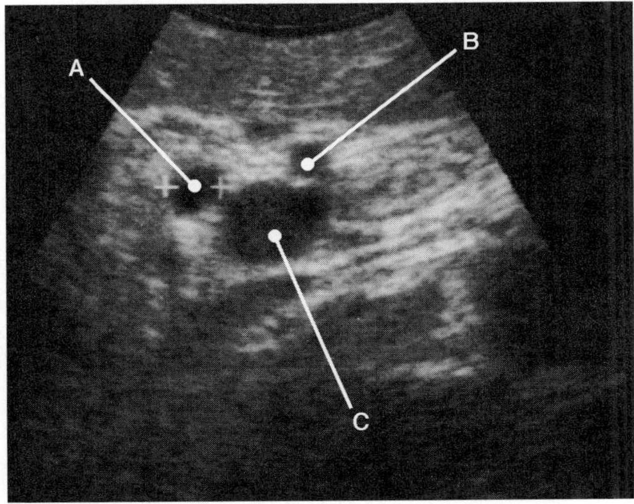

a. Common bile duct.
b. Portal vein.
c. Right hepatic artery.
d. Common hepatic artery.

Ref.: 5, 6

COMMENTS: A general principle of ultrasonography is that any structure visualized in one plane should also be examined in a second plane at a 90-degree angle to the first view to ascertain where and what the structure is. Intraoperative ultrasonography (US), whether laparoscopic or open, is an accurate method for assessing the bile duct for stones during cholecystectomy. The longitudinal and transverse scans of the hepatoduodenal ligament in Questions 5 and 6 depict typical anatomy. In the longitudinal plane, the common bile duct appears as a hypoechoic, tubular structure parallel and anterior to the portal vein. The normal upper limit diameter of the duct at this location is 6 mm by US criteria. In other words, a nondilated duct should not exceed one-half the diameter of the neighboring portal vein. The right hepatic artery most commonly crosses behind the bile duct and is viewed in cross section on the longitudinal scan. In the transverse plane, the structures of the hepatoduodenal ligament have a "Mickey Mouse" configuration. The cross sections of the bile duct and common hepatic artery appear as smaller hypoechoic circles anterior to the larger portal vein.

ANSWER:
Question 5: A-a; B-d; C-c; D-b
Question 6: A-a; B-d; C-b

7. With regard to the composition of hepatic bile, which of the following statements is/are true?

A. It contains 90% water.
B. Concentration of bicarbonate is lower than in plasma.
C. The primary organic solute is conjugated bilirubin.
D. Osmolarity of hepatic bile is similar to that of plasma.

Ref.: 2, 3, 7

COMMENTS: Hepatic bile is composed of 90% water and 10% electrolytes and organic solutes. The inorganic electrolyte composition is similar to that of plasma, although the concentration of sodium, potassium, calcium, and bicarbonate is somewhat higher and that of chloride is somewhat lower. The osmolarity of hepatic bile is approximately 300 mOsm, which is also similar to that of plasma. Bile acids comprise approximately two-thirds of the organic solute composition; the remainder is approximately 20% phospholipid, 4–5% cholesterol, 4–5% proteins, and less than 1% bilirubin, which is predominantly in conjugated form. Other organic solutes, including drugs, hormones, and dyes, may be present as well.

ANSWER: A, D

8. For which of the following functions is bile essential?

A. Triglyceride absorption.
B. Vitamin D absorption.
C. Bilirubin excretion.
D. Cholesterol excretion.
E. Lipase transport.

Ref.: 3

COMMENTS: Bile has a number of critical functions pertaining to the digestion and absorption of fats and the elimination of various endogenous and exogenous substances. Bile interacts with pancreatic lipase and co-lipase in the intraluminal hydrolysis of dietary triglycerides. It subsequently solubilizes the monoglycerides and fatty acids produced by triglyceride metabolism by forming mixed micelles. These micelles facilitate mucosal uptake of triglycerides by permitting transport across the water barrier adjacent to the enterocyte membrane. Although bile therefore plays an important role in triglyceride absorption, a substantial amount of triglycerides can be absorbed even in the absence of bile because of the long length of the intestine. The same is not true for fat-soluble vitamins A, D, E, and K, which are minimally water-soluble and are not absorbed in any substantial amount in the absence of micelles. Patients with long-standing cholestasis generally require supplementation of these fat-soluble vitamins to prevent the clinical effects of deficiency. Bile is the sole pathway for elimination of bilirubin and cholesterol from the body. Bilirubin is secreted into hepatic bile by an active transport mechanism following hepatic uptake and conjugation. Cholesterol is eliminated, both by synthesis of bile acids from cholesterol and by solubilization of cholesterol in bile during secretion.

ANSWER: B, C, D

9. What change(s) in bile flow would be expected in a patient with an external biliary fistula?

A. Increased total canalicular flow.
B. Decreased bile acid-dependent canalicular flow.
C. Increased bile acid-dependent canalicular flow.
D. Decreased bile acid-independent canalicular flow.
E. Increased bile acid-independent canalicular flow.

Ref.: 2, 3

COMMENTS: Approximately 600 ml of hepatic bile is produced daily. Seventy-five percent of hepatic bile is formed by bile canaliculi, and the remainder is secreted by the ducts. **Canalicular** bile can be divided into approximately equal bile acid-dependent and bile acid-independent fractions. The **bile acid-dependent** fraction results from active secretion of bile acids by the hepatocyte. This secretion depends on intestinal absorption and enterohepatic circulation of bile acids. Patients with external bile losses therefore have reduced bile acid-dependent canalicular flow and therefore reduced total canalicular flow. The **bile acid-independent** portion of canalicular flow is the result of secretion of inorganic electrolytes. **Ductular secretion** modifies canalicular bile flow by adding fluid and inorganic electrolytes.

ANSWER: B

10. Which of the following is/are primary bile acids in humans?

A. Cholic acid.
B. Deoxycholic acid.
C. Chenodeoxycholic acid.
D. Lithocholic acid.
E. Ursodeoxycholic acid.

Ref.: 1–3, 8

COMMENTS: The primary bile acids *cholic acid* and *chenodeoxycholic acid* are synthesized from cholesterol in the liver. The secondary bile acids *deoxycholic acid* and *lithocholic acid* are formed in the intestine as the result of bacterial enzyme activity. 7-Ketolithocholic acid is also a secondary bile acid; it is converted to the tertiary bile acid ursodeoxycholic acid in the liver.

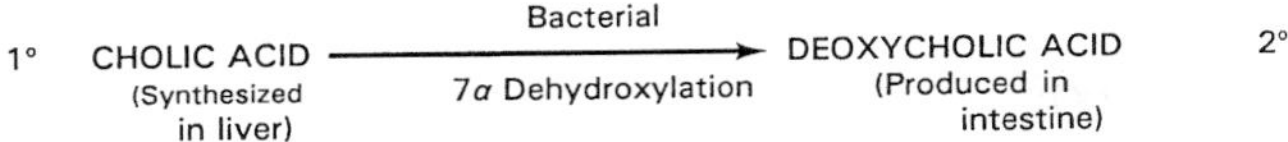

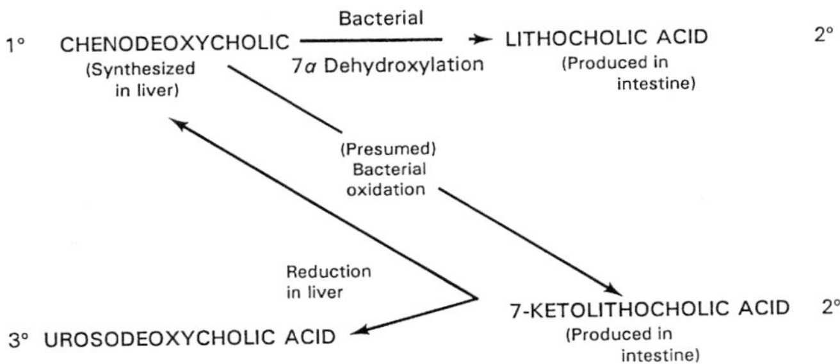

ANSWER: A, C

11. Match each metabolic step of enterohepatic bile acid circulation in the left column with the appropriate anatomic site or sites in the right column.

A. Bile acid conjugation with glycine or taurine	a. Liver
B. Bile acid deconjugation	b. Bile ducts
C. Conversion of primary bile acids to secondary bile acids	c. Gallbladder
D. Active intestinal transport of bile acids	d. Small intestine
E. Passive intestinal resorption of bile acids	e. Colon

Ref.: 1, 3, 4, 5

COMMENTS: See Question 12.

12. With regard to enterohepatic circulation of bile acids, which of the following is/are true?

A. Bile secreted by the liver contains both primary and secondary bile acids.
B. Ninety-five percent of bile acids are reabsorbed in the intestine.
C. Interruption of enterohepatic circulation increases hepatocyte secretion of bile acids.
D. Bile acid deficiency results in vitamin C malabsorption.

Ref.: 1–3, 8

COMMENTS: Enterohepatic cycling of bile acids begins at the hepatocyte level. Bile acids are conjugated in the liver with glycine or taurine, secreted into the biliary system, concentrated and stored in the gallbladder, and then delivered to the duodenum after gallbladder contraction. Most bile acids are efficiently resorbed in the intestine; the site and mechanism of intestine absorption differs according to the form of the bile acid and its corresponding lipid solubility. Conjugated bile acids are predominantly ionized in the intestinal pH range and are relatively lipid insoluble. Conjugated forms are therefore absorbed by an active transport mechanism in the terminal ileum; this mechanism accounts for approximately 70–80% of the enterohepatic circulation. Bacterial deconjugation of bile acids occurs in the colon and small intestine, as does conversion of primary bile acids to secondary forms. Deconjugation raises the pKa of bile acids and enables resorption by passive nonionic diffusion, which occurs predominantly in the colon but to some extent in the small intestine as well. Both primary and secondary bile acids are resorbed and taken back to the liver; unconjugated forms are then reconjugated and resecreted. Hepatic bile therefore contains both primary and secondary bile acids, with the primary bile acids normally constituting 60–90% of the total bile pool. Hepatic synthesis of new bile acids approximates fecal losses of 300–600 mg/day. The bile acid pool cycles four to eight times per day, and hepatic secretion is dependent on enteral return; disruption of this cycle therefore diminishes bile acid secretion. Clinical conditions that might be associated with bile acid malabsorption include ileal disease or resection, small bowel dysmotility or obstruction, and blind-loop syndrome. Clinical consequences of this disordered physiology may include fat malabsorption, deficiencies of fat-soluble vitamins (A, D, E, K), choleretic diarrhea caused by impaired colonic water absorption by bile acids, and of course gallstones.

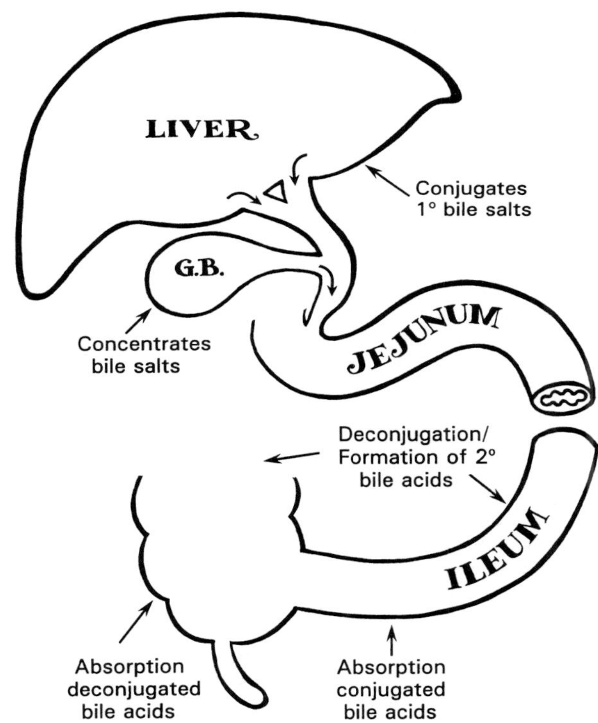

ANSWER:
Question 11: A-a; B-d,e; C-d,e; D-d; E-d,e
Question 12: A, B

13. Normal functions of the gallbladder epithelium include all of the following *except*:

A. Absorption of water.
B. Absorption of sodium and chloride.
C. Absorption of conjugated bile acids.
D. Secretion of hydrogen iron.
E. Secretion of glycoproteins.

Ref.: 1, 8

COMMENTS: The primary functions of the gallbladder are to concentrate and store bile between feedings. The gallbladder epithelium absorbs solutes and water across concentration gradients by both active and passive mechanisms. The main concentrating force is active absorption of sodium (coupled to chloride transport), which leads to passive absorption of water. Abnormalities in gallbladder absorption are part of the pathophysiologic process of gallstone formation. Absorption of organic solutes is normally minimal and depends on their lipid solubility. Unconjugated bile acids are more lipid-soluble than their conjugated forms. Absorption of unconjugated bile acids that form in the presence of bacteria or inflammation damages the mucosa, thereby promoting absorption of other solutes and destabilizing cholesterol in solution. The gallbladder epithelium is also secretory. Secretion of hydrogen ion lowers the pH of gallbladder bile compared to hepatic bile. Mucin glycoproteins secreted by the mucosa may have both protective function and a critical role as a nucleating factor during gallstone formation.

ANSWER: C

14. Which of the following usually produces gallbladder contraction?

A. Cholinergic stimulation.
B. Adrenergic stimulation.
C. Cholecystokinin (CCK).
D. Vasoactive intestinal peptide (VIP).
E. Somatostatin.

Ref.: 1

COMMENTS: Gallbladder function is subject to many neurohormonal influences. Historically, parasympathetic vagal nerves have been considered responsible for gallbladder contraction, and stimulation of sympathetic nerves from the celiac ganglion has been thought to cause gallbladder relaxation. Regulation of gallbladder function is actually a much more complex process that involves the interaction of various neural, hormonal, and peptidergic stimuli on various receptors located on the gallbladder muscle, blood vessels, and nerves. Cholinergic stimuli (including vagal) and CCK cause contraction. CCK receptors can be found on both gallbladder smooth muscle cells and intrinsic cholinergic nerves. Adrenergic stimulation (sympathetic) usually causes relaxation, but selective stimulation of certain adrenergic receptors can cause concentration. VIP and somatostatin inhibit gallbladder contraction, which can account for clinical biliary manifestations in patients with tumors that secrete those substances or in patients being administered somatostatin antagonists. Many other peptides, hormones, and neurotransmitters may also affect gallbladder function, although their clinical significance is unknown.

ANSWER: A, C

15. Gallbladder emptying is influenced by all of the following *except*:

A. Sphincter of Oddi resistance.
B. Common bile duct peristalsis.
C. Postprandial CCK.
D. Fasting motilin.

Ref.: 1, 8

COMMENTS: Bile flow in the biliary tract varies according to the *fasting* or *fed* state of the individual. CCK, which is released by the duodenum in response to ingestion of food substances, is the most important postprandial stimulant to gallbladder contraction and to relaxation of the sphincter of Oddi, permitting bile delivery to the intestine. Normal contraction of the gallbladder in response to meals results in approximately 80% emptying in 2 hours. The common bile duct is, for the most part, a passive conduit in humans and is not thought to play an active role in biliary motility. Filling of the gallbladder after it has emptied depends on neural and hormonal factors that relax the gallbladder and increase resistance of the sphincter of Oddi. During the interdigestive period, the gallbladder gradually fills, but it is interrupted by cyclic periods of emptying, during which time approximately one-third of the gallbladder volume is dispensed. This cyclic pattern during fasting correlates with the interdigestive myoelectric migratory complex of the intestine and seems to be related to increased levels of plasma motilin. Motilin is a 21-amino-acid peptide, and plasma motilin levels vary cyclically during the fasting period.

ANSWER: B

16. Which of the following levels of enzyme activity is most likely to be present in a nonobese individual with cholesterol gallstones?

A. Increased 3-hydroxy-3-methylglutaryl coenzyme A (HMG-CoA) reductase activity.
B. Decreased HMG-CoA reductase activity.
C. Increased 7α-hydroxylase activity.
D. Decreased 7α-hydroxylase activity.

Ref.: 3

COMMENTS: Cholesterol solubility in bile depends on the concentration of cholesterol relative to bile acids and phospholipids. Whereas an increase in hepatocyte cholesterol synthesis and secretion has been implicated in obese patients with gallstones, a relative deficiency of bile acid secretion is thought to be responsible for gallstone formation in many nonobese patients. HMG-CoA reductase catalyzes the conversion of HMG-CoA to mevalonate and is the early rate-limiting enzyme in cholesterol synthesis. The primary bile acids are formed from cholesterol, and the rate-limiting enzyme in this process is 7α-hydroxylase. Relative imbalances in the activities of these enzymes therefore affect cholesterol solubility in bile.

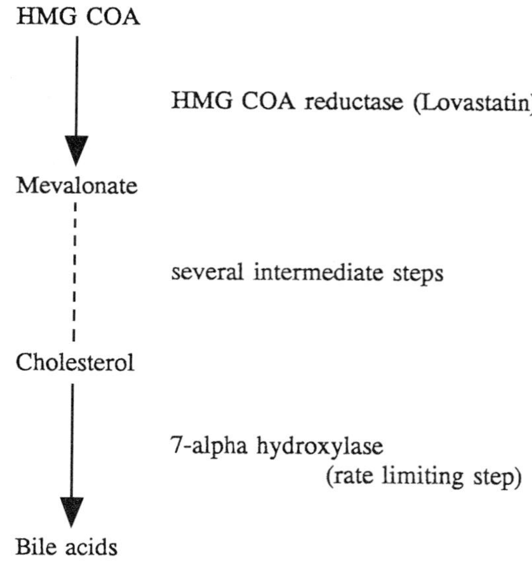

ANSWER: D

17. Which of the following is/are decreased following cholecystectomy?

A. Size of the bile acid pool.
B. Rate of enterohepatic recycling.
C. Rate of bile acid secretion.
D. Cholesterol solubility in bile.

Ref.: 2

COMMENTS: The total size of the bile acid pool is diminished by cholecystectomy as a result of loss of the gallbladder reservoir. However, cholecystectomy produces a more continuous flow of bile into the intestine, which increases the frequency of enterohepatic cycling and stimulates bile acid secretion. For these reasons, even though the size of the bile acid pool is diminished, cholecystectomy improves cholesterol solubility in bile. The solubility of cholesterol in bile depends on the relative molar concentration of cholesterol in relation to the concentrations of bile acids and the phospholipid lecithin. This relation, described by Admirand and Small in 1963, is graphically depicted by this familiar diagram:

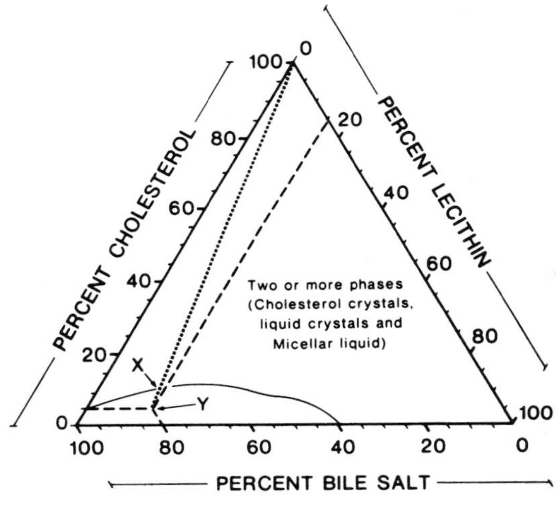

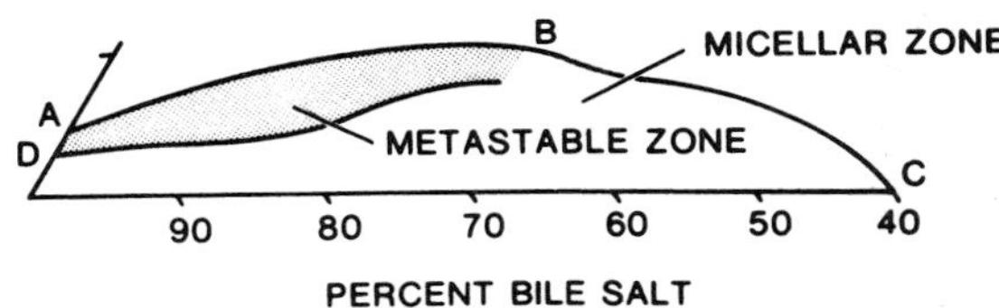

The three biliary lipids plotted as mole percentages on triangular coordinates. On the upper diagram, point Y represents a bile with 15% phospholipid (lecithin), 80% bile salt, and 5% cholesterol and is within the micellar zone. The dotted line connecting Y to the apex of the triangle intersects at point X the line of maximum solubility of cholesterol as defined by Admirand and Small. To calculate the saturation index of the bile represented by Y, the actual mole percent cholesterol (5) is divided by the mole percent cholesterol at point X (9), to give a value of 0.56. The expanded lower diagram shows a line DBC that indicates the true equilibrium solubility line of bile. Bile with a lipid composition, represented by a point between ABC and DBC, lies within a metastable zone where cholesterol may require nucleating factors to precipitate from solution. It is usual to calculate the saturation index using the line DBC and not ABC. (From Way LW, Pellegrini CA: *Surgery of the Gallbladder and Bile Ducts*. WB Saunders, Philadelphia, 1987.)

ANSWER: A

18. Which of the following is the primary form in which cholesterol is transported in bile?

A. Dissolved as free cholesterol.
B. Dissolved as conjugated cholesterol.
C. Attached to a protein carrier.
D. Solubilized in mixed micelles.
E. Solubilized in phospholipid vesicles.

Ref.: 1, 8

COMMENTS: Cholesterol is insoluble in water, and bile is a solution composed of 90% water. The solubility of cholesterol in bile depends on the presence of bile acids and the phospholipid lecithin. These molecules aggregate into physicochemical structures that shelter cholesterol within a nonpolar, hydrophobic center and thus permit dissolution. For many years the mixed micelle was recognized as the structure principally responsible for cholesterol solubility. Subsequently, it has been found that most cholesterol is usually solubilized in larger bilayered lipid structures known as vesicles. The balance between micelles and vesicles is a dynamic process. Recognition of these vesicles is particularly important because crystallization of cholesterol to form stones is thought to occur from this phase.

ANSWER: E

19. Which of the following is/are *not* part of the process of cholesterol gallstone formation?

A. Cholesterol supersaturation of bile.
B. Bilirubin deconjugation.
C. Crystal nucleation.
D. Glyocalyx production.
E. Stone growth.

Ref.: 1, 2, 7, 8

COMMENTS: Cholesterol gallstone formation is a complex physicochemical process. The requisite steps in the genesis of cholesterol stones can be conceptually simplified as: cholesterol saturation, nucleation, and stone growth. The cholesterol content of bile must exceed the capacity for bile to solubilize cholesterol in vesicles and micelles. Cholesterol supersaturation alone, however, is not sufficient to cause stones as this process can occur in normal individuals. Nucleation must also take place; that is, cholesterol monohydrate crystals must form and aggregate. Finally, the crystals must enlarge by fusion or continued solid deposition to produce a stone large enough to be clinically relevant. Bacterial infection is thought to be an important pathogenetic factor in the development of some pigment stones but not generally in cholesterol stones. Bacterial infection is associated with deconjugation of bilirubin and subsequent formation of insoluble calcium bilirubinate complexes. Bacterial infection can also result in the production of glycocalyx, an adhesive glycoprotein that may play a role in pigment stone formation.

ANSWER: B, D

20. Nucleation during cholesterol gallstone formation appears to involve all of the following *except*:

A. Mixed micelles.
B. Biliary vesicles.
C. Biliary calcium.
D. Gallbladder stasis.
E. Mucus secretion.

Ref.: 1, 8

COMMENTS: Nucleation, the formation and aggregation of solid cholesterol monohydrate crystals, is a critical step in gallstone formation. Although the process is not entirely understood, it has been determined that there are important factors that promote nucleation and some antinucleating factors that may protect against stone formation. Mucin glycoproteins secreted by the gallbladder epithelium are thought to be key nucleating factors. Increased mucus secretion occurs whenever there is stasis, which precedes the development of crystals. Prostaglandins stimulate mucus production in animal models, and prostaglandin inhibitors can prevent stones. Nucleation appears to be associated with the vesicular fraction of bile rather than with the mixed micelles. Biliary calcium also plays a role in the formation of both cholesterol and pigment stones. Calcium levels in gallbladder bile are increased during cholesterol stone formation. Calcium affects the absorptive function of the gallbladder epithelium and may also promote nucleation from vesicles. An understanding that the events of vesicle fusion, nucleation, and stone growth occur *in* the gallbladder is a basic foundation for cholecystectomy as definitive treatment for cholesterol gallstone disease.

ANSWER: A

21. Which of the following is/are associated with an increased incidence of cholesterol gallstone formation?

A. Obesity.
B. Rapid weight loss.
C. Total parenteral nutrition.
D. Exogenous estrogen.
E. Ileal resection.

Ref.: 1, 2

COMMENTS: Changes in bile composition that either increase the relative concentration of cholesterol or decrease the relative concentration of bile acids favor cholesterol gallstone formation. Situations that lead to increased hepatocyte cholesterol secretion include obesity, rapid weight loss, diets high in calories and polyunsaturated fats, and estrogen therapy. Drugs that inhibit HMG-CoA reductase are used to treat hypercholesterolemia and may prevent gallstone formation. Theoretically, a relative decrease in the size of the bile acid pool would predispose a person to cholesterol gallstone formation in situations in which there were excessive bile acid losses (e.g., ileal disease or resection) or decreased bile acid synthesis (e.g., decreased 7α-hydroxylase activity). Stones associated with ileal disease or resection are of the pigment type, however. Total parenteral nutrition is also associated with pigment gallstones in a high proportion of patients, depending on the duration of therapy.

ANSWER: A, B, D

22. Which of the following is the main chemical component of pigment gallstones?

A. Cholesterol.
B. Calcium bilirubinate.
C. Calcium carbonate.
D. Calcium phosphate.
E. Calcium oxalate.

Ref.: 2, 8

COMMENTS: Pigment gallstones are composed primarily of calcium precipitated with bilirubin, carbonate, phosphate, or palmitate anions. Two relatively distinct types of pigment gallstones are recognized: black-pigment gallstones and brown-pigment gallstones. There are differences between black- and brown-pigment gallstones in terms of gross appearance, chemical composition, pathogenesis, and clinical implications. **Black-pigment gallstones** are small and spiculated; they contain calcium bilirubinate primarily in polymerized form, as well as calcium carbonate or phosphate. **Brown-pigment gallstones** are soft and yellow-brown, are composed primarily of calcium bilirubinate also, but contain more calcium palmitate (fatty acid derived from lecithin) and cholesterol than black stones. The oxalate salts of calcium play no role in gallstone disease.

ANSWER: B

23. Match each item in the left column with the appropriate item in the right column.

A. Associated with cirrhosis
B. Most commonly associated with bile infection
C. Found more often in the common bile duct than the gallbladder
D. Surgical treatment requires drainage procedure

a. Black-pigment gallstones
b. Brown-pigment gallstones
c. Both
d. Neither

Ref.: 1, 2, 8

COMMENTS: There are some important clinical differences between patients with black-pigment gallstones and those with brown-pigment gallstones. It is postulated that these stones form by different pathogenic mechanisms. Stasis and infection are critical factors in the formation of **brown-pigment gallstones**. Positive bile cultures can be demonstrated in most patients with brown-pigment gallstones, and scanning electron microscopy demonstrates bacterial colonies or casts within the stones. Brown-pigment gallstones are found more frequently in the common bile duct than in the gallbladder; they occur in older patients with stasis and in postcholecystectomy patients. **Black-pigment gallstones** are thought to have a metabolic etiology. They typically occur in patients with cirrhosis or hemolysis. The precise role of stasis and infection in black stone formation remains unclear. Approximately 20% of patients with black-pigment gallstones have positive bile cultures, and some investigators have demonstrated bacteria in black stones. A subset of patients with gallstones have combined features of both black- and brown-pigment gallstones. The important therapeutic implication in differentiating black- from brown-pigment gallstones is that patients with brown-pigment gallstones may require a definitive biliary drainage procedure to prevent recurrence, whereas patients with black-pigment gallstones may not.

ANSWER: A-a; B-b; C-b; D-b

24. Which of the following sonographic findings are necessary to diagnose gallstones?

A. Hyperechoic intraluminal structure.
B. Movement of structure.
C. Posterior shadowing.
D. Posterior acoustic enhancement.

Ref.: 5

COMMENTS: External ultrasonography has a sensitivity of about 95% for the diagnosis of gallstones. The three sonographic criteria for gallstones are (1) the presence of a hyperechoic intraluminal focus, (2) shadowing posterior to that focus, and (3) movement of the focus with positional changes of the patient. Problems in interpretation arise when all of these criteria are not fulfilled. For example, small stones may not shadow well, and impacted stones do not move. Ultrasonography may also fail to diagnose stones if the gallbladder cannot be visualized well because it is contracted or close to excessive bowel gas. For an optimal elective ultrasound scan, the gallbladder should be examined after the patient has fasted for about 6 hours. Posterior acoustic enhancement is a sonographic feature of hypodense structures such as cysts. The signals behind the structure are "whiter" because the sound wave energy is less attenuated as it passes through. The gallbladder itself is a cystic structure and demonstrates this phenomenon, whereas gallstones do the opposite.

ANSWER: A, B, C

25. Ultrasonography reveals gallstones in an asymptomatic 50-year-old woman. Which of the following is the recommended treatment?

A. Observation.
B. Laparoscopic cholecystectomy.
C. Open cholecystectomy.
D. Ursodeoxycholic acid (UDCA).
E. Extracorporeal shock wave lithotripsy (ESWL).

Ref.: 1, 2, 7, 8

COMMENTS: The appropriate management of asymptomatic cholelithiasis is controversial. First, the physician must determine whether the patient is in fact asymptomatic, because gastrointestinal complaints other than pain may be attributable to biliary tract disease. It was formerly thought that most patients with silent gallstones would eventually develop symptoms and that the risk of subsequent complications was high. Subsequent studies suggest that symptoms develop in about 1–2% of patients each year, and that serious complications are relatively infrequent. The morbidity, mortality, and cost of intervention in these patients may exceed that of expectant therapy. The availability of laparoscopic cholecystectomy has not yet changed the basic indications for surgery, although it likely has altered the symptomatic threshold for surgical referral. The validity of laparoscopic cholecystectomy for asymptomatic patients has not been established. Nonoperative pharmacologic dissolution and ESWL are neither definitive nor cost-effective. Currently, therefore, the incidental finding of asymptomatic cholelithiasis is not an indication for therapy in most situations. Circumstances that may be exceptions and that merit consideration on an individual basis include (1) transplant patient with anticipated immunosuppression because of the risk of sepsis; (2) anticipated long-term parenteral nutrition, because of associated stasis and sludge formation; (3) anticipated pregnancy because of the possibility of becoming symptomatic as gallbladder emptying is impaired and because of the potential risk imposed on both mother and fetus if complicated cholelithiasis occurs; (4) concurrent abdominal operation for an unrelated problem because of the relative ease and safety of incidental cholecystectomy in most situations and in consideration of the potential for postoperative cholecystitis otherwise; and (5) coincident with antiobesity surgery because of the high incidence of gallstones associated with obesity and during rapid weight loss. In patients requiring massive intestinal resection, concomitant cholecystectomy has been recommended even when the gallbladder is normal because disease will likely develop during parenteral nutrition.

ANSWER: A

26. For which of the following conditions is early elective cholecystectomy for symptomatic gallstones indicated?

A. Elderly status.
B. Diabetes mellitus.
C. Child's C cirrhosis.
D. Total parenteral nutrition (TPN)-induced gallstones.
E. None of the above.

Ref.: 1

COMMENTS: Patients with certain medical conditions are often considered to be at higher risk for morbidity and mortality from gallstone disease. Elderly patients more frequently develop complications of cholelithiasis, such as sepsis, perforation, and choledocholithiasis; they also have a higher mortality rate during emergent operations. Elective cholecystectomy can usually be performed safely in the elderly and is recommended for symptomatic patients. Although the supportive evidence has not always been conclusive, diabetics may also be at increased risk particularly if emergency intervention is required and therefore should be considered for early elective cholecystectomy. A high proportion of patients on long-term TPN develop gallstones, and reports suggest that complications, emergency operations, and mortality are more frequent in this population as well. Early cholecystectomy is therefore indicated. Patients with hepatic cirrhosis, on the other hand, have high morbidity and mortality rates related to cholecystectomy. This is particularly true for patients with more advanced hepatocellular dysfunction and portal hypertension. Cholecystectomy should be approached with great caution under these circumstances and is usually reserved for patients with complications of cholelithiasis or for patients with substantial symptoms and less advanced hepatic disease.

ANSWER: A, B, D

27. A patient with episodic abdominal pain has a cholecystokinin (CCK)-stimulated HIDA scan that demonstrates 25% gallbladder emptying. Ultrasonography of the gallbladder is normal. What is *true* regarding cholecystectomy in this situation?

A. Not indicated, as persistent or recurrent symptoms are likely.
B. Indicated only if duodenal drainage yields cholesterol crystals or bilirubinate granules.
C. Can alleviate symptoms in most patients if pain is episodic and in the right upper quadrant.
D. Improves symptoms in most patients, regardless of pain location or characteristics.

Ref.: 1, 9

COMMENTS: Surgeons are often confronted with the challenge of evaluating patients for abdominal pain that may or may not be of biliary origin. If the symptoms are typical of biliary "colic" and ultrasonography (US) demonstrates gallstones, the situation is straightforward. However, when the symptoms are less typical (even the presence of gallstones) or when US does not identify any abnormality, further evaluation is necessary to determine whether cholecystectomy is warranted. Certainly, other diagnoses must be excluded and any number of additional investigations may be appropriate depending on the specific circumstances (e.g., esophagogastroduodenoscopy, CT scan, endoscopic retrograde cholangiopancreatography, gastrointestinal contrast studies, colonoscopy). CCK-stimulated cholescintigraphy can be useful for identifying patients who may have symptoms due to motility disorders of the gallbladder. However, the test does not always reliably predict the long-term outcome of cholecystectomy. If the symptoms are more typical of biliary origin, and CCK scintigraphy is abnormal (<30% ejection), data suggest that most patients (>70%) can benefit from cholecystectomy. Pathologic abnormalities of the gallbladder are found in a reasonable number of these patients. If the symptoms are less typical, the results of cholecystectomy cannot be expected to be as favorable, even though emptying is abnormal. Additional specific tests for the gallbladder such as repeated ultrasonography, duodenal drainage with CCK cholecystography, or even oral cholecystocystography are sometimes useful for evaluating these patients.

ANSWER: C

28. Laparoscopic cholecystectomy is most strongly contraindicated in which of these situations?

A. Pregnancy.
B. Prior upper abdominal surgery.
C. Known common bile duct stones.
D. Chronic obstructive pulmonary disease.
E. Gallbladder cancer.

Ref.: 1, 10, 11

COMMENTS: When laparoscopic cholecystectomy was first introduced worldwide during the late 1980s, there were a number of circumstances in which it was more or less strongly contraindicated. Today most contraindications are relative, and in fact the laparoscopic approach is preferred when possible in certain situations that were initially considered contraindications (acute cholecystitis, choledocholithiasis, obesity). Basically, the surgeon must be adequately trained and the patient reasonably fit for an operation and give informed consent that includes the possibility of laparotomy. Although usually performed under general anesthesia, the operation has even been accomplished with thoracic epidural anesthesia. It must be recognized that there are patients for whom the potential physiologic consequences of a CO_2 pneumoperitoneum are more important but the presence of underlying disease itself does not prohibit a laparoscopic approach. In fact, laparoscopic cholecystectomy may be more beneficial to the postoperative course of a compromised patient. Pregnancy is not a contraindication with appropriate precautions, although the physiologic effects on the fetus are not completely known. Perhaps the strongest contraindication currently is in the patient with suspected or known gallbladder cancer because of the risk of dissemination.

ANSWER: E

29. Most major bile duct injuries during laparoscopic cholecystectomy occur in patients under which one of the following circumstances?

A. Acute cholecystitis.
B. Gallstone pancreatitis.
C. Choledocholithiasis.
D. Elective cholecystectomy.
E. Laparoscopic procedure converted to open procedure.

Ref.: 12, 13

COMMENTS: There are several risk factors for bile duct injury during laparoscopic cholecystectomy. Pathologic risk factors include severe acute or chronic inflammation. Several studies have found a statistical correlation between the rate of duct injury and the presence of acute cholecystitis. Bleeding has long been implicated as a factor predisposing to duct injury during open or laparoscopic cholecystectomy. Injuries are sometimes attributed to the "anomalous" anatomy of the bile ducts. More often than not, however, "anomalies" are simply common anatomic variations the surgeon must recognize to prevent injury (see Question 2). Surgeon experience, or the "learning curve," is clearly a risk factor, as higher rates of duct injury have been well documented among less experienced surgeons. Interestingly, there is no convincing evidence that duct injury is more frequent during cases involving laparoscopic management of common bile duct stones possibly because these procedures are performed by more experienced surgeons. Unfortunately, most major bile duct injuries during laparoscopic cholecystectomy have occurred in elective and otherwise uncomplicated cases. Despite the presence or absence of risk factors, the primary problem resulting in duct injury is misidentification of the anatomy. The most frequent mechanism of injury is when a major bile duct is mistaken for the cystic duct and is clipped and cut. This pitfall is best avoided by correct operative strategy (i.e., appropriate retraction and adequate dissection) and by the surgeon's alertness to the visual misperceptions that can occur during laparoscopic cholecystectomy.

ANSWER: D

30. You encounter difficulty during an elective laparoscopic cholecystectomy in a healthy 25-year-old woman and open the patient. The 4 mm common hepatic duct has been transected 1 cm below the bifurcation. Choose your therapy.

A. Perform duct-to-duct anastomosis over a T-tube.
B. Perform duct-to-duct anastomosis without a stent.
C. Perform Roux-en-Y hepaticojejunostomy.
D. Perform hepaticoduodenostomy.
E. Place drains and transfer patient to referral center.

Ref.: 12, 13

COMMENTS: When a transection or resection injury of the extrahepatic biliary tree is discovered at the time of cholecystectomy, the surgeon must make some careful decisions. Repair at the time would be preferable, provided a successful repair could be ensured. Unfortunately, the body of evidence indicates that most primary repairs by the initial operating surgeon have failed, necessitating repeat operations and other interventions. The first repair of a major duct injury has the best chance for long-term success. Therefore, unless the surgeon is experienced with anastomosis of nondilated ducts, most would advise that it is in the patient's best interest not to attempt a definitive repair. Rather, place drains and arrange transfer to an appropriate hepatobiliary surgeon. If repair at the time is appropriate, the standard reconstruction for this type of injury is a Roux-en-Y hepaticojejunostomy. Duct-to-duct repairs virtually always fail in this situation. Hepaticoduodenostomy is not recommended for an injury at this level.

ANSWER: C or E

31. The bile duct injury described above in Question 30 would be classified as a:

A. Bismuth type 1.
B. Bismuth type 2.
C. Bismuth type 3.
D. Bismuth type 4.
E. Bismuth type 5.

Ref.: 3

COMMENTS: The Bismuth level classification of bile duct injuries and strictures essentially relates the site of injury to the bifurcation of the main right and left hepatic ducts. Higher injuries are more difficult: They require a greater degree of technical skill and expertise to reconstruct and have a lower long-term success rate. Many of the injuries resulting from laparoscopic cholecystectomy have been higher than those seen with open cholecystectomy. Also many injuries, initially lower, end up being higher when repaired because of the need to débride unhealthy ductal tissue consequent to ischemia or inflammation and infection caused by bile leakage. With a type 1 injury, 2 cm or more of the common hepatic duct is preserved below the bifurcation. With a type 2 injury, less than 2 cm remains. A type 3 injury involves the hilum with preserved continuity between the right and left sides. A type 4 injury involves destruction of the hepatic confluence with separation of the right and left hepatic ducts. A type 5 injury involves a separate inserting sectoral duct with or without injury of the common duct.

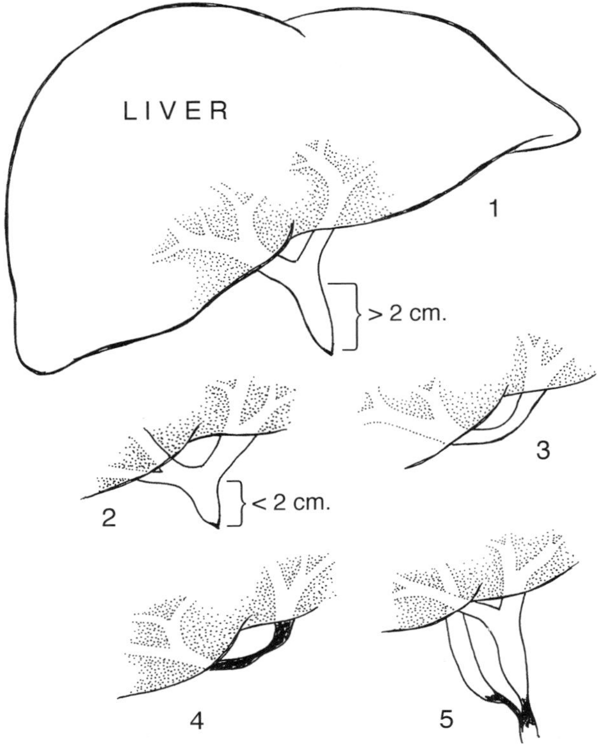

ANSWER: B

32. On the second postoperative day after elective laparoscopic cholecystectomy, a 40-year-old woman complains of nausea and abdominal pain. Examination shows a temperature of 100°F, pulse 100, mild abdominal distension and moderate right upper quadrant tenderness. What should be done next?

A. Ultrasonography (US) of the abdomen.
B. CT scan.
C. HIDA scan.
D. Endoscopic retrograde cholangiopancreatography (ERCP).
E. Percutaneous transhepatic cholangiography (PTC).

Ref.: 13, 14

COMMENTS: Serious delays in the postoperative diagnosis of bile duct injuries can compound a patient's problems. A patient should be investigated promptly when the clinical course suggests anything other than the anticipated straightforward recovery that most patients experience. The primary concern is development of a bile leak, which occurs in 1–2% of patients. Other problems such as retained bile duct stones or intestinal injury can occur as well, although they are less frequent. The various imaging studies can provide complementary information. A HIDA scan shows an ongoing bile leak and is often the most reasonable initial investigation after the patient is examined. A US or CT scan can demonstrate fluid collections or intrahepatic bile duct dilatation. If a fluid collection is seen, percutaneous aspiration can determine whether the fluid is bile. If a bile leak is confirmed, cholangiography is necessary to establish the site of leakage and to help determine further therapy. Endoscopic cholangiography is generally the first choice and may be all that is necessary for bile leaks that originate from lateral injuries, the cystic duct stump, or the gallbladder fossa. Percutaneous transhepatic cholangiography is necessary for complete anatomic definition in patients with transection or resection injuries or injuries to sectoral hepatic ducts that may not be in continuity with the rest of the extrahepatic bile ducts.

ANSWER: C

33. A stable patient has this endoscopic cholangiogram following laparoscopic cholecystectomy two days previously. What should be done next?

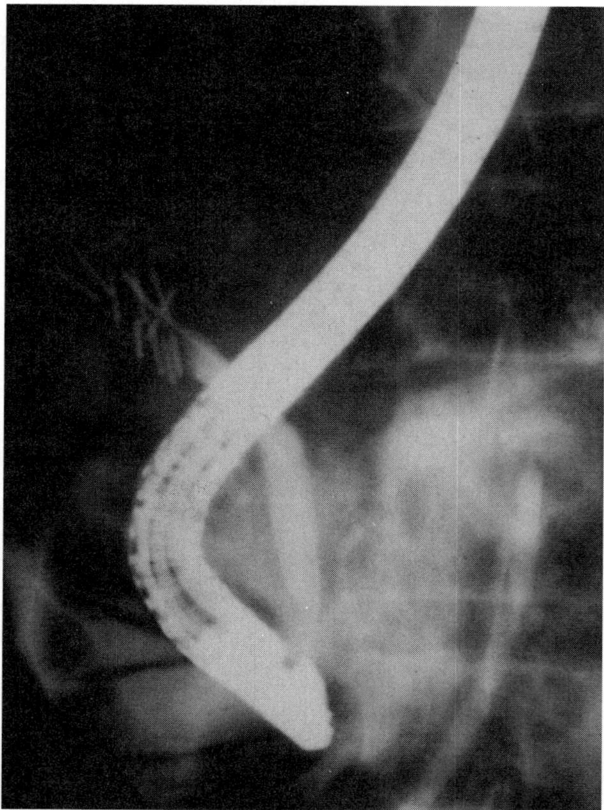

A. Attempt endoscopic balloon dilatation and stent placement.
B. Percutaneous transhepatic cholangiography.
C. Urgent reoperation for bile drainage.
D. Urgent reoperation for bile duct reconstruction.

Ref.: 12, 13

COMMENTS: The endoscopic cholangiogram demonstrates complete occlusion of the supraduodenal common bile duct without extravasation of dye. A classic mechanism of major bile duct injury during laparoscopic cholecystectomy involves clipping the distal common bile duct and resecting a portion of the extrahepatic ductal system. The proximal level of injury is variable but typically high. Patients present with bile leak or obstruction depending on the status of the proximal ducts. The first priority when managing these injuries is to control sepsis and ensure adequate drainage of any bile leak. Generally this can be accomplished by nonoperative percutaneous or endoscopic methods. Urgent reoperation for bile drainage is not typically necessary. Complete cholangiographic definition of the injury is essential prior to definitive repair. For resection or transection injuries, as depicted here, PTC is required to assess the status of the proximal ducts. Endoscopic cholangiography alone may be adequate for lateral injuries when the continuity of the ducts is preserved. Occasionally, a "fistulagram" done through a percutaneous drainage catheter may visualize the proximal ducts. After complete cholangiography, long-term success is best achieved by an elective, expert reconstruction.

ANSWER: B

34. Which of the following is/are true regarding the role of intraoperative cholangiography (IOC) in bile duct injury during laparoscopic cholecystectomy?

A. IOC prevents duct injury.
B. IOC increases the rate of duct injury.
C. IOC can limit the severity of injury.
D. IOC increases the diagnosis of injury.

Ref.: 15

COMMENTS: So long as there are imaging studies to assess the bile ducts intraoperatively, the debate between proponents of routine versus selective use of such studies will continue. Proponents of IOC argue that its routine or liberal use can be advantageous in terms of bile duct injury, but there is no convincing evidence that IOC actually lowers the rate of duct injury. Certainly, cholangiograms can be incomplete or misinterpreted or injuries can occur after an IOC has been done. Likewise, properly performed IOC does not lead to duct injuries. There is a compelling argument that IOC may limit the severity of duct injury, for example when IOC allows a surgeon to recognize that the cholangiogram catheter has been placed in the common duct and not into the cystic duct prior to the common duct being transected. Some evidence suggests that the number of high ductal injuries and of anastomotic repairs required to remedy duct injuries have been lower when IOC was performed. The use of IOC clearly appears to increase the rate of intraoperative recognition of injury. About 70–90% of injuries have been identified intraoperatively when IOC has been performed compared to only 15–25% when IOC has not been done. Failure to interpret the IOC correctly can account for missed injuries. The two primary reasons for misinterpreting an IOC are failure to completely visualize the proximal ducts (including both right anterior and posterior ducts) and extravasation of dye of uncertain origin.

ANSWER: C, D

35. Which of the following is/are *not* considered primary events in the pathophysiology of acute calculous cholecystitis?

A. Increased biliary lysolecithin.
B. Gallbladder ischemia.
C. Bacterial infection.
D. Cystic duct obstruction.

Ref.: 1, 7, 8

COMMENTS: Acute cholecystitis is thought to be initiated by gallbladder obstruction and activation of various inflammatory mediators, which leads to mucosal damage, gallbladder distension, and eventual ischemia. Bacteria can be identified in the bile of about 50% (30–70%) of patients with acute cholecystitis, *but* bacterial infection is a secondary phenomenon. The primary pathophysiology depends on biochemical events. Some of the mediators that may be involved in the inflammatory process of acute cholecystitis are bile acids, lithogenic bile, pancreatic juice, prostaglandins, phospholipids, and lysolecithin. Lysolecithin is formed from lecithin by the enzyme phospholipase, and levels are elevated in acute cholecystitis. The role of prostaglandins as mediators in this process has also received considerable attention.

ANSWER: B, C

36. Which of the following is most accurate in the diagnosis of acute cholecystitis?

A. Plain abdominal radiograph.
B. Ultrasonography.
C. Oral cholecystography.
D. Technetium 99m pertechnetate (^{99m}Tc) iminodiacetic acid scan.

Ref.: 1, 2, 7

COMMENTS: Radionuclide scanning with ^{99m}Tc iminodiacetic acid agents normally allows visualization of the liver, gallbladder, and extrahepatic biliary tree. In the presence of acute cholecystitis, the gallbladder cannot be seen because of cystic duct obstruction; this finding is present in approximately 98% of patients with acute cholecystitis. Cholescintigraphy is not necessary in most patients with acute cholecystitis, as the diagnosis is founded on clinical examination and demonstration of gallstones by ultrasonography. However, it can be quite useful in less typical situations and to exclude acute cholecystitis (by normal gallbladder uptake) in patients with other diagnoses. Ultrasonography of acute cholecystitis may demonstrate gallstones, pericholecystic fluid, thickening of the gallbladder, intramural edema, or a positive sonographic Murphy's sign; but the morphologic findings are not specific. Although oral cholecystography fails to allow visualization of the gallbladder in acute cholecystitis, this finding is not as diagnostically reliable as a radioisotope study because of the high frequency of gallbladders that cannot be visualized as a result of impaired dye absorption or hepatic uptake or because chronic cholecystitis is present. Plain abdominal radiographs reveal up to 15% of gallstones and demonstrate emphysematous cholecystitis but otherwise play no specific role in the diagnosis of acute cholecystitis.

ANSWER: D

37. A ^{99m}Tc iminodiacetic acid scan in a fasting patient demonstrates the following: normal liver activity, no gallbladder visualization at 60 minutes, intestinal activity present at 60 minutes, gallbladder visualization at 120 minutes. These findings are most consistent with which of the following situations?

A. A normal study.
B. Acute calculous cholecystitis.
C. Acute acalculous cholecystitis.
D. Chronic cholecystitis.
E. Partial bile duct obstruction.

Ref.: 1, 2

COMMENTS: Since the mid-1970s technetium-labeled derivatives of iminodiacetic acid (i.e., HIDA, PIPIDA, DISIDA) have been important in the evaluation of biliary tract disease. After intravenous injection these radioisotopes are taken up by the liver and excreted into the biliary tract. Characteristics of a normal study include visualization of the gallbladder within 60 minutes in fasting patients and the appearance of radioisotope in the duodenum by about the same time. In nonfasting patients, gallbladder visualization may be delayed. The hepatic phase of the study may demonstrate mass lesions or diminished uptake when there is hepatic dysfunction; such results are similar to those of a liver scan. With both calculous and acalculous acute cholecystitis, the gallbladder is not visualized owing to cystic duct obstruction. No visualization or delayed visualization are common with chronic cholecystitis; the distinction between acute and chronic cholecystitis therefore depends on the clinical presentation, not simply an abnormal scan. Bile duct obstruction may cause delayed or absent clearance of isotope from the liver or delayed hepatic uptake. Radioisotope scans can be useful in the clinical assessment of disorders other than cholecystitis, including biliary motility, biliary enteric anastomosis, bile fistulas or leaks, and enterogastric relfux.

ANSWER: D

38. The preferred treatment for acute calculous cholecystitis is:

A. Early laparoscopic cholecystectomy.
B. Delayed laparoscopic cholecystectomy.
C. Early open cholecystectomy.
D. Delayed open cholecystectomy.

Ref.: 1, 2, 7

COMMENTS: The former debate over early versus late cholecystectomy for acute cholecystitis has for the most part been put to rest. Prospective studies have demonstrated that early cholecystectomy is not associated with higher morbidity or mortality, and delayed treatment requires longer hospitalization, is more expensive, and risks recurrent biliary problems prior to definitive therapy. Most patients are effectively treated by stabilization, administration of antibiotics, and prompt operation. From a technical standpoint, cholecystectomy is often easier during the first day or two of the patient's illness when the inflammation tends to be more edematous than necrotic and hyperemic, as it becomes when the process progresses. Laparoscopic cholecystectomy is the preferred treatment in most circumstances, although conversion to an open procedure is required more often (20–30%) than when performed electively for nonacute symptoms (5%).

ANSWER: A

39. With regard to acalculous cholecystitis, which of the following statements is/are true?

A. It most commonly affects elderly patients in an outpatient setting.
B. Primary pathophysiology involves gallbladder stasis.
C. HIDA scan is usually normal.
D. Ultrasonogram of the gallbladder is usually normal.
E. Treatment requires cholecystectomy.

Ref.: 1, 2, 7

COMMENTS: Approximately 5–10% of acute cholecystitis cases occur in patients without gallstones. The primary predisposing factor is gallbladder stasis with subsequent distension and ischemia. Acalculous cholecystitis typically develops in hospitalized patients, often after trauma, unrelated surgery, or other critical illnesses. Factors present in these patients that may contribute to biliary stasis include hypovolemia, intestinal ileus, absence of oral nutrition, multiple blood transfusions, narcotic use, and positive-pressure ventilation. Because of the clinical situation in which acute acalculous cholecystitis occurs, the diagnosis may not be readily apparent. The patient may present with fever or unexplained sepsis, and abdominal signs may not be initially appreciated. Imaging studies are generally abnormal; HIDA scan fails to allow visualization of the gallbladder as a result of stasis and functional obstruction of the cystic duct; and ultrasonography may demonstrate sludge, gallbladder wall thickening, or pericholecystic fluid. None of these findings is specific to the presence of acute acalculous cholecystitis, however, and the diagnosis must rely on clinical suspicion. Standard surgical treatment consists of cholecystectomy (or cholecystostomy for patients who are too infirm to withstand general anesthesia). Percutaneous cholecystostomy can be a valuable technique for establishing gallbladder decompression in these critically ill patients; later cholecystectomy may not be required if stones are not present and if subsequent cholangiography demonstrates a patent cystic duct. Cholecystectomy is the only effective treatment if the gallbladder is necrotic or gangrenous.

ANSWER: B

40. The pertinent area of a plain x-ray film of the abdomen obtained on a 78-year-old diabetic man with severe right upper quadrant pain is shown. Which of the following is the appropriate next step?

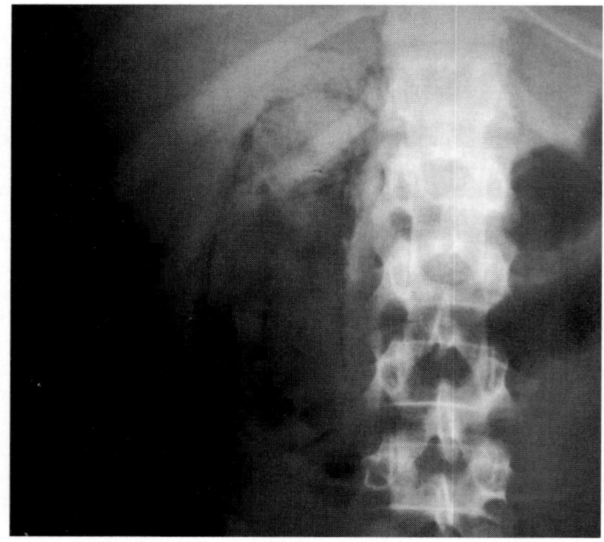

A. Ultrasonography of the gallbladder.
B. CT scan.
C. HIDA scan.
D. Cholecystectomy.
E. ERCP.

Ref.: 1, 2, 7

COMMENTS: Emphysematous cholecystitis occurs most typically in elderly diabetic men. Curvilinear lucencies in the right upper quadrant have the configuration of the gallbladder, are in the location of the gallbladder, and are diagnostic for gas in the gallbladder wall. In their totality, they are pathognomonic of emphysematous cholecystitis. Gas may also be seen in the gallbladder lumen. This condition is associated with a high incidence of gallbladder necrosis, perforation, and sepsis. Unnecessary diagnostic examinations would only delay prompt surgical therapy and possibly affect the outcome adversely. Urgent operation is needed. An ultrasound study of an emphysematous gallbladder would show highly reflective shadows as a result of the gas. Differentiation from bowel gas might be difficult, although usually the diagnosis is evident. About one-third of patients do not have stones. A CT scan would show the abnormal gas in the gallbladder wall, lumen, or both. HIDA scans would fail to allow visualization of the gallbladder. ERCP is unnecessary.

ANSWER: D

41. With regard to choledocholithiasis, which of the following statements is/are true?

A. Common duct stones are present in one-third of patients undergoing cholecystectomy.
B. The incidence of common duct stones is highest in elderly patients.
C. Most common duct stones are composed of calcium bilirubinate.
D. Common duct stones are found more frequently when cholecystectomy is performed for chronic cholecystitis than for acute cholecystitis.

Ref.: 1, 2, 7

COMMENTS: Somewhere around 8–18% of patients with symptomatic gallstones have choledocholithiasis, which has a spectrum of clinical presentations. Approximately 6% of patients undergoing cholecystectomy have common bile duct stones that were completely unsuspected. Proper recognition of common duct stones is important because of the associated risk of biliary tract obstruction and cholangitis. The incidence of choledocholithiasis increases with each decade over age 60. Most common duct calculi originate in the gallbladder and are therefore of the cholesterol variety. Friable "earthy" stones (brown-pigment gallstones) contain calcium complexed with bilirubinate and other anions and arise de novo in the common duct in association with biliary stasis and infection. Choledocholithiasis occurs as often with acute cholecystitis as with chronic cholecystitis; therefore appropriate evaluation of the patient for potential choledocholithiasis is mandatory.

ANSWER: B

42. Which of the following is the best indication for preoperative ERCP in a patient with gallstones?

A. Obstructive jaundice.
B. Gallstone pancreatitis.
C. History of jaundice.
D. Elevated alkaline phosphatase to twice normal.
E. A 10 mm common bile duct seen on ultrasonography.

Ref.: 16

COMMENTS: The rationale for preoperative ERCP is to identify and remove common bile duct stones so patients might subsequently undergo laparoscopic cholecystectomy and hopefully avoid the need for an open operation or for operative treatment of the common bile duct. Endoscopic evaluation of the bile duct has its own risks, however, so it should be selected for patients at the highest risk for choledocholithiasis. Unfortunately, there are no absolute predictors of common bile duct stones. The yield of ERCP in identifying common bile duct stones is highest in patients presenting with obstructive jaundice or clinical cholangitis or when a duct stone is actually seen on the ultrasound scan. In all other circumstances most patients have negative endoscopic cholangiograms, and the examination was not necessary for most of these patients. As the number of parameters suggestive of common bile duct stones increases, however, so does the likelihood of finding stones. There is no substitute for good clinical judgment in the utilization of preoperative ERCP. It is an unquestionably valuable tool for diagnosing and removing common bile duct stones, but its *overuse* is dangerous and must be discouraged.

ANSWER: A

43. An intraoperative cholangiogram obtained during laparoscopic cholecystectomy shows several 2- to 3-mm filling defects in the distal common duct. What should be done next?

A. Complete laparoscopic cholecystectomy and perform ERCP postoperatively.
B. Open the patient and perform common bile duct exploration.
C. Administer glucagon and flush the common bile duct.
D. Laparoscopically dilate the cystic duct and perform transcystic choledochoscopy.
E. Laparoscopic choledochotomy.

Ref.: 17

COMMENTS: Choledocholithiasis discovered intraoperatively can often be managed laparoscopically depending on a number of considerations, such as the size, number, and location of the stones and the size and anatomy of the bile ducts. When approaching common bile stones laparoscopically, one should start with simple techniques and progress to more complex maneuvers as necessary. Small stones can often be cleared by flushing the common duct through a transcystic catheter after glucagon has been given to relax the choledochoduodenal sphincter. Other transcystic manipulations can be used if the cystic duct is dilated or dilatable (with hydrostatic balloons) and providing there is a relatively direct course between the cystic duct and the common bile duct. These techniques include retrieval with balloon catheters or stone baskets under fluoroscopic or choledochoscopic visualization. Experienced laparoscopic surgeons can perform choledochotomy when the common bile duct is sufficiently large and when simpler efforts have failed. In general, the surgeon should not leave common duct stones untreated but may elect to terminate the procedure when (1) the stones are very small or questionable; (2) the common bile duct is narrow; (3) laparoscopic clearance is not feasible; and (4) the morbidity of an open common bile duct exploration is judged to be too high for a particular patient. Intraoperative endoscopic retrieval of common bile duct stones has been successful but may be logistically impractical. Relying on postoperative endoscopy for intentionally neglected stones carries the risk that endoscopic removal may fail. A traditional open common bile duct exploration is a safe, reliable fallback for most patients when laparoscopic methods are unsuccessful and the duct is not too small.

ANSWER: C

44. In general, which of the following is the best treatment for a patient with choledocholithiasis 3 years after cholecystectomy?

A. Transhepatic infusion of monooctanoin.
B. Percutaneous transhepatic stone extraction.
C. Endoscopic sphincterotomy and stone extraction.
D. Common bile duct exploration and T-tube placement.
E. Common bile duct exploration and choledochoduodenostomy.

Ref.: 1, 2, 7

COMMENTS: Most common bile duct stones found in patients after cholecystectomy can be successfully treated by nonoperative methods. Stone extraction through a T-tube or endoscopically after endoscopic sphincterotomy if the patient does not have a T-tube in place results in successful duct clearance with a low complication rate in more than 90% of patients. By definition, bile duct stones occurring more than 2 years after cholecystectomy are considered primary common duct stones. These are pigment gallstones related to biliary stasis and infection rather than the typical cholesterol stones found in the gallbladder. In addition to stone removal, some type of ductal drainage procedure therefore also is indicated in most of these patients to prevent stone recurrence. When performed by experienced clinicians, endoscopic sphincterotomy is successful in more than 90% of patients and, when combined with endoscopic extraction with the use of balloon catheters or baskets, results in stone clearance in 85–90% of patients. Contact dissolution of duct stones with monooctanoin is successful in certain patients with retained cholesterol stones, but this medium-chain diglyceride is not an effective solvent for pigment stones. Duct stones have been successfully removed via the percutaneous transhepatic route when endoscopic approaches are unsuccessful. Neither transhepatic instillation of contact solvents nor transhepatic extraction alone provides long-term biliary drainage, however. A number of situations may make endoscopic clearance of bile duct stones difficult or unsuccessful, including large impacted stones, the presence of a distal bile duct stricture, previous gastrectomy with gastroenterostomy or Roux-en-Y anastomosis, complications of endoscopic sphincterotomy before stone extraction, or the presence of a duodenal diverticulum. If access to the bile duct can be achieved endoscopically, adjuvant modalities such as intracorporeal fragmentation techniques (i.e., mechanical, electrohydraulic, or laser lithotripsy) or extracorporeal shock wave lithotripsy may allow successful removal of even difficult stones. Reoperation on the biliary tract for clearance of duct stones is reserved for physiologically fit patients in whom other extraction techniques are unsuccessful.

ANSWER: C

45. Which of the following is the most appropriate initial test for the evaluation of obstructive jaundice?

A. HIDA scan.
B. Ultrasonography.
C. CT scan.
D. Percutaneous transhepatic cholangiography (PTC).
E. Endoscopic retrograde cholangiopancreatography (ERCP).

Ref.: 1, 2, 7

COMMENTS: All of the above imaging modalities may be useful for evaluating a patient with obstructive jaundice. Overall, ultrasonography is the most cost-effective initial examination; it permits identification or visualization of ductal dilatation, suggests the level of obstruction, and provides information about the liver, pancreas, and the presence or absence of calculous disease. **CT or magnetic resonance imaging (MRI)** may best delineate the anatomy of mass lesions in the hepatobiliary pancreatic region and assist in the preoperative assessment of resectability. MR cholangiography can provide precise delineation of the ductal anatomy and is increasingly important in the evaluation of malignant disease. **PTC** can demonstrate the **proximal** extent of obstruction and is useful for assessing the suitability of the proximal hepatic ducts for anastomosis. **ERCP** is particularly useful in cases of **distal** biliary tract obstruction and allows evaluation of the ampullary region. Both PTC and ERCP allow cytologic or histologic sampling, and both can be used to place catheters to decompress the obstructed biliary tract. Although ^{99m}Tc iminodiacetic acid scans can demonstrate ductal obstruction, they do not provide sufficient anatomic definition to determine etiology or assist in making therapeutic decisions.

ANSWER: B

46. Two weeks following hepaticojejunostomy for treatment of a benign bile duct stricture, a patient has a serum bilirubin level of 6 mg/dl. The patient was jaundiced for 4 weeks before the operation and had a preoperative serum bilirubin level of 12 mg/dl. Which of the following is the most likely explanation for this current serum bilirubin level?

A. Anastomotic stricture.
B. Persistent delta-bilirubinemia.
C. Postoperative hepatitis.
D. Normal expected decline after relief of any obstructive jaundice.

Ref.: 3, 7

COMMENTS: After relief of biliary obstruction, there is a prompt increase in bile flow, and normal bile acid secretion resumes within several days. Serum bilirubin levels decline approximately 50% by 36–48 hours after surgery and 8% per day thereafter. This rate varies depending on the duration of jaundice. Delta-bilirubin is a form of bilirubin that is covalently bonded to albumin and is measured as a part of the direct bilirubin fraction. As such, it is not filtered by the kidney and has the same serum half-life as albumin, approximately 18 days, which accounts for the slow decline in serum bilirubin levels observed in patients following relief of long-standing jaundice. Whereas 90% of patients who had jaundice for 1 week or less have a normal serum bilirubin level 3–4 weeks postoperatively, only one-third of patients who had jaundice for 4 weeks or longer obtain normal levels by the same time. Anastomotic stenosis does not usually present early during the postoperative period. Postoperative hepatocellular dysfunction as a result of hepatitis or other causes can certainly occur early in the postoperative period, but it is a less likely cause of hyperbilirubinemia in a patient whose serum bilirubin levels are gradually declining and who would be anticipated to have persistent delta-bilirubinemia.

ANSWER: B

47. Which of the following statements is the most likely explanation for a serum bilirubin level of 40 mg/dl in a patient with obstructive jaundice?

A. Patient has complete biliary obstruction.
B. Duration of obstruction has exceeded 2 weeks.
C. Patient has associated renal dysfunction.
D. Patient has malignant biliary obstruction.

Ref.: 3

COMMENTS: In the presence of complete biliary obstruction, serum bilirubin levels generally plateau at 25–30 mg/dl; at this point the daily bilirubin load equals that excreted by the kidneys. Situations in which even higher bilirubin levels can be found include renal insufficiency, hemolysis, hepatocellular disease, and rarely a bile duct–hepatic vein fistula. Hyperbilirubinemia tends to be more pronounced in patients with obstruction caused by malignant disease compared with obstruction as a result of benign causes; however, malignant obstruction in the absence of the previously enumerated factors does not produce this degree of hyperbilirubinemia.

ANSWER: C

48. The pathophysiology of acute renal failure in a patient with biliary obstruction is related to which of the following conditions?

A. Systemic hypotension.
B. Hyperbilirubinemia.
C. Endotoxemia.
D. Bile acidemia.

Ref.: 3

COMMENTS: Acute renal failure is a common and commonly fatal complication of biliary sepsis. A number of factors contribute to the development of this complication. Renal hypoperfusion occurs as a result of bacteremia, systemic hypotension, and hypovolemia. Circulating bacterial endotoxins also are nephrotoxic. Patients with biliary obstruction are at higher risk for renal failure than patients with sepsis from other causes. Evidence suggests that circulating bile acids themselves may induce tubular damage and exacerbate the effects of renal ischemia. Therapy of patients with biliary sepsis must focus on adequate fluid and vasopressor support, antibiotic coverage, and biliary decompression to prevent renal failure. Additional treatment such as the administration of bile acids to minimize gut absorption of bacterial endotoxins has also been used. Little evidence exists to support renal damage by bilirubin, even though it may predispose the tubular cells for ischemia.

ANSWER: A, C, D

49. Which of the following conditions is usually associated with the highest incidence of positive bile cultures?

A. Acute cholecystitis.
B. Chronic cholecystitis.
C. Choledocholithiasis.
D. Postoperative bile duct stricture.
E. Bile duct malignancy.

Ref.: 2, 3

COMMENTS: The recognition of clinical situations in which bacteria are likely to be present in bile is important because the presence of bacteria in the bile correlates with the risk of postoperative infectious complications. Prophylactic antibiotics have decreased infectious morbidity in patients older than 50 years of age and in those with jaundice, acute cholecystitis, or choledocholithiasis and cholangitis. Bile cultures are positive in approximately 5–40% of patients with chronic cholecystitis, 30–70% of patients with acute cholecystitis, 60–80% of patients with choledocholithiasis, and nearly all patients with bile duct stricture. Bacterial infection of bile occurs in 25–50% of patients with malignant obstruction. Bile cultures are expected to be positive in any patient with an indwelling biliary tube.

ANSWER: D

50. Which of the following organisms is/are most commonly isolated from bile?

A. *Escherichia coli.*
B. *Clostridium* species.
C. *Bacteroides fragilis.*

D. *Pseudomonas* species.
E. *Enterococcus* species.

Ref.: 2, 3, 7, 8

COMMENTS: All of the above organisms are found in the biliary tract, but gram-negative aerobic organisms, particularly *E. coli* and *Klebsiella*, are found most frequently. Other gram-negative aerobic bacteria that can be cultured are *Proteus*, *Pseudomonas*, and *Enterobacter* species. Gram-positive organisms, especially the *Enterococcus* species and *Streptococcus faecalis*, are also frequently observed. Anaerobes are now recognized in 25–30% of cases, most commonly *B. fragilis*, followed by *Clostridium* species. Polymicrobial infection occurs in approximately 60%. Effective prophylactic or therapeutic antibiotic therapy must be effective against the anticipated organisms. Serious biliary sepsis is usually treated with broad-spectrum or combination antibiotics that are effective against gram-negative organisms, anaerobes, and enterococci.

ANSWER: A

51. Which of the following is the most common mechanism leading to bacterial infection in the bile?

A. Ascending infection from the duodenum.
B. Hematogenous portal venous spread.
C. Hematogenous arterial spread.
D. Lymphatic spread.

Ref.: 2, 3

COMMENTS: Bile is usually sterile. There are various routes by which bacteria can reach the biliary tract; and although not proved, dissemination from the portal venous system via the liver is currently favored as the most common mechanism. Ascending infection from the duodenum does not occur to a significant extent. Also, evidence suggests that the direction of lymphatic flow is from the liver downward rather than in the reverse direction. Hematogenous dissemination via hepatic arterial flow is a mechanism of hepatic abscess formation and may lead to bactibilia but is thought to be less common than portal venous spread.

ANSWER: B

52. Which of the following conditions is alone sufficient to cause cholangitis with bacteremia?

A. Bacteria in bile.
B. Partial bile duct obstruction.
C. Complete bile duct obstruction.
D. None of the above.

Ref.: 2, 7, 8

COMMENTS: The pathophysiology of cholangitis requires both bacterial infection of bile and bile duct obstruction with elevated intraductal pressure. Neither the presence of bacteria in bile nor biliary obstruction alone is sufficient to produce bacteremia. When bacteria are present in the bile and common duct pressures exceed 20 cm H_2O, cholangiovenous and cholangiolymphatic reflux occur, resulting in systemic bacteremia. Partial or complete bile duct obstruction may produce cholangitis if bacteria are present; in fact, cholangitis occurs more commonly with partial obstruction because it is more frequently associated with stone disease, whereas complete obstruction is more often found with malignancy. Calculous disease is the most common etiology of cholangitis, which is understandable because it is associated with both bile duct obstruction and bacterial infection.

ANSWER: D

53. If an antibiotic is effective against the bacteria present in the bile, which of the following is the most important consideration for effective therapy of biliary tract infection?

A. Serum concentration of the antibiotic.
B. Bile concentration of the antibiotic in an unobstructed biliary tract.
C. Bile concentration of the antibiotic in an obstructed biliary tract.
D. Potential renal toxicity of the antibiotic.

Ref.: 2, 3

COMMENTS: The most important pharmacologic considerations pertaining to selection of antimicrobial agents for the treatment of biliary sepsis are the antibacterial activity spectrum of the agent and the achievement of adequate serum levels of the drug. Therapy cannot be adequate if the agents selected are not effective against the anticipated organisms (i.e., gram-negative Enterobacteriaceae, enterococci, anaerobes) or if dosing does not produce sufficient serum levels. The significance of biliary levels of antibiotics is often discussed, but they are of little clinical importance. High bile levels of an antibiotic are meaningless if the agent is not effective against the bacteria present. Moreover, agents that achieve high concentrations in the normal biliary tract may not reach such levels in the presence of biliary obstruction. The aminoglycoside gentamicin, for example, has traditionally been an effective agent against the gram-negative organisms that cause biliary sepsis, but it is not concentrated in the bile. The potential nephrotoxicity of an antibiotic is an important consideration, because the risk of renal compromise already exists in a patient with sepsis and biliary obstruction. This has encouraged the use of nonaminoglycoside drugs for gram-negative coverage, but this consideration is not as important as the activity spectrum and adequate serum levels of the drugs.

ANSWER: A

54. Which of the following is/are necessary in the initial treatment of a patient with acute cholangitis?

A. Intravenous antibiotics.
B. Percutaneous transhepatic drainage.
C. Endoscopic sphincterotomy and drainage.
D. T-Tube decompression of the common bile duct.
E. Choledochoduodenostomy.

Ref.: 2, 7, 8

COMMENTS: Charcot's triad, which consists of fever, jaundice, and upper abdominal pain, is the clinical hallmark of acute cholangitis. When accompanied by shock and changes in mental status, it is referred to as Reynold's pentad. Cholangitis varies widely in severity, and treatment must be individualized according to the patient's condition. Initial therapy consists of fluid resuscitation and antibiotics that are effective against gram-negative organisms, enterococci, and anaerobes. Approximately 5–10% of patients present with severe toxic cholangitis and the manifestations of Reynold's pentad. Patients who fail to improve or who deteriorate despite antibiotic and fluid support require urgent biliary decompression. This generally can be accomplished nonoperatively by percutaneous transhepatic or endoscopic approaches, depending on the suspected location of the obstruction based on ultrasonographic findings and on the availability of local expertise in these procedures. The ability to decompress the biliary tract nonoperatively in these cases has been advantageous because it not only allows stabilization of a high percentage of patients but permits diagnostic cholangiography to be performed when the patient has stabilized. When initial operative decompression of the biliary tract was the only approach for these critically ill patients, the mortality rate was high, and there was a frequent need for subsequent reoperation on the biliary tract because of the inability to identify or deal with the underlying pathology at the time of the initial operation. If effective nonoperative drainage of the biliary tract is not possible, surgery should not be delayed in these critically ill patients. T-Tube decompression of the common bile duct is performed. Choledochoduodenostomy is not performed in critically ill patients but can be considered if the common bile duct is dilated to 15 mm or more, the patient is physiologically stable, and other conditions permit a safe anastomosis. The current mortality rate of acute cholangitis is approximately 5%. Poor prognostic factors include renal failure, liver abscess, cirrhosis, and proximal malignant obstruction.

ANSWER: A

55. A 30-year-old woman is found at the time of cholecystectomy to have hydrops of the gallbladder and a firm, yellow nodule in the cystic duct. Which of the following is the most likely diagnosis?

A. Cholesterolosis.
B. Carcinoid tumor.
C. Adenocarcinoma.
D. Granular cell myoblastoma.
E. Sarcoidosis.

Ref.: 2

COMMENTS: Benign tumors of the gallbladder include papillary adenomas, nonpapillary adenomas, and a host of relatively uncommon neoplasms derived from various connective tissues. These lesions are usually incidental findings in patients who are undergoing cholecystectomy. Granular cell myoblastomas are neuroectodermally derived benign tumors that can occur at many sites. In the biliary tract they occasionally occur in the gallbladder, common duct, or obstruction of the gallbladder with symptoms indistinguishable from those of cholelithiasis. No treatment beyond cholecystectomy is required. Cholesterolosis is a condition in which deposits of cholesterol are found in macrophages known as foamy histiocytes in the lamina propria of the gallbladder wall. This condition is often referred to as "strawberry gallbladder" because of the gross appearance of speckled, yellow cholesterol deposits on the background of an erythematous mucosa. Cholesterolosis is often generalized, although a localized collection may form a "cholesterol polyp." Carcinoid tumors may occur in the gallbladder, but they are rare and usually incidental findings and are not associated with the carcinoid syndrome. Adenocarcinoma of the gallbladder usually occurs in elderly individuals and grossly does not appear as a yellow nodule. Sarcoidosis is a systemic disorder that may produce granulomatous inflammation of the liver but is not associated with a specific biliary tract lesion.

ANSWER: D

56. Ultrasonography of the gallbladder demonstrates a single hyperechoic focus along the gallbladder wall that does not move or shadow and that has a "comet tail" echo pattern behind it. The most likely diagnosis is:

A. Adenomatous polyp.
B. Cholesterol polyp.
C. Gallstone.
D. Adenomyomatosis.
E. Fibroxanthogranulomatous inflammation.

Ref.: 5

COMMENTS: The term hyperplastic cholecystosis describes a group of benign proliferative conditions of the gallbladder, including cholesterolosis and adenomyomatosis, or adenomatous hyperplasia. These conditions can be symptomatic and are often diagnosed based on their sonographic features. **Cholesterolosis** consists of deposits of cholesterol in foamy histiocytes in the gallbladder wall. A localized collection of such cholesterol-laden cells covered by a normal layer of epithelium and connected to the mucosa by a small pedicle is known as a cholesterol polyp. Ultrasonography shows hyperechoic foci with an "comet tail" artifact. Unlike gallstones, the foci do not move or produce acoustic shadowing. **Adenomatous hyperplasia** is a proliferative lesion characterized by increased thickness of the mucosa and muscle with mucosal diverticula known as Rokitansky-Aschoff sinuses. Segmental, diffuse, and localized forms of adenomyomatous hyperplasia have been described. Of these, a localized form involving the fundus of the gallbladder is most frequently encountered. Ultrasonography demonstrates a mass lesion or "pseudotumor." **Adenomatous polyps** are true neoplasms derived from the glandular epithelium of the gallbladder. **Fibroxanthogranulomatous inflammation** is a condition in which foamy histiocytes are found in conjunction with inflammatory cells and a fibroblastic vascular reaction, often with mucosal ulceration.

ANSWER: B

57. With regard to adenomyomatosis, which of the following statements is/are true?

A. It can be a premalignant lesion.
B. It results from chronic inflammation.
C. It may cause right upper quadrant pain in the absence of gallstones.
D. It is rarely associated with cholelithiasis and cholecystitis.

Ref.: 1, 2

COMMENTS: Adenomyomatosis is a hyperplastic abnormality of the gallbladder that is not related to inflammation or neoplasia. Approximately one-half or more of patients with adenomyomatosis also have cholelithiasis and cholecystitis, but the relation is not causal. Adenomyomatosis is not a premalignant lesion. The hyperplastic conditions of adenomyomatosis and cholesterolosis may be associated with functional abnormalities of the gallbladder, as evidenced by motility disturbances or hyperconcentration during oral cholecystography. These abnormalities may be the cause of biliary tract symptoms in patients with hyperplastic cholecystoses in the absence of cholelithiasis. Cholecystectomy can relieve symptoms in these patients.

ANSWER: C

58. Of the fistulas in the left column select the most common type of biliary enteric fistula, and match it with its most common etiology in the right column.

A. Cholecystocolic	a. Cholelithiasis
B. Cholecystoduodenal	b. Malignancy
C. Cholecystoduodenocolic	c. Peptic ulcer
D. Choledochoduodenal	d. Congenital
E. Choledochogastric	e. Traumatic

Ref.: 2, 3, 7

COMMENTS: Almost all internal biliary fistulas are acquired communications between the extrahepatic biliary tree and the intestinal tract. In rare instances, acquired or congenital bronchobiliary or acquired pleurobiliary fistulas occur. Biliary enteric fistulas most commonly involve the gallbladder and the duodenum (70–80% of cases) and are the result of chronic inflammation caused by gallstone disease. The second most common fistula occurs between the gallbladder and colon; infrequently, the stomach or multiple sites (cholecystoduodenocolic) are involved. Occasionally, the biliary site of the fistula is the common bile duct. Choledochoduodenal fistulas are most frequently caused by penetrating peptic ulcers, but they might occur in patients with choledocholithiasis and prior cholecystectomy. Other, less common causes of biliary enteric fistulas are malignancy and penetrating trauma.

ANSWER: B-a

59. With regard to the management of a patient with gallstone ileus, which of the following statements is/are true?

A. Initial tube decompression and nonoperative management allows spontaneous stone passage in one-third of patients.
B. Operative treatment attempts to displace the stone into the colon without enterotomy.
C. Operative treatment is by enterotomy proximal to the site of obstruction.
D. Cholecystectomy and fistula repair at the time of stone removal are contraindicated.
E. Standard treatment is initial laparotomy for stone removal and mandatory reoperation for cholecystectomy when the patient is stable.

Ref.: 2, 3, 7

COMMENTS: Gallstone ileus is mechanical obstruction of the gastrointestinal tract caused by a gallstone that has entered the intestine via an acquired biliary enteric fistula. Although gallstone ileus accounts for only 1–3% of all small bowel obstructions, it is associated with a higher mortality rate than other nonmalignant causes of bowel obstruction because it tends to occur in the elderly population, and typical cases are characterized by diagnostic delay due to waxing and waning of symptoms ("tumbling obstruction"). Pathopneumonic radiologic features include a gas pattern of small bowel obstruction with pneumobilia and an opaque stone outside the expected location of the gallbladder. Not all of these radiologic features are usually present, however. The most common site of obstruction is in the terminal ileum; infrequently, sigmoid obstruction occurs in an area narrowed by intrinsic colonic disease. Initial therapy is appropriate resuscitation followed by surgery. Spontaneous passage is a rare phenomenon, and nonoperative management is associated with a prohibitive mortality rate. Stone removal is best accomplished by an enterotomy placed proximal to the site of obstruction. Care must be taken to search for additional intestinal stones, which are present in 10% of patients. Attempts to extraluminally crush the stone or to milk it distally are contraindicated because they may cause bowel injury. In rare instances, small bowel resection is necessary if there is ischemic compromise or bleeding at the site of impaction. The main controversy regarding surgical treatment of gallstone ileus is whether a definitive biliary tract operation with cholecystectomy, fistula repair, and possible common duct exploration should be performed at the time of stone removal. This decision must be based on sound surgical judgment, considering the underlying physiologic status of the patient and the anatomic status of the right upper quadrant. Up to one-third of patients who do not undergo definitive biliary surgery experience recurrent biliary symptoms, including cholecystitis, cholangitis, and recurrent gallstone ileus. Furthermore, the rate of spontaneous fistula closure is open to question. For these reasons, a definitive one-stage procedure should be considered in physiologically fit patients if the right upper quadrant dissection does not prove unduly hazardous from a technical standpoint, particularly if residual stones can be demonstrated in the right upper quadrant. In properly selected patients, a definitive one-stage procedure is not associated with higher operative morbidity or mortality rates. However, because most of these patients are elderly and have a high incidence of co-morbid disease, surgical therapy has been limited to stone removal in most instances. Interval cholecystectomy should be considered for patients with postoperative biliary symptoms and for those with residual right upper quadrant stones, provided they are physiologically fit. In reality, because of the compromised underlying status of many of these patients, interval elective procedures are not commonly performed.

ANSWER: C

60. Which of the following is the preferred management of a type I choledochal cyst?

A. Cyst excision.
B. Cyst duodenostomy.
C. Cyst jejunostomy.
D. External drainage.
E. Endoscopic sphincterotomy.

Ref.: 2, 7

COMMENTS: Cystic disease of the biliary tract may involve the intrahepatic ducts, extrahepatic ducts, or both. The most common form of involvement is a cystic dilatation of the extrahepatic bile duct (type I). Combined intrahepatic and extrahepatic cysts (type IV) are next in frequency of occurrence. A diverticulum of the common bile duct (type II), a "choledochocele" extending from the distal duct into the duodenum (type III), and cystic disease confined to the intrahepatic ducts (type V) are less common. Bile duct cysts may be associated with jaundice, abdominal pain, and cholangitis in both adult and pediatric patients. Furthermore, their association with biliary tract malignancy and with anomalous relations between the pancreatic duct and bile duct are well recognized. For these reasons, complete cyst excision with Roux-en-Y hepaticojejunostomy is the preferred treatment. Internal drainage procedures are followed by a high rate of recurrent jaundice, cholangitis, and stricture. In some instances, because of the intrahepatic or retroduodenal extent of disease or because of technical considerations, complete excision may not be feasible, and the surgeon may have to settle for partial excision.

Endoscopic treatment by sphincterotomy or resection is occasionally appropriate for the rarely occurring choledochocele.

ANSWER: A

61. With regard to balloon dilatation of biliary strictures, which of the following statements is/are true?

A. Dilatation can be performed by the transhepatic or endoscopic route.
B. Repeat dilatations are not often required.
C. Bleeding and sepsis are the most frequent complications.
D. Better success is obtained with primary duct strictures than with anastomotic strictures.
E. The long-term success rate is better than that with surgical repair.

Ref.: 1, 2

COMMENTS: Nonoperative dilatation of biliary strictures via endoscopic or percutaneous transhepatic access is an alternative to surgery that may be appropriate for some patients. Repeat dilatations are often required, but overall success rates of 70–80% at 2–3 years of follow-up have been reported. Success has generally been somewhat higher for patients with primary ductal strictures than for those with strictures of biliary enteric anastomoses. Bleeding and sepsis have been the most frequent complications and can be life-threatening. Data on long-term results are limited. Comparison between balloon dilatation and surgery has demonstrated better long-term results (approximate mean follow-up at 5 years) with surgery, with no difference in overall morbidity, hospitalization, or cost between the two therapies. It cannot be ensured that treatment groups are comparable, however. Nonoperative dilatation of biliary strictures may be appropriate as initial treatment for a strictured biliary anastomosis or for patients in whom surgical repair is deemed excessively difficult or dangerous. The decisions about how a biliary stricture is initially treated and when nonoperative maneuvers are abandoned in favor of surgery should be made in consultation with a skilled endoscopist, interventional radiologist, and an experienced hepatobiliary surgeon.

ANSWER: A, C, D

62. A 40-year-old man presents with fluctuating jaundice, pruritus, and fatigue. Liver enzymes demonstrate cholestasis. Ultrasonography does not show gallstones or bile duct dilatation. What diagnostic test should be obtained next?

A. Serum antimitochondrial antibodies.
B. CT scan.
C. HIDA scan.
D. ERCP.
E. Liver biopsy.

Ref.: 1, 2, 3, 7

COMMENTS: The described presentation is fairly typical for sclerosing cholangitis, which also can be discovered in asymptomatic patients based on their cholestatic liver enzyme levels. Sclerosing cholangitis is a disease of undetermined etiology characterized by inflammatory fibrosis and stenosis of the bile ducts. The process can be considered primary when no specific etiologic factor is identified or secondary when associated with specific causes such as bile duct stones, operative trauma, hepatic arterial infusion of chemotherapeutic agents, or intraductal instillation of various irritants for the treatment of echinococcal disease. Primary sclerosing cholangitis may be an isolated finding or may occur in conjunction with a variety of other disease processes, most commonly ulcerative colitis and pancreatitis. Although the etiology of primary sclerosing cholangitis is unknown, most attention has focused on an autoimmune or infectious cause. Evidence of an autoimmune etiology is largely inferential and is based on the association of sclerosing cholangitis with a variety of autoimmune diseases. Abnormal immunologic parameters can be found in the serum of some patients with sclerosing cholangitis, but there are no specific serologic markers for the disease. Antimitochondrial antibodies are generally associated with primary biliary cirrhosis. The diagnosis is usually made following ERCP showing multiple strictures and dilatations, giving a "beaded" appearance to the ducts. Typically, sclerosing cholangitis is a diffuse process affecting both the intrahepatic and extrahepatic bile ducts. In some cases, more limited involvement of the distal bile duct, the intrahepatic ducts, or the area of the bifurcation can be seen. Liver biopsy may show fibroobliterative cholangitis or cirrhosis as the disease progresses.

ANSWER: D

63. Definitive treatment for a patient with sclerosing cholangitis and biliary cirrhosis involves which of the following?

A. Ursodeoxycholic acid.
B. Corticosteroids.
C. Endoscopic balloon dilatation and stenting.
D. Extrahepatic bile duct resection and transhepatic stenting.
E. Hepatic transplantation.

Ref.: 1, 2, 3, 7

COMMENTS: Once sclerosing cholangitis has progressed to cirrhosis, the only definitive treatment is hepatic transplantation. The results of transplantation are generally similar to those obtained when it is performed for other indications. Prior to the development of cirrhosis, a number of medical and surgical therapies have been tried. Pharmacologic approaches have included the use of immunosuppressants, bile acid binding, and antifibrotic and antimicrobial drugs. Unfortunately, there is little evidence that any medical therapy has been effective in slowing progression. Some hopeful results have been reported with ursodeoxycholic acid, which may improve liver enzyme tests and liver histology. Dominant strictures can be treated operatively or by nonoperative dilatation via endoscopic or percutaneous transhepatic approaches. The long-term efficacy of nonoperative approaches has often been limited, however. Selected patients with predominantly extrahepatic or bifurcation strictures have been successfully treated with bile duct resection followed by Roux-en-Y reconstruction and long-term anastomotic stenting.

ANSWER: E

64. Adenocarcinoma of the gallbladder extending into the subserosa is discovered incidentally following cholecystectomy. Recommended treatment includes which of the following?

A. Nothing further at this time.
B. External beam irradiation.
C. Irradiation and chemotherapy.
D. Reoperation for liver resection and lymphadenectomy.

E. Reoperation for performance of pancreaticoduodenectomy.

Ref.: 18, 19

COMMENTS: When gallbladder cancer is discovered postoperatively during pathologic examination of the specimen, the depth of tumor invasion is an important determinant of further therapy. Recall the layers of the gallbladder wall (see Question 1). Tumors limited to the mucosa (pT1a) or muscular layer (pT1b) are usually cured by cholecystectomy alone. (It should be noted, however, that recurrence and death have occasionally been reported following cholecystectomy alone for pT1b lesions, so further treatment could be considered in this situation depending on the individual circumstances.) Patients with tumors extending into the subserosal connective tissue layer (pT2) are those most likely to benefit from resection of the adjacent liver segments (IV and V) and hepatoduodenal lymphadenectomy. A substantial proportion of patients with pT2 lesions can be found to have positive lymph nodes or residual disease. Reoperation may increase the 5-year survival to 70–90% compared to 40% for cholecystectomy alone. More extensive invasion through the serosa (pT3) or more than 2 cm into the liver (pT4) with or without adjacent organ invasion would hopefully be recognized by the surgeon at the time of cholecystectomy although not necessarily. Cholecystectomy is inadequate for cure of these lesions. Radical resection of these cancers may certainly benefit some patients, but the morbidity and mortality may be high, and conclusive evidence of benefit to many patients is lacking. Other pathologic findings in the gallbladder specimen that favor reoperation are a positive cystic duct margin (in which case bile duct resection must be considered) or a positive cystic duct lymph node. Irradiation and chemotherapy have generally been ineffective for treatment of gallbladder cancer.

ANSWER: D

65. Ultrasonography demonstrates a 15 mm polypoid lesion in the gallbladder of an asymptomatic 60-year-old patient. Which of the following best describes the recommended treatment?

A. Observation with repeat ultrasonography in 6 months.
B. Cholecystectomy.
C. Cholecystectomy if the patient is female.
D. Cholecystectomy only if symptoms develop.
E. Cholecystectomy only if the patient also has gallstones.

Ref.: 20, 21

COMMENTS: Polypoid lesions of the gallbladder may be benign, premalignant, or malignant. Inflammatory polyps and cholesterol polyps are benign, non-neoplastic lesions. Benign adenomas are neoplasms that have a malignant potential similar to that of adenomas arising in other areas of the gastrointestinal tract. Polypoid lesions are typically diagnosed by ultrasonography and occasionally by other imaging modalities such as CT scanning. The indications for cholecystectomy to treat a polypoid lesion are (1) symptoms and (2) possible malignancy. The risk of malignancy is related to the size of the lesion and is higher for lesions that are 10 mm or larger and quite substantial for lesions of 15 mm. Therefore cholecystectomy is performed if the patient has biliary tract symptoms, regardless of polyp size, or the presence or absence of gallstones, or if the lesion is larger than 10 mm. Polypoid lesions in patients 60 years of age or older are also more frequently malignant. The use of laparoscopic cholecystectomy for polypoid lesions is controversial. Proponents hold that the laparoscopic approach is appropriate, as most polyps are benign and even limited cancers may be cured by cholecystectomy alone. However, gallbladder leakage is common during laparoscopic cholecystectomy, and consequent dissemination of otherwise "curable" early cancers has been reported. The long-term results of radical resection following laparoscopic cholecystectomy for gallbladder cancers are unknown. Until more information becomes available, it is generally advised that open cholecystectomy be performed for patients considered at risk for gallbladder cancer.

ANSWER: B

66. Which of the following is/are contraindications for resection of the bile duct cancer?

A. Tumor location in distal common bile duct.
B. Tumor location at bifurcation of bile duct.
C. Peritoneal metastases.
D. Invasion of right portal vein and right hepatic artery.
E. None of the above.

Ref.: 1, 3

COMMENTS: Cancers of the extrahepatic bile ducts usually carry a poor prognosis because these tumors are often beyond the confines of surgical resection at the time of diagnosis. Substantial palliation often can be achieved by therapy directed at the relief of biliary obstruction. Prognosis is related to tumor location, resectability, and histologic pattern. Proximal lesions at or near the hepatic bifurcation are most common but also are least often resectable and therefore have a less favorable prognosis. In some centers, aggressive resection of proximal lesions, usually including hepatic resection, has produced improved survival with morbidity not exeeding that of nonoperative treatment. Hilar cancers are considered unresectable if there is metastatic disease, bilateral vascular involvement, or bilateral extension of the tumor to second-order biliary radicles. Hepatic transplantation for otherwise unresectable tumors has had poor results. Distal lesions resectable by pancreaticoduodenectomy have the best prognosis, with a 5-year survival rate of approximately 30%. Palliative decompression can be achieved by surgical anastomosis, surgical intubation, or endoscopic or percutaneous catheter placement. The most appropriate method of palliative decompression for a particular patient depends on the tumor location and extent, the patient's underlying condition, the expertise of the surgeon, and the anticipated complications of each technique. Nonoperative decompression is preferred for patients who can be demonstrated to have metastasis or otherwise unresectable disease prior to operation.

ANSWER: C

67. A contusion of the gallbladder from blunt abdominal trauma is best managed by:

A. Drain placement.
B. Cholecystostomy tube.
C. Suture imbrication of contusion.
D. Cholecystectomy.

Ref.: 7

COMMENTS: The gallbladder may be injured as a result of blunt or penetrating trauma; penetrating injury is the most common. Most injuries of the gallbladder and extrahepatic biliary tree are associated with involvement of other organs, such as liver, small bowel, and colon. Blunt injuries, including contusion, avulsion, and rupture, are treated by cholecystectomy. Penetrating injuries occasionally cause isolated injury to the gallbladder; the treatment in such instances usually is cholecystectomy, although cholecystostomy or simple closure and drainage are conceivable. In general, the prognosis following a nonoperative injury of the biliary tract is related to the significance of the associated injuries.

ANSWER: D

REFERENCES

1. Greenfield LJ: *Surgery: Scientific Principles and Practice*, 2nd ed. Lippincott-Raven, Philadelphia, 1997.
2. Sabiston DC Jr: *Textbook of Surgery*, 15th ed. WB Saunders, Philadelphia, 1997.
3. Blumgart LH: *Surgery of the Liver and Biliary Tract*, 2nd ed. Churchill-Livingstone, Edinburgh 1994.
4. Yoshida J, Chijiwa K, Yamaguchi K, et al: Practical classification of the branching types of the biliary tree: an analysis of 1,094 consecutive direct choler programs. *J Am Coll Surg* 182:37–40, 1996.
5. Deziel DJ: Hepatobiliary ultrasound. *Probl Gen Surg* 14:13–24, 1997.
6. Staren ED, Arregui ME: *Ultrasound for the Surgeon*. Lippincott-Raven, Philadelphia, 1997.
7. Schwartz SJ, Shires GT, Spencer FC: *Principles of Surgery*, 7th ed. McGraw-Hill, New York, 1994.
8. O'Leary JP: *The Physiologic Basis of Surgery*, 2nd ed. Williams & Wilkins, Baltimore, 1996.
9. Canfield AJ, Hetz SP, Schriver JP, et al: Biliary dyskinesia: a study of more than 200 patients and review of the literature. *J Gastrointest Surg* 2:443–448, 1998.
10. Fong Y, Brennan MF, Turnbulla A, et al: Gallbladder cancer discovered during laparoscopic surgery. *Arch Surg* 128:1050–1054, 1993.
11. Shirai Y, Ohtani T, Hatakeyama K: Is laparoscopic cholecystectomy indicated for early gallbladder cancer? *Surgery* 122:120–121, 1997.
12. Stewart L, Way LW: Bile duct injuries during laparoscopic cholecystectomy: factors that influence the results of treatment. *Arch Surg* 130:1123–1129, 1995.
13. Lillemoe KD, Martin SA, Cameron JL, et al: Major bile duct injuries during laparoscopic cholecystectomy. *Ann Surg* 225:459–471, 1997.
14. Deziel DJ: Complications of cholecystectomy. *Surg Clin North Am* 74:809–823, 1994.
15. Woods MS, Traverso LW, Kozarek RA, et al: Biliary tract complications of laparoscopic cholecystectomy are detected more frequently with routine intraoperative cholangiography. *Surg Endosc* 9:1076–1080, 1995.
16. Barkun AN, Barkun JS, Fried GM, et al: Useful predictors of bile duct stones in patients undergoing laparoscopic cholecystectomy. *Ann Surg* 220:32–39, 1994.
17. Petelin J: Laparoscopic approach to common duct pathology. *Am J Surg* 165:487–491, 1993.
18. Shirai Y, Yoshida K, Tsukada K, Muto T: Inapparent carcinoma of the gallbladder: an appraisal of a radical second operation after simple cholecystetomy. *Ann Surg* 215:326–331, 1992.
19. Bartlett DL, Fong Y, Fortner JG, et al: Long-term results after resection for gallbladder cancer: implications for staging and management. *Ann Surg* 224:639–646, 1996.
20. Kubota K, Bandai Y, Noie T, et al: How should polypoid lesions of the gallbladder be treated in the era of laparoscopic cholecystectomy? *Surgery* 117:481–487, 1995.
21. Shirai Y, Ohtani T, Hatakeyama K: Is laparoscopic cholecystectomy recommended for large polypoid lesions of the gallbladder [letter]? *Surg Laparosc Endosc* 7:435, 1997.

CHAPTER 35

Pancreas

1. The embryologic ventral pancreas forms which area(s) of the fully developed gland?

A. Superior head.
B. Neck.
C. Uncinate process.
D. Body.
E. Tail.

Ref.: 1, 2, 3

COMMENTS: The pancreas is formed from two outpouchings of the primitive gut. The dorsal pancreas originates from the duodenum; the ventral pancreas begins as a bud from the hepatic diverticulum, which itself is an outpouching of the duodenum. Other outgrowths from the hepatic diverticulum mature into the liver, gallbladder, and bile ducts. During normal fetal development the ventral pancreas rotates along with the primitive gut and fuses with the dorsal component. The ventral pancreas constitutes the uncinate process and the inferior portion of the head of the gland in the fully developed state, and the dorsal pancreas forms the remainder of the gland. Abnormalities in this developmental process result in recognized congenital anomalies that can be clinically important. An understanding of this embryology is also important when it comes to recognizing the relation of the pancreas to adjacent vascular structures during pancreatic operations.

ANSWER: C

2. Which of the following correctly describe(s) the anatomic location of the uncinate process of the pancreas?

A. Ventral to portal vein.
B. Ventral to aorta.
C. Ventral to left renal vein.
D. Dorsal to superior mesenteric artery.
E. Caudal to third portion of duodenum.

Ref.: 1, 2, 3, 4, 5

COMMENTS: The pancreas can be divided into various parts: head, uncinate, neck, body, and tail. The uncinate process is the portion of the gland that extends to the left behind the portal vein and superior mesenteric artery and in front of the aorta and inferior vena cava. The uncinate process is located below and ventral to the left renal vein and above the distal duodenum. Understanding the extent and location of the uncinate is important during resection of the head of the pancreas. The blood supply of the uncinate is from numerous short branches of the superior mesenteric artery and portal vein; bleeding from these branches must be carefully controlled during resection.

ANSWER: B, C, D

3. With regard to the vascular relations of the pancreas, which of the following statements is/are true?

A. The portal vein is formed by the confluence of the splenic vein and the inferior mesenteric vein behind the pancreatic neck.
B. The portal vein generally has no anterior tributaries behind the neck of the pancreas.
C. The arterial supply of the pancreatic head is derived primarily from the splenic artery.
D. The inferior pancreaticoduodenal artery is the first branch of the superior mesenteric artery.
E. Anomalous hepatic and middle colic arteries may be intimately associated with the pancreatic head.

Ref.: 1, 2, 3, 5

COMMENTS: The relation of the pancreas to neighboring organs and to critical vascular structures is of great surgical significance. The arterial supply to the head of the gland is derived from both the gastroduodenal and superior mesenteric arteries via anterior and posterior pancreaticoduodenal arcades. For the most part, the head of the pancreas and the duodenum have a shared blood supply, so they generally must be resected together. However, techniques for "duodenal sparing" resection of the pancreatic head or "pancreatic-sparing" duodenectomy are appropriate in select circumstances. The body and tail of the gland receive their blood supply mainly from multiple branches of the splenic artery, which also connect with superior mesenteric sources. Variations in major arteries—such as the origin of the right hepatic artery from the superior mesenteric artery and origin of the middle colic artery from the superior mesenteric artery or dorsal pancreatic artery—place these vessels in close proximity to the head and neck of the pancreas, where they are subject to injury during pancreatectomy. The junction of the splenic vein and superior mesenteric vein to form the portal vein lies behind the neck of the pancreas. Usually these vessels do not have large anterior tributaries in this area, but appropriate caution must nonetheless be exercised when developing this plane during pancreatic operations.

ANSWER: B, D, E

4. Which of the following statements regarding heterotopic pancreas is/are true?

A. Can be histologically distinguished from normally located pancreatic tissue based on the absence of islet cells.
B. Most patients with heterotopic pancreas have no related symptoms.
C. Heterotopic pancreas is associated with an increased risk of pancreatic cancer.
D. Resection of heterotopic pancreas is appropriate when it is discovered coincidentally at operation.

Ref.: 1, 2, 5

COMMENTS: Heterotopic pancreas refers to pancreatic tissue located at sites other than the normal location of the gland. Ectopic pancreatic tissue has been described at many anatomic locations but typically is found in the stomach, duodenum, or a Meckel's diverticulum. Theories of origin include metaplasia (favored) and transplantation. Histologic findings range from those of a rudimentary structure to a fully formed gland. Most heterotopic rests contain ducts, and both endocrine and exocrine elements may be present. This entity is not uncommon, being described in 1–2% of autopsies; it is usually asymptomatic. When symptoms occur, they are related to the location of the ectopic site and include obstruction (due to intussusception), ulceration, and bleeding. Although malignancy has been reported, there is no evidence that heterotopic pancreatic tissue is predisposed. The typical gross appearance is a submucosal nodule often with a central umbilication. Resection is indicated for symptomatic lesions and is appropriate diagnostically for incidental lesions discovered during operations for other reasons.

ANSWER: B, D

5. Recommended treatment of an adult with duodenal obstruction caused by annular pancreas is:

A. Endoscopic division of associated duodenal web.
B. Gastrojejunostomy.
C. Duodenojejunostomy.
D. Surgical division of annular tissue.
E. Pancreaticoduodenectomy.

Ref.: 1, 2, 5

COMMENTS: Annular pancreas is a congenital anomaly involving a band of pancreatic tissue encircling the second portion of the duodenum. The annular tissue appears to originate from the embryologic ventral pancreas. Causal theories include abnormal fixation of the ventral pancreatic primordium (extramural type) or development of heterotopic pancreatic tissue in the duodenum (intramural type). Approximately one-half of these cases are diagnosed in infants and the remainder in adults, with a peak during the fourth decade. Most patients are asymptomatic. Clinical presentations are obstruction in infants and children and obstruction, ulceration, or pancreatitis in adults. Associated anomalies include duodenal stenosis or atresia and Down syndrome. Treatment of symptomatic patients is surgical bypass by duodenoduodenostomy or duodenojejunostomy. Gastrojejunostomy can also alleviate obstruction but risks marginal ulceration. Resection or division of the annular band is not advised, as it risks pancreatic fistula and may fail to relieve the obstruction.

ANSWER: C

6. Which of the following developmental anomalies *best* characterizes pancreas divisum?

A. Aplasia of the dorsal pancreatic anlage.
B. Aplasia of the ventral pancreatic anlage.
C. Incomplete rotation of the ventral pancreatic anlage.
D. Failed fusion of the ventral and dorsal pancreatic parenchyma.
E. Failed fusion of the ventral and dorsal pancreatic ducts.

Ref.: 1, 2, 4

COMMENTS: See Question 7.

7. The diagnosis of pancreas divisum can be made by which one or more of the following?

A. Ultrasonography.
B. Computed tomography (CT) scan.
C. Pancreatic scintigraphy.
D. Endoscopic retrograde cholangiopancreatography (ERCP).
E. Glucose tolerance testing.

Ref.: 2

COMMENTS: Pancreas divisum currently refers to congenital variations of the pancreatic ducts that result from failed or incomplete fusion of the embryologic ventral and dorsal ductal systems. (Historically, the term may also refer to the rare failure of parenchymal fusion.) There may be complete separation of the ducts, an absent or minimal ventral duct, or only a few meager connections between the systems. As a consequence, most of the pancreatic duct drainage is through the dorsal duct joining the duodenum at the minor papilla. Any existing ventral ducts (Wirsung) drain only the uncinate process and the caudal head of the gland rather than draining the bulk of the gland at the major papilla as when normally developed. Some variation of pancreas divisum is present in about 10% of the population. In some individuals it is clinically significant if the relatively stenotic minor papilla imposes an obstruction to ductal flow. This can potentially result in recurrent abdominal pain, acute pancreatitis, or even chronic pancreatitis. The diagnosis of pancreas divisum requires ERCP to visualize the ductal anatomy.

ANSWER:
Question 6: E
Question 7: D

8. Which of the following might be appropriate treatment(s) for a patient with pancreas divisum, chronic abdominal pain, a dilated dorsal pancreatic duct, and an enlarged, calcified pancreatic head?

A. Endoscopic dorsal sphincterotomy.
B. Endoscopic dorsal duct stenting.
C. Operative dorsal sphincterotomy.
D. Longitudinal pancreaticojejunostomy.
E. Pancreaticoduodenectomy.

Ref.: 1, 2

COMMENTS: The true relation between the anatomic diagnosis of pancreas divisum and any clinical symptoms is difficult to determine. Symptomatic patients with pancreas divisum require thorough evaluation of the nature of their symptoms and for any other causes of abdominal pain or pancreatitis. When it is reasonable to suspect that a stenotic lesser papilla is the cause of recurrent abdominal pain or recurrent acute pancreatitis, therapeutic considerations include endoscopic sphincterotomy or stenting (or both) or operative sphincterotomy/sphincteroplasty. The long-term results of endoscopic treatment have not always been encouraging, and operative sphincterotomy is considered definitive intervention when sphincter ablation is appropriate. Occasionally, there are patients (as described in this question) with established findings of chronic pancreatitis and pancreas divisum. Sphincter operations are not indicated in this setting. Rather, surgical treatment when indicated must be directed at pancreatic decompression or resection, both of which might be appropriate for the patient described.

ANSWER: D, E

9. Which of the following is/are more characteristic of pancreatic centroacinar cells than acinar cells?

A. Carbonic anhydrase.
B. Zymogen granules.
C. Golgi apparatus.
D. Rough endoplasmic reticulum.
E. Contractile proteins.

Ref.: 2, 4

COMMENTS: The twofold function of the exocrine pancreas—to secrete bicarbonate-rich fluid and to synthesize digestive enzymes—is accomplished by different cell types. The **acinar cells**, which elaborate and secrete digestive enzymes, are designed for protein synthesis. They contain abundant rough endoplasmic reticulum, Golgi apparatus, and secretory zymogen granules. Contractile proteins also are abundant near the apical membrane of the cell to facilitate exocytosis of the enzyme bundles into the ductal lumen. The **centroacinar cells** are part of the ductal system. They secrete bicarbonate and therefore contain carbonic anhydrase, which dissociates carbonic acid into bicarbonate and hydrogen ion: $H_2O + CO_2 \rightarrow H^+ + HCO_3^-$. Some ductal cells also contain synthetic and secretory organelles for production of mucoproteins.

ANSWER: A

10. Which of the following is/are true regarding regulation of pancreatic fluid and electrolyte secretion?

A. Secretin is the primary stimulant.
B. Cholecystokinin is the primary stimulant.
C. Bicarbonate concentration increases with the secretory rate.
D. Bicarbonate concentration decreases with the secretory rate.
E. Sodium and potassium concentrations are relatively constant.

Ref.: 1, 3, 4

COMMENTS: The centroacinar cells secrete a bicarbonate-rich solution by an active transport mechanism primarily in response to secretin. Cholecystokinin is the primary stimulant of enzyme secretion from the acinar cells. The bicarbonate and chloride contents of pancreatic juice are reciprocally related. As ductal flow rates increase, bicarbonate concentration increases and chloride concentration decreases. This is the result of two processes: (1) changes in passive exchange of intraductal bicarbonate for intracellular chloride, and (2) changes in the relative contribution of acinar cell secretion. Acinar cells secrete fluid high in chloride in addition to digestive enzymes. In contradistinction to anion concentrations, the concentrations of sodium and potassium in pancreatic duct secretion remain relatively constant despite the flow rate and are similar to the concentrations in plasma.

ANSWER: A, C, E

11. Which of the following normally activates pancreatic trypsinogen?

A. Pancreatic amylase.
B. pH >7.0.
C. Lysosomal hydrolase.
D. Duodenal enterokinase.
E. Pancreatic enterokinase.

Ref.: 1, 3, 4, 5

COMMENTS: The pancreatic acinar cells secrete digestive enzymes for fats, carbohydrates, and proteins. With the exception of amylase, these enzymes are secreted in inactive forms to protect the pancreas from autodigestion. Activation of the proenzyme trypsinogen to trypsin is the primary event that leads to activation of the other various proteases and phospholipases. It occurs in the duodenum via the action of enterokinase. Trypsinogen activation can also occur in acidic environments (pH <7.0). With acute pancreatitis, intraglandular activation can occur when the inactive enzymes are exposed to lysosomal hydrolases.

ANSWER: D

12. Match the islet cell type in the left-hand column with the peptide hormone produced in the right-hand column.

A. A cell	a. Pancreatic polypeptide
B. B cell	b. Glucagon
C. D cell	c. Insulin
D. F cell	d. Somatostatin

Ref.: 1, 3, 4, 5

COMMENTS: See Question 13.

13. Match the pancreatic peptide in the left-hand column with the physiologic effect(s) in the right-hand column. Each answer may be used more than once or not at all.

A. Insulin	a. Stimulates lipolysis
B. Glucagon	b. Inhibits lipolysis
C. Somatostatin	c. Inhibits pancreatic exocrine secretion
D. Pancreatic polypeptide	d. Marker for pancreatic endocrine tumors

Ref.: 1, 3, 4, 5

COMMENTS: The endocrine pancreas is composed of various cells located in the islets of Langerhans, approximately one million of which are interspersed with the acinar and ductal elements throughout the gland. The hormonal peptides that the islets produce effect a wide range of metabolic and physiologic actions. The primary function of the endocrine pancreas is to regulate glucose homeostasis. The B cells, which are the most numerous, produce insulin. Insulin promotes glucose transport, stimulates protein synthesis, and inhibits glycogenolysis and lipolysis. The A cells secrete glucagon, which counterbalances insulin by stimulating hepatic glycogenolysis, gluconeogenesis, ketogenesis, and lipolysis. Glucagon also inhibits intestinal motility and gastric acid and pancreatic exocrine secretion. Somatostatin, produced by the D cells, has a broad range of inhibitory effects on the gastrointestinal tract, including inhibition of secretion of other pancreatic peptides; inhibition of gastric, biliary, intestinal, and pancreatic exocrine secretions; and inhibition of gastrointestinal motility. The F, or PP, cells are the source of pancreatic polypeptide. Pancreatic polypeptide inhibits pancreatic exocrine secretion and biliary motility; and it may play a role in glucose homeostasis, although its physiologic function has not been fully elucidated. Clinically, deficiency of pancreatic polypeptide has been linked to diabetes following resection of the pancreatic head or chronic pancreatitis. Pancreatic polypeptide has been used as a marker for pancreatic endocrine tumors. Postprandial secretion of pancreatic polypeptide is dependent on vagal innervation, so it has been used to assess completeness of vagotomy.

ANSWER:
Question 12: A-b; B-c; C-d; D-a
Question 13: A-b; B-a,c; C-c; D-c,d

14. Which is the principal cell type located at the center of the islets of Langerhans?

A. A cell.
B. B cell.
C. D cell.
D. F cell.
E. Varies according to the location of the islet in the pancreas.

Ref.: 1, 3

COMMENTS: Each islet of Langerhans is composed of an average of 3000 cells, with the major types as listed above and discussed in the preceding comments. The B cells are located at the core and comprise about 70% of the islet. The other cell types are located at the periphery of the islet. This cellular anatomy has potential functional implications that are as yet not well understood. The distribution of cell types within the islet varies in different areas of the gland. Islets in the uncinate process derived from the embryologic ventral pancreas contain F cells but few A cells. Islets in the body and tail of the gland have abundant A cells but no F cells.

ANSWER: B

15. Which of the following statements is/are true regarding the microvasculature of the pancreas?

A. The islet cells receive a greater proportion of pancreatic blood flow than exocrine elements.
B. Cholecystokinin (CCK) and secretin regulate secretion by altering blood flow.
C. Fragile anastomotic networks predispose the gland to ischemia.
D. Arterioles supply both the islets and the acinar tissue.
E. Blood draining from islets perfuses acinar tissues.

Ref.: 2, 3, 4

COMMENTS: The microcirculation of the pancreas is complex and has important correlations with the endocrine and exocrine functions of the gland. The rich anastomotic supply from different sources makes pancreatic ischemic unusual. The islets receive a disproportionately large amount of total pancreatic blood flow (10–25%) relative to their mass (1–2%). Both the islets and the exocrine tissue have arteriolar blood supply. The acinar tissue is also perfused by blood that drains from the islets, which is referred to as the islet-acinar or insuloacinar portal system; it is the structural basis for endocrine regulation of exocrine function. Insulin receptors are present on acinar cells, and the density of receptors is higher on acini located near the islets. The islets themselves often have a central to peripheral pattern of perfusion so that insulin from the centrally located B cells can influence the other peripheral islet cell types. Also, some islets are apparently perfused in a peripheral to central pattern. CCK and secretin have relatively little effect on blood flow and so exert their stimulatory effects independently. Pancreatic blood flow is also maintained relatively constant despite changes in arterial pressure.

ANSWER: A, D, E

16. Which of the following events occur in the acinar cell with acute pancreatitis?

A. Accelerated extrusion of zymogen granules.
B. Impaired extrusion of zymogen granules.
C. Fusion of lysosomes and zymogen granules.
D. Fusion of mitochondria and zymogen granules.
E. Impaired protein synthesis.

Ref.: 2, 3, 4

COMMENTS: The pathogenesis of pancreatitis involves intrapancreatic activation of digestive enzymes that normally are secreted in inactive form. It results in "autodigestion" of the gland. Although the mechanisms by which the various etiologies of clinical pancreatitis leading to this state are incompletely understood, experimental observations have identified certain derangements in acinar cell biology that may be the underlying common pathway to pancreatic injury. The primary defects involve blocked extrusion of zymogen granules containing inactive digestive enzymes and alterations in intracellular transport that result in fusion of zymogen granules with lysosomes to form large cytoplasmic vacuoles. This sequence results in co-localization of digestive enzymes and lysosomal hydrolases. Lysosomal enzymes, such as cathepsin B, activate trypsinogen and initiate a cascade of intracellular digestive enzyme activation. Amino acid uptake and protein synthesis are not impaired during this process. These cellular events have been observed in experimental models of acute pancreatitis. To what extent they reflect the cellular change that occurs in human acute pancreatitis is not known.

ANSWER: B, C

17. The mechanism of alcohol-induced acute pancreatitis is thought to involve which of the following?

A. Pancreatic ductal obstruction.
B. Pancreatic exocrine hypersecretion.
C. Hypertriglyceridemia.
D. Acetaldehyde toxicity.
E. Impaired trypsin inhibition.

Ref.: 1, 3

COMMENTS: Ethanol is the prevalent etiologic factor in acute pancreatitis. The precise mechanisms by which alcohol-induced pancreatic injury occur are not known, but there are several plausible theories. Ethanol causes pancreatic ductal hypertension by increasing ampullary resistance and by intraductal deposition of stone proteins. Concomitantly, ethanol stimulates gastric acid secretion and increases pancreatic exocrine secretion via secretin release. The combination of ductal obstruction with stimulated secretion may result in enzyme extravasation. Acetaldehyde, the metabolic product of ethanol, injures acinar cells by increasing membrane permeability and disrupting the microtubule structure. Elevated levels of serum triglycerides induced by alcohol are a source of cytotoxic free fatty acids. Alcohol also impairs normal trypsin inhibition and reduces pancreatic blood flow. All of these effects may contribute to intraglandular enzyme activation and the development of acute alcoholic pancreatitis.

ANSWER: A, B, C, D, E

18. Hyperamylasemia is diagnostic of acute pancreatitis when associated with which of the following laboratory findings?

A. Hyperlipasemia.
B. Increased urinary amylase.
C. Amylase/creatinine clearance ratio greater than 5%.
D. Hypocalcemia.
E. None of the above.

Ref.: 1, 2, 3, 5

COMMENTS: The diagnosis of acute pancreatitis is based on the clinical presentation, supported by biochemical findings and morphologic abnormalities on imaging studies such as CT scans. No biochemical feature is pathognomonic for acute pancreatitis. Hyperamylasemia, hyperlipasemia, and elevations in urinary amylase and in the amylase/creatinine clearance ratio are typical of acute pancreatitis but are not specific or sensitive, and they can occur with other abdominal and extraabdominal disorders. Hypocalcemia may occur as a consequence of pancreatitis, but it also is nonspecific. There is no absolute level of serum amylase or lipase that is diagnostic of acute pancreatitis. Marked elevations are more indicative of pancreatitis but, again, are not themselves diagnostic. Both amylase and lipase may be elevated in a number of conditions that can be confused with acute pancreatitis, such as acute cholecystitis, perforated peptic ulcer, and intestinal infarction. Moreover, severe pancreatitis can occur without substantial elevations in these serum enzymes.

ANSWER: E

19. A patient with abdominal pain is found to have a serum amylase level of 1200 IU/L, normal urinary amylase level, and an amylase/creatinine clearance ratio of less than 2%. Based on these findings, the likely diagnosis is which of the following conditions?

A. Acute pancreatitis.
B. Chronic pancreatitis.
C. Renal failure.
D. Choledocholithiasis without pancreatitis.
E. Macroamylasemia.

Ref.: 2

COMMENTS: Elevations in serum and urinary amylase and in the amylase/creatinine clearance ratio (ACCR), as determined by the following equation, are typical of acute pancreatitis. ACCR = $U_{amy}/S_{amy} \times S_{cr}/U_{cr} \times 100$, where U = urine; S = serum; amy = amylase; and cr = creatinine. Elevation of the ACCR above the normal 2–5% range is not specific for pancreatitis, but a normal ratio in the presence of hyperamylasemia suggests that the hyperamylasemia results from something other than pancreatitis. Serum and urinary amylase and the ACCR may be normal in the presence of chronic pancreatitis or elevated during an acute exacerbation. Renal disease may be associated with low urinary amylase and an elevated ACCR. Common duct stones may produce hyperamylasemia without true pancreatitis; the urinary amylase is elevated, although the ACCR may be normal. With macroamylasemia, amylase forms complexes with serum proteins too large for glomerular filtration. Serum amylase is therefore elevated, but urinary amylase and the ACCR are low. The diagnosis can be confirmed by electrophoresis. Abdominal pain has been reported in more than one-half of patients with macroamylasemia, although the biochemical abnormality probably is not etiologically related to the pain. Hyperamylasemia predominantly caused by salivary amylase also may be associated with a low urinary amylase and ACCR because the salivary isoenzyme is cleared more slowly by the kidneys than the pancreatic isoenzyme.

ANSWER: E

20. Which of the following conditions are unfavorable prognostic criteria for acute alcoholic pancreatitis?

A. White blood cell (WBC) count higher than 16,000/ml.
B. Serum calcium level of less than 8 mg/dl during the initial 48 hours.
C. Serum amylase on admission of more than 1200 IU/L.
D. Serum lipase level more than three times normal.
E. Serum BUN elevation over 2 mg/dl during the initial 48 hours.

Ref.: 1, 2, 3

COMMENTS: Several prognostic systems have been devised to gauge the severity of acute pancreatitis. These systems involve multiple clinical, biochemical, and sometimes radiologic criteria. The most widely used system in the United States, developed by Ranson, was based on retrospective analysis and subsequent prospective verification. Ranson's criteria include 11 parameters determined at the time of admission or during the subsequent 48 hours. Patients with three or more criteria have more severe disease and are at increased risk of septic complications and death. The criteria reflect the patient's underlying status, the severity of the retroperitoneal inflammatory process, and the effects on renal and respiratory function. Ranson's criteria originally were developed for alcoholic pancreatitis and have been modified somewhat for gallstone pancreatitis. For example, a rise in serum BUN of more than 2 mg/dl is one of the 10 criteria for gallstone pancreatitis, but the rise must be more than 5 mg/dl to meet the criteria for alcoholic pancreatitis (a subtle point). Other physiologic scoring systems such as the APACHE II may also be useful prognostically although not designed to be specific to acute pancreatitis.

ANSWER: A, B

21. Routine, initial treatment of a patient with alcoholic pancreatitis and five Ranson's criteria should include which of the following measures?

A. Gastric decompression.
B. Intravenous antibiotics.
C. Peritoneal lavage.
D. Octreotide.
E. Laparotomy.

Ref.: 1, 2

COMMENTS: The diagnosis of acute pancreatitis initially is a presumptive one. Patients presenting with acute abdominal symptoms require careful clinical, biochemical, and radiologic evaluation to exclude other intraabdominal problems, such as bowel obstruction, perforated viscus, mesenteric ischemia, cholecystitis, and others. Immediate laparotomy may be indicated. In the patient with acute pancreatitis, the initial treatment is nonoperative and focuses on fluid resuscitation; maintenance of ventilation, oxygenation, and renal perfusion; and prevention of complications. • Gastric decompression is indicated because of associated paralytic ileus and delayed gastric emptying. Although decompression may theoretically decrease pancreatic stimulation, controlled studies have not shown that decompression alters the course of alcoholic pancreatitis. • Controlled studies also have failed to demonstrate the benefit of routine antibiotics in the prevention of infectious complications, but these trials included patients with mild pancreatitis. Patients with more severe pancreatitis based on established indices (more than three of Ranson's signs) are at greater risk for pancreatic infection, and experienced pancreatic surgeons generally advocate antibiotics in these patients. A randomized study of intravenous imipenem has shown that it produced decreased pancreatic sepsis in treated patients. Selective decontamination of the gut has also been reported to decrease mortality in patients with severe pancreatitis. Antibiotics are commonly used in patients with biliary pancreatitis. • Various inhibitors of pancreatic enzymes and secretion have been tried without benefit. Octreotide, a long-acting analogue of somatostatin, has received attention in clinical trials but has not been proved beneficial and could potentially be detrimental by decreasing pancreatic blood flow. • Peritoneal lavage can decrease the early mortality of severe pancreatitis in patients who do not respond to standard supportive measures. A small study suggested that longer periods of lavage (up to 2 weeks) may decrease septic complications and overall mortality. • Planned early operative intervention to accomplish pancreatic resection in patients with acute pancreatitis has a higher mortality than nonoperative therapy; operation is therefore delayed unless prompted by complications such as infection or hemorrhage.

ANSWER: A, B

22. The leading cause of death in acute pancreatitis is:

A. Hemorrhage.
B. Pseudocyst rupture.
C. Secondary pancreatic infection.
D. Biliary sepsis.
E. Renal failure.

Ref.: 6

COMMENTS: Formerly, death from acute pancreatitis often occurred early in the course of the disease owing to the acute effects of hypovolemia and inadequate resuscitation. In the current era, about 80% of deaths are attributed to secondary pancreatic infection, which develops in about 10% of patients with acute pancreatitis. Fatal pancreatic sepsis typically progresses to multisystem organ failure, and deaths occur later in the course of the disease. To have an impact on this disease therapeutic efforts have therefore focused on the prevention and early diagnosis of pancreatic infection and on more effective methods of surgical therapy.

ANSWER: C

23. Which of the following complications of acute pancreatitis is associated with the highest mortality rate?

A. Peripancreatic abscess.
B. Infected pancreatic pseudocyst.
C. Infected pancreatic necrosis.
D. Sterile pancreatic necrosis.

Ref.: 2, 6

COMMENTS: Retroperitoneal infection is a serious, often fatal complication of acute pancreatitis. Early literature pertaining to the local infectious sequelae of pancreatitis may be confusing because of the nonselective use of the term "pancreatic abscess" to describe infectious complications, which vary in severity. "Pancreatic abscess" best describes a localized collection of drainable pus in or around the pancreas. Pancreatic abscess and infected pseudocyst can be treated effectively by external drainage; anticipated mortality for each is about 5%. Pancreatic necrosis is a manifestation of severe pancreatitis. When accompanied by infection it has been associated with a mortality rate that may exceed 40%, which is higher than the mortality rate for noninfected necrosis. Infected pancreatic necrosis is treated by operative débridement and open or closed retroperitoneal drainage. Patients with sterile necrosis may require operative intervention as well but are generally treated nonoperatively with intensive support so long as their condition permits.

ANSWER: C

24. An alcoholic patient has acute pancreatitis with five of Ranson's criteria. He gradually improves over a 14-day hospitalization but then develops a pulse of 120 bpm, a temperature of 39°C, and abdominal distension. A CT scan is obtained; results are shown below. The next most appropriate therapy is which of the following measures?

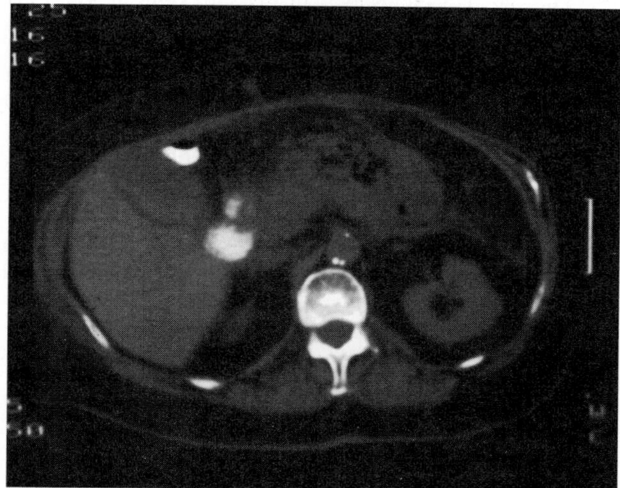

A. Antibiotics.
B. Percutaneous catheter drainage.

C. Peritoneal lavage.
D. Laparoscopy.
E. Operative drainage.

Ref.: 2, 6

COMMENTS: Pancreatic infection complicating acute pancreatitis should be suspected based on the clinical course of any patient who fails to improve following supportive medical therapy or improves but then demonstrates deterioration. Pancreatic infection occasionally occurs early during the chronologic course of the disease, but typically it presents later, as in the patient described. CT scanning is the best method for imaging the pancreas; it should be used serially in patients with severe pancreatitis. Results of CT of this patient demonstrate air in the pancreas, which is characteristic of pancreatic infection. The technique of dynamic pancreatography can identify ischemic areas of pancreas and is useful for evaluating patients who may have pancreatic necrosis. Dynamic pancreatography is performed by serially imaging the pancreas after bolus injection of an intravenous contrast medium. Percutaneous needle aspiration of fluid collections or necrotic areas found on CT imaging can be performed to identify the presence of infection and guide therapeutic decisions about the need for drainage. When pancreatic infection is present, operative drainage and débridement are indicated. Percutaneous catheter drainage does not permit adequate egress of necrotic tissue. Interest has focused on the selection of closed or open methods of operative drainage and on whether nonoperative or operative therapy is best for patients with noninfected pancreatic necrosis.

ANSWER: E

25. Most patients with acute gallstone pancreatitis are best treated by which of the following measures?

A. Urgent (within 24 hours) cholecystectomy and common bile duct exploration.
B. Urgent endoscopic retrograde cholangiopancreatography (ERCP) and subsequent laparoscopic cholecystectomy.
C. Initial supportive therapy with cholecystectomy during the same admission.
D. Initial supportive therapy with cholecystectomy within 6–8 weeks.
E. Initial supportive therapy, with cholecystectomy only if symptoms recur.

Ref.: 1, 2

COMMENTS: Gallstone pancreatitis is related to passage of stones through the ampulla of Vater. Patients with smaller gallstones have an increased risk of developing this manifestation. Cholecystectomy is indicated because gallstone pancreatitis is a recurrent problem for 30–50% of patients if surgery is not performed. The traditional controversy has been in regard to the timing of operation. Proponents of immediate intervention have found a higher incidence of choledocholithiasis but have not demonstrated that this approach is safer than delayed operation or that it is necessary for most patients. Most surgeons advise initial nonoperative therapy until the patient's signs and symptoms subside (most do within 2–3 days) and then elective cholecystectomy with cholangiography and common duct exploration, as necessary, during the same hospitalization. Laparoscopic cholecystectomy is a safe, effective treatment. Operative evaluation of the common bile duct with intraoperative cholangiography, laparoscopic ultrasonography, or both should be undertaken. The role of urgent ERCP and endoscopic sphincterotomy for management of biliary pancreatitis has been controversial. Remember that most (97%) patients with gallstone pancreatitis have only mild pancreatitis that improves rapidly. ERCP finds common duct stones in only a small percentage of patients and is *not* indicated routinely. Some randomized trials comparing urgent ERCP and sphincterotomy to traditional treatment have suggested benefit for patients with severe pancreatitis, but this has not been consistently observed. ERCP can understandably be useful in patients with pancreatitis and concomitant and persisting biliary obstruction or in patients deemed unfit for surgery. For the small proportion of patients with severe biliary pancreatitis, early cholecystectomy should be avoided. Treatment in this group is directed at resolution of the pancreatitis and its complications. When pancreatitis has subsided, delayed cholecystectomy is indicated.

ANSWER: C

26. Which one or more of the following forms of nutritional support should be avoided in a patient with acute alcoholic pancreatitis?

A. Enteral fat.
B. Parenteral hypertonic dextrose.
C. Parenteral fatty acids.
D. Parenteral amino acids.
E. Parenteral combination of amino acids, glucose, and fat.

Ref.: 2, 7

COMMENTS: Nutritional support is an important component to the successful management of patients with moderate or severe pancreatitis; the mortality rate is lowered for patients achieving a positive nitrogen balance. Effects of specific nutrients and administration routes have been studied. Feeding fat into the stomach and duodenum stimulates pancreatic exocrine secretion and should be avoided. Jejunal feeding of nutrients does not produce the same degree of stimulation. Parenteral administration of fats, glucose, and amino acids alone or in combination does not stimulate the exocrine pancreas. Total parenteral nutrition with intravenous lipid infusions has not been associated with a detrimental outcome and has been critical for reversing nutritional defects and preventing essential fatty acid deficiency. In patients with acute pancreatitis due to hyperlipidemia, however, there is scarce information about the effect of intravenous lipid administration.

ANSWER: A

27. In North America, chronic pancreatitis is most commonly related to chronic alcohol ingestion. Which of the following is the second most common etiology?

A. Gallstone disease.
B. Drug-related.
C. Infectious.
D. Malnutrition.
E. Idiopathic.

Ref.: 3

COMMENTS: In the Western world, alcohol use accounts for about 75% of cases of chronic pancreatitis; approximately 20% of cases are considered idiopathic. In parts of Africa and

Asia, protein malnutrition is an important etiologic factor. Other, less common causes of chronic pancreatitis include pancreatic duct obstruction (stenosis, pancreas divisum), hyperparathyroidism, trauma, cystic fibrosis, and hereditary causes. Unlike acute pancreatitis, calculous biliary disease is not a typical cause of chronic pancreatitis. Certain infections (particularly viral) and drugs are among the many factors that can produce acute, rather than chronic, pancreatitis.

ANSWER: E

28. With regard to histologic characteristics of chronic pancreatitis, all of the following are observed *except*:

A. Increased interstitial connective tissue.
B. Loss of acinar cells.
C. Loss of islet cells.
D. Decrease in nerve tissue.
E. Damaged perineurium.

Ref.: 2

COMMENTS: Chronic pancreatitis is characterized on histologic examination by loss of exocrine acinar cells and a marked increase in interstitial fibrous connective tissue. The islets of Langerhans are preserved and constitute a relatively greater proportion of pancreatic tissue. Hyperplasia of islet cells also is seen. The size and number of nerves are increased, but the protective perineural sheath is damaged and nerves are found in proximity to inflammatory foci. There appear to be selective increases in certain peptidergic nerves. These histologic observations may be related to the etiology of pain in chronic pancreatitis.

ANSWER: C, D

29. Pain is the predominant clinical manifestation of chronic alcoholic pancreatitis. Most patients also have which of the following associated manifestations?

A. Clinical diabetes mellitus.
B. Hypoglycemia.
C. Steatorrhea.
D. Subclinical fat malabsorption.
E. Hepatic cirrhosis.

Ref.: 1, 3, 5

COMMENTS: Recurrent or persistent abdominal pain is the predominant symptom of chronic pancreatitis. Patients usually have variable degrees of nausea, anorexia, and weight loss. Mechanisms that may contribute to pain include ductal obstruction, parenchymal hypertension, acute inflammation, and perineural inflammation. About two-thirds of patients have abnormal glucose tolerance tests and subclinical fat malabsorption, whereas overt diabetes is present in perhaps 30–50% and frank steatorrhea in only 10–15%. Endocrine and exocrine insufficiency progresses during the course of the disease. Diabetes mellitus may be related to impaired insulin release because the islet cells themselves are relatively preserved. Despite the common etiologic factor of ethanol, most patients with chronic pancreatitis do not have hepatic cirrhosis.

ANSWER: D

30. Appropriate management of frank steatorrhea may include all except which of the following choices?

A. Fat restriction to 75 gm/day.
B. Nonencapsulated pancreatic enzymes.
C. Encapsulated pancreatic enzymes.
D. Nonencapsulated pancreatic enzymes and an H_2-blocker.
E. Encapsulated pancreatic enzymes and an H_2-blocker.

Ref.: 2, 3

COMMENTS: Gross steatorrhea and diarrhea occur when pancreatic exocrine function is reduced to about 10% of normal. Therapy involves limitation of fat intake and administration of adequate amounts of exogenous pancreatic enzyme preparations to provide at least 10% of normal lipolytic activity in the duodenum at the time the food substrate is present. Various commercial formulations of pancreatic enzymes are available. Nonencapsulated forms may improve the malabsorption but can be ineffective due to inactivation in the stomach when the pH falls below 4. The addition of H_2-blockers may then be useful. Enteric-coated preparations release their enzymes at a pH above 5; therefore they are useful in patients whose gastric pH remains low so the enzyme is not released until it reaches the duodenum. Use of encapsulated forms with H_2-blockers is counterproductive because the enzyme is released in the stomach and is then inactivated if pH falls. In addition, enteric-coated preparations are microspheres of varying size; the larger ones do not empty into the duodenum until after the food substrate does.

ANSWER: E

31. A 58-year-old woman with jaundice had an endoscopic retrograde cholangiopancreatogram (ERCP) (results shown below) as part of her diagnostic workup. On the basis of this radiograph, what diagnosis is considered the most likely?

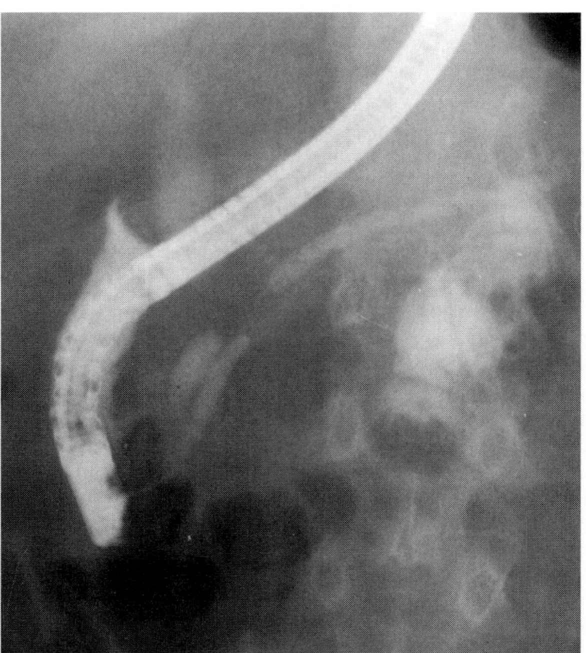

A. Chronic pancreatitis.
B. Pancreatic neoplasm.

C. Cholangiocarcinoma.
D. Pancreas divisum.

Ref.: 1, 5

COMMENTS: This ERCP study shows the classic "double duct sign": dilatation of the biliary system above an area of abrupt narrowing and abrupt termination of the main pancreatic duct. These findings place the primary abnormality in the geographic location of the pancreatic head, and it is not uncommon for a **pancreatic neoplasm** to involve both ducts. **Chronic pancreatitis** may cause biliary obstruction, but the obstruction in the biliary systems is usually more distal. Likewise, no coexistent changes are present in this patient, such as irregular beading of the pancreatic duct, to suggest that there has been chronic pancreatitis. **Cholangiocarcinoma** may be responsible for the stenosis in the biliary system, but cholangiocarcinomas rarely become so grossly large as to involve the pancreatic duct. With **pancreas divisum**, injection of the major papilla opacifies only a short, tapering ventral duct draining the caudal portion of the pancreatic head and uncinate process; injection of the minor papilla demonstrates the dorsal duct draining the major portion of the gland.

ANSWER: B

32. A 45-year-old nondiabetic patient with chronic alcoholic pancreatitis and intractable abdominal pain has a 10 mm pancreatic duct. Which of the following choices constitute(s) the best treatment?

A. Sphincteroplasty.
B. Lateral pancreaticojejunostomy.
C. Caudal (tail) pancreatectomy.
D. Total pancreatectomy.
E. Continued nonoperative therapy.

Ref.: 1, 2, 8

COMMENTS: Pain is the primary indication for surgery in patients with chronic pancreatitis. Selecting the best operation for a particular patient must include consideration of the anatomy of the gland, preexisting endocrine or exocrine dysfunction, compliance and the rehabilitative capacity of the patient, postoperative endocrine or exocrine deficiency, and the likelihood of postoperative pain relief. Patients with a dilated duct (>6 mm) are treated by ductal drainage, with lateral pancreaticojejunostomy being the best choice of these procedures. It is important to achieve adequate decompression of the pancreatic head and uncinate process during drainage procedures. Sphincteroplasty does not have a role in the management of patients with established chronic pancreatitis. Patients with small duct disease are treated by resection if surgery is necessary. Resection of the pancreatic head in properly selected patients generally has yielded better long-term results for pain relief than tail resection. The head of the pancreas is often enlarged and bulky in chronic pancreatitis and has been considered to be the "pacemaker" of the disease. A number of operative techniques are available for pancreatic head resection. Total or near-total 95% resections have higher long-term morbidity and mortality rates related to postoperative endocrine insufficiency. Autotransplantation is investigational for chronic pancreatitis. Although endocrine and exocrine function tends to deteriorate with time in chronic pancreatitis, some evidence suggests that pancreaticojejunostomy halts or delays this decline better than nonoperative therapy.

ANSWER: B

33. Biochemical characteristics of pancreatic ascites include which of the following laboratory values?

A. Fluid amylase level higher than serum amylase level.
B. Fluid amylase level lower than serum amylase level.
C. Fluid protein level higher than 3 gm/dl.
D. Fluid protein level lower than 3 gm/dl.

Ref.: 1, 5

COMMENTS: Pancreatic ascites can be differentiated from ascites of other causes by the characteristic high amylase and protein content of the peritoneal fluid. Pancreatic ascites and pleural effusion are the results of a disruption in the pancreatic duct usually consequent to pancreatitis. The ascites may resolve with conservative management consisting of paracentesis (thoracentesis), total parenteral nutrition, and administration of a somatostatin analogue to inhibit pancreatic exocrine secretion. Otherwise, an operation is required for internal drainage of the pancreatic duct fistula or pseudocyst.

ANSWER: A, C

34. CT scan demonstrates a 5 cm peripancreatic fluid collection in a patient 3 weeks after an episode of acute pancreatitis. The patient is eating and does not have clinical signs of infection. Recommended treatment is:

A. Expectant management without intervention.
B. NPO and total parenteral nutrition.
C. Percutaneous catheter drainage of fluid collection.
D. Operation for external drainage of fluid collection.
E. Operation within 3 weeks for internal drainage of fluid collection.

Ref.: 1, 2, 9

COMMENTS: Peripancreatic fluid collections can be found in about 20% of patients with acute pancreatitis. Many of them resolve spontaneously and should not be mistaken for pancreatic pseudocysts. If the patient is stable, can eat, and does not have clinical evidence of infection or other complications, expectant management is indicated. The fluid collection can be followed with ultrasonography or CT scans in 1–3 months. If the patient has persistent pain and is unable to eat, parenteral nutrition may be instituted for several weeks to allow resolution or maturation of the collection into a pseudocyst. If the patient has a symptomatic or complicated fluid collection that requires early intervention, some method of external drainage must be used. If the fluid is thin, percutaneous catheter drainage may suffice. Operative drainage is preferred if there is substantial necrotic debris, as there often is, or if there is concern about infection.

ANSWER: A

35. Which of the following is the most important determinant of the need for drainage of a pancreatic pseudocyst?

A. Pseudocyst symptoms.
B. Pseudocyst size.
C. Pseudocyst duration.
D. Associated chronic pancreatitis.

Ref.: 1, 2, 9

COMMENTS: Historically, pancreatic pseudocysts larger than 5 to 6 cm in size and present for longer than 6 weeks were thought to have a low rate of spontaneous resolution and a high rate of complications; they were therefore treated by operative drainage. Current understanding of the natural history of pseudocysts is that the rate of spontaneous resolution is higher and the rate of complications lower than previously thought. Pseudocyst size and duration are therefore no longer absolute criteria for intervention. Rather, pseudocyst-related symptoms are the primary indication for treatment. Large pseudocysts are more likely to be symptomatic and less likely to resolve spontaneously than small pseudocysts. Also, pseudocysts in patients with chronic pancreatitis are unlikely to resolve but may not require intervention if they are stable, asymptomatic, and uncomplicated.

ANSWER: A

36. A patient with chronic pancreatitis is unable to eat because of persistent postprandial pain. The CT scan is shown. Recommended treatment is:

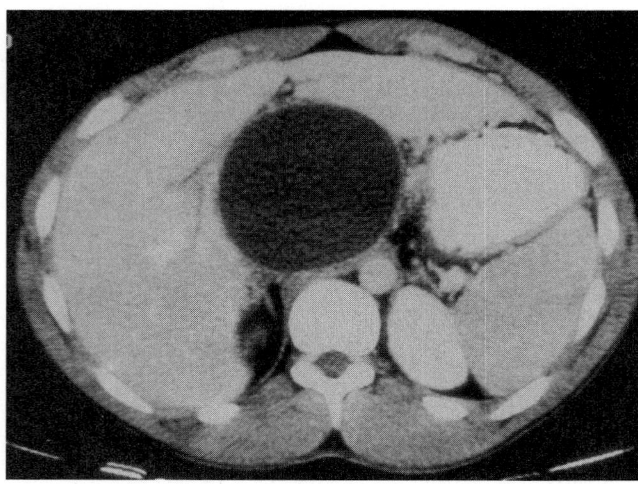

A. NPO and total parenteral nutrition for 4–6 weeks.
B. Percutaneous catheter drainage.
C. Endoscopic drainage.
D. Operative internal drainage.
E. Operative external drainage.

Ref.: 1, 2, 9

COMMENTS: Pseudocysts that develop in patients with chronic pancreatitis can be considered mature when they are discovered unless there also has been a recent episode of acute pancreatitis. The indications for treatment of a pancreatic pseudocyst are (1) persistent symptoms (pain, inability to eat, biliary or gastrointestinal obstruction); (2) enlargement; or (3) onset of a pseudocyst-related complication (infection, hemorrhage, rupture). Operative internal pseudocyst drainage into the stomach, jejunum, or duodenum is generally the preferred treatment depending on the location of the pseudocyst. In patients with chronic pancreatitis, it is critical also to evaluate the pancreatic duct to determine whether a concomitant duct drainage procedure is necessary. Cyst gastrostomy can be accomplished laparoscopically in some situations. Pseudocysts in the tail of the gland are sometimes best treated with distal pancreatectomy. Percutaneous or endoscopic drainage of established pseudocysts is still much debated. These techniques can successfully treat pseudocysts in some circumstances but have definite limitations and potential complications. Selection of the most appropriate approach depends on numerous considerations.

ANSWER: D

37. Which of the following risk factors is most strongly associated with ductal adenocarcinoma of the pancreas?

A. Chronic pancreatitis.
B. Diabetes mellitus.
C. Cigarette smoking.
D. Coffee consumption.
E. Alcohol consumption.

Ref.: 1, 2, 3

COMMENTS: Epidemiologic studies have identified numerous demographic, medical, environmental, and dietary factors that have some relation to pancreatic cancer. The most firmly established risk factor is cigarette smoking; experimentally, nitrosamines have been found to be carcinogenic. Also, carcinogens in cigarettes have been related to K-*ras* oncogene mutations, which are frequent in pancreatic cancer. Alcohol has not been demonstrated conclusively to be a risk factor independent of cigarettes. The previously reported association of pancreatic cancer with coffee consumption is questionable. Diets high in fats and meat may be associated with pancreatic cancer, whereas diets high in fruits and vegetables may be protective. Certain occupational and industrial exposures have an increased risk. There may be some association with diabetes mellitus and certain forms of chronic pancreatitis, but the relation is not considered causal. Prior gastrectomy has been associated with an increased risk, whereas tonsillectomy may be protective.

ANSWER: C

38. A jaundiced, otherwise healthy patient has a 3 cm mass in the head of the pancreas on CT scan. No other disease is apparent. Which of the following is the most appropriate next step?

A. Endoscopic placement of a biliary stent.
B. Operative exploration for resection.
C. Percutaneous fine-needle aspiration.
D. Angiography.
E. Endoscopic ultrasonography.

Ref.: 1, 2, 5

COMMENTS: When the clinical situation suggests a resectable pancreatic neoplasm in a good risk patient with biliary obstruction, operation for potential resection is generally indicated without additional tests. Routine preoperative biliary decompression is not advantageous in this setting and may increase the morbidity associated with resection. Endoscopic biliary decompression is invaluable, of course, for palliation of obstruction in patients deemed inoperable or if operation must be delayed for treatment of a serious concomitant medical problem. Percutaneous pancreatic biopsy is unnecessary for patients who are to be explored and should be discouraged. Although percutaneous fine-needle aspiration is usually safe, it occasionally causes complications that could prohibit curative resection. Angiography was formerly popular for preoperative staging of pancreatic cancer, but its accuracy for determining resectability has limitations and it generally adds little to good quality contrast-enhanced CT scans. Endoscopic ultrasonography has emerged as an adjunct to CT for assessing vascular invasion and can be useful for identifying small tumors that are inapparent on CT. Some surgeons would perform laparoscopy prior to laparotomy on the patient described to identify small liver or peritoneal metastases (which would eliminate resection). Laparoscopic ultrasonography has also become a useful tool for improving the accuracy of laparoscopic staging. If it is determined that the patient is best served by operative palliation because the tumor is found to be unresectable, laparoscopy is unnecessary, although skilled laparoscopic surgeons can perform cholecystojejunostomy and gastrojejunostomy without laparotomy.

ANSWER: B

39. In which one or more of the following situations is resection of a pancreatic tumor contraindicated?

A. Patient age greater than 70 years.
B. Tumor located in body of pancreas.
C. Inability to verify malignancy histologically prior to resection.
D. Tumor invading portal vein.
E. Presence of small peritoneal metastases.

Ref.: 1, 2, 3, 5

COMMENTS: Resection of a pancreatic malignancy offers the only chance for cure. Most commonly, resection of ductal carcinomas involves pancreaticoduodenectomy, as most potentially resectable tumors are located in the head or uncinate process of the gland. Tumors originating in the body or tail of the pancreas are often not diagnosed until they are beyond the confines of surgical resection. However, location alone does not contraindicate resection because, stage for stage, tumors in the body have the same survival as tumors in the head. Resection is indicated for physiologically fit patients (age alone is not a contraindication) who do not have metastases beyond the field of resection. Histologic or cytologic confirmation of malignancy can often be obtained intraoperatively but is not necessary prior to resection if the clinical circumstances suggest cancer and the surgeon is appropriately experienced. Tumors with local vascular invasion are often considered unresectable, but en bloc resection with reconstruction of involved vessels is appropriate for some patients if a tumor-free resection can be accomplished. Positive lymph nodes outside the resection site, peritoneal metastases, and liver metastases contraindicate resection for adenocarcinoma of the exocrine pancreas. However, tumor "debulking" and resection of liver metastases can be beneficial for patients with functioning tumors of the endocrine pancreas.

ANSWER: E

40. Which of the following operations would not be appropriate for a 3 cm adenocarcinoma in the head of the pancreas?

A. Pancreaticoduodenectomy (Whipple) with hemigastrectomy.
B. Pancreaticoduodenectomy (Whipple) with preservation of stomach and pylorus.
C. Duodenum-sparing pancreaticoduodenectomy.
D. Total pancreaticoduodenectomy.

Ref.: 1, 2, 3, 5

COMMENTS: A standard Whipple-type resection with gastrectomy or a pyloric and gastric-preserving resection is indicated for a resectable cancer in the head of the pancreas. Each of these operations yields a long-term survival rate of approximately 15–20%. There is a higher incidence of initial delayed gastric emptying with pyloric-preserving operations. However, long-term studies demonstrate normal emptying and good nutritional outcomes. Likewise, the postprandial gastrin and acid responses are normal despite the loss of duodenal inhibitory factors; and marginal ulcer has not been a prohibitive problem. Additional advantages of the pyloric-preserving technique are shorter operative time and lower operative blood loss. Of course, preservation of the stomach and most proximal duodenum is not appropriate for patients with tumors in close proximity if the margins would be compromised. Duodenum-sparing resection of the pancreatic head has been used in some centers for patients with chronic pancreatitis and has been reported to better maintain enteropancreatic hormonal relations and glucose homeostasis. This operation is not indicated for cancer. Total pancreaticoduodenectomy is not advocated for pancreatic cancers that can be resected otherwise. It has been used based on the grounds that it produces better clearance of lymph nodes and possible multicentric disease and avoids a pancreatic anastomosis. However, long-term survival is not improved and total pancreatectomy is associated with a higher rate of both early and late complications. Extended pancreaticoduodenectomy involves removal of more retroperitoneal soft tissue and regional lymph nodes. Some centers have favored this procedure, but improved survival has not yet been conclusively demonstrated and operative complications may be higher.

ANSWER: C, D

41. At laparotomy a jaundiced patient is found to have an unresectable pancreatic cancer obstructing the bile duct. Which of the following statements regarding biliary decompression is/are correct?

A. Preferred management is to close the patient and place an endoscopic stent postoperatively.
B. Cholecystectomy and T-tube placement is preferred management.
C. Choledochoduodenostomy is contraindicated.
D. Cholecystojejunostomy should not be performed if the patient has cholelithiasis.
E. Roux-en-Y choledochojejunostomy is not appropriate because of limited life expectancy.

Ref.: 1, 2, 3, 5

COMMENTS: Most patients with pancreatic cancer do not have resectable disease. Palliative treatment is directed to relieve obstruction of the bile duct and duodenum and to alleviate pain. For lesions demonstrated to be unresectable prior to laparotomy, nonoperative relief of biliary obstruction can be achieved by the endoscopic (preferred) or transhepatic route. Surgical bypass with some form of biliary enteric anastomosis generally provides more durable relief with less need for further intervention; it is preferred for patients when unresectability is determined at the time of laparotomy. Cholecystojejunostomy, choledo(hepatico)jejunostomy, and choledochoduodenostomy are each appropriate for management of distal bile duct obstruction. If there is extensive disease at the porta hepatis, the left hepatic duct is sometimes useful for anastomosis. Otherwise, transhepatic U-tubes can be placed, or nonoperative decompression can be attempted. T-Tubes are inadequate when the obstruction is proximal. **Choledochojejunostomy** usually provides the most durable relief, although it is somewhat more involved technically. A Roux-en-Y configuration is preferred by many surgeons, although a simple loop (with or without distal enteroenterostomy) also suffices. **Cholecystojejunostomy** is relatively simple but should be avoided if the gallbladder is diseased or when cystic duct patency cannot be demonstrated or may be jeopardized by tumor proximity. It is sometimes taught that **choledochoduodenostomy** should be avoided with malignant obstruction because of possible tumor growth and eventual reobstruction. In reality, choledochoduodenostomy can be an effective solution provided the common bile duct is sufficiently dilated and the duodenum is pliable.

ANSWER: D

42. When should gastrojejunostomy be performed at the time of biliary bypass in a patient with unresectable pancreatic cancer?

A. Always.
B. Never.
C. Only if symptomatic duodenal obstruction is present at the time of operation.
D. Selectively based on tumor extent and anticipated life expectancy.

Ref.: 1, 2, 3, 5

COMMENTS: In addition to biliary obstruction, pancreatic cancers can obstruct the duodenum. Traditionally, many surgeons have favored routine "double bypass" for operated patients because the rate of duodenal obstruction that develops later in patients treated by biliary bypass alone has been cited to be 5–30%. However, most patients do not develop duodenal obstruction, and gastrojejunostomy is sometimes associated with serious problems, such as bleeding or delayed gastric emptying. The selective approach therefore seems appropriate. Certainly, patients with obstructive symptoms or impending obstruction due to tumor location should undergo gastrojejunostomy. Gastrojejunostomy is probably also advisable for patients with an anticipated longer survival, such as those whose lesions are not resected because of local tumor invasion rather than because of hepatic or peritoneal metastases.

ANSWER: D

43. A 45-year-old woman who is not an alcoholic presents with a septated 10 cm cystic mass in the head of the pancreas. Which of the following statements constitute appropriate advice?

A. The lesion is benign and requires no intervention.
B. The lesion is malignant and likely incurable.
C. Pancreaticoduodenectomy is indicated.
D. Percutaneous needle biopsy is indicated.
E. Drainage by Roux-en-Y cyst jejunostomy is indicated.

Ref.: 1, 2, 3, 5

COMMENTS: Cystadenoma and cystadenocarcinoma are cystic neoplasms of the pancreas that most commonly present as mass lesions in middle-aged women. Serous and mucinous types are recognized, and the risk of malignancy is significant in the mucinous variety. Cystadenoma is more common than its malignant counterpart, but malignant transformation may occur; without resection, exclusion of malignancy can be difficult. Internal drainage of cystic neoplasms is not appropriate therapy. Complete excision should be carried out whenever possible. Five-year survival after resection of cystadenocarcinoma is approximately 50%. Occasionally, islet cell tumors, ductal adenocarcinomas, or other unusual tumors (such as papillary and cystic pancreatic neoplasms) present with cystic components.

ANSWER: C

44. Whipple's triad includes which of the following characteristics?

A. Fasting hypoglycemia (<50 mg/dl).
B. Symptoms of hypoglycemia.
C. Jaundice.
D. Hyperamylasemia.
E. Symptoms of hypoglycemia relieved by glucose administration.

Ref.: 1, 3, 5

COMMENTS: See Question 45.

45. Which of the following is/are true regarding the diagnosis of insulinoma?

A. Whipple's triad is pathognomonic.
B. The serum insulin/glucose ratio exceeds 0.3.
C. An oral glucose tolerance test permits differentiation from reactive hypoglycemia.
D. The tolbutamide test is useful for excluding factitious hyperinsulinemia.
E. A CT scan is the most accurate preoperative method for tumor localization.

Ref.: 1, 3, 5

COMMENTS: Whipple's triad clinically establishes hypoglycemia, the differential diagnosis of which requires further evaluation. The biochemical diagnosis of insulinoma is based on the findings of fasting hypoglycemia (<50 mg/dl) and hyperinsulinemia (>20 μU/ml), yielding an insulin/glucose ratio higher than 0.3. The use of tolbutamide or leucine as a provocative test to release insulin may be dangerous and is not required. C-peptide is cleaved from insulin prior to its release, and determination of C-peptide levels may be useful for excluding factitious hyperinsulinemia. Serial blood sampling results following oral glucose administration and subsequent fasting demonstrate persistent hypoglycemia and hyperinsulinemia in the case of organic hyperinsulinism. With reactive hypoglycemia, insulin levels initially rise and glucose falls, but the levels become normal after several hours. Most insulinomas are small; arteriography or selective venous sampling may provide useful preoperative localization. Endoscopic and intraoperative ultrasonography also can aid identification.

ANSWER:
Question 44: A, B, E
Question 45: B, C

46. Which of the following statements is/are true regarding the treatment of insulinoma?

A. Diazoxide, which inhibits insulin release, is the preferred initial method of management.
B. Simple enucleation is acceptable for localized pancreatic lesions.

C. Because most lesions are multiple or diffuse, total or near-total pancreatectomy is usually necessary.
D. Because most lesions are malignant, adjuvant streptozocin is usually indicated.
E. Parathyroid adenoma should be excluded or treated prior to pancreatic resection.

Ref.: 1, 3, 5

COMMENTS: Insulinomas are usually single and benign and are rarely ectopic. Localization of an insulinoma can be difficult, and preoperative imaging along with thorough mobilization and exploration of the pancreas are mandatory; intraoperative ultrasonography is indispensable. For localized lesions, simple enucleation is the preferred treatment, but the integrity of the pancreatic duct must be ascertained. If the lesion cannot be identified and the biochemical basis of the diagnosis is firm, blind distal pancreatic resection with careful histologic examination of the specimen may be necessary. Intraoperative monitoring of serum glucose levels also has been used. Diazoxide inhibits insulin release from beta cells and is occasionally used for preoperative control or for patients with recurrent postoperative hypoglycemia. For patients with metastatic malignant insulinoma, tumor debulking may be beneficial, as is the use of streptozocin and 5-fluorouracil. Gastrinoma, not insulinoma, is the most common pancreatic adenoma associated with multiple endocrine adenomatosis type I (MEA-I) syndrome. Parathyroid disease should be excluded or treated prior to surgical intervention for gastrinoma.

ANSWER: B

47. Match each item in the left-hand column with the appropriate response in the right-hand column to compare the characteristics of Zollinger-Ellison syndrome with those of Verner-Morrison syndrome.

A. Diarrhea	a. Zollinger-Ellison syndrome
B. Decreased gastric acid secretion	b. Verner-Morrison syndrome
C. Increased gastric acid secretion	c. Both
D. Hypercalcemia	d. Neither
E. Malignancy	

Ref.: 1, 3, 5

COMMENTS: Both of these syndromes are produced by islet cell tumors, which in the case of Zollinger-Ellison syndrome secrete gastrin and in the case of Verner-Morrison syndrome secrete vasoactive intestinal peptide. Zollinger-Ellison syndrome is associated with a marked increase in gastric acid secretion and with diarrhea; hypercalcemia may occur because of associated parathyroid abnormalities. The Verner-Morrison syndrome is characterized by watery diarrhea, hypokalemia, and achlorhydria. Hypercalcemia may occur, but the parathyroids are usually normal. Both syndromes are frequently associated with malignant tumors.

ANSWER: A-c; B-b; C-a; D-c; E-c

48. Which of the following is/are characteristic of the clinical syndrome associated with glucagon-producing islet cell tumors?

A. Skin rash.
B. Diabetes.
C. Seizures.
D. Hypoglycemia.
E. Anemia.

Ref.: 1, 3, 5

COMMENTS: Patients with glucagon-secreting tumors present with diabetes, anemia, weight loss, venous thrombosis, glossitis, and a characteristic cutaneous lesion known as "necrolytic migratory erythema." The lesion is rare and often metastatic at the time of diagnosis. Treatment is directed at achieving as complete a resection as possible. Postoperatively, chemotherapy with dacarbazine (DTIC) or streptozocin may be useful for residual or recurrent disease.

ANSWER: A, B, E

49. Which of the following statements is/are true about pancreatic trauma?

A. It most often occurs secondary to blunt abdominal injury.
B. It is the most common cause of pancreatic pseudocyst.
C. Hyperamylasemia is pathognomonic.
D. Negative peritoneal tap effectively excludes a diagnosis of significant pancreatic injury.
E. Exclusion requires exploration of all central retroperitoneal hematomas.

Ref.: 1, 3, 5

COMMENTS: Most pancreatic injuries are the result of penetrating trauma, although the gland is vulnerable to blunt trauma because of its fixed position anteriorly over the vertebral column. The presence of significant pancreatic injury following blunt trauma is not always immediately apparent. Hyperamylasemia in the serum or peritoneal fluid suggests the diagnosis, but a negative peritoneal tap does not exclude significant retroperitoneal injury. Retroperitoneal hematomas in the upper abdomen should be explored to exclude pancreatic ductal injury. Pancreatitis is the most common cause of pseudocyst, although about 25% occur as a result of trauma.

ANSWER: E

50. During surgical exploration for blunt abdominal injury, a patient is found to have complete transection of the pancreatic neck. There is no associated injury. Appropriate treatment includes which of the following items?

A. Drainage alone.
B. Distal pancreatectomy, oversewing of the proximal duct.
C. Roux-en-Y pancreaticojejunostomy to the distal pancreas, oversewing of the proximal duct.
D. Roux-en-Y pancreaticojejunostomy of both proximal and distal segments.
E. Pancreaticoduodenectomy with Roux-en-Y pancreaticojejunostomy to the distal duct.

Ref.: 1, 3, 5

COMMENTS: Pancreatic contusions or lacerations without ductal disruption are managed by drainage alone. The pancreatic neck is a frequent site of pancreatic injury when it occurs with blunt trauma. Distal pancreatectomy with identification and closure of the proximal duct and drainage is safe, and resections involving up to 80% of an otherwise normal gland can be accomplished without subsequent endocrine insufficiency. Roux-en-Y pancreaticojejunostomy may be desirable in theory to preserve pancreatic tissue but is not advisable for the management of acute injuries because of the risk of a pancreatic anastomosis and the need to open the gut. Pancreaticoduodenectomy is indicated only for patients with severe combined duodenal, pancreatic, and bile duct injuries.

ANSWER: B

REFERENCES

1. Sabiston DC Jr: *Textbook of Surgery: The Biological Basis of Modern Surgical Practice*, 15th ed. WB Saunders, Philadelphia, 1997.
2. Howard J, Idezuki Y, Ihse I, Prinz R: *Surgical Diseases of the Pancreas*, 3rd ed. Williams & Wilkins, Baltimore, 1998.
3. Greenfield LJ, Mulholland M, Oldham KT, et al: *Surgery: Scientific Principles and Practice*, 2nd ed. Lippincott-Raven, Philadelphia, 1997.
4. O'Leary JP: *The Physiologic Basis of Surgery*, 2nd ed. Williams & Wilkins, Baltimore, 1996.
5. Schwartz SI, Shires GT, Spencer FC, et al: *Principles of Surgery*, 7th ed. McGraw-Hill, New York, 1999.
6. Sarr MG: Acute necrotizing pancreatitis. *Probl Gen Surg* 13(4), 1996.
7. Pisters PWT, Ranson JHC: Nutritional support for acute pancreatitis. *Surg Gynecol Obstet* 175:275, 1992.
8. Prinz, RA, Deziel DJ: Chronic pancreatitis. *Probl Gen Surg* 15(1), 1998.
9. Deziel DJ, Prinz RA: Drainage of pancreatic pseudocysts: indications and long-term results. *Dig Surg* 13:101–108, 1996.

CHAPTER 36

Spleen

1. Regarding the surgical anatomy of the spleen, which of the following statements is/are true?

   A. The embryologic origin is in the ventral mesogastrium.
   B. The suspensory ligaments, with the exception of the gastrosplenic ligament, normally are avascular.
   C. The spleen is fixed in the left upper quadrant and cannot be safely mobilized.
   D. Accessory spleens are most commonly located along the greater omentum.

Ref.: 1, 2

COMMENTS: Embryologically, the spleen arises from mesenchymal differentiation in the dorsal mesogastrium next to the anlagen of the left gonad. The remnants of the embryologic ventral mesogastrium are the gastrohepatic ligament and the falciform ligament. • The spleen is the second largest organ in the reticuloendothelial system. In adults the spleen weighs 75–100 gm and resides in the posterior aspect of the left upper quadrant adjacent to the diaphragm, colon, stomach, and left kidney. It is suspended by several ligaments, including the gastrosplenic, gastrocolic, splenorenal, and phrenosplenic ligaments, which have some complex relation with the peritoneal reflections in this region. The suspensory ligaments are usually avascular except for the gastrosplenic ligament containing the short gastric vessels. Transection of these suspensory ligaments superiorly, laterally, and inferiorly allows mobilization of the spleen from its position in the left upper quadrant to the midline. In certain disease states, such as portal hypertension or myeloproliferative disorders, the ligaments become replete with vessels and can be a significant source of operative hemorrhage. • The splenic pedicle enters the hilum of the spleen and contains artery, vein, lymphatics, and often the tail of the pancreas. The arterial supply is furnished by the celiac artery via the splenic artery (a direct branch off the celiac) and via the short gastric arteries, which originate off the gastroepiploic, and occasionally the splenic artery. The artery divides into six segmental branches that are end-arteries and form the anatomic basis for partial splenectomy. • Accessory spleens occur in 15–35% of individuals (the percentage is higher in the presence of hematologic disease). The most common location is in the splenic hilum followed by, in decreasing frequency, the gastrosplenic, splenocolic, gastrocolic, and splenorenal ligaments, the greater omentum, and the mesentery. Uncommonly, accessory splenic tissue is found in the pelvis along the left ureter or adjacent to the left gonad.

ANSWER: B

2. With regard to splenic blood supply and microscopic anatomy, which statement is/are true?

   A. The blood supply of the spleen enters the splenic capsule circumferentially.
   B. The blood supply is a segmental end-artery type blood supply.
   C. Because of intervening splenic cords, splenic pulp pressure is isolated from the pressure in the portal venous circulation.
   D. Splenic venous drainage is isolated from the portal circulation via the inferior mesenteric vein.

Ref.: 1, 2

COMMENTS: The spleen has a 1–2 mm thick capsule. At the splenic hilum trabeculae extend from the capsule into the splenic parenchyma, enclosing the splenic pulp into small communicating compartments. Each of these small compartments is divided into three areas or zones: **inner white pulp**, **interfacing marginal zone**, and **outer red pulp**. Arterial branches follow the trabeculae (as trabecular arteries) and enter the white pulp as central arteries. Venous and lymphatic vessels draining the pulp follow these trabeculae peripherally to leave the spleen at the hilum. The central artery branches into various arterioles, some ending in the white pulp, some ending in the marginal zone, and some terminating in the red pulp where they form branching, thin-walled vessels known as splenic sinuses. These sinuses are separated by cords of reticular connective tissue forming splenic cords (or pulp cords). Blood can directly enter these cords via pores in the walls of the splenic sinuses creating an "open" circulation. Approximately 90% of splenic blood flow enters the open circulation of the red pulp. Only 10% passes directly into the venous circulation. Blood from the pulp cords and sinuses drain into pulp veins, which coalesce into trabecular veins. These trabecular veins coalesce to form the splenic vein before entering the portal circulation. Splenic pulp pressure therefore reflects the pressure throughout the portal venous system.

ANSWER: B

3. Which of the following statements is/are true regarding the microanatomy of the spleen?

   A. White pulp serves a phagocytic function.
   B. Red pulp serves an immunologic function.
   C. Microcirculation is predominantly a closed system with direct arteriovenous channels.

D. Cellular elements of the blood pass directly from red pulp cords to sinuses.

Ref.: 1, 2

COMMENTS: The unique microanatomy of the spleen provides the basis for its immunologic and phagocytic functions. The spleen is made up of white pulp, red pulp, and trabeculae that surround and invaginate the pulp. **White pulp**, composed of lymphatic follicles and periarterial lymphatic sheets, serves an immunologic function. Adjacent to the white pulp is a **marginal zone** with lymphocytes, macrophages, and sinuses that filter material from the white pulp. The **red pulp** peripheral to the marginal zone is made up of cords and sinuses through which cellular elements of the blood travel; the red pulp serves primarily a phagocytic function. **Trabecular arteries** bring blood to the central artery of the white pulp from which branches are oriented nearly perpendicular so the plasma is "skimmed off" while the cellular elements of the blood pass through to the red pulp cords. For red blood cells (RBCs) to pass from cords to sinuses where they are subsequently collected for venous drainage, the cells must be deformable. Hence, this is the site for removal of cells with abnormal membrane characteristics. Approximately 90% of blood cells pass through this "open circulation," whereas 10% go through direct arteriovenous connections.

ANSWER: D

4. Normal splenic functions in the human include which one or more of the following items?

A. Reservoir for platelets, RBCs, and white blood cells (WBCs).
B. A site of hematopoiesis throughout life.
C. Removal of abnormal intracellular erythrocyte particles and maturation of reticulocytes.
D. Removal of erythrocytes with abnormal membranes.
E. Production of tuftsin and opsonins.

Ref.: 1, 2

COMMENTS: The spleen has a number of important functions, particularly its immunologic and phagocytic activities. It normally is a reservoir for circulating platelets but is not normally an important reservoir for RBCs or lymphocytes and reticulocytes except in some disease states. In the presence of splenomegaly, as occurs in the presence of portal hypertension, RBC pooling with increased destruction can occur. Normally, an RBC survives 120 days, 2 days of which are spent passing through the spleen. The intraparenchymal trabeculae of the spleen have smooth muscles that can contract and release stored platelets into the systemic circulation. In the fetus the spleen is one of the primary sites of hematopoiesis; this function decreases after birth but can become significant again in the presence of certain pathologic conditions such as myeloid metaplasia. Because of the microvascular anatomy of the spleen, it is an effective filter for old or damaged blood elements and for bacteria and particulate antigens. In concert with its filtering ability, it is important in the phagocytosis of these elements. This phagocytic function is provided by the splenic reticuloendothelial tissue located in the splenic cords. Cell morphology, surface characteristics, and splenic pulp pressure affect the spleen's filtering/phagocytic function. *Pitting* is the process by which the spleen removes abnormal intracellular particles such as Howell-Jolly bodies (nuclear remnants), Heinz bodies (denatured hemoglobin), and Pappenheimer bodies (iron granules) from RBCs with deformable membranes. *Culling* is the removal of RBCs with abnormal, less deformable membranes. **Immunologically**, the spleen produces *opsonins* including *tuftsin* (a peptide that stimulates phagocytosis of leukocytes) and *properdin* (involved in the alternative pathway of complement). The spleen also produces antibodies (particularly immunoglobulin M and other substances). The spleen also has a role in recycling iron released from destroyed RBCs.

ANSWER: C, D, E

5. Which of the following statements regarding the spleen is/are true?

A. Lack of Howell-Jolly bodies after splenectomy suggests an accessory spleen or splenosis.
B. The splenic white pulp, consisting mainly of sinusoids instead of capillaries, has a pressure that reflects the portal venous pressure.
C. Levels of properdin and tuftsin fall after splenectomy.
D. The spleen can only remove cells coated with immunoglobulin A (IgA).

Ref.: 1, 2

COMMENTS: The spleen contains macrophages that are part of the reticuloendothelial system; they function to remove *Pappenheimer bodies* (iron granules), *Heinz bodies* (denatured hemoglobin), and *Howell-Jolly bodies* (nuclear remnants); RBCs 100–120 days old are removed as well. • **Accessory spleens** (mesenchymal splenic remnants that did not fuse) are found in 15–30% of people. • **Splenosis** results from autotransplantation of splenic fragments from a traumatized spleen; these neospleens are capable of performing some reticuloendothelial function. It should be noted, however, that accessory spleens and splenic remnants or transplants do not necessarily perform all, or even part, of the functions of the whole spleen. Evidence suggests that 30–50% of normal splenic volume is required for full function, including protection from postsplenectomy sepsis. • The *splenic pulp* consists of three zones: red pulp, white pulp, and marginal zone. The *red pulp* is an open splenic microcirculation consisting of venous sinuses with pores designed to filter cells in passage. The *white pulp* consists of various leukocytes arranged in a periarteriolar pattern. The marginal zone interfaces these two areas. The venous sinuses, open to the venous circulation, reflect the portal pressure into which they drain. • Properdin and tuftsin are important opsonins manufactured in the spleen. *Properdin* helps initiate the alternative pathway of complement activation, which helps destroy bacteria and other invaders. • The spleen removes cells coated with IgG or IgM. Therefore, autoimmune diseases such as autoimmune hemolytic anemia, immune thrombocytic purpura, and probably Felty syndrome lead to cell destruction in the spleen. The spleen is also the site of clearance of antibody-coated bacteria and is the initial site of IgM synthesis in response to bacteria.

ANSWER: A, C

6. True or False: Bacteria without preexisting antibody are primarily cleared by hepatic reticuloendothelial cells independent of splenic activity.

Ref.: 1, 2

COMMENTS: The reticuloendothelial cells of the spleen are highly effective in removing bacteria and foreign cells coated with antibodies or opsonized protein. The spleen is the major site for clearance of bacteria for which the host lacks preexisting antibodies. The spleen is also the site for initial IgM synthesis against these bacteria. Encapsulated bacteria resist antibody binding. Whereas the reticuloendothelial system of the liver can clear most well opsonized and well antibody-bound bacteria, the spleen is the primary site for removal of poorly opsonized bacteria. Because encapsulated bacteria resist antibody binding, removal of these organisms depends on splenic function. Encapsulated bacteria are ineffectively removed in asplenic individuals.

ANSWER: False

7. Regarding the ruptured spleen, which of the following statements is/are true?

A. The spleen is the organ most commonly injured during blunt abdominal trauma.
B. The spleen is the organ most commonly injured during penetrating abdominal trauma.
C. Spontaneous rupture is most commonly associated with hematologic, rather than infectious, disease.
D. Nonoperative management of splenic injury has increased the frequency of delayed splenic rupture.

Ref.: 1, 2

COMMENTS: The spleen is the most frequently injured organ during blunt trauma to the abdomen or lower thorax. In up to 70% of cases there is associated injury to other organ systems including, in decreasing order of frequency, the ribs, kidney, spinal cord, and liver. Penetrating trauma, however, results in small bowel and liver injuries far more commonly than splenic injuries. • **Spontaneous** splenic rupture is most often caused by complications of malaria and infectious mononucleosis, but it also can occur with sarcoidosis, leukemia, hemolytic anemia, and polycythemia vera. General signs of splenic rupture include pain at the left shoulder as a result of diaphragmatic irritation (Kehr's sign) and a mass or fixed dullness in the left upper quadrant (Ballance's sign). Kehr's sign is elicited by manual compression of the left upper quadrant after placing the patient in Trendelenburg position for several minutes. Kehr's sign is inconsistent, occurring in 15–70% of patients. Ballance's sign is rare. In patients with a ruptured spleen the hematocrit is usually 10–30% below normal, and there is mild leukocytosis. Diagnostic peritoneal lavage, ultrasonography and computed tomography (CT) are accurate tools; of these, CT is probably the most accurate. • "**Delayed**" rupture of the spleen was thought to occur in 10–15% of cases of blunt splenic trauma. The length of the delay, as originally described by Baudet in 1907 (*period de latence*) was less than 2 weeks in 75% of these cases. Delayed rupture represents bleeding confined to the subcapsular area until it ruptures at a later time. This is swiftly becoming less common as newer and more accurate radiologic diagnostic capabilities enable the surgeon to detect and address this type of injury much earlier. • Approximately 30–50% of vascularized splenic tissue is necessary for normal splenic functions. This is pertinent when trying to salvage inadequate fragments of a traumatized spleen; in such instances, total splenectomy is more expeditious and safer.

ANSWER: A

8. Regarding hemolytic anemias, which of the following statements is/are true?

A. They develop because of defects intrinsic to the red blood cell (RBC).
B. They develop because of extracellular factors affecting normal RBCs.
C. Technetium-labeled sulfur colloid is used to determine RBC life-span.
D. Hemolytic anemia develops early because of the limited ability of the bone marrow to increase RBC production.
E. The jaundice associated with hemolytic anemia is caused by elevated levels of conjugated bilirubin.

Ref.: 1, 2

COMMENTS: Hemolytic anemia develops as a result of increased RBC destruction. Congenital hemolytic anemia is a result from defects intrinsic to the RBC. Acquired hemolytic anemias occur when an extracorpuscular factor develops that affects the life-span of normal RBCs. Technetium-labeled sulfur colloid is used to image the reticuloendothelial cells of the liver and spleen. Chromium 51 is used to label RBCs for RBC survival studies. Chromium 51-labeled RBC studies can also be used to detect sites of RBC destruction when evaluating patients with hemolytic anemia. The bone marrow can increase RBC production six- to eightfold. Hemolysis may be severe before anemia develops. The jaundice associated with hemolysis is caused by an excess of unconjugated (free) bilirubin, which is reflected in an increase in the indirect fraction of bilirubin.

ANSWER: A, B

9. Which of the following congenital hemolytic anemias is/are caused primarily by RBC membrane defects?

A. Thalassemia.
B. Sickle cell anemia.
C. Hereditary spherocytosis.
D. Hereditary elliptocytosis.
E. Hereditary pyropoikilocytosis.

Ref.: 1, 2

COMMENTS: **Thalassemia** and **sickle cell anemia** are hereditary disorders of hemoglobin synthesis. **Hereditary spherocytosis, elliptocytosis**, and **pyropoikilocytosis** are abnormalities of RBC membrane synthesis. **Hereditary spherocytosis** is primarily an autosomal-dominant inherited disorder, although 20–25% of cases appear spontaneously. The membrane defect results from a deficiency in *spectrin* (a compound of the RBC membrane skeleton). The severity of its presentation is variable, characterized by anemia, jaundice, cholelithiasis (in up to 55% of patients), and moderate splenomegaly. Diagnosis is made by the presence of spherocytes in the peripheral blood, reticulocytosis, increased osmotic fragility, and a negative Coombs' test. Splenectomy is indicated in all patients and usually can be deferred until age 4. Preoperative ultrasonography should be done to rule out gallstones. Cholecystectomy combined with splenectomy should be performed in patients with gallstones. • **Hereditary elliptocytosis** is characterized by an abundance of elliptical RBCs and is caused by defects in the cell membrane skeleton. Impaired spectrin chain association and a deficiency of protein 4.1 have been identified in these patients. It usually produces a mild anemia, with most patients being asymptomatic. Clinical and laboratory findings in symptomatic patients are similar to those in patients with hereditary spherocytosis except the RBCs are elliptical in appearance.

Results of splenectomy in symptomatic patients is uniformly good. • **Hereditary pyropoikilocytosis** is rare. It is associated with severe alterations of RBC morphology. It occurs primarily in African-Americans. The RBCs are severely deformed, and nearly all RBCs are affected. As with hereditary spherocytosis and elliptocytosis, jaundice is frequently present. Splenectomy reduces hemolysis.

ANSWER: C, D, E

10. Which of the following congenital hemolytic anemias are caused by molecular enzyme alterations?

A. Pyruvate kinase (PK) deficiency.
B. Glucose-6-phosphate dehydrogenase (G6PD) deficiency.
C. Hereditary hydrocytosis.
D. Hereditary xerocytosis.

Ref.: 1, 2

COMMENTS: **PK deficiency** is an example of an enzymopathy involving the Embden-Meyerhof pathway of anaerobic glycolysis. It is inherited as an autosomal recessive trait. RBC energy needs exceed the production capability and lead to increased cell destruction primarily in the spleen. These patients often have splenomegaly. Splenectomy can help, but hemolysis and mild anemia persist. In patients with **G6PD deficiency**, hemolysis is precipitated by infection, certain drugs, and fava beans. Splenomegaly is rare, and splenectomy is not indicated. **Hereditary hydrocytosis** and **hereditary xerocytosis** are rare. They result from altered RBC membrane monovalent cation permeability. Hydrocytosis occurs when the defect allows sodium gain to exceed potassium loss. The cells swell and show increased osmotic fragility. Splenectomy reduces but does not eliminate hemolysis in these patients. Xerocytes form when the defect allows potassium loss to exceed sodium gain, and the cells become dehydrated and develop resistance to osmotic lysis. Hemolysis is rarely severe in these patients, and splenectomy is seldom required.

ANSWER: A, B

11. For which of the following congenital hemolytic anemias is splenectomy most commonly indicated?

A. Thalassemia.
B. Hereditary spherocytosis.
C. Pyruvate kinase deficiency.
D. Glucose-6-phosphate dehydrogenase deficiency.
E. Sickle cell anemia.
F. Hereditary elliptocytosis.

Ref.: 1, 2

COMMENTS: Splenectomy is the sole effective therapy for **hereditary spherocytosis**, which is the most common congenital anemia for which splenectomy is indicated. This disorder is transmitted as an autosomal dominant trait and is characterized by anemia, reticulocytosis, jaundice, and splenomegaly. Cholelithiasis (pigment stones) is seen in up to 55% of patients and should be sought by ultrasonography prior to splenectomy; if identified, concomitant cholecystectomy is appropriate. An erythrocyte membrane defect caused by a lack of spectrin, a major component of the cell membrane skeleton, causes increased osmotic fragility and susceptibility to destruction by the spleen. Splenectomy can generally be delayed until the fourth year of life, at which time the risk of postsplenectomy sepsis is decreased. • Splenectomy can also be an effective therapy for **hereditary elliptocytosis**. This disorder usually is harmless but can become symptomatic when ovalocytes constitute 50–90% of the RBC population. In such cases splenectomy is indicated. • The **thalassemias** have defective hemoglobin synthesis with intracellular precipitates that lead to increased RBC destruction. The patient presents with anemia, splenic infarctions, intercurrent infection, leg ulcers, and gallstones. Splenectomy may be beneficial in decreasing the rate of hemolysis and consequent transfusion requirements and may be indicated in some cases of splenic infarction with pain and infection. • Deficiences in RBC enzymes such as **pyruvate kinase** and **glucose-6-phosphate dehydrogenase** (G6PD) result in hemolysis because the RBCs are unable to utilize glucose. Because the spleen is not always the primary site of hemolysis, the benefit from splenectomy is not predictable and so usually is not required. In severe cases of pyruvate kinase deficiency splenectomy may be worthwhile, but it is not beneficial in G6PD deficiency. • Splenectomy usually is not necessary for **sickle cell anemia** because of the splenic infarction and "autosplenectomy" that eventually occurs in many of these patients. Occasionally, however, patients with sickle cell diseases other than sickle cell anemia (e.g., sickle thalassemia or sickle cell disease) may develop chronic hypersplenism; here, if increased RBC sequestration can be demonstrated, splenectomy may be helpful.

ANSWER: B

12. Regarding thalassemia and sickle cell disease, which of the following statements is/are true?

A. Thalassemia is transmitted as an autosomal dominant trait and occurs in a major (homozygous) and a minor (heterozygous) form.
B. Thalassemia major is characterized by an increase in hemoglobin A and F with abnormal hemoglobins and subsequent splenic sequestration of RBCs necessitating splenectomy.
C. Heterozygons α-thalassemia is associated with severe and debilitating symptoms as compared to heterozygons β-thalassemia.
D. Splenectomy usually is not indicated for sickle cell disease.
E. Patients with sickle cell disease have an increased risk of infectious complications due to autosplenectomy from splenic infarction.

Ref.: 1, 2

COMMENTS: Gene pairs are responsible for synthesis of alpha, beta, gamma, and delta chains of the hemoglobin molecule. Reduction in the production of one of these chains leads to an imbalance in these units, with resultant unstable hemoglobin molecules. Reduction in the beta chain of β-thalassemia is the most common form. **Thalassemia major** (homozygous thalassemia) is the most common form transmitted as an autosomal dominant trait. It becomes apparent during the first year of life and is characterized by pallor, retarded body growth, and enlargement of the head. The characteristic features of this disease are persistence of hemoglobin F (fetal hemoglobin) and decreased hemoglobin A. With thalassemia major, splenectomy occasionally lessens the hemolytic process. In a few patients, splenomegaly or symptomatic repeated splenic infarction constitutes an indication for splenectomy. Most patients with thalassemia major die by the second decade of life from hemosiderosis (iron excess), in contradistinction to patients with **thalassemia minor** (heterozygous thalassemia), who generally are able to lead normal lives and accommodate to a slightly reduced level of hemoglobin. **α-thalassemia** may present in a homozygous or heterozygous form. Homozygous **α-thalassemia** is not compatible with life, although symptoms from heterozygous α- and β-thalassemia are minor and similar. • In **sickle cell disease**, normal hemoglobin A is replaced by abnormal sickle hemoglobin (hemoglobin S). Under conditions of reduced oxygen tension, hemoglobin S undergoes crystallization, producing sickling of RBCs, in turn leading to increased blood viscosity and microvascular stasis. Repeated episodes of stasis may produce splenic infarction, which may lead eventually to autosplenectomy with subsequent symptoms of hyposplenism, including increased risk of infectious complications. Rarely, in patients with sickle cell anemia (homozygous state for hemoglobin S), excessive splenic sequestrations of RBCs can be eliminated by splenectomy. • Although drainage is occasionally suitable therapy for a splenic abscess associated with sickle cell anemia, splenectomy generally is the correct procedure.

ANSWER: A, D, E

13. Regarding the management of patients with idiopathic (immune) thrombocytopenic purpura (ITP), which of the following statements is/are true?

A. Splenectomy is indicated for patients who fail to improve with initial therapy with steroids.
B. Splenectomy is more often necessary in children with ITP than it is for adults.
C. Splenectomy is not indicated in the absence of splenomegaly.
D. Preoperative platelet transfusions are recommended for patients with platelet counts under 50,000/mm^3.
E. The sole reason for splenectomy in ITP is to remove the source of platelet phagocytization.

Ref.: 1, 2

COMMENTS: Although there is no established etiology, it is believed that **idiopathic** (immune) **thrombocytopenic purpura (ITP)** is an autoimmune disease. As such, the initial treatment is with steroids. Splenectomy is recommended for patients who do not respond, for those whose required dose for response is excessive even for a few months, or for those requiring chronic steroid therapy (1 year or longer). Only 25% of adults respond to medical management; up to 88% have relief after splenectomy. • Spontaneous remission occurs in most children (85%), and few need splenectomy. • The diagnosis of ITP is one of exclusion, which requires careful search for possible precipitating factors, such as drugs. The diagnosis also requires a normal to hypercellular megakaryocyte count in the bone marrow. • Splenomegaly is rare in ITP, its presence suggesting another source for thrombocytopenia, such as hemolytic disease. • Generally, platelet transfusions are not required, despite low platelet counts, unless they are needed to control bleeding. Platelets should be withheld intraoperatively until just after the spleen is removed; if given before this time they simply are consumed and confer minimal benefit. • Splenectomy is useful not only for removing the organ responsible for phagocytizing platelets but also for decreasing the *immunologic* response causing the ITP in the first place, as evidenced by the lower IgG levels (especially antiplatelet antibody levels) seen following splenectomy.

ANSWER: A

14. The primary pathophysiology of thrombotic thrombocytopenic purpura (TTP) involves which one of the following characteristics?

A. Circulating antiplatelet antibodies.
B. Venous thrombosis.
C. Arteriolar and capillary occlusion.
D. Intravascular activation of the coagulation cascade.

Ref.: 1, 2

COMMENTS: Thrombotic thrombocytopenic purpura (TTP) is characterized by occlusion of arterioles and capillaries by hyalin deposits composed of aggregated platelets and fibrin; presumably this occurs on an immunologic basis. The classic clinical features include the pentad of fever, purpura, anemia, neurologic manifestations, and renal dysfunction. Unchecked, the disease runs a fulminant course resulting in death, most commonly secondary to intracerebral hemorrhage or renal failure. Current primary therapy of TTP involves high-volume plasmapheresis with fresh-frozen plasma replacement and often with corticosteroids as well; it can result in survival for approximately 50% of patients. Splenectomy no longer is an initial treatment modality, but in patients who fail to respond to plasmapheresis it can be salvage therapy in combination with steroids and dextran as an antiplatelet agent.

ANSWER: C

15. With regard to hypersplenism, which of the following statements is/are true?

A. Hypersplenism is a syndrome of multiple splenic implants, generally seen after traumatic rupture of the spleen.
B. The thrombocytopenia resulting from secondary hypersplenism caused by hepatic disease generally requires splenectomy.
C. Primary hypersplenism rarely responds to steroids, and splenectomy is curative.
D. Gaucher's disease and Felty syndrome may cause secondary hypersplenism.

Ref.: 1, 2

COMMENTS: Hypersplenism is any combination of neutropenia, anemia, and thrombocytopenia caused by splenic cellular sequestration. It is characterized by marrow hyperplasia and splenomegaly. The diagnosis of **primary hypersplenism** is one of exclusion and is confirmed by a clinical response to splenectomy; corticosteroids rarely affect the course of this disease. **Secondary hypersplenism** is most often the result of hepatic disease or extrahepatic portal vein obstruction leading to anemia, leukopenia, or thrombocytopenia, singly or in any combination. In this circumstance, no correlation exists between the degree of cellular depression and symptoms. Splenectomy usually is not necessary in those with liver disease, especially in light of their frequent lack of symptoms (e.g., petechiae). • **Gaucher's disease** (familial disorder characterized by disordered lipid metabolism leading to splenomegaly) and **Felty syndrome** (splenomegaly, hepatomegaly, and adenopathy associated with rheumatoid arthritis) are examples of diseases causing secondary hypersplenism. Secondary hypersplenism also can be caused by work hypertrophy from an immune response and RBC destruction, venous congestion, myeloproliferation, infiltration, and neoplastic proliferation within the spleen. **Splenosis** is the term used to refer to the condition of multiple splenic implants, generally following traumatic injury to the spleen.

ANSWER: C, D

16. Match the anatomic involvement with Hodgkin's disease in the left column with the appropriate clinical stage of the disease in the right column.

A. Right axillary lymph nodes
B. Epigastric lymph nodes; liver
C. Left cervical lymph nodes; right mediastinal lymph nodes
D. Left cervical lymph nodes; epigastric lymph nodes; spleen
E. Left cervical lymph nodes; left axillary lymph nodes with an adjacent extranodal focus

a. Stage I
b. Stage II
c. Stage III
d. Stage IV
e. Stage IIE

Ref.: 1, 2

COMMENTS: The treatment and prognosis of Hodgkin's disease is related to the histologic type and clinical stage at the time of presentation. Hodgkin's disease is commonly staged as follows (Ann Arbor classification): stage I—one area or two contiguous areas of lymph node involvement on the same side of the diaphragm; stage II—two noncontiguous areas on the same side of the diaphragm; stage III—involvement on each side of the diaphragm (for purposes of this classification the spleen is considered a lymph node); stage IV—involvement of liver, bone marrow, lung, or any other non-lymph-node tissue, exclusive of the spleen. The superscript E signifies involvement adjacent to involved lymph nodes. There are those who believe that even rather extensive lung parenchymal disease can be considered stage IIE rather than stage IV disease because of the often good prognosis associated with lung presentations. In addition to staging the disease anatomically, the system is modified to allow distinction between patients who are asymptomatic ("A" patients) and those who have constitutional symptoms such as night sweats, fever (temperature higher than 38°C), or 10% weight loss within 6 months ("B" patients).

ANSWER: A-a; B-d; C-b; D-c; E-e

17. Regarding staging laparotomy of patients with Hodgkin's disease, which of the following statements is/are true?

A. Lymphangiography and computed tomography (CT) scanning used together have eliminated the need for a staging laparotomy in most patients.
B. The operative technique of a staging laparotomy is different for women than it is for men.
C. Partial splenectomy is adequate for staging and has helped lower the incidence of postsplenectomy sepsis.
D. Laparotomy for purposes of splenectomy described in statement C is indicated, because it enhances the quality and duration of response to chemotherapy.
E. Staging laparotomy results in a change in the stage of Hodgkin's disease in 30–40% of cases.

Ref.: 1, 2

COMMENTS: Accurate staging is critical if one is to avoid the consequences of over- or undertreatment. Although CT scanning, lymphangiography, and other noninvasive tests may obviate the need of laparotomy for staging select patients, such noninvasive means of clinical staging occasionally are inaccurate. This is particularly true when assessing upper abdominal lymph nodes, spleen, and liver. In most reported clinical series, the preoperative stage of the disease changes in 30–40% of patients following laparotomy; slightly more cases are up-staged (and need more aggressive therapy) than are down-staged. It should be stated that in few of these reports are *all* patients studied by CT. This fact notwithstanding, several groups of patients do not require a staging laparotomy: Those with stage IA disease (especially with lesions of nodular sclerosing histology, with isolated high cervical lymph nodes) do not because the likelihood of subdiaphragmatic disease is exceedingly remote. Patients with clearly advanced disease (stage III or IV), as determined by lymphangiography and CT scan or bone marrow biopsy, likewise do not require a staging laparotomy because their treatment includes systemic chemotherapy. • Symptomatic patients with stage I or II disease ("B" patients) require staging laparotomy to search for occult visceral or intraabdominal involvement if they are to avoid systemic therapy (chemotherapy). Similarly, patients with an equivocal lymphangiogram or CT scan probably should be staged by laparotomy. The controversy centers on patients with stage 1A or 2A disease (other than those with isolated high cervical node involvement). In this group, laparotomy provides the most accurate staging but, unless there is symptomatic splenomegaly, carries with it the risk of an unnecessary operation. • In women of childbearing age wishing to remain fertile, oophoropexy (repositioning the ovaries to the midline) should be performed to move them away from the radiation field in the event irradiation of the iliac lymph nodes becomes necessary. • Partial splenectomy is not sufficiently accurate for staging to justify its use. • Certain splenic involvement (as can be determined with noninvasive tests) does not necessarily constitute an indication for splenectomy; in most series the morbidity associated with radiation therapy and chemotherapy as treatment in these patients is not significantly increased. However, if at the time of staging celiotomy Hodgkin's disease is identified at extrasplenic sites, the spleen should be removed, even if it is not involved. On occasion, splenectomy other than that associated with staging is necessary in patients with advanced disease, purely for relief of symptoms. • Finally, there is a fairly prominent school that holds that staging laparotomy is never necessary.

ANSWER: B, E

18. In which one or more of the following disorders does splenectomy clearly have a beneficial influence on survival?

A. Chronic lymphocytic leukemia.
B. Chronic myeloid leukemia.
C. Non-Hodgkin's lymphoma.
D. Hairy cell leukemia.
E. Myeloid metaplasia.

Ref.: 1, 2

COMMENTS: Hairy cell leukemia, so named because of the characteristic cellular appearance under a light microscope, was thought best treated initially by splenectomy, with good expectation for long-term survival. This view, however, is probably no longer held universally. Instead, splenectomy has been supplanted by interferon therapy, which induces a stable remission in most patients. The cytotoxic agents deoxycoformycin and 2-chlorodeoxyadenosine also have this potential.

Splenectomy is best reserved for those who fail to improve after such medical management. Splenectomy is primarily palliative for the remainder of the disorders that follow. • **Chronic lymphocytic leukemia**, characterized by abnormal lymphocytes, lymphadenopathy, splenomegaly, and lymphocytosis, often follows an indolent course. Splenectomy is performed primarily for the hematologic consequences of hypersplenism or for palliation in symptomic splenomegaly. • This is also true for **non-Hodgkin's lymphoma**. Because most patients with non-Hodgkin's lymphoma have disseminated disease at the time of diagnosis, splenectomy is performed much less often as a staging procedure and more often for palliation. • **Chronic myeloid leukemia**, with its high leukocyte counts and characteristic Philadelphia chromosome, may require splenectomy to alleviate thrombocytopenia, anemia, or pain from splenomegaly. Death often is from myeoblastic crisis. Splenectomy again is palliative and does not delay blastic transformation, improve life after transformation, or generally prolong survival. • The course of **myeloid metaplasia** is likewise not altered by splenectomy, although significant palliation may be obtained.

ANSWER: D

19. Regarding the role of splenectomy in the treatment of acquired immune hemolytic anemias, which of the following statements is/are true?

A. Splenectomy is indicated only after failure of steroid therapy.
B. Splenectomy may be indicated for warm antibody-type immune hemolytic anemia.
C. Splenectomy may be indicated for cold antibody-type acquired immune hemolytic anemia.
D. Splenectomy is contraindicated for acquired immune hemolytic anemias.
E. Postoperative thromboembolic complications are more common when splenectomy is performed for acquired immune hemolytic anemias.

Ref.: 1, 2

COMMENTS: Splenectomy may be *beneficial* for *certain* acquired immune hemolytic anemias just as it is beneficial for certain congenital anemic disorders. The acquired immune hemolytic anemias can be divided into cold and warm antibody types. With the **warm antibody type**, IgG antibody binds to cell membranes, and the RBCs are subsequently removed by the spleen. There is no complement fixation or direct hemolysis. Corticosteroids constitute the first line of therapy, but 30–40% of patients do not respond, or they sustain relapse; approximately 80% of them respond to splenectomy. Splenectomy is *not* indicated for treatment of the **cold antibody type** immune hemolytic anemias; these anemias are mediated by IgM antibody and complement fixation to direct intravascular cell lysis. *Postoperative morbidity* following splenectomy for acquired hemolytic anemia is no higher than that with other hematologic disorders. An increase in thromboembolic complications has been observed, however, following splenectomy for myeloproliferative disorders.

ANSWER: A, B

20. Regarding postsplenectomy sepsis, which of the following statements is/are true?

A. It is the most common complication of splenectomy for hematologic disease.
B. The onset is typically characterized by sudden high fevers.
C. It is more common in adults than in children.
D. It is more commonly fatal in children than in adults.
E. It is more common after splenectomy for hematologic disease than for trauma.

Ref.: 1, 2

COMMENTS: Overwhelming postsplenectomy sepsis is an uncommon but well recognized potential complication of splenectomy. The risk of postsplenectomy sepsis depends on the age of the patient and the reason for splenectomy. It occurs in 0.3% of adults and 0.6% of children and is more common when splenectomy is performed for hematologic disease. Postsplenectomy sepsis is uncommon in adults undergoing splenectomy for trauma. The mortality of postsplenectomy sepsis exceeds 50% in children and approximates 30% in adults. Most episodes occur within the first 2 years after splenectomy, although it can occur later. The typical onset of this clinical syndrome is often insidious, marked by nonspecific symptoms of malaise, headache, nausea, and confusion; it can progress rapidly to shock and death within 48–72 hours. The most common organisms are encapsulated bacteria, such as *Streptococcus pneumoniae* (50% of cases), *Haemophilus influenzae*, *Neisseria meningitidis*, *Escherichia coli*, β-hemolytic streptococci, and *Pseudomonas*.

ANSWER: D, E

21. Appropriate steps to prevent postsplenectomy sepsis include which one or more of the following measures?

A. Administration of polyvalent vaccines if the splenectomy is for a child.
B. Avoidance of splenectomy in children under 4 years of age.
C. Routine prophylactic antibiotics after splenectomy.
D. Splenic preservation by splenorrhaphy when possible.
E. Autotransplantation of splenic fragments when splenectomy is necessary.

Ref.: 1, 2

COMMENTS: Preventive measures against postsplenectomy sepsis include the use of Pneumovax, which should be given before splenectomy if possible. *Haemophilus* flu vaccine is now given to *all* children as part of routine immunization. *Meningococcus* vaccine is *not* routinely given. Prophylactic antibiotics are recommended for children under age 10 years (but compliance is often inadequate). Prophylactic antibiotics also should be considered for patients with immunosuppression. The administration of antibiotic prophylaxis in other individuals has not been shown to decrease the risk of postsplenectomy sepsis. • Because the risk of this syndrome is greatest in children, elective splenectomy should be postponed if possible until the child is 4 years old. Concerted attempts at splenic preservation, by nonoperative therapy or splenorrhaphy for young children with splenic injury, also are appropriate. • Perhaps one of the most important methods for preventing postsplenectomy sepsis is to evaluate patients having splenectomy and have them seek prompt medical consultation with the first signs of illness. Although our understanding of the precise requirements for relatively normal splenic function is incomplete, experimental findings permit certain observations. Evidence suggests that with partial splenectomy at least one-third of functioning splenic tissue is necessary for immunologic protection. Blood flow is also critical in that immunologic protection is lost following splenic artery ligation. Finally, it should be kept in mind that although it is laudable to attempt splenic preservation to avoid postsplenectomy sepsis, this syndrome is uncommon. Excessive concern with preservation should not compromise the welfare of the trauma patient during the operation. • Autotransplantation of splenic fragments has been investigated as an attempt to preserve critical splenic function. Following autotransplantation, immunologic function in the form of increases in IgM and serum complement can be demonstrated, as has resumption of filtering function by disappearance of target cells and Howell-Jolly bodies. These functions are apparently subnormal, however, and do not provide protection against postsplenectomy sepsis.

ANSWER: A, B, D

22. Which of the following hematologic or immunologic changes is/are anticipated following splenectomy?

A. Increased RBC volume and RBC survival.
B. Increased number of circulating WBCs and platelets.
C. Abnormal circulating RBC forms.
D. Increased serum IgM.
E. Decreased antibody response to intravenous antigens.

Ref.: 1, 2

COMMENTS: Based on the spleen's filtering, phagocytic, and immunologic functions, a number of changes can be expected related to loss of these functions following splenectomy. Hematologically, circulating RBCs with abnormal forms (target cells) and abnormal cytoplasmic inclusions (e.g., Howell-Jolly bodies) are seen. However, RBC survival may improve dramatically in hereditary spherocytosis and warm antibody acquired hemolytic anemia, whereas RBC volume and survival generally remain unchanged. Sometimes the RBC volume increases because more reticulocytes are permitted to remain in the circulation. There are increases in the number of circulating WBCs and platelets. Immunologically, decreases in serum IgM, tuftsin, opsonin, and properdin are seen. Bacterial clearance and antibody response to intravenous antigens are impaired. T cell function also may be altered.

ANSWER: A, B, C, E

23. During the performance of a left hemicolectomy, an actively bleeding 2 cm laceration at the inferior pole of the spleen is discovered. Appropriate initial management includes which one or more of the following measures?

A. Splenorrhaphy with topical hemostatic agents, suture repair, or both.
B. Partial splenectomy.
C. Splenectomy.
D. Drainage of the left upper quadrant.

Ref.: 1, 2

COMMENTS: Iatrogenic splenic injuries incurred during the course of unrelated abdominal operations are particularly amenable to splenorrhaphy rather than splenectomy because of the generally limited nature of such injuries. An additional concern has been the increased risk of postoperative complications and even long-term septic sequelae reported in patients undergoing incidental splenectomy. Simple techniques such as compression, cautery, and the use of topical hemostatic agents alone or in combination with simple suture repair are adequate for more than 90% of mild or moderate splenic injuries, including most iatrogenic injuries. Partial splenectomy is reserved for a small percentage of patients in whom a substantial segment of spleen can be salvaged in an otherwise extensively injured organ. Most iatrogenic injuries, because of their limited nature, should not require splenectomy. However, if the surgeon is not able to control the bleeding, splenectomy may be necessary. Complications related to splenorrhaphy following splenic injury are uncommon; the overall rate of rebleeding following splenorrhaphy for any reason is less than 2%. Drainage of the left upper quadrant generally is not necessary.

ANSWER: A

24. Partial, rather than total, splenectomy may be the correct operation for which of the following conditions?

A. Felty syndrome.
B. Gaucher's disease.
C. Splenic sarcoidosis.
D. Splenic hemangioma.

Ref.: 1, 2, 3

COMMENTS: **Gaucher's disease** is an inherited metabolic disorder in which deficiency of acid β-glucosidase activity results in the accumulation of glycosyl ceramide in reticuloendothelial cells of the liver, bone, and spleen. Traditionally, splenectomy has been the therapy for patients with this condition, who develop hypersplenism or mechanical symptoms due to splenomegaly. More recent experience has shown that partial splenectomy can be beneficial for these patients. Also, because accelerated bone disease and an increased risk of malignancy have been observed in patients with Gaucher's disease following total splenectomy, it has been suggested that partial splenectomy may be the procedure of choice. **Felty syndrome** describes the clinical association of rheumatoid arthritis, splenomegaly, and neutropenia. Patients are plagued by recurrent infections. Because neutropenia is secondary to both antibody and splenic destruction, a good and lasting response to total splenectomy can occur. Granulomatous involvement of the spleen by **sarcoidosis** can produce anemia and thrombocytopenia and occasionally requires total splenectomy. **Splenic hemangiomas** constitute the most common benign neoplasms of the spleen. For the most part, they are asymptomatic and require no therapy. If the hemangioma is large, it may be associated with thrombocytopenia and pancytopenia or even rupture; in these instances total splenectomy is appropriate.

ANSWER: B

REFERENCES

1. Sabiston DC Jr: *Textbook of Surgery*, 15th ed. WB Saunders, Philadelphia, 1997.
2. Schwartz SI, Shires GT, Spencer FC: *Principles of Surgery*, 7th ed. McGraw-Hill, New York, 1999.
3. Fleshner PR, Aufses AM Jr, Grabowski GA, Elias R: A 27-year experience with splenectomy for Gaucher's disease. *Am J Surg* 161:69–75, 1991.

CHAPTER 37

Hernia, Abdominal Wall, and Retroperitoneum

1. Match each item in the left column with the corresponding item in the right column.

Abdominal Wall Layers	***Spermatic Cord Layers***
A. Subcutaneous tissue	a. Cremasteric muscle
B. Transversalis fascia	b. Internal spermatic fascia
C. External oblique	c. Obliterated processus vaginalis
D. Internal oblique	d. Dartos muscle (in the scrotum)
E. Parietal peritoneum	e. External spermatic fascia

Ref.: 1, 2, 3

COMMENTS: During descent of the testicle from its original retroperitoneal position to the scrotum, it passes through the abdominal wall. Understanding the anatomic continuations of the abdominal wall layers onto the spermatic cord is essential for the proper performance of herniorrhaphy.

ANSWER: A-d; B-b; C-e; D-a; E-c

2. Which of the following statements is/are true regarding the iliopubic tract?

   A. Extends from the anterosuperior iliac spine to the pubis.
   B. Is a condensation of the transversalis fascia.
   C. Is of anatomic interest but has little clinical significance.
   D. Is synonymous with the shelving portion of Poupart's ligament.
   E. None of the above.

Ref.: 2, 3

COMMENTS: The transversalis fascia is the portion of the endoabdominal fascia that underlies the transversus abdominis muscle. It has several thickenings, the most important of which is the iliopubic tract arising from the iliopectineal arch, inserting on the anterosuperior iliac spine, and extending over the femoral vessels to the pubis. Proper utilization of the transversalis fascia during repair of an inguinal hernia is important to the success of operations not utilizing prosthetic materials.

ANSWER: A, B

3. Which of the following statements is/are true regarding Hesselbach's triangle?

   A. Defines the boundaries of a low lumbar hernia.
   B. Defines the inguinal floor in the region of a direct inguinal hernia.
   C. Is found in a single plane of the inguinal floor and is bounded by the inferior epigastric artery, inguinal ligament, and rectus sheath.
   D. Is bounded medially by the inferior epigastric vessels.
   E. None of the above.

Ref.: 1, 2, 3

COMMENTS: A direct inguinal hernia projects through the inguinal floor in the region of Hesselbach's triangle. The boundaries of this anatomic triangle are generally considered to be the inguinal ligament inferiorly, the inferior epigastric artery laterally, and the lateral border of the rectus sheath medially. This definition is not anatomically precise, however, because none of the borders is in the same abdominal wall layer, and all are superficial to the floor of the inguinal canal. The inferior epigastric vessels may be useful landmarks for differentiating groin hernias because indirect hernias originate lateral to these vessels and direct hernias originate medial to them. Large indirect hernias disrupt the posterior inguinal wall medial to the epigastric vessels, thereby extending to the region of Hesselbach's triangle. Because surgical treatment of most adult inguinal hernias (direct or indirect) requires some repair or mesh replacement of the floor, the concept of the triangle is more an aid to teaching anatomy.

ANSWER: B

4. Which of the following statements is/are true regarding the incidence of abdominal wall hernias?

   A. The indirect inguinal hernia is the most common hernia in either gender.
   B. Femoral hernias are more common in females than in males.
   C. Direct hernias are unusual in females.
   D. Hernias generally occur with equal frequency in males and females.
   E. None of the above.

Ref.: 1, 2, 3

COMMENTS: Approximately three-fourths of all abdominal wall hernias occur in the inguinal region, and roughly two-thirds of them are indirect inguinal hernias. In general, hernias are considered to be at least five times more common in males than in females; the most common hernia in each gender is the indirect variety. It has been estimated that 25% of males and only 2% of females develop inguinal hernias during their lifetime. Hernias therefore constitute a significant economic problem in terms of loss of time from work.

ANSWER: A, B, C

5. Which of the following statements is/are true regarding direct inguinal hernias?

A. The most likely etiology is acquired wear and tear.
B. Direct hernias should be repaired promptly because of the risk of incarceration.
C. A direct hernia may be a sliding hernia involving a portion of the bladder wall.
D. A direct hernia may pass through the external inguinal ring.
E. None of the above.

Ref.: 1, 2, 3

COMMENTS: Direct inguinal hernias generally are acquired from the "wear and tear" of daily life; other factors, such as chronic straining to urinate or defecate, chronic coughing, and heavy lifting, have been implicated as well. Because generally there is a diffuse weakness in the area of Hesselbach's triangle without a narrow-necked sac, the risk of incarceration is low. Rarely, incarceration results when the direct hernia passes through the external ring posterior to the cord structures. The involvement of the urinary bladder as a sliding component on the medial wall of a direct hernia sac usually does not cause a problem because the sac can be simply reduced unopened.

ANSWER: A, C, D

6. A sliding inguinal hernia on the right side is likely to involve which of the following?

A. Ileum composing the posterior wall of the sac.
B. Ovary and fallopian tube in a female infant.
C. A loop of small bowel fixed by adhesions.
D. Cecum composing the posterior wall of the sac.
E. Cecum composing the anteromedial wall of the sac.

Ref.: 1, 2, 3

COMMENTS: A sliding hernia is one in which the visceral peritoneum of an organ makes up a part of the wall of the hernia sac. If the hernia is indirect, it most commonly involves the cecum on the right or the sigmoid colon on the left. In females, especially infants and children, portions of the female genital tract often are involved. Recognition of the presence of a sliding hernia and the position of the visceral component is important to avoid injury of the involved organs during repair.

ANSWER: B, D

7. Which of the following statements is/are true regarding groin hernias in females?

A. Femoral hernias are more common than inguinal hernias.
B. A mass within a hernia in a female infant is usually a nonfunctioning ovary.
C. An ovary present within a hernia should be returned to the abdominal cavity before repair is completed.
D. During repair of an indirect inguinal hernia, the round ligament should be preserved.
E. Biopsy should be performed on any abnormal-appearing gonad found in a hernia sac.

Ref.: 1, 2, 3

COMMENTS: Although femoral hernias are found more often in females than in males, inguinal hernias are still more common than femoral hernias. The round ligament is usually adherent to the hernial sac when an indirect hernia is present; the round ligament can simply be divided, and recurrence of an indirect hernia in females is extremely unusual. A solid mass palpable within the hernia of a female infant is usually a normal ovary that simply is returned to the abdominal cavity. The internal ring can be closed completely after retiring the ovary and fallopian tube to the abdominal cavity. If the gonad appears abnormal or resembles a testicle, however, biopsy must be performed to rule out testicular feminization. Most patients with this syndrome have inguinal hernias.

ANSWER: C, E

8. Correct statements regarding the management of an incarcerated groin hernia include which of the following?

A. Intravenous sedation and attempted reduction of an inguinal hernia are appropriate.
B. Successful reduction eliminates the possibility of obstruction.
C. Operation is indicated only after repeated attempts at reduction have failed.
D. If reduction is successful, delayed repair may be performed in 2–3 days.
E. Opening of the hernial sac prior to reduction at the time of operation is essential.

Ref.: 1, 2, 3

COMMENTS: Incarceration and subsequent strangulation of small bowel are serious complications of groin hernias, particularly femoral hernias, which have a narrow neck and greater likelihood of trapping bowel segments. If the patient has an incarcerated inguinal hernia and strangulation is not suspected, an attempt at reduction by using sedation, Trendelenburg's positioning, and gentle sustained pressure over the groin mass is appropriate. Vigorous repetitive attempts at reducing an incarcerated hernia are ill-advised and may produce "reduction en masse," wherein the entire hernial sac and its contents are reduced so that even though the external bulge is gone the incarceration within the sac remains. If there is any indication of strangulation, reduction should not be attempted preoperatively. Rather, the sac should first be opened prior to reduction to inspect the viability of the contents. Delayed repair following successful reduction may permit resolution of edema.

ANSWER: A, D, E

9. Which of the following statements about the management of inguinal hernias in infants and children is/are true?

A. Repair should be delayed until the child is 2 years of age.
B. Repair usually requires only high ligation of the hernial sac.
C. The distal sac should be removed to prevent formation of a secondary hydrocele.
D. Contralateral inguinal exploration is indicated routinely because of the high risk of bilaterality.
E. None of the above.

Ref.: 1, 2, 3

COMMENTS: Inguinal hernias in infants and children are nearly always indirect, resulting from failure of obliteration of the processus vaginalis. Effective treatment requires only high ligation and transection of the sac with or without excision of the distal component. Repair need not be delayed unless the infant has associated medical problems. In fact, bowel obstruction and gonadal or intestinal infarction as a result of strangulation are most likely to occur during the first 6 months of life; therefore repair should be performed soon after the diagnosis is made. Exploration of the opposite side in children who present with a unilateral inguinal hernia is controversial. The incidence of a contralateral hernia following unilateral inguinal herniorrhaphy in children has been reported to be 10–30%. Contralateral exploration should be performed routinely in the subset of patients most likely to have a clinically occult hernia: patients less than 2 years old, females less than 3 years old (higher bilateral rate), patients with ventriculoperitoneal shunts, and patients less than 2 years with a *left*-sided hernia. This last recommendation is based on the fact that most (60%) pediatric hernias are *right*-sided. Intubation of the clinically apparent hernia sac with a laparoscope is one method of examining the contralateral side.

ANSWER: B

10. Which of the following statements is/are true regarding the preperitoneal or posterior approach for the repair of groin hernias?

A. It may be appropriate for repair of both direct and indirect inguinal hernias.
B. It may be appropriate for repair of femoral hernias.
C. It is performed through the same skin incision as for the anterior approach.
D. When performing a Cooper's ligament repair via a preperitoneal approach, a transition suture is not required.
E. None of the above.

Ref.: 2, 3

COMMENTS: The preperitoneal approach, utilizing a horizontal skin incision three fingerbreadths above the pubic tubercle, has been especially successful in the repair of femoral hernias. Both direct and indirect inguinal hernias also can be approached in this manner, although many surgeons have reported higher recurrence rates for direct hernias when using this approach. A Cooper's ligament repair is carried out in the same way as for an anterior approach: The ligament is approximated to the transversus abdominis aponeurosis medially with a transition suture between the transversus aponeurosis, the iliopubic tract, and Cooper's ligament, with completion laterally by approximation of the iliopubic tract and transversus aponeurosis. This approach, as originally described, has not achieved widespread use. Modifications of the preperitoneal approach utilizing prosthetic material have become more popular, particularly for repair of recurrent hernias. General or regional anesthesia is necessary. Postoperative paralytic ileus is not infrequent.

ANSWER: A, B

11. Match the type of hernia repair in the left column with the appropriate statement in the right column.

A. McVay repair
B. Bassini repair
C. Preperitoneal repair
D. Shouldice repair
E. Lichtenstein repair

a. Variation of Bassini repair with overlap of transversalis plane with four lines of continuous suture
b. Transversus abdominis aponeurosis approximated to Cooper's ligament
c. Transversus abdominis aponeurosis approximated to Poupart's ligament
d. Posterior approach to hernia repair
e. Tension-free replacement of transversalis fascia with mesh

Ref.: 1, 2

COMMENTS: The **Bassini** repair and its modifications is accomplished by suturing the conjoined tendon of the transversus abdominis and the internal oblique muscles to the inguinal (Poupart's) ligament. The **McVay** (Cooper's ligament) operation is used for large inguinal hernias and recurrent hernias, and it is ideally suited to repairing femoral hernias. Beginning at the pubic tubercle, the conjoined tendon is sutured to Cooper's ligament; at the femoral canal a transition is made whereby the conjoined tendon is sutured to the inguinal ligament laterally. A relaxing incision is required if mesh is not used. Complications include femoral vein injury. The **Shouldice** repair utilizes a multilayer, imbricated repair of the inguinal canal floor with running sutures. The **Lichtenstein** repair utilizes a segment of prosthetic material sutured medially to the pubic bone, inferiorly to Poupart's ligament, and superiorly to the conjoined tendon. Laterally the mesh is split, wrapped around the spermatic cord, and the tails sutured together.

ANSWER: A-b; B-c; C-d; D-a; E-e

12. Which of the following hernias is most likely to recur after primary repair?

A. Umbilical hernia.
B. Spigelian hernia.
C. Incisional hernia.
D. Indirect inguinal hernia.
E. Femoral hernia.

Ref.: 1, 2, 3

COMMENTS: Despite the use of prosthetic material to reduce tension, the rates of recurrence after incisional hernia repair remain at 10% or higher. This may be the result of a lack of success in correcting some of the predisposing factors to incisional hernia, such as obesity, chronic debilitating illness, advanced age, and smoking. The recurrence rates after the other listed hernia repairs should all be 5% or less.

ANSWER: C

13. Which of the following statements is/are true regarding recurrence after repair of groin hernias?

A. Most indirect recurrences are attributed to an inadequate repair of the inguinal floor.
B. Indirect hernias at any age have a lower recurrence rate than either direct or femoral hernias.
C. Most recurrent hernias are direct.
D. Recurrence rates are higher following bilateral simultaneous herniorrhaphy in adults.
E. None of the above.

Ref.: 1, 2, 3

COMMENTS: Recurrence rates for groin hernias vary between 2% and approximately 30%; 3–10% is a reasonable estimate. True recurrence rates are difficult to establish because of inadequate patient follow-up. Recurrence is more common with direct or femoral hernias than with indirect hernias. Repair of recurrent hernias is associated with even higher rates of recurrence. High recurrence rates have been associated with failure to recognize and treat chronic respiratory problems, urinary tract obstruction, chronic constipation, anorectal disease, and ascites. Because most recurrences take place after 1 year, the etiology is probably tissue dysfunction related to excessive tension. Relaxing incisions or the use of prosthetic material may be helpful for reducing tension on repairs involving fascial tissue. With attenuated tissue and large defects, the selective use of prosthetic materials has been demonstrated to result in low recurrence rates. The most popular prosthetic materials are Marlex (polypropylene), Mersilene, and Gore-Tex (polytetrafluoroethylene). Many surgeons routinely use prosthetic material when performing herniorrhaphy in adults in an effort to reduce tension on the repair, tighten the internal ring, and thus reduce recurrences. Recurrence of an indirect inguinal hernia is the result of failure to remove the hernia sac or failure when repairing the dilated internal ring. Higher recurrence rates after simultaneous bilateral repair in adults may be reduced by repairs utilizing a tension-free mesh technique.

ANSWER: B, C, D

14. The anatomic boundaries of the orifice of the femoral canal include which of the following structures?

A. Cooper's ligament.
B. Inguinal ligament.
C. Iliopubic tract.
D. Femoral vein.
E. Lacunar ligament.

Ref.: 1, 2, 3

COMMENTS: Femoral hernias are located in the femoral canal, the entrance to which is bounded superiorly and medially by the iliopubic tract, inferiorly by Cooper's ligament, and laterally by the femoral vein. The inguinal ligament is more superficial; it is a common misconception that the medial boundary of the femoral canal is formed by the recurved fibers of the inguinal ligament known as the lacunar ligament.

ANSWER: A, C, D

15. Which of the following is/are true statements regarding umbilical hernias?

A. They are the embryologic equivalent of a small omphalocele.
B. Prompt repair of even small defects in infants is indicated because of the risk of incarceration.
C. Repair in asymptomatic adults is not indicated.
D. The "vest-over-pants" type of repair is stronger than simple approximation of fascial margins.
E. They are most common in African-American infants.

Ref.: 1, 2, 3

COMMENTS: Umbilical hernias are the result of a patent umbilical ring, whereas an omphalocele is the result of failure of abdominal wall closure in the midline during early intrauterine life. Umbilical hernias are said to be present in 40–90% of African-American infants. Incarceration is rare in infants; unless the defect is large, most surgeons defer repair until the child is approximately 4 years of age, because spontaneous closure does occur. In adults, however, repair should be carried out promptly because of the risk of incarceration. There is no convincing evidence that a "vest-over-pants" type of repair is structurally superior to simple approximation of fascial margins. Repair in adults may require use of a prosthetic material such as Marlex, Mersilene, or Gore-Tex if the fascial defect is large, or if there is tension.

ANSWER: E

16. Most umbilical hernias are associated with which of the following structures?

A. Patent urachus.
B. Patent omphalomesenteric duct.
C. Patent vitelline duct.
D. Patent ligamentum venosum.
E. None of the above.

COMMENTS: Umbilical hernias result when the umbilical ring remains patent after birth. Other abnormalities may be present at the umbilicus in the form of draining sinuses, fistulas, or cysts as a result of the persistence of embryologic structures such as the urachus or the omphalomesenteric (vitelline) duct. This association with umbilical hernia, however, is coincidental rather than causal.

ANSWER: E

17. Match the hernia listed in the left column with the most appropriate statement listed in the right column.

A. Spigelian hernia	a. Noncircumferential incarceration of bowel wall
B. Richter's hernia	b. Latissimus dorsi, external oblique, iliac crest
C. Littre's hernia	c. Incarcerated Meckel's diverticulum
D. Petit's hernia	d. Howship-Romberg sign
E. Grynfelt hernia	e. Twelfth rib, internal oblique
F. Obturator hernia	f. Lateral border of rectus at linea semicircularis

Ref.: 1, 3

COMMENTS: All of the above refer to unusual anatomic locations of abdominal or lumbar hernias except for Richter's and Littre's hernias, which represent incarceration of a limited portion of the small bowel. It is important to recognize these two types of hernia because vascular compromise may occur without evidence of intestinal obstruction.

ANSWER: A-f; B-a; C-c; D-b; E-e; F-d

18. Testicular atrophy following inguinal hernia repair most likely results from which of the following circumstances?

A. Overly tight closure of the internal ring, compromising the arterial supply.
B. Trauma to the inferior epigastric vessels at the internal ring.
C. Dissection of the distal component of the indirect sac.
D. Accidental division of external spermatic vessels.
E. None of the above.

Ref.: 1, 2, 3, 4

COMMENTS: Testicular atrophy is a relatively unusual but distressing sequela of inguinal hernia repair. The atrophy results from thrombosis of veins of the spermatic cord following surgical dissection of the cord. This potential trauma can be reduced by minimizing dissection of the distal component of indirect hernia sacs. A snug closure of the internal ring is important for preventing recurrence of an indirect hernia. It is extremely difficult to compress the small-diameter internal spermatic artery with this closure. Ligation and division of the inferior epigastric vessels are not associated with undesirable consequences. Ligation and division of the external spermatic vessels may produce anesthesia as the result of division of the accompanying genital branch of the genitofemoral nerve.

ANSWER: C

19. Which of the following is/are true regarding laparoscopic hernia repair?

A. Operative approach is primarily performed through either a transabdominal preperitoneal or a total extraperitoneal approach.
B. Staples placed below the lateral iliopubic tract risk injury to the genitofemoral and ilioinguinal nerve.
C. Staples should not be placed below the internal ring, between the ductus deferens and the spermatic vessels.
D. This approach is best suited for recurrent and bilateral hernias.

Ref.: 1

COMMENTS: Laparoscopic techniques have gained acceptance for the repair of inguinal hernias and may offer advantages in terms of reduced pain, faster return to full activities, and better cosmesis. Although there is controversy regarding its use for unilateral, newly diagnosed hernias, it seems ideally suited for recurrent and bilateral hernias where the disability and technical difficulty associated with open (conventional) repairs cannot be overlooked. Laparoscopy can be performed totally extraperitoneally by dissecting within the rectus sheath or transabdominally. In either case, a preperitoneal repair is performed. Staples placed below the lateral iliopubic tract risk injury to the genitofemoral nerve and the lateral femoral cutaneous nerve. Stapling is also avoided just below the internal inguinal ring in an area known as the *triangle of doom.* This triangle is bordered laterally by the spermatic vessels and medially by the ductus deferens; located within this triangle are the external iliac artery and vein and the femoral nerve.

ANSWER: A, C, D

20. Which of the following items represents the optimal convalescent period required before returning to work after inguinal herniorrhaphy?

A. 6–8 weeks.
B. 4 weeks.
C. 1 week.
D. Unknown.

Ref.: 1, 2

COMMENTS: Traditionally, patients who engage in strenuous work activities have been allowed periods of 6–8 weeks to recuperate after *traditional* open herniorrhaphy. Recent studies have shown that collagen maturation and tensile strength in a hernia wound require months to reach maximal states. *Tension-free* repair utilizing *prosthetic materials* has allowed patients to return to normal activities sooner. These repairs allow patients to perform any activity they choose as soon as they feel comfortable, which is usually within 1–3 weeks. *Laparoscopic mesh* repair therefore may allow even earlier return to strenuous activity because postoperative discomfort is said to be much less marked.

ANSWER: D

21. A 42-year-old man has an uneventful Shouldice repair of an inguinal hernia. On the day following surgery he complains of pain atypically severe for a routine herniorrhaphy. His pain continues for the next 6 months, resulting in multiple office visits. Which of the following statements is/are applicable to his care?

A. The pain may be due to osteitis of the pubic bone.
B. Local infiltration of the ilioinguinal nerve may be therapeutic and diagnostic.
C. Paravertebral block at L1 and L2 may be therapeutic and diagnostic.
D. Inadvertent division of the iliohypogastric nerve is the likely cause.

Ref.: 5

COMMENTS: Chronic groin pain following inguinal hernia repair is frustrating for both the patient and the surgeon. The pain may result from injury to nerves during the surgical procedure, the **ilioinguinal nerve** being most commonly involved. Its anterior location makes it prone to entrapment by sutures used for the repair, whereas adherence to the external oblique aponeurosis may predispose it to inadvertent division. The **iliohypogastric nerve** is usually not entrapped or divided because of its more medial location, but care must be exercised when utilizing a relaxing incision in the more medially situated rectus sheath or when anchoring prosthetic material. The surgical significance of the **genitofemoral nerve** is commonly not appreciated. The genital branch of the genitofemoral nerve passes through the inguinal ring and lies adjacent to the external spermatic vessels as they enter the cremaster muscle. The nerve may be divided while "mobilizing" the cord, or it can be entrapped by a suture during the repair. This nerve is particularly in jeopardy with a Shouldice repair. Some surgeons routinely dissect this nerve and provide a separate foramen for it in a mesh repair. Relief of pain by ilioinguinal nerve block suggests ilioinguinal nerve involvement. Relief by paravertebral block at the L1 and L2 levels suggests genitofemoral nerve origin. The ilioinguinal nerve can be released if it is entrapped by the repair, or it can be divided lateral (proximal) to the repair. The genitofemoral nerve can be divided by a retroperitoneal approach. Although anesthesia is common following division of sensory nerves during a hernia repair, the symptoms are mild and usually not disabling because the overlap of sensory distribution of these nerves decreases the disability. Occasionally, however, a troublesome causalgia may result from division of a sensory nerve.

ANSWER: B, C

22. Which of the following statements regarding the anatomy of the rectus sheath is/are true?

A. The anterior sheath is complete throughout (from xiphoid to pubis).
B. The anterior sheath is composed of external oblique and internal oblique fasciae.
C. The transverse tendons of the rectus sheath adhere to the anterior and posterior surfaces of the rectus muscle.
D. The linea semicircularis is between the umbilicus and the xiphoid.
E. Caudal to the linea semicircularis there is no internal oblique fascia behind the rectus muscle.

Ref.: 1, 2, 6

COMMENTS: Each rectus muscle is contained within a sheath that has anterior and posterior components. The *anterior sheath* is continuous from xiphoid to pubis and is composed of the external oblique and internal oblique aponeurosis. The *posterior sheath* anatomy varies above and below the linea semicircularis, which is the point at which the inferior epigastric artery enters the rectus sheath. Above this point the posterior sheath is strong and is composed of internal oblique fascia, the transversus abdominis muscle, and the transversalis fascia. Below the linea semicircularis the posterior sheath is lacking, as the internal oblique fascia passes anterior to the rectus muscle. Consequently, the rectus muscle is covered posteriorly by only a thin, transparent layer of transversalis fascia. Bleeding into the sheath at this level may produce symptoms that mimic an acute abdomen. The transverse tendons of the rectus sheath adhere only to the anterior sheath.

ANSWER: A, B, E

23. Which of the following statements is/are true regarding hematomas of the rectus sheath?

A. They usually result from rupture of the epigastric vessels.
B. The only recognized etiologic factor is trauma.
C. They are characterized by a palpable mass that is not influenced by tensing of the rectus abdominis muscle (Fothergill's sign).
D. Their treatment is usually nonoperative.
E. They occur three times more often in women.

Ref.: 1, 2

COMMENTS: Although rectus sheath hematomas most commonly follow trauma, they also can follow minor straining or as a result of certain infectious diseases (e.g., typhoid fever), collagen vascular diseases, blood dyscrasias, coagulopathies, and anticoagulation therapy. They usually are the result of rupture of the epigastric artery or vein rather than a tear of the rectus muscle. In addition to **Fothergill's sign**, a bluish discoloration to the skin is also diagnostic, but it may take a few days to develop. Sonography can be helpful for establishing the diagnosis. Treatment usually is nonoperative. Operation may be indicated in cases of an expanding hematoma or if the diagnosis is in doubt, in which case evacuation without entering the peritoneal cavity and closure without drains are standard.

ANSWER: A, C, D, E

24. Which of the following statements is/are true regarding desmoid tumors?

A. They occur more commonly in women.
B. They are benign fibrous growths often found within or deep to the lower anterior abdominal musculature.
C. Because of their benign nature, they are unlikely to recur following excision.
D. If located within the abdominal wall, the proper treatment is wide resection.
E. They are found in conjunction with Gardner syndrome.

Ref.: 1, 2

COMMENTS: Desmoid tumors fall in the middle of a spectrum of fibromatoses ranging from benign fibroma to aggressive fibrosarcoma. Although considered "benign," they have the malignant property of local invasiveness; and when excised incompletely they have a propensity to recur. They usually present as a painless mass within or deep to the anterior abdominal wall musculature. They occur most frequently in women of childbearing age, and are seen as well in patients with Gardner syndrome for reasons that are not clear. In these cases, the desmoids are located within the small bowel mesentery and may cause obstructive symptoms and potentially death. Although local irradiation may have a role in the therapy of some abdominal wall desmoid tumors, the appropriate treatment is wide resection to include the contiguously invaded structures. Nonsteroidal antiinflammatory drugs and antiestrogens have achieved tumor regression. Indomethacin combined with ascorbic acid has also caused regression. The mesenteric desmoids found with Gardner syndrome are capable of acting in a highly aggressive fashion. Because of their propensity to grow rapidly following surgery, resection is not advised. Instead, these desmoids are treated with clinoril, tamoxifen, or both. In refractory or extremely aggressive cases, cytotoxic chemotherapy may be indicated.

ANSWER: A, B, D, E

25. Which of the following statements characterizes retroperitoneal fibrosis?

A. A hypersensitivity reaction to the antiserotonin drug methysergide has been implicated.
B. It is two to three times more common in women.
C. Symptoms generally are related to partial inferior vena caval obstruction.
D. The most definitive noninvasive diagnostic test is intravenous pyelography (IVP).

Ref.: 1, 2

COMMENTS: Retroperitoneal fibrosis is one of a constellation of processes of "systemic idiopathic fibrosis" that can involve the mediastinum, the thyroid gland (Riedel's struma), or the biliary tract (sclerosing cholangitis). Hypersensitivity to methysergide is one of the few identified etiologic factors. Its incidence is two to three times higher in men than in women. Although the inferior vena cava may be compressed by the fibrotic stage of the process, symptoms usually relate to genitourinary tract involvement (specifically, entrapment of the ureters) and lymphatic obstruction. The characteristic findings of hydronephrosis and medial deviation of the ureters on IVP is highly diagnostic of this entity. The disease is usually bilateral and symmetrical. High grade ureteral obstruction accompanied by infection may require urgent nephrostomy. Otherwise, mild disease is treated with cessation of potentially responsible medications and institution of corticosteroid therapy. Surgery is indicated when renal function is compromised; options include freeing the encased ureters and wrapping them with omentum or renal autotransplantation.

ANSWER: A, D

26. Which of the following statements is/are true regarding mesenteric lymphadenitis?

A. It occurs more commonly in children than in adults.
B. It is easily distinguished clinically from appendicitis.
C. Culture specimens taken at the time of operation usually show the presence of coliform bacteria.
D. The disease process tends to be self-limiting, and it rarely recurs.

Ref.: 1, 2

COMMENTS: A disease primarily of children and adolescents, mesenteric lymphadenitis is characterized by vague and at times migratory abdominal pain. Frequently it is difficult to distinguish from appendicitis; the inability to localize the site of maximal tenderness exactly and the change in that site often are helpful signs. The small amount of free peritoneal fluid found in these patients is usually sterile. The disease process is self-limiting, although approximately one-fourth of patients have additional episodes during their childhood years.

ANSWER: A

27. Tumors of the mesentery are characterized by which one or more of the following statements?

A. Primary and metastatic tumors of the mesentery occur with approximately equal frequency.
B. Of the primary mesenteric tumors, most are cystic.
C. Of the solid primary tumors of the mesentery, most are malignant.
D. Malignant mesenteric tumors tend to occur near the root of the mesentery, whereas benign tumors are more often peripheral in location.

Ref.: 2

COMMENTS: Most tumors within the mesentery represent metastases to the mesenteric lymph nodes. Primary mesenteric tumors are rare and are more often cystic than solid, frequently representing developmental defects of embryonic rests. Among the solid primary tumors, most are benign and frequently are found in the periphery of the mesentery. Malignant mesenteric tumors (most often liposarcoma and leiomyosarcoma) are usually found near the root of the mesentery, which significantly increases both the hazards of resection and the likelihood of subsequent recurrence.

ANSWER: B, D

28. Regarding retroperitoneal tumors in general, which of the following statements is/are true?

A. They are tumors of young adulthood.
B. Malignant tumors predominate, the most common of which is rhabdomyosarcoma.
C. Patient complaints usually are vague, but on clinical examination a palpable mass almost always is present.
D. Ultrasonography or computed tomography (CT) scanning gives valuable information.

Ref.: 1, 2

COMMENTS: Considering all histologic types of retroperitoneal tumors, it tends to be a disease of the fifth and sixth decades, although 15% of these lesions are found in children. Malignant tumors predominate over benign ones, the most common being lymphoma, followed by liposarcoma, fibrosarcoma, and then the other sarcomas. The clinical history usually is one of vague back or abdominal pain. Because the tumor is palpable only when it reaches significant size, surgeons rely heavily on imaging techniques, and so CT scanning and ultrasonography have been valuable for delineating the extent of the tumor and its relation to contiguous structures.

ANSWER: D

29. Which of the following statements accurately characterize retroperitoneal sarcomas?

A. The operative approach to them is best achieved through a flank incision.
B. These tumors have a well defined capsule and can easily be shelled out of the tumor bed with excellent results.
C. Fewer than 25% can be resected totally.
D. Local recurrence rates range from 30% to 50%.
E. The 5-year disease-free survival rate is in the range of 10%.

Ref.: 1, 2

COMMENTS: Retroperitoneal sarcomas can grow to a large size and typically invade contiguous structures. They are surrounded by a pseudocapsule; and although the tumors can be shelled out along this capsular plane, in such instances there is virtually always residual tumor. Avoiding this situation requires wide excision—frequently en bloc excision with the attached organs (e.g., kidney, bowel, abdominal wall). Because of the frequent proximity of these tumors to nonresectable structures, complete excision is possible in only about 25% of patients. For the same reasons, local recurrence rates may be as high as 50%. This, and their potential for distant metastasis, result in 5-year disease-free survival rates as low as 10%.

ANSWER: C, D, E

30. Tumors of the omentum are characterized by which of the following statements?

A. All omental cysts are postinflammatory in nature.
B. Omental cysts usually are asymptomatic.
C. The most common solid omental tumor is metastatic carcinoma.
D. Primary solid tumors of the omentum are fairly common and most often malignant.
E. Omentectomy for metastatic carcinoma has a role in the management of certain tumors.

Ref.: 1, 2

COMMENTS: Omental cysts may be "true cysts" (presumably caused by congenital lymphatic obstruction) or neoplastic dermoid cysts, or they may be pseudocysts resulting usually from fat necrosis, trauma, or a foreign body reaction. Unless they undergo torsion, most are asymptomatic; the rest produce vague, nondescript symptoms. Most solid omental tumors represent metastatic carcinoma; and in the case of ovarian carcinoma, omentectomy can contribute to improved disease control despite the presence of metastases elsewhere. Primary solid omental tumors are rare, and only one-third are malignant. Ultrasonography can be valuable for bolstering a clinical diagnosis and determining a tumor's cystic or solid nature. At present, percutaneous needle or catheter drainage of presumed omental cysts is too hazardous.

ANSWER: B, C, E

31. Regarding the physiology of the peritoneal membrane, which of the following is/are true?

A. Intraperitoneal isotonic saline is absorbed at a rate of 30–35 ml/hr.
B. Intraperitoneal blood is generally not absorbed; the few red blood cells that are absorbed are nonviable.
C. Intraperitoneal hypertonic fluids can cause a large shift of fluid from the intravascular space (300–500 ml/hr), causing hypotension and possible shock.
D. The following substances can be removed by peritoneal dialysis: ammonia, calcium, iron, lead, lithium.
E. The following substances are not removed by peritoneal dialysis: opiates, digitalis, diazepam, antidepressives, hallucinogens.

Ref.: 1, 2

COMMENTS: After an initial equilibration phase, isotonic saline is absorbed at a rate of 30 to 35 ml/hr. The presence of a hypertonic solution, however, causes movement of fluid from the intravascular space into the peritoneal cavity; such movement is driven by the osmolar gradient. Flow rates up to 300 to 500 ml/hr have been described and can cause hypotension and shock. Approximately 70% of intraperitoneal blood is absorbed, albeit at a slower rate than above, and occurs primarily through fenestrated lymphatic channels on the undersurface of the diaphragm. Absorbed red blood cells have a normal survival time in the circulation. Leaving blood in the peritoneal cavity is not advised since it may potentiate infection. Peritoneal dialysis is capable of removing a variety of medications and elements including those listed; however, it is not capable of eliminating some medications that carry potential morbidity from overdose.

ANSWER: A, B, D, E

32. Study this intraperitoneal view of the left inguinal area, and match the anatomic names listed below (A–G) with the illustrated structures (lower case letters).

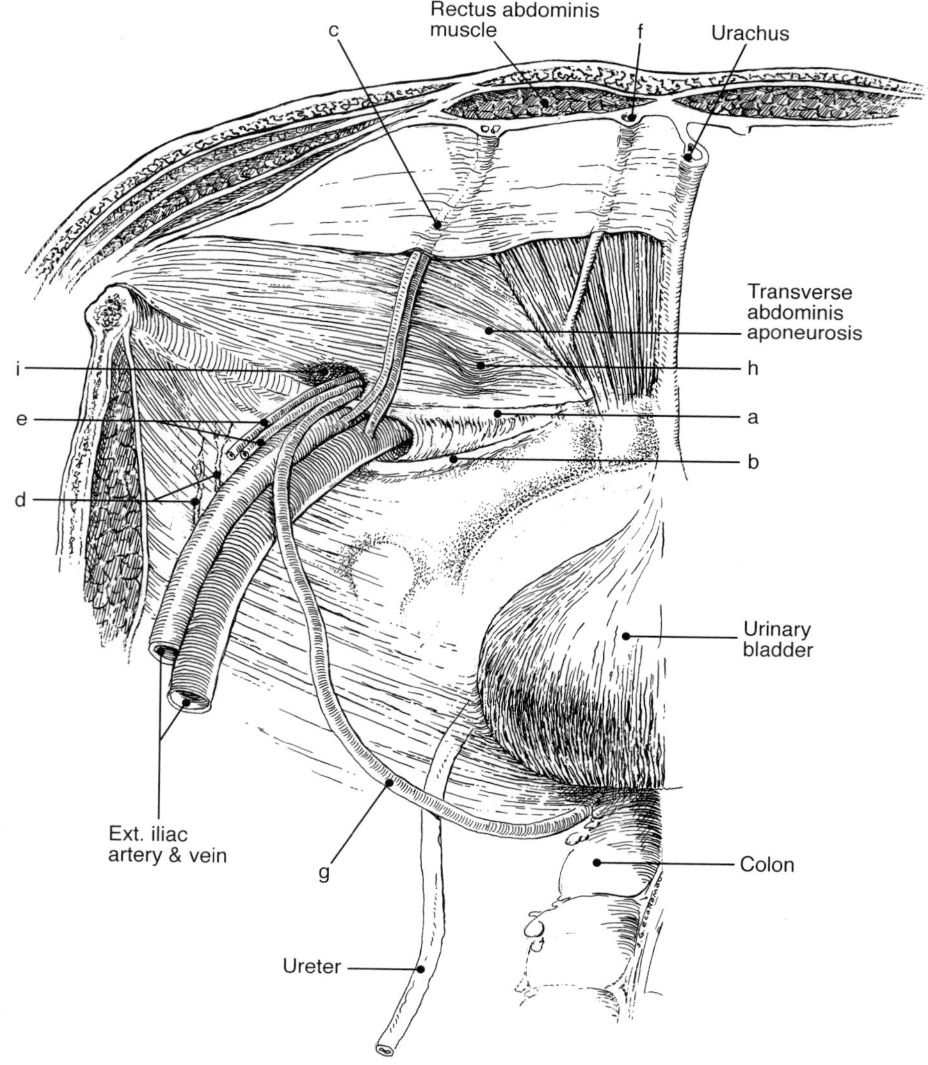

A. Medical umbilical ligament.
B. Spermatic vessels.
C. Cooper's ligament.
D. Inferior epigastric vessels.
E. Vas deferens.
F. Iliopubic tract.
G. Lateral femoral and genitofemoral nerves.

Ref.: 7

COMMENTS: See Question 33.

33. In the same illustration, match the appropriate statement below (A–F) with the illustrated structure or area (lower case letters).

A. Neuralgia.
B. Lower margin of direct defect.
C. Direct hernia.
D. May lead to testicular atrophy.
E. Congenital hernia.
F. Inferior border of femoral hernia.

Ref.: 7

COMMENTS: Hernia surgery, especially when performed through the laparoscopic approach, requires a clear understanding of the anatomy of the lower abdominal wall. The posterior wall of the inguinal canal consists of the transversus abdominis muscle, its aponeurosis, and the transversalis fascia (musculopectineal orifice of Fruchaud). Transperitoneal inspection of the lower third of the abdomen wall permits identification of the *medial umbilical ligament* (in the figure, f) as the most prominent landmark medially. Laterally, the *epigastric vessels* (c) exit from the *external iliac* artery and vein and form the medial border of the *internal ring* (i), the site of an indirect (congenital) hernia. The area between the *vas deferens* (g) and the *spermatic vessels* (e) has been named the "triangle of doom" because underneath it lie the iliac vessels and the *femoral nerve*. Lateral to them but inferior to the ileopubic tract, the *genitofemoral* and *lateral femoral cutaneous nerve* (d) can be easily injured by injudicious application of staples or sutures in that area, giving rise to a chronic neuralgia that may necessitate nerve block or even nerve division. *Cooper's ligament* (b) can be easily identified by dissecting the properitoneal layer at the confluence of the epigastric vessels, iliac vessels, and the *spermatic cord* (e) as it exits through the *internal ring* (i). The glossy white firm structure, Cooper's ligament, constitutes the inferior border of a femoral hernia. Direct inguinal hernias are acquired and occur because of a weakness in *Hesselbach triangle* (h). The *ileopubic tract* (a) forms the lower border of the direct inguinal hernia, and the transversus abdominis arch constitutes the upper border.

ANSWER:
Question 32: a-F; b-E; c-B; d-C; e-G; f-A; g-D
Question 33: a-D; b-A; c-H; d-E; e-I; f-B

REFERENCES

1. Sabiston DC Jr: *Textbook of Surgery*, 15th ed. WB Saunders, Philadelphia, 1997.
2. Schwartz SI, Shires GT, Spencer FC: *Principles of Surgery*, 7th ed. McGraw-Hill, New York, 1999.
3. Nyhus LM, Condon RE: *Hernia*, 3rd ed. JB Lippincott, Philadelphia, 1989.
4. Wantz GE: Testicular atrophy as sequela of inguinal herniorrhaphy. *Int Surg* 71:159–163, 1986.
5. Lichtenstein IL, Shulman AG, Amid PK, Montllor MM: Cause and prevention of post-herniorrhaphy neuralgia: a proposed protocol for treatment. *Am J Surg* 155:786–790, 1988.
6. Williams PL, Warwick R, Dyson M, Bannister LH: *Gray's Anatomy*, 37th ed. Churchill Livingstone, New York, 1989.
7. Rutkow IM: Groin hernia surgery. *Surg Clin North Am* 78:1156–1921, 1998.

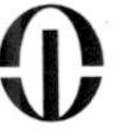

CHAPTER 38

Pediatric Surgery

1. Which of the following fluid regimens provides the most appropriate fluid and electrolyte *maintenance* for a 6 kg infant?

A. Lactated Ringer's solution at 15 ml/hr.
B. Dextrose 5% in water (D_5W), 0.5% normal saline + potassium chloride (KCl) 20 mEq/L at 15 ml/hr.
C. D_5W, 0.25% normal saline + KCl 20 mEq/L at 25 ml/hr.
D. D_5W, 0.5% normal saline + KCl 15 mEq/L at 25 ml/hr.
E. D_5W, 0.25% normal saline + KCl 15 mEq/L at 50 ml/hr.

***Ref.*:** 1, 2, 3

COMMENTS: Understanding maintenance fluid and electrolyte requirements is critical for management of infant surgical patients. Free water maintenance requirements include replacement of insensible losses from the skin and lungs and the free water necessary to clear metabolic solutes in the urine. It does not include treatment for preexisting deficits or ongoing fluid losses. Numerous formulas are applicable to the calculation of maintenance requirements. The most widely used formula is based on weight, although the one based on body surface is equally accurate. The 24-hour requirement is approximately 100 ml/kg for infants up to 10 kg, plus an additional 50 ml/kg for those 10–20 kg, plus an additional 20 ml/kg in those over 20 kg. Estimations based on body surface area give equivalent results. Daily electrolyte requirements include sodium (Na) 2–5 mEq/kg and potassium (K) 2–3 mEq/kg. For term infants during the first week of life the maintenance needs are less, ranging from 50 to 90 ml/kg/day. Dextrose is administered to provide a glucose substrate; complete caloric support without enteral supplement requires parenteral nutrition solutions.

ANSWER: C

2. A 5-week-old boy has a history of vomiting for 5 days and a weight loss of 0.4 kg (from 4.0 kg to 3.6 kg). On examination his anterior fontanelle is found to be flattened, and his mucous membranes are dry. Laboratory data are as follows (mEq/L): Na 132, K 3.2, Cl 91, and CO_2 28; his capillary pH is 7.48. Which of the following statements about this infant is/are likely true?

A. It is crucial to determine if the emesis is bilious.
B. Palpation of the abdomen might reveal the diagnosis.
C. Ultrasonography of the abdomen might confirm the diagnosis.
D. The diagnosis is intussusception.
E. The condition should be corrected promptly by operation.

***Ref.*:** 1, 2, 3

COMMENTS: Age at the time of symptom manifestation is important in the pediatric population. Duodenal atresia, for example, manifests only in newborns; pyloric stenosis typically produces symptoms in infants between 3 and 12 weeks of age; intussusception, in contrast, most commonly occurs in children between 3 and 18 months of age. • The symptoms of pyloric stenosis usually start with nonbilious vomiting, which progressively becomes projectile in nature. Dehydration and electrolyte imbalance are usually a function of the length of time the baby has been symptomatic: If the condition is diagnosed early, fluid and electrolytes are mostly normal; if it is diagnosed late, infants are more likely to present with a hypochloremic, hypokalemic alkalosis and more severe dehydration. Physical examination often reveals an olive-sized mass in the upper abdomen to the right of the midline that is pathognomonic. Sometimes gastric waves are seen through the abdominal wall. If the pyloric mass cannot be palpated by an experienced examiner, ultrasonography, an upper gastrointestinal series with contrast, or both may be undertaken to confirm the diagnosis. Preoperative preparation to correct fluid and electrolyte imbalances is important. When—but not before—correction is achieved, surgery can be performed. The Ramstedt pyloromyotomy is the preferred treatment; laparoscopic pyloromyotomy is an *alternative* approach.

ANSWER: A, B, C

3. The laboratory data of the infant described in Question 2 reflect which of the following?

A. Normal acid-base balance.
B. Metabolic alkalosis.
C. Respiratory alkalosis.
D. Combined metabolic and respiratory alkalosis.
E. Compensated metabolic alkalosis.

***Ref.*:** 1, 3

COMMENTS: Gastric outlet obstruction with sufficient loss of gastric contents produces a hypochloremic, hypokalemic metabolic alkalosis. The ability to compensate by hypoventilation is limited; in fact, infants and children who are crying are hyperventilating and have additional respiratory alkalosis.

ANSWER: B

4. Which of the following solutions is/are appropriate for initial intravenous therapy of the baby described in Question 2?

   A. Lactated Ringer's solution at 25 ml/hr.
   B. D_5W, 0.5% normal saline + KCl 20 mEq/L at 15 ml/hr.
   C. D_5W, 0.25% normal saline + KCl 30 mEq/L at 30 ml/hr.
   D. D_5W, 0.5% normal saline + KCl 30 mEq/L at 25 ml/hr.
   E. D_5W + 0.1% normal hydrochloride (HCl) at 30 ml/hr.

Ref.: 1, 2, 3

COMMENTS: Appropriate fluid therapy in this situation requires maintenance in addition to replacement for estimated deficit and for ongoing losses. Estimated initial volume replacement for the first 24 hours includes maintenance of 100 ml/kg = 360 cc/24°C and replacement of approximately half of the estimated deficit. Weight loss is 40 gm or 10% dehydration 360 cc/24°C + 200 cc/24°C. The initial rate of fluid replacement is only an estimate, however, and should be adjusted to maintain urine output of 1–2 ml/kg/hr. An initial bolus of normal saline 20 ml/kg may be appropriate for severely dehydrated patients. As far as electrolytes are concerned, sodium, potassium, and chloride must be supplied for both maintenance and replacement of gastric losses. They can be supplied by a solution of 5% dextrose with 0.5% normal saline and KCl (approximately 30 mEq/L). Ongoing assessment of serum electrolytes should be performed and electrolyte replacement adjusted as necessary. The operation should proceed only after appropriate fluid and electrolyte correction.

ANSWER: D

5. With regard to sacrococcygeal teratomas, which of the following statements is/are true?

   A. Approximately 90% are benign at birth.
   B. They have great potential to become malignant.
   C. α-Fetoprotein is a good tumor marker.
   D. Affected children require close follow-up observation for years.
   E. The coccyx is not, in truth, connected with the tumor.

Ref.: 1, 3

COMMENTS: Sacrococcygeal teratoma is a lesion encountered mostly during the first year of life, and it predominates among females (80–85%). In 90% of cases, there is an exophytic component that makes the diagnosis obvious at birth. The other 10% grow within the pelvis or abdominal cavity, making the diagnosis more difficult unless they are suspected and sought. The behavior of such tumors is unique among childhood tumors. When identified and operated on before infants are 2 months of age, 90% of these tumors qualify as benign teratomas. If they are removed after infants are 2 months of age, the pathologic diagnosis in 90% of cases is a malignant teratoma. • Because of the attachment of the tumor to the coccyx, coccygectomy should always be part of the surgical technique for removal of the tumor. Malignant lesions do not respond well to radiotherapy or chemotherapy. α-Fetoprotein is the marker used to make the diagnosis in utero as well as during the follow-up period after operation. Because of late recurrence, affected infants should be observed closely throughout their entire childhood.

ANSWER: A, B, C, D

6. A 2-month old boy is brought to the emergency room with a history of an acute, nonreducible mass in the right groin. Which of the following are possible diagnoses?

   A. Incarcerated inguinal hernia.
   B. Acute hydrocele.
   C. Torsion of the testis.
   D. Inguinal lymphadenopathy.
   E. Testicular teratoma.

Ref.: 1, 2, 3

COMMENTS: When an infant presents with an acute inguinoscrotal mass, it should be diagnosed as soon as possible. An **incarcerated inguinal hernia** in an infant can usually be reduced if the infant is placed in a warm, calm environment and adequately sedated. After successful reduction, the child is admitted to the hospital, and herniorrhaphy is performed within 24–48 hours. If the hernia cannot be reduced, an emergency operation is obviously indicated. Incarceration of an inguinal hernia risks not only intestinal ischemia but testicular ischemia and subsequent atrophy as well. In females the hernia sac may contain the ovary and tube, but ovarian ischemia is not common unless there is associated torsion. **Testicular torsion** usually manifests suddenly as a mass in the scrotal area with swelling and edema of that side of the scrotum. The testis on that side rides high and is extremely tender. The differential diagnosis usually is epididymitis or torsion of the appendix testis. A nuclear scan can be helpful; but if there is any doubt, immediate surgical exploration via scrotol raphe is indicated. If testicular torsion is found, orchidopexy should be performed (for both the affected testis and contralateral testis). If differentiation between nonreducible indirect inguinal hernia and **acute hydrocele** is unclear, prompt surgical exploration and repair should be performed. Not infrequently, acute **inguinal lymphadenopathy** manifests as a nonreducible inguinal mass and may be difficult to differentiate from an incarcerated indirect inguinal hernia. Of all the conditions listed, only **testicular teratoma** does not have an acute onset.

ANSWER: A, B, C, D

7. With regard to the treatment of unilateral inguinal hernia in infants, which of the following statements is/are true?

   A. Operation should be delayed until patients are 1 year of age because spontaneous obliteration of the processus vaginalis may occur.
   B. High ligation of an indirect hernia sac without formal repair of the floor is sufficient.
   C. Removal of the distal hernia sac is always indicated to prevent postoperative hydrocele.
   D. Contralateral exploration is always indicated because of the high incidence of bilaterality.

Ref.: 1, 2, 3

COMMENTS: Inguinal hernias in children nearly always are caused by failure of the processus vaginalis to close. Repair is recommended at the time of diagnosis because there is a significant risk of incarceration. The exception is the premature infant weighing less than 2 kg. These infants are observed in the hospital and treated for their other problems related to prematurity. Hernia repair is then done prior to discharge or at 2 kg to decrease anesthetic risk and risk of injury to inguinal structures. A patent processus vaginalis is not always associated with a clinical hernia, however, and some closure must occur during postnatal development in view of the fact that the patency rates are lower in adults. In infants with indirect inguinal hernia, simple high ligation and excision of the hernia sac at the internal ring is adequate treatment; routine repair of the inguinal floor should be avoided because it is unnecessary and carries the risk of injury to important fascial structures. It is not necessary to remove the entire distal hernia sac, and it should be left in place if its dissection might jeopardize cord structures. The role of exploration of clinically normal contralateral groins in infants is controversial. The latest data provided via laparoscopic exploration does not support routine contralateral exploration; 25–30% of all infants have a contralateral hernia. Use of the laparoscope allows appropriate selection for repair.

ANSWER: B

8. A mass in the mesentery of the ileum adjacent to the bowel wall may be which of the following entities?

A. Intestinal duplication.
B. Meckel's diverticulum.
C. Mesenteric cyst.

Ref.: 2, 3

COMMENTS: Intestinal duplications are a **misnomer**; most are enteric cysts and occur most commonly within the abdomen. They manifest as cystic or tubular masses next to the bowel wall between the mesenteric leaves and contain elements of intestinal wall. Mesenteric cysts are also located within the mesentery, but they do not contain any muscular wall. Meckel's diverticulum is a type of omphalomesenteric duct remnant and, although found in the terminal ileum, is located on the antimesenteric side of the bowel.

ANSWER: A, C

9. Which of the following entities is the most common childhood malignancy?

A. Lymphoma.
B. Leukemia.
C. Wilms' tumor.
D. Neuroblastoma.
E. Rhabdomyosarcoma.

Ref.: 1, 2, 3

COMMENTS: Malignancy is second only to trauma as the leading cause of death during childhood. In infants, malignant disease is the third most frequent cause of death after prematurity and congenital anomalies. Approximately 40% of childhood malignancies are leukemias. The most common solid tumor in children under 2 years of age is neuroblastoma; in children older than 2 years, it is Wilms' tumor.

ANSWER: B

10. With regard to hepatoportoenterostomy (Kasai procedure) for treatment of biliary atresia, which of the following statements is/are true?

A. Hepatoportoenterostomy is most successfully performed after patients are 3 months of age, when the bile ducts are larger.
B. When successful, hepatoportoenterostomy is rarely complicated by cholangitis.
C. Hepatoportoenterostomy is no longer indicated as the initial surgical procedure if hepatic transplantation is available.
D. Hepatic cirrhosis and portal hypertension remain problems despite successful hepatoportoenterostomy.

Ref.: 1, 2, 3

COMMENTS: Biliary atresia occurs as part of a spectrum of anomalies known as **infantile obstructive cholangiopathy**. Although the etiology of these anomalies is unknown, it has been related to in utero viral infection. A hepatic HIDA scan and ultrasonography of the bile ducts are the mainstays among imaging tests to support the diagnosis. Variable patterns of ductal involvement may occur, although the extrahepatic bile ducts are commonly obliterated and replaced by fibrous cords. Both the intrahepatic and extrahepatic biliary tree may be involved, although in only 10% of patients is the disorder solely extrahepatic. The goals of treatment are to provide biliary drainage and prevent late complications of biliary cirrhosis with secondary hepatic failure. **Hepatoportoenterostomy** is most successful in establishing bile drainage when performed during the patient's first 2 months of life. The success rate falls dramatically after 3 months of age. Cholangitis, biliary cirrhosis, hepatic failure, and portal hypertension remain as late problems despite the fact that bile drainage is achieved. **Hepatic transplantation** has been successful in the treatment of this problem but has not replaced an attempt at biliary enteric anastomosis as the initial procedure. An unsuccessful hepatoportoenterostomy does not preclude later hepatic transplantation. Attempts to minimize later cholangitic complications include prompt use of antibiotics coupled with steroids during the initial phase of recovery to minimize inflammation and infection.

ANSWER: D

11. With regard to imperforate anus, which of the following statements is/are true?

A. This anomaly is defined as high or low, according to the relation between the rectum and the anal sphincter complex.
B. High anomalies are associated with a perineal fistula.
C. Most affected female infants require an initial colostomy.
D. Imperforate anus may be associated with esophageal atresia and tracheoesophageal fistula.
E. Pull-through techniques are successful in preserving continence in low lesions.

Ref.: 1, 2, 3

COMMENTS: Imperforate anus is a type of anorectal agenesis in which the anus is absent and the rectum ends at varying levels in relation to the puborectalis muscle. The blind rectum may end in a fistula which, with *high* lesions, usually opens into the prostatic urethra in males and the vagina in females. *Low* lesions manifest with a perineal fistula, which often is seen in the median scrotal raphe of males and in the posterior vaginal fourchette of females. • The level of the anomaly is the critical determinant of the type of correction required. *High* lesions are initially treated by colostomy, followed by a definitive reconstructive procedure aimed at bringing the rectum through the anal sphincter complex to achieve continence. *Low* lesions, which are suspected in the presence of a perineal fistula, can be corrected by a simple perineal approach. Most cases of imperforate anus in females are of the low variety. • The posterior sagittal anoplasty (described by Penã) achieves continence in all those with low lesions and in 65–75% of those with high lesions. • Imperforate anus may be part of the VATER syndrome (**v**ertebral anomalies, imperforate **a**nus, **t**racheoesophageal fistula, **e**sophageal atresia, and **r**adial and **r**enal anomalies). These, as well as associated genitourinary and occasional cardiac anomalies, must be evaluated before reparative surgery is undertaken.

ANSWER: A, D, E

12. Which of the following entities always requires surgical correction during infancy?

A. Imperforate anus.
B. Hypoplastic left colon.
C. Meconium plug syndrome.
D. Hirschsprung's disease.
E. Meconium ileus.

Ref.: 1, 2, 3

COMMENTS: Choices A–E above present as distal bowel obstruction. Large bowel obstruction cannot be differentiated from small bowel obstruction in infants based on plain radiographs because of the lack of haustral markings. **Hirschsprung's disease** is caused by congenital absence of colonic ganglion cells and should be suspected whenever an infant fails to pass meconium within the first 24 hours of life. The rectum and rectosigmoid areas are the regions most commonly affected, although longer segments may be involved; in rare cases, total colonic aganglionosis may be present. All types require surgical correction. **Hypoplastic left colon syndrome** is often seen in infants of diabetic mothers; infants with **meconium plug** syndrome may have clinical and radiographic characteristics similar to those of Hirschsprung's disease. Both of these conditions usually can be treated with hypertonic water-soluble radiographic contrast enemas. The diagnosis of **cystic fibrosis** must be considered in patients with **meconium ileus** and an associated microcolon (unused colon). In 80–90% of cases a Gastrografin enema relieves the obstruction without need for operation. **Anorectal anomalies** rarely present with neonatal intestinal obstruction because 80% present with a fistula to the genitourinary tract; all require surgical intervention.

ANSWER: A, D

13. With regard to Hirschsprung's disease, which of the following statements is/are true?

A. It is more common in males.
B. It may be complicated by enterocolitis.
C. Barium enema studies may be normal.
D. It is best diagnosed by rectal biopsy.
E. The initial treatment may involve colostomy.

Ref.: 1, 2, 3

COMMENTS: The primary clinical manifestation of Hirschsprung's disease is that of intestinal obstruction with failure to pass meconium in newborn male infants or chronic constipation in older infants and children. Infants with Hirschsprung's disease are prone to develop enterocolitis, which although not pseudomembranous still carries a high mortality rate if not recognized and treated promptly. In newborns, in whom dilatation of the bowel proximal to the aganglionic segment may not yet have developed, a barium enema study may be normal. Anal manometry demonstrates a characteristic failure of sphincter relaxation in a response to rectal distension. This finding, however, is not diagnostic. A definitive diagnosis is based on the rectal biopsy, which demonstrates an absence of ganglion cells in the *Aurbach's* and *Meisrer's* plexi, hypertrophied nerve endings, and an abundance of acetylcholinesterase by histochemical techniques. Infants with Hirschsprung's disease may be treated with 1-degree pull-through if full term with no enterocolitis present. All others are treated with colostomy at the level of ganglionosis followed by pull-through 3–6 months later. Anastomosis of normally innervated colon to the anus is the basis of all three pull-through procedures (***Swanson, Duhamel, Soave***).

ANSWER: A, B, C, D, E

14. A 3-week-old infant, heretofore apparently well, exhibits sudden onset of bilious vomiting. Which of the following is the most likely diagnosis?

A. Pyloric stenosis.
B. Tracheoesophageal fistula, H type.
C. Hirschsprung's disease.
D. Duodenal atresia.
E. Malrotation of midgut.

Ref.: 1, 2, 3

COMMENTS: See Question 15.

15. With regard to the infant described in Question 14, which study is most useful for making the diagnosis?

A. Abdominal radiography.
B. Computed tomography (CT) scan.
C. Upper gastrointestinal series.
D. Barium enema.
E. Esophageal pH studies.

Ref.: 1, 2, 3

COMMENTS: In any infant with the sudden onset of bilious vomiting, **malrotation of the midgut** with **volvulus** should be assumed to be the cause until proven otherwise. In 50% of children with malrotation and volvulus, the presentation is during the first few weeks of life. Immediate treatment is mandatory if the risk of complete necrosis of the midgut is to be lessened. **Pyloric stenosis** is seldom present with bilious vomiting. Infants with **tracheoesophageal fistula**, **H type**, also seldom vomit; the main symptoms usually are difficulty feeding and recurrent pneumonia. The main symptom of **Hirschsprung's disease** is constipation, but the disease may progress to bowel obstruction with bilious emesis. **Duodenal atresia** may mimic malrotation in the first 24–48 hours of life, but at 3 weeks of age duodenal atresia should have been already diagnosed and treated. There is a strong association between duodenal atresia and malrotation of the midgut. • If immediately available, an upper gastrointestinal series may be done since malrotation is suggested by a cutoff at the duodenum or absence of the ligament in Treitz in the left upper quadrant. A barium enema can be misleading in the presence of malrotation because the cecum may look normally placed. As soon as a diagnosis is made, the infant should be taken immediately to surgery to undergo resuscitation and operation simultaneously. If studies cannot be done immediately, an operation is justified on clinical suspicion alone, inasmuch as delay only increases the chances of intestinal necrosis.

ANSWER:
Question 14: E
Question 15: C

16. Operation for midgut volvulus with viable bowel should include detorsion and which of the following procedures?

A. Cecopexy in the right lower quadrant.
B. Appendectomy.
C. Repositioning the small bowel in the right side of the abdomen.
D. Repositioning the colon in the left side of the abdomen.

Ref.: 1, 2, 3

COMMENTS: The operative management of malrotation involves counterclockwise reduction of a midgut volvulus when present; nonviable bowel is resected. If viability is in question or the presence of necrosis not certain, the bowel may be returned to the abdomen in the hope that some or all of it will survive and bowel length may be preserved. In this case, a second-look laparotomy should be performed 24 hours later to reassess and treat the intestine appropriately. Peritoneal bands (Ladd's bands) between the cecum and the abdominal wall are divided, and the duodenum is mobilized so the small bowel can be positioned in the right side of the abdomen and the colon in the left side of the abdomen. Appendectomy is routinely performed. Intraluminal duodenal obstruction can occur with malrotation as a result of an associated web or stenosis. Ability to pass a nasogastric tube into the proximal duodenum and, after injection of saline through the tube, rapid filling of the jejunum usually rule out an intrinsic duodenal obstruction.

ANSWER: B, C, D

17. Match each clinical characteristic in the left column with the appropriate diagnosis or diagnoses in the right column.

A. Anterior mediastinal mass	a. Esophageal duplication
B. Respiratory distress	b. Bronchogenic cyst
C. Middle mediastinal mass	c. Mediastinal teratoma
D. Benign	d. Thoracic neuroblastoma
E. Posterior mediastinal mass	

Ref.: 1, 2, 3

COMMENTS: Respiratory distress and dysphagia are symptoms common to all mediastinal masses regardless of location. Masses in the anterior mediastinum are much more frequently **teratomas** than thymic tumors. They are or may become malignant and should always be resected. The younger the child at the time of resection of teratomas, the better the prognosis. **Esophageal duplication** and **bronchogenic cysts** are of a benign nature but are removed for obstructive symptoms and the risk for malignant degeneration. In newborns both entities can be responsible for airway obstruction, usually resulting from a mass. Bronchogenic cysts may arise within the wall of the bronchus and produce life-threatening respiratory distress without producing an obvious mass. Neuroblastomas, like teratomas, are or may become malignant. Masses arising from the posterior mediastinum are almost exclusively **neuroblastomas** or **ganglioneuromas**.

ANSWER: A-c; B-a,b,c,d; C-b,c; D-a,b; E-d

18. Advice to parents of an infant with a unilateral undescended testicle should include which of the following statements?

A. The problem should be corrected promptly.
B. Descent may occur spontaneously; but if this has not happened by age 2 years, descent should be performed surgically.
C. Orchiopexy should be performed to prevent malignancy.
D. Orchiopexy may prevent infertility.

Ref.: 1, 2, 3

COMMENTS: An undescended testicle must first be differentiated from a retractile testicle, which on careful examination can be brought into the scrotum and does not require surgical treatment. In instances of bilateral undescended testicles, serum gonadotropins and chromosomal studies may be helpful for establishing the presence of testicular tissue. In many infants with undescended testicles, descent occurs spontaneously during the first year or so of life; if not, an orchiopexy should be performed by the time the child is 2 years old. There is evidence that in patients with undescended testicles after the age of 2 years, spermatogenesis is impaired. Orchiopexy before this time may lessen the chance of infertility, although among patients with bilateral cryptorchidism in particular the incidence of infertility continues to be high. Cryptorchidism is associated with an increased risk of testicular cancer (predominantly seminoma). Orchiopexy, however, does not diminish this risk, and affected patients require periodic examination throughout their adolescent years. Approximately 10% of testicular tumors arise in undescended testicles, but the chances that an undescended testicle will undergo malignant transformation is approximately 1 in 4000. Additional reasons to perform orchiopexy include psychological considerations, an increased incidence of testicular torsion, and the possibility of testicular trauma when the testicle is at the level of the pubic tubercle.

ANSWER: B, D

19. At the time of a scheduled orchiopexy in a 2-year-old child, the undescended testicle cannot be brought down into the scrotum. Which of the following procedures would be appropriate treatment?

A. Orchiectomy.
B. Attachment to the pubic tubercle and reoperation in 1 year.
C. Division of the spermatic artery and vein to provide additional length.
D. Termination of the procedure and treatment with chorionic gonadotropin.

Ref.: 1, 2, 3

COMMENTS: In most cases of cryptorchidism, particularly if the testicle is palpable, the testicle can be brought down into the scrotum without difficulty. The approach is through a herniorrhaphy incision; the cord is carefully dissected, and an associated hernia sac, which is usually present, is dissected free and ligated at the internal ring. The testicle is secured in a subcutaneous pouch in the scrotum after passage through the dartos fascia. For the occasional instance in which the testicle is in a higher retroperitoneal position and adequate length cannot be obtained for scrotal positioning, different approaches have been used, including staged orchiopexy with reoperation in 6 months and division of the spermatic vessels, preserving the testicular blood supply along the vas deferens. In postpubertal teenagers with this condition, orchiectomy is the appropriate treatment. Human chorionic gonadotropin has been used as a nonoperative method of producing testicular descent. It is more successful in patients with bilateral undescended testicles than in those with unilateral undescended testicles, but the success rate is nevertheless modest.

ANSWER: B, C

20. With regard to jejunoileal atresia, which of the following statements is/are true?

A. The etiology is failure of embryologic recanalization of the gut, and therefore the atresias usually are multiple.
B. Passage of meconium does not exclude the diagnosis.
C. Associated anomalies are more common with jejunoileal atresia than with duodenal atresia.
D. Disparity in lumen size is common but is rarely a technical problem.

Ref.: 1, 2, 3

COMMENTS: Intestinal atresia is thought to result from an in utero vascular accident; in approximately 10% of patients the atresias are multiple. A variety of forms may be seen, ranging from a simple web or stenosis to complete separation of bowel ends with varying degrees of mesenteric defect. With the most severe type, most of the small bowel mesentery is absent and the remaining distal small bowel is supplied by the ileocolic artery. Intestinal atresia usually manifests with bilious vomiting and abdominal distension. The passage of meconium does not exclude the diagnosis. There may be a considerable disparity in size between the proximal bowel and the distal bowel. This has led to the development of a number of operative techniques for achieving a functional anastomosis. Associated anomalies are not seen as commonly as they are with duodenal atresia, which in as many as one-third of cases are associated with trisomy 21 (Down syndrome).

ANSWER: B, D

21. Eight hours after birth an infant exhibits excessive drooling and mild respiratory distress. An abdominal radiograph shows complete lack of air in the gastrointestinal tract. Which is the most likely diagnosis?

A. Hirschsprung's disease.
B. Tracheoesophageal fistula, H type.
C. Pyloric atresia.
D. Choanal atresia (bilateral).
E. Esophageal atresia without tracheoesophageal fistula.
F. Esophageal atresia with distal tracheoesophageal fistula.

Ref.: 1, 2, 3

COMMENTS: See Question 22.

22. With regard to the diagram, which is the most common type of esophageal atresia and tracheoesophageal fistula?

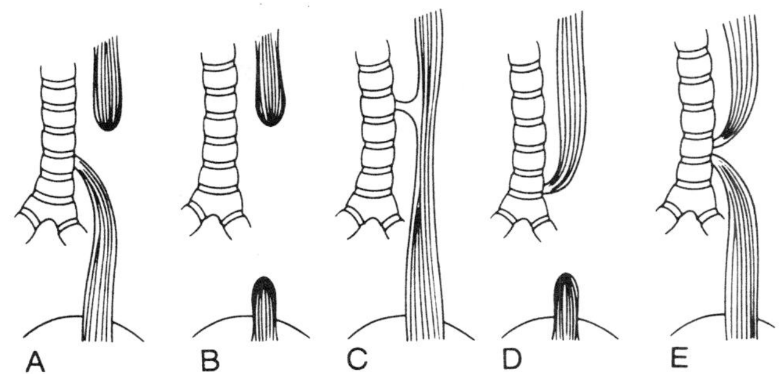

Ref.: 1, 2, 3

COMMENTS: It is necessary to remember that at birth neonates have a completely gasless gastrointestinal tract. Soon after birth they start swallowing air, and within 6–12 hours this air reaches the colon. A **tracheoesophageal fistula** of any type does not prevent swallowed or inspired air from reaching the stomach and small bowel. About 85–90% of patients with esophageal atresia and tracheoesophageal fistula have a blind proximal pouch with a distal tracheoesophageal fistula. Esophageal atresia without an associated fistula is the second most common form. Esophageal atresia is suggested when an infant has excess saliva or spits up during attempted feedings. In the presence of esophageal atresia, a fistula manifests as air in the gastrointestinal tract, respiratory symptoms with feedings, or both. When an orogastric tube is passed in an infant with esophageal atresia, a chest radiograph shows the tube coiled in the blind pouch. Contrast studies and bronchoscopy may be useful in selected cases to confirm the diagnosis and demonstrate the location of a tracheoesophageal fistula. Recognition of the anatomy of the anomaly is important for establishing appropriate initial treatment and definitive repair. **Hirschsprung's disease** is characterized by congenital lack of ganglion cells in the wall of the bowel, most commonly in the distal colon; and so air should be present in the stomach and small bowel. **Pyloric atresia**, a rare congenital anomaly, prevents air from going to the duodenum and small bowel, but radiography shows extreme distension of the stomach with air-fluid levels. Neonates, being obligatory nasal breathers, have major respiratory problems when born with **bilateral choanal atresia** but do not have any difficulty swallowing air.

ANSWER:
Question 21: E
Question 22: A

23. For a 3000-gm infant with esophageal atresia and distal tracheoesophageal fistula, if there is no respiratory distress or associated anomaly, which of the following is the preferred treatment?

A. Gastrostomy, cervical esophagostomy, and delayed repair.
B. Gastrostomy, sump tube drainage of proximal pouch, and delayed repair.
C. Fistula ligation and delayed esophageal repair.
D. Division of the fistula with primary esophageal anastomosis.
E. Primary repair with colon interposition.

Ref.: 1, 2, 3

COMMENTS: The timing of surgical intervention for esophageal atresia and tracheoesophageal fistula is influenced by the maturity of the infant and the presence or absence of associated cardiorespiratory problems or other congenital anomalies. Mortality from primary repair is directly related to the risk group to which the infant belongs. Otherwise healthy infants weighing more than 2500 gm are treated by primary repair with fistula division, closure of its tracheal end, and end-to-end anastomosis of the esophageal segments. Infants who are not well enough for primary repair are treated by gastrostomy and drainage of the blind proximal pouch. Repair is accomplished after complicating cardiorespiratory problems have been corrected. The presence of the tracheoesophageal fistula can cause problems with dissipation of ventilatory pressure into the stomach or allow aspiration of gastric contents into the lung.

ANSWER: D

24. Which of the following is/are complications of esophageal atresia and tracheoesophageal fistula repair?

A. Esophageal stricture.
B. Anastomotic leakage.
C. Gastroesophageal reflux.
D. Recurrent fistula.
E. Empyema.

Ref.: 1, 2, 3

COMMENTS: Gastroesophageal reflux is a common complication after operation for esophageal atresia and tracheoesophageal fistula in infants and frequently requires later fundoplication. The etiology of reflux may relate to underlying esophageal dysmotility and to dysfunction of the lower esophageal sphincter, which often is displaced cephalad after repair. Stricture or anastomotic leakage and subsequent recurrent fistula can also occur but are less common. The morbidity of potential anastomotic leakage can be minimized by use of an extrapleural approach; if leakage does occur, it remains extrapleural.

ANSWER: A, B, C, D, E

25. A premature infant with respiratory distress at birth has been successfully weaned from the ventilator and now is being fed oral formula. Abdominal distension develops, and blood-streaked stool is passed. Appropriate management includes which of the following?

A. Anoscopy for probable neonatal fissure.
B. Barium enema to rule out intussusception.
C. Restriction of oral intake to clear fluids to prevent mucosal injury.
D. Antibiotics only if specific pathogens are cultured from the stool.
E. Cessation of all oral feedings and institution of nasogastric drainage, intravenous antibiotics, total parenteral nutrition, and serial abdominal examinations and radiography.

Ref.: 1, 2, 3

COMMENTS: See Question 26.

26. Which of the following are indications for operation in an infant with necrotizing enterocolitis (NEC)?

A. Pneumatosis intestinalis.
B. Portal venous gas.
C. Pneumoperitoneum.
D. Erythema and edema of the abdominal wall.
E. Progressive acidosis and thrombocytopenia.
F. Abdominal mass with fixed bowel loops.

Ref.: 1, 2, 3

COMMENTS: The diagnosis of NEC should be considered whenever a premature infant exhibits the findings listed above, and it is the most likely diagnosis in this infant. NEC is a disease of premature infants and infants subjected to neonatal stress. The pathophysiologic processes involve mucosal ischemia, bowel necrosis, perforation, peritonitis, and sepsis. NEC nearly always occurs in affected infants after the start of oral feedings. Clinical manifestations initially are intolerance of formula, abdominal distension, blood-streaked stools with progression to frank peritonitis, and signs of systemic sepsis including acidosis, disseminated intravascular coagulation, and thrombocytopenia. • Initial treatment is directed at the prevention of both further mucosal injury and septic complications. The initial therapy for NEC is medical: Oral feedings are stopped, tube decompression is instituted, broad-spectrum antibiotics are administered, and fluid and electrolyte support is provided. Close monitoring is mandatory, involving not only physical examination but also serial radiographs every 6–8 hours and serial biochemical assessment to detect signs of deterioration. • *Pneumatosis intestinalis* is a characteristic radiographic finding in NEC caused by invasion of the bowel wall by gas-forming organisms. Similarly, portal venous gas indicates the presence of gas-forming organisms that have been transported in the portal circulation to the liver. Neither of these radiographic findings alone, however, is an absolute indication for operation. • **Indications for surgical intervention are** signs of perforation, peritonitis, and progressive clinical deterioration despite nonoperative therapeutic measures. These signs include pneumoperitoneum, an abdominal mass with fixed bowel loops that may be suggestive of abscess, tenderness, erythema and edema of the abdominal wall, and progressive acidosis or thrombocytopenia. When operation is performed, necrotic bowel is resected, abscesses are drained, and the ends of the retained bowel are brought out as enterostomies. • Persistent acidosis and decreased platelet counts are signs of a poor outcome. The mortality rate associated with NEC ranges from 30% to 60%, according to different reports.

ANSWER:
Question 25: E
Question 26: C, D, E, F

27. Which of the following may be required during treatment of an infant with congenital diaphragmatic hernia?

A. Tube thoracostomy.
B. Extracorporeal membrane oxygenation (ECMO).
C. Nitric oxide.
D. High-frequency oscillatory ventilation (HFOV).
E. Immediate operation.
F. Repair via abdominal approach.
G. Patches of synthetic material for repair.

Ref.: 1, 2, 3

COMMENTS: The primary physiologic disturbance in infants with respiratory distress caused by congenital posterolateral diaphragmatic hernia is related to pulmonary hypoplasia and the high resistance that develops in the pulmonary vasculature because of constriction of pulmonary arterioles. The initial resuscitation must be rapid to avoid stress such as hypoxia, metabolic acidosis, and hypothermia, which increase pulmonary vasoconstriction. High resistance in the pulmonary circulation produces right-to-left shunting via the patent ductus arteriosus, further compromising the infant's cardiopulmonary status. Initial treatment involves endotracheal intubation in infants experiencing respiratory distress, placement of an orogastric tube with suction, and maintenance of adequate vascular volume. Ventilated infants are prone to develop pneumothorax, and tube thoracostomy may be required. Inhaled nitric oxide is a pulmonary vascular dilator and the primary treatment along with HFOV when required to provide gentle ventilation while recruiting alveoli. The use of ECMO has salvaged infants who have remained critically ill despite conventional ventilator support. • Definitive surgical repair is usually carried out via an abdominal approach. Synthetic material such as Gore-Tex may be used to repair the deficit if insufficient diaphragm muscle is present. The possibility of mortality depends on the severity of lung hypoplasia and persistent pulmonary hypertension. Resuscitation and stabilization of pulmonary status are attempted before surgical repair.

ANSWER: A, B, C, D, F, G

28. Which one or more of the following entities characteristically manifests with respiratory distress at birth?

A. Diaphragmatic hernia.
B. Pulmonary sequestration.
C. Tracheoesophageal fistula.
D. Congenital lobar emphysema.

Ref.: 1, 2, 3

COMMENTS: Persistence of the pleuroperitoneal canal of Bochdalek produces the common **congenital diaphragmatic hernia**. Displacement of the abdominal contents into the chest results in pulmonary hypoplasia and high-resistance pulmonary arterioles. Infants often present with low Apgar scores and respiratory distress at birth. Some of these infants initially remain stable and then deteriorate. Other causes of immediate respiratory distress after delivery include pneumothorax, airway obstruction, and aspiration. • With **congenital lobar emphysema** immediate respiratory distress may occur, but progressive respiratory distress more commonly develops as a result of overexpression of the affected lobe. • Patients with **tracheoesophageal fistula** may have difficulty handling salivary secretions because of esophageal atresia, and respiratory symptoms commonly develop with attempted feeding. • The usual complication of **pulmonary sequestration** is infection.

ANSWER: A, C, D

29. Match each clinical characteristic in the left column with the appropriate abdominal wall defect or defects in the right column.

A. Associated anomalies	a. Omphalocele
B. May close spontaneously	b. Gastroschisis
C. Requires operation in the newborn	c. Umbilical hernia
D. Associated heat and fluid losses	d. None of the above
E. Closure may require prosthetic material	
F. Midline lesion	
G. Lateral to umbilical cord	
H. Absence of sac	

Ref.: 1, 2, 3

COMMENTS: Despite the similarities among these lesions, there are also major differences. **Omphalocele** results from failure of embryonic development of a portion of the anterior abdominal wall; it manifests as a truly midline sac-covered defect and frequently is associated with other anomalies. The umbilical cord always forms part of the omphalocele sac. An omphalocele always is covered by a sac devoid of skin and may be ruptured at birth. If the omphalocele is large it is not unusual for a major portion of the liver to protrude into the sac, although this is unusual with gastroschisis. If the omphalocele is small, primary closure usually is possible. If it is large, a silo of Dacron sheet coated with Silastic (Silon) or of Gore-Tex sheet is fashioned around the sac; at subsequent sessions the silo is progressively made smaller until the contents are reduced. In contrast, **gastroschisis** is thought to occur as the result of an umbilical vein vascular accident and manifests with eviscerated bowel through a defect without a sac; it usually appears on the right side of a normal cord. The exposure of the extraperitoneal viscera to amniotic fluid and subsequently to the postnatal environment results in a burn-type physiology with significant fluid and heat losses that must be compensated for during resuscitation of the infant. Gastroschisis can be repaired in one stage, but if this is not possible a Silastic or Gore-Tex silo similar to that for an omphalocele can be used. **Umbilical hernias** result from failure of closure of the linea alba at the umbilical ring and may close spontaneously. If spontaneous closure has not occurred, herniorrhaphy is performed usually when patients are older than 3 years.

ANSWER: A-a; B-c; C-a,b; D-a,b; E-a,b; F-a,c; G-b; H-b

30. A 6-month-old infant has a history of acute onset of crampy abdominal pain and leg withdrawal of 12 hours' duration. Rectal examination shows guaiac-positive stool. Which of the following is the most likely diagnosis?

A. Bleeding Meckel's diverticulum.
B. Acute appendicitis.
C. Kidney stone.
D. Infected urachal cyst.
E. Intussusception.

Ref.: 2, 3

COMMENTS: See Question 32.

31. With regard to the operative management of intussusception, which of the following statements is/are true?

A. Resection should be performed without an attempt at intraoperative reduction if reduction by barium enema has been unsuccessful.
B. Primary ileocolic anastomosis may be performed if bowel resection is necessary.
C. After successful reduction by barium enema, delayed operation should be performed because of the risk of recurrence.
D. After successful reduction by barium enema in a child over 3 years of age, exploration is indicated to rule out associated pathologic processes.

Ref.: 2, 3

COMMENTS: See Question 32.

32. Which of the following are contraindications to attempted barium enema reduction of an intussusception in a child?

A. Pneumoperitoneum.
B. Peritonitis.
C. "Currant jelly" stool.
D. Recurrence after previous hydrostatic reduction.
E. Patient's age over 5 years.

Ref.: 1, 2, 3

COMMENTS: Ileocolic intussusception should be strongly suspected in a child between the ages of 3 and 18 months with the symptoms described in Question 30. Barium enema should be performed promptly for diagnosis and for reduction of the intussusception by hydrostatic pressure. It is successful in approximately 80% of children, usually being the only therapy necessary. An attempt at hydrostatic reduction is contraindicated, however, in the presence of perforation or peritonitis. In such instances prompt operation is indicated. When nonviable bowel is encountered at the time of exploration for intussusception, resection is carried out without an attempt at reduction. Otherwise, reduction by gentle digital pressure pushing intussusceptum proximally is attempted; resection is performed if the intussusception is not reducible by this means. Primary anastomosis can generally be performed. In cases of successful manual reduction at operation, an appendectomy is usually performed. Contrast studies usually are sufficient to rule out significant associated pathologic processes that would require operation in older children. The passage of the characteristic "currant jelly" stool seen with intussusception may occur as the result of mucosal venous congestion and does not necessarily indicate necrosis; thus it does not contraindicate an attempt at nonoperative reduction. Recurrence (in 5% of patients after hydrostatic or open reduction) is no longer considered an absolute indication for surgery, and a second and third attempt at hydrostatic reduction should be attempted and may be successful. Age alone does not mandate operation, although a leading point such as a polyp, Meckel's diverticulum, or tumor (lymphoma) is more likely to be found in older children and is more likely to necessitate an operation. **Acute appendicitis** and **nephrolithiasis** can occur in this age group but are extremely rare. Infected **urachal cyst** is also infrequent, and symptoms are mainly related to sepsis. Bleeding **Meckel's diverticulum** usually is painless, and frank red blood is seen in the stools.

ANSWER:
Question 30: E
Question 31: B
Question 32: A, B

33. Which of the following is the most common complication of a cystic hygroma?

A. Infection.
B. Hemorrhage.
C. Respiratory distress.
D. Malignancy.

Ref.: 1, 2, 3

COMMENTS: Cystic hygroma is a congenital lymphangiomatous malformation commonly occurring in the posterior region of the neck or the axilla, groin, or mediastinum. These lesions can reach large size, and all of the complications listed above have been described except malignant degeneration. Infection, however, is the most common complication.

ANSWER: A

34. Progressive abdominal distension and bilious vomiting develop in a newborn. Radiography reveals distended bowel loops of varying size with air-fluid levels and a "soap suds" appearance in the right lower quadrant. Which of the following procedures should be performed next?

A. Laparotomy.
B. Sweat chloride test.
C. Gastrografin lower gastrointestinal radiography.
D. Gastrografin upper gastrointestinal radiography.
E. Paracentesis.

Ref.: 1, 2, 3

COMMENTS: The postnatal development of signs of intestinal obstruction with classic radiographic findings described above suggests a diagnosis of **meconium ileus**. Nearly all affected infants have cystic fibrosis with a deficiency of pancreatic enzymes, which produces a thick, tenacious meconium plug that causes obstruction in the distal ileum (associated meconium ileus develops in only 10% of children with cystic fibrosis). With uncomplicated meconium ileus, as described in this clinical presentation, administration of a Gastrografin enema may be both diagnostic and therapeutic. The detergent and hyperosmolar effects of the contrast material may relieve the obstruction. Operation is indicated if the obstruction does not respond to the Gastrografin enema or if complications such as peritonitis or perforation are present. In such instances, the usual operative treatment entails resection of impaired bowel and creation of an external vent to allow postoperative irrigation with N-acetylcysteine (Mucormyst); later, gastrointestinal continuity is reestablished. • A sweat chloride test should be performed in all of these infants. • Paracentesis or lavage may be helpful for diagnosing perforated NEC, a condition mandating prompt operation.

ANSWER: C

35. In a newborn undergoing abdominal radiography, the "double-bubble" sign can be seen with which of the following conditions?

A. Duodenal atresia.
B. Normal newborn right after delivery.
C. Malrotation of the midgut.
D. Annular pancreas.
E. Meconium ileus.

Ref.: 1, 2, 3

COMMENTS: The double-bubble sign has always been thought to be pathognomonic of duodenal atresia, but other entities manifest with a similar picture and it is difficult to differentiate them. Infants are born with a gasless abdomen. After taking the first few breaths, they start swallowing air. This column of air usually takes 6–12 hours to reach the distal colon. Therefore, an abdominal film taken a few minutes after delivery might show a double-bubble and yet be normal. • **Annular pancreas** and **duodenal atresia** are clinically similar entities, and though they both necessitate surgical repair they are not operative emergencies. • In contrast, and most important, a double-bubble on a radiograph might be indicative of **malrotation of the midgut with volvulus**, in which case an operation is mandatory as soon as the diagnosis is made; any delay increases the chance of vascular obstruction and necrosis of the entire small bowel. Radiographic assessment of high obstruction in neonates can be performed with simple injection of air into the stomach; contrast dyes are usually not necessary. • **Meconium ileus** is a distal small bowel obstruction in neonates with cystic fibrosis. The radiographic findings are multiple, variably sized loops of small bowel—"soapsuds" appearance—in the right lower quadrant.

ANSWER: A, B, C, D

36. Which of the following entities is the most common cause of duodenal obstruction at birth?

A. Duodenal atresia.
B. Choledochal cyst.
C. Malrotation.
D. Annular pancreas.

Ref.: 1, 2, 3

COMMENTS: Vomiting within the first 24 hours of life in the absence of abdominal distension suggests high obstruction in the neonate. Among the various causes of duodenal obstruction beyond neonatal age, malrotation is the most common and potentially the most serious. The duodenal obstruction generally is caused by extrinsic compression by the peritoneal bands that extend from the abdominal wall to the anomalously located cecum in the right upper quadrant. The catastrophic complication of malrotation is midgut volvulus and intestinal infarction, which occurs because of torsion about the narrow mesenteric pedicle by which the midgut is suspended. Choledochal cyst and annual pancreas may cause duodenal obstruction but are rare.

ANSWER: A

37. Which of the following is the treatment of choice for duodenal atresia?

A. Duodenojejunostomy.
B. Gastrojejunostomy.
C. Roux-en-Y enterostomy.
D. Duodenostomy with delay repair.
E. Duodenoduodenostomy.

Ref.: 1, 2, 3

COMMENTS: Once diagnosis is made, surgery can be deferred until all other pertinent systems can be studied and other anomalies excluded. Duodenoduodenostomy is the preferred operation because it provides physiologic continuity to the gastrointestinal tract. A windsock diaphragm and intraluminal or partial webs should be sought; otherwise, the obstruction may persist. It is mandatory to identify the common bile duct and the ampulla of Vater to obviate any damage to these structures. Postoperatively, the infant is kept on gastric suction until peristalsis resumes, after which oral feedings can be started. Excellent results (in 95% of patients) can be expected from this operation.

ANSWER: E

38. Match each characteristic in the left column with the appropriate pediatric hepatic tumor or tumors in the right column.

A. More common	a. Hepatoblastoma
B. Better prognosis	b. Hepatocarcinoma
C. Bimodal age distribution	
D. Primary treatment surgical	

Ref.: 1, 2, 3

COMMENTS: Hepatoblastoma and hepatocarcinoma are the two most common types of hepatic malignancy in pediatric age groups. Hepatoblastoma is found most frequently in children under 3 years of age; hepatocarcinoma occurs in young infants and during late childhood to early adolescence. Hepatoblastoma is the more common of the two lesions and has the more favorable prognosis (overall 5-year survival rate of 30–50%), whereas the rate of survival with hepatocarcinoma is approximately 15%. α-Fetoprotein is a useful biochemical marker for hepatic malignancies. Therapy of these tumors involves a multimodality approach, although surgical resection offers the best chance of cure.

ANSWER: A-a; B-a; C-b; D-a,b

39. With regard to gastroesophageal reflux in children, which of the following statements is/are true?

A. It has been reported as a primary cause for sudden infant death syndrome.
B. Aspiration pneumonia is a common associated finding.
C. Nissen fundoplication (or its variations) is the preferred surgical treatment.
D. Gastroesophageal reflux is commonly found after repair of esophageal atresia.
E. Cerebral palsy is one of the most common associated diseases.

Ref.: 1, 2, 3

COMMENTS: Sudden infant death syndrome is thought to be caused, at least in part, by gastroesophageal reflux with pulmonary aspiration that triggers apnea in a specific subgroup of infants. The presence of recurrent pneumonia in a young child should alert the clinician to the possibility of aspiration as a result of such reflux. Nissen fundoplication is the preferred surgical therapy for this condition; and good results have been obtained in approximately 85% of patients. Gastroesophageal reflux with aspiration is one of the most common complications after repair of esophageal atresia; Nissen fundoplication is necessary in 20–25% of those infants. Children with cerebral palsy constitute the largest group of patients undergoing operation for this diagnosis in most pediatric hospitals. The relation of the two diseases is not well understood, but they seem to have a central nervous origin, in contrast to gastroesophageal reflux in otherwise normal children, in whom the problem is thought to be related to the gastroesophageal sphincter.

ANSWER: A, B, C, D, E

40. Which of the following tests is the most reliable for establishing the diagnosis of gastroesophageal reflux in pediatric patients?

A. Esophagram.
B. Upper gastrointestinal series.
C. Nuclear scan after ingestion of radioactive milk.
D. Esophagoscopy with biopsy.

E. Monitoring the pH of the esophagus for 12–24 hours.

Ref.: 1, 2, 3

COMMENTS: All of the studies listed above are used for diagnosis of gastroesophageal reflux, but there is no doubt today that the test of choice is the 12- to 24-hour pH monitoring of the esophagus.

ANSWER: E

41. Match each characteristic in the left column with the appropriate pediatric solid tumor or tumors in the right column.

A. More common during first 2 years of life
B. Usually manifests as an asymptomatic mass
C. Calyceal distortion on intravenous pyelography (IVP)
D. Elevated vanillylmandelic acid (VMA) level
E. Primary treatment is surgical
F. Overall 5-year survival rate >75%

a. Wilms' tumor
b. Neuroblastoma

Ref.: 1, 2, 3

COMMENTS: Neuroblastoma and nephroblastoma (Wilms' tumor) are common solid malignancies in children. Neuroblastoma is the second most common solid tumor after brain tumors. The clinical presentation is often similar for abdominal involvement, the most common site for both; the diseases manifest as an asymptomatic mass in children during the first years of life. **Wilms' tumor**, which is an embryonal tumor arising from the kidney, typically produces distortion of the renal collecting system as seen on IVP. The lungs are the most common site of metastatic disease. **Neuroblastoma** arises from cells of neural crest origin, typically occurring in the adrenal or posterior mediastinum. IVP differentiates adrenal neuroblastoma from Wilms' tumor by demonstrating renal displacement but not calyceal distortion. Neuroblastoma may extend through the intervertebral foramen, and because of this feature magnetic resonance imaging of the spine should be performed on all these patients. Because of continued catecholamine turnover, VMA levels are elevated in most patients with neuroblastoma and have been a useful biochemical marker. Horner syndrome is a common finding in children with cervical neuroblastoma, attributed to the origin of this tumor at the site of the stellate ganglia. Neuroblastoma most commonly metastasizes to the liver and bone. The primary treatment of both of these lesions is complete surgical excision, which is more often possible with Wilms' tumor. Both chemotherapy and radiotherapy are used but have been more useful for enhancing the survival of patients with Wilms' tumor than those with neuroblastoma. The overall cure rate for Wilms' tumor is approximately 80%, compared with 30% for neuroblastoma. Younger children with neuroblastoma have a better prognosis, however, and infants under 1 year of age may attain a survival rate of 80%.

ANSWER: A-b; B-a,b; C-a; D-b; E-a,b; F-a

42. Daily fluid requirements vary by age and weight. Which of the following statements are true?

A. Premature infants weighing less than 2 kg may require up to 150 ml/kg/day.
B. Neonates and infants of 3–10 kg require 200 ml/kg/day.
C. Infants and children of 10–20 kg require 1000 ml/day + 30 ml/kg/day for every kilogram over 10.
D. Children over 20 kg require 1500 ml/day + 20 ml/kg/day for every kilogram over 20.

Ref.: 1, 2, 3

COMMENTS: Premature infants require up to 150 ml/kg/day because of their inability to achieve conservation of heat and high insensible losses through immature skin. Newborn term infants during the first 24 hours of life require 80–90 ml/kg/day due to hypervolemia from transfusion of fluid via placenta at birth. Diuresis occurs during the first week of life. Neonates less than 30 days of age then require 110 ml/kg/day. Infants more than 30 days of age to adulthood require 100 ml/kg/day for the first 10 kg, plus 50 ml/kg/day for 10–20 kg, plus 20 ml/kg/day for every kilogram over 20.

ANSWER: A, D

43. Match the appropriate kilocalories and protein requirement to age.

Age (years)	***Kilocalories (kcal/kg)/ Protein (g/kg)***
A. 0–1	a. 30–60/1.5
B. 1–7	b. 60–75/2.0
C. 7–12	c. 90–120/2.5–3.5
D. 12–18	d. 75–90/2.0–2.5

Ref.: 1, 2, 3

COMMENTS: Infants require an average of 110 kcal/kg/day; and if stressed they may require protein up to 2.5–3.5 gm/kg/day. Appropriate weight gain for a neonate is 1% body weight per day. As children age their caloric needs decrease, as do their protein needs, so by the time they reach adolescence they require approximately 50% of their neonatal needs.

ANSWER: A-c; B-d; C-b; D-a

44. A 3-year-old boy is brought to the emergency room via ambulance after being extricated from a motor vehicle accident. He was an unrestrained rear-seat passenger. He is crying and struggling. His pulse is 150 bpm, blood pressure 90/50 mm Hg, respiratory rate 40 breaths per minute, and weight 15 kg. His initial management should include:

A. Placement of oral airway, auscultation of breath sounds, 300 ml crystalloid bolus via peripheral intravenous infusion, diagnostic peritoneal gavage to rule out intraabdominal bleeding in light of unstable hemodynamics.
B. Fentanyl 15 mg for pain and sedation, intubation for airway control, CT scan of head and abdomen, monitoring of airway, oxygen administration via face mask.
C. Crystalloid bolus 150 ml via central venous line.
D. Administration of oxygen, placement of nasogastric tube, auscultation of breath sounds, 300 ml crystalloid bolus via peripheral intravenous infusion.

Ref.: 1, 2, 3

COMMENTS: Sedation should be used for trauma resuscitation only after a primary survey including neurologic disability. Observation and maintenance of the airway is the first step in management while maintaining cervical spine precautions. Although it is normal for a child to struggle and cry while being restrained by strangers, during trauma resuscitation these signs should be read as potential hypoxemia, and oxygen administration by face mask should be initiated with pulse oximetry monitoring. Intubation may be required if hypoxemia persists. Placement of a nasogastric tube is appropriate to empty the stomach and reduce the risk of aspiration from emesis and to relieve the gastric distension resulting from air swallowing with crying. This measure helps reduce respiratory distress in infants who are "abdominal breathers." Breath sounds are assessed to relieve life-threatening pneumothorax prior to chest radiography. The fluid bolus is given via a peripheral intravenous infusion if possible at 20 ml/kg using warmed lactated Ringer's solution, lessening the risk of hyperchloremic metabolic acidosis. If peripheral access is not easily obtained, an intraosseous needle is placed—a safer, more expedient method then central venous access. Vital signs must be monitored for a response to the fluid bolus. In a 15 kg 3-year-old boy who is crying, a pulse of 150 bpm may reflect agitation but should be presumed to be hypovolemia in the setting of trauma. Blood pressure is normally 100/60 mm Hg in this age range; and if an appropriate increase with the bolus is not observed, a second bolus of lactated Ringer's solution (20 ml/kg) should be given. CT is the diagnostic test of choice for the child with stable hemodynamics and suspected head and abdominal injuries.

ANSWER: D

45. Which of the following statements concerning branchial cleft sinuses is/are true?

A. A branchial cleft sinus is a small pairless opening in the anterior border of the sternocleinomastoid muscle and may be associated with a cyst or infection.
B. The first branchial cleft sinus routinely drains into the internal auditory canal and is associated with chronic otitis media.
C. Second branchial cleft sinuses, when complete, track through the carotid bifurcation and into the tonsillar fossa.
D. Differential diagnosis includes cystic hygroma, dermoid, lipoma, neurofibroma, lymphadenitis.

Ref.: 1, 2, 3

COMMENTS: The first branchial cleft sinus routinely ends in the external auditory canal if complete. When it is infected it is associated with a draining sinus located anterior to the ear. During excision, risk includes injury to the facial nerve.

ANSWER: A, C, D

REFERENCES

1. Sabiston DC Jr: *Textbook of Surgery*, 15th ed. WB Saunders, Philadelphia, 1997.
2. Schwartz SI, Shires GT, Spencer FC: *Principles of Surgery*, 7th ed. McGraw-Hill, New York, 1999.
3. Rowe MI, O'Neill JA, Grosfied JL, et al: *Essentials of Pediatric Surgery*. Mosby, St. Louis, 1995.

CHAPTER 39

Vascular

A. Principles

1. Which of the following is/are the most common cause(s) of late failure of reversed saphenous vein grafts?

A. Smoking.
B. Progression of atherosclerosis proximal to the graft.
C. Progression of atherosclerosis distal to the graft.
D. Hypercoagulable states.
E. Vein graft atherosclerosis.

Ref.: 1, 2, 3

COMMENTS: Smoking is the single most important risk factor that determines the late success of any percutaneous or operative interventions. Continued smoking decreases long-term patency rates for both operative bypass and balloon angioplasty by almost 50%. Whereas early failure of saphenous vein grafts is attributed to technical error, late failure is usually related to progressive atherosclerosis of the arterial inflow or the outflow. Other pathogenic changes that may lead to late failure include valve stenosis due to fibrosis, and atherosclerosis of the vein graft itself.

ANSWER: A

2. Which of the following characterize claudication?

A. The term claudication originated from the Greek ruler Claudius, who suffered from a disabling form of this condition.
B. Without intervention, the risk of limb loss approaches 50% at 5 years.
C. It can be alleviated significantly with pentoxifylline, cilostazol or verapamil.
D. It can be managed successfully without arteriography, balloon angioplasty, or operation in most cases.
E. The optimal treatment is cessation of smoking and exercise consisting of 1 hour of walking per day.

Ref.: 1, 2, 3, 4, 5

COMMENTS: Claudication is derived from the Latin root meaning "to limp." The risk of limb loss for all claudicants is only 5% over 5 years. The risk of limb loss drops substantially, from 12% to 2%, if a patient successfully stops smoking. Claudication usually can be treated safely with medication. Several medications, including pentoxyphylline, cilostazol and verapamil have been shown to improve walking distance. "Stop smoking and keep walking" are five words that sum up the treatment strategy for most patients. A regular, organized walking program generally doubles walking distance.

ANSWER: C, D, E

3. Which one or more of the following describes chronic leg ulcers?

A. The etiology of ulcers often can be diagnosed by their location on the leg.
B. Venous ulcers are seldom located on the foot.
C. Arterial ulcers are seldom located on the leg.
D. Leg ulcers affect diabetic patients less often than other patient groups.

Ref.: 1, 2, 3

COMMENTS: Chronic venous insufficiency causes characteristic skin changes including hyperpigmentation, thickened skin, and ulceration in the gaiter region, named for the ski clothing that covers the leg from the ankle to the knee. **Venous** ulcers usually occur at the malleoli but seldom extend below the ankles. **Arterial** ulcers form at the distal aspect to the region that has compromised arterial circulation. It usually results in ulcers of the toes or foot, but islands of ischemia can occur more proximally on the leg, especially the anterior leg. Diabetic patients can form **neurotrophic** ulcers. The neuropathy that afflicts patients with long-standing diabetes causes wasting of the muscles of the foot and collapse of the standard architecture of the foot, causing pressure points between the toes and at the metatarsal heads. Strict non-weight-bearing is important if one is to heal these pressure ulcers when the arterial circulation is adequate. If the arterial circulation is compromised, these patients usually need arterial leg bypass operations, rather than balloon angioplasty to heal these ulcers.

ANSWER: A, B

4. Which of the following is/are characteristic of ischemic extremity rest pain?

A. Occurs mostly at night.
B. Can be relieved by placing the involved extremity in the dependent position.
C. Is usually located at the toes.
D. Can be relieved by intravenous heparin.
E. Can be relieved with pentoxyphylline.

F. Is characterized as nocturnal calf cramping.

Ref.: 1, 2, 4, 5

COMMENTS: Extremity angina occurs most commonly at night because when patients with severe lower extremity arterial insufficiency lie supine, they lose the added benefit of gravity for perfusing the lower extremity. Patients with nocturnal ischemic rest pain quickly discover that walking, standing, or sleeping in a chair relieves this pain, which is centered over the metatarsal heads, not the toes. Pain in the toes suggest gout or an infection. Intravenous heparin causes vasodilation by promoting the release of nitric oxide, thereby improving extremity arterial circulation. Intravenous heparin can relieve rest pain until the arterial circulation can be improved with a bypass operation. Pentoxifylline improves claudication-impaired distance walking but has not been shown to be effective for treating ischemic rest pain. Nocturnal calf cramping afflicts one in five adults and is not indicative of extremity ischemia.

ANSWER: A, B, D

5. Which of the following characteristics of leg swelling due to venous insufficiency or lymphedema is/are true?

A. Lymphedema usually involves the feet and toes (boxcar toes), whereas swelling due to venous insufficiency usually does not involve the toes.
B. Venous insufficiency causes pigmentation and hypertrophic changes in the skin over the ankle, but lymphedema does not.
C. Lymphedema causes elephantiasis.
D. Operative intervention can treat venous insufficiency but not lymphedema.

Ref.: 2, 3, 5

COMMENTS: Lymphedema is found in the toes, feet, ankle, and leg, in that order. The squaring off of the toes found with lymphedema (boxcar toes) is not found with isolated venous insufficiency. Hyperpigmentation and cicatrix formation in the gaiter region (legs from ankle to knees) is pathognomonic of venous insufficiency and is caused by the breakdown of extravascular red blood cells and subcutaneous scar tissue (liposclerosis). With severe cases of untreated chronic venous insufficiency, this scar tissue formation can cause local destruction of leg lymphatics and cause secondary formation of lymphedema. Any severe hypoproteinemia can cause lymphedema. Operations for lymphedema are generally not performed. Operation for venous insufficiency include perforator vein ligation, varicose vein ligation and stripping, and deep vein valve transplant. Lymphedema can be associated with hyperpigmentation, but it is not as severe as is seen with venous insufficiency. Elephantiasis is caused by a parasitic infection that results in blockage of extremity lymphatics.

ANSWER: A, D

6. A patient underwent aortobifemoral bypass grafting 9 months ago and now has purulent drainage from the left side of the groin. Along with the administration of intravenous antibiotics, appropriate treatment includes which one or more of the following?

A. Surgical drainage of the left side of the groin.
B. High ligation and excision of the left limb of the graft and, if necessary, extraanatomic bypass.
C. Removal of the entire prosthesis and bilateral axillofemoral bypass.
D. Ligation of the left femoral artery and, if necessary, amputation.

Ref.: 1, 2, 3

COMMENTS: The general approach to the treatment of infected prosthetic grafts involves antibiotics, removal of the entire prosthesis, and reestablishment of vascular continuity through noncontaminated fields. In select circumstances, local drainage and intravenous antibiotics alone may be adequate to control infection, particularly if the anastomotic suture line is not involved and viable tissue can be rotated to cover the exposed prosthetic material. The options available depend critically on the extent of infection along the prosthesis and the previous operative sites. Extraanatomic routes of axillofemoral or femorofemoral grafts permit revascularization through a clean field distal to the original site, but often they are not applicable when the femoral artery anastomosis is infected. In the case described, infection at the femoral anastomosis precludes left repeated common femoral artery grafting. If the graft above the inguinal ligament is uninvolved, the aortic and right-limb portions could be salvaged, and either obturator bypass from the right-limb graft to the left superficial femoral artery or left axillosuperficial femoral artery or left axillopopliteal artery bypass brought laterally to avoid the contaminated groin could be performed. In situations requiring revascularization through a contaminated area, autologous tissue using superficial femoral vein can be used. Autologous tissue, however, can also become infected; and for that reason a route for revascularization that avoids the area of contamination is always preferable. If the patient's life is in jeopardy from systemic sepsis, femoral artery ligation and amputation is an unpleasant but acceptable alternative treatment ("life before limb").

ANSWER: A, B, C, D

7. The *early* objective diagnosis of compartmental syndrome is *best* verified by which of the following?

A. Tense fullness of the compartment.
B. Absence of distal pulses.
C. Paralysis of compartmental nerves.
D. Compartmental pain.
E. Compartmental pressure higher than 40 mm Hg.
F. None of the above.

Ref.: 2, 3, 4

COMMENTS: Compartmental syndromes occur whenever tissue pressure within a confined anatomic space becomes sufficiently elevated to impair venous return. It can be due to bleeding within a compartment or to reperfusion edema. There is no absolute pressure above which the syndrome invariably occurs. Tissue blood flow diminishes rapidly as the venous pressure approaches the tissue pressure, which is approximately 30 mm Hg. Successful treatment is based on early, accurate diagnosis. All the aforementioned symptoms and signs are important, and compartmental syndromes are best diagnosed by a high index of suspicion. Pulses may be palpated even in the presence of developing compartment syndrome.

ANSWER: F

8. In a low resistance arterial vascular system, at which percent diameter reduction does a stenosis become flow limiting?

A. 10%.
B. 20%.
C. 40%.
D. 50%.
E. 80%.

Ref.: 2, 6

COMMENTS: In low resistance arterial systems, such as the internal carotid artery, total blood flow across a stenosis does not decrease until the diameter is reduced by approximately 50%. This corresponds to a 75% reduction in cross-sectional area. Total blood flow is maintained by increasing the velocity. Shear stress (drag) and viscosity limit further increases in velocity once the diameter reduction exceeds 50%. This hemodynamic fact is the reason for not repairing short stenoses of less than 50%, as total blood flow is not altered. A longer stenosis increases the shear stress and causes a lesser degree of stenosis over a long length to be flow-limiting.

ANSWER: D

9. Which of the following characterize duplex ultrasound imaging?

A. Duplex is a combination of Doppler and B-mode ultrasonography.
B. Lower frequencies (e.g., 3 MHz) are better suited for deep abdominal imaging, and higher frequencies (e.g., 7 MHz) are better for more superficial structures, such as in situ vein grafts.
C. High-frequency ultrasound waves have higher energy than low-frequency ultrasound waves.
D. Diagnosis of deep venous thrombosis (DVT) is best done without color flow imaging.
E. Calcification within a diseased artery usually is severe enough to prevent an adequate vascular ultrasound examination.

Ref.: 2, 3, 6

COMMENTS: Duplex ultrasonography consists of the B-mode image (picture) and Doppler shift, which measures the velocity of the flowing blood. High-frequency transducers (7–10 MHz) are used for superficial structures such as saphenous vein mapping and in situ vein bypasses or pedal bypasses. These higher frequency transducers have greater resolution but lower energy and cannot penetrate deeper tissues as can lower frequency, higher energy transducers (3 or 5 MHz). Venous flow velocity is slower than arterial flow, so artifacts can be more easily introduced by transducer movement when performing a venous examination, especially to rule out a DVT. For these reasons, a more accurate venous examination to look for a DVT is one without color. The black and white image allows better assessment of vein compressibility and is not confused by an artifact introduced by transducer movement. Arterial wall calcium occasionally interferes with vascular ultrasound scans by blocking ultrasound wave transmission, but it is unusual that one cannot perform an adequate vascular examination of the carotid or other structure because of severe calcification.

ANSWER: A, B, D

10. The advantages of lower extremity arterial Doppler examinations performed with waveform analysis compared to the ankle-brachial index (ABI) alone include which of the following?

A. Calcification of the artery by diseases such as diabetes mellitus and chronic renal failure make the arterial wall incompressible, causing the ABI to be artificially elevated and unreliable.
B. Inflow disease can be recognized by the delay in the upstroke of the waveform.
C. The loss of reversal of flow—when the arterial waveform transforms from triphasic to biphasic—is observed with exercise or with moderate atherosclerosis.
D. The ABI can be used to diagnose an arteriovenous fistula.
E. The ABI can be used to diagnose a deep vein thrombosis (DVT).

Ref.: 2, 3, 6

COMMENTS: The ABI is a measurement for quantifying extremity ischemia. The assumption behind using the ABI to quantify the degree of extremity ischemic is that the flow in the limb is proportional to the blood pressure in the limb. The ABI is obtained with a blood pressure cuff and a hand-held Doppler instrument. The cuff is applied at the point the pressure measurement is desired. The Doppler device is placed over any vessel distal to the cuff, but routinely it is the radial artery in the upper extremity or the posterior tibial or dorsal pedal artery in the lower extremity. The cuff is inflated to a pressure greater than the systolic pressure. The pressure at which the arterial Doppler signal returns as the cuff is deflated is the pressure used to calculate the ABI. Diabetes and renal failure cause calcification of the axial extremity arteries, which makes the arteries noncompressible; the ABI is artificially elevated with these conditions. When the ABI is unreliable (ABI >1.2), one must depend on the Doppler waveform to assess the degree of extremity ischemia. Waveforms become monophasic in diseased arteries regardless of whether the vessels are compressible. The degree of arterial inflow disease (above the inguinal ligament) can be assessed by examining the femoral artery waveform. An arterial upstroke prolonged to more than 180 ms is consistent with significant iliac disease. Digital artery pressures are useful for quantifying ischemia in patients with diabetes and renal failure, as these vessels are usually compressible even in these conditions. Toe pressures of less than 30 mm Hg are consistent with severe ischemia in nondiabetic patients, and those less than 50 mm Hg are consistent with severe ischemia in diabetic patients. Reversal of blood flow direction is caused by vascular resistance. Exercise causes vasodilation in the muscular beds and decreases resistance, resulting in the loss of flow. The first change one observes in waveform morphology due to mild atherosclerotic disease is the loss of flow reversal, when the waveform goes from triphasic to biphasic. Duplex imaging is required to diagnose arteriovenous fistulas and deep venous thrombosis; the ABI alone is inadequate to diagnose these conditions.

ANSWER: A, B, C

11. While performing duplex imaging of the carotid arteries, what factors help distinguish the external carotid artery from the internal carotid artery?

A. The internal carotid artery has continuous forward flow. The external carotid artery has reversal of flow during diastole.
B. The external carotid artery is larger.
C. The internal carotid artery is generally seen first.
D. The superior thyroid artery is the first branch of the internal carotid artery and aids in identifying the internal carotid artery.

Ref.: 2, 3

COMMENTS: The external carotid artery is usually found anteromedially, whereas the internal carotid artery is usually found posterolaterally on the Duplex examination. The external carotid artery is usually the first artery seen; it has triphasic flow, not continuous flow as is found in the internal carotid artery. The first branch of the external carotid artery is the superior thyroid artery. The internal carotid artery has monophasic continuous flow because it feeds the brain, a low resistance system. The external carotid artery has triphasic flow with flow reversal because it feeds the face and its musculature, all high resistance systems. Both arteries are approximately the same size in their proximal aspects. The internal carotid has no branches in the neck in contrast to the external carotid artery.

ANSWER: A

12. Which of the following statements regarding percutaneous transluminal balloon angioplasty (PTA) for the treatment of occlusive atherosclerotic arterial blockages or stenoses is/are true?

A. The rates for intimal hyperplasia following PTA in a small artery (<5 mm) exceed the rates observed following operative repair of arteries of a similar size.
B. The short- and long-term results of balloon angioplasty for lesions longer than 10 cm are better than the results for operative intervention.
C. Balloon angioplasty has demonstrated excellent results for stenotic lesions of the common iliac artery, but the results that are not as good for occlusive lesions of the external iliac artery.
D. Complications of PTA include dissection, thrombosis, and atheroembolization.

Ref.: 2, 3, 6

COMMENTS: PTA is performed via the percutaneous intravascular passage of balloon-tipped catheters. During balloon dilation the atherosclerotic intima is ruptured and compressed, allowing the media to become overstretched. PTA works best for short stenoses or occlusions in large arteries, such as may be found in the common iliac artery. The success rates for PTA of the common iliac artery are 80% at 1 year. The results of PTA of the external iliac artery fall off to approximately 55% at 2 years. • Myointimal hyperplasia affects all blood vessels that have undergone intervention, but this process exerts its greatest influence on small arteries with diameters less than 5 mm. Stents have been introduced to combat this problem, but they have not eliminated this complication of PTA. Myointimal hyperplasia can lead to failure rates of up to 40% at 6 months for small arteries that have undergone PTA, with the outcome being recurrent stenosis or thrombosis. PTA of long superficial femoral artery lesions has a success rate of only 22% at 1 year, whereas femoropopliteal bypass has a patency rate of 90% at 1 year. PTA of the renal artery works well for fibromuscular dysplasia but not as effectively for atherosclerotic lesions. The patency rates following PTA of the renal artery is only 60% at 2 years. Atheroembolization, dissection, and thrombosis can complicate any attempted percutaneous intervention and can lead to limb loss.

ANSWER: A, C, D

13. What is the most common cause of a *congenital* hypercoagulable disorder?

A. Protein S deficiency.
B. Protein C deficiency.
C. Antithrombin III deficiency.
D. Activated protein C resistance (APC-R) (factor V Leiden mutation).
E. Homocysteinemia.

Ref.: 2, 3, 6

COMMENTS: Hemostasis is a finely tuned balance between coagulation and fibrinolysis. The existence of a congenital defect in the procoagulant or anticoagulant proteins can shift this balance and cause increased bleeding or increased thrombotic tendencies, respectively. Hypercoagulable states are the most common cause of early bypass graft failure in young adults who require vascular interventions for limb salvage. More than 50% of patients under the age of 50 who require a lower extremity bypass and experience early graft thrombosis have a hypercoagulable state. • Protein C, protein S, and antithrombin III deficiency have been known to exist for years, but until recently a specific inherited hypercoagulable state could not be identified in as many as 80% of patients. • We now know that **activated protein C resistance (APC-R)** is the most common inherited hypercoagulable state, existing in more than 50% of patients with inherited thrombosis tendencies. The etiology of APC-R is an amino acid substitution in factor V of glutamine for arginine 506. Patients with activated protein C resistance have a poor anticoagulant response to activated protein C, a vitamin K-dependent and anticoagulant protein. When protein C is activated, it normally degrades activated clotting factors Va and VIIa. The altered factor V, or Leiden mutation (named for the Belgium city where it was first found), is resistant to the degrading action of APC. The altered, activated factor V retains its procoagulant activity, and the hemostatic balance is shifted toward thrombosis. • **Antithrombin III** is the major plasma inhibitor of thrombin. Heparin performs its anticoagulant function by forming a trivalent molecule of heparin–antithrombin III–thrombin to inactivate thrombin. This deficiency is rare, with an incidence of only 1:5000. Thrombotic events are usually triggered by trauma, operation, or pregnancy. • **Proteins C and S** are both vitamin K-dependent *anticoagulant* proteins synthesized by the liver. The incidence of congenital protein C deficiency is 1:200. Protein C and S deficiencies are found in 20% of patients under the age of 50 with arterial thrombosis, but the combined incidence is much less than the incidence of APC-R. • The treatment for antithrombin III, protein C, and protein S deficiency is lifelong warfarin anticoagulation. Heparin must be given before initiating warfarin anticoagulation in these patients to protect against warfarin-induced skin necrosis. *All* patients with thrombosis who are to receive warfarin therapy should receive heparin during the first 3–4 days of warfarin therapy because the half-life of the anticoagulation protein C is much less, as it is degraded much faster than the procoagulant vitamin K-dependent factors II, IX, and X. • **Mild homocysteinemia exists in 5–7%** of the population. Elevated levels of homocysteine occur because of a defect in the pathway that metabolizes methionine. The treatment for homocysteinemia is the B vitamin folate 1–5 mg/day.

ANSWER: D

14. What is the most common cause of an *acquired* hypercoaguable state?

A. Smoking.
B. Heparin-induced thrombocytopenia.
C. Antiphospholipid antibody (e.g., lupus anticoagulant).
D. Warfarin.
E. Oral contraceptives.

Ref.: 2, 3, 6

COMMENTS: **Smoking** is the most common cause of acquired hypercoagulability. Smoking is the most important factor that determines the short- and long-term results of any vascular intervention. The mechanisms of action of smoking are multiple and include both vasoconstriction and a measurable elevation of plasma fibrinogen levels, which itself is a risk factor for thrombosis. • The next most common cause of acquired hypercoaguability is **heparin-induced thrombocytopenia (HIT)**. This condition affects 2–3% of all patients who receive heparin. Antibodies form to heparin because it is obtained from bovine or porcine sources. The clinical manifestations are a falling platelet count, increasing resistance to anticoagulation with heparin, and new paradoxical thrombotic events while receiving heparin treatment. Although low-molecular-weight heparin has a lower incidence of HIT than standard heparin, 25% of patients with HIT who receive low-molecular-weight heparin manifest the heparin allergy. The treatment for HIT is cessation of all heparin. Warfarin-induced skin necrosis is unusual so long as heparin is given for the first 3 days that warfarin is given. • **The antiphospholipid syndrome (APS)** is common, affecting 1–5% of the population. Specific types are lupus anticoagulant and anticardiolipin antibodies. The incidence of APS increases with age, so 50% of patients over the age of 80 have APS. This syndrome is recognized by prolongation of the baseline partial thromboplastin time (PPT). Brain thromboplastin is the reagent used for triggering the intrinsic clotting system when the PTT is measured. Patients with APS have serum antibodies that consume this reagent, resulting in a prolonged PTT. This is an unforgiving hypercoagulable state with an incidence of thrombotic complications approaching 50%. • **Warfarin** and **oral contraceptives** are less common causes of hypercoagulability.

ANSWER: A

REFERENCES

1. Sabiston DC Jr: *Textbook of Surgery*, 15th ed. WB Saunders, Philadelphia, 1997.
2. Moore WS: *Vascular Surgery*, 5th ed. WB Saunders, Philadelphia, 1998.
3. Yao STJ, Pearce WH: *Practical Vascular Surgery*. Appleton & Lange, Stamford, CT, 1999.
4. Schwartz SI, Shires GT, Spencer FC: *Principles of Surgery*, 7th ed. McGraw-Hill, New York, 1999.
5. Ernst CB, Stanley JC: *Current Therapy in Vascular Surgery*, 3rd ed. Mosby, St. Louis, 1995.
6. Porter JM, Taylor LM Jr: *Basic Data Underlying Clinical Decision Making in Vascular Surgery*. Quality Medical Publishing, St. Louis, 1994.

Vascular

B. Cerebrovascular

1. The most common cause of cerebral ischemia involves which one of the following?

   A. Extracranial arterial stenosis.
   B. Intracranial arterial thrombosis.
   C. Arterioarterial embolization (atheroembolization).
   D. Cardioarterial embolization.

Ref.: 1, 2

COMMENTS: Atherosclerosis is the most common cause of ischemic stroke. Arterioarterial embolization of plaque fragments from degenerative plaques or platelet fibrin aggregates from a thrombogenic plaque surface are believed to be responsible for the neurologic injury. A small proportion of ischemic strokes may be caused by processes other than atherosclerosis, such as emboli from cardiac sources, fibromuscular hyperplasia, occlusive arteritis of the aortic arch vessels (Takayasu's disease), dissecting thoracic aortic aneurysms, and trauma.

ANSWER: C

2. What percentage of patients with cerebral ischemia have a surgically accessible lesion?

   A. 95%.
   B. 75%.
   C. 50%.
   D. 25%.
   E. 5%.

Ref.: 2

COMMENTS: Of the patients with cerebrovascular ischemia who are studied by four-vessel angiography (common carotid and vertebral arteries), 75% are found to have significant extracranial disease that is surgically accessible. In the carotid vessels, lesions characteristically involve the carotid bifurcation and the proximal 1–2 cm of the internal carotid artery. In patients with vertebral basilar insufficiency, plaques or stenotic lesions characteristically occur near the origin of the vertebral arteries from the subclavian vessels. Because stroke is the third leading cause of death in the United States and because the responsible lesions are often surgically accessible, endarterectomy benefits a significant proportion of patients with symptoms of cerebral ischemia.

ANSWER: B

3. In patients with at least a 60% diameter stenosis site, for which one or more of the following situations is carotid endarterectomy a generally accepted form of treatment?

   A. Acute stroke, rapid recovery, negative head computed tomography (CT) scan.
   B. Acute stroke, totally occluded internal carotid artery.
   C. Transient neurologic deficit (<24 hours).
   D. Completed stroke, mild deficit, ulcerated carotid plaque.
   E. Completed stroke, totally occluded internal carotid artery.

Ref.: 1, 2

COMMENTS: Among patients with symptoms of cerebrovascular ischemia, those with transient ischemic attacks (TIAs) are optimal candidates for carotid endarterectomy, because their risk of subsequent stroke is significantly decreased by operative intervention. Endarterectomy may also benefit patients with a completed stroke if the neurologic deficit is not severe and there is no evidence of a stroke on CT scan. A large stroke evident on CT scans means the patient should wait 6 weeks for endarterectomy. There is no benefit to performing endarterectomy of the internal carotid artery for a completed stroke with total occlusion of the internal carotid artery, because restoration of flow does not restore neurologic function. The role of carotid endarterectomy in an acute or evolving stroke is controversial. Restoration of flow is usually not indicated in patients with acute, fixed deficits and may in fact worsen symptoms and produce death by causing hemorrhage in the area of infarction. In patients with an evolving stroke (so called crescendo TIAs) and fluctuating neurologic deficit, emergent endarterectomy may be of benefit.

ANSWER: A, C, D

4. The presence of a cervical bruit is correlated with which one or more of the following?

   A. Risk of stroke.
   B. Presence of carotid stenosis.
   C. Degree of carotid stenosis.
   D. Presence of ulcerated carotid stenosis.
   E. Risk of coronary artery disease.

Ref.: 2

COMMENTS: Cervical bruits reflect disturbances of flow and may result from carotid or noncarotid sources, such as cardiac valvar disease. The presence of a bruit is not a reliable indicator of hemodynamically significant stenosis. Whereas half of all patients with hemodynamically significant lesions have a cervical bruit, only one-third of patients with bruits have hemodynamically significant lesions. The other two-thirds of patients with bruits have stenoses of at least 40%. The stroke rate has been higher than expected when bruits were detected. Studies have demonstrated a strong correlation between cervical bruits and subsequent risk of coronary artery disease. Despite the poor correlation between the mere presence of a cervical bruit and ipsilateral cerebral ischemia, bruits should not be ignored and should prompt a noninvasive evaluation to rule out significant carotid lesions.

ANSWER: A, B, E

5. Which of the following is the best screening test for significant carotid stenosis in a patient with an asymptomatic bruit?

A. Magnetic resonance angiography.
B. Four-vessel cerebral angiography.
C. Digital subtraction angiography.
D. CT brain scan with infusion.
E. Duplex scanning.

Ref.: 1, 2

COMMENTS: Because of their sensitivity, safety, and repeatability, noninvasive cerebrovascular studies provide the best means of screening patients with asymptomatic bruits to detect significant stenotic lesions. **Duplex scanning** (real-time B-mode ultrasonography), which combines ultrasonography and frequency spectrum analysis, provides a noninvasive method for quantifying the degree of stenosis and assessing morphologic characteristics. As such, it is the single best screening test for evaluating carotid disease. **Angiography** is the definitive method of evaluating carotid anatomy in most centers, but it is not advocated as a screening procedure because it carries a 0.5–1.0% combined risk of mortality and major neurologic injury. **Digital subtraction angiography** has been evaluated as a screening tool in asymptomatic patients but has been found to have limited usefulness. **CT scan** of the brain and **electroencephalography** rarely are indicated for screening.

ANSWER: E

6. With regard to asymptomatic carotid stenosis, which of the following statements is/are true?

A. If symptoms eventually develop, they invariably involve TIAs, not stroke.
B. The incidence of subsequent TIAs is higher among patients with stenosis than in those without stenosis.
C. The incidence of subsequent stroke is higher among patients with stenosis than in those without stenosis.
D. Cerebral ischemic events can be decreased by prophylactic carotid endarterectomy in patients with as little as 40% stenosis.

Ref.: 1, 2, 3

COMMENTS: The value of prophylactic carotid endarterectomy in patients with asymptomatic stenosis is predicated on a progressive natural history of the disease process and the ability to perform endarterectomy with morbidity and mortality rates of less than 2%. Several studies have shown that among *asymptomatic* patients with hemodynamically significant carotid stenosis (exceeding 60%) the percentage of cerebral ischemic events is higher than among patients without stenosis, and that carotid endarterectomy in a prophylactic setting probably decreases the expected risk of cerebral ischemic events. No data to date, however, support the use of endarterectomy in patients with a less than 60% asymptomatic stenosis.

ANSWER: B, C

7. Of the following changing factors that contribute to flow through a stenotic artery, which is the most important?

A. Diameter of stenosis.
B. Length of stenosis.
C. Blood viscosity.
D. Blood pressure.

Ref.: 1

COMMENTS: Stenosis is usually considered hemodynamically significant if the diameter of the lumen is reduced by 50% or more, which corresponds to a 75% decrease in cross-sectional area. Blood flow is best described by Poiseuille's law, written as $Q = \Delta P \pi r^4/8Ln$, where Q is flow, P is pressure, r is radius, L is length, and n is viscosity. Flow is proportional to pressure and inversely proportional to the length of the stenosis and to the blood viscosity, but flow is directly related to the fourth power of the radius. The radius is the most important factor when determining total blood flow.

ANSWER: A

8. A patient with symptomatic (85%) carotid stenosis is found to have 50% stenosis of the contralateral carotid artery that is asymptomatic. Appropriate initial treatment includes which of the following?

A. Simultaneous bilateral carotid endarterectomy.
B. Staged bilateral carotid endarterectomy with a 1-week interval between stages.
C. Carotid endarterectomy on the symptomatic side only.
D. Carotid endarterectomy on the side with the greatest stenosis, regardless of symptoms.

Ref.: 3

COMMENTS: The long-term risk of asymptomatic carotid stenosis is not fully defined. The Toronto Asymptomatic Bruit Trial observed an 18% annual incidence of neurologic events in patients with 75% stenosis. Evaluation of patients with symptomatic disease who are found to have asymptomatic stenosis on the contralateral side suggests that in 10–15% of patients TIAs related to the asymptomatic lesion may develop, and approximately 1% of patients suffer stroke. The latter rate occurs among patients whose lesions have 50–75% stenosis. The risk for patients with more significant narrowing is not known and may be higher. It therefore appears that patients with asymptomatic contralateral disease can be managed expectantly and that cerebral ischemic symptoms, when they do develop, are predominantly in the form of TIAs, which can be treated when they manifest.

ANSWER: C

9. After elective carotid endarterectomy, a patient is noted to exhibit a new neurologic deficit while in the recovery room. Appropriate management of this perioperative neurologic deficit includes which of the following?

A. Immediate return of the patient to the operating room for neck exploration.
B. Noninvasive studies in the operating room to determine flow within the operated carotid artery.
C. Cerebral angiography.

D. Observe patient overnight.

Ref.: 3

COMMENTS: The overriding concern in this patient is to be certain that no technical error has been made during surgery. (The most common technical error is creation of an intimal flap.) This possibility can be determined most effectively by immediately returning the patient to the operating room for a neck exploration. The patient should be heparinized once the neck is opened, and the artery is checked for a pulse, a thrill, or intracarotid thrombosis. If the pulse is diminished or there is evidence of thrombosis, the artery is reopened to examine it for thrombosis or flap elevation. If there are no signs of a carotid problem when the neck is opened, an intraoperative duplex scan should be considered to identify intraluminal debris. Intraoperative angiography also may be a useful maneuver in this desperate situation. Intraoperative thrombolytic therapy with urokinase has been used for acute thrombotic emboli seen on intraoperative arteriography.

ANSWER: A, B

10. With regard to long-term results of carotid endarterectomy, which of the following statements is/are true?

A. The rate of restenosis is 10–15%.
B. Restenosis most commonly manifests as stroke.
C. Ischemic cerebral events are the main cause of late death.
D. Restenosis rates are higher when endarterectomy is performed for symptomatic disease than when it is performed for asymptomatic disease.

Ref.: 2

COMMENTS: The combined operative morbidity and mortality rate for carotid endarterectomy should be less than 5%. Coronary artery disease is the main cause of both immediate and late postoperative death. There is a significant rate of restenosis (10–15%) after carotid endarterectomy, although many of these lesions are asymptomatic and not hemodynamically significant. It is therefore recommended that patients undergo annual B-mode duplex scanning to look for restenosis.

ANSWER: A

11. With regard to symptoms of vertebral basilar insufficiency (VBI) ischemia, which of the following statements is/are correct?

A. They include diplopia, ataxia, vertigo, and tinnitus.
B. They are usually indistinguishable from those of carotid insufficiency.
C. They usually reflect unilateral vertebral disease.
D. They are most commonly caused by emboli.

Ref.: 2

COMMENTS: Stenosis of the vertebral artery usually involves a localized segment near the origin from the subclavian artery. Unlike carotid plaques, the stenotic lesions are usually smooth and nonulcerated, and ischemia is generally attributed to decreased flow rather than to an embolic phenomenon. Although one vertebral artery is usually dominant, unilateral vertebral stenosis rarely produces symptoms; symptoms generally reflect bilateral disease. Associated atherosclerotic involvement of the basilar artery is also common. Symptoms of VBI ischemia are the same as those of brain stem ischemia and produce a characteristic clinical syndrome (diplopia, dysarthria, vertigo, tinnitus) quite distinct from the cerebral hemispheric ischemia produced by carotid disease.

ANSWER: A

12. Most patients with "subclavian steal" syndrome have which of the following conditions?

A. Reversal of flow in the involved vertebral artery.
B. Disabling neurologic symptoms.
C. Upper extremity claudication.
D. Decreased systolic blood pressure in the ipsilateral arm.

Ref.: 1, 2

COMMENTS: "Subclavian steal" syndrome results from occlusion of a subclavian artery, rarely the innominate, with decreased systolic pressure distal to this obstruction. This causes blood to flow up the contralateral vertebral area, across the basilar artery (from which more blood is "stolen") as it courses down (in a retrograde manner) the ipsilateral vertebral to help supply that subclavian artery. Most patients with this phenomenon are asymptomatic and do not require intervention, although limb weakness and paresthesias or symptoms of VBI may occur, in which case intervention is appropriate.

ANSWER: A, D

13. Amaurosis fugax is brought about by occlusion of which of the following arteries?

A. Facial artery.
B. Occipital artery.
C. Retinal artery.
D. Posterior auricular artery.

Ref.: 1, 2

COMMENTS: About 75% of patients who suffer a stroke have had a previous TIA. Amaurosis fugax, one type of TIA (lasting minutes to hours) manifests as ipsilateral blindness, described by the patient as being like a window shade being pulled across the eye. It is caused by emboli traveling via the ophthalmic artery—the first intracerebral branch of the internal carotid artery—that lodge in the retinal artery. These emboli may be seen on funduscopic examination and are called Hollenhorst plaques. The other arteries listed are branches of the external carotid artery. There are eight branches of the external carotid artery: superior thyroid, lingual, facial, ascending pharyngeal, occipital, posterior auricular, superficial temporal, and maxillary.

ANSWER: C

14. Carotid body tumors most commonly manifest with which of the following?

A. Hypertension.
B. Painless neck mass.
C. Cranial nerve deficit.
D. Horner syndrome.
E. Cerebral ischemia.

Ref.: 1,2

COMMENTS: The carotid body is 3–4 mm in size and located within the adventitial tissue of the carotid bifurcation. It arises from paraganglionic cells of neural crest origin. Carotid body tumors (chemodectomas) are uncommon, slow-growing (they may even remain stationary for long periods), and usually manifest as a painless mass. There are two types of carotid body tumors: *sporadic* (5% of which are bilateral) and *autosomal dominant familial* (32% of which are bilateral). The criteria for malignancy are controversial, influenced by the tumor's location, biologic behavior, or evidence of local invasion or distal spread. The definitive treatment is excision.

ANSWER: B

REFERENCES

1. Sabiston DC Jr: *Textbook of Surgery*, 15th ed. WB Saunders, Philadelphia, 1997.
2. Schwartz SI, Shires GT, Spencer FC: *Principles of Surgery*, 7th ed. McGraw-Hill, New York 1999.
3. Ernst CB, Stanley JC: *Current Therapy in Vascular Surgery*, 3rd ed. Mosby, St. Louis, 1995.

Vascular

C. Thoracic

1. With regard to ascending aortic aneurysms, which of the following statements is/are true?

A. They are most often caused by connective tissue abnormalities.
B. They may be related to earlier venereal disease.
C. Most dissecting aneurysms begin in the ascending aorta.
D. They are usually associated with aortic insufficiency.
E. Death usually is caused by rupture with resulting pneumothorax.

Ref.: 1, 2

COMMENTS: Etiologic factors involved in aortic aneurysms vary according to the location of the aneurysm. In the ascending aorta a connective tissue abnormality, recognized histologically as cystic medial necrosis, is the most common underlying abnormality and is the defect seen in aneurysms associated with Marfan syndrome. • Other known causes such as syphilitic aneurysms are steadily decreasing in frequency, and atherosclerotic aneurysms of the ascending aorta are relatively uncommon. • Most dissecting aneurysms do originate in the ascending aorta. • Aortic insufficiency occurs only when there is associated annular dilatation or when one or more aortic cusps are sheared off by an acute dissection. • Death from an ascending aortic aneurysm is usually caused by cardiac failure secondary to chronic untreated aortic insufficiency or to rupture into the pericardium with pericardial tamponade.

ANSWER: A, B, C

2. With regard to the clinical characteristics and management of ascending aortic aneurysms, which of the following statements is/are true?

A. Most ascending aortic aneurysms are asymptomatic and are detected primarily by routine chest radiography.
B. Valvar murmurs are rare.
C. Aortography is contraindicated because of the risk of causing dissection of the aneurysm with the catheter.
D. Operative management with placement of a composite graft of aortic conduit and aortic valve is the treatment of choice for all ascending aortic aneurysms.
E. Computed tomography (CT) scanning with contrast is a good noninvasive modality with which to delineate the size and extent of an aortic aneurysm.

Ref.: 1, 2

COMMENTS: Although the relatively uncommon ascending aortic aneurysm may manifest as a mass in the anterior chest wall, patients are usually asymptomatic, in which case the aneurysm is likely to be detected on routine chest radiography. Aneurysms can be localized (saccular) or more generalized (fusiform). When symptoms are present, they are commonly related to congestive heart failure caused by dilatation of the aortic annulus, resulting in aortic insufficiency and its characteristic murmur (an early diastolic murmur at the second interspace along the right sternal border). This murmur often is present even in asymptomatic patients. Rupture and cardiac failure are the most common causes of death in patients with thoracic artery aneurysms. • Aortography confirms the diagnosis and is important for defining the dimensional extent of the aneurysm and its relation to the rest of the aorta, its major branches, and the coronary ostia. • Although surgical correction is clearly the treatment of choice, debate persists over the routine use of a composite valve/conduit graft. The composite is widely used, however, for aneurysms that are associated with massive dilatation of aortic root, the aortic annulus, and the aortic leaflets (Bentall operation). • CT scanning with intravenous contrast and magnetic resonance imaging (MRI) are excellent noninvasive modalities that delineate the extent and size of an aneurysmal aorta; they cannot, however, take the place of aortography during the preoperative evaluation.

ANSWER: A, E

3. Superior vena cava (SVC) syndrome is characterized by which one or more of the following?

A. Bronchogenic carcinoma with invasion into the mediastinum is the leading cause of SVC syndrome.
B. Venous pressures in the SVC rarely exceed 15 mm Hg.
C. Acute obstruction of the SVC is rarely clinically significant because of the large number of collateral vessels available.
D. Occlusion of the SVC between the azygos vein and the right atrium is better tolerated than occlusion above the azygos vein.
E. Surgical correction is rarely indicated.

Ref.: 1, 2

COMMENTS: More than 90% of SVC obstructions are caused by malignant tumors, most often mediastinal invasion by bronchogenic carcinoma. When obstruction occurs, venous pressures rise to levels of 20–50 mm Hg. • *Acute complete* obstruction allows little time for the formation of collateral vessels and therefore can produce significant edematous laryngeal obstruction and even fatal cerebral edema. A more *gradual* onset of obstruction results in the characteristic clinical picture of facial swelling and dilatation of the collateral veins of the head and neck, arm, and upper thoracic areas. • Obstruction between the azygos vein the the right atrium is less disabling because the azygos vein provides a large collateral venous channel for drainage of the SVC system into the inferior vena caval system. Obstruction above the azygos vein eliminates this collateral channel and is not as well tolerated. • The treatment of choice for obstruction caused by associated malignancy is prompt *radiation* therapy, often in association with diuretics and chemotherapy. Surgery rarely is indicated for management of SVC obstruction because of the technical difficulties associated with vena caval grafts, the underlying poor prognosis in patients with malignant conditions, and the usual adequacy of collateral venous circulation in the rare instances of slowly developing obstruction caused by benign conditions. The only indication for operation is the unusual instance of a benign problem in which collateral circulation does not relieve the symptoms. In this case, a composite saphenous vein graft is appropriate.

ANSWER: A, D, E

4. Match each type of aneurysm in the left column with its most likely etiology in the right column.

A. Ascending aorta	a. Cystic medial necrosis
B. Transverse aortic arch	b. Atherosclerosis
C. Descending thoracic aorta	c. Syphilis
D. Thoracoabdominal aorta	d. Posttraumatic factors

Ref.: 1, 2

COMMENTS: Thoracic aneurysms are classified as ascending, transverse, descending, and thoracoabdominal. The ascending type is the most common (40%) followed by the descending type (35%) and the transverse type. The most common cause of ascending aortic arch aneurysm is cystic medial necrosis (seen in Marfan syndrome). Syphilis was a common cause in the past but is a relatively rare cause in the United States today. The most common etiologic factor associated with transverse, descending, and thoracoabdominal aneurysm is atherosclerosis. Although transverse and thoracoabdominal aneurysms rarely are attributable to causes other than atherosclerosis, descending aortic aneurysms can be posttraumatic or—probably of historical interest—postsyphilitic. Aneurysmal dilatation of chronic aortic dissection is another etiology of a diffuse aneurysm involving the entire thoracoabdominal aorta.

ANSWER: A-a; B-b; C-b; D-b

5. With regard to thoracic trauma, match each statement in the left column with the appropriate item in the right column.

A. Aortography should be performed in most stable patients.	a. Penetrating chest injury.
B. Cardiac tamponade is a major cause of death.	b. Deceleration chest injury.
C. Fatal hemorrhage is sometimes prevented by the aortic adventitia.	c. Both.
D. Thoracotomy may be indicated.	d. Neither.

Ref.: 1, 2

COMMENTS: Both penetrating and deceleration injuries of the thoracic aorta are commonly fatal. When the patient is in extremis from exsanguination, thoracotomy in the emergency room to control hemorrhage may be indicated, even though success is unlikely. In clinically stable patients, aortography is indicated for both types of injury to define the anatomy of the injury because it may influence the choice of surgical approach. With penetrating injuries, pericardial tamponade, in addition to exsanguination, is a major cause of death. With deceleration injuries, complete disruption of the aorta is nearly always fatal. In some instances, however, the adventitia remains intact, confining the hemorrhage and allowing time for surgical correction. With severe blunt trauma to the chest, the possibility of aortic injury must be suspected, and aortography should be used liberally. Mediastinal widening (>8.0 cm) with loss of the aortic window contour remains the key to diagnosis. CT scans and MRI are currently being evaluated as noninvasive screening tests, but they have not been shown to be as valuable as aortography for establishing the diagnosis.

ANSWER: A-c; B-a; C-b; D-c

6. Traumatic thoracic aortic aneurysms are characterized by which of the following?

A. They result from partial aortic transection caused by closed chest trauma.
B. Survival without repair beyond 2 months after the injury is rare.
C. Most traumatic thoracic aortic aneurysms arise just distal to the origin of the left subclavian artery.
D. Hoarseness may be a presenting complaint.
E. Emergency operation is indicated once the diagnosis is made.

Ref.: 1, 2

COMMENTS: Traumatic thoracic aortic aneurysms are false aneurysms, most commonly resulting from horizontal deceleration injury. The most common site of origin of traumatic thoracic aortic aneurysm is just distal to the origin of the left subclavian artery. It is at this point that the aorta is fixed (and prone to tears during rapid deceleration) by the *ligamentum arteriosum*. Unlike aneurysms from other causes, traumatic thoracic aneurysms may enlarge slowly and manifest 10–20 years after the traumatic event. Only 2% of patients with acute aortic dissection survive long enough for a false aneurysm to develop. Elective repair is indicated in most patients. Enlargement of the aneurysm may result in compression of the left recurrent laryngeal nerve, the left main stem bronchus, or the esophagus, producing hoarseness, dyspnea, or dysphagia. Unlike aneurysms from other causes, traumatic thoracic aneurysms enlarge slowly or may remain unchanged for 10–20 years. Nonetheless, there is an ever-present risk of rupture; approximately 10% of patients with traumatic aneurysms seen more than 10 years after injury die of rupture within 5 years after diagnosis. It is impossible to predict which aneurysm will rupture.

ANSWER: A, C, D

7. With regard to aortic dissection, match each item in the left column with the appropriate item or items in the right column.

A. Related to Marfan syndrome.
B. Readily accessible to surgical excision.
C. Early causes of death are cardiac tamponade and acute aortic insufficiency.
D. Multiple points of entry and reentry.
E. Primarily treated surgically.

a. Type A.
b. Type B.
c. Type C1.
d. Type C2.

Ref.: 1, 2

COMMENTS: Aortic dissections have been classified according to their site of origin and extent of aortic involvement. **Type A** originates in the ascending aorta and dissects throughout the entire thoracic and abdominal aorta. **Type B** originates in the ascending aorta but is confined to that segment of the aorta and is the type commonly seen in Marfan syndrome. **Type C1** originates distal to the left subclavian artery but remains confined to the descending thoracic aorta; it is readily accessible to surgical excision. **Type C2** originates distal to the left subclavian artery but dissects down into the abdominal aorta, which complicates its surgical repair. Definition of the origin and extent of aortic dissection is of paramount importance because these considerations dictate therapy. Most dissections occur in the inner third or half of the aortic wall; the underlying defect is the destruction of the media from an unknown cause. Hypertension is present in 80–90% of patients and in well over 95% of those with dissection of the descending aorta. Dissections originating in the ascending aorta most commonly occur through the entire length, whereas those originating distal to the subclavian artery occur distal to this point. Multiple entry and reentry points are seen in type A dissections. • After initial presentation and diagnosis, antihypertensive therapy (nitroprusside) should be instituted. Nearly all patients with ascending aortic dissection (types A and B) should be operated on immediately. Early causes of death in patients with type A and B dissections are rupture, cardiac tamponade, and acute aortic insufficiency. The goal of operation is to correct aortic insufficiency and to graft the ascending aorta with obliteration of the false lumen. Dissections of the descending aorta require prompt operation if signs of visceral ischemia are present or if rupture has occurred. In the absence of the aforementioned indications, operation can be postponed. Thirty percent of such patients ultimately require an operation because of an enlarging aneurysm.

ANSWER: A-b; B-c; C-a,b; D-a; E-a,b,c,d

8. With regard to blunt traumatic rupture of the aorta, which of the following statements is/are correct?

A. The most common site of rupture is distal to the left subclavian artery at the point of insertion of the ligamentum arteriosum.
B. Nearly 90% of patients die at the scene of the accident.
C. The intima provides nearly 60% of the strength of the thoracic aorta and must remain intact for the patient to survive.
D. There is still a high risk of free aortic rupture, even in patients who survive the first 6 weeks after injury.
E. Bypass support is mandatory for its correction.

Ref.: 1, 2

COMMENTS: About 85–90% of patients who sustain an aortic rupture die at the scene of the accident. Patients who sustain rupture of the ascending aorta rarely reach the hospital alive. In most patients who survive, the rupture is located at the aortic isthmus (immediately distal to the origin of the left subclavian artery). The aortic adventitia provides 60% of the tensile strength of the thoracic aorta; for someone to survive blunt trauma to the aorta, this layer must remain intact to prevent a free rupture and exsanguinating hemorrhage. Of the patients who initially survive and are merely observed because the pathologic process is not recognized or some other reason, 20% die within 6 hours and 72% die within 1 week. If a patient survives 6–8 weeks after injury, the risk of free aortic rupture is low. There is evidence that if an operation is performed expeditiously with appropriate monitoring of somatosensory potentials to prevent paraplegia, with adequate physiologic support, and with control of blood pressure with nitroprusside, simple aortic clamping without bypass is equally safe, and the operative time and blood loss are significantly less.

ANSWER: A, B

9. With regard to thoracoabdominal aneurysms, which of the following statements is/are true?

A. They are considerably less common that aortic aneurysms below the renal arteries.
B. They are usually palpable because of their large size.
C. They can become quite large before symptoms develop.
D. Repair by placing an intraluminal graft is the treatment of choice for symptomatic or significantly enlarging aneurysms.
E. Paraplegia is a recognized complication of repair.

Ref.: 1, 2

COMMENTS: Thoracoabdominal aneurysms occur primarily in older patients with extensive atherosclerosis and are infrequent in comparison with infrarenal aortic aneurysms. The cephalad location of the abdominal component frequently precludes palpation because of the overlying pancreas and the stomach. Thirty percent of patients in a large series were asymptomatic, and the condition was first diagnosed on routine chest radiography, which revealed dilatation of the aorta at the diaphragm. A major advance in the treatment of these aneurysms was made by E. Stanley Crawford, who developed the intraluminal graft technique; this procedure has significantly reduced rates of morbidity and mortality associated with surgical repair. Technical difficulties during surgical repair, including the need to reimplant the celiac, superior mesenteric, and renal arteries, increase the risk of this operation sufficiently that repair is usually warranted only for symptomatic or significantly enlarging aneurysms. Paraplegia, resulting from temporary or permanent loss of spinal cord blood flow, can occur in 20–40%. The frequency can be decreased by somatosensory potential monitoring of the spinal cord. Distal aortic pressure above 60 mm Hg, rather than flow rate, is the key to perfusion of the spinal cord. Reattachment of large lumbar vessels has helped lower the incidence of paraplegia to 15%.

ANSWER: A, C, D, E

10. With regard to transverse aortic arch aneurysms, which of the following statements is/are true?

A. Cystic medial necrosis is a major cause.
B. Repair of these aneurysms is associated with the highest operative mortality rate of any of the aortic aneurysms.
C. Differentiation from mediastinal tumors is usually possible on standard chest radiography.
D. Deep hypothermia with circulatory arrest and cardiopulmonary bypass have significantly reduced the mortality rate due to repair of these aneurysms.

Ref.: 1, 2

COMMENTS: Transverse aortic arch aneurysms are almost always the result of atherosclerosis. In asymptomatic individuals they are most often detected on routine chest radiography. Aortography and CT, however, are required to differentiate them from mediastinal tumors and to define the vascular anatomy before repair. Concomitant association with coronary and cerebrovascular disease, together with the need to disrupt flow to the brain temporarily during repair, has resulted in an operative mortality rate that exceeds that for repair of other aortic aneurysms. The introduction of cardiopulmonary bypass and hypothermic circulatory arrest has significantly reduced this operative mortality rate.

ANSWER: B, D

11. Radiographic signs of aortic injury secondary to blunt chest trauma include which of the following?

A. Widening of the mediastinum.
B. Blunting of the aortic knob.
C. Left apical capping.
D. Depression of the left main bronchus.

Ref.: 1, 2

COMMENTS: Blunt injury to the thoracic aorta may occur without clinical signs or symptoms that such an injury is present. Often the mechanism of injury (sudden deceleration from vehicular accidents, falls) and a high index of suspicion obligate the examining physician to rule out aortic trauma by aortography. Radiographic signs of aortic injury, when present, include blunting of the aortic knob, widening of the mediastinum (to 8.0 cm), deviation of the trachea to the right, left apical blunting, and depression of the left main bronchus. Even when these radiographic signs are present, aortography is required to define precisely the anatomy and the extent of the vascular injury.

ANSWER: A, B, C, D

12. With regard to aortic dissections, which of the following statements is/are correct?

A. DeBakey type I aortic dissection begins in the proximal aorta.
B. Stanford type B aortic dissection is limited to the descending thoracic aorta.
C. Hypertension is found in up to 30% of patients with aortic dissection.
D. Atherosclerosis is the most common cause of aortic dissection.
E. Aortic regurgitation is present in 50–75% of patients with acute proximal aortic dissection.

Ref.: 1, 2, 3

COMMENTS: *Dissection* is the most common catastrophic event affecting the aorta and is approximately two to three times more frequent than *rupture* of an abdominal aortic aneurysm. The most commonly accepted classifications are those of DeBakey and Stanford. With the Stanford classification, a type A dissection is one involving the ascending aorta, regardless of the site of origin or the distal extent of the process. Dissection of the descending thoracic aortic is designated type B. • With the DeBakey classification, type I begins in the proximal aorta and involves most of the entire vessel. Type II involves only the ascending aorta. Dissection of the descending thoracic aorta is termed type III. • Most authors believe atherosclerosis is coincidental rather than causative of aortic *dissection*. This is different from thoracic aortic *aneurysms*, in which atherosclerosis is considered a causative factor. *Hypertension* is found in 60–90% of patients presenting with aortic dissection and is more commonly seen with type B (90%) than with type A (60%) dissection. *Aortic valve cusps* prolapse in aortic dissection involving the proximal aorta. The aortic valve can usually be repaired by resuspension of the cusps of the valve; preservation of the native valve is possible in 70–90% of patients with acute type A dissections. Postoperative freedom from the need of valve replacement at 10 years is 90%. In contrast, patients with dilated aortic roots or with Marfan syndrome require composite root replacement, rather than resuspension or repair of the aortic valve.

ANSWER: A, B, E

13. With regard to diagnosis and treatment of aortic dissection, which of the following statements is/are true?

A. Aortography and coronary angiography are essential before surgery for type A acute aortic dissection.
B. Transesophageal echocardiography is highly accurate for diagnosing acute aortic dissection.
C. Type B acute aortic dissection is treated primarily medically.
D. Surgical treatment of acute type A dissection is similar in patients with or without Marfan syndrome.
E. With chronic type B dissection the indications for surgery are related to the size of the aneurysm, symptoms of pain, and the development of visceral, renal, and neurological ischemia.

Ref.: 1, 2, 3, 4

COMMENTS: Coronary angiography prior to emergency repair of acute proximal aortic dissection is not recommended. Even in the presence of moderate coronary artery disease, early repair of the dissection has precedence over other procedures. Since its introduction in 1984, the use of transesophageal echocardiography to diagnose aortic dissection has gained acceptance by many surgeons. It has a sensitivity and specificity of 99% and 98%, respectively. It can be performed in the emergency room or the operating room and so does not require transferring the patient to a separate area, as for angiography. It can also assess the function of the left ventricle, the aortic valve, and the mitral valve. • Type B aortic dissection is treated primarily medically by instituting strict control of hypertension. Indications for surgery of acute type B dissection are limited to prevention or relief of life-threatening complications (i.e., aortic rupture, ischemia of limbs and organ systems, persistent pain, or uncontrolled hypertension). • Patients with Marfan syndrome have more extensive tissue pathology, which makes the dissection process more extensive. There is general agreement that a composite root replacement rather than an interposition graft is the surgical treatment of choice for patients with Marfan syndrome.

ANSWER: B, C, E

14. A 50-year-old man involved in a deceleration-type motor vehicle accident is brought to the emergency room. He has a systolic blood pressure of 90 mm Hg. Chest radiography reveals a widened mediastinum. He has a bilateral pelvic fracture and a tender abdomen. Which of the following statements is/are true about this patient?

A. Management should begin with aortography to evaluate the widened mediastinum.
B. The most common site of traumatic aortic rupture is distal to the left subclavian artery.
C. Repair of this type of injury virtually always requires cardiopulmonary bypass.
D. Rarely does this type of injury present 10 years after the accident.
E. The risk of paraplegia following repair of the thoracic aorta can be avoided if certain precautions are taken.

Ref.: 1, 2, 4

COMMENTS: Patients with multiple injuries and suspected aortic tear should have certain associated injuries addressed first (e.g., extensive pelvic fractures or intraabdominal injuries). In this patient, diagnostic peritoneal lavage or immediate abdominal CT scanning should be done before evaluating the widened mediastinum. The most common site of an aorta tear is just distal to the left subclavian artery. Although cardiopulmonary bypass may be required in certain patients with an extensive aortic tear, most tears can be treated by a partial shunt between the left atrium or ascending aorta and the descending aorta. Although patients with a thoracic aorta tear can have a successful repair, many patients with this injury die at the accident scene. Some arrive at the hospital and die during initial resuscitation. Rarely, such patients present with chronic dissection up to 15 years after the accident. • Paraplegia following repair of the thoracic aorta remains one of the most distressing complications associated with the operation. Aortic cross-clamp time, distal aortic pressure monitoring, and cerebrospinal fluid drainage by spinal tap have been utilized. However, none of these steps has proved reliable for eliminating the risk of postoperative paraplegia, which is 3–10%.

ANSWER: B, D

REFERENCES

1. Sabiston DC Jr: *Textbook of Surgery*, 15th ed. WB Saunders, Philadelphia, 1997.
2. Schwartz SI, Shires GT, Spencer FC: *Principles of Surgery*, 7th ed. McGraw-Hill, New York, 1999.
3. Edmunds LH (ed): *Cardiac Surgery in the Adult*. McGraw-Hill, New York, 1997.
4. Crawford ES, et al: Thoracoabdominal aortic aneurysms: preoperative and intraoperative factors determining immediate and long-term results of operations in 605 patients. *J Vasc Surg* 3:389–404, 1986.

Vascular

D. Abdominal Aorta

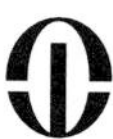

1. Which one or more of the following may be acceptable treatment for occlusive aortoiliac disease?

A. Thromboendarterectomy.
B. Aortofemoral bypass.
C. Axillofemoral bypass.
D. Percutaneous balloon angioplasty.

Ref.: 1, 2, 3

COMMENTS: The basic goal of arterial revascularization for occlusive arterial disease is to reestablish adequate blood flow to the tissue being supplied. In patients with occlusive aortoiliac disease who require surgery, a variety of techniques are applicable, depending on the site and extent of obstruction, the presence or absence of aneurysmal disease, and the patient's underlying medical condition (Table 1). **Thromboendarterectomy** (TEA) is appropriate for some patients with disease confined to the distal aorta and common iliac arteries. Results of TEA are similar to those with aortofemoral bypass grafting. TEA is contraindicated in the presence of aneurysmal disease and disease that extends to the external iliac arteries. Most patients are managed by **aortofemoral bypass grafting**, which produces excellent results in terms of immediate and long-term patency and relief of claudication. The long-term patency rates are reported to be 65–90%. **Axillofemoral** and **thoracofemoral** bypass grafts have been successful in patients in whom an abdominal operation may pose excessive risk, including those with infected aortic prosthetic grafts, those with previously occluded aortofemoral grafts, and those with a "hostile" abdomen. **Femorofemoral** and **ileofemoral** bypass grafts are used when only one iliac artery is diseased. **Percutaneous balloon angioplasty** is successful for isolated short-segment lesions of the iliac arteries in patients with good distal runoff. This may yield 5-year patency rates as high as 60%. Angioplasty can also be used to dilate an iliac stenosis prior to a subsequent, more distal bypass. The addition of intraluminal stents has broadened the number and location of lesions amenable to balloon angioplasty and has increased the technical success rates of these procedures. Disadvantages of percutaneous angioplasty include a lower rate of overall success in patients with poor distal runoff or limb-threatening ischemia and the potential complications of intimal dissection, vascular occlusion or rupture, and distal embolization.

ANSWER: A, B, C, D

2. Which of the following is the most common graft-related late complication of aortic bypass grafts?

A. Graft occlusion caused by progressive atherosclerosis.
B. Suture line pseudoaneurysm.
C. Aortoenteric fistula.
D. Distal embolization.
E. Infection caused by transient bacteremia.

Ref.: 2

COMMENTS: The long-term patency rates of aortofemoral bypass grafts are reported to range from approximately 65% to 90%. The most common graft-related late complication is **graft occlusion**, which develops in 10–35% of cases. The most common cause of graft occlusion is progressive atherosclerosis, usually occurring at or just beyond the distal anastomosis. Other late complications include **anastomotic pseudoaneurysm** (1–5%) and **graft infection** (1%), both of which occur more often when a femoral anastomosis is involved. **Aortoenteric fistula** is rare but carries a high mortality rate (50%); therefore it should be a primary consideration in any patient with a previous abdominal aortic graft who has gastro-

Table 1

Procedure	Indications	Contraindications
Thromboendarterectomy	Short stenotic segment of distal aorta on iliac artery	Concomitant aneurysmal disease
Aortofemoral bypass	For the usual aortoiliac involvement To provide inflow or outflow (or both) for concomitant endarterectomy	Short stenosis (relative contraindication)
Axillofemoral, femorofemoral bypass	Infected aortic aneurysm Infected aortic prosthetic graft Poor risk for abdominal operation	Less successful patency, so not appropriate unless conditions at left present
Percutaneous balloon angioplasty with stent placement	Short segment involvement with good distal runoff To provide inflow for a more distal femoropopliteal bypass	Intimal dissection (with occlusion, rupture, distal embolization)

intestinal bleeding. Most often there is bleeding into the third portion of the duodenum from the proximal aortic suture line.

ANSWER: A

3. What is the most common cause of death after recovery from successful aortic bypass graft?

A. Rupture of pseudoaneurysm.
B. Acute graft thrombosis.
C. Cerebrovascular accident.
D. Coronary artery disease.
E. Complications of peripheral vascular disease.
F. Renal failure.

Ref.: 1, 3

COMMENTS: Associated **coronary artery disease** is the leading cause of death after aortic reconstruction. Predictive risk factors for postoperative cardiac events include age over 70 years, previous myocardial infarction (MI), history of ventricular arrhythmias, diabetes mellitus, and angina pectoris. The dipyridamole thallium stress test has an excellent negative predictive value for postoperative cardiac complications. Combining clinical markers with dipyridamole thallium stress testing increases the specificity of dipyridamole thallium alone. Aggressive preoperative cardiac evaluation is justified to define a patient's operative risk and to identify patients who would benefit from further invasive cardiac evaluation and therapy.

ANSWER: D

4. Which of the following is the most common manifestation of an abdominal aortic aneurysm?

A. Incidental finding on physical examination or by computed tomography (CT) scan done for unrelated disease.
B. Back or abdominal pain.
C. Acute rupture.
D. Spontaneous thrombosis with peripheral ischemia.
E. Peripheral embolization.

Ref.: 1, 2, 4

COMMENTS: Approximately three-fourths of all abdominal aortic aneurysms are discovered incidentally and are asymptomatic. The most common complaint in patients with symptoms is vague abdominal pain. Patients may also note back or flank pain. Abdominal aortic aneurysms may expand without symptoms, erode into the adjacent vertebral bodies, partially obstruct the duodenum or ureters (inflammatory aneurysms), embolize, thrombose, or rupture. Rare manifestations include aortoenteric fistula and aortocaval fistula, the latter which present with an abdominal bruit, venous hypertension, and high-output cardiac failure. Rupture may mimic other acute intraabdominal emergencies such as diverticulitis and renal colic and may manifest with acute abdominal pain followed by transient hypotension and eventual vascular collapse. Signs and symptoms of acute ischemia in the lower extremities may follow thrombosis or embolization from an abdominal aneurysm.

ANSWER: A

5. Which of the following is the most common associated manifestation of atherosclerotic disease seen in patients with abdominal aortic aneurysms?

A. Thoracic aortic aneurysm.
B. Occlusive peripheral vascular disease.
C. Coronary artery disease.
D. Carotid stenosis.
E. Renovascular hypertension.

Ref.: 1, 2

COMMENTS: Atherosclerosis is the etiology of most abdominal aortic aneurysms. Other, less common causes include trauma, acute and chronic infection, cystic medial necrosis, late sequela of aortic dissection, connective tissue disorders, anastomotic pseudoaneurysms, inflammatory aneurysms, and syphilis. More than half of all deaths in patients with abdominal aortic aneurysms are due to cardiac complications. Up to 30% of patients with abdominal aortic aneurysms have severe correctable coronary artery disease. Elevated systemic blood pressure is present in up to 40% of patients with atherosclerosis, but only uncommonly is the etiology renovascular in origin. Associated aneurysms may be found concomitantly in the thoracic aorta (4%), femoral arteries (3%), and popliteal arteries (4%). It is essential that patients with abdominal aortic aneurysms undergo a thorough preoperative cardiovascular evaluation.

ANSWER: C

6. Which of the following are acceptable indications for operation on an abdominal aortic aneurysm?

A. Any abdominal aortic aneurysm.
B. Symptomatic aneurysms of any size.
C. Symptomatic aneurysm larger than 5 cm in diameter.
D. Asymptomatic aneurysm larger than 5 cm in diameter.
E. Asymptomatic 4.5 cm aneurysm involving the renal arteries.

Ref.: 2, 4

COMMENTS: The natural history of most abdominal aortic aneurysms is progressive enlargement. The risk of rupture is directly related to the size of the aneurysm. This relates to the law of Laplace, according to which the mean tension (T) in the wall of a vessel is directly proportional to the product of the radius (R) and the intraluminal pressure (P). Therefore an increase in radius (expansion) or pressure (hypertension) results in an increase in wall tension: $T = P \times R$. Approximately one-half of deaths in patients with untreated abdominal aortic aneurysms are caused by rupture. The risk of rupture of an aneurysm 5–6 cm in diameter is approximately 25% within 5 years. Ruptured aneurysms carry a 50% mortality among patients who reach the hospital alive; therefore any patients with symptoms suggestive of impending rupture should be operated on immediately. Ultrasonography provides a reliable noninvasive method for observing patients with small asymptomatic aneurysms. The anticipated growth rate is 0.4 cm per year. Diastolic hypertension and severe chronic obstructive pulmonary disease are thought to be predictors of expansion and rupture, especially for large aneurysms. The decision to operate must therefore be based on considerations of size, shape (saccular is more ominous than fusiform), presence of symptoms, cardiac risk, and presence of cerebrovascular or chronic obstructive pulmonary disease. The mortality rate of elective repair is approximately 4–5%. A juxtarenal position of an asymptomatic aneurysm does not change the indication for elective repair; although the potential problems associated with renal artery involvement are increased, the risk of complications from elective aneurysmectomy with revascularization of the kidney is even greater.

ANSWER: B, C, D

7. The initial diagnosis of a suspected abdominal aortic aneurysm is best made by which one or more of the following?

   A. Magnetic resonance imaging (MRI).
   B. Computed tomography (CT).
   C. Arteriography.
   D. Ultrasonography.
   E. Digital venous subtraction arteriography.

Ref.: 1, 2, 3

COMMENTS: An abdominal aortic aneurysm should be suspected in a patient in whom the palpated abdominal aortic pulsation is greater than 2.5 cm in diameter at a level above the umbilicus. Radiographic confirmation and delineation of anatomic characteristics can be accomplished with ultrasonography, CT scan, MRI, or arteriography. **Ultrasonography** is reliable, noninvasive, and relatively inexpensive and thus is the preferred method for making the initial diagnosis and observing patients with small aneurysms. Ultrasonography can also be used to assess renal and visceral flow. The success of its use is technician-dependent, and its applicability is limited by obesity and overlying bowel gas in patients. Its major drawback is its inability to image the quality of the distal arterial anatomy. **CT scans** are highly predictive of aneurysm size and produce no false-negative results, which makes them the preferred noninvasive method for preoperative evaluation of an abdominal aortic aneurysm. They allow definition of thrombus within the aneurysm, provide information on renal status, define suspected inflammatory aneurysms, define relations to the inferior vena cava and other venous anomalies, and identify leaking or ruptured aneurysms. **Arteriography** is most useful for evaluating associated distal occlusive disease, the patency of renal, celiac, and visceral vessels, the presence of suprarenal aneurysmal disease, and associated other aneurysmal disease. Because a thrombus may be present within the aneurysm, contrast visualization of the lumen alone may not yield an accurate assessment of the true size of the aneurysm. The lateral projection of biplane aortography is useful for demonstrating the presence of an abdominal aortic aneurysm despite an anterior view that demonstrates a normal diameter of contrast. The lateral view shows anterior displacement of the contrast column off the spine by a laminated thrombus located posteriorly within the aneurysm sac. **MRI** has superior capabilities in three-dimensional reconstruction, assessment of arterial flow, and composition of the aortic wall.

ANSWER: D

8. With regard to the operative technique of abdominal aortic aneurysm repair, which of the following statements is/are true?

   A. Bifurcation grafts are preferred to straight grafts, even if the iliac vessels are not involved.
   B. An endoaneurysmal approach is most commonly used today.
   C. Bleeding lumbar vessels are routinely ligated from within the aneurysm sac.
   D. The inferior mesenteric artery is routinely reimplanted in elderly patients to prevent ischemia of the left colon.
   E. Flow should first be restored to the external iliac vessels when the crossclamps are removed.
   F. To avoid tissue necrosis and risk of infection, most of the aneurysm wall is resected before closure.

Ref.: 1, 2, 4

COMMENTS: Details of the operative technique for repair of abdominal aortic aneurysms vary somewhat, depending on individual circumstances, but several general principles should be emphasized. Proximal control is established distal to the renal vessels after identifying the left renal vein. • Manipulation of the aorta is kept to a minimum to prevent embolization of aneurysm contents. • After the proximal and distal clamps are applied, the aneurysm is opened and the thrombus evacuated. • The lumbar vessels are ligated from within the aneurysm sac. • The inferior mesenteric artery (IMA) can usually be safely ligated precisely at its origin, thereby avoiding any collateral vessels within the mesentery of the left colon. If backflow from the inferior mesenteric artery is poor, consideration should be given to reimplanting the artery to the side of the prosthesis. Some surgeons evaluate backflow by viewing the IMA orifice from inside the opened aneurysm; others measure the IMA stump pressure and find that a pressure of less than 40 mm Hg is a reason to reimplant. • Flow to at least one hypogastric artery should be preserved to maintain collateral flow to the colon via the middle hemorrhoidal arteries. • If ischemic injury to the left colon is suspected, a second-look laparotomy should be performed 24 hours later. • Because most of the aneurysm sac is preserved, the posterior suture lines consist of a double thickness of aorta. This provides more suture line strength and hemostasis because the graft is sutured to the aorta from within the aneurysm sac in an end-to-end manner. • A tube graft is preferable to a bifurcation graft when the common iliac arteries are uninvolved; tube grafts avoid the need for an additional anastomosis, avoid an increased risk of dissection, and avoid the increased incidence of infection associated with anastomosis performed in the groin. • In some instances in which the aneurysm is extensive, the celiac, superior mesenteric, and renal arteries are involved. These aneurysms require more complex revascularization procedures, including reimplantation of the vessels previously mentioned. • After graft placement, proper techniques of aortic flushing and sequential unclamping are important to minimize the risk of hypotension, declamping shock, and distal embolization. The latter is accomplished by adequate flushing before completing the distal anastomosis and opening the circulation first into the internal iliacs and then into the external iliacs. • The surgeon should control the systemic arterial pressure with finger pressure on the graft until appropriate volume replacement has been accomplished. • Hypotension after removal of the aortic crossclamp is believed to occur on the basis of washout of acidic metabolites and vasoactive substances from the ischemic lower extremities, third-space loss into permeable distal tissues, and sudden flow into vasodilated beds, as well as vascular steal secondary to reactive hyperemia in the lower extremities. • The aneurysm sac is not extensively resected and is closed over the prosthetic graft to isolate the graft from the duodenum and to minimize the risk of erosion and fistulization.

ANSWER: B, C

9. Two days after an uncomplicated repair of an abdominal aortic aneurysm, bloody diarrhea develops in the patient, who is still receiving antibiotics. The differential diagnosis includes which of the following?

A. Coagulopathy.
B. Pseudomembranous colitis.
C. Ischemic colitis.
D. Aortoenteric fistula.
E. Acute hepatic failure.

Ref.: 1, 2, 3

COMMENTS: The main concern in this situation is that **ischemic colitis** may have developed as a result of interruption of flow to the inferior mesenteric artery without adequate collateral blood supply from the superior mesenteric or hypogastric artery (or both) to the sigmoid colon. It is important to realize that diarrhea, whether Hemoccult positive or negative, is one of the first signs of ischemic colitis. Less commonly, ischemic colitis can also develop on the basis of embolization of atheromatous debris into the mesenteric circulation during aneurysm repair. The reported incidence of clinically significant ischemia reported is at 1–2%. Additional risk factors related to ischemia include duration and placement of cross-clamping, hypotension, and cardiac arrhythmias. It occurs more commonly in patients with prior colon resection and those undergoing total redo aortic grafting. Immediate proctosigmoidoscopy is important during the initial evaluation of such a patient to assess colonic viability. The rectum is usually spared; and ischemic changes, seen through the sigmoidoscope as pale, patchy areas with membranes, can be visualized 10–20 cm from the anal verge. Ischemic colitis may be limited to the mucosa or may be transmural. Management must be individualized: The presence of associated increasing abdominal tenderness, peritoneal signs, fever, and elevated white blood cell count point to a transmural process that necessitates operation. Resection of the descending and sigmoid colon with Hartmann's pouch and end-colostomy is required for transmural necrosis to prevent gross spillage and graft contamination. **Pseudomembranous enterocolitis** associated with antibiotic use is also a consideration, although it occurs somewhat later during the postoperative course. Evaluation of the possibility of pseudomembranous colitis includes proctosigmoidoscopy with biopsy and examination of stool for *Clostridium difficile* toxin. Treatment involves supportive measures and the administration of vancomycin or metronidazole enterally. **Aortoenteric fistula** is a late complication of aortic aneurysm repair, resulting from erosion of a false aneurysm at the proximal aortic suture line into the duodenum or, on occasion, the sigmoid colon; it is not a likely diagnosis in this clinical scenario. **Coagulopathy** usually does not manifest as bloody diarrhea, but hepatic function and the coagulation profile should be promptly assessed if a bleeding diathesis is suspected.

ANSWER: B, C

10. With regard to rupture of an abdominal aortic aneurysm, which of the following statements is/are true?

A. It is the most common cause of death in patients with an untreated abdominal aortic aneurysm.
B. The rate of associated operative mortality is 30–50%.
C. The highest salvage rate is obtained by prompt left thoracotomy for proximal control.
D. Renal failure is the leading cause of late postoperative death.

Ref.: 1, 2

COMMENTS: Rupture of an abdominal aortic aneurysm is a catastrophic complication that may be heralded by abdominal, back, or flank pain followed by vascular collapse. It is the most common cause of death among patients with *untreated* abdominal aneurysm, with a mortality rate of 30–50%, although nearly that many patients die of associated atherosclerotic problems, including cardiac, cerebral, or renal disease. The mortality rate associated with elective resection is 5% or less. The mortality rate of a *ruptured* abdominal aortic aneurysm is also correlated with hypotension, transfusion requirements, operative time, and the time interval before operative intervention. Immediate operation and obtaining control of the proximal aorta is mandatory if these patients are to survive; these procedures are accomplished best transabdominally at a level just below the diaphragm. Because left thoracotomy is occasionally required for control, access to the chest and the abdomen should be provided for when the patient is prepared in the operating room. Renal failure is a leading cause of late death. Cardiac complications remain the leading cause of *early* mortality; renal failure is the leading cause of *late* death.

ANSWER: A, B, D

11. Which one of the following complications occurs most commonly after successful repair of an abdominal aortic aneurysm in a 58-year-old man?

A. Sexual dysfunction.
B. Ischemic colitis.
C. Renal failure.
D. Peripheral embolization.
E. Leg paralysis.

Ref.: 1, 2, 4

COMMENTS: All of these complications may occur after repair of an abdominal aortic aneurysm, but with appropriate operative technique most of them are uncommon except for changes in sexual function. Retrograde ejaculation has been reported in as many as two-thirds and loss of potency in as many as one-third of such patients. These changes may result from injury to the autonomic nerve fibers overlying the anterior aorta near the origin of the inferior mesenteric artery or injury to those fibers overlying the proximal left common iliac artery and aortic bifurcation. Avoiding excessive aortic dissection in this region can help minimize this complication. Documentation that sexual dysfunction existed preoperatively is of obvious importance in aortoiliac surgery, inasmuch as the incidence of impotence in men of this age with no aortoiliac occlusive disease is considerable. Unilateral, isolated iliac artery obstruction in men is often best treated with femorofemoral bypass to avoid the potential for postoperative impotence. Revascularization of the internal iliacs at the time of aortoiliac reconstruction for occlusive disease can reverse vasculogenic impotence in patients with distal obstructive disease.

ANSWER: A

12. With regard to inflammatory abdominal aortic aneurysms, which of the following statements is/are true?

A. Fewer than 1% of abdominal aortic aneurysms are considered inflammatory.
B. There is a characteristic gross appearance, consisting of a thick, white fibrotic retroperitoneal process with adherence of the aneurysm to the duodenum and inferior vena cava.
C. An infectious etiology is responsible for the inflammatory process.

D. The operative approach is the same as for the usual atherosclerotic aneurysm.
E. Most inflammatory abdominal aortic aneurysms occur in a suprarenal location.

Ref.: 2, 3, 4

COMMENTS: Inflammatory abdominal aortic aneurysms represent 2.5–15.0% of all abdominal aortic aneurysms. There is a male predominance. This type of aneurysm is infrarenal and characterized by an intense adventitial fibroplastic reaction with adherence of the aneurysm to the third and fourth portions of the duodenum and inferior vena cava. Ureteral entrapment is present in 25% of patients. No infectious etiology has been found, and the inflammatory process is thought to be autoimmune. Abdominal and back pain, weight loss, and an elevated erythrocyte sedimentation rate (ESR) in a patient with abdominal aortic aneurysm suggest this diagnosis. Abdominal CT scanning with contrast is the most definitive examination for securing a preoperative diagnosis. This scan demonstrates aortic wall thickening outside the rim of aortic calcification. In contrast to a leaking abdominal aortic aneurysm, the inflammatory process is enhanced with contrast and demonstrates less attenuation than does blood. The operative strategy includes proximal aortic control above the left renal vein and the use of ureteral catheters if the inflammatory process extends to the iliac vessels; dissecting off adherent structures (duodenum) should be avoided. Ureterolysis is rarely necessary. The risk of rupture is lower than that seen with the usual atherosclerotic aneurysm. After aneurysmorrhaphy with graft placement, the inflammatory process gradually resolves, and the ESR returns to normal.

ANSWER: B

13. A patient who had an abdominal aortic aneurysm (AAA) repaired 5 years previously now presents with fever and positive blood cultures. Which of the following statements are true?

A. CT scan is the preferred initial imaging technique for suspected graft infection.
B. Published mortality rates following surgery for infected aortic grafts range between 5% and 10%.
C. Graft infections identified within 4 months of AAA repair are associated with a more virulent course than later infections.
D. *Staphylococcus epidermidis* is the most common infecting pathogen.
E. Upper gastrointestinal bleeding is the most common initial presentation of an infected abdominal aortic graft.

Ref.: 4

COMMENTS: Diagnosis of an infected aortic graft is often a difficult task. Clinical symptoms can be as subtle as a prolonged ileus, abdominal pain or tenderness, or unexplained sepsis. The patient should be examined closely for anastomotic pseudoaneurysms or signs of septic embolization. CT scanning with intravenous contrast is the preferred initial imaging technique for patients with suspected aortic graft infection. Fluid or gas around the graft, obliteration of the normal retroperitoneal tissue planes, and pseudoaneurysm formation suggest a graft infection. Published mortality rates range between 10% and 50%, with subsequent amputation rates ranging from 15% to 60%. The reasons for the high mortality rates are stump blow-out and persistent sepsis. Graft infections diagnosed within 4 months are more virulent than those diagnosed later. *Staphylococcus aureus* and gram-negative bacteria are the pathogens mainly implicated in early graft infection. Gram-negative bacteria are particularly virulent because the endotoxins (elastase and alkaline protease) they produce can lead to compromise of the structural integrity of the anastomosis. *Staphylococcus aureus* was the most prevalent pathogen in infected aortic grafts, although the incidence of *Staphylococcus epidermidis* infections is on the rise. *Staphylococcus epidermidis* infection is more chronic and insidious in nature and is usually diagnosed more than 4 months postoperatively.

ANSWER: A, C, D

14. Which of the following statements is/are correct regarding endovascular repair of infrarenal abdominal aortic aneurysms (AAA)?

A. The most common complication with this technique is endoleak.
B. An infrarenal neck 5 mm in length is essential to the use of this technique.
C. Iliac stenosis is an absolute contraindication to endoluminal repair.
D. Use of this technique is more likely to be feasible on large aneurysms.

Ref.: 4, 5

COMMENTS: Complications following endovascular repair of AAAs include endoleaks, microembolization, improper or incomplete placement of the stent, graft migration, and graft thrombosis. An endoleak is defined as persistent arterial supply of the aneurysmal sac. Although the natural history of endoleaks has not been studied, most authors believe that an aneurysm that has been incompletely excluded does not protect the patient from aortic rupture. The incidence of this complication has been reported to be between 0 and 40%. Treatment of endoleaks varies. Some leaks can be managed conservatively, but others require treatment with further endovascular stenting or conversion to the open technique. Type I leaks occur at the proximal or distal anastomosis or involve a defect in the graft. Type II leaks involve persistent blood flow into the sac from the inferior mesenteric artery or lumbar arteries. Favorable anatomic characteristics for endovascular repair include a proximal neck at least 15 mm in length and no more than 28 mm in diameter. The distal neck should be at least 10 mm in length and no more than 28 mm in diameter. Patients with iliac stenosis can have stent placement that precedes endovascular repair of the aneurysm, thus not making it a contraindication to repair. The smaller the aneurysm, the more likely it is to have a proximal and distal neck, and the less likely it is to have mural thrombus formation. About 60% of aneurysms less than 60 mm in diameter fulfill the anatomic criteria for endovascular repair, a number that drops to 50% if all aneurysms are considered.

ANSWER: A

15. Which of the following statements regarding ruptured abdominal aortic aneurysm (AAA) is/are true?

A. The preferred exposure is via the retroperitoneal technique.
B. For the unstable patient the best diagnostic test is abdominal ultrasonography.

C. Control of the proximal aorta can be accomplished endoluminally.
D. The highest mortality rates occur in patients with preexisting coronary disease.
E. In a stable patient, CT scanning with intravenous contrast is the gold standard for confirming the diagnosis.

Ref.: 3, 4

COMMENTS: Although there are proponents of the retroperitoneal exposure for surgical management of a ruptured AAA, most surgeons believe that a midline incision allows better exposure and control of the ruptured abdominal aorta. The best diagnostic test for a patient with a suspected ruptured AAA is operative exploration and repair of the aneurysm. If the patient does not have a clear history of an AAA and is stable, ultrasonography is a very good test to confirm the presence of an aneurysm, but not necessarily if it has ruptured. CT scan has been used in patients who are hemodynamically stable to determine if there is a contained rupture. Signs of contained rupture on CT scan include loss of clear tissue planes in the retroperitoneal space, extraluminal contrast, and the presence of a retroperitoneal hematoma or fluid. Control of the aorta is a critical issue. With free abdominal rupture or retroperitoneal rupture above the renal vein, manual compression of the aorta can be used at the level of the crus of the diaphragm for control. Infrarenal control can then be obtained the same way control is obtained during an elective aneurysm repair. A left thoracotomy with control of the aorta in the chest is a rarely used technique that is especially useful in cases where the patient has undergone previous upper abdominal surgery. A large Foley or Fogarty catheter can be placed in the aneurysm and inflated to achieve immediate control. The most significant predictors of mortality are the presence of preoperative hypotension and a low hematocrit. Other factors include age, intraperitoneal rupture, transfusion requirements, and gender (females have a higher mortality rate). The presence of preexisting coronary disease is not the most significant preoperative factor in the mortality due to a ruptured AAA.

ANSWER: C, E

16. Retroperitoneal repair of an abdominal aortic aneurysm (AAA) is:

A. Technically more difficult than the anterior transperitoneal approach.
B. Associated with fewer postoperative complications.
C. The preferred approach for suspected ruptured AAA.
D. An alternative approach often used in patients with previous abdominal operations.
E. Contraindicated when there is bilateral iliac artery involvement.

Ref.: 4

COMMENTS: The retroperitoneal exposure for repair of an AAA is an alternative to the traditional transabdominal approach. It is no easier or more difficult in the hands of surgeons who use this approach with regularity. No studies have shown one approach to have a lower complication rate than the other. Although some surgeons do use the retroperitoneal approach for repair of ruptured AAAs, most use the transabdominal approach. Often the aorta has ruptured into and is contained by the retroperitoneum, and opening the retroperitoneal space relieves the tamponade and makes control more difficult. The transabdominal approach also allows rapid manual control of the supraceliac aorta. Although exposure of the right iliac artery is difficult in a patient who undergoes retroperitoneal exposure of the AAA, it is not impossible.

ANSWER: D

17. With regard to infected (mycotic) abdominal aneurysms (AAAs), which of the following is/are true?

A. Infected aneurysms account for 5% of all AAAs.
B. Most infected aneurysms develop when septic emboli infect an artery.
C. *Salmonella* is the most commonly isolated bacterial pathogen.
D. Negative intraoperative Gram stain excludes the diagnosis of an infected AAA.
E. Most patients are treated with aneurysm excision and in situ aortic reconstruction.

Ref.: 1, 3, 4

COMMENTS: Infected (mycotic) aneurysms are a rare subset of AAAs, comprising only 0.1–1.5%. Most infected aneurysms are caused by the spread of hematogenous bacteria that infect nonaneurysmal but atherosclerotic arteries, leading to aneurysmal degeneration. Other causes include arterial trauma leading to false aneurysm formation with concomitant bacterial contamination, septic emboli of cardiac origin, or infection of a preexisting aneurysm. *Salmonella* has been identified in almost 40% of patients with infected AAAs. Infections with gram-negative organisms are less common but are associated with a higher incidence of aneurysm rupture. The most common symptoms of patients with infected aneurysms are fever and abdominal or back pain. Laboratory data lack sensitivity and specificity when considered alone. Blood cultures are positive in approximately 35–50% of patients. CT scanning is the preferred diagnostic study and may reveal an enhancing and eccentric periaortic mass, an aneurysm at an atypical location, periaortic fluid or gas, retroperitoneal soft tissue edema, prominent periaortic lymphadenopathy, and evidence of aneurysm rupture. When the diagnosis of infected AAA is entertained, broad-spectrum antibiotics and prompt surgical intervention are mandatory. Aneurysm excision with débridement of all involved tissues, secure aortic stump closure, and extraanatomic reconstruction, such as axillofemoral bypass, is recommended in most cases. Following surgery, patients are placed on parenteral antibiotics for 4–6 weeks depending on the virulence of the organism, the extent of infection, and the method of arterial reconstruction. Aneurysm excision with in situ aortic reconstruction may be performed in cases with minimal infection and low-virulence organisms, such as *Staphylococcus epidermidis*. After in situ aortic graft reconstruction, lifelong oral antibiotics are advised.

ANSWER: C

18. With regard to prosthetic aortic graft infections, which of the following is/are true?

A. Infected prosthetic aortic grafts occur more commonly after aortofemoral bypass than after aortoiliac bypass.
B. *Staphylococcus aureus* is the most commonly isolated pathogen from infected prosthetic aortic grafts.
C. Ultrasonography is the preferred diagnostic modality to confirm prosthetic aortic graft infection.
D. Most prosthetic aortic graft infections are diagnosed more than 1 year after implantation.

E. Graft excision, secure aortic stump closure, and extraanatomic reconstruction are required for all infected prosthetic aortic grafts.

Ref.: 1, 3, 4

COMMENTS: Infected prosthetic aortic bypass grafts have an incidence of approximately 1% following aortoiliac bypass and 1.5–2.0% following aortofemoral bypass. Mortality from infected grafts is as high as 50% in reported series. The most common pathogen isolated from infected prosthetic aortic grafts is *Staphylococcus epidermidis*. Factors that contribute to graft infection include contact between the graft and skin during insertion, break in sterile technique, extension of contaminated wounds, contaminated lymphatics, arterial wall infection, and early transient bacteremia. CT scanning has proved to be the most sensitive tool for diagnosing infected prosthetic grafts. Changes on the CT scan suggestive of infected grafts include perigraft fluid or gas, soft tissue swelling, focal bowel wall thickening, increased soft tissue between the graft and the wrap, and false aneurysm formation. Radionuclide techniques have similar sensitivity but high false-positive rates due to labeling techniques especially after graft implantation. Ultrasonography provides limited information. MRI is limited by its inability to differentiate between infected and sterile fluid especially during the early postoperative period. Most prosthetic graft infections are diagnosed more than 1 year after implantation. Early infection (<4 months) is associated with emergent operation for ruptured AAA, impaired immunocompetence states, concomitant remote infection, and postoperative colon ischemia. Most infected prosthetic aortic grafts are treated with graft excision, wide débridement of infected tissues, secure aortic stump closure, and extraanatomic reconstruction. Those patients with late graft infections of low virulence (*S. epidermidis*) without gross contamination may be treated with segmental graft excision and in situ graft replacement. Regardless of the technique of reconstruction, patients are placed on long-term antibiotics and are subjected to close follow-up.

ANSWER: A, D

19. Which of the following is/are acceptable treatment options for the patient with late aortic graft limb occlusion?

A. Nonoperative therapy.
B. Thrombolytic therapy.
C. Graft limb thrombectomy.
D. Femorofemoral bypass.
E. Redo aortofemoral bypass.
F. Thoracofemoral bypass.

Ref.: 1, 3

COMMENTS: The most common graft-related complication following aortofemoral bypass is thrombosis of one limb. Graft limb occlusion occurs in 10–20% of patients depending on the duration of follow-up. Late graft limb occlusion is most commonly due to progressive atherosclerotic disease at or just beyond the distal anastomosis. Other causes include worsening disease of the outflow vessels, commonly the proximal profunda femoris artery, thrombosis of an anastomotic aneurysm, arterial embolus from a cardiac source, low-output states, hypercoagulable states, and iatrogenic injury to the graft or native vessels following cardiac catheterization or diagnostic angiography. Except in cases of profound limb ischemia, preoperative angiography should be performed in all patients. In high risk or inactive patients without evidence of limb-threatening ischemia, a **nonoperative** approach may be the most prudent course. **Thrombolytic therapy** has been used in patients with acute graft thrombosis. Its use is limited in patients with severe limb-threatening ischemia. Significant complications such as bleeding, distal embolization, and worsening ischemia may occur. Furthermore, surgical revision of the graft is usually required in most patients. Therefore its use is limited to patients with acute occlusion and non-limb-threatening ischemia, particularly high risk patients. Most patients with graft limb occlusion are treated with an operative approach. In patients with graft limb occlusion of short duration, absence of proximal aortic disease, and unilateral occlusion, **graft limb thrombectomy** has been shown to be 90% successful. To prevent further thrombosis, repair of the distal anastomosis may be required if a defect is present. Advantages of this approach include the use of a unilateral groin incision and the fact that the procedure may be done under local or regional anesthesia. A common procedure for those with unilateral limb occlusion is a **femorofemoral bypass**. This procedure is usually not excessively time-consuming, may be done under local or regional anesthesia, and is technically easier than aortic re-operation. In patients with proximal aortic disease, anastomotic complications, or significant degeneration or dilation of the original prosthesis, **redo aortofemoral bypass** grafting is the preferred approach. In patients with multiple occluded grafts or "hostile" abdomens in whom the other less formidable options are contraindicated, extraanatomic reconstructions, such as **axillofemoral** or **descending thoracic aorto to femoral** bypass, may be utilized. Regardless of the technique used, revision of the outflow tract must be accomplished if necessary. It may require profundaplasty, graft limb extension, and bypass to the popliteal or tibial level. Distal grafts are required in 25–50% of all procedures for graft limb occlusion.

ANSWER: A, B, C, D, E, F

REFERENCES

1. Sabiston DC Jr: *Textbook of Surgery*, 15th ed. WB Saunders, Philadelphia, 1997.
2. Schwartz SI, Shires GT, Spencer FC: *Principles of Surgery*, 7th ed. McGraw-Hill, New York, 1999.
3. Ernst CB, Stanley JC: *Current Therapy in Vascular Surgery*, 2nd ed. CV Mosby, St. Louis, 1991.
4. Rutherford RB: *Vascular Surgery*, 4th ed. WB Saunders, Philadelphia, 1995.
5. D'Ayala M, Hollier LH, Marin ML: Endovascular grafting for abdominal aortic aneurysms. *Surg Clin North Am* 78:845–862, 1998.

Vascular

E. Peripheral

1. With regard to the clinical manifestations of arterial occlusive disease of the lower extremities, which of the following statements is/are true?

A. Claudication is a virtually diagnostic symptom of chronic arterial occlusion.
B. Pain during rest usually occurs in the same muscle groups affected by claudication and is often relieved by dependent positioning of the affected extremity.
C. Nutritional changes such as hair loss and nail brittleness generally precede symptoms of claudication.
D. Tissue necrosis is more likely in the presence of multilevel distal arterial disease.
E. Arterial ulcerations, like those of venous insufficiency, characteristically begin near the malleoli.

Ref.: 1, 2

COMMENTS: Chronic arterial occlusion of the lower extremities is the result of atherosclerotic disease of the aorta and its branches and can be diagnosed from characteristic signs and symptoms. The classic symptom, intermittent claudication, is cramping pain in specific muscle groups that occurs when blood flow is inadequate for meeting the demands of exercise. The pain usually occurs below the level of occlusion; hence claudication of the buttock and thigh muscles is suggestive of aortoiliac obstruction, and calf claudication is suggestive of femoral artery obstruction. As chronic ischemia progresses, trophic changes such as hair loss, nail brittleness, and muscular atrophy occur. Ischemic pain during rest is a manifestation of end-stage disease and characteristically involves the more distal aspects of the arterial circulation, such as the toes and feet. Pain is typically felt across the metatarsal heads. Associated physical findings include exacerbation of pain with extremity elevation, relief of pain by dependent positioning of the extremity, and dependent rubor caused by reactive hyperemia. Tissue necrosis usually signifies multilevel disease of the distal arterial tree inasmuch as chronic proximal occlusion alone is associated with the development of collateral circulation, which normally is adequate for preventing necrosis and gangrene. Most ulcers resulting from arterial insufficiency involve the toes or plantar surface of the foot and are painful, whereas venous ulcers are less painful and typically occur near the malleoli.

ANSWER: A, D

2. Which of the following is the most common site for atherosclerotic occlusion in the lower extremities?

A. Aortic bifurcation.
B. Common femoral artery.
C. Profunda femoris artery.
D. Proximal superficial femoral artery.
E. Distal superficial femoral artery.

Ref.: 2

COMMENTS: Although atherosclerotic disease frequently involves the area of arterial bifurcations, such as the aortic, iliac, and common femoral bifurcations, the most common site of occlusion on the lower extremities is the distal superficial femoral artery. The occlusion occurs in the adductor canal proximal to the popliteal fossa and may be related to the anatomic relation of the artery to the adductor magnus tendon at this site. Affected patients frequently have disease at several levels, however, which emphasizes the need for accurate angiographic assessment before revascularization procedures. Involvement of the superficial femoral artery alone is usually associated with intermittent claudication but not generally with tissue loss or pain during rest. The profunda femoris artery is usually not occluded in this situation and serves as an important source of collateral blood flow. Distal tibioperoneal disease is characteristically found in diabetic patients.

ANSWER: E

3. With regard to aortoiliac disease, which of the following statements is/are correct?

A. Impotence is a common finding that results from decreased blood flow through the external iliac vessels.
B. Thigh or buttock claudication (or both) is typical; toe ulceration or gangrene secondary to atherosclerotic emboli is occasionally present.
C. Lower extremity hair loss and nail brittleness occur in 60% of patients.
D. Concomitant coronary artery disease is the principal cause of death after aortoiliac reconstruction.
E. Balloon angioplasty of iliac lesions only occasionally relieves symptoms.

Ref.: 1, 2

COMMENTS: Thrombotic occlusion of the aortic bifurcation has characteristic manifestations. A significant thrombotic component is often associated with the atherosclerotic process, particularly in young patients. The common clinical manifestations are intermittent claudication of the thigh or buttock and impotence, caused by hypogastric arterial occlusion, which reduces blood flow through the internal pudendal artery and the corpora cavernosa. Femoral, popliteal, and pedal pulses are diminished or absent; and there may be lower limb atrophy. With aortoiliac involvement alone, however, trophic changes are not present because collateral flow originating from the lumbar arteries is preserved. Nutritional changes, when present, signify additional distal disease. Although distal tissue necrosis is often suggestive of more distal occlusive disease, the possibility of emboli from atherosclerotic plaques in the aortoiliac vessels must always be considered. This has been referred to as the "blue-toe syndrome" and can occur even in the absence of occluding lesions. Approximately 10% of patients with occlusive aortoiliac disease have an associated aortic aneurysm. The principal cause of death in this group of patients is coronary artery disease. Iliac angioplasty is particularly successful with short-segment iliac disease and when multilevel disease necessitates conventional distal bypass techniques only after adequate inflow is established with balloon angioplasty.

ANSWER: B, D

4. Any patient with intermittent calf claudication should be advised of which of the following?

A. Angiography is indicated to determine the extent of arterial disease.
B. Surgical reconstruction should be performed to prevent progression of disease and the development of pain at rest with gangrene.
C. Nonoperative treatment is sufficient for 75% of patients.
D. Sympathectomy may alleviate the symptoms.
E. Claudication progresses to gangrene at a rate of 2–3% of patients per year.

Ref.: 1, 2

COMMENTS: The goals of therapy for occlusive arterial disease of the lower extremities are to relieve pain, prevent limb loss, and maintain bipedal gait. Most patients with intermittent claudication alone remain stable or even improve with appropriate conservative management. Prophylactic surgical intervention is therefore not indicated. Claudicators have a low rate of progression to gangrene. In fact, more than 75% of these patients remain stable; the amputation rate is less than 7% in patients treated nonoperatively and observed for up to 8 years. In patients with severe claudication and marked involvement of the tibial vessels, the disease progresses to gangrene in 2–3% of patients annually. In contradistinction, patients with pain at rest, ulceration, or gangrene are at risk for limb loss and should be evaluated for revascularization procedures. Surgical intervention may be indicated in the presence of claudication alone for patients whose life style or livelihood is impaired by their symptoms and who do not otherwise have limiting cardiac disease. Arteriography is indicated only for patients who are considered candidates for operation. Sympathectomy is of little value in the treatment of claudication.

ANSWER: C, E

5. With regard to nonoperative treatment of occlusive atherosclerotic disease of the lower extremities, which of the following statements is/are true?

A. Exercise to the point of claudication leads to improved muscle performance due to adaptive changes made in muscle enzymes, leading to more efficient oxygen extraction.
B. Cessation of cigarette smoking reduces claudication and decreases the risk that gangrene will develop.
C. Foot protection is important because even minor trauma may lead to gangrene.
D. Anticoagulant therapy with warfarin (Coumadin) or heparin promotes healing of arterial ulcers.

Ref.: 1, 2

COMMENTS: Most patients in whom intermittent claudication is the only manifestation of peripheral vascular disease respond to conservative measures consisting of abstinence from tobacco and a graduated exercise program. Continued tobacco use has been associated with an increased risk of gangrene and a higher rate of premature graft failure after reconstructive procedures. For patients with more advanced ischemia, protection of the lower extremity is critical. Patients should avoid temperature extremes, improper footwear, or overly aggressive trimming of nails and calluses. It is not uncommon for relatively minor trauma to result in gangrene and eventual amputation of an already compromised foot. There is evidence that regular low-dose therapy with acetylsalicylic acid may be of benefit in preventing thrombosis in patients with atherosclerotic disease, but therapy with heparin or warfarin sodium has not proved beneficial.

ANSWER: A, B, C

6. Occlusive tibioperoneal disease occurs commonly in patients with which of the following entities?

A. Buerger's disease.
B. Raynaud's phenomenon.
C. Diabetes mellitus.
D. Arterial emboli.
E. Hyperlipidemia.

Ref.: 2

COMMENTS: Whereas the common pattern of atherosclerotic occlusive disease involves the femoral artery or the more proximal aortoiliac system, diabetic patients characteristically acquire a pattern of distal occlusive disease involving the distal popliteal artery and its branches. This type of distal involvement may also be seen in patients with Buerger's disease or arterioarterial embolism. The cause of this particular distribution of arterial occlusion is unknown. Patients with tibioperoneal involvement often present with advanced ischemia rather than simple claudication, and arterial reconstruction may necessitate grafts extended to the ankle or proximal foot.

ANSWER: A, C, D

7. With regard to the diabetic foot, which of the following statements is/are true?

A. Foot pain resulting from diabetic neuropathy usually is relieved by dependent positioning.
B. Trophic ulcers rarely occur if pedal pulses are palpable.
C. Débridement of infected tissue should be avoided until revascularization is accomplished because of the risk of nonhealing.
D. Surgical revascularization distal to the popliteal artery may be required to control infection and allow healing if there is arterial occlusion.
E. The ankle brachial index in a diabetic with an ischemic foot is often higher than 1.0 because of calcified vessels.

Ref.: 1, 2

COMMENTS: Diabetic patients are at risk for foot disorders caused by diabetic neuropathy, occlusive arterial disease, and infection. Diabetic neuropathy has generally adverse consequences: **Sensory** neuropathy renders the foot susceptible to trauma because of analgesia; **motor** neuropathy causes imbalances in the intrinsic musculature of the foot, leading to ventral subluxation of the metatarsal heads and pressure necrosis of the plantar tissue; and **autonomic** neuropathy may alter the microcirculation, further exacerbating tissue ischemia. Ischemic pain during rest, unlike pain secondary to neuropathy, may be relieved by dependent positioning. Trophic ulcers, which are painless, often occur on the plantar surface over the metatarsal heads as the result of pressure necrosis and often occur in the presence of palpable pedal pulses. Such lesions provide sites of entry for infection, to which the diabetic foot is markedly susceptible. Control of infection requires aggressive initial débridement of all necrotic tissue, systemic antibiotics, and arterial revascularization if there is occlusive disease. Arterial reconstruction in diabetic patients usually involves the tibioperoneal vessels and plays an important role in limb salvage. The ankle brachial index in diabetic patients is typically higher than 1.0 and does not reflect the degree of occlusive disease. Doppler velocity waveforms and those utilizing pulse volume recordings are a better guide to the degree of ischemia and are flattened in diabetics with peripheral ischemia.

ANSWER: D, E

8. With regard to femoropopliteal bypass, which of the following statements is/are true?

A. The patency of prosthetic grafts is nearly equal to that of autologous vein grafts in both above- and below-knee bypasses.
B. Patency rates are higher when bypass is performed for claudication than when done for limb salvage.
C. Continued cigarette smoking adversely affects graft patency.
D. Diabetes adversely affects graft patency.
E. Patency rates are unaffected by vein size.

Ref.: 1, 2

COMMENTS: The reversed saphenous vein autograft has been the most successful arterial bypass graft below the inguinal ligament and is the standard against which the success of prosthetic grafts is measured. Controversy exists with regard to the primary use of polytetrafluoroethylene (PTFE) for above-knee popliteal bypasses. The autologous vein is clearly the first choice for bypasses below the knee. Patency rates for saphenous vein grafts are approximately 80–90% at 1 year and approximately 75% at 5 years. • Patency rates generally are higher when bypass is performed for claudication than when done for salvage of the limb because of the extent of the underlying pathologic process. • Patency is adversely affected by grafts performed below the knee, continued tobacco use, poor distal runoff, and small vein size (<4 mm). Small vein size and size mismatch can be corrected through the in situ technique. • Associated risk factors, such as diabetes, hypertension, and coronary artery disease, have not been shown to exert a detrimental effect on long-term graft patency. Limb salvage rates generally exceed graft patency rates. If healing is *complete* after distal bypasses and the bypass subsequently becomes occluded, limb salvage is maintained in more than 50% of patients.

ANSWER: B, C

9. Which one or more of the following may be used for femoropopliteal bypass as an alternative to reversed saphenous vein graft?

A. PTFE graft.
B. Basilic and cephalic arm vein autografts.
C. In situ saphenous vein graft.
D. Umbilical vein allograft.
E. Lesser saphenous vein graft.

Ref.: 1, 2

COMMENTS: In approximately 25% of individuals the ipsilateral saphenous vein is inadequate for use as an arterial bypass graft because of small size, previous disease, or prior removal. In this setting a number of techniques have been used, although none has proved superior to saphenous vein grafting. At 36 months **PTFE** grafts have patency rates equivalent to those obtained with saphenous vein for above-knee femoropopliteal bypass, but PTFE grafts are significantly less successful when used below the knee. **Umbilical** vein grafts have success rates similar to those of PTFE grafts; however, enthusiasm about umbilical vein grafts has waned with the recognition that late aneurysm formation contributes to an unacceptably high rate of thrombosis. **Arm vein autografts** have produced results comparable to those seen with prosthetic materials and offer a potential alternative for distal bypass when the saphenous vein is unavailable. They are particularly useful for composite or sequential grafting. Their use is often limited because of lack of veins in arms, which is a consequence of thrombosis resulting from repeated in-hospital use in chronically ill patients. Dacron, PTFE, or the umbilical vein can be successfully employed as the proximal portion of a composite bypass graft when only a short segment of the saphenous vein is available. **In situ bypasses** offer the advantages of maintaining a physiologically active endothelium that maximizes the availability of a vein, with the ability to match a small distal outflow artery to a small distal saphenous vein. The 5-year patency rate approaches 75% for femorotibial bypasses performed for limb salvage. These bypasses require meticulous attention to detail and are time-consuming. Furthermore, their patency rates for proximal infrainguinal bypasses are no better than those of bypasses with reversed saphenous vein grafts; thus their use typically is reserved for distal bypasses.

ANSWER: A, B, C, D, E

10. Indications for tibioperoneal bypass grafting include which one or more of the following?

A. Necrotizing infection (in which case revascularization should be combined with local débridement).
B. Foot claudication.
C. Pain during rest.
D. Ischemic ulceration.
E. Gangrene involving the proximal and distal plantar surface of the foot.

Ref.: 2

COMMENTS: Revascularization procedures performed below the knee to the level of the proximal calf or to the ankle are indicated *only* for limb salvage. Intermittent foot claudication alone is not an acceptable indication. Revascularization should be considered, however, when there is ischemic pain during rest, progressive ischemic gangrene of the forefoot, necrotizing infection (in which case revascularization should be combined with débridement), or a nonhealing wound. A foot in which gangrene of the sole extends proximally past the midtarsal level is not generally considered suitable for weight-bearing; and the amputation level, which would likely be at the below-knee level, is not changed by distal arterial reconstruction.

ANSWER: A, C, D

11. Long-term patency of bypass grafts to the tibioperoneal vessels is influenced by which one or more of the following?

A. Diabetes.
B. Concomitant endarterectomy.
C. Previous attempts at revascularization.
D. Presence of a patent pedal arch.
E. Level of distal anastomosis.

Ref.: 1, 2, 3

COMMENTS: Bypass graft procedures distal to the knee are typically performed only for limb salvage and therefore are less successful than bypasses performed for claudication. Patency is better when the pedal arch is angiographically intact, but absence of a pedal arch is not a contraindication to surgery. Grafts to the anterior or posterior tibial arteries are therefore preferred, but grafts to the peroneal artery are also useful. Continuity with a patent pedal arch is of paramount importance for graft survival and limb salvage. Concomitant endarterectomy of vessels in the upper calf has produced results similar to those seen with venous bypass alone. The presence of diabetes does not significantly adversely affect patency on bypasses to the popliteal or tibial levels. Diabetes is, however, a significant risk factor in the development of tibioperoneal occlusive disease. Previously performed operative procedures have not adversely affected early or long-term patency rates or limb salvage. The role of sequential grafts, the addition of an arteriovenous fistula to a bypass graft, and the use of postoperative antiplatelet drugs or anticoagulants in improving graft patency rates are difficult to assess. The level of the distal anastomosis does not influence graft patency; however, the quality of the distal runoff is a primary factor.

ANSWER: D

12. Sudden pain and weakness in the left leg develop in a patient with a history of coronary artery disease and atrial fibrillation. Examination reveals a cool, pale extremity with an absence of pulses below the groin and a normal contralateral leg. Which of the following is the most likely diagnosis?

A. Cerebrovascular accident.
B. Arterial thrombosis.
C. Arterial embolism.
D. Acute thrombophlebitis.
E. Dissecting aortic aneurysm.

Ref.: 1, 2

COMMENTS: See Question 14.

13. For the initial evaluation of the patient described in Question 12, which of the following tests is/are mandatory?

A. Electrocardiography.
B. Venography.
C. Arteriography.
D. Abdominal ultrasonography.
E. Chest radiography.

Ref.: 1, 2

COMMENTS: See Question 14.

14. If the patient described in Question 12 had a history of intermittent left calf claudication and if examination showed, in addition, diminished pulses on the contralateral leg and trophic skin changes bilaterally, which of the following would be true?

A. Arteriography is of great value for differentiating thrombosis from embolism.
B. Venography is mandatory for ruling out phlegmasia alba dolens.
C. Indications for surgical intervention are unchanged.
D. Anticipated surgical procedure is unchanged.

Ref.: 1, 2

COMMENTS: The classic signs of acute arterial occlusion are pain, pallor, absence of pulse, paralysis, and paresthesia (the five P's). The common causes of acute arterial occlusion are embolism, thrombosis, and trauma. In the patient described in Question 12, the history of atrial fibrillation coupled with the classic findings of acute arterial occlusion make arterial embolism the most likely diagnosis. • Clinical findings that suggest arterial thrombosis rather than embolism as the cause include an absence of cardiac disease commonly associated with embolization phenomena, symptoms of underlying occlusive atherosclerotic disease, and physical findings suggestive of chronic ischemia. It can be difficult, however, to differentiate embolism from thrombosis on clinical grounds alone; embolism can certainly occur in patients with underlying peripheral vascular disease. • Prompt operative intervention is indicated, regardless of etiology, when there is acute limb-threatening ischemia. It is important, however, to distinguish arterial emoblism from arterial thrombosis superimposed on an atherosclerotic plaque because the extent of operation may vary considerably. Whereas embolism may be successfully treated by simple embolectomy and extraction of the thrombus that forms distal to the embolism, effective treatment of arterial thrombosis can be much more difficult, sometimes requiring arterial reconstruction. Arteriography is helpful for differentiating between embolic and thrombotic occlusions. A careful history and physical examination permit a diagnosis of embolic occlusions in most cases; arteriography is not always necessary and should not be performed if it will delay operative reestablishment of blood flow. Patients with arterial embolism should undergo electrocardiography and radiography of the chest because of the high association with intrinsic cardiac disease and its potential for myocardial infarction. • Acute arterial occlusion can be differentiated from acute thrombophlebitis, because thrombophlebitis is usually associated with edema, preservation of peripheral pulses, and superficial venous distension. Severe venous obstruction produces phlegmasia cerulea dolens; when this is associated with arterial thrombosis and spasm, phlegmasia alba dolens may occur. • In rare instances, an aortic dissection mimics acute embolism by producing loss of peripheral pulses, but the diagnosis may be suspected because of the presence of back or chest pain and hypertension. • Acute arterial occlusion that rapidly produces paralysis and paresthesia may be mistaken for a stroke; however, the physical examination should direct attention toward the compromised extremity and eliminate stroke from the differential diagnosis. • Prompt diagnosis of arterial occlusion is critical because irreversible muscular necrosis necessitating amputation may occur within 4–6 hours.

ANSWER:
Question 12: C
Question 13: A, E
Question 14: A, C

15. For an acute arterial embolus to the lower extremity with limb-threatening ischemia, appropriate initial treatment includes which one or more of the following?

A. Intravenous 5,000- to 10,000-unit heparin bolus followed by continuous-drip administration.
B. Delay heparinization until anesthesia is administered because heparinization precludes spinal anesthesia.
C. Routine preoperative trial of vasodilators.
D. Routine trial of fibrinolytic therapy such as streptokinase or urokinase.

Ref.: 1, 2

COMMENTS: Treatment of arterial embolism must be initiated promptly to prevent irreversible ischemic damage. Intravenous heparin should be administered to prevent formation and propagation of thrombus distal to the embolus and is the most important first step. Heparinization should not be delayed, particularly because most embolectomies can be performed with the use of local anesthesia; furthermore, the degree of distal thrombus is an important determinant of surgical success and limb salvage. Although arterial spasm accompanies acute arterial occlusion, the routine use of vasodilators is not advocated. Fibrinolytic agents have an important role in the treatment of patients with acute thrombosis superimposed on chronic ischemia. Their routine use to treat acute arterial embolus with limb-threatening ischemia is not advocated, however, particularly because timely intervention is of utmost importance. Because patients with arterial embolism often have associated cardiac disease and may be compromised further by the metabolic effects of ischemic tissue, preoperative attention must be given to careful physiologic monitoring and to the fluid balance, electrolyte balance, and arterial blood gas status of the patient.

ANSWER: A

16. With regard to operative management of lower extremity arterial embolism, which of the following statements is/are true?

A. Embolectomy can be performed in most cases.
B. Aortoiliac emboli should be removed through an abdominal approach.
C. Brisk back-bleeding is a reliable indicator of successful complete distal embolectomy.
D. Wide fasciotomy should be avoided in heparinized patients because of the risk of hemorrhage.

Ref.: 1, 2

COMMENTS: In most cases, **thromboembolectomy** can be performed with the use of balloon catheters introduced through arteriotomies proximal to the embolic site. **Aortoiliac emboli** can be removed successfully via bilateral femoral arteriotomies. **Back-bleeding** does not necessarily indicate adequate removal of the embolus distally because it may originate from an arterial branch proximal to the thrombus that remains. For this reason, restoration of distal pulses and intraoperative arteriography comprise the gold standard used to assess completeness of thromboembolectomy. **Fasciotomy** is an important concomitant procedure if the limb has been subjected to ischemia for 4–6 hours or longer if increased muscle turgor is present preoperatively; fasciotomy should be performed even in heparinized patients. Compartmental syndromes can develop after reperfusion of an ischemic limb, and close postoperative attention is thus required.

ANSWER: A

17. While a patient is in the recovery room after femoral embolectomy, a palpable pedal pulse disappears. The patient's leg is pale and swollen. Appropriate treatment includes which of the following?

A. Venography.
B. Fibrinolytic therapy.
C. Arteriography.
D. Immediate reexploration.
E. Fasciotomy.

Ref.: 1, 2

COMMENTS: During the immediate postoperative period, therapy focuses on maintenance of peripheral perfusion, treatment of the patient's underlying cardiac disease, and treatment of the potential metabolic complications after resumption of perfusion of an ischemic limb. Frequent evaluation of peripheral pulses by palpation and by Doppler ultrasonography and of limb temperature and color is mandatory. Any change that indicates ischemia warrants *immediate reexploration.* If swelling threatens the viability of peripheral musculature, *fasciotomy* is indicated. *Fibrinolytic* therapy has been used for arterial thrombosis but is contraindicated in patients who have undergone a recent operation because of the risk of hemorrhage at the operative site.

ANSWER: D, E

18. After undergoing femoral embolectomy and fasciotomy, a patient becomes oliguric, and the urine is brownish red. Immediate treatment includes which of the following?

A. Cessation of intravenous administration of heparin.
B. Determination of serum potassium level.
C. Intravenous administration of sodium bicarbonate and mannitol.
D. Renal arteriography.

Ref.: 1

COMMENTS: When an extremity has been subjected to ischemia and muscular necrosis occurs, reperfusion can result in metabolic acidosis and profound hyperkalemia. Rhabdomyolysis releases myoglobulin, which precipitates in acid urine and produces brownish red urine that is free of red blood cells. Treatment of patients in this situation requires prompt reversal of hyperkalemia to prevent cardiac arrest (intravenous insulin and glucose), administration of sodium bicarbonate to alkalinize the urine and to treat the systemic metabolic acidosis, and osmotic diuresis with mannitol to prevent renal tubular obstruction. Fasciotomy is indicated if it has not already been performed. Continuation of anticoagulation therapy is critical because the patient remains at significant risk of recurrent embolism from the underlying cardiac disease. Fewer than 10%

of arterial emboli involve the renal vessels, and renal arteriography is not indicated in this case.

ANSWER: B, C

19. Most arterial emboli originate from which one of the following sites?

A. Cardiac valves.
B. Left atrium.
C. Left ventricle.
D. Thoracic aorta.
E. Abdominal aorta.

Ref.: 1, 2

COMMENTS: By far, most arterial emboli originate in the heart; fewer than 10% arise from ulcerated plaques in the aorta, carotid arteries, or subclavian arteries. The most common intracardiac site is the left atrium, in which thrombi form as the result of stasis in patients with atrial fibrillation, mitral valvular disease, or both. A rare source of left atrial emboli is a left atrial myxoma. Left ventricular thrombi are a potential source of embolism in patients with myocardial infarction, left ventricular aneurysm, congestive heart failure, or cardiomyopathy. Valvular sources of emboli include vegetative endocarditis and thrombi formed on mechanical prosthetic heart valves. Paradoxical emboli arising from the venous system may reach the arterial circulation through a patent foramen ovale.

ANSWER: B

20. Cardioarterial emboli most frequently produce occlusion of which one of the following?

A. Cerebral vessels.
B. Distal aorta.
C. Common femoral artery.
D. Superficial femoral artery.
E. Popliteal artery.

Ref.: 1, 2

COMMENTS: Arterial emboli usually lodge proximal to arterial bifurcations and most commonly involve the lower extremities. One-third to one-half of arterial emboli obstruct the common femoral artery. This tendency for obstruction to occur proximal, rather than distal, to major bifurcations results in significant interruption of potential collateral flow and dangerous ischemic consequences.

ANSWER: C

21. After undergoing brachial artery catheterization for coronary angiography, a patient complains of hand numbness, and the previously present radial pulse is noted to be absent. Which of the following is the appropriate treatment?

A. Administration of systemic vasodilators.
B. Surgical exploration and topical application of papaverine.
C. Percutaneous balloon dilatation of brachial artery.
D. Brachial artery exposure with direct repair of the injured segment.
E. Arteriography to determine the presence of thrombus at the catheterization site.

Ref.: 1

COMMENTS: Iatrogenic arterial injuries may result from placement of needles and catheters for radiographic studies or monitoring purposes. Arterial occlusion usually occurs as the result of thrombus in association with intimal injury. Treatment consists of prompt exploration with arteriotomy and thrombectomy. Intimal damage may be treated by segmental excision with direct anastomosis. Surgery should not be delayed by attributing ischemia associated with arterial injury to arterial "spasm." Arteriography to confirm what is already clinically apparent delays the required surgical exploration and usually is not indicated.

ANSWER: D

22. Which of the following is the most common symptom of thoracic outlet syndrome?

A. Raynaud's phenomenon.
B. Pain or paresthesia in the C8 to T1 nerve distribution.
C. Pain or paresthesia in the radial nerve distribution area.
D. Ischemia or pain caused by arterial compression.
E. Arm edema caused by venous obstruction.

Ref.: 1, 2

COMMENTS: Anatomic compression of the brachial plexus, subclavian-axillary vessels, or both may occur at the thoracic outlet by a variety of mechanisms at several specific sites. The primary symptoms depend on which anatomic structures are compressed. Most patients have pain or paresthesias as a result of brachial plexus compression. Pain and paresthesias may affect any part of the shoulder or upper extremity but most commonly are noted in the C8 to T1, or ulnar nerve distribution, area. Symptoms of arterial compression, such as ischemic pain, fatigue, and decreased temperature are less common. Embolic events may produce digital gangrene or Raynaud's phenomenon. Symptoms of venous compression occur even less frequently than those of arterial compromise and may include edema, venous distension, and discoloration. In rare instances so-called effort thrombosis of the subclavian vein (Paget-von Schroetter syndrome) may occur. Nerve conduction studies, arteriography, and dynamic computed tomography (CT) scans may aid in the diagnosis of thoracic outlet syndrome: Physician maneuvers aimed at detecting a pulse deficit have low specificity. Resection of a cervical rib or a first rib and anterior scalenectomy are performed to decompress the thoracic outlet. Associated subclavian-axillary arterial lesions are corrected. A transaxillary, transclavicular or supraclavicular approach may be used.

ANSWER: B

23. With regard to Buerger's disease, which of the following statements is/are correct?

A. It is most frequently found in African-American men 20–40 years of age.
B. Recurrent migratory superficial phlebitis often predates arterial involvement.
C. Sympathectomy is effective in 50% of patients, but arterial reconstruction offers better long-term results.
D. Cessation of cigarette smoking is the primary therapy.
E. Can be successfully treated with anticoagulants, vasodilators, and steroids.

Ref.: 1, 2

COMMENTS: Buerger's disease (thromboangiitis obliterans) is an inflammatory process of uncertain etiology that produces thrombosis of medium-sized and small arteries and veins. The disease typically affects young men who are heavy smokers; it is rare in African-Americans. Recurrent migratory superficial thrombophlebitis involving the pedal veins often predates arterial involvement by several years. Both upper and lower extremities can be affected, and ischemic gangrene frequently results. Complete cessation of tobacco use is the most important aspect of treatment and may produce remission; simply decreasing the frequency of tobacco use is ineffective. Arterial reconstruction usually is not possible, because distal small vessels are frequently involved. Cervical or lumbar sympathectomy is useful in 50% of patients. No pharmacologic treatment has proved widely successful.

ANSWER: B, D

24. True statements regarding anterior tibial compartmental syndrome include which of the following?

A. May be caused by severe exertion.
B. Pain is the dominant symptom, with pain elicited on palpation of the calf.
C. The dorsalis pedis pulse is always absent.
D. Unlike other compartment syndromes, fasciotomy is rarely needed.

Ref.: 2

COMMENTS: The anterior tibial compartmental syndrome is related to pressure from tissue fluid within the closed compartment. The syndrome may be secondary to arterial trauma or arterial embolism and may be seen as a complication of cardiopulmonary bypass or femoropopliteal bypass. It may also be caused by severe exertion with no proven anatomic lesion. Pain is characteristically the first and dominant symptom and is located over the anterior compartment. As with other compartmental syndromes, the presence of pulses does not negate the diagnosis. Early fasciotomy before neuromuscular necrosis is the treatment of choice and produces excellent results.

ANSWER: A

25. With regard to the appropriate management of peripheral aneurysms, which of the following statements is/are true?

A. Popliteal artery aneurysms should be managed conservatively if less than 3 cm long, asymptomatic, and stable.
B. Multiple peripheral artery aneurysms are common; bilateral popliteal aneurysms occur in 70% of patients.
C. Proximal and distal ligation with bypass graft is the procedure of choice for popliteal artery aneurysms.
D. Their presence should heighten suspicion for associated aneurysms in the abdomen and thorax.

Ref.: 2

COMMENTS: Peripheral aneurysms are primarily atherosclerotic in origin, associated with hypertension, and frequently multiple. Popliteal artery aneurysms are the most common, are bilateral in 25–50% of patients, and frequently are associated with proximal femoral or aortoiliac aneurysm. (This is particularly true in patients with bilateral popliteal artery aneurysm.) Patients therefore require thorough assessment to rule out other associated aneurysms. Peripheral aneurysms present a high risk of limb loss as a result of thrombosis or embolus. Popliteal aneurysms should be operated on even when small, with diameters of 1.5–2.0 cm as a useful guideline; proximal and distal ligation with bypass grafting is the procedure of choice. On occasion, if the aneurysm is small and the artery is tortuous, excision with end-to-end anastomosis is possible.

ANSWER: C, D

26. With regard to Raynaud's disease/phenomenon, which of the following statements is/are correct?

A. It is characterized by upper extremity sequential phases of pallor, cyanosis, and rubor, which are initiated by exposure to heat or emotional stress.
B. It is most frequently seen in elderly women.
C. It is characterized by a pathologic mechanism that mainly involves vasospasm with a reduction in the dermal circulation.
D. Calcium channel blockers often yield good symptomatic control.
E. Cervical sympathectomy is usually the primary therapy.

Ref.: 2

COMMENTS: Raynaud's disease/phenomenon is the most common vasospastic disorder and most commonly affects young women (90% of patients are less than 40 years old). It may exist as a primary disorder (Raynaud's disease), or it may be a secondary manifestation (Raynaud's phenomenon) of disorders such as scleroderma, Buerger's disease, or thoracic outlet syndrome. The classic pattern of pallor, cyanosis, and rubor occurs after exposure to cold or stress. Vasospasm with a decrease in dermal circulation results in pallor. Cyanosis occurs as a result of sluggish flow of blood. Reactive hyperemia then occurs as the vasospasm subsides. Avoidance of initiating factors is often adequate; calcium channel blockers comprise the initial drug of choice.

ANSWER: C, D

27. Appropriate management of frostbite includes which of the following?

A. Rapid rewarming with dry heat rather than rapid rewarming with warm water.
B. Rapid rewarming with warm water.
C. Slow rewarming at room temperature if heparin or dextran is administered.
D. Thorough débridement of blisters and devitalized tissue.
E. Sympathectomy in the presence of tissue necrosis may minimize the extent of necrosis and prevent late vasomotor sequelae.

Ref.: 2

COMMENTS: The cold-injured extremity is best treated by rapid rewarming in warm water (40°–42°C). This results in less tissue damage than treatment by slow rewarming (i.e., at room temperature). Dry heat or water at higher temperature risks additional thermal injury because of decreased sensation of the injured part. The extremity should be elevated and exposed. Antibiotics are given if there is an open wound; tetanus prophylaxis is administered as indicated. Opening blisters and débridement of apparently devitalized tissue are contraindicated. True demarcation of nonviable tissue requires many weeks and should be allowed to develop spontaneously. The initial use of vasodilating drugs or antithrombotic agents such as heparin and low-molecular-weight dextran have not been shown conclusively to be effective. Sympathectomy may be useful for treatment of the chronic sequelae of frostbite such as paresthesia, hyperhidrosis, and coldness but does not minimize the amount of tissue necrosis.

ANSWER: B

28. With regard to popliteal entrapment syndrome, which of the following is/are true?

A. The syndrome commonly affects men before the age of 40.
B. Limb-threatening ischemia is the most common presentation.
C. Fibrous bands of the popliteus muscle most commonly cause arterial impingement.
D. Magnetic resonance imaging (MRI) is the diagnostic procedure of choice.
E. Symptoms are usually treated with exercise and antiplatelet medications.

Ref.: 3, 4

COMMENTS: The popliteal artery entrapment syndrome most commonly affects men before the age of 40. The most common presentation is mild, intermittent claudication. Arterial thrombosis or occlusion is rare. Other, less common causes of claudication in young adults include premature atherosclerosis caused by malignant hyperlipidemia, medial cystic degenerative disease, chronic exertional compartment syndrome, and vasculitis secondary to collagen vascular disorders. Physical examination typically reveals a loss of tibial pulses with plantar flexion. Noninvasive blood flow studies and duplex scanning may reveal the abnormality when done in conjunction with plantar flexion. The most sensitive diagnostic study is MRI, which can delineate the musculotendinous structures of the popliteal fossa and document their dynamic relation with the popliteal vessels. The most common abnormality encountered is medial deviation of the popliteal artery around the medial head of the gastrocnemius muscle. Five other anatomic variants have been described. Surgical repair is the only effective treatment of symptomatic patients. Resection or release of the variant musculotendinous structures is performed. Arterial reconstruction is necessary when stenotic or aneurysmal lesions are present. Surgical repair is also recommended for asymptomatic patients who are noted to have anatomic variants on the opposite side to prevent the development of secondary vascular complications.

ANSWER: A, D

29. With regard to atheroembolic disease of the lower extremities, which of the following is/are true?

A. Atheroemboli commonly cause acute occlusion of the common femoral bifurcation.
B. Normal pedal pulses are commonly found in patients with atheroembolic disease.
C. The most common source of atheroemboli is aortoiliac atherosclerotic disease.
D. Medical therapy is associated with a low rate of recurrence.
E. Aortofemoral bypass, femoropopliteal bypass, extraanatomic bypass with aortic exclusion, and localized endarterectomy are indicated for management of atheroembolic disease.

Ref.: 1, 2, 3, 4

COMMENTS: The term atheroemboli describes cholesterol or atherothrombotic microemboli. Both aneurysms and atherosclerotic plaque may be the source of microemboli. Aortoiliac atherosclerotic disease is the most common source of lower extremity microemboli. Whereas macroemboli from cardiac sources tend to lodge at the bifurcations of large vessels, microemboli commonly lodge in distal small vessels, such as the digital arteries of the toes. Cholesterol debris is often found on pathologic review of patients with atheroemboli. Patients typically present with the sudden appearance of painful, mottled areas on the toes. Microemboli may lodge in the capillaries of the skin leading to livedo reticularis of the knees, thighs, and buttocks. Typically, patients have palpable pedal pulses. If the superficial femoral artery is the source, a bruit or thrill may be present. Duplex scans may help define atherosclerotic lesions, but biplane angiography is the most sensitive diagnostic method for determining the source of emboli. Medical management with antiplatelet agents, steroids, aspirin, or warfarin is associated with a high rate of recurrence. Warfarin may lead to exacerbation of the condition due to plaque destabilization. Surgical intervention is indicated to remove the embolic source and reconstruct the arterial tree if necessary. Aortofemoral bypass, femoropopliteal bypass, extraanatomic bypass with aortic exclusion, and localized endarterectomy may all be indicated depending on the location and extent of disease.

ANSWER: B, C, E

REFERENCES

1. Sabiston DC Jr: *Textbook of Surgery*, 15th ed. WB Saunders, Philadelphia, 1997.
2. Schwartz SI, Shires GT, Spencer FC: *Principles of Surgery*, 7th ed. McGraw-Hill, New York, 1999.
3. Rutherford RB: *Vascular Surgery*, 4th ed. WB Saunders, Philadelphia, 1995.
4. Ernst EB, Stanley JE: *Current Therapy in Vascular Surgery*, 3rd ed. CV Mosby, St. Louis, 1995.

Vascular

F. Renal

1. With regard to the pathophysiology of renovascular hypertension, which of the following statements is/are true?

A. The relation between unilateral renal artery stenosis and hypertension was established by Goldblatt.
B. Activation of the renin-angiotensin system depends on intact aortic and carotid arch baroreceptors.
C. In response to reduced renal blood flow and pressure, the juxtaglomerular apparatus produces angiotensin I.
D. Angiotensin II elevates blood pressure by increasing peripheral vascular resistance and aldosterone production.
E. Saralasin competitively inhibits angiotensin II and is routinely used to screen for patients with hypertension caused by renin excess.

Ref.: 1, 2

COMMENTS: Renovascular hypertension is the elevation of diastolic and systolic pressures in association with renal artery occlusive disease. Goldblatt's classic experiment in 1934 confirmed a renovascular source for hypertension. Renovascular hypertension caused by renal artery stenosis (specifically decreased mean arterial perfusion pressure) stimulates the release of renin, a proteolytic enzyme, from the juxtaglomerular apparatus. Renin interacts with renin substrate, an α_2-globulin named angiotensinogen (synthesized in the liver), to produce angiotensin I. Converting enzymes (located primarily in the lung) convert angiotensin I (an inactive, labile decapeptide) to angiotensin II (an active octapeptide). • Angiotensin II, with a half-life of 4 minutes, increases blood pressure by its direct vasoconstrictor properties and by stimulating the release of aldosterone from the zona glomerulosa of the adrenal cortex. The latter effect increases sodium and water resorption in the renal tubules, leading to increased plasma volume. Establishment of normal renal artery blood flow can restore normal levels of renin production. Parenchymal lesions caused by infarction (secondary to emboli, thrombus, or trauma), disease of the distal renal artery branches, arteriolar nephrosclerosis, infrarenal aneurysms, spontaneous dissection, and renal artery occlusion with insufficient collateralization can also produce hypertension via renin-angiotensin stimulation. • Saralasin is a specific inhibitor of angiotensin II at the level of the arteriolar receptor site but has not proved reliable for screening patients with presumed renovascular hypertension.

ANSWER: A, D

2. With regard to surgically correctable hypertension, which of the following statements is/are true?

A. Surgically correctable hypertension, by definition, represents disease of the renal blood vessels and parenchyma.
B. It should be suspected when there is the sudden onset of severe hypertension before the age of 35 or when severe hypertension develops after age 55 in the absence of a family history of hypertension.
C. It should be suspected when easily controllable hypertension becomes labile.
D. It should be suspected in children, adolescents, and premenopausal women with hypertension.

Ref.: 1, 2

COMMENTS: Approximately 5–15% of cases of hypertension are surgically correctable. Although lesions of the renal artery are the most common cause of surgically correctable hypertension, a number of other causes amenable to surgical correction exist. They include pheochromocytoma, various causes of Cushing syndrome (adrenal hyperplasia, cortical adenoma, adrenal carcinoma), primary hyperaldosteronism, coarctation of the aorta (upper extremity hypertension), and unilateral renal parenchymal disease such as renal cell carcinoma associated with renin production. The diagnostic screens of these surgically correctable causes of hypertension include physical examination, family history of multiple endocrine adenomatosis, serum potassium (three determinations), urinary 17-hydroxyketosteroids and 17-ketosteroids, catecholamines, vanillylmandelic acid, ketosteroids, renal arteriography, and selective renin sampling.

ANSWER: B, C, D

3. With regard to atherosclerosis and renovascular hypertension, which of the following statements is/are true?

A. Atherosclerosis accounts for up to 80% of renal artery occlusions that produce hypertension.
B. Renovascular hypertension occurs equally in men and women between the ages of 55 and 75.
C. The lesions are most commonly located near the origin of the renal artery, are segmental, and often are less than 1 cm in length.
D. These lesions are the most common source of emboli to the kidney.
E. Up to one-third of affected patients have bilateral disease.

Ref.: 1, 2

COMMENTS: Atherosclerosis is the most common cause of renovascular hypertension, accounting for 95% of reported cases; fibromuscular dysplasia is another cause. Renovascular hypertension affects primarily men between the ages of 55 and 75 and is often a segmental defect of the proximal renal artery. The stenosis is most commonly on the left. Up to three-fourths of affected patients have bilateral disease. Renal artery atherosclerosis may be associated with renal artery aneurysms and renal emboli. Most renal emboli, however, originate from the heart. Hypertension that appears suddenly or that is difficult to control in patients with other stigmata of atherosclerosis is highly suggestive of the diagnosis. The more severe the hypertension, the more likely there is a correctable cause. Bruits over the kidneys are common but may represent transmission of sounds from nonrenal arterial stenosis. Renal bruits in essential hypertension are unusual. Arterial fibrodysplasia includes intimal fibroplasia, medial fibroplasia, and perimedial dysplasia. Medial fibroplasia is the most common and accounts for 85% of dysplastic renal artery disease.

ANSWER: A, C, E

4. A 14-year-old child who complains of headaches presents with marked diastolic hypertension and a soft to-and-fro bruit heard at the right costovertebral angle. Which of the following is/are the most likely diagnoses?

A. Coarctation of the aorta.
B. Spontaneous segmental renal infarction.
C. Intimal fibromuscular dysplasia.
D. Medial fibromuscular dysplasia.

Ref.: 1, 2

COMMENTS: Most asymptomatic children with mildly elevated blood pressure have essential hypertension. However, children with symptoms and a diastolic blood pressure above 100–110 mm Hg usually have secondary hypertension caused by either a renal parenchymal disorder (such as glomerulonephritis) or a neurovascular lesion. One of the common causes of renovascular hypertension in children is **fibromuscular dysplasia**. Fibromuscular dysplasia causes approximately 5% of all cases of renovascular hypertension. It is a disease primarily of children and premenopausal women. The lesions are classified according to the site (intimal, medial, adventitial) and type (hyperplastic, fibrosing, or both) of involvement. The most common lesions in children are *intimal* and *medial* dysplasias of unclear etiology. In women, medial fibrodysplasia is most common and may be caused by repeated renal artery stretching during pregnancy, causing damage to the vasa vasorum and mural ischemia, or by the effect of estrogens, which are known to cause medial degeneration. The right renal artery is affected in 85% of patients; in comparison, the left renal artery is involved most commonly with atherosclerotic lesions. Medial fibroplasia can be a systemic process with the internal carotid and external iliac arteries most often affected. The lesions frequently are multiple, creating the angiographic "string of beads" appearance. Medial fibromuscular dysplastic lesions may lend themselves to dilatation, whereas intimal and adventitial lesions do not. In 15% of patients, the lesions progress or new lesions are formed after treatment. **Coarctation** is usually associated with brachial femoral pulse discrepancies and a chest radiograph showing rib notching usually after age 11. Physical examination also reveals a palpable thrill or a hum heard on auscultation over the upper back from well developed intercostal collateral vessels. Unilateral blood pressure elevation suggests anomalous origin or stenosis of a subclavian artery. Due to distal renal hypoperfusion there may be a renin-angiotensin component to the hypertension as well.

ANSWER: C, D

5. With regard to the workup of patients in whom renovascular hypertension is suspected, which of the following statements is/are true?

A. Split-renal function studies provide the most accurate assessment for the presence of renovascular hypertension.
B. Renal artery stenosis demonstrated on arteriogram is sufficient indication for surgical correction in hypertensive patients.
C. Intravenous pyelography (IVP) is considered the diagnostic procedure of choice for evaluating patients in whom renovascular hypertension is suspected.
D. Systemic renin assays are the screening procedure of choice for patients in whom renovascular hypertension is suspected.
E. Renal vein renin ratios are currently the best means for determining the site of physiologically significant renal artery stenosis.

Ref.: 1, 2

COMMENTS: The goal of the workup for renovascular hypertension is to establish a relation between an identifiable renal abnormality and altered renin-angiotensin function. In other words, the functional significance of an angiographically demonstrated renal artery stenosis must be evaluated as well. The use of **IVP** to screen these patients has some drawbacks. There is a 75% rate of false-negative findings in children and a 20% rate of false-negative findings in adults with atherosclerosis. Delayed opacification, reduced kidney size, and ureteral notching are considered positive findings. IVP is limited for identifying segmental or arterial branch lesions, bilateral parenchymal disease of unequal severity, and bilateral arterial disease. **Intravenous digital subtraction angiography** may miss fibromuscular lesions, does not enable examination of branch vessels, and requires a large amount of contrast fluid. **Intraarterial digital subtraction angiography** offers better detail with less contrast fluid. **Arteriography** remains the definitive procedure for localization of significant renal artery lesions in patients suitable for operation or percutaneous intervention. Because **peripheral venous renin** activity is variable, it is not considered a reliable screening test. **Bilateral renal vein renin** activity, used alone or in combination with peripheral vein renin activity (the ratio of renal vein renin/systemic renin), is of central importance to the preoperative evaluation. A renal vein/peripheral vein renin ratio greater than 1.5 is considered positive. The patient must be on a low sodium diet and off β-adrenergic blockade before renin levels are determined. Captopril may be used to amplify the difference in renin activity between the normal and abnormal kidney. Before renin assays were available, **split-renal function studies** were used to assess the physiologic significance of renal lesions; they are no longer in wide use because of the high incidence of technical failure, complications, and unreliability. The advantages of split-renal function studies over plasma renin studies are that the former can assess the viability of the ischemic kidney, and it assesses the worse of the two sides when there is bilateral renal artery stenosis.

ANSWER: E

6. With regard to the selection and preparation of patients for surgery to correct renovascular hypertension, which of the following statements is/are true?

A. Most patients with renovascular hypertension are hypovolemic and require careful preoperative hydration.
B. Surgery clearly is superior to medical management of hypertension caused by renal artery occlusive disease.
C. Patients with renin levels that are nonlateralizing should not undergo operation.
D. Patients with generalized atherosclerosis and renovascular hypertension do best with surgery because hypertension is tolerated least by these patients.

Ref.: 1, 2

COMMENTS: Many patients with renovascular hypertension are hypovolemic and hypokalemic, usually because of diuretic therapy. These deficits must be carefully corrected before surgery. The importance of discontinuing antihypertensive therapy before operation is debatable. A diagnosis of renovascular hypertension can truly be made only in retrospect when correction of a renal artery stenosis leads to correction of the hypertension. • Most patients with unilateral stenosis and lateralizing renin values are helped by surgery. (False-negative results may result from problems with the screening technique or from the presence of unsuspected bilateral disease.) Medical therapy may control renovascular hypertension, but patients managed medically require close supervision and must comply with the regimen because renovascular hypertension seems to have a more aggressive course than does any other underlying atherosclerosis. Also, many patients with renovascular hypertension treated with angiotensin-converting enzyme (ACE) inhibitors exhibit deterioration in the glomerular filtration rate, as evidenced by a rising creatinine level. • It is clearly established that renal artery reconstruction provides long-term correction of hypertension. The same is true in women with fibromuscular dysplastic disease. The patients with atherosclerosis in whom disease is confined to the renal artery are the ones who do best with reconstruction. • In patients with generalized atherosclerosis and involvement of other organs, surgery may be best reserved for those who fail medical management or in whom renal failure develops as a result of progressive renal artery occlusion.

ANSWER: A

7. With regard to the choice of procedure for correction of renovascular hypertension, which of the following statements is/are correct?

A. Endarterectomy is rarely indicated because of the risk that emboli will cause parenchymal ischemia and further renin activation.
B. The internal iliac artery is the most common graft used for aortorenal bypass.
C. Partial nephrectomy rather than revascularization may be curative for hypertension caused by segmental infarction, renal artery branch lesions, intrarenal aneurysms, or isolated arteriovenous malformations.
D. Medial fibromuscular dysplasia and renal artery occlusion by plaques originating in the aortic wall next to the renal artery are lesions most amenable to transluminal angioplasty.

Ref.: 1, 2

COMMENTS: There are many surgical options for the treatment of renovascular hypertension. The most frequent is aortorenal bypass with the use of the saphenous vein. There is a tendency for the vein graft to dilate in children, so internal iliac artery grafts are used in pediatric patients. • Selected bilateral atherosclerotic lesions are amenable to transaortic endarterectomy with good results. • A growing experience with the technique of transluminal renal angioplasty suggests a technical success rate of up to 90% with proper selection of patients and preprocedure vascular surgery consultation. Fibromuscular dysplasia responds best to dilatation, whereas occlusion by atheromas originating in the aorta is least amenable. Restenosis after dilatation occurs more frequently in patients with atherosclerosis. • Small branch disease may be treated by benchwork surgery with the use of cold perfusion and ex vivo surgical repair, followed by reimplantation. • In general, surgical treatment of carefully selected patients with renovascular hypertension is 80–90% successful.

ANSWER: C

8. Considerations for the patient undergoing renal vein renin assay include which of the following?

A. Low-sodium diet.
B. Continuation of antihypertensive medications, especially β-blockers.
C. Contrast injection to confirm venous catheter placement into the left renal vein and not the adrenal, gonadal, or lumbar veins.
D. Supine position before and during the initial sampling procedure.

Ref.: 2, 3

COMMENTS: Erroneous results may be obtained during sampling procedures for renal vein renins. It is important, therefore, that the patient follow a low-sodium diet for 2 weeks before sampling procedures. Sodium restriction plus diuretic therapy stimulates the renin-angiotensin system and improves the sensitivity of the test. Antihypertensives, specifically β-blockers and α-methyldopa, may blunt renin release and should be stopped. It is preferable that a dual-catheter sampling technique be used and the catheter position be confirmed at the time of the sampling. Because position affects renin release, the patient should be supine 4 hours before and during the study. The values can be compared to the contralateral kidney level or to systemic renin levels. The renal vein renin ratio (RVRR) is the venous renin activity from the affected kidney divided by the renin activity from the contralateral kidney. A RVRR of more than 1.48 indicates significant renovascular stenosis. The renal/systemic renin index (RSRI) is the difference between systemic venous renin activity and individual renal vein renin activity divided by systemic venous renin activity. In the setting of renovascular hypertension, an RSRI over 0.24 for the affected kidney is present. The normal contralateral kidney demonstrates suppression of renin production with an RSRI of less than 0.24.

ANSWER: A, C, D

9. Which of the following lesions are best treated by percutaneous transluminal angioplasty (PTA)?

A. Renal artery occlusion.
B. Transplant renal artery stenosis.
C. Congenital hypoplasia of the renal arteries.
D. Orificial, atherosclerotic renal artery stenosis.
E. Bilateral renal artery stenosis.

Ref.: 4, 5

COMMENTS: Percutaneous transluminal angioplasty (PTA) of significant renal artery stenosis is a growing trend in the treatment of renovascular hypertension and renal insufficiency. The introduction of stents has led to a lower incidence of restenosis especially for the treatment of orificial, atherosclerotic disease. The etiology of the stenosis is an important predictor of success. PTA has become first-line therapy for renal transplant arterial stenosis. Acceptable results following PTA have been found with nonorificial atherosclerotic disease, unilateral disease, and fibromuscular disease (intimal and medial dysplastic stenosis). Less favorable results occur with PTA in patients with branch vessel disease, aneurysmal disease, renal artery occlusion, and congenital renal artery hypoplasia. The consequences of stent placement should be considered prior to intervention. These include myointimal hyperplasia, obstruction of a suitable target site for future bypass, and protrusion of the stent into the aortic lumen creating the potential for thrombus formation and distal embolization or difficulty with subsequent angiographic interventions. Complications due to PTA occur in a small percentage of cases. Proximal renal artery dilation can result in intimal disruption with preservation of the flexible elastic media found in this portion of the vessel. Distal renal artery dilation results in medial disruption due to greater stiffness of this layer in this portion of the vessel. Myointimal hyperplasia leads to recurrent stenosis after PTA. Stenting has improved the patency of percutaneous interventions involving the renal arteries. An initial trial of flexible stents in the renal arteries to reduce myointimal hyperplasia led to greater in-stent restenosis. Rigid stents are now the configuration of choice for the renal arteries.

ANSWER: B

10. Which of the following suggests nephrectomy or partial nephrectomy as the treatment of choice for patients with severe hypertension?

A. Complete renal artery occlusion with a kidney length of less than 7 cm, poor collateralization, and a normal contralateral kidney.
B. Complete renal artery occlusion with a kidney length of 9 cm or more and urographic visualization of the kidney.
C. Segmental renal infarction.
D. Severe arteriolar nephrosclerosis.
E. Intrarenal aneurysms associated with hypertension.

Ref.: 1, 2

COMMENTS: Patients with severe hypertension secondary to advanced parenchymal disease may undergo nephrectomy or partial nephrectomy especially when the kidney is contributing little to overall renal function. Such is the situation in which overall renal length is less than 7 cm in the presence of minimal collaterals and good contralateral renal function. Segmental arterial disease or infection may be amenable to partial nephrectomy for treatment of hypertension. Intrarenal aneurysms, arteriovenous malformation, segmental renal hypoplasia may be treated in a similar manner. Potentially salvageable renal parenchyma is suggested by an overall renal length of 9 cm or more, collateral vessels (lumbar, capsular, ureteral), and filling of the distal arterial tree. Also helpful are lateralizing renal vein renins.

ANSWER: A, C, D, E

REFERENCES

1. Sabiston DC Jr: *Textbook of Surgery*, 15th ed. WB Saunders, Philadelphia, 1997.
2. Schwartz SI, Shires GT, Spencer FC: *Principles of Surgery*, 7th ed. McGraw-Hill, New York, 1999.
3. Moore WS: *Vascular Surgery: A Comprehensive Review*. WB Saunders, Philadelphia, 1998.
4. Greenfield LJ, Mulholland M, Oldham KT, et al: *Surgery: Scientific Principles and Practice*. Lippincott-Raven, Philadelphia, 1997.
5. Kidney DD, Deutsch LS: The indications and results of percutaneous transluminal angioplasty and stenting in renal artery stenosis. *Semin Vasc Surg* 9:188–197, 1996.

Vascular

G. Visceral

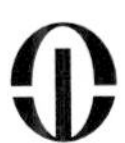

1. With regard to the mesenteric circulation, which of the following statements is/are true?

   A. The splanchnic vascular blood flow receives 25–30% of the cardiac output.
   B. Normal portal venous pressure is approximately 12–15 cm H_2O as a result of valves in the portal system.
   C. The ileum has more vascular arcades than does the jejunum.
   D. The presence of several sources of collateral blood supply to the superior mesenteric system minimizes the risk of bowel infarction when there is an acute occlusion of the superior mesenteric artery.
   E. The artery of Drummond, also known as the arch of Riolan or meandering mesenteric artery, provides an important collateral pathway between the celiac and superior mesenteric arteries.

Ref.: 1

COMMENTS: Under resting conditions, the splanchnic vascular bed receives up to 30% of the cardiac output and contains as much as one-third of the total blood volume. This represents a large potential reservoir of blood from which the patient is "autotransfused" in situations of severe hypovolemia. Normal portal venous pressure is between 12 and 15 cm H_2O. The portal vein contains no valves, and therefore blood flows within the portal vein based on the pressure gradient between the portal and systemic venous systems. Blood from the superior mesenteric artery reaches the small bowel via numerous arterial arcades; and although they become progressively greater in number and complexity in the more distal portion of the small bowel, it does not enhance the ability of the ileum to withstand acute occlusion of the superior mesenteric artery. Also, although collateral flow does exist between the superior mesenteric and celiac circulations (via the gastroduodenal and the pancreaticoduodenal arteries) and between the superior mesenteric and inferior mesenteric circulations (via the arch of Riolan and the marginal artery of Drummond), these sources of collateral flow only rarely are sufficient to maintain bowel viability in the event of acute occlusion of the superior mesenteric artery. Occlusion of the celiac or inferior mesenteric artery are much better tolerated and usually asymptomatic.

ANSWER: A, C

2. With regard to mesenteric vascular occlusion, which of the following statements is/are true?

   A. Occlusion of the inferior mesenteric artery usually causes severe colonic ischemia.
   B. Occlusion of the superior mesenteric artery occurs most often at its origin or at the origin of the middle colic artery.
   C. Intestinal infarctions are caused more often by arterial occlusion than by venous occlusion.
   D. Venous occlusions most often are embolic rather than thrombotic.

Ref.: 1, 2

COMMENTS: Although acute occlusion of the inferior mesenteric artery can produce symptoms of colonic ischemia, collateral supply from the superior mesenteric system via the marginal artery of Drummond and the branches of the middle and inferior hemorrhoidal arteries from the internal iliac arteries is usually sufficient to preserve the viability of the left colon. Acute and chronic occlusion of the superior mesenteric artery occurs most often at its origin or near its second branch, the middle colic artery. Approximately 50% of clinically significant mesenteric vascular accidents are caused by primary arterial occlusion, and 20% are caused by primary venous thrombosis. The remaining cases are considered nonocclusive, as in low-flow states, spasm, hemoconcentration, and hypovolemia.

ANSWER: B, C

3. Which one or more of the following statements accurately characterize(s) acute occlusion of the superior mesenteric artery?

   A. Sudden complete occlusion is more often caused by embolism than by thrombosis.
   B. Emboli most commonly arise from atheromatous plaques within the aorta.
   C. Abdominal pain classically is out of proportion to physical findings (e.g., guarding, tenderness).
   D. Acute occlusion of the superior mesenteric artery usually results in complete foregut infarction.
   E. The right and left colon are generally spared as a result of sparing of the middle colic artery.

Ref.: 1, 2

COMMENTS: Arterial emboli are the most common cause of sudden complete occlusion of the superior mesenteric artery. These emboli most often arise from the heart, either as mural thrombi from recent myocardial infarction or as auricular thrombi in patients with atrial fibrillation. Other cardiac arrhythmias, cardiac tumors such as atrial myxoma, and paradoxical emboli through a patent foramen ovale may also be a source of arterial emboli. One-fourth of the patients report previous embolic events. The initial abdominal pain is severe, often refractory to narcotics, and often out of proportion to the physical findings. The physical signs of peritonitis imply transmural ischemia and therefore, when present, represent a late stage in the evolution of this process. Acute occlusion of the superior mesenteric artery results usually in midgut infarction (ligament of Treitz to splenic flexure of the colon). The proximal jejunum, however, is often spared during acute superior mesenteric artery obstruction because of the location of the embolus beyond the first branch of the artery and the collateral vessels (middle colic artery) and because of the dual supply by the celiac axis system and the peripancreatic collateral vascular bed. The latter is formed by anastomosis between the superior pancreaticoduodenal artery (celiac-based) and the inferior pancreaticoduodenal artery (first branch of the superior mesenteric artery).

ANSWER: A, C

4. With regard to the diagnosis and management of acute occlusion of the superior mesenteric artery, which of the following statements is/are true?

A. Early arteriography can be of both diagnostic and therapeutic value.
B. Most patients can avoid operation if arterial infusion of papaverine is begun early during the clinical course.
C. Papaverine lyses thrombi and dilates the smaller mesenteric vessels.
D. As much as 70% of the small intestine can be resected without creating incapacitating digestive problems.
E. Clinical assessment, Doppler flowmeter analysis, and fluorescein staining are equally accurate for determining intestinal viability.

Ref.: 1, 2

COMMENTS: Early arteriography not only confirms the diagnosis and assists in determining the etiology; it also provides a route by which intraarterial papaverine can be administered. Papaverine, a potent vasodilator, assists in dilating the more peripheral mesenteric bed, which frequently is severely constricted as a reflex response to the more proximal mechanical occlusion. Despite these beneficial effects, most patients require laparotomy. • Serious gastrointestinal disturbances are uncommon if more than 30% of the small bowel can be preserved; the likelihood of a good result is enhanced if the terminal ileum and ileocecal valve are preserved as well. • Fluorescein dye may be administered intravenously, and assessment of fluorescein staining of the bowel by a woods lamp may be used to evaluate viability. The fluorescence pattern is significantly more reliable than either clinical judgment or the Doppler flowmeter for assessing bowel viability in borderline cases at the time of laparotomy. Reestablishment of the circulation should be attempted before bowel resection is undertaken. When long segments of intestine are of questionable viability, they are best left in place and reexamined at a second operation 24 hours later to ensure the maximal length of viable intestine.

ANSWER: A, D

5. Which of the following statements correctly characterize a nonocclusive mesenteric infarction?

A. It occurs more frequently but carries a lower mortality rate than does occlusive mesenteric infarction.
B. It is usually related to a low cardiac output state and may be exacerbated by digoxin.
C. It is often accompanied by a markedly elevated hematocrit as a result of polycythemia.
D. Arteriography with intraarterial infusion of papaverine can be effective in selected cases.

Ref.: 2

COMMENTS: Only 20–30% of cases of small bowel infarction are caused by nonocclusive phenomena. It is the most lethal form of acute mesenteric ischemia. The "final common pathway" of nonocclusive infarction appears to be a low cardiac output state, which may accompany numerous processes, including primary cardiac disease as well as septicemia and hypovolemia. Digoxin induces mesenteric vasoconstriction and therefore worsens the ischemic process. Papaverine, isoproterenol, and glucagon are vasodilating agents and may be therapeutically beneficial when accompanied by efforts to correct the low-flow state. Often, however, laparotomy is necessary because of refractory hypotension, because the diagnosis is in question, or because there are signs of peritonitis. The elevated hematocrit frequently seen in this disease process is caused by third-space loss of serum, not polycythemia. Early use of arteriography to distinguish occlusive from nonocclusive mesenteric ischemia can lead to therapeutic intervention with intraarterial papaverine. This approach, however, is contraindicated in patients in shock because the vasodilation of the splanchnic bed due to papaverine aggravates the hypovolemia. Correction of underlying and associated conditions is paramount to the survival of these patients.

ANSWER: B, D

6. With regard to mesenteric venous occlusion, which of the following statements is/are true?

A. Inflammatory conditions such as appendicitis or diverticulitis can be predisposing factors.
B. Patients with polycythemia vera, those with antithrombin III deficiency, and those taking oral contraceptives may be at increased risk for mesenteric venous occlusion.
C. Bloody diarrhea occurs less commonly with venous occlusion than with arterial occlusion.
D. Shorter segments of intestine are usually involved in venous occlusion in comparison with arterial occlusion.
E. Because of the frequent need for reoperation, heparin is contraindicated in these patients.

Ref.: 2

COMMENTS: Often subacute in its presentation, mesenteric venous occlusion may be idiopathic or secondary to a number of conditions, including appendicitis, diverticulitis, pelvic abscess, hematologic conditions, the postsplenectomy state in some patients (myeloproliferative disorders), use of oral contraceptives, extrinsic compression by tumor, venous trauma, acute portal vein thrombosis, polycythemia vera, and antithrombin III deficiency. All of these conditions bring into play various pathophysiologic mechanisms predisposing to clotting, including hypercoagulability, inflammatory or mechanical damage to the endothelium of veins, and low flow resulting from a variety of causes. Bowel wall edema may be seen on plain films. Computed tomography may show thrombus within the portal vein or the superior mesenteric vein. Mesenteric vein thrombosis is not often diagnosed intraoperatively. • Bloody diarrhea is seen more commonly with venous occlusion but tends to be a later finding than with arterial occlusion. The site of venous occlusion tends to be more peripheral within the mesentery than is the site of arterial occlusion, and therefore shorter segments of intestine are involved. Resection should encompass involved bowel and mesentery until grossly normal veins are encountered; otherwise, extension of residual clot leads to further gangrene. Anticoagulation with heparin should be started promptly. Because of a 30–40% recurrent thrombosis rate in untreated patients, lifelong anticoagulation is generally recommended. A second-look operation should be performed after 24 hours because of the common recurrence of thrombosis.

ANSWER: A, B, D

7. In which of the patients in the following clinical situations is surgical correction of the splanchnic artery aneurysm indicated?

A. A 25-year-old man with an asymptomatic 3 cm splenic artery aneurysm.
B. A 50-year-old man with a 3 cm splenic artery aneurysm and left upper quadrant pain.
C. A 20-year-old woman with a splenic artery aneurysm.
D. A 30-year-old ballerina with an asymptomatic hepatic artery aneurysm.
E. A 55-year-old woman about to undergo an open cholecystectomy who has an asymptomatic 3 cm splenic artery aneurysm.

Ref.: 2

COMMENTS: Because rupture occurs in only approximately 2% of splenic artery aneurysms, most affected patients can be managed conservatively. Patients who are symptomatic, however, should undergo aneurysmectomy, as should any women in their childbearing years because of the increased hazard of rupture during pregnancy. The overall mortality from splenic artery aneurysm rupture is 25%; rupture during pregnancy leads to death in more than half of the women and more than 90% of the fetuses. Aneurysms of the other splanchnic arteries should be repaired in patients with acceptable surgical risks, regardless of the absence of symptoms, because the incidence of rupture among these aneurysms approaches 50%.

ANSWER: B, C, D

8. With regard to intestinal angina, which of the following statements is/are true?

A. This term is a misnomer because it bears no pathophysiologic similarity to cardiac angina or claudication.
B. It is usually characterized by insidious weight loss, food aversion, and postprandial abdominal pain.
C. Anteroposterior aortography is invaluable for visualizing the origins of the visceral vessels and for demonstrating the large collateral vessels that develop in response to chronic visceral artery occlusion.
D. Operative correction is almost always indicated even if only one vessel is diseased.
E. The operative approach involves primarily transaortic endarterectomy or aortovisceral grafting (antegrade or retrograde).

Ref.: 1, 2

COMMENTS: As with angina pectoris and claudication, intestinal angina represents an imbalance between the metabolic needs of an organ (the intestines) and the blood supply available to meet these needs. Postprandial abdominal cramping is characteristic and is often accompanied by weight loss (11 kg on average) from food aversion rather than malabsorption. Although the diagnosis is suggested clinically, *anteroposterior and lateral aortography* is essential for delineating arterial anatomy before operation. Only lateral views can demonstrate the origins of the visceral vessels. A long, meandering artery is often demonstrated on the left side of the abdomen; it results from the collateral circulation between the inferior mesenteric and superior mesenteric arteries through the artery of Drummond (if lateral) and the arch of Riolan (if medial in location). Noninvasive ultrasonic imaging of the celiac and mesenteric vessels is developing as an important screening tool for patients presenting with weight loss and postprandial pain. Symptoms typically are not present unless two or more vessels are involved. Because of the difficulty of exposing the origins of the superior mesenteric and celiac arteries, most surgeons prefer to use bypass grafting for operative correction of these vascular abnormalities. Antegrade conduits of either prosthetic material or autogenous saphenous vein are preferred. Trap door aortotomy and endarterectomy may be appropriate in the presence of multiple proximal visceral and renal artery stenoses. Percutaneous angioplasty has been performed on a selective basis, although large series and long-term follow-up are lacking.

ANSWER: B

9. Compression of the celiac artery by the median arcuate ligament is characterized by which of the following statements?

A. It is always caused by an embryologic anomaly of the diaphragmatic fibers of the median arcuate ligament.
B. A bruit is classically present over the epigastrium.
C. Chronic abdominal pain, diarrhea, weight loss, and occasional nausea are the usual presenting symptoms.
D. Treatment should include transection of the median arcuate ligament to ensure celiac axis patency.
E. Direct arterial reconstruction to ensure celiac axis patency should be avoided, as the pathologic process involves the abnormal median arcuate ligament.

Ref.: 1, 2

COMMENTS: Compression of the celiac artery by the median arcuate ligament may be caused by an abnormal proximal origin of the celiac artery or abnormally low positioning of the median arcuate ligament. Chronic abdominal pain, diarrhea, weight loss, and occasional nausea are characteristic symptoms. The weight loss may be severe because patients stop eating to avoid the fairly predictable postprandial pain. Classically, a bruit is heard over the epigastrium, but its absence does not negate the diagnosis. If initial transection of the median arcuate ligament and surrounding neural tissue does not result in restoration of proper blood flow, direct arterial reconstruction may be necessary to ensure celiac axis patency. Irritation of neural tissue around the origin of the celiac axis by the accurate ligament may represent another pathophysiologic mechanism for this pain syndrome.

ANSWER: B, C, D

10. Accepted principles of management of traumatic injury to the visceral blood vessels include which of the following?

A. Mesenteric vascular injuries secondary to stab wounds of the abdomen are commonly associated with bowel or visceral damage.
B. When indicated, ligation of the inferior mesenteric artery and smaller branches of the superior mesenteric artery and veins can be accomplished, usually with impunity.
C. If possible, the hepatic artery and portal vein should be repaired rather than ligated.
D. Bullet injuries to visceral vessels may be repaired primarily only if there is a minimal "clean" injury.

Ref.: 2

COMMENTS: Patients with penetrating trauma to the abdomen should undergo surgical exploration whenever there is evidence of peritonitis or ongoing hemorrhage. When there is injury to visceral blood vessels, associated injuries to the bowel or solid viscera are common. Whereas smaller branches of the superior mesenteric artery can be ligated, the trunk of the superior mesenteric artery must be repaired. Collateral flow through the marginal artery is usually sufficient to permit ligation of the inferior mesenteric artery. Arterial and portal venous blood flow to the liver should be preserved if possible. Bullet injuries of mesenteric vessels are accompanied by adjacent trauma from the explosive characteristics of the trauma and can never be considered "clean" and confined to only what is visible to the naked eye. Primary repair of the laceration therefore is wrong.

ANSWER: A, B, C

11. Of the following causes of intestinal infarction, which has been estimated to be the most common?

A. Mesenteric venous thrombosis.
B. Acute embolic arterial occlusion.
C. Acute thrombotic arterial occlusion.
D. Nonocclusive mesenteric ischemia.

Ref.: 1, 2, 3, 4

COMMENTS: Acute mesenteric ischemia is most often secondary to acute embolic arterial occlusion of the superior mesenteric artery (30-degree take-off from the abdominal aorta creates the most accessible visceral vessel for embolic events) at the take-off of the middle colic artery. Approximately 50% of cases of acute mesenteric ischemia are secondary to arterial emboli. Thrombotic arterial occlusion is the next most frequent cause, accounting for 25%. The occlusion usually involves the origin of the superior mesenteric artery, dissimilar to an embolic occlusion. Nonocclusive mesenteric ischemia comprises 20% of cases of acute intestinal ischemia and is found most often in patients with advanced heart failure requiring aggressive diuresis and inotropic support. Mesenteric venous occlusion is the least frequent cause of acute mesenteric ischemia (5%).

ANSWER: B

REFERENCES

1. Sabiston DC Jr: *Textbook of Surgery*, 15th ed. WB Saunders, Philadelphia, 1997.
2. Schwartz SI, Shires GT, Spencer FC: *Principles of Surgery*, 7th ed. McGraw-Hill, New York, 1999.
3. Greenfield LJ, Mulholland M, Oldham KT, et al: *Surgery: Scientific Principles and Practice*. Lippincott-Raven, Philadelphia, 1997.
4. Moore WS: *Vascular Surgery: A Comprehensive Review*. WB Saunders, Philadelphia, 1998.

CHAPTER 40

Vascular-Peripheral Venous and Lymphatic Disease

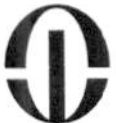

1. A 28-year-old overweight woman comes to the emergency room with a slightly reddened, painful "knot" 8 cm above the medial malleolus. Examination in the standing position demonstrates a palpable vein above and below a tender 2 cm mass. The patient is afebrile and has no other abnormalities on physical examination. Which of the following is the most likely diagnosis?

   A. Early deep vein thrombosis.
   B. Superficial venous thrombosis.
   C. Suppurative thrombophlebitis.
   D. Cellulitis.
   E. Hematoma.
   F. Insect bite.

Ref.: 1, 2, 3

COMMENTS: Superficial venous thrombi may be associated with thrombophlebitis, which is an acute, nonbacterial inflammation producing pain, redness, and swelling. Thrombi, however, may form without producing any signs or symptoms. **Superficial thrombophlebitis** usually appears as a localized process over the known course of a superficial vein. It occurs in association with intravenous catheters in the upper extremity and is usually seen at the site of varicose veins in the lower extremity. Distended varicosities above and below the lesion aid in the diagnosis. The diagnosis usually is easy via the history and physical examination. Lack of blood flow through the vein can be confirmed with Doppler ultrasonography, but this test usually is unnecessary unless there is concern about a deep venous thrombosis. Venography is not indicated and may even exacerbate the condition. The diagnoses of cellulitis, insect bite, subcutaneous hematoma, and traumatic ecchymosis must be considered when evaluating these lesions. An **insect bite** frequently is associated with itching. The presence of a hematoma or ecchymosis might indicate **trauma** as the cause. **Suppurative thrombophlebitis** also must be considered, especially in the presence of fever and leukocytosis. Suppurative thrombophlebitis is characterized by purulence within the vein and usually is a complication of intravenous cannulation. The presence of increased redness, pain, fluctuance, fever, and leukocytosis is more typical of bacterial infection than of superficial thrombophlebitis.

ANSWER: B

2. In a patient with superficial thrombophlebitis associated with varicose veins, the treatment plan may include which of the following measures?

   A. Excision of the entire vein and administration of intravenous antibiotics.
   B. Iodine 125 (^{125}I)-labeled fibrinogen scan, hospitalization, heparinization.
   C. Ligation of the vein proximal and distal to the mass, bed rest, intravenous antibiotics.
   D. Bed rest, elastic support hose, leg elevation, antibiotics.
   E. Warm moist packs, elastic support hose, nonsteroidal antiinflammatory drugs, ambulation with limited sitting or standing.

Ref.: 1, 2

COMMENTS: The usual aim when treating superficial thrombophlebitis is to relieve symptoms. The inflammation is nonbacterial, and antibiotics are not necessary unless there is evidence of secondary infection. These thrombi almost never embolize to the lungs unless they have propagated to the deep venous system. Fortunately, superficial venous thrombosis does not usually progress to deep vein thrombosis. Anticoagulation therefore is not necessary. Ligation is reserved for superficial lesions in the greater saphenous system above the knee near its junction with the femoral vein and for lesions of the lesser saphenous system near the popliteal fossa, locations from which a thrombus might more easily extend to the deep venous system. • Superficial phlebitis in these locations is best evaluated with duplex scanning. Unlike the recommendations made for deep venous thrombosis, with superficial thrombosis the risk of propagation of the thrombus is lessened by preventing venous stasis. This is accomplished by frequent walking, use of elastic stocking support, and keeping the leg elevated above the level of the heart when in the supine position. In other words, the patient should either walk or lie down with elevation of the leg; sitting and standing still for extended periods should be avoided whenever possible. Superficial thrombophlebitis is an acute problem, and symptoms from it usually resolve in several weeks. Antiinflammatory drugs are of variable effectiveness; aspirin usually suffices. Recurrent superficial thrombophlebitis may respond to proximal ligation followed by vein stripping.

ANSWER: E

3. Match the site of thrombosis in the left column with the appropriate signs and symptoms in the right column.

A. Calf vein
B. Femoral vein
C. Ileofemoral vein
D. Pelvic vein
E. Subclavian vein

a. Left side more frequently involved; severe swelling associated with cyanosis and pain
b. No swelling
c. Ankle and calf swelling; venous pressure two to five times normal
d. Minimal swelling; venous pressure normal
e. Swelling in a patient with a central venous catheter

Ref.: 1, 2

COMMENTS: The signs and symptoms of deep vein thrombosis (DVT) vary according to the vein involved. The most frequent site of thrombus is the calf, with the lesion usually arising in the sinuses of the soleus muscle. **Calf vein thrombi** usually produce pain and localized tenderness. Little swelling occurs (generally less than 1.5 cm diameter difference between the calves, although it is entirely absent in 30% of patients), and normal venous pressure is present. **Femoral vein thrombi** produce pain in the calf, popliteal region, or adductor canal. Swelling generally is present up to the midcalf, and venous pressure is elevated. **Ileofemoral thrombi** often are localized but may extend to the calf. The left leg is involved twice as often as the right, probably because of the longer course of the left iliac vein and its compression by the right iliac artery. As the venous pressure becomes elevated, the leg becomes painful, edematous, swollen, and pale (*phlegmasia alba dolens*). In this condition the blanched appearance of the limb is the result of edema and not arterial spasm, as previously thought. More extensive ileofemoral venous thrombosis, in which clot is propagated distally and into the ileofemoral venous tributaries, can obstruct all venous drainage and impair arterial inflow, producing ischemia and threatened loss of the limb. This condition, *phlegmasia cerulea dolens*, is a surgical emergency. **Pelvic vein thrombus** can occur in women with pelvic inflammatory disease or in men with prostatic infections. The condition is detected by pelvic examination; there are few leg signs. Venous thrombosis is less frequent in the upper extremity than in the lower extremity; and most commonly it is the result of **subclavian vein thrombosis** from an indwelling catheter. **Upper extremity DVT** may occur in patients also with heart failure or cancer. In otherwise normal patients, it has been termed the Paget-Von Schroetter syndrome or ''effort thrombosis'' and is a subclavian axillary vein thrombosis resulting from injury of the vein at the thoracic outlet. It presents as arm swelling and heaviness with discomfort made worse by activity.

ANSWER: A-d; B-c; C-a; D-b; E-e

4. Increased risk of DVT is associated with which of the following factors?

A. Blood group type O.
B. Diabetes mellitus.
C. Pregnancy.
D. General anesthesia.
E. Knee joint replacement.

Ref.: 3

COMMENTS: Venostasis of the lower extremities is associated with prolonged bed rest, standing, or sitting. It is also associated with the immobilization and muscular paralysis associated with trauma and general and spinal anesthesia. The most significant risk factor is a previous deep vein thrombosis (DVT). Additional risk factors include advanced age, obesity, diabetes mellitus, and the presence of malignancy. Patients with blood group type O are at low risk for DVT, whereas patients with group A blood are at higher risk for it; in both instances the reason is unknown. • Oral contraceptives and pregnancy are associated with increased levels of fibrinogen and factors VII, VIII, IX, and X; and both are associated with increased risk of DVT. • The incidence of DVT in surgery patients is 20–50%. The incidence in patients with hip fractures or those undergoing knee or hip replacement may exceed 50%.

ANSWER: B, C, D, E

5. Regarding the workup of patients with DVT, which of the following statements is/are true?

A. Venography as the initial test largely has been replaced by the use of noninvasive tests.
B. Many prefer duplex scanning with B-mode ultrasonography as the initial test.
C. Doppler ultrasonography and impedance plethysmography are equally useful for diagnosing femoral, popliteal, and major calf vein thrombosis.
D. Doppler ultrasonography and impedance plethysmography are equally sensitive for diagnosing ileofemoral venous occlusion.
E. Isotope scans cannot differentiate between active thrombosis and inflammatory fibrous exudate.
F. Venography is considered the definitive test for the diagnosis of DVT.

Ref.: 1, 2, 3

COMMENTS: **Isotope scans** with ^{125}I-human fibrinogen are used to detect clot formation or thrombus propagation. Studies of even the sickest patient are possible using portable instrumentation. Isotope scanning is not useful in patients with superficial thrombophlebitis, overlying recent incisions, traumatic injuries, hematomas, cellulitis, active arthritis, or primary lymphedema because it cannot differentiate between active inflammatory fibrous exudate and thrombus formation. Upper thigh and pelvic lesions are often confused by the high background counts of the isotope within the pelvic organs. An isotope scan can be 90% accurate for detecting the onset of thrombus when performed serially (daily) in high risk patients. Isotope scanning is now almost never used for a routine clinical diagnosis and is reserved for serial studies of patients in research studies. It is 80% accurate when testing for suspected established venous thrombosis and generally is reserved for such patients. **Doppler ultrasonography** is useful for detecting occlusions of major venous channels. It can also detect incompetence of the deep and perforator veins, but it cannot differentiate between old and new thrombi; nor can it help diagnose small, nonobstructing thrombi. **B-mode ultrasonography/duplex scanning** is the most recent and most promising of the noninvasive studies for DVT. This test can reliably differentiate extrinsic venous compression from DVT and new thrombi from old; and it can determine valvular competence. Superficial and deep veins of the calf and thigh as well as the iliac veins and inferior vena cava also can be visualized. These tests are increasingly viewed as the preferred initial tests for

DVT. **Impedance plethysmography** is more accurate than Doppler ultrasonography for diagnosing femoral, popliteal, and major calf vein thromboses but less accurate than duplex scanning. **Venography** is still considered the definitive test for the diagnosis of DVT and is used to resolve equivocal results obtained by the noninvasive techniques.

ANSWER: A, B, E, F

6. Which of the following statements is/are true regarding the prevention of venous thrombosis?

A. Elastic stockings have not been shown to influence the incidence of thrombus formation.
B. To be effective, pneumatic calf compression must be used for at least 3 days after an operation.
C. Injury to the intima of veins is an important cause of venous thrombosis.
D. Sequential pneumatic calf compression and low dose heparinization are essentially equally effective in preventing venous thrombosis.
E. Low-molecular-weight heparin is less effective than low-dose heparin in preventing deep vein thrombosis.

Ref.: 1, 2

COMMENTS: Prophylaxis is critical in averting venous thrombosis, and a variety of techniques have been used to accomplish this. Attention to technical detail when handling veins so as not to injure their intima and avoidance of leg veins when infusing hypertonic or irritating solutions are two examples of ways to help minimize the risk of thrombosis. Leg elevation and leg exercises during the postoperative period decrease venous stasis and its predisposition to thrombus formation. ^{125}I-fibrinogen scans have demonstrated the usefulness of pneumatic compression stockings in decreasing the incidence of thrombus formation. Pneumatic stockings work by generating fibrinolysin and antithrombin III and, as such, are effective even when placed on an arm rather than the legs. Sequential pneumatic devices are more effective than nonsequential devices; and in at least one study they have been shown to be as effective as low dose heparinization. Low dose heparinization (i.e., 5000 units subcutaneously) given 2 hours preoperatively and continued twice daily until the seventh postoperative day has been shown to decrease the incidence of DVT. There is evidence, however, that it may increase the rate of postoperative bleeding and wound complications. Its impact on the incidence of postoperative pulmonary emboli has not been clearly defined. Low-molecular-weight heparin has been shown to be superior to low-dose heparin to prevent deep vein thrombosis for patients undergoing both general and orthopedic surgery. Although no single method of prophylaxis has been shown to be clearly superior, some form of prophylaxis is important, whether it is aimed at preventing venous stasis physically or includes the use of anticoagulants.

ANSWER: C, D

7. Regarding the medical treatment of DVT, which of the following statements is/are true?

A. Bed rest is recommended to decrease venous pressure and thus lessen the risk of embolism.
B. Heparin is given to prevent thrombus attachment to the venous wall.
C. Platelet counts lower than 75,000/mm^3 imply active clot formation and inadequate levels of heparin.
D. Anticoagulation should be continued for 1–6 months after the acute event, depending on the site of involvement.
E. Streptokinase and urokinase are contraindicated within 10 days of major operations or trauma.

Ref.: 1, 2

COMMENTS: The prevention of embolization from existing thrombi and the inhibition of new thrombus formation are the goals of medical therapy for DVT. **Bed rest with leg elevation** decreases venous pressure and prevents fluctuations of pressure in the deep venous system. This allows the thrombus already present to become firmly attached to the vessel wall, minimizes venous distension, and reduces edema and pain. Elastic support is not needed if there is adequate elevation, but it should be used when ambulation is started. **Heparin** prevents propagation of the thrombus: It inhibits thrombin by inactivating the thrombin in the presence of antithrombin III (now called antithrombin). A partial thromboplastin time (PTT) that is two times normal indicates adequate heparinization. Giving heparin by continuous intravenous infusion is the preferred method, but intravenous or subcutaneous administration as a bolus can be used. Heparinization is continued for at least 7 days. Some patients receiving heparin therapy develop platelet clots in the arterial and venous system (heparin-induced thrombocytopenia), which can be a catastrophic complication. Therefore a platelet count that falls to less than 75,000/mm^3 is thought by some to be a reason to consider discontinuing heparin. Antiplatelet antibody levels should be evaluated in these patients. Alternative anticoagulation medications should be used. Warfarin (Coumadin) derivatives are begun prior to stopping the heparin to allow anticoagulant therapy to be continued on an outpatient basis. Treatment usually is continued for 1–3 months until the risk of recurrence diminishes. In cases of ileofemoral thrombosis, anticoagulation is continued for 6 months to allow time for the development of adequate collateral circulation, which decreases the risk of recurrence. **Streptokinase** and **urokinase** are capable of lysing thrombi via activation of plasminogen to plasmin. Their use in combination with heparin may reduce the incidence of late postphlebitic complications when compared with heparin alone. Both agents are most effective when given to patients with DVT of less than 5–7 days' duration, and the best results are obtained in patients who have had symptoms of less than 48 hours' duration. Pyrogenic, allergic, and bleeding complications occur with both agents, and their use is contraindicated within 10 days of major operations or injury. Bleeding complications occur two to five times more frequently than in patients treated with heparin alone, and intracranial bleed may occur in 1% of patients. Thus thrombolytic treatment of lower extremity DVT bosis is best limited to severe cases. The value of antiplatelet drugs such as aspirin is still undefined; however, inhibition of platelet adherence and aggregation with platelet-inhibiting agents does not stop clotting once it has begun. Such drugs therefore appear to be more useful for prophylaxis than for treatment.

ANSWER: A, D, E

8. Which of the following statements is/are true? Which is/are false?

A. The major indication for deep venous thrombectomy is recurrent pulmonary emboli.
B. Thrombectomy for ileofemoral DVT uniformly results in less swelling, pain, and venous stasis than does conservative therapy.

C. Thrombectomy is contraindicated for phlegmasia cerulea dolens.
D. Ileofemoral thrombosis from a pelvic infection is best treated with thrombectomy.
E. Caval interruption should always precede ileofemoral thrombectomy.

Ref.: 1, 2

COMMENTS: The role of surgery in the treatment of acute DVT is limited because of the effectiveness of medical management, the high incidence of residual or recurrent venous obstruction, and valvular incompetence that occurs after operative correction. Operation usually is reserved for major obstruction of the subclavian, iliac, or femoral vein and when the immediate- or long-term function of the limb is in jeopardy. Clinical studies have not demonstrated that thrombectomy leads to less swelling, pain, and venostasis than nonoperative therapy. Progression of ileofemoral thrombosis to the stage of near-total occlusion, with tenderness, massive edema, and cyanosis (*phlegmasia cerulea dolens*) may lead to venous gangrene. When it occurs, failure of the patient to respond promptly to treatment with leg elevation and heparinization or thrombolytic therapy (or both) is an indication for thrombectomy. • Although there is a theoretic advantage to caval interruption prior to thrombectomy, ileofemoral thrombectomy can be safely performed without caval interruption. • Septic ileofemoral thrombi (usually as a result of pelvic infection) is a contraindication to thrombectomy. • Operations for subclavian vein thrombosis should include resection of the first rib, cervical rib, or clavicle because most thrombi originate at the point where the clavicle crosses the first rib; failure to resect these structures is associated with a high rate of postoperative recurrence. • Success of venous thrombectomy depends on early operation, good technique, and complete removal of the thrombus. Surgery is not useful after 7–10 days; the best results occur when thrombectomy is performed within 48 hours of symptoms. • Pulmonary emboli that recur despite proper medical therapy are best treated with a caval filter.

ANSWER: A-false; B-false; C-false; D-false; E-false

9. Which of the following statements regarding the evaluation of patients with suspected pulmonary emboli is/are true?

A. The triad of dyspnea, pain, and hemoptysis is present in more than 60% of patients.
B. Normal serum glutamic-oxaloacetic transaminase (SGOT) in the presence of elevated serum bilirubin and lactate dehydrogenase (LDH) is seen in more than 50% of patients.
C. Pulmonary arteriography requires cardiac catheterization.
D. The arterial blood gas value is characterized by hypoxemia and normal to decreased PCO_2.
E. Ventilation-perfusion scans must be compared with a recent chest radiograph to be of value.

Ref.: 1, 2

COMMENTS: Surgeons must have a low threshold for suspecting pulmonary emboli in postoperative patients. About 85% of pulmonary emboli arise from the lower extremity, 10% from the right atrium, and 5% from the pelvic veins, vena cava, or arms. Up to 30% of patients with pulmonary embolism are free of symptoms, and only one-third of patients with pulmonary emboli have physical evidence of deep vein thrombosis (DVT) at the time of diagnosis. Emboli produce symptoms either by the direct effects of arterial obstruction or by secondary bronchospasm and vasoconstriction. The most common symptoms are dyspnea and pleuritic chest pain, and the most common signs are tachypnea, tachycardia, and rales. The classic triad of dyspnea, pain, and hemoptysis is present in fewer than 25% of patients. In fact, hemoptysis is indicative of frank pulmonary infarction and is uncommon. The classic biochemical triad of a normal SGOT with elevated LDH and bilirubin now is considered unreliable. Few patients show diagnostic electrocardiographic (ECG) changes other than tachycardia. Wedge-shaped defects on chest radiographs are seen only if infarction occurs. Decreased vascularity, pulmonary artery distension, and pleural fluid may be detected. Pulmonary arteriograms are the most specific tests for diagnosis and are performed by contrast infusion through a right atrial or main pulmonary artery catheter. On ventilation-perfusion scans, areas of the lungs that are normally ventilated but not perfused and that appear normal on chest radiographs should be considered to have pulmonary emboli. These scans are safe, convenient, and reliable if they are strongly positive or normal; in most patients they are generally preferred to arteriography as an initial study. The arterial blood gas result typically demonstrates hypoxemia and decreased PCO_2. This is the opposite of what is expected with "deadspace" disease (i.e., normal ventilation with decreased perfusion), wherein PO_2 is normal and PCO_2 usually is elevated. This paradox is explained by a (presumably) chemically mediated right-to-left shunt induced by pulmonary embolus and tachypnea leading to a normal or slightly decreased PCO_2.

ANSWER: D, E

10. Match each location and blood flow pattern in the left column with the appropriate superficial venous system in the right column.

A. Ultimately joins the femoral vein in the thigh
B. Ultimately joins the popliteal vein behind the knee
C. Anterior and posterior branch in the calf; lateral and medial branch in the thigh
D. Receives blood from the deep system via perforators
E. Blood flows into the deep system via the perforators
F. Perforators are located posterior and superior to the malleoli

a. Greater saphenous
b. Lesser saphenous
c. Both
d. Neither

Ref.: 1, 2

COMMENTS: An understanding of normal venous anatomy and blood flow is essential when considering chronic venous insufficiency and its sequelae. Normal veins of the lower extremity contain valves that direct the flow of blood centrally toward the heart and from the superficial into the deep venous system. Competent valves resist the force of gravity, which in the erect position tends to pool blood at the ankle. Forward flow is provided by the action of the left ventricle and compression of the veins as a result of muscular contraction. During muscular relaxation, deep venous pressure falls, leading to increased emptying of the superficial veins into the deep veins with a resultant fall in superficial venous pressures to below resting levels. Incompetence of the valves of the deep veins (usually the result of previous venous thrombosis) allows blood pooling and ineffective muscular pumping. Incompetence of the perforator valves (as a direct result of venous thrombosis or the result of dilation by back pressure from a valveless deep system) allows transmission of this increased deep venous pressure to the superficial system. When this occurs, the sequelae of venous stasis develop (brawny, nonpitting edema, brown pigmentation, dermatitis, and venous ulceration). Venous ulcers usually occur over the perforators, which are located dorsal and cephalad to the medial and lateral malleoli. Superficial venous incompetence, perforator incompetence, and deep vein abnormalities have the potential of causing these changes; and each may occur alone or in combination with the others.

ANSWER: A-a; B-b; C-a; D-d; E-c; F-a

11. Which one or more of the following patients is a candidate for an inferior vena cava filter?

A. A 33-year-old woman, 6 weeks pregnant, with a documented deep vein thrombosis (DVT) of the femoral vein and a ventilation-perfusion (V/Q) scan suggestive of a small pulmonary embolism (PE).
B. A 65-year-old man, after bilateral total knee replacement, with bilateral femoral DVT.
C. A 50-year-old woman, after total abdominal hysterectomy, with angiographically confirmed PE that occurred despite adequate anticoagulation.
D. A 26-year-old man with an ileofemoral DVT and massive thigh swelling, on heparin, and with a platelet count remaining stable at 90,000/mm^3.
E. A 70-year-old woman with evidence of right ileofemoral DVT and a large, loose thrombus in the infrarenal inferior vena cava (IVC).

Ref.: 3

COMMENTS: The primary therapy for PEs in most patients is anticoagulation. The precise role of thrombolytic agents is still evolving. For certain patients caval interruption may be indicated: patients in whom heparin therapy is contraindicated, those with recurrent emboli despite adequate anticoagulation, and those with free-floating ileofemoral thrombi. • Caval interruption may be used prophylactically in high risk patients (e.g., prior to major pelvic surgery in those with a history of previous DVT or PE). In addition, caval interruption is indicated for some patients with septic pulmonary emboli whose condition is refractory to heparin and antibiotics. Caval interruption may be complete or partial; recurrence of PEs after complete interruption is possible through new collaterals, although rare. Recurrence also results from thrombi arising from the ovarian veins, the cava between the ligature and the renal veins, the right atrium, the right ventricle, and veins of the head and neck. Chronic leg swelling, recurring phlebitis, and the sequelae of deep venous obstruction (edema, discoloration, ulceration) are more common after complete caval interruption and have been reported to occur with a frequency as high as 35%. Experience with transvenously placed devices that totally occlude the cava has shown the incidence of these complications to be low (5%) in patients who can be maintained on anticoagulants after caval interruption. Also, the presence of preexisting deep venous obstruction and chronic venous insufficiency strongly influences late results after caval interruption. Devices that partially interrupt the cava produce a lower incidence of postphlebitic sequelae, a higher incidence of nonfatal emboli (7% versus 4%), and a similar incidence of fatal emboli (about 1%). Caval filters can migrate and have also been associated with injury to adjacent retroperitoneal structures. • Patients with massive PEs producing hypotension who survive the acute event are candidates for pulmonary embolectomy, which is performed using a median sternotomy, cardiopulmonary bypass, and open clot extraction. An alternative to median sternotomy may be percutaneous catheter embolectomy. • Warfarin is contraindicated during pregnancy because of its teratogenic potential. Although a pregnant patient with a PE may be treated with long-term therapy with low-molecular-weight heparin, an alternative is a caval filter, especially if the patient is unable to administer subcutaneous heparin.

ANSWER: C, E

12. A 56-year-old man presents with a history of heaviness, tiredness, and aching of the left lower leg for the past several months. The symptoms are relieved by leg elevation. He mentions that he is awakened from sleep because of calf and foot cramping, but it is relieved by walking or massage. On physical examination, he has thick, darkly pigmented skin, nonpitting edema bilaterally and a superficial ulcer 2 cm in diameter, 5 cm above and behind the medial malleolus, that is slightly painful. The differential diagnosis includes which of the following?

A. Arterial insufficiency with ulceration.
B. Isolated symptomatic varicose veins.
C. Varicose veins associated with incompetent perforator veins.
D. Deep venous insufficiency with incompetent perforator veins.
E. Diabetic ulcer.

Ref.: 1, 2

COMMENTS: The most common symptoms associated with venous insufficiency are aching, swelling, and night cramps of the involved leg; the symptoms often occur after periods of sitting or inactive standing. Leg elevation frequently provides relief. Although the **edema** of venous insufficiency can occur with varicose veins alone, usually it is associated with deep venous abnormalities and incompetent perforating veins. **Night cramps** are the result of sustained contractions of the calf and foot muscles and are relieved by massage, ambulation, and proper management of the underlying venous insufficiency. **Brawny, nonpitting edema** is the result of increased connective tissue in the subcutaneous tissue. **Brown discoloration** is the result of hemosiderin deposition. **Ulceration** is most common in patients with deep venous abnormalities and incompetent perforators. In such cases the ulcers usually are located above and posterior to the malleoli (medial more than lateral), reinforcing their relation with perforator abnormalities. When patients with a history of DVT are followed beyond 10 years, up to 20% ultimately develop ulcers. • In contrast to arterial ulcers, venous ulcers are superficial and rarely penetrate the fascia. The pain of arterial insufficiency often is increased with leg elevation. Ulcers associated with arterial insufficiency may occur anywhere on the lower leg but usually occur distally, often involving the toe first. Arterial ulcers have an associated blue erythematous border and are more painful than venous ulcers. Patients with diabetes mellitus may develop shallow ulcers of the ankle that closely resemble venous stasis ulcers. Treating them as venous stasis ulcers (i.e., leg elevation, Unna boot, and other measures) may be disastrous because of the associated arterial insufficiency. The diabetic ulcer often occurs on the calf or ankle but is *not* associated with the edema and other skin changes seen with venous stasis ulcers. These ulcers result from arterial insufficiency and often begin with minor trauma to the affected area.

ANSWER: C, D

13. You have performed a Trendelenburg test on the patient described in Question 12 and determine that he has incompetent varicose veins associated with incompetent perforating veins. You interpret this as a:

A. Negative/negative Trendelenburg test.
B. Negative/positive Trendelenburg test.
C. Positive/negative Trendelenburg test.
D. Positive/positive Trendelenburg test.

Ref.: 1, 2

COMMENTS: There are several tests for diagnosing venous insufficiency. The **Trendelenburg test** is a two-part test used to delineate the competence of the superficial and perforating veins. While in the supine position, the patient elevates the legs until the superficial veins empty. **Part I**: The saphenofemoral junction is then occluded digitally, and the patient is asked to stand. The superficial veins are observed for 30 seconds. This action allows assessment of the competence of the perforator veins: Slow, ascending, incomplete filling of the superficial veins during compression is a negative (normal) result, whereas rapid filling is a positive result, indicating incompetence of the deep and perforating veins. **Part II**: The saphenofemoral occlusion is now released while the veins are kept under observation. This action allows assessment of the competence of the superficial veins: Continued slow ascending filling after saphenofemoral release is a negative (normal) result. Rapid retrograde filling is a positive result, indicating incompetence of the valves of the superficial system. **Percussion test**: This test is performed by tapping the superficial veins near the saphenofemoral junction while palpating over the knee for transmitted pulses. It can also be used to examine the lesser saphenous system. Transmission of a pulse suggests incompetent valves. **Venous pressure** studies help delineate abnormalities in the normal venous pressure relations during exercise. **Functional phlebography** is performed in patients before and after a standard active exercise and can demonstrate important pathologic and physiologic abnormalities. The **Perthes' test** involves application of elastic wraps to a leg with varicosities (to occlude the superficial venous system) before the patient is asked to exercise; pain during exercise suggests obstruction of the deep venous system.

ANSWER: D

14. Your therapeutic plan for the patient in Question 12 should include which of the following measures?

A. Varicose vein ligation and stripping as soon as possible.
B. Ligation of his medial perforating veins as soon as possible.
C. Initial treatment with appropriate leg wraps, leg elevation, and ambulation with avoidance of prolonged sitting or standing still.
D. Ulcer débridement, vein stripping, and skin graft.

Ref.: 1, 2

COMMENTS: Operative treatment of venous insufficiency in most instances is an adjunct to aggressive conservative management. Leg elevation, active exercise, and elastic compression form the cornerstones of nonoperative management. The goals of compression are to relieve symptoms and reduce swelling. When ulcers are present, local medications should be avoided unless evidence of infection exists. Ulcers smaller than 3 cm in diameter often heal with the above treatment. The indications for superficial vein ligation and stripping are moderate to severe symptoms without other signs of venous insufficiency, venous insufficiency with recurrent ulceration despite aggressive medical management, and occasionally severe varicosities without symptoms. Ligation of incompetent perforators can be an important addition to the treatment of venous insufficiency, particularly if done before ulceration develops. Ligation is most often performed through a longitudinal incision placed posterior and superior to the malleoli, as first described by Linton. Subfascial endoscopic techniques have recently reduced the morbidity of this technique. When present, incompetent superficial veins should be stripped as part of the procedure. Postoperatively, conservative measures must be continued aggressively. Obstructions of ileofemoral or femoropopliteal veins have been bypassed using the ipsilateral (femoropopliteal occlusions) or contralateral (ileofemoral occlusions) saphenous veins.

ANSWER: C

15. Which of the following statements is/are true regarding lymphatic anatomy?

A. The limb lymphatic vessels are valveless.
B. The lymphatic system begins just below the dermis as a network of fine capillaries.
C. Red blood cells, bacteria, and proteins readily enter lymphatic capillaries.
D. Extrinsic factors (muscle contraction, arterial pulsations, respiratory movement, massage) aid in the movement of lymph flow.

Ref.: 1, 2

COMMENTS: The lymphatic system begins as a network of valveless capillaries in the superficial dermis. There is a second valved plexus in the deep or subdermal layer that joins with the first to form the lymphatic vessels, and their course parallels that of the major blood vessels. The lymphatic vessels also are valved, and lymph flow toward the heart is aided by massage, arterial pulsations, respiratory movement, and muscle contraction. Intradermal lymphatics can be evaluated by the intradermal injection of patent blue dye. The capillaries normally become visible as a fine network 30–60 seconds after injection. Lymphangiography is rarely used to visualize the lymphatic vessels, as it may make lymphedema worse. Unlike veins, these vessels appear to be of uniform caliber throughout their course. • Lymphatic vessels are entered readily by proteins present in the extracellular fluid. Red blood cells and lymphocytes enter lymphatic vessels by separating the endothelial cells at their junctions. • Lymphedema occurs when the lymphatics are obstructed, too few in number, or nonfunctional, which results in the retention of interstitial fluid with a high protein concentration. Tissue oncotic pressure increases, and fluid is drawn into the interstitium. Measurement of the protein content of edema fluid (normally less than 1.5 mg/dl) can be used to assess the status of lymphatic function in the edematous extremity.

ANSWER: C, D

16. Which of the following statements is/are true regarding the etiology and complications of lymphedema?

A. Primary lymphedema appears at birth, is more common in females, and occurs in the right leg more often than the left.
B. Milroy's disease is a form of primary lymphedema that is sex-linked.
C. A lymphangiogram usually demonstrates a point of obstruction of the lymphatics in primary lymphedema.
D. Primary lymphedema almost always progresses to involve both lower extremities.
E. The major complication of lymphedema is the later development of lymphangiosarcoma.

Ref.: 1, 2

COMMENTS: Primary lymphedema is caused by abnormal development resulting in aplasia, hypoplasia, or varicosities of the lymphatic vessels. **Congenital lymphedema** (Milroy's disease) is present at birth and has a familial, sex-linked incidence; but the family history is present in fewer than 5% of patients. Primary lymphedema usually appears in individuals during their teens, more commonly in females; it often develops insidiously. The left limb is more frequently involved than the right (3:1); and often only one limb is involved. **Secondary lymphedema** is the result of obstruction or destruction of normal lymphatic channels and can be caused by tumor, repeated infection, or parasitic infection (particularly filariasis); or it can occur following lymph node dissection. Lymphangiography often demonstrates a discrete obstruction. Recurrent infections of venous stasis ulcers can destroy lymphatic vessels and lead to lymphedema. • The inability to clear proteins leads to edema formation that gradually increases over time and becomes woody because of fibrous tissue in the subcutaneous tissue. Repeated infection hastens formation of this fibrous tissue accumulation. Some patients develop blisters containing edema fluid or chyle. The major complication of lymphedema is recurrent attacks of cellulitis or lymphangitis, often following minor injury. β-Hemolytic streptococci are the responsible organisms, and the infection spreads rapidly because the protein-containing edema fluid is an excellent culture medium. • Lymphangiosarcoma is a rare complication of longstanding lymphedema, most frequently described in patients following radical mastectomy (Stewart-Treves syndrome). It presents as a blue or purple nodule with a satellite lesion. Metastases develop early, primarily to the lung. • Rarely, patients with lymphedema develop a protein-losing enteropathy that has been attributed to lymphatic obstruction of the small bowel.

ANSWER: B

17. Regarding the treatment of lymphedema, which of the following statements is/are true?

A. More than 50% of patients ultimately require an operation.
B. Diuretics have a crucial role in the conservative management of early lymphedema.
C. Pneumatic compression devices can damage the remaining lymphatics and should not be used.
D. Microsurgically constructed lymphovenous shunts are far more effective than are excisional procedures.
E. All surgical procedures have significant failure rates.

Ref.: 1, 2

COMMENTS: The mainstay of management of lymphedema is conservative and nonoperative; fewer than 5% of patients require an operation. The goals of therapy are the prevention of infection and the reduction of subcutaneous fluid volume. Fluid volume is reduced by elevating the extremity during sleep, the use of pneumatic compression devices, and carefully fitted elastic support stockings. Diuretics are not used routinely but may be useful in women who retain fluid during the premenstrual period. Patients prone to recurrent lymphangitis require intermittent long-term antibiotic therapy at the first sign of infection. The drug of choice is penicillin because streptococci are the usual infecting organisms. Secondary lymphedema requires treatment of the underlying cause, such as giving diethylcarbamazine for filariasis and appropriate antibiotics for tuberculosis or lymphogranuloma venereum. Edema that is excessive and interferes with normal activity and the presence of severe recurrent cellulitis are indications for operation. Patients with minimal edema, gross obesity, and progressing disease are not candidates for surgery. Excisional procedures include removal of skin, subcutaneous tissue, and fascia followed by split-thickness skin graft reconstruction (the Charles operation); excision of strips of skin and subcutaneous tissue followed by primary closure; and creation of buried dermal flaps. Physiologic procedures to restore or enhance lymphatic drainage include insertion of silk, Teflon, or polystyrene threads into the subcutaneous tissue; construction of pedicle grafts from the involved limb to the trunk; and microsurgical lymphovenous shunts using dilated lymphatics or the capsule and efferent channels of isolated lymph nodes anastomosed to neighboring veins. All procedures are associated with significant failure rates.

ANSWER: E

18. Manifestations of acquired peripheral arteriovenous fistula include which of the following?

A. Bacterial endarteritis.
B. Distal embolization.
C. Peripheral arterial insufficiency.
D. Congestive heart failure.
E. Venous aneurysm formation.

Ref.: 2, 3, 4

COMMENTS: Acquired arteriovenous fistula is most commonly the result of penetrating trauma, which causes injury to an adjacent artery and vein. The upper and lower extremities are the most common sites. Other causes include suture-ligation of adjacent vessels, vessel catheterization for diagnostic or therapeutic study, erosion of an adjacent vein by an atherosclerotic aneurysm, periarterial abscess, or neoplasm. Another cause is a remnant fistula following an in situ peripheral artery bypass. Small fistulas may close spontaneously. Fistulas that persist lead to dilation and ectasia of the proximal artery, and the adjacent vein becomes thick-walled, dilated, and aneurysmal. The intimal damage that occurs leads to an increased risk of infection and bacterial endarteritis. Depending on the size and location of the fistula, significant flow may lead to arterial insufficiency distal to the fistula ("steal phenomenon"). Venous congestion, chronic venous stasis changes, edema, and venous varicosities may also occur. In young children a peripheral fistula may lead to limb length inequality if it is present before closure of the epiphyseal plate. If the fistula is large, patients may develop signs and symptoms of high-output congestive heart failure. Temporary compression of the fistula may elicit a Branham-Nicoladoni sign with a rise in diastolic blood pressure and decreased heart rate. Peripheral arteriovenous fistulas do not cause thrombosis or distal embolization.

ANSWER: A, C, D, E

19. With regard to the diagnosis and treatment of peripheral acquired arteriovenous fistula, which of the following is/are true?

A. Acquired arteriovenous fistulas are rarely diagnosed by physical examination.
B. Angiography is the initial preferred diagnostic study.
C. Most arteriovenous fistulas can be observed without surgical intervention.
D. Proximal arterial ligation is the surgical procedure required for repair of most arteriovenous fistulas.
E. Percutaneous techniques such as detachable balloons and embolization are used to treat arteriovenous fistulas.

Ref.: 1, 3, 4

COMMENTS: Most arteriovenous fistulas (AVFs) are easily detected with a careful history and physical examination. A history of penetrating trauma is usually elicited. Physical findings may include a continuous (''machinery'') murmur heard over the site; a palpable thrill; distended, tortuous, or varicose veins; chronic venous stasis changes; elevated skin temperature; and the changes seen with congestive heart failure. Duplex scanning is useful for establishing a diagnosis. Arteriography is the preferred diagnostic study to document an AVF. The fistula is identified by the presence of a dilated afferent artery with early venous filling and simultaneous visualization of both arteries and veins. There is also diminished contrast distally. Duplex scanning is useful to diagnose AVF formation in the groin after catheterization injury. In this instance it may be the only test required prior to surgical repair. Most acquired AVFs should be repaired soon after diagnosis because of the low rate of spontaneous closure and the long-term sequelae. The goals of surgical repair include complete closure of the arteriovenous connection and restoration of normal arterial and venous flow. It may require placement of an interposition arterial graft. Autogenous vein is preferred when the repair is in the extremity. Most often the venous defect is repaired with a lateral suture. Repair with proximal arterial ligation leads to early distal ischemia and long-term persistence of the fistula due to collateral circulation. In certain instances, surgical repair is not possible owing to the location or technical difficulties. Percutaneous embolization with emboligenic materials or detachable balloons is useful in these situations. Both surgical repair and percutaneous embolization can lead to distal ischemia, infarction, and closure of an undesired artery. After repair of a long-standing AVF long-term surveillance is required because of the risk of arterial aneurysmal degeneration.

ANSWER: E

20. With regard to axillary-subclavian vein thrombosis (Paget-Schroetter syndrome), which of the following is/are true?

A. It is commonly associated with thoracic outlet compression syndrome.
B. Severe pain in the affected extremity is usually the presenting symptom.
C. Venography is the gold standard for making the diagnosis.
D. Surgical thrombectomy is highly successful for treating acute disease.
E. Patients treated with thrombolytic and anticoagulation therapy alone have a high rate of recurrence.

Ref.: 3, 4

COMMENTS: Spontaneous thrombosis of the axillary-subclavian vein is termed *effort thrombosis* or Paget-Schroetter syndrome. There is a strong male predominance. Thrombosis typically follows upper extremity exertion. Patients invariably develop swelling and complain of heaviness and discomfort in the arm that is exacerbated with activity and relieved with rest. Severe pain is a rare complaint. As many as 80% of patients who present with effort thrombosis have an associated thoracic outlet compression syndrome. As many as 25–75% of patients develop symptoms of disabling venous hypertension if not treated appropriately. Venography remains the gold standard for diagnosis. Computed tomography scans, magnetic resonance imaging, and arteriography are often required when planning surgical decompression of the thoracic outlet. Treatment with thrombolytic therapy and anticoagulation is highly successful for short-term treatment of this disease. Diagnosis and staged treatment of thoracic outlet compression is mandatory because of the high rate of rethrombosis in those treated with thrombolytic and anticoagulation therapy alone.

ANSWER: A, C, E

REFERENCES

1. Sabiston Jr DC: *Textbook of Surgery*, 15th ed. WB Saunders, Philadelphia, 1997.
2. Schwartz SI, Shires GT, Spencer FC: *Principles of Surgery*, 7th ed. McGraw-Hill, New York, 1999
3. Rutherford RB: *Vascular Surgery*, 4th ed. WB Saunders, Philadelphia, 1995.
4. Ernst EB, Stanley JE: *Current Therapy in Vascular Surgery*, 3rd ed. CV Mosby, St. Louis, 1995.

CHAPTER 41

Lung, Chest Wall, and Mediastinum

1. Which one or more of the following indicates that the patient is at high risk for respiratory failure following pulmonary resection?

   A. Preoperative 1-second forced expiratory volume (FEV_1) = 800 ml.
   B. Preoperative $PaCO_2$ = 38 mm Hg.
   C. Ventilation/perfusion (V/Q) scan shows 30% perfusion to operative side.
   D. Predicted postoperative FEV_1 = 1.1 liters.
   E. Maximum O_2 consumption (MVO_2) = 10 ml/kg/min.

Ref.: 1, 2, 3

COMMENTS: During the evaluation of a patient for pulmonary resection, many aspects of pulmonary physiology must be considered. If the preoperative FEV_1 is 800 ml, or the predicted postoperative FEV_1 is 800–1000 ml, the patient may have inadequate ventilatory reserve for pulmonary resection. Elevated arterial carbon dioxide tension ($PaCO_2$) suggests serious abnormalities in alveolar ventilation. The ventilation/perfusion (V/A) scan is a useful test to predict what the FEV_1 of the remaining lung will be after pneumonectomy. In marginal patients a maximal oxygen consumption (MVO_2) of less than 10 ml/kg/min is associated with a 29% mortality and 43% morbidity. No mortality occurs with MVO_2 over 20 ml/kg/min.

ANSWER: A, E

2. With regard to surgical anatomy of the lung, which of the following statements is/are true?

   A. The volumes of the right and left lung are approximately equal.
   B. The left main stem bronchus is longer than the right.
   C. The trachea is approximately 20 cm in length.
   D. The right pulmonary artery has a greater length than the left before giving off its first segmental branch.
   E. The angle of takeoff of the right main stem bronchus is the same as that of the left main stem bronchus.

Ref.: 1, 2

COMMENTS: The volume of the left lung is approximately 45%, and that of the right 55%, of the total pulmonary volume. The right main stem bronchus is 1.2 cm in length, and the left main stem bronchus is 4–6 cm in length. The trachea is 10–13 cm in length measured from the cricoid cartilage through the takeoff of the left main stem bronchus. The right pulmonary artery passes from the left side of the mediastinum to the right pleural cavity before giving off a segmental branch. The left tracheal bronchial angle is sharper than on the right, resulting in more frequent aspiration of material to the right than to the left.

ANSWER: B, D

3. For which one or more of the following is flexible fiberoptic bronchoscopy preferred to rigid bronchoscopy?

   A. Yttrium aluminum garnet (YAG) laser therapy.
   B. Massive hemoptysis.
   C. Transcarinal needle biopsy.
   D. Bedside aspiration.
   E. Stent placement.

Ref.: 1, 2, 3

COMMENTS: **YAG laser** débridement of endobronchial neoplasms is more efficiently accomplished with the rigid bronchoscope. Special open-tube bronchoscopes with channels for aspiration and biopsy have been developed for this technique. Pieces of tissue can be removed, bleeding is more easily controlled, and time for the procedure is reduced with the rigid bronchoscope. In patients with **massive hemoptysis**, the rigid bronchoscope accommodates the use of larger suction tubing and easier clearing of the airway. The lens of the flexible bronchoscope, on the other hand, frequently is covered with fresh blood, preventing visualization of the tracheobronchial tree. **Transcarinal** and **transtracheal biopsy** of mediastinal lymph nodes is best accomplished with the flexible bronchoscope. A special needle-tip catheter is inserted through the channel of the flexible bronchoscope, and selective positioning of the flexible bronchoscope directs the needle to the previously identified mediastinal lymph node. The flexible bronchoscope greatly facilitates the ease and comfort of **bedside aspiration**. **Stent placement** frequently requires stricture dilatation or tumor débridement. On occasion, the stent must be repositioned. All of these maneuvers are more easily accomplished with the rigid bronchoscope.

ANSWER: C, D

4. Which of the following is the most common complication following pulmonary lobectomy?

A. Retained secretions and atelectasis.
B. Bronchopleural fistula.
C. Persistent air leakage from the surface of the operated lung.
D. Empyema.
E. Persistent symptomatic air space.

Ref.: 1, 2

COMMENTS: The most common complication following pulmonary lobectomy is related to retained bronchial secretions and consequent atelectasis. This occurs in 10–30% of patients and is related to reflex splinting of the chest, shallow breathing, and an impaired cough mechanism. Air leakages, if not from the bronchial stump closure, usually close early. A small, persistent air space may occur, but it usually causes no problems. An asymptomatic air space gradually disappears with reabsorption of the air within the space. Bronchopleural fistula and empyema are uncommon after a lobectomy.

ANSWER: A

5. In patients who have sustained blunt trauma to the chest, which of the following would most likely be the cause of acute cardiopulmonary collapse?

A. Hemothorax.
B. Pulmonary contusion.
C. Acute adult respiratory distress syndrome (ARDS).
D. Pneumothorax.
E. Rib fractures.

Ref.: 1, 2

COMMENTS: Rib fractures are the most common injuries to the chest wall, but unless there is a flail segment they usually do not cause respiratory insufficiency. Hemothorax can cause respiratory insufficiency but is less common than pneumothorax. Pulmonary contusion causes delayed ARDS as a result of increased alveolar edema. Pneumothorax can cause sudden cardiorespiratory collapse if not treated.

ANSWER: D

6. Which of the following is the most common malignant primary tumor of the chest wall?

A. Chondrosarcoma.
B. Plasmacytoma.
C. Osteogenic sarcoma.
D. Ewing's sarcoma.
E. Fibrosarcoma.

Ref.: 1, 2

COMMENTS: Primary tumors of the chest wall are malignant in 60–90% of reported cases. **Chondrosarcoma** is the most common primary chest wall tumor, occurring in 35–40% of patients. It commonly occurs in 10- to 40-year-olds and usually in the sternum or adjacent costocartilages. It occurs more frequently in males and has a favorable cure rate when wide and complete resection is accomplished. **Plasmacytoma** or **myeloma** is a somewhat common tumor of the chest wall and often presents as a painful rib lesion without a palpable mass. It is most common in 40- to 60-year-olds and more frequently affects males. Solitary myeloma of the rib is a harbinger of the development of manifestations of the systemic disease of myeloma. **Osteogenic sarcoma** accounts for 6% of primary bone tumors and is most common in males younger than age 20. Osteogenic sarcoma presents as an enlarged, painful mass, and the radiologic appearance is that of the typical "sunburst" pattern. **Ewing's sarcoma** occurs most frequently in males younger than age 20 and accounts for 8% of primary bone tumors; it is associated with fever, malaise, anemia, and an increased erythrocyte sedimentation rate. The typical "onion-skin" appearance on the surface of the bone is caused by elevation of the periosteum and multiple layers of new bone formation. **Fibrosarcomas** commonly occur in adults aged 50–70. They are frequently slightly painful, slowly enlarging masses and can arise in previously irradiated fields.

ANSWER: A

7. Which of the following is the most common primary tumor of the anterior mediastinal compartment in adults?

A. Thyroid goiter.
B. Thymoma.
C. Teratoma.
D. Lymphoma.
E. Neurogenic tumor.

Ref.: 1, 2

COMMENTS: **Thyroid goiter** extends into the anterior mediastinum in about 15% of patients with goiter and, in fact, is not considered a true primary mediastinal tumor. **Thymoma** is the most common primary anterior mediastinal tumor, followed by **lymphoma** and rarely **teratoma**. **Neurogenic tumors** are one of the most common primary tumors of the mediastinum but occur in the posterior mediastinum.

ANSWER: B

8. Which of the following is the most common cause of acute mediastinitis?

A. Perforation of the esophagus secondary to instrumentation.
B. Postoperative infection following median sternotomy for open heart surgery.
C. Traumatic injury to the mediastinum and mediastinal structures.
D. Intrathoracic leak of an anastomotic suture line.
E. Erosion of a foreign body from the tracheobronchial tree or esophagus.

Ref.: 1, 2

COMMENTS: Currently, the most common setting of mediastinitis is cardiac surgery performed through a median sternotomy incision. Prolonged perfusion time, poor cardiac output postoperatively, and postoperative bleeding of sufficient magnitude to require reexploration are common predisposing factors. Perforation of the esophagus, anastomotic leaks, and traumatic injuries can rapidly lead to a fulminating illness. The standard treatment is appropriate antibiotic therapy, drainage of the contaminated area, and repair or exclusion of the esophagus.

ANSWER: B

9. Which one or more of the following tumors has an increased incidence in asbestos workers?

A. Cancer of the lung.
B. Pleural mesothelioma.
C. Cancer of the esophagus.
D. Cancer of the stomach.

Ref.: 1, 2

COMMENTS: All of the neoplasms listed above occur more commonly in asbestos workers. There is usually a long latent period (15–35 years) between exposure to asbestos and the development of tumors. Among asbestos workers, 6–7% of all deaths are due to mesothelioma and 20% are due to carcinoma of the lung. The death rate from carcinoma of the esophagus is 2.5 times higher than expected; the incidence of deaths from stomach cancer is 1.5 times higher.

ANSWER: A, B, C, D

10. In a patient with a malignant pleural effusion, which of the following is/are considered effective therapy?

A. Thoracentesis.
B. Thoracoscopy with instillation of a sclerosing agent.
C. Tube thoracostomy with instillation of a sclerosing agent.
D. Pleurectomy.
E. Irradiation.

Ref.: 1, 2

COMMENTS: For treatment of a malignant effusion, **thoracentesis** alone has a 98–99% failure rate. **Closed-tube thoracostomy** alone also has a high failure rate. **Closed-tube thoracostomy and instillation** of a sclerosing agent involve the principle of total removal of the fluid and obliteration of the space between the pleura and the lung. Obliteration of the pleural space can usually be accomplished by injecting a sclerosing agent such as bleomycin, doxycycline, or talc into the pleural space through the chest tube. This can be accomplished by thorascopy. Occasionally, **parietal pleurectomy** is necessary to obliterate the space. Complications are frequent, and mortality rates are significant with pleurectomy. **Pleuroperitoneal shunt** is a recent technique that can be effective for unresolving benign and malignant pleural effusions. **Irradiation** alone is not effective in controlling malignant effusion.

ANSWER: B, C, D

11. Empyema thoracis can be caused by which one or more of the following?

A. Pneumonia with subsequent pyogenic infection of the associated effusion.
B. Infections associated with a surgical procedure on the lung.
C. Penetration of the pleural space by a foreign body.
D. Extension from a subphrenic abscess.
E. Secondary to systemic sepsis.

Ref.: 1, 2

COMMENTS: Most commonly, empyema is secondary to infection of parapneumonic effusion. It occurs less frequently now with the early use of antibiotics for pneumonia. Any trauma, especially penetration of the chest with a nonsterile foreign body, can lead to an empyema. In one series patients with subphrenic abscess after abdominal surgery or disease constituted 10% of a group of patients who developed empyema. Empyema also occasionally results from systemic sepsis in immunocompromised patients, trauma victims, and patients who have had cardiac surgery.

ANSWER: A, B, C, D, E

12. Which of the following methods is/are useful for treatment of empyema thoracis?

A. Antibiotic therapy combined with thoracentesis.
B. Video-assisted thoracoscopy with tube drainage.
C. Dependent open drainage of the empyema cavity.
D. Decortication and pulmonary resection.
E. Muscle flap transposition.

Ref.: 1, 2, 3

COMMENTS: Antibiotic therapy without additional management of the empyema cavity is ineffective. If the effusion is still fluid, rather than viscid, thoracentesis with aggressive antibiotic therapy may abort the process. Video-assisted thoracoscopy with drainage may also be used during the early empyema stage with improved success. Frequently, however, it is not possible to remove all the fluid from the pleural space, and so the empyema progresses. With a well established empyema, initial drainage is established by closed-tube thoracostomy, followed by dependent open drainage achieved by a rib resection, or possibly an Eloesser flap. Early decortication may be necessary for the cavity of a chronic empyema in which the lung does not reexpand after 4–6 weeks of the standard treatment. Decortication is also indicated for the acute empyema that has not responded to nonoperative therapy. Mobilization with a vascular pedicle and transposition of chest wall muscles, omentum, or, occasionally abdominal wall muscles is used to obliterate postpneumonectomy and postlobectomy empyema spaces with or without bronchopleural fistula in patients who otherwise are stable.

ANSWER: A, B, C, D, E

13. Which of the following is the most common primary tumor involving the trachea?

A. Adenoid cystic carcinoma.
B. Squamous cell carcinoma.
C. Carcinoid.
D. Mucoepidermoid carcinoma.
E. Spread of malignant tumor from adjacent structures.

Ref.: 2

COMMENTS: Squamous cell carcinoma remains the most common *primary* tumor of the trachea, accounting for approximately two-thirds of primary tracheal tumors. Adenoid cystic carcinoma (formerly called cylindroma) accounts for one-fourth of primary tracheal tumors. *Secondary* involvement of the trachea by carcinoma of the esophagus, lung, thyroid gland, or larynx is far more common than are primary tumors of the trachea.

ANSWER: B

14. Which one or more of the following can cause lung abscesses?

A. Aspiration in an alcoholic or debilitated patient.
B. Aspiration secondary to esophageal disease.
C. Infection of a structural abnormality in the lung.

D. Hematogenous spread of bacteremia.
E. Hemothorax.

Ref.: 1, 2

COMMENTS: Aspiration from any cause, but especially in alcoholics and debilitated patients, is a frequent cause of lung abscess. Anaerobic bacterial organisms are most commonly responsible. Hematogenous spread of bacteria tends to cause multiple abscesses and has a high rate of morbidity and mortality. Achalasia, esophageal reflux, and cricopharyngeal diverticula may lead to pulmonary infection as a consequence of aspiration of esophageal contents. Pulmonary sequestration often presents as an abscess. Hemothorax left undrained may become infected, but the result is empyema rather than parenchymal lung abscess.

ANSWER: A, B, C, D

15. The standard therapy for pulmonary abscess includes which one or more of the following?

A. Antibiotics.
B. Bronchoscopy.
C. Early surgical resection of the involved area of the lung.
D. Catheter drainage of abscess cavity.
E. Muscle flap transposition.

Ref.: 1, 2

COMMENTS: Treatment of pulmonary abscesses consists of (1) diagnostic bronchoscopy to remove any foreign bodies, evaluate for bronchial stenosis or obstruction, and collect secretions for culture and cytology; and (2) administration of the appropriate antibiotics. With adequate therapy, complete collapse of the abscess cavity wall and complete healing generally take place in 10–14 weeks. Failure of an abscess cavity to heal should alert the physician to a possible underlying carcinoma. Patients who have persistent cavities or cavities that are initially 6 cm or larger are candidates for an operation. Massive bleeding or empyema also necessitates surgery, which should include resection of the entire lobe. Tube drainage is done only if the abscess cavity is adherent to the pleura. Muscle flap transposition procedures are not normally used for treatment unless a large empyema cavity occurs as a postoperative complication of surgical resection of a persistent large abscess cavity.

ANSWER: A, B

16. Match each of the lung volume measurements in the left column with the appropriate definition of airflow resistance in the right column.

A. Vital capacity (VC)	a. Volume in the lungs after a maximal inspiration
B. Total lung capacity (TLC)	b. Volume in the lungs after a normal expiration
C. Functional residual capacity (FRC)	c. Volume of a spontaneous breath
D. Residual volume (RV)	d. Volume remaining in the lungs after maximal expiration
E. Tidal volume (TV)	e. Maximum volume that can be expired after a maximal inspiration

Ref.: 1, 2

COMMENTS: **VC** can be measured as slow or forced, with the forced maneuver producing a lower volume in a patient with chronic obstructive pulmonary disease (COPD). **FRC** is determined by inspiration of an inert gas or plethysmography. **RV** is determined by subtracting the expiratory RV (the volume that can be expired from normal end-expiration) from the FRC. **TV** is easily determined and is a commonly used measurement for management of patients with mechanical ventilators. **TLC** is determined by adding the VC and RV.

ANSWER: A-e; B-a; C-b; D-d; E-c

17. Which of the following are the three most common drugs used to treat infection with *Mycobacterium tuberculosis*?

A. Isoniazid.
B. Ethambutol.
C. Rifampin.
D. Streptomycin.
E. Paraaminosalicylic acid.

Ref.: 1, 2

COMMENTS: Isoniazid, ethambutol, and rifampin are considered first-line drugs for treatment of *M. tuberculosis* infection. Single-drug treatment is discouraged because early development of bacterial resistance occurs. Resistance is frequently prevented when two or more drugs are used in combination. Streptomycin is less frequently used because it needs to be administered by injection. All the others are second-line drugs and are used when resistance to the first-line drug develops.

ANSWER: A, B, C

18. Which of the following is the most common cause of spontaneous pneumothorax?

A. Tuberculosis.
B. Rupture of small blebs.
C. Emphysema and chronic bronchitis.
D. Various pulmonary neoplasms.
E. Endometriosis.

Ref.: 1, 2

COMMENTS: The most common cause of spontaneous pneumothorax is **rupture of small blebs** generally located in the apex of the lung in persons without underlying lung disease. The highest incidence is in tall, thin individuals 20–40 years of age. Men are affected five to six times more frequently. **Emphysema** and **chronic bronchitis** account for 10% of cases of spontaneous pneumothorax. Before there was effective drug therapy for **tuberculosis**, it was thought to be the most common cause of spontaneous pneumothorax. **Metastatic sarcoma** is known to erode through the visceral pleura, causing a spontaneous pneumothorax. **Endometriosis** may cause pneumothorax with menses (catamenial pneumothorax).

ANSWER: B

19. Which of the following is/are indications for surgical intervention in a patient with spontaneous pneumothorax?

A. Recurrent spontaneous pneumothorax.
B. A persistent air leak at the end of a 3-day trial of closed drainage of a spontaneous pneumothorax.

C. Complete collapse of the lung in a patient with an initial spontaneous pneumothorax.
D. Initial pneumothorax in a commercial airline pilot.
E. Pregnancy.

Ref.: 1, 2

COMMENTS: Recurrence of a spontaneous pneumothorax is generally considered an indication for its operative repair. The incidence of recurrence after an initial pneumothorax is 15–20%; the incidence of a subsequent spontaneous pneumothorax after recurrence is 70–80%. Operative repair is suggested for a patient with an initial spontaneous pneumothorax whose occupation entails immediate responsibility for the safety of other persons (e.g., an airplane pilot) or who lives in a remote area. Operative repair of persistent air leaks from spontaneous pneumothorax is not considered until at least 7–10 days of closed therapy. Other indications for early operation are massive air leakage preventing lung reexpansion, hemopneumothorax, or a large solitary bulla. Treatment should be conservative in a pregnant woman until after delivery when the indications are as otherwise noted.

ANSWER: A, D

20. Which one or more of the following disease processes can lead to massive hemoptysis?

A. Bronchogenic carcinoma.
B. Bronchiectasis.
C. Broncholith.
D. Tuberculosis.
E. Lung abscess.

Ref.: 1, 2

COMMENTS: Lung abscess, tuberculosis, and bronchiectasis can frequently lead to massive hemorrhage, that is, more than 600 ml of blood in 24 hours. Both active tuberculosis and chronic cavitary tuberculosis can present with massive exsanguinating hemorrhage. Although bronchogenic carcinoma can present with major hemorrhage if the tumor erodes into a major pulmonary artery or vein, this occurrence is less frequent. Broncholiths almost never cause massive hemorrhage; the quantity of blood may vary from 1 to 50 ml.

ANSWER: A, B, D, E

21. A 62-year-old female cigarette smoker underwent a mastectomy 6 years earlier for adenocarcinoma of the right breast. Although asymptomatic, she now has a routine chest radiograph that demonstrates a 2 cm soft-tissue nodule in the anterior segment of the right upper lobe. Which one or more of the following is/are useful for further evaluation?

A. Contrast infusion computed tomography (CT) scanning of the chest.
B. Magnetic resonance imaging (MRI) scanning.
C. Prior chest radiography.
D. Transthoracic percutaneous lung biopsy.
E. Bronchoscopy.

Ref.: 1, 2

COMMENTS: Not all patients with a prior extrathoracic malignancy who have a soft-tissue nodule in the lung can be presumed to have metastatic disease without further evaluation. Indeed, in the scenario described above, the chance that the lung nodule is metastatic is about 50%. If the extrathoracic malignancy is controlled, the lung abnormality should be approached as if it were a primary neoplasm. Comparison with any previous chest radiograph would be the next step in the evaluation. If the nodule was present on prior radiographs (more than 2 years old) and it is unchanged in size and appearance, by definition it is benign and no further workup is required. If the nodule is new or has enlarged or if previous films are not available, the abnormality should be investigated as if it were a primary lung nodule. **Radiographs of the chest** (posteroanterior and lateral views) are the least expensive but also the least sensitive. In this case, **CT** scanning of the chest would be the next diagnostic procedure to determine if calcification is present within the peripheral nodule. CT scans are quite sensitive and can identify 50% more nodules than can lung tomograms. CT has the advantage of also allowing evaluation of the mediastinum, hila, and remaining lung. **MRI** scanning does not image small lung nodules with the same sensitivity as CT and cannot detect calcifications. **Percutaneous biopsy** is not generally indicated because a negative result does not ensure the absence of malignancy and therefore does not change the need for surgery for diagnosis and treatment if the other tests are not conclusive. It would be unlikely that a bronchoscopic examination would provide histologic diagnosis of a 2 cm peripheral nodule in the anterior segment of the right upper lobe. The likelihood of confirming a malignant diagnosis is less than 25% for peripheral lesions of the lung. Bronchoscopy is done at the time of pulmonary resection to make certain the tracheobronchial tree is free of pathology. The role of the newer positron emission tomography (PET) scan is currently being defined and may prove useful in the future.

ANSWER: A, C, E

22. Which of the following is the most common type of "bronchial adenoma"?

A. Adenoid.
B. Carcinoid.
C. Mucoepidermoid.
D. Hamartoma.

Ref.: 1, 2

COMMENTS: The term "bronchial adenoma" is of historical interest only; currently, these tumors are identified as bronchial carcinoids, adenoid cystic carcinoma, and mucoepidermoid carcinoma. Carcinoid adenomas account for approximately 85% of all "bronchial adenomas." Adenoid cystic carcinoma (in the past called cylindroma) accounts for 10–15% of "adenomas." These tumors are more malignant than carcinoid adenomas and have a poorer prognosis. All other "adenomas" are rare. Hamartoma is not a bronchial adenoma but, rather, a tumor consistent of a disorganized arrangement of tissues normally present in the lung.

ANSWER: B

23. Which of the following characterizes respiratory movements?

A. Elevation of the ribs by the intercostal muscles only during labored respiration.
B. A greater increase in the anteroposterior and bilateral dimensions of the chest than in the superoinferior dimension during unlabored respiration.

C. The movement of the diaphragm accounts for 50% of pulmonary ventilation during quiet respiration.
D. The abdominal wall does most of the work when additional muscles are required to aid inspiration.
E. There is diaphragmatic excursion of 1–2 cm during normal respiration.

Ref.: 1, 2

COMMENTS: During quiet respiration the diaphragm and intercostal muscles are responsible for thoracic volume changes, with the contraction of the diaphragm constituting 80%. The increase in the superoinferior dimensions of the chest by diaphragmatic flattening is greater than the anteroposterior and bilateral dimensions even though the diaphragm excursion is only 1–2 cm during quiet respiration. Elevation of the ribs with an increase in anteroposterior and bilateral dimensions is accomplished during normal inspiration completely by the intercostal muscles. During labored inspiration, however, accessory muscles are required, including the sternocleidomastoid, serratus posterior, and levatores. Arm and shoulder movement may also contribute to a small increase in thoracic dimension when needed, with contraction of deltoid, trapezius, pectoral, and latissimus dorsi muscles. Abdominal wall muscle contraction facilitates forced expiration during activities such as shouting and singing.

ANSWER: E

24. Which of the following is/are absolute contraindications to surgical resection of a lung tumor?

A. Vagus nerve involvement as evidenced by ipsilateral cord paralysis.
B. Pleural effusion.
C. Chest wall invasion of the tumor.
D. Liver metastases.
E. Mediastinal node involvement on the ipsilateral side.
F. Superior sulcus tumor.

Ref.: 1, 2

COMMENTS: **Vagus nerve involvement** is usually betrayed by left vocal cord paralysis and indicates invasion of the left recurrent nerve in the aorticopulmonary window; tumor in this area is generally considered nonresectable. Occasionally, however, the left vagus nerve is involved above the aortic arch by direct invasion of the mediastinum. Although this is classified as stage III disease, it is not an absolute contraindication to resection. **Pleural effusion** that contains malignant cells makes the disease noncurable by operation. Such an effusion, however, must be shown cytologically to be malignant before such a patient is denied an operation. **Chest wall invasion** and superior sulcus tumor, although constituting stage III disease, can be resected for cure with reasonable survival rates. **Mediastinal lymph node involvement** on the ipsilateral side, particularly with squamous cell carcinomas, can likewise be resected for cure and with the expectation of reasonable survival rates. **Liver metastases** constitute an absolute contraindication to pulmonary resection because under these conditions the lung cancer is categorically noncurable.

ANSWER: D

25. Which of the following extrapulmonary manifestations of carcinoma of the lung is/are associated with small-cell (oat cell) carcinoma?

A. Cushing syndrome.
B. Excessive production of antidiuretic hormone.
C. Hypertrophic pulmonary osteoarthropathy.
D. Hypercalcemia.
E. Carcinomatous neuromyopathy.

Ref.: 1, 2

COMMENTS: **Hypercalcemia** is most frequently associated with squamous cell carcinoma. **Hypertrophic pulmonary osteoarthropathy** occurs with equal frequency among non-small-cell cancers but does not occur in small-cell cancer. **Cushing syndrome** and **excessive production of antidiuretic hormone** are usually associated with small-cell carcinoma. **Carcinomatous neuromyopathies** are the most frequent (15% incidence when closely looked for) extrathoracic nonmetastatic manifestations of lung cancer; the most common are a myasthenia-like syndrome and polymyositis. About 50% of the patients have small-cell cancer.

ANSWER: A, B, E

26. With regard to the pathophysiology of adult respiratory distress syndrome (ARDS), which of the following statement is/are true?

A. The initial injury is characterized by pneumocyte injury and leakage of surfactant, causing interstitial edema.
B. Neutrophils have little to do with the initiation of ARDS but are important in reversal of the acute changes and lung healing.
C. Type II cells are particularly sensitive to injury during the early phases of ARDS.
D. Increases in the number of type II pneumocytes, pulmonary fibrosis, and vascular obliteration characterize the proliferative phase of ARDS.
E. There is little or no resolution of pulmonary fibrosis in ARDS patients, and marked reduction in pulmonary function in survivors of the disease is usually demonstrated.

Ref.: 1, 2

COMMENTS: Activation of neutrophils by various mechanisms with adherence to the pulmonary capillary endothelial surface appears to be one of the key initiating factors of ARDS. The endothelial cells are injured by release of various enzymes and substances from neutrophils, including toxic oxygen radicals, resulting in an increased gap between endothelial cells and leakage of fluid protein and cells into the interstitium. Alveolar flooding occurs when the capacity of the interstitium is exceeded and the sensitive type I pneumocytes, which cannot replicate, are destroyed. These events result in loss of function of the alveolar–capillary interface and characterize the early or exudative phase of the illness. The proliferative phase follows, characterized by the proliferation of type II cells and activation of interstitial fibroblasts with resulting pulmonary fibrosis and obliteration of alveoli, interstitium, and capillaries. Fortunately, not all ARDS progresses to destruction of the pulmonary system. In patients who recover, the type II pneumocytes evolve into type I pneumocytes. Interstitial fibrosis may resolve to a remarkable degree, and patients examined 6 months to 1 year after recovery have near-normal pulmonary function tests.

ANSWER: D

27. In the general population, what percentage of non-symptom-producing solitary pulmonary nodules are carcinoma?

A. 5%.
B. 20%.
C. 35%.
D. 50%.
E. 75%.

Ref.: 1, 2

COMMENTS: In the general population, only 5% of "coin" lesions discovered on routine screening chest radiographs are carcinomas, most being granulomas. In patients older than 50 years of age who have undergone resection of such a "coin" lesion, however, the incidence of cancer is 50%. In those 80 years of age or older, the rate of malignancy of these lesions increases to almost 100%.

ANSWER: A

28. With regard to the gas exchange area of the lung, which of the following statements is/are true?

A. Adjacent alveoli have no direct communication
B. Type I alveolar cells constitute 50% of the alveolar surface and are more numerous than type II cells.
C. Type II alveolar cells secrete surfactant and have a cuboidal shape.
D. The connective tissue, fibroblasts, and fluid of the interstitium between alveolar and capillary basement membranes are of relatively constant thickness under normal conditions.
E. Surfactant increases the surface tension at the air–liquid interface of the alveoli.

Ref.: 1, 2

COMMENTS: The alveolar surface comprises two main cellular elements. **The type I pneumocytes** are broad, thin cells that cover 95% of the alveolar surface, although they are 30% less numerous than type II pneumocytes. **The type II cells** are cuboidal in shape and cover only 5% of the alveolar surface; but they have the important function of surfactant production. The interstitium between the alveolar and capillary basement membrane varies greatly in amount and thickness. At some points it is absent, with fusion of the two basement membranes. These areas are particularly important for gas exchange. In some areas the alveolar septum is interrupted by the pores of Kahn, which provide direct air exchange between adjacent alveoli. Surfactant has two main characteristics: the ability to lower surface tension at the air–liquid interface of the alveoli and the ability to vary the surface tension depending on the amount of inflation of the alveoli.

ANSWER: C

29. What is the overall 5-year survival rate of patients with carcinoma of the lung?

A. 10%.
B. 20%.
C. 30%.
D. 40%.
E. 50%.

Ref.: 1

COMMENTS: The 5-year survival rate of all patients who develop carcinoma of the lung is 8–10%. The 5-year salvage rate after surgical resection is 20–35%. However, for patients who have T1 lesions without nodal involvement and no distant metastasis, the survival rate can be as high as 80%. Accurate staging is required in all patients to allow one to arrive at a meaningful prognosis.

ANSWER: A

30. Which of the following factors is/are suspected to contribute to the development of lung cancer?

A. Cigarette smoking.
B. Asbestos mining and use.
C. Exposure to hydrocarbons.
D. Radioactive ore mining.
E. Polluted urban air.

Ref.: 1, 2

COMMENTS: All of the agents listed above are reported to increase the incidence of carcinoma of the lung. Cigarette smoking appears to be the major contributing factor in the development of lung carcinoma. Cessation of smoking appears to reduce the risk of developing carcinoma of the lung, but the risk may never be reduced to that of a person who has never smoked.

ANSWER: A, B, C, D, E

31. A patient being followed after apparently successful treatment of a squamous cell cancer of the head and neck is found to have a new solitary pulmonary nodule. Which of the following is the most likely diagnosis of this lesion?

A. Solitary metastasis.
B. Granuloma.
C. Primary lung carcinoma.
D. Benign lung tumor.

Ref.: 1, 2

COMMENTS: Chest radiographs should be evaluated for new lung lesions in the context of the time frame in which a patient is at risk from a previous malignancy. In general, a new lung lesion in a patient who had had a known primary head and neck tumor, especially a squamous cell carcinoma, is most likely a new primary cancer rather than a solitary metastasis. In a patient who previously had a melanoma or sarcoma, however, a solitary lesion in the lung is more likely to be a metastasis. In patients with known cancers of the gastrointestinal tract, genitourinary tract, or breast, a solitary pulmonary nodule has an equal chance of being a metastasis or a new primary lung cancer.

ANSWER: C

32. A metastasis to the lung from a known malignant tumor elsewhere should not be resected in which of the following situations?

A. The primary tumor is not controlled.
B. There are bilateral metastases.
C. There is metastatic disease in organs in addition to the lung.
D. There are multiple unilateral metastases.

E. The cell type is melanoma.

Ref.: 1, 2

COMMENTS: Before resection of a metastatic neoplasm to the lung, the primary tumor must be under control, and there must be assurance that no other organ is involved with metastasis. The planned operation must be able to remove all known tumor, and the patient must be able to tolerate removal of involved lung tissue. Therefore whether the lesions are multiple or bilateral, these lesions should be resected only if the unresected lung tissue permits adequate pulmonary function. Several other factors influence the decision to operate, including histologic type, disease-free interval, tumor doubling time, and the presence of secondary nodal metastasis. Each of these factors has been shown to influence survival, but none of these unfavorable situations is an absolute contraindication to resection.

ANSWER: A, C

33. When performing a posterolateral thoracotomy, which of the following muscles is/are usually divided?

A. Pectoralis major.
B. Latissimus dorsi.
C. Serratus anterior.
D. Serratus posterior.

Ref.: 1

COMMENTS: When performing a posterolateral thoracotomy, the *latissimus dorsi* and *serratus anterior* muscles are both divided. If the incision is carried far posteriorly, the *trapezius* and *rhomboids* are also divided. This standard thoracotomy incision provides wide exposure to all intrathoracic structures. It is, however, associated with significant postoperative pain because of the large mass of muscle divided. A lateral thoracotomy incision is better tolerated yet affords less exposure. Neither the pectoralis major nor the serratus posterior muscles are divided during a posterolateral thoracotomy.

ANSWER: B, C

34. Patients with ARDS respond favorably to therapeutic interventions such as increased concentration of inspired oxygen and positive end-expiratory pressure (PEEP) by which of the following mechanisms?

A. Increasing the functional residual capacity (FRC).
B. Increasing alveolar oxygen saturation.
C. Increasing venous return to the right heart.
D. Correction of alveolar closing volume.

Ref.: 1

COMMENTS: All multiply injured patients and those with ARDS have reduced lung volume, reduced pulmonary compliance, and a diminished FRC. The main therapeutic effect of PEEP is to bring the FRC back to normal and to open collapsed alveoli. PEEP has the positive effect of *improving oxygenation*, stabilizing the airway, and maintaining alveolar structure by preventing collapse. Negative effects of PEEP, however, especially at high levels (>12 cm H_2O) *decrease venous filling* of the right heart and can impair cardiac output. Barotrauma and tension pneumothorax are other potential complications of PEEP. Increasing the concentration of inspired oxygen *increases alveolar oxygen saturation*, making more oxygen available for gas exchange across the alveolar–capillary membrane.

ANSWER: A, B, D

35. Match each of the organisms causing lung infection in the left column with the appropriate clinical statement in the right column.

A. Actinomycosis
B. Histoplasmosis
C. Blastomycosis
D. Aspergillosis

a. Cutaneous and pulmonary infections often occur together
b. Drainage from the abscess or sinus looks like sulfur granules
c. Has propensity to colonize a preexisting pulmonary cavity, forming a fungus ball
d. Endemic to Mississippi River basin; is the most common systemic fungal infection in the United States

Ref.: 1, 2

COMMENTS: **Actinomycosis**, unlike the other three infections listed above, is caused by a microaerophilic bacterium; it is often incorrectly called a fungus. Abscesses and sinus tracts caused by actinomycosis drain a yellow-brown material resembling sulfur granules. Histoplasmosis, blastomycosis, and aspergillosis are caused by fungi. **Histoplasmosis** is the most common systemic fungal infection in the United States and is endemic to the Mississippi River basin. Calcified lymph nodes in the mediastinum are often the result of a past infection caused by histoplasmosis. **Blastomycosis** is caused by the organism *Blastomyces dermatitidis*. As the name implies, the cutaneous and pulmonary infections are often seen together. The organism can readily be cultured from the margins of the skin ulcers it causes. **Aspergillosis** is usually caused by colonization of a preexisting pulmonary cavity, leading to what is called a "fungus ball," or aspergilloma.

ANSWER: A-b; B-d; C-a; D-c

36. Which of the following is/are characteristic of chyle?

A. Resistant to infection.
B. High erythrocyte count.
C. Low lymphocyte count.
D. High triglyceride level.

Ref.: 1

COMMENTS: A chyle leak is most often the result of operative injury to the thoracic duct. It is less often associated with malignancy and obstruction of lymphatic channels. Normal daily chyle flow in the thoracic duct can range from 1.5 to 2.5 L/day and varies considerably with diet. Chyle characteristically has a high lymphocyte count and thus is quite resistant to infection. Few erythrocytes are found in chyle. It has an extremely high triglyceride level, often 10 times that of serum.

ANSWER: A, D

37. A 57-year-old man presents to the emergency room with shortness of breath. **Scenario 1**: A posteroanterior portable view of the chest demonstrates complete opacification of the right hemithorax. The heart and mediastinum are *shifted toward* the right side. Which of the following is indicated for further evaluation?

A. Thoracentesis.
B. Bronchoscopy.
C. CT scan of the chest with infusion.
D. Ultrasound scan of the chest.

Ref.: 1, 2, 3

COMMENTS: See Question 38.

38. **Scenario 2**: If the radiograph of the patient in Question 37 had demonstrated complete hemithorax opacification and a *midline* heart and mediastinum, which of the following would be indicated for further evaluation?

A. Thoracentesis.
B. Bronchoscopy.
C. CT scan of the chest with infusion.
D. Ultrasound scan of the chest.

Ref.: 1, 2, 3

COMMENTS: **Scenario 1**: The most important radiographic observation in such a setting is the position of the heart and the mediastinum. The *shift* of the heart and the mediastinum *toward* the opaque hemithorax, as in this case, indicates lung collapse and volume loss, most likely secondary to a central obstructing process. If the heart and mediastinum are *shifted away* from the abnormally opaque hemithorax, it indicates a space-occupying process, most likely pleural effusion, although an accompanying neoplasm cannot be excluded. In this clinical setting, lung collapse is the most likely possibility, and bronchoscopy would yield the most diagnostic information quickly. **Scenario 2**: The radiographic findings described indicate either a combination of balanced lung collapse and pleural effusion or an abnormal process *fixing* the mediastinum in the *midline*, such as a neoplasm or chronic inflammation. In this setting, further imaging of the chest is essential to plan appropriate diagnostic and therapeutic maneuvers. **Ultrasound** scans of the chest are usually not valuable because normally aerated lung is an effective sound barrier. However, with an opaque hemithorax secondary to fluid or collapsed lung, the ultrasound scan can be valuable for distinguishing the component of pleural effusion from an associated solid component. It can be done quickly and inexpensively and may serve as a guide for follow-up thoracentesis. **Thoracentesis** performed without radiographic or fluoroscopic guidance may yield fluid positive for malignancy but may not yield a positive diagnosis and could interfere with further imaging. **Bronchoscopy** would probably have even less yield in this setting.

ANSWER:
Question 37: B
Question 38: C

39. A 53-year-old man presents with Horner syndrome and left arm pain. A posteroanterior chest radiograph demonstrates a 4 cm soft-tissue mass in the left apex. Which of the following would be useful for evaluating this patient?

A. CT scanning of the chest with infusion.
B. MRI scanning.
C. Percutaneous transthoracic needle biopsy.
D. Bronchoscopy

Ref.: 1, 2

COMMENTS: A left apical mass on a chest radiograph with this clinical presentation is characteristic of a superior sulcus tumor. With this neoplasm **bronchoscopy** is usually of little or no value in the diagnosis because the abnormal tissue is located far peripherally. MRI is better than CT for showing the fine details of vascular and neural structures but is not superior for detecting and assessing mediastinal adenopathy, which is a key aspect during the evaluation of any lung cancer. The standard evaluation includes a CT scan. If there is evidence of neural or vascular involvement, MRI is useful. **Percutaneous needle aspiration biopsy** is mandatory to establish a diagnosis of cancer with the typical presentation and radiographic findings. These neoplasms are commonly treated with preoperative radiation, and a histologic diagnosis is required.

ANSWER: A, B

40. With regard to myasthenia gravis, which of the following statements is/are true?

A. It is characterized clinically by abnormal fatigability of voluntary muscles on repetitive activity with recovery after rest.
B. It is associated with an increased number of postsynaptic acetylcholinesterase (ACh) receptors of the neuromuscular junction.
C. It is thought to be related to complement-mediated damage to ACh receptors initiated by circulating antibodies to the receptors.
D. It has no palliative or curative medical or surgical treatment.
E. It is probably of infectious etiology.

Ref.: 1

COMMENTS: Myasthenia gravis is a neuromuscular disorder probably of autoimmune etiology clinically characterized by abnormal fatigability of voluntary muscles on repetitive activity and recovery with rest. The ocular muscles are often the first group in which clinical manifestations are seen. The thymus has been implicated in the disease by producing antibodies to postsynaptic ACh receptors at the neuromuscular junction. The number of receptors is decreased, and there is alteration in structures, probably as a result of complement-mediated damage of the receptors. Treatment includes immunosuppressive drugs, steroids, cholinesterase inhibitors, and in severe cases plasmapheresis. Complete thymectomy can be palliative or even curative.

ANSWER: A, C

41. With regard to thymoma, which of the following statements is/are true?

A. Determination of whether a lesion is benign or malignant is usually based on histologic evidence.
B. Fifty percent of patients with thymoma have myasthenia gravis.
C. Fifty percent of patients with myasthenia gravis have thymoma.
D. Ninety percent of patients with thymoma are asymptomatic.
E. Radiation therapy plays no role in the care of patients with thymoma.

Ref.: 1, 2

COMMENTS: Thymomas are notoriously difficult to define as benign or malignant by histologic examination. Encapsulation and invasion into adjacent structures determined at the time of surgery constitute the major criteria for classifying them as benign or malignant. Of patients with thymoma, 50% have myasthenia gravis. In contrast, only 10–15% of patients with myasthenia gravis have thymoma. About one-half of patients with thymoma present with local symptoms, most commonly chest pain, shortness of breath, and cough. Radiation therapy is commonly used after excision of all but the most benign-appearing thymomas and appears to have a beneficial effect on recurrence and survival.

ANSWER: B

42. A 69-year-old smoker presents with hemoptysis. The CT scan reveals a tumor in the right upper lobe bronchus with distal pneumonia and enlarged (> 1 cm) right hilar and paratracheal lymph nodes. The next step should be:

A. Bronchoscopy.
B. Mediastinoscopy.
C. Thoracotomy and resection.
D. Refer to oncologist for chemotherapy.
E. Refer for radiation therapy.

Ref.: 1, 2, 3

COMMENTS: An accurate diagnosis with proper staging is important in patients with bronchogenic carcinomas. Bronchoscopy usually produces a diagnosis at this proximal site. With enlarged mediastinal nodes it is important to differentiate between metastatic disease and simple hyperplastic inflammatory nodes, so mediastinoscopy is indicated for diagnostic staging. If the tumor is a non-small-cell carcinoma and positive ipsilateral nodes are found, it is at stage IIIA and is probably best treated with induction chemotherapy and irradiation followed by surgical resection. Positive contralateral nodes indicate a stage IIIB tumor, which is surgically unresectable. The patient with small-cell lung cancer is best referred to an oncologist for chemotherapy.

ANSWER: A

43. Which of the following studies best predict the potential for malignant tracheoesophageal fistula from carcinoma of the esophagus.

A. Chest radiography.
B. CT scanning of the chest.
C. Esophagography.
D. Esophagoscopy.
E. Bronchoscopy.

Ref.: 1, 2, 3

COMMENTS: About 95% of respiratory-esophageal fistulas secondary to carcinoma of the esophagus occur in the trachea or proximal main bronchi. All patients with lesions involving these areas should undergo bronchoscopy to evaluate for possible invasion. If invasion is present, approximately 60% of these patients develop a fistula during radiation/chemotherapy treatment. Irregularity of the posterior tracheal wall as seen on the lateral chest radiography or CT scan also has a high fistula rate. Esophagography or esophagoscopy aids in outlining the location and extent of the tumor but rarely helps in predicting fistula formation.

ANSWER: E

44. A patient who underwent transhiatal esophagectomy developed a chylothorax postoperatively. Which is/are the appropriate method(s) of treatment?

A. Multiple thoracentesis.
B. Tube thoracostomy.
C. Low fat diet.
D. Parenteral nutrition.
E. Thoracic duct ligation

Ref.: 1, 2, 3

COMMENTS: Diagnostic thoracentesis is performed initially to identify the effusion as chyle. Once diagnosed, chest tube drainage is initiated to evacuate all fluid and allow full lung expansion. A low fat diet provides long chain triglycerides, which are absorbed in the intestine and produce more chyle. Adequate nutrition must be maintained while minimizing chyle production. This is best done by parenteral nutrition, although a strict medium-chain triglyceride diet is used by some. Conservative treatment may last up to 2 weeks with a success rate of 50–70%. Thoracic duct ligation is performed if the chyle leak persists and has an expected 80% success rate. A pleuroperitoneal shunt may be useful for refractory or recurrent cases.

ANSWER: B, D, E

45. A 20-year-old white man presents with chest pain and a large bulky anterior mediastinal mass on chest CT. An appropriate initial workup should include:

A. Fine-needle biopsy.
B. Incisional biopsy.
C. Human chorionic gonadotropin-β (hCGβ) assay.
D. α-Fetoprotein (AFP) assay.
E. Thoracotomy/sternotomy.

Ref.: 1, 2, 3

COMMENTS: This presentation in a young white man is highly suspicious of a malignant germ cell tumor. It is important to distinguish between a seminoma and a nonseminomatous germ cell tumor (NSGCT). A fine-needle biopsy often gives an accurate diagnosis. If nondiagnostic, an incisional biopsy can be done. Fully 90% of NSGCTs produce an elevation in AFP and hCG-β. Seminomas, which rarely produce hGB-β and never produce AFP, are highly radiosensitive. NSGCTs are rarely radiosensitive and are treated by multiagent chemotherapy. Open excision is rarely possible and is reserved for small local tumors and posttherapy residual disease.

ANSWER: A, C, D

REFERENCES

1. Sabiston Jr DC: *Textbook of Surgery*, 15th ed. WB Saunders, Philadelphia, 1997.
2. Schwartz SI, Shires GT, Spencer FC: *Principles of Surgery*, 7th ed. McGraw-Hill, New York, 1999.
3. Sabiston DC Jr, Spencer FC: *Surgery of the Chest*, 6th ed. WB Saunders, Philadelphia, 1995.

CHAPTER 42

Cardiac Surgery

A. Congenital Defects

1. Which of the following statements is/are true regarding fetal circulation?

   A. Blood flows through the ductus arteriosus from the pulmonary artery to the aorta.
   B. Less than 25% of the cardiac output flows through the lungs.
   C. Unoxygenated blood is in the ductus venosus.
   D. The atrial septum is intact.
   E. The right side of the heart pumps against lower resistance than the left side.

Ref.: 1, 2

COMMENTS: The circulation in utero differs markedly from postnatal circulation. Gas exchange occurs in the placenta, which receives blood from the umbilical arteries. Oxygenated blood then returns through the ductus venosus, which joins the inferior vena cava at the level of the hepatic veins. This blood is mixed with the venous return from the superior vena cava in the right atrium. Blood in the right atrium may be shunted across the foramen ovale to the left atrium, where it goes to the left ventricle and is pumped into the circulation. Blood in the right atrium may also go to the right ventricle and be pumped into the pulmonary artery. Pulmonary vascular resistance is very high in utero, and much of the blood pumped into the pulmonary artery goes through the ductus arteriosus and into the descending aorta. Because the ductus arteriosus is large and communicates with the aorta, the pressure in the pulmonary artery is the same as in the aorta (systemic). After birth the umbilical cord is cut, decreasing the ductus venosus return to zero, which causes the ductus venosus to constrict and obliterate. Pulmonary vascular resistance drops with expansion of the lungs, causing pulmonary blood flow to increase. Because return to the left atrium is increased, left atrial pressure causes the foramen ovale to close. Increased oxygen tension causes the ductus arteriosus to constrict and close. The pulmonary and systemic circulations at this point become separate.

ANSWER: A, B

2. Match each of the defects in the left column with its pathophysiologic effect in the right column.

A. Obstructive lesions	a. Decreased pulmonary blood flow
B. Right-to-left shunt	b. Increased pulmonary blood flow
C. Left-to right shunt	c. Increased ventricular work

Ref.: 1, 2

COMMENTS: Congenital heart defects can be divided into four categories, each associated with distinct physiologic abnormalities. **Obstructive lesions** (pulmonary stenosis, aortic stenosis, coarctation of the aorta) restrict the flow of blood and increase the workload of the obstructed ventricle. Without an associated lesion, there is no shunting or mixing of blood between the pulmonary and systemic circulations. **Left-to-right shunts** occur in the setting of a communication between the pulmonary and systemic circulations at the level of the atria (e.g., atrial septal defect), ventricles (e.g., ventricular septal defect), or great vessels (e.g., patent ductus arteriosus). When there is no obstruction to pulmonary blood flow, these communications usually result in flow of blood across the defect from the systemic to the pulmonary circuit. The amount of pulmonary blood flow per minute may be as much as four or five times as great as the amount that flows in the systemic circulation. **Right-to-left shunts** occur in the setting of a similar communication but where there is obstruction to pulmonary blood flow. Obstruction of pulmonary blood flow causes blood to flow from the right to left side without having passed through the lungs. If a sufficient amount of desaturated blood goes into the systemic circuit without passing through the lungs, the patient becomes cyanotic. Complex lesions include defects such as transposition of the great arteries or hypoplastic left heart syndrome where the pathophysiology cannot be so easily described. A child with a complex lesion may suffer from cyanosis, pulmonary overcirculation, and obstructive lesions simultaneously.

ANSWER: A-c; B-a; C-b

3. With regard to increased pulmonary blood flow (left-to-right shunts), which of the following statements is/are true?

   A. A shunt becomes physiologically important when pulmonary blood flow is 1.5–2.0 times as great as systemic flow.
   B. High pulmonary artery pressures preclude surgical correction of the defect.

C. Delivering 100% oxygen to the patient during cardiac catheterization may provide crucial information for determining if the patient is an operative candidate.
D. The rapidity with which pulmonary vascular disease develops depends on the magnitude of the shunt regardless of the anatomic location of the defect.
E. Increased fixed pulmonary vascular resistance precludes surgical correction of the defect.

Ref.: 1, 2

COMMENTS: Large left-to-right shunts have, by definition, an increased amount of pulmonary blood flow. There is often elevated pulmonary artery pressures and elevated left atrial pressures. The combination of these factors causes increased extravascular fluid in the pulmonary parenchyma and thus congestive heart failure. A shunt where the pulmonary blood flow is less than 1.5 times systemic flow is unlikely to produce symptoms and usually does not represent an indication for surgical repair. If a patient has a large communication at the level of the ventricles or the great vessels, the pulmonary artery pressures are systemic, as there is free communication between the systemic pressures and the pulmonary artery. This does not necessarily imply that the patient has pulmonary vascular disease; high pulmonary artery pressure with a large pulmonary flow (Qp)/systemic flow (Qs) (e.g., Qp/Qs $\geq$3) implies low pulmonary vascular resistance, making the child an appropriate candidate for repair. If a child has high pulmonary artery pressures at cardiac catheterization and a relatively low pulmonary blood flow (Qp/Qs $<$2), pulmonary vascular resistance is high and the child may not tolerate surgical correction. Oxygen 100% is a potent pulmonary vasodilator; if the shunt significantly increases with the administration of 100% oxygen, it implies that the pulmonary vascular disease is reversible and the child may yet be a candidate for surgical correction. Because development of pulmonary vascular disease depends on pressure as well as flow, patients with large atrial level shunts uncommonly develop severe pulmonary vascular obstructive disease, whereas patients with large ventricular or arterial level shunts usually do.

ANSWER: A, C, E

4. True or False: Resolution of congestive heart failure without surgical correction in a patient who has had a large left-to-right shunt is a sign of improving prognosis.

Ref.: 1, 2

COMMENTS: The natural history of a large left-to-right shunt (especially at the ventricular or arterial level) is progressive pulmonary vascular obstructive disease. There is considerable variations regarding the progression of pulmonary vascular disease. A child with a large VSD will usually develop pulmonary vascular disease at 2–4 years of age. A child with a large left-to-right shunt may have considerable congestive heart failure during the first year of life. However, as pulmonary vascular obstructive disease progresses, the left-to-right shunt decreases as the pulmonary vascular resistance approaches systemic vascular resistance. During this period the child's symptoms may improve; chest radiographic findings of cardiomegaly and pulmonary plethora may also improve. However, this finding is grave because the pulmonary vascular disease is usually progressive at this point despite surgical correction or any other currently available therapies. Pulmonary vascular disease progresses until the pulmonary vascular resistance exceeds systemic vascular resistance. Shunting ceases to be left-to-right and becomes right-to-left, resulting in the patient becoming cyanotic; it is referred to as Eisenmenger syndrome. This process usually continues until it results in the patient's death. Most patients who succumb from the Eisenmenger syndrome die during their teens or twenties.

ANSWER: False

5. With regard to obstructive congenital heart lesions, which of the following statements is/are true?

A. The most common obstructive lesions are pulmonary valve stenosis, aortic valve stenosis, and coarctation of the aorta.
B. Obstructive congenital heart lesions produce "systolic" overloading and concentric hypertrophy.
C. Concentric hypertrophy produces marked cardiac enlargement, detected by physical examination and routine chest radiography.
D. Electrocardiographic (ECG) changes occur only after there is marked enlargement of the cardiac silhouette.
E. Angina pectoris, arrhythmia, a predisposition to sudden death, and end-stage cardiac failure result from progressive obstruction.

Ref.: 1, 2

COMMENTS: The concentric hypertrophy of obstructive congenital heart lesions is not easily detected by chest radiography. Auscultation may give some indication of the severity of aortic or pulmonary stenosis. Coarctation of the aorta may be indicated by differences in the pulses and blood pressures between the arms and legs. The ECG and echocardiogram with Doppler examination are additional noninvasive tests useful for assessing chamber size, degree of obstruction, and function. Although often not necessary, cardiac catheterization is the definitive modality for assessing the gradient across obstructive lesions. Aortic stenosis causes increased myocardial oxygen demand while reducing supply, especially to the subendocardium. This may lead to myocardial ischemia with all its sequelae.

ANSWER: A, B, E

6. True or False: Lesions that produce large left-to-right shunts are often symptomatic during the newborn period.

COMMENTS: Large left-to-right shunting occurs because of a communication between the pulmonary and systemic circuits combined with lower resistance in the pulmonary circuit. Blood is directed toward the lower resistance. The pulmonary vascular resistance of newborns is at systemic levels and then falls during the first few weeks of life. Thus there is no left-to-right shunting in the newborn despite the presence of typical lesions, such as a large ventricular septal defect (VSD). There are none of the typical signs of VSD, including no murmur, no tachypnea, and no hepatomegaly. As the pulmonary vascular resistance falls the shunt becomes greater in magnitude, and signs and symptoms of left-to-right shunting appear.

ANSWER: False

7. With regard to right-to-left shunts, which of the following statements is/are true?

A. The degree of cyanosis depends on both the severity of anoxia and the blood hemoglobin concentration.
B. Systemic emboli are common because the polycythemia may lead to venous thrombosis, which may get shunted through the ventricular septal defect.
C. Cardiac catheterization is mandatory to determine the degree of pulmonary stenosis and the suitability of the patient for surgery.
D. A PO_2 of 45 mm Hg is life-threatening and requires immediate surgical treatment if it cannot be increased.

Ref.: 1, 2

COMMENTS: Cyanosis is present when the amount of desaturated hemoglobin present in the systemic circulation exceeds 5 gm/dl. Thus cyanosis is dependent on both the oxygen saturation and the hemoglobin level. A patient with severe hypoxia who also has a relatively low hemoglobin level may be minimally cyanotic. Conversely, patients with a similar oxygen saturation may appear profoundly cyanotic if they are polycythemic. Polycythemia is a physiologic response to cyanosis and can lead to a hematocrit of more than 60%. A high hematocrit increases blood viscosity and predisposes individuals to venous thrombosis. Systemic emboli, particularly cerebral emboli, may be life-threatening. In particular, children with right-to-left shunts are at risk for cerebral abscesses. Most children who have right-to-left shunts can be well evaluated with echocardiography alone. Cardiac catheterization is reserved for patients who require better delineation of small pulmonary arteries. Children tolerate saturations down to around 75%, which corresponds to a PO_2 of 40 mm Hg. A child who chronically has a PO_2 around 45 mm Hg usually does well while waiting for an elective operation.

ANSWER: A, B

8. Match each of the congenital defects in the left column with its associated radiographic change in the right column.

A. Tetralogy of Fallot	a. Egg-shaped heart
B. Transposition of great vessels	b. Sabot-shaped heart
C. Total anomalous pulmonary venous drainage	c. Figure-of-eight abnormality
D. Atrial septal defect (ASD)	d. Left atrial and ventricular enlargement
E. Mitral insufficiency	e. Right atrial and ventricular enlargement
F. Ventricular septal defect (VSD)	
G. Ebstein's malformation	

Ref.: 1, 2

COMMENTS: The chest radiograph plays an important role in the evaluation of congenital heart disease. The right ventricular hypertrophy of tetralogy of Fallot tends to produce a "boot"-shaped heart with an upturned apex. With transposition of the great arteries, the great arteries usually overlie each other, leaving a narrow mediastinum. The heart looks like an "egg on a string." Supracardiac total anomalous pulmonary venous return (TAPVR) has a large vertical vein and large innominate vein, which make a wide mediastinum and a figure-of-eight contour. ASDs cause right-sided enlargement because of the atrial level shunt. VSDs cause left-sided heart enlargement (blood goes through the VSD to the pulmonary artery, left atrium, left ventricle, and then back through the VSD—hence the *left* atrial and ventricular enlargement). Atrioventricular valve regurgitation also causes enlargement on its respective side (Ebstein's anomaly of the tricuspid valve on the right, mitral valve on the left) secondary to the volume overload.

ANSWER: A-b; B-a; C-c; D-e; E-d; F-d; G-e

9. Which of the following statements is/are true regarding Blalock-Taussig shunts?

A. They join one of the great vessels with the pulmonary artery, either directly or by means of a prosthetic graft.
B. They are used to increase pulmonary blood flow in patients with tetralogy of Fallot.
C. Because less blood goes to the body, the pulse pressure is narrowed after shunt placement.
D. A successful shunt may make definitive surgery unnecessary.
E. A shunt may be used in a cyanotic infant to delay definitive surgery until the patient is older.

Ref.: 1, 2

COMMENTS: Blalock-Taussig shunts are part of the broader classification of systemic-pulmonary artery shunts. Although other kinds of shunt connections were made in the past, most shunts today consist of Gore-Tex grafts between the aorta or one of the great vessels (e.g., innominate artery) and the pulmonary artery. Pulmonary blood flow may be increased to relieve severe hypoxia. A shunt may delay the need for definitive surgery in young patients with complex heart disease. Shunt physiology is inherently inefficient, as the blood going through the lungs via the shunt is already partly oxygenated. Thus a shunt is never considered the final repair except in complex cases where definitive repair is not possible. Because there is runoff through the shunt into the low resistance pulmonary circuit during diastole, systemic diastolic pressures tend to be low, making pulse pressures wide.

ANSWER: A, B, E

10. Match each of the comments/pathologies in the left column with the associated auscultatory finding in the right column.

A. Most common form of "innocent" murmur	a. Systolic murmurs
B. Infrequent but when present a significant finding	b. Increased second heart sound (S_2)
C. Pulmonary hypertension	c. Diastolic murmurs
D. Pulmonary stenosis or atresia	d. Widely split and "fixed" S_2
E. Atrial septal defect (ASD)	e. Continuous murmur
F. Appearance at 4 weeks of age consistent with a ventricular septal defect (VSD)	f. Decreased S_2
G. Patent ductus arteriosus (PDA)	

Ref.: 1, 2

COMMENTS: Proper auscultation of the heart often leads to the correct diagnosis of a congenital cardiac abnormality. The S_2 is heard best at the left upper sternal border and should be evaluated in terms of its degree of splitting and relative intensity. The degree of splitting of S_2 normally varies with respirations (increases with inspiration and decreases or becomes single with expiration). An abnormal S_2 may be in the form of: (1) wide splitting; (2) narrow splitting; (3) single S_2; (4) abnormal increase/decrease in the pulmonary component of the second sound (P_2); and (5) paradoxical splitting of S_2. Systolic murmurs occur between S_1 and S_2 and may be (1) ejection (through stenotic semilunar valves or due to increased flow through normal semilunar valves) or (2) regurgitant (pansystolic or holosystolic). The latter are associated with a VSD, mitral regurgitation, or tricuspid regurgitation. Diastolic murmurs may occur because of an incompetent semilunar valve or increased flow through an atrioventricular valve. Diastolic murmurs are virtually always pathologic. Continuous murmurs begin during systole and continue through S_2 into all or part of diastole. They are caused by aortopulmonary or arteriovenous connection (PDA, arteriovenous fistula, after a systemic-pulmonary shunt), flow disturbance in veins (venous hum), or arteries (coarctation, peripheral pulmonary artery stenosis).

ANSWER: A-a; B-c; C-b; D-f; E-d; F-a; G-e

11. With regard to echocardiography for the evaluation of congenital heart disease, which of the following statements is/are true?

A. It is the most accurate method by which to delineate intracardiac anatomy.
B. It may precisely define pulmonary artery anatomy.
C. It may indicate whether the right ventricular pressure is at or well below systemic pressures.
D. It may indicate the gradient across a valve.
E. Coronary arteries cannot be assessed.

Ref.: 1, 2

COMMENTS: Echocardiography has become the dominant imaging modality for congenital heart disease. It is the most accurate method by which to delineate intracardiac anatomy, and nearly all diagnoses are determined by echocardiography. Doppler echocardiography measures velocities across valves and outflow tracts, and these velocities may be translated into gradients by the formula: $\Delta P = 4 \times V^2$ (V is velocity). The velocity of a small amount of tricuspid regurgitation may be translated into the right ventricular/right atrial (RV-RA) gradient and be a good estimate of RV pressure. Pulmonary artery distortion may be difficult to assess by echocardiography, and better delineation is often needed by cardiac catheterization. Coronary arteries may be assessed with a good deal of accuracy, although the images obtained do not always yield definitive information.

ANSWER: A, C, D

12. With regard to pulmonic stenosis, which of the following statements is/are true?

A. The most common morphology is hypoplasia of the pulmonic valve annulus.
B. The physiologic abnormality is obstruction of flow from the right ventricle, with secondary concentric hypertrophy.
C. The intervention of choice is a surgical commissurotomy.
D. The most common symptom is dyspnea on exertion.
E. Echocardiography accurately delineates the anatomy and severity of obstruction.

Ref.: 1, 2

COMMENTS: Pulmonic stenosis accounts for 10% of congenital abnormalities. It most commonly involves fusion of the cusps of the pulmonary valve, poststenotic dilatation of the main pulmonary artery, and concentric hypertrophy of the right ventricle. Less common morphologies include hypoplasia of the pulmonary valve annulus, supravalvar stenosis, or subvalvular obstruction from hypertrophied muscle (infundibular stenosis). The condition is usually asymptomatic; however, when symptoms are present, the most common is dyspnea on exertion. Echocardiography accurately delineates the nature and severity of the obstruction by visualizing the anatomy and measuring the velocity of the jet across the obstruction. The current treatment of choice is balloon valvotomy, which works in most cases that do not have hypoplasia of the valve annulus. Surgical therapy is reserved for patients who have annular hypoplasia, infundibular obstruction, or failed balloon valvuloplasty.

ANSWER: B, D, E

13. With regard to coarctation of the aorta, which of the following statements is/are true?

A. The lesion involves narrowing of the descending aorta just distal to the left subclavian artery.
B. Early left ventricular failure requiring surgical correction is common when coarctation presents in a neonate.
C. Coarctation is one of the causes of surgically correctable hypertenison.
D. Arm hypertension, decreased or absent leg pulses, and a systolic murmur over the left hemithorax are the typical physical findings.
E. Late recoarctation occurs in a certain percentage of cases regardless of the repair technique.

COMMENTS: Coarctation of the aorta accounts for 10–15% of congenital heart defects and occurs twice as frequently in males. It usually occurs distal to the left subclavian artery in association with the ligamentum arteriosum. When severe, coarctation presents in neonates with severe left ventricular failure, requiring immediate surgical correction. Patients who present later in childhood often are without symptoms but have severe arm hypertension. Differential pulses or blood pressures between the arms and legs strongly suggests the diagnosis. Because collateral flow via the intercostal arteries is sufficient, ischemic symptoms of the lower body are uncommon when the patient presents after the neonatal period. The findings on physical examination and an ECG showing left ventricular hypertrophy establish the diagnosis. Coarctation is one of the classic causes of surgically correctable hypertension (others include pheochromocytomas, aldosterone secreting tumor, and renal artery stenosis). Postoperative hypertension may continue to exist, even after adequate surgical repair. Repair may be accomplished by several means, including resection with end-to-end anastomosis, left subclavian flap, and patch aortoplasty. All are associated with a small but definite percentage of late recoarctation.

ANSWER: A, B, C, D, E

14. With regard to valvar aortic stenosis, which of the following statements is/are true?

A. Aortic stenosis predisposes to sudden death, even in children.
B. There is no valve replacement that grows as the patient grows.
C. Gradient alone is an indication for intervention, even without symptoms.
D. Surgical or balloon valvotomy for aortic stenosis has a high likelihood of causing aortic regurgitation.
E. A bicuspid aortic valve is virtually always stenotic.

Ref.: 1, 2

COMMENTS: Valvar aortic stenosis may develop from a bicuspid or tricuspid aortic valve. Newborns may be affected with critical aortic stenosis, or the stenosis may progress with time and manifest at any time in the patient's life. Newborns with critical aortic stenosis present with severe cardiomegaly and heart failure. The symptoms and indications for surgery for older children are similar as for adults. Symptoms of congestive heart failure, angina, and syncope may develop. A gradient of over 50 mm Hg is thought to be a risk for sudden death. The presence of symptoms or an asymptomatic gradient over 50 mm Hg are thought to be indications for intervention. Unlike adults, aortic stenosis in children usually does not involve calcified leaflets; therefore valvuloplasty (surgical or balloon) is an option. Valvuloplasty has produced good results in terms of relieving stenosis so long as the annulus is adequate, but a high rate of postvalvuloplasty aortic regurgitation is encountered which often results in valve replacement at a future date. An increasingly common valve replacement option is the pulmonary autograft (Ross procedure). In addition to not requiring anticoagulation, the pulmonary autograft grows as the child grows. A bicuspid valve constitutes a common underlying morphology for aortic valve stenosis. However, most people who have a bicuspid aortic valve do not suffer from clinically significant aortic stenosis.

ANSWER: A, C, D

15. Which of the following statements is/are true regarding subaortic stenosis?

A. It is usually caused by diffuse narrowing of the subaortic area.
B. A turbulent bloodstream may hit the aortic valve, causing inflammation and valvar aortic stenosis.
C. The indications for operation are the same as for valvar aortic stenosis.
D. Subvalvar aortic stenosis is not ammenable to balloon valvuloplasty.
E. The area of resection of subaortic stenosis is adjacent to the conduction tissue.

Ref.: 1, 2

COMMENTS: Subaortic stenosis can occur as a discrete membrane or as a diffuse tunnel-like narrowing, but it is more commonly discrete. Surgery involves removal of the membrane with or without septal myotomy to further widen the outflow tract. Because valve replacement is rarely necessary and because the jet from the subaortic stenosis may precipitate aortic regurgitation, the threshold for surgery on a subaortic stenosis is far less than for valvar aortic stenosis. Because the membrane requires resection with subaortic stenosis, transcatheter interventions have little role. Despite the fact that the membrane directly overlies the conduction tissue, careful resection of a subaortic membrane rarely leads to heart block.

ANSWER: D, E

16. True or False: Hypertrophic cardiomyopathy is a diffuse disease of the myocardium, and so surgery has little role.

COMMENTS: Hypertrophic cardiomyopathy (also known as idiopathic hypertrophic subaortic stenosis) is a diffuse, inherited myocardial disease. Patients generally develop asymmetric hypertrophy of the ventricular septum, which may result in dynamic left ventricular outflow tract obstruction. There are four surgical options for patients with hypertrophic cardiomyopathy. The first is dual-chambered pacing. The mechanism of action of cardiac pacing is unclear, but it is thought to work by changing the pathway of spread of the electrical signal throughout the ventricle. By doing this the contraction of various parts of the outflow tract may be less coordinated, and there is less dynamic obstruction. The second option is septal myotomy. This technique reduces the obstruction by physically removing some of the hypertrophied muscle to enlarge the outflow tract. The third option is mitral valve replacement to improve outflow tract obstruction or mitral regurgitation. The fourth option is cardiac transplantation.

ANSWER: False

17. Which of the following statements is/are true regarding aortic regurgitation?

A. Discrete subaortic stenosis or ventricular septal defect may be responsible for producing aortic regurgitation.
B. Symptoms are those of congestive heart failure.
C. Echocardiography accurately estimates the degree of regurgitation and the chamber sizes.
D. Because effective cardiac output is reduced the pulses are weak and the pulse pressure is narrowed.
E. Operation is indicated when symptoms develop.

Ref.: 1, 2

COMMENTS: Aortic regurgitation causes volume overload on the left ventricle, which eventually results in left ventricular dilatation and left ventricular failure. There is increased stroke volume because of the regurgitant fraction, resulting in bounding pulses and wide pulse pressure. Symptoms are those of congestive heart failure. Angina may occur as a late finding; syncope is generally not associated with aortic regurgitation as it is with aortic stenosis. The diagnosis is accurately made and the case followed by echocardiography. Indications for surgery include the onset of symptoms or increased left ventricular dimensions even before symptoms occur. Aortic regurgitation may occur as the primary valve pathology, secondary to valvuloplasty for aortic stenosis, or after damage to a normal aortic valve caused by discrete subaortic stenosis or a ventricular septal defect. The possibility of creating aortic insufficiency is one of the indications for repair of subaortic stenosis and ventricular septal defects.

ANSWER: A, B, C, E

18. Match each of the indications for surgery for bacterial endocarditis on the left with the appropriateness of the indication on the right.

A. Severe congestive heart failure
B. Endocarditis of a bicuspid aortic valve
C. Heart block
D. Positive blood culture 10 days after starting antibiotics
E. Vegetation >1 cm
F. Fungal endocarditis
G. Hypotension upon presentation requiring pressors
H. Multiple emboli

a. Absolute indication
b. Relative indication
c. Not an indication by itself

Ref.: 1, 2

COMMENTS: The primary treatment for bacterial endocarditis is medical therapy; surgery is reserved for the complications of endocarditis. The most common indications for surgical intervention for bacterial endocarditis are severe congestive heart failure (from valvular regurgitation) and sepsis refractory to medical therapy. Several other indications for surgery exist as well: a significant abscess (often manifesting as heart block), multiple emboli, and endocarditis due to refractory organisms. Fungal endocarditis is considered to be an absolute indication for surgery, and gram-negative endocarditis is a strong relative indication. There is a relation between the size of a vegetation and many of the accepted indications, and some surgeons have described operating on all cases of endocarditis over a certain diameter. Endocarditis of a bicuspid aortic valve is not, by itself, an indication for surgery.

ANSWER: A-a; B-c; C-a; D-a; E-b; F-a; G-c; H-a

19. With regard to atrial septal defects, which of the following statements is/are true?

A. The magnitude of the shunt is determined by the difference in compliance between the ventricles.
B. The left ventricle frequently becomes enlarged.
C. Patients may develop increased pulmonary vascular resistance.
D. An atrial septal defect should be surgically corrected before the patient is 1 year of age to avoid pulmonary hypertension.
E. Surgical closure with cardiopulmonary bypass is the only option for closure.

Ref.: 1, 2

COMMENTS: Atrial septal defects (ASDs) may produce large left-to-right shunts without high pulmonary artery pressures. The magnitude of the shunt is determined by the differences in compliance between the two ventricles. The shunt occurs during diastole, when blood goes from the atria to the ventricles. Because of the defect the atria have equal pressures, and so the filling pressures for the two ventricles are similar. The amount of blood that goes to each side depends on the amount that each ventricle distends given that filling pressure. Because the right ventricle is more compliant, blood from the left atrium has a tendency to cross the defect and enter the right ventricle, creating the left-to-right shunt. Pulmonary artery pressures may be normal or near-normal, as there is no communication between the two sides during systole. Congestive heart failure eventually develops in about 25% of individuals with ASDs, usually during the third to fourth decade of life, if the ASD if left untreated. Pulmonary vascular obstructive disease occurs in about 10% if the ASD is left untreated. Because symptoms rarely occur during the first decade of life, repair is entirely elective. Repair is usually done when the child is at a preschool age (3–4 years), when he or she is large enough for easy closure but has few psychological effects from undergoing the surgery. During the current era, many defects are now closed with transcatheter devices by interventional cardiologists.

ANSWER: A, C

20. Which of the following statements is/are true regarding total anomalous pulmonary venous return (TAPVR)?

A. TAPVR is categorized as supracardiac, cardiac, infracardiac, or mixed.
B. The pathology occurs when the pulmonary veins fail to empty into the left atrium and, instead, connect directly to the right atrium or one of the large systemic veins.
C. The connection between the pulmonary veins and the systemic veins may be obstructed with equal frequency regardless of whether the connection is supracardiac, cardiac, or infracardiac.
D. When a patient has obstructed TAPVR there is reduced pulmonary blood flow, leaving the lungs relatively dark on a chest radiograph.
E. An atrial septal defect (ASD) must be present for survival.

Ref.: 1, 2

COMMENTS: During embryologic development the four pulmonary veins form a confluence that merges with the back of the left atrium. TAPVR is an anomaly where this connection fails to occur. The pulmonary venous flow then goes through an anomolous vessel that most commonly connects to the innominate vein (supracardiac), the coronary sinus (cardiac), or the portal vein (infracardiac). Supracardiac TAPVR occurs in approximately 50% of cases, cardiac TAPVR in 25% of cases, infracardiac TAPVR in 20% of cases, and 5% are mixed. Because both the systemic and pulmonary venous return goes to the right side of the heart, an ASD must be present to allow blood into the left side of the heart and the systemic circulation. The blood returning to the atrium distributes itself between the right and left ventricles according to their relative compliances, as with any large ASD. Because the right ventricle has greater compliance than the left ventricle there is more pulmonary flow than systemic flow. This is equivalent to a large left-to-right shunt. A serious complication of TAPVR occurs when the connection between the pulmonary venous confluence and the systemic veins is obstructed. With infracardiac TAPVR obstruction is the rule because the pulmonary venous return must go through the hepatic capillary bed. With supracardiac TAPVR obstruction occurs in only a few patients, and with cardiac TAPVR obstruction is rare. When obstruction occurs, pulmonary venous pressure is high, causing severe pulmonary edema.

ANSWER: A, B, E

21. Match each of the clinical comments in the left column with the associated heart defect in the right column.

A. More commonly associated with Down syndrome	a. Secundum atrial septal defect (ASD)
B. Frequently causes symptoms during infancy	b. Ostium primum defect
C. An endocardial cushion defect	c. Both secundum ASD and ostium primum defect
D. Long-term risk for mitral insufficiency	d. Neither secundum ASD or ostium primum defect
E. Uncommonly causes increased pulmonary vascular resistance	
F. Left axis division	

Ref.: 1, 2

COMMENTS: Secundum ASDs and primum atrial septal defects have in common right-to-left shunting at the atrial level, but are different malformations. Because of their similar atrial level shunting, they rarely cause symptoms during infancy and generally require elective repair at 1–4 years of age. Secundum ASDs rarely cause any residual problems after closure. However, primum ASDs are truly part of the spectrum of atrioventricular (AV) canal defects (endocardial cushion defects). Therefore the AV valves are abnormal; and frequently the left AV valve (mitral valve) becomes insufficient with time. Long-term insufficiency requiring valve repair or replacement is a well known complication. Patients with primum ASDs also may develop left ventricular outflow tract obstruction. Patients with primum ASDs have left axis deviation on their ECGs, which also distinguishes them from secundum ASDs. Children with Down syndrome have a high incidence of endocardial cushion defects, although secundum ASDs and typical ventricular septal defects may be found as well.

ANSWER: A-b; B-d; C-b; D-b; E-c; F-b

22. With regard to partial anomalous pulmonary venous drainage, which of the following statements is/are true?

A. All patterns of partial anomalous pulmonary venous drainage require surgical correction.
B. The pathophysiology is similar to that of an atrial septal defect (ASD) (atrial level left-to-right shunt).
C. Fifty percent of partial anomalous pulmonary veins are associated with an ASD.
D. Partial anomalous pulmonary veins arise more commonly from the right lung.
E. Balloon septostomy is used to palliate infants with partial anomalous pulmonary venous drainage.

Ref.: 1, 2

COMMENTS: Only rarely are partial anomalous pulmonary veins found with an intact atrial septum; they usually arise from a single lung, most commonly the right. Right anomalous pulmonary veins entering the superior vena cava are usually associated with a high secundum ASD known as sinus venosus defect. Single anomalous pulmonary veins (from one lobe of the lung) may result in a small shunt (Qp/Qs <1.5) and require no treatment. Because pulmonary venous blood enters the right atrium instead of the left atrium, the end result is physiology similar to other atrial level left-to-right shunts. Balloon septostomy is virtually never required for palliation, as the atrial septum is usually open and the left pulmonary veins directly empty into the left atrium. Surgical repair involves closing the ASD with a patch that also covers the anomalous pulmonary vein, such that the pulmonary venous return is kept on the left side of the patch.

ANSWER: B, D

23. With regard to ventricular septal defects (VSDs), which of the following statements is/are true?

A. Moderate-to-large defects usually become symptomatic at about 1 year of age.
B. Defects less than 2 cm in diameter are generally well tolerated.
C. Irreversible pulmonary vascular obstructive disease is uncommon before 1 year of age.
D. Banding of the pulmonary artery is the operation of choice in infants younger than 2 years of age.
E. Many small VSDs will close spontaneously.

Ref.: 1, 2

COMMENTS: VSDs account for 20–30% of congenital heart defects. Associated anomalies are common (patent ductus arteriosus, coarctation, ASD, aortic insufficiency). Defects less than 4–5 mm in diameter are associated with pulmonary blood flow less than two times the systemic flow, with few adverse physiologic consequences. Larger defects can produce cardiac failure, pulmonary hypertension, and death. VSDs are usually asymptomatic during the newborn period; pulmonary vascular resistance is high, which keeps left-to-right shunting and pulmonary overcirculation minimized. At 1–2 months of age the pulmonary vascular resistance decreases, allowing a large left-to-right shunt, which produces symptoms of congestive heart failure. In symptomatic infants with large lesions, surgical correction is indicated. If such infants are left untreated, increased pulmonary vascular resistance may become irreversible by the age of 2 years. It is rare for irreversible pulmonary vascular resistance to occur before 1 year of age. Up to 40% of VSDs close spontaneously by 2 years of age. Pulmonary artery banding, once widely used in infants with significant VSDs, is now rarely used with the increasing success of definitive closure in younger patients.

ANSWER: C, E

24. True or False: The preferred approach for repair of most ventricular septal defects (VSDs) is the transatrial approach.

Ref.: 1, 2

COMMENTS: Repair of a VSD was traditionally performed via ventriculotomy. Advances in operative technique now allow most defects to be closed through the right atrium with retraction of the tricuspid valve. This procedure avoids disruption of the ventricular wall and potential coronary artery damage. Some defects, particularly muscular defects, may still require ventriculotomy.

ANSWER: True

25. True or False: Eisenmenger syndrome is a classic conduction defect resulting from inappropriate repair of a VSD.

Ref.: 1, 2

COMMENTS: Eisenmenger syndrome is the end-stage that results from a large left-to-right shunt with fixed pulmonary hypertension secondary to irreversible pulmonary vascular resistance. It can occur with VSD, patent ductus arteriosus, AV canal defects, transposition of the great arteries, truncus arteriosus, and rarely in association with a large ASD. The increased pulmonary vascular resistance from the left-to-right shunt eventually exceeds systemic vascular resistance, causing reversal of the original left-to-right shunt and producing cyanosis.

ANSWER: False

26. With regard to patent ductus arteriosus (PDA), which of the following statements is/are true?

A. It produces a left-to-right shunt at the level of the great arteries.
B. Irreversible, increased pulmonary vascular disease generally occurs only in association with another defect.
C. Because of low cardiac output, children with PDA tend to have narrow pulse pressures.
D. Indomethacin can be used to close PDAs in term infants but not in premature babies.
E. The presence of cyanosis is a contraindication to closure.

Ref.: 1, 2

COMMENTS: PDA is an abnormal communication between the descending aorta and the pulmonary artery. The ductus arteriosus ordinarily closes after birth in response to rising oxygen tension and numerous other hormonal factors. PDA in premature babies usually involves a structurally normal ductus that fails to close because of the low oxygen tension and surrounding mediators (e.g., increased prostaglandins) that maintain ductus patency. By changing the hormonal environment with indomethacin (blocks prostaglandin production), a PDA in a premature infant may be closed. In a term baby a patent ductus is caused by a structurally abnormal ductal wall; indomethacin therefore has little effect on term infants. If a PDA is large, there is a large left-to-right shunt, with the pulmonary artery being exposed to systemic pressures. These children experience the same course of congestive heart failure followed by increased pulmonary vascular resistance as do children with a large VSD. Like children with a large VSD, children with a large PDA may develop Eisenmenger syndrome. Cyanosis from Eisenmenger syndrome is a contraindication to closure of a PDA. Because of runoff from the aorta into the low-resistance pulmonary artery during diastole, the diastolic pressure in children with a PDA tends to be low with large pulse pressures.

ANSWER: A, E

27. True or False: Prostaglandins may be indicated to maintain ductal patency in right-sided obstructive lesions (e.g., tetralogy of Fallot) but not in left-sided obstructive lesions (e.g., interrupted aortic arch).

Ref.: 1, 2

COMMENTS: Prostaglandins (PGE_1) are useful for maintaining ductal patency in the newborn. The indications may be for either right- or left-sided obstructive lesions. If a patient has a right-sided obstructive lesion (e.g., pulmonary atresia) pulmonary blood flow may be duct-dependent. Prostaglandins may be used to keep the ductus patent until a surgically created systemic–pulmonary artery shunt or definitive repair can be accomplished. With left-sided lesions, such as an interrupted aortic arch, blood flow to parts of the systemic circulation may be duct-dependent; that is, before repair can be undertaken the ductus is the only means by which part of the systemic circulation can receive blood flow. Ductal closure is lethal in the setting of a severe left-sided obstruction, such as an interrupted aortic arch. In this situation, blood through the ductus flows from the pulmonary artery to the aorta.

ANSWER: False

28. Which of the following statements is/are true regarding complete atrioventricular (AV) canal defects?

A. It is associated with Down syndrome.
B. There is one AV orifice instead of separate mitral and tricuspid valves.
C. Because most of the shunting occurs at the ventricular level, the natural history of the disease is virtually identical to that of a VSD.
D. The decompression through the atrial part of the defect protects against pulmonary vascular disease.
E. Recurrent ventricular-level shunting is the most common long-term complication of repair.

Ref.: 1, 2

COMMENTS: Common AV canal defects involve abnormal endocardial cushion development. The central point at which the atrial septum, ventricular septum, and AV valves should join fail to meet. The patient is usually left with a large defect in the inferior atrial septum and inlet ventricular septum. Instead of the usual mitral and tricuspid valves, there is one large AV valve that separates both atria from both ventricles. Most patients with complete AV canal defects also have Down syndrome. The pathophysiology is that of a large left-to-right shunt, as with a VSD. Pulmonary vascular disease develops somewhat faster with an AV canal than a VSD, partly because the shunt is both atrial and ventricular and partly because Down syndrome children have a tendency to develop early vascular disease. Patients may develop significant postoperative AV valve regurgitation, usually of the left-sided AV (mitral) valve. The incidence of reoperation for left-sided AV valve regurgitation is approximately 10–15% at 10 years.

ANSWER: A, B

29. With regard to tetralogy of Fallot, which of the following statements is/are true?

A. Cyanosis occurs because of the septal defect associated with the right ventricular hypertrophy.
B. A right-to-left shunt occurs because of the septal defect associated with the right ventricular outflow tract obstruction.
C. Patients often become anemic.
D. Patients learn to squat because it lowers their pulmonary artery pressures.
E. The aorta is overriding, which exacerbates the right-to-left shunt.

Ref.: 1, 2

COMMENTS: The classic congenital abnormality producing a right-to-left shunt is tetralogy of Fallot—a combination of a VSD, pulmonary stenosis, overriding of the aorta, and right ventricular hypertrophy. The amount of shunting across the VSD is related to the amount of pulmonary stenosis. In patients with little pulmonary stenosis, the shunting may be left-to-right, as with an uncomplicated VSD. Most patients with tetralogy of Fallot have enough pulmonary stenosis that some of the desaturated blood in the right ventricle goes through the VSD to the systemic circulation. Because of the chronic cyanosis, patients may develop polycythemia with hemoglobin values that exceed 20 mg/dl. Patients will learn to squat if the problem remains uncorrected past a few years of age. Squatting increases systemic vascular resistance, forcing more blood to go to the lungs. Squatting does nothing directly to the pulmonary vasculature.

ANSWER: B

30. True or False: Most patients with tetralogy of Fallot require palliative surgery (Blalock-Taussig shunt) prior to complete repair.

Ref.: 1, 2

COMMENTS: About 15–20 years ago most patients with tetralogy of Fallot underwent palliation with a Blalock-Taussig shunt followed by complete repair at 3–6 years of age. At that time, complete repair during infancy carried significant morbidity/mortality. Since then, improvements in surgical, anesthetic, and perfusion techniques have allowed single-stage correction during infancy for most patients with tetralogy of Fallot. Elective repair is usually performed at approximately 6 months of age. Earlier repair may be done if a child is too cyanotic to wait until 6 months. A staged approach may still be performed. One such circumstance is in a patient with very small pulmonary arteries. VSD closure may cause the right ventricular pressures to become suprasystemic trying to pump blood through the small pulmonary arteries. A staged approach may allow time for pulmonary artery growth and a definitive repair at a later date.

ANSWER: False

31. True or False: A child with tetralogy of Fallot who presents with a hypercyanotic spell usually responds to medical (nonsurgical) treatment.

Ref.: 1, 2

COMMENTS: Hypercyanotic spells ("tet spells") are well known occurrences in children with uncorrected tetralogy of Fallot. The pathophysiology is thought to result from increased dynamic obstruction of the right ventricular outflow tract (RVOT). An inciting event may or may not be identified, although dehydration may be a cause. As RVOT obstruction increases, more blood is shunted through the VSD and cyanosis may transiently increase. Hyperpnea is thought to perpetuate the hypoxic spell. Hyperpnea increases systemic venous return. Because pulmonary blood flow is fairly fixed, increased systemic venous return results in more right-to-left shunting. The increasing hypoxia continues to exacerbate the process. Maneuvers that decrease the dynamic obstruction of the right ventricular outflow tract tend to alleviate the spell. Medical treatment includes oxygen, fluids, morphine, propranolol, and vasopressors (Neo-Synephrine). Medical treatment is the treatment of choice acutely for a spell. However, once a patient is stabilized, semiurgent surgery is recommended because patients have a tendency to have spells with increasing frequency.

ANSWER: True

32. The repair of tetralogy of Fallot may include which of the following:

A. Repair of aortic override.
B. Closure of the ventricular septal defect (VSD).
C. Division of muscle bundles in the right ventricular outflow tract (RVOT).
D. Patch augmentation of the pulmonary annulus.
E. Resection of the endocardium of the right ventricle to alleviate right ventricular hypertrophy.

Ref.: 1, 2

COMMENTS: Repair of tetralogy of Fallot involves closure of the VSD and relief of the RVOT obstruction. It is usually necessary to resect or divide the thick muscle bundles in the infundibulum to open the subvalvar area of the outflow tract. If the pulmonary annulus is hypoplastic, the annulus may require augmentation with a transannular patch. The aortic override is not repaired; the VSD patch is tilted anteriorly at its superior end to accommodate the aortic override. The right ventricular hypertrophy subsides when the right ventricle is no longer subjected to systemic pressures.

ANSWER: B, C, D

33. With regard to transposition of the great vessels, which of the following statements is/are true?

A. The aorta arises from the right ventricle and carries unoxygenated blood to the body.
B. The pulmonary artery arises from the left ventricle and carries unoxygenated blood to the lung.
C. A patent ductus arteriosus (PDA), a ventricular septal defect (VSD), or an atrial septal defect (ASD) is necessary for survival (before definitive correction).
D. Pulmonary stenosis occurs in approximately 10% of patients.
E. VSD occurs in approximately 25% of patients.

Ref.: 1, 2

COMMENTS: Transposition of the great arteries is a common form of complex cyanotic heart disease. The aorta arises from the right ventricle, carrying unoxygenated blood to the body; the pulmonary artery arises from the left ventricle carrying oxygenated blood to the lungs. For any oxygen to be delivered to the body there must be mixing between the systemic and pulmonary circuits; this mixing is necessary for survival. The common points of mixing are an ASD, a VSD, and a PDA. If the patient has an intact ventricular septum and a small ASD, it may be necessary to use a large balloon-tipped catheter to enlarge the atrial septum to stabilize the child preoperatively. Transposition of the great arteries has many associated defects, the most common being VSDs and pulmonary stenosis (i.e., left ventricular outflow tract obstruction). Other associations include interrupted aortic arches, coarctation of the aorta, and hypoplastic ventricles. The associated lesions may greatly affect prognosis and treatment.

ANSWER: A, C, D, E

34. Which of the following statements regarding the arterial switch operation for transposition of the great arteries is/are true?

A. The arterial switch involves redirecting flow from the inferior/superior vena cavae to the left ventricle.
B. Switching the coronary arteries often provides the greatest source of morbidity.
C. The presence of a ventricular septal defect (VSD) is a contraindication for the arterial switch operation.
D. The presence of pulmonary stenosis is a contraindication for the arterial switch operation.
E. The arterial switch operation is generally performed at 6 months of age.

Ref.: 1, 2

COMMENTS: The usual surgical treatment for transposition of the great arteries is the arterial switch operation. This operation involves transecting the great vessels just above the semilunar valves and "switching" their positions, such that the aorta would come off the left ventricle and the pulmonary artery off the right ventricle. The difficulty of the arterial switch involves switching the coronary arteries. The small coronary arteries of a newborn may twist and obstruct when being transferred; the morbidity associated with this procedure has been greatly reduced as the combined surgical experience with this operation has taught surgeons how the coronaries need to be transferred. Approximately one-third of patients with transposition have abnormal coronary artery branching patterns. Some of these branching patterns are difficult to switch and dramatically increase the risk of the procedure. The presence of a VSD does not change one's plan to do an arterial switch; the VSD is closed as part of the procedure. The presence of pulmonary stenosis does preclude an arterial switch because after a switch the patient would be left with aortic stenosis, which would be poorly tolerated. Before arterial switch procedures were developed most patients were treated with atrial switch operations (Mustard or Senning procedures). They involved redirecting the systemic and pulmonary venous return with baffles inside the atrium, which left the right ventricle still pumping blood to the body and the left ventricle pumping blood to the lungs. This procedure has been largely abandoned because of the incidence of long-term failure of the right ventricle. The arterial switch is performed during the neonatal period; if one waits longer, the left ventricle becomes unable to pump against systemic pressure.

ANSWER: B, D

35. Which of the following statements is/are true regarding the Fontan procedure (total cavopulmonary anastomosis)?

A. It involves a direct connection between both venae cavae and the pulmonary artery.
B. It is used in patients with a single functioning ventricle.
C. The Fontan procedure allows the central venous pressure (CVP) to be normal (5–10 mm Hg).
D. Children with moderately elevated pulmonary vascular resistance may not be candidates for a Fontan operation.
E. The Fontan procedure is performed as soon as the diagnosis is made.

Ref.: 1, 2

COMMENTS: The issue with patients with single-ventricle physiology is how to provide pulmonary blood flow. Options include the Fontan procedure and a systemic–pulmonary artery shunt. The Fontan procedure (total cavopulmonary anastomosis) is an operation used for patients with single-ventricle physiology; it has been in existence since the mid-1970s. There are a number of techniques for making the connection, but the Fontan procedure in any of its forms involves a connection between the venae cavae and the pulmonary artery. Blood flow through the pulmonary capillary bed is driven only by the CVP. After going through the lungs, blood is returned to the single ventricle and is pumped to the body. Patients remain fully saturated without an extra volume load on the heart. Neither of these goals is satisfied by providing pulmonary blood flow with a systemic–pulmonary artery shunt. The problem with a Fontan operation is that patients rarely tolerate a CVP of more than 15 mm Hg. For the CVP to drive blood through the lungs at an acceptable CVP level, the patient must have excellent "Fontan" hemodynamics: pulmonary arteries without stenosis, low pulmonary vascular resistance, no pulmonary venous obstruction, no atrioventricular valve regurgitation, and low ventricular filling pressures. Because the pulmonary resistance is elevated in infants, a Fontan operation is generally not performed until 18–24 months of age.

ANSWER: A, B, D

36. Which of the following statements is/are true of vascular rings?

A. They may cause decreased perfusion to the lower extremities.
B. The most common form is a double aortic arch.
C. A vascular ring may manifest as recurrent respiratory infections.
D. Repair of a vascular ring requires a bypass graft.
E. Dysphagia may be a sign of a vascular ring.

Ref.: 1, 2

COMMENTS: A vascular ring is an encirclement of the trachea and esophagus by an abnormal formation of the arch and great vessels. The most common form is a double aortic arch. During early development fetuses all have two aortic arches: a right (posterior) arch and a left (anterior) arch. These arches encircle the forming trachea and esophagus. Ordinarily, the right arch regresses. If both arches persist, the trachea and esophagus become encircled. A double aortic arch may be asymptomatic, but it often causes compression symptoms. The trachea is more often affected, and there may be recurrent respiratory infections. Esophageal compression may be present with or without tracheal symptoms. Although they may present at any age, symptoms usually develop during infancy or early childhood. Repair consists of dividing the smaller of the two arches as determined by ultrasonography, magnetic resonance imaging, or at the time of surgery. Repair is generally performed through a left thoracotomy and does not involve cardiopulmonary bypass. A bypass graft is not necessary for repair. There are other vascular rings in addition to the double aortic arch; and their clinical manifestations, natural history, and principles of repair are similar.

ANSWER: B, C, E

REFERENCES

1. Baue AE, Geha AS, Hammond GL, et al: *Glenn's Thoracic and Cardiovascular Surgery*. Appleton & Lange, Stamford, CT, 1996.
2. Kirklin JW, Barratt-Boyes BG: *Cardiac Surgery*. Churchill Livingstone, New York, 1993.

Cardiac Surgery

B. Acquired Diseases

1. A 60-year-old man is successfully resuscitated after an episode of sudden cardiac death. Appropriate evaluation and treatment might include which of the following?

A. Cardiac catheterization and coronary angiography.
B. If significant coronary stenoses or left ventricular aneurysm is identified, surgical intervention directed at these targets can achieve satisfactory control of the arrhythmia.
C. Automatic implantable cardioverter defibrillator (AICD) in patients whose ventricular tachycardia cannot be mapped or medically/surgically controlled.
D. Electrophysiologic studies (EPS) to determine the mechanism, origin, inducibility, and suppressibility of the arrhythmia.
E. EPS-directed resection.

Ref.: 1, 2

COMMENTS: Sudden cardiac death is a major cause of morbidity and mortality in the United States: Most cases are thought to be of arrhythmogenic origin. The number of survivors is increasing as a result of the rising number of lay people trained in cardiopulmonary resuscitation as well as improved prehospital and emergency medical care. Survivors, however, have a 60% chance of recurrence during the first 2 years after hospitalization, resulting in sudden death. During evaluation of these patients, one must include the following: EPS to determine the mechanism of the arrhythmia (automatic vs. reentrant), to identify the origin of the arrhythmia, and to identify the inducibility and assess the suppressibility of induced arrhythmias by various pharmacologic agents. Cardiac catheterization and coronary angiography should be performed to identify significant coronary stenoses and the presence of a ventricular aneurysm, which may be the arrhythmogenic focus. However, coronary revascularization alone fails to control the arrhythmia, and blind aneurysmectomy (non-EPS directed) often fails because the endocardial origin of the arrhythmia may be distant from the border of the aneurysm. EPS-directed endocardial resection and encircling endocardial ventriculotomy with or without adjunctive cryoablation have success rates in the range of 90%. For inpatients whose arrhythmia cannot be mapped or controlled medically and surgically, the AICD is a last alternative. The AICD is a device that senses ventricular tachycardia/fibrillation through an epicardial or endocardial sensing lead and delivers a high-energy defibrillating pulse between two epicardial electrode patches or between a patch and a transvenous coil electrode in the superior vena cava.

ANSWER: A, C, D, E

2. Which of the following is the maximum amount of time extracorporeal circulation can be tolerated before significant risk of physiologic injury and metabolic defects occurs?

A. 2–4 hours.
B. 6–8 hours.
C. 10–12 hours.
D. 14–16 hours.
E. 18–20 hours.

Ref.: 1, 3

COMMENTS: Tolerance of extracorporeal circulation is variable. Six to eight hours is an acceptable range, although physiologic injury may occur earlier; occasionally patients undergo longer perfusion with relatively few consequences. With proper myocardial preservation, the heart can be safely arrested for up to 4 hours. Physiologic defects observed with extracorporeal circulation include progressive sludging of blood elements in the capillary microcirculation, red blood cell hemolysis, coagulation defects, denaturation of plasma proteins, and fibrinolysis.

ANSWER: B

3. Which of the following is/are complications of prolonged extracorporeal circulation?

A. Postoperative bleeding.
B. Pancreatitis.
C. Respiratory insufficiency.
D. Psychosis.
E. Hepatic insufficiency.

Ref.: 3

COMMENTS: The physiologic and metabolic injuries resulting from prolonged extracorporeal circulation are exhibited in several ways. Postoperative bleeding may occur owing to dilution of clotting factors, destruction of platelets, impairment of platelet function, and improper titration of protamine to reverse systemic heparinization. The coagulation defect may be transient and usually resolves within the first 12 hours following perfusion. The importance of meticulous surgical hemostasis is apparent. Both renal and respiratory insufficiency are usually transient and often require only supportive treatment. Hepatic insufficiency is usually not problematic. A variety of central nervous system changes may occur. These changes have both metabolic and organic causes and may be manifested by localized or generalized deficit of variable severity and duration. With prolonged nonpulsatile cardiopulmonary bypass and hypothermia, some patients have an elevation of serum amylase, which fortunately is less frequently associated with signs and symptoms of pancreatitis.

ANSWER: A, B, C, D

4. Following aortic valve replacement for calcific aortic stenosis, a patient experiences seizures. Which of the following are the most likely causes?

A. Air embolism.
B. Calcium emboli.
C. Emboli from a left atrial thrombus.
D. Emboli from aortic atherosclerosis.
E. Extracorporeal circulation.

Ref.: 3

COMMENTS: Seizures may occur as a manifestation of focal injury to the central nervous system. Air embolism is a result of incomplete evacuation of air from the cardiac chambers following open heart surgery. Evacuation may be facilitated by use of a left ventricle vent, an aortic vent, or both; the vents are left in place until after the heart is beating. During this time, cardiopulmonary bypass is gradually reduced, the patient is rotated, and the heart is manipulated to assist in removing air from within the cardiac chambers. Calcium fragments may embolize after removal of calcific debris from a diseased aortic valve. Cannulation or clamping a diseased aorta may result in dislodgement of arteriosclerotic debris. Left atrial thrombi are another potential source of cerebral emboli, usually seen in patients with mitral stenosis. The usual neurologic deficit observed following prolonged extracorporeal circulation is a transient generalized depression of cerebral function related to sludging of blood elements in the cerebral capillaries, resulting in focal areas of stasis and hypoperfusion of the microcirculation.

ANSWER: A, B, D

5. Indications for coronary artery bypass (CABG) include which of the following?

A. Severe triple-vessel occlusive disease.
B. Stenosis of the left main coronary.
C. Severe double-vessel occlusive artery disease.
D. Acute myocardial infarction.
E. Patients who develop complications during percutaneous coronary angioplasty (PTCA).

Ref.: 4

COMMENTS: Surgical revascularization provides relief of angina in more than 90% of patients and improves survival in selected groups. Patients are referred to as having single-, double-, or triple-vessel disease if there are significant stenoses in one, two, or all three of the major coronary arteries. Numerous studies have concluded that patients with significant triple-vessel disease, especially with impaired left ventricular function, are best treated with surgery. Left main disease is also a well accepted indication. Most surgeons and cardiologists agree that double-vessel disease is not always an indication for surgery unless the left anterior descending (LAD) artery is involved with a severe (>50%) proximal stenosis. Acute myocardial infarction is not an unequivocal indication for surgery. Finally, approximately 3% of patients undergoing PTCA develop complications requiring surgery.

ANSWER: A, B, E

6. Contraindications to coronary artery bypass include which of the following?

A. Severely depressed left ventricular ejection fraction (<0.20).
B. Age greater than 70 years.
C. Angiographic inability to visualize a patent distal vessel.
D. Acute myocardial infarction.
E. Refractory congestive heart failure.

Ref.: 1, 3

COMMENTS: Most authorities consider congestive heart failure with pulmonary hypertension (in the absence of mechanical defects, such as left ventricular aneurysm, mitral regurgitation, ventricular septal defect) the only cardiac contraindications to bypass grafting. With current techniques of myocardial preservation and revascularization, bypass can be successfully performed in patients who, for various reasons, were once considered excessive-risk candidates. Angiographic visualization depends on technique and the collateral circulation and is not a reliable criterion of operability. Revascularization may be beneficial in the face of an acute, evolving myocardial infarction if the patient can be operated on within the first 3–6 hours. The role of surgery in relation to balloon angioplasty and thrombolytic therapy in this setting has not yet been fully defined.

ANSWER: E

7. The operative mortality rate of coronary artery bypass is approximately 10% in which of the following situations?

A. Elective operations.
B. Revision of failed coronary artery bypass surgery.
C. Emergency coronary artery bypass surgery.
D. Severely impaired left ventricular function.
E. None of the above.

Ref.: 1, 3

COMMENTS: Improvement in anesthetic and surgical techniques and methods of myocardial protection have reduced the mortality rate of elective coronary artery bypass to approximately 2%. The risk is somewhat higher in certain groups of patients, but even in higher-risk categories, in situations of emergency coronary artery bypass surgery, or during revision of failed surgery the risk rarely exceeds 3–5%.

ANSWER: E

8. With regard to the prognosis of coronary artery disease, which of the following statements is/are true?

A. Most patients die within 1–2 years of the onset of congestive heart failure.
B. Ventricular function influences survival more than does the extent of vessel involvement.
C. Mortality associated with acute myocardial infarction is approximately 50%.
D. Acute myocardial infarction is the most common cause of sudden cardiac death.

Ref.: 3

COMMENTS: Manifestations of coronary occlusive disease include angina pectoris, myocardial infarction, congestive heart failure, arrhythmias, and sudden death. Sudden death is often the result of ventricular fibrillation without demonstrable infarction. The current mortality due to acute myocardial infarction is approximately 10%. With destruction of significant left ventricular muscle mass, chronic congestive heart failure occurs and the prognosis is poor. Data suggest that although both the extent of coronary vessel involvement and the status of the left ventricle are important prognostically it is left ventricular function that allows the most accurate prediction of long-term survival.

ANSWER: A, B

9. Following a documented acute myocardial infarction (MI), surgery is indicated in which of the following situations?

A. Postinfarction angina with anatomic lesions not amenable to percutaneous transluminal coronary angioplasty (PTCA).
B. Ventricular septal defect (VSD).
C. Acute mitral regurgitation.
D. Free wall rupture.

Ref.: 4

COMMENTS: Postinfarction angina occurs in 10–15% of patients, with the incidence increasing to 30% if a thrombolytic agent was used. It generally indicates residual myocardial tissue at risk for subsequent cell death and infarct extension. In this setting, cardiac angiography is indicated, with PTCA or surgery depending on the anatomy. VSDs occur in about 2% of patients following MI, generally 3–5 days after MI. Early surgical intervention is indicated. Acute mitral regurgitation resulting from papillary muscle infarction and rupture occurs in fewer than 2% of patients. Surgery leads to a better survival than medical therapy. Ventricular free wall rupture occurs 3–6 days following transmural MI. Although the exact incidence is not known, medical therapy almost certainly leads to death, leaving surgical repair as the only therapeutic option.

ANSWER: A, B, C, D

10. A 70-year-old woman in the coronary care unit develops refractory angina 2 days after being hospitalized for acute myocardial infarction (MI). With regard to coronary artery bypass in this situation, which of the following statements is/are true?

A. It should be performed only if there is left main coronary disease.
B. Operative mortality and long-term survival rates are poor compared with those in patients who have unstable angina not precipitated by MI.
C. It should be preceded by thrombolytic therapy if multivessel disease is also present.
D. The operative mortality rate is less than 5%.

Ref.: 1

COMMENTS: Unstable angina is preceded by MI in approximately one-half of patients. The initial treatment of patients with unstable angina involves intensive medical therapy with β-blockers, nitrates, and calcium channel blockers. Patients with refractory angina should undergo emergent percutaneous transluminal coronary angioplasty (PTCA) or coronary artery bypass grafting (CABG). PTCA may be tried for one- and two-vessel disease, but significant left main artery disease should be approached surgically. Most trials have demonstrated reduced in-hospital and 1-year mortality rates when thrombolytic therapy has been effective in reestablishing flow to ischemic tissue within 4 hours. PTCA has been used alone and in conjunction with thrombolytic therapy with a 90% successful reperfusion rate, 10% in-house mortality rate, and 10–30% reocclusion rate within 6 months. These modalities have been less effective for multivessel disease and in older patients, those in cardiogenic shock, women, and those with poor left ventricular function. CABG has a 4% mortality rate in patients with unstable angina, with approximately 80% of patients surviving 10 years and 80% experiencing long-term relief of angina.

ANSWER: D

11. A patient develops angina 5 years after coronary artery bypass grafting (CABG). Angiography most likely reveals which of the following?

A. Vein graft thrombosis.
B. Progressive atherosclerosis in the vein graft.
C. Progressive atherosclerosis in the coronary arteries.
D. A dominant right coronary system.

Ref.: 1, 3

COMMENTS: The rate of recurrence of angina following CABG is approximately 5–7% per year. Surgery, unfortunately, does not slow the progression of atherosclerosis, which is the primary cause of recurrent symptoms. Graft occlusion may also occur as a result of thrombosis, intimal fibrosis, or fibrous endarteritis. Vein grafts may also be involved with atherosclerosis, which usually occurs later during the postoperative course. Overall, the rate of vein graft patency is approximately 80% after 5 years. Internal mammary artery grafts have significantly higher long-term patency and improved event-free survival compared to vein grafts.

ANSWER: C

12. Ventricular aneurysms usually have which of the following characteristics?

A. They result from myocardial infarction.
B. They involve the posterior left ventricle.
C. They present with peripheral emboli from a mural thrombosis.
D. They cause death because of rupture.
E. Ventricular arrhythmias are uncommon.

Ref.: 1, 3

COMMENTS: Most ventricular aneurysms result from transmural infarction. They frequently involve the anterior left ventricle in the distribution of the left anterior descending artery. The most common complication is congestive heart failure, followed by arrhythmias and angina. Peripheral emboli may occur but are infrequent. Death due to rupture of a ventricular aneurysm is an unusual event.

ANSWER: A

13. Indications for surgical resection of a left ventricular aneurysm includes which of the following?

A. Angina.
B. Congestive heart failure.
C. Systemic arterial emboli.
D. Ventricular tachyarrhythmias refractory to drug therapy.

Ref.: 2, 4

COMMENTS: See Question 14.

14. With regard to surgical treatment of ventricular aneurysm, which of the following statements are true?

A. Preservation of the left anterior descending artery is mandatory.
B. All aneurysms should be excised due to the progressive nature of this lesion and the poor prognosis if untreated.
C. Complete aneurysmectomy is preferred.
D. Concomitant coronary bypass is generally performed.

Ref.: 1, 2

COMMENTS: Clinical manifestations of ventricular aneurysm resulting from transmural myocardial infarction include those mentioned in Question 13. Ventricular aneurysms may also be totally asymptomatic in which case observation rather than resection is usually indicated. Preservation of the LAD is preferred if possible to provide blood flow to the septum, but preservation is not mandatory. Small aneurysms are generally asymptomatic and can be observed. During surgical resection, total scar removal is generally not performed, but rather, a rim of scar tissue is left by the surgeon to facilitate closure of the defect. Because of the high incidence of concomitant multivessel coronary occlusive disease, approximately 75% of patients considered for aneurysm resection also have coronary bypass. Actual rupture of a true ventricular aneurysm is rare.

ANSWER:
Question 13: A, C, D
Question 14: D

15. Treatment of acute pyogenic pericarditis may require which of the following?

A. Parenteral antibiotics active against *Streptococcus* and *Mycobacterium*.
B. Serial pericardial aspiration.
C. Subxiphoid pericardiotomy.
D. Radical pericardiectomy.

Ref.: 1, 3

COMMENTS: Pyogenic pericarditis is rare. Today it is usually seen in infants or young children, in whom it is associated with a high mortality rate. *Staphylococcus* and gram-negative species are the most common organisms in adults, whereas *Staphylococcus* and *Haemophilus influenzae* predominate in infants and children. Parenteral antibiotics combined with serial pericardial aspiration and occasional intrapericardial instillation of antibiotics are usually adequate treatment. Surgical drainage may be necessary, but radical pericardiectomy is not indicated.

ANSWER: B, C

16. With regard to chronic constrictive pericarditis, which of the following statements is/are true?

A. It is usually caused by a previous streptococcal infection.
B. It is characterized by equalization of right- and left-sided pressures.
C. It is best treated with a combination of diuretics and β-blocking agents.
D. Pericardiectomy is successful in 50% of patients.

Ref.: 1, 3

COMMENTS: Chronic constrictive pericarditis often occurs secondary to a viral infection, although in most cases the true cause is unknown. Tuberculosis was once thought to be the most frequent cause. The disease is marked by progressive edema, ascites, hepatic enlargement, and dyspnea on exertion. Hemodynamic findings include elevation of the right ventricular end-diastolic, right atrial, and central venous pressures to levels equal to those of the pulmonary artery wedge and left ventricular end-diastolic pressures. Pericardiectomy is the treatment of choice and is successful in 90% of cases if adequate resection is performed.

ANSWER: B

17. Following open heart surgery, a patient experiences chest pain, fever, tachycardia, and a pericardial friction rub. Which of the following statements is/are true?

A. The most likely diagnosis is postoperative mediastinitis.
B. Primary treatment should include surgical exploration.
C. The patient most likely responds well to antibiotics.
D. There is usually an associated leukocytosis or lymphocytosis.
E. This syndrome is usually accompanied by pleural effusion and shortness of breath.

Ref.: 1, 3

COMMENTS: Following procedures in which the pericardium is entered, transient pericardial inflammation known as the postpericardiotomy syndrome may occur. Clinical manifestations include fever, pericarditis, pleuritis, and sometimes a pericardial friction rub. The syndrome usually appears 2–4 weeks postoperatively, and the erythrocyte sedimentation rate is elevated. There is also leukocytosis with an increase in lymphocytic cells. Patients usually respond well to a short course of an antiinflammatory agent, although some cases require the use of a corticosteroid.

ANSWER: D

18. Three hours after aortic valve replacement, a patient suddenly becomes hypotensive. The cardiac index has decreased from 2.5 L/min to 1.6 L/min. Central venous pressure is 19 mm Hg with a pulmonary artery wedge pressure of 20 mm Hg. Mediastinal drainage over the last hour has been minimal. Immediate treatment should include which of the following?

A. Echocardiogram to assess prosthetic valve function.
B. Volume resuscitation to increase cardiac output.
C. Afterload reduction with nitroprusside.
D. Preload reduction with nitroglycerin.
E. Mediastinal exploration.

Ref.: 1, 3

COMMENTS: Hypotension and low cardiac output following open heart surgery necessitate prompt, careful evaluation. Specific causes include inadequate blood volume, occult bleeding, cardiac tamponade, arrhythmias, myocardial insufficiency, and acidosis. The finding of elevated filling pressures with equalization of right- and left-sided pressures suggests the diagnosis of cardiac tamponade, in which case immediate reoperation is mandatory. Substantial elevation of filling pressures in association with low cardiac output may also be indicative of cardiac failure, which may be treated with inotropic agents, digitalis, and intraaortic balloon counterpulsation. Chest radiography is of variable diagnostic value, occasionally allowing detection of occult accumulation of blood in a pleural space.

ANSWER: E

19. Aortic stenosis presenting in an adult may result from which of the following?

A. Congenital bicuspid valve.
B. Marfan syndrome.
C. Rheumatic fever.
D. Syphilis.
E. Bacterial endocarditis.

Ref.: 1, 3

COMMENTS: Aortic stenosis presenting in an adult may result from rheumatic fever or from a congenital valvular deformity. A congenital bicuspid *valve* may remain asymptomatic for many years, but the deformed valve is susceptible to endocarditis and eventually develops calcification and symptomatic stenosis. Aortic insufficiency commonly follows bacterial endocarditis. Aortic insufficiency may also result from dilatation of the aortic annulus due to an ascending aortic aneurysm, as seen with Marfan syndrome or, more rarely, syphilis.

ANSWER: A, C

20. Clinical manifestations of severe aortic valve stenosis include which of the following?

A. Syncope.
B. Angina pectoris.
C. Dyspnea on exertion.
D. Atrial fibrillation.

Ref.: 1, 3

COMMENTS: Characteristically, patients with aortic stenosis remain asymptomatic for many years but deteriorate rapidly once symptoms begin. About two-thirds of patients develop angina pectoris. Left ventricular hypertrophy, increased left ventricular diastolic volume, and prolongation of the isometric contraction phase and systolic ejection time are compensatory mechanisms to allow a longer period for ventricular emptying. However, the duration of diastolic coronary perfusion to the hypertrophied ventricle is decreased, which gives rise to angina pectoris even in the absence of primary coronary artery disease. Syncope, present in one-third of patients, also reflects impaired cardiac output but in some patients is related to a conduction abnormality due to calcification of the atrioventricular node. Signs of left ventricular failure and atrial fibrillation resulting in elevated left atrial pressures are evidence of more advanced disease.

ANSWER: A, B, C, D

21. With regard to the prognosis of adults with aortic stenosis, which of the following statements is/are true?

A. Intensity of the murmur correlates with severity of disease and therefore prognosis.
B. Sudden death accounts for most fatalities.
C. Symptomatic patients have a greater risk of sudden death than do asymptomatic patients.
D. Left ventricular failure signifies a worse prognosis than does syncope or chest pain.

Ref.: 1, 3

COMMENTS: Once patients with aortic stenosis develop symptoms, the prognosis is poor. With angina or syncope, the average life expectancy of untreated patients is 2–3 years; death occurs 1–2 years after left ventricular failure. Sudden death occurs more frequently with aortic stenosis than with any other valvular lesion. It accounts for approximately 20% of deaths from aortic stenosis and is always a risk, but it occurs more frequently in symptomatic patients. The loudness of the classic systolic diamond-shaped ejection murmur heard over the aortic area and the apex does not have prognostic significance.

ANSWER: C, D

22. Indications for operation in patients with aortic stenosis include which of the following?

A. All symptomatic patients.
B. Systolic pressure gradient greater than 50 mm Hg in asymptomatic patients.
C. Valvular cross-sectional area smaller than 1 cm^2.
D. Serial radiographic evidence of rapid cardiac enlargement.

Ref.: 1, 3

COMMENTS: All symptomatic patients require prompt valve replacement because of the high risk of sudden death and deterioration. Peak systolic gradients across the valve of more than 50 mm Hg and cross-sectional areas of 0.8–1.0 cm^2 are generally found with moderate to severe aortic stenosis and are indications for valve replacement, even if symptoms are absent. Serial radiographic evidence of rapid cardiac enlargement is an ominous sign in patients with aortic stenosis and is an urgent indication for operation. Severe stenosis (based on the cross-sectional area) but a low transvalvular gradient may result from compromised ventricular function, which increases the risk of valve replacement. The 5-year survival rate following aortic valve replacement is approximately 80%.

ANSWER: A, B, C, D

23. With regard to the selection of prosthetic heart valves, which of the following statements is/are true?

A. Free aortic homograft valves have a lower incidence of infective endocarditis than porcine valves.
B. Bioprosthetic valves should be avoided in patients with chronic renal failure.
C. Mechanical valves should be avoided in children.
D. Mechanical valves have better durability than bioprosthetic valves.
E. Reconstructed mitral valves have limited durability and offer no advantage over valve replacement.

Ref.: 1, 5

COMMENTS: The ideal prosthetic heart valve has yet to be developed; selection is based on patient characteristics, operative findings, and the surgeon's preference. **Bioprosthetic** valves (glutaraldehyde-fixed porcine heterografts or bovine pericardium) have a low rate of associated thromboembolism, and therefore these patients do not require long-term anticoagulation. The problem with bioprosthetic valves, however, is long-term durability; the rate of valve failure is 2–5% yearly, and the rate increases after the first 6 years. These valves are contraindicated in children, in patients younger than 20–30 years of age, and in those with chronic renal failure who require hemodialysis because of rapid calcific degeneration. • **Mechanical heart valves** are more durable, but their usefulness is limited by the need for permanent anticoagulation, which is contraindicated in certain clinical states (e.g., pregnancy, coagulopathy, ulcer disease). Thromboembolic complications occur at an annual rate of 2–5% even in patients who are adequately anticoagulated. Patients with mechanical valves require permanent anticoagulation therapy, which carries a mortality rate of approximately 1% per year. The risk of prosthetic valve endocarditis is about 1–2% per year for both bioprosthetic and mechanical valves; because of the low recurrence rate of endocarditis, free aortic **homograft valves** are advantageous in the setting of active endocarditis. Even with small valves there is virtually no gradient across the homograft valve and a markedly decreased incidence of valve cusp calcification in young patients. • Mitral valve reconstruction is preferred to replacement whenever possible because of the freedom from prosthetic valve complications; chronic anticoagulant therapy is not needed, and endocarditis is rare. Durability has been satisfactory, with approximately 90% of patients remaining free from the need of late valve replacement at 5 years after operation.

ANSWER: A, B, D

24. Cardiac catheterization of a 50-year-old man with a recent history of dyspnea on exertion, hemoptysis, and paroxysmal nocturnal dyspnea demonstrates a left atrial pressure of 28 mm Hg. The primary determinants of this pressure include which of the following?

A. Pulmonary artery pressure.
B. Cross-sectional area of the mitral opening.
C. Cardiac output.
D. Heart rate.
E. Size of the left atrium.

Ref.: 1, 3

COMMENTS: The primary physiologic consequences of mitral stenosis are increased left atrial pressure, decreased cardiac output, and increased pulmonary vascular resistance. The clinical manifestations of these changes include the typical symptoms of congestive heart failure, pulmonary edema, and right-sided heart failure, as well as atrial fibrillation and arterial embolism. The left atrial pressure is determined by the size of the mitral orifice, cardiac output, and heart rate. The severity of disease is best classified by calculating the cross-sectional area of the valve, which takes into consideration both pressure gradient and cardiac output. A mitral valve area (MVA) of approximately 1 cm^2 or less is indicative of significant stenosis, although low flow rates and the presence of mitral regurgitation may influence calculations. When left atrial pressures exceed the plasma oncotic pressure (24–30 mm Hg), pulmonary edema develops.

ANSWER: B, C, D

25. Indications for valve replacement in patients with significant mitral stenosis include which of the following?

A. Congestive heart failure.
B. Pulmonary hypertension.
C. Atrial fibrillation.
D. Asymptomatic patients.
E. Systemic embolization.

Ref.: 1

COMMENTS: See Question 26.

26. With regard to results of surgical treatment for symptomatic mitral stenosis, which of the following statements is/are true?

A. Survival rate is increased compared with that after medical therapy.
B. Commissurotomy decreases the risk of systemic embolization and endocarditis.
C. Pulmonary vascular resistance usually diminishes following valve replacement or commissurotomy.
D. Ten-year survival rate exceeds 90%.

Ref.: 1

COMMENTS: The natural history of mitral stenosis is one of progressive symptomatology. Treatment of mitral stenosis is a judicious combination of medical and surgical therapy. Most asymptomatic patients are treated medically and observed. Symptomatic patients with only medical treatment eventually die from their cardiac disease. Indications for operative intervention include congestive heart failure (with New York Heart Association class III or IV symptoms), onset of atrial fibrillation with significant mitral stenosis, pulmonary hypertension, systemic embolization, and infective endocarditis. Surgical therapy is also recommended for patients who have mild symptoms and a severe reduction in valvular area. In this situation mitral commissurotomy is initially indicated. It produces physiologic and clinical improvement, but these benefits tend to deteriorate. Recurrent valvular dysfunction that necessitates treatment is almost always best treated by valve replacement.

ANSWER:
Question 25: A, B, C, E
Question 26: A, B, C, D

27. Which of the following is the most common cause of mitral insufficiency?

A. Bacterial endocarditis.
B. Rheumatic fever.
C. Marfan syndrome.
D. Silent myocardial infarction.
E. Rupture of chordae tendineae.

Ref.: 1, 3

COMMENTS: See Question 28.

28. With regard to patients with mitral regurgitation compared with those mitral stenosis, which of the following statements is/are true?

A. Left ventricular failure is more common.
B. Atrial fibrillation rarely develops.
C. Systemic emboli are less common.
D. Postoperative prognosis is generally poorer.

E. Pulmonary hypertension usually fails to resolve following valve replacement.

Ref.: 1

COMMENTS: Rheumatic fever is the most common cause of both mitral regurgitation and mitral stenosis. Although mitral stenosis almost exclusively results from rheumatic fever, mitral regurgitation may have other causes, including mitral valve prolapse, idiopathic calcification, bacterial endocarditis, chordae rupture, and ischemic heart disease. A cause other than rheumatic fever is often suspected on the basis of the history and clinical presentation. The physical signs of pulmonary hypertension and right heart failure produced by mitral regurgitation are similar to those seen with mitral stenosis. Unlike patients with mitral stenosis, however, moderate to severe mitral regurgitation can be tolerated for many years with minor symptoms until left ventricular failure ultimately develops as a result of chronic overload. Atrial fibrillation is a common manifestation of mitral regurgitation; embolization does occur, but it is less common than with mitral stenosis. The natural history of mitral regurgitation and the results of operative correction are somewhat more variable than those of mitral stenosis because of the different etiologic factors that may produce mitral incompetence; clinical severity depends on the degree of regurgitation, the status of left ventricular function, and the course of the valve disease. In cases of infective endocarditis, trauma, or chordae rupture, emergency operation therapy is required and can be life-saving; operation is avoided, however, in patients with ischemic mitral regurgitation and poor ventricular function and in elderly patients with severe associated conditions. Pulmonary hypertension usually resolves after successful valve replacement. In most studies, success of valve replacement for mitral insufficiency is less durable than that for isolated mitral stenosis.

ANSWER:
Question 27: B
Question 28: A, C, D

29. A 75-year-old man with a history of dyspnea on exertion, palpitations, and episodes of severe diaphoresis has a high-pitched diastolic murmur along the left sternal border. Expected findings include which of the following?

A. Systolic ejection murmur.
B. Enlargement of both the left atrium and the left ventricle on chest radiographs.
C. Atrial fibrillation.
D. History of syphilis.
E. Bounding peripheral pulses.

Ref.: 3

COMMENTS: Common symptoms of aortic insufficiency include angina, progressive dyspnea, palpitations, and peripheral vasomotor changes. Signs of pulmonary congestion occur later as left ventricular failure develops. Findings on physical examination include a normal cardiac rhythm and bounding peripheral pulses due to the widened pulse pressure. The classic decrescendo diastolic murmur is present and is accentuated when the patient leans forward. A systolic ejection murmur may also be heard but usually represents aortic stenosis. Enlargement of the left ventricle is seen on chest radiographs or echocardiogram but generally not atrial enlargement.

ANSWER: A, E

30. The indications for operative intervention to correct aortic insufficiency include which of the following?

A. Progressive symptoms.
B. Loudness and length of diastolic murmur.
C. Increasing left ventricular size.
D. Magnitude of regurgitation as measured during catheterization.

Ref.: 1, 3

COMMENTS: Patients with aortic insufficiency generally remain asymptomatic for many years, although there is substantial variability. Progressive symptoms of heart failure or ischemia and increasing left ventricular size on chest radiography or echocardiography are considered indications for operation. The loudness of the diastolic murmur does not correlate with the severity of the disease. The length of the murmur reflects to some extent the patient's physiologic status in that a longer murmur reflects a greater degree of regurgitation. Short murmurs may be heard, however, in patients with early disease and minimal regurgitation and those with end-stage disease and elevated left ventricular end-diastolic pressures. Measurement of regurgitation is possible during cardiac catheterization, but it has not yet proved useful for selecting patients for operation.

ANSWER: A, C

31. Which one or more of the following statements commonly applies to tricuspid valvular disease?

A. Cause is rheumatic fever.
B. Cause is right ventricular dilatation.
C. Manifests as insufficiency.
D. Manifests as stenosis.

Ref.: 1, 3

COMMENTS: **Insufficiency** is the most common hemodynamic abnormality of the tricuspid valve. Most often it is a functional disorder secondary to right ventricular dilatation, which is due to mitral disease, pulmonary hypertension, or other causes of right ventricular failure. Organic causes of tricuspid insufficiency, such as rheumatic fever, endocarditis, and carcinoid syndrome, are less common. Tricuspid **stenosis** is infrequent, usually of rheumatic origin, and most often accompanied by mitral valve involvement. Treatment of serious tricuspid insufficiency or stenosis generally involves valve repair or replacement. Isolated organic disease of the tricuspid valve is most commonly seen as a result of endocarditis secondary to intravenous drug abuse. Total valve excision without replacement has occasionally been an alternative in this difficult situation but is not well tolerated long term.

ANSWER: B, C

32. A 30-year-old man arrives in the emergency room following a high-impact automobile accident. Initial chest radiograph demonstrates a widened mediastinum. Which of the following statements is/are true?

A. Despite a normal blood pressure, the patient should be explored to drain the hemopericardium before impending tamponade occurs.
B. The finding of normally palpable femoral pulses makes aortic rupture unlikely, and the patient should be managed medically with β-blocking agents.

C. Despite a normal blood pressure, the patient should undergo urgent aortography.
D. The most common site of aortic disruption is the proximal arch, which should be approached through a left thoracotomy.
E. Surgical repair of traumatic aortic rupture carries a 15–20% incidence of paraplegia, but it is the only effective therapy.

Ref.: 3, 5

COMMENTS: Traumatic rupture of the aorta requires urgent diagnosis and therapy. Most patients with this lesion do not reach the hospital alive. The history of a sudden deceleration injury along with chest radiographic findings of a widened mediastinum and loss of the aortic knob contour are strongly suggestive of the diagnosis. Aortography demonstrates the site of injury. Ninety-five percent of traumatic disruptions occur in the proximal descending aorta, just distal to the left subclavian artery, and are best approached through a left thoracotomy. Surgical repair is the only effective therapy and is associated with paraplegia in approximately 5% of patients. Many surgeons prefer simple cross-clamping during repair, and others employ techniques to provide distal perfusion during clamping such as a Gott shunt. The superiority of either method remains controversial.

ANSWER: C

33. Which cardiac chamber is most frequently injured by penetrating trauma?

A. Left ventricle.
B. Right ventricle.
C. Left atrium.
D. Right atrium.

Ref.: 1, 3

COMMENTS: The right ventricle is the most anterior chamber of the heart and consequently is the area most susceptible to penetrating injury. Cardiac injury may produce exsanguination, cardiac tamponade, and rarely cardiac failure secondary to damage to a major coronary artery, a valve, or the conduction system. The key to saving patients who arrive in the emergency room with cardiac injury is prompt recognition and treatment of tamponade while other resuscitative measures are instituted. Pericardiocentesis can be life-saving as well as diagnostic while the operating room is made ready. Most penetrating injuries can be treated without the need to resort to pump support. Nonpenetrating cardiac trauma usually produces diffuse contusion, which warrants cardiac monitoring.

ANSWER: B

34. Which of the following is the most common primary cardiac neoplasm?

A. Myxoma.
B. Rhabdomyoma.
C. Sarcoma.
D. Lymphoma.
E. Metastatic sarcoma.

Ref.: 1, 3

COMMENTS: The most common cardiac neoplasms are metastatic. Primary cardiac tumors are rare, with an incidence of 0.33% on postmortem studies. Most primary cardiac neoplasms are benign, and of them myxoma is the most common, followed by rhabdomyoma. Approximately 20% of primary tumors are malignant; they are almost always rhabdomyosarcomas and angiosarcomas, and they generally have systemic metastases at the time of diagnosis. The clinical manifestations of cardiac tumors are due to local invasion, mass effect, embolization, or systemic constitutional signs such as fever, malaise, weight loss, and autoimmune phenomena, particularly associated with atrial myxomas. Echocardiography is the initial diagnostic technique of choice, followed by computed tomography (CT), magnetic resonance imaging (MRI), and transesophageal echocardiography. Myxomas constitute 50% of benign primary cardiac tumors. They are most frequently found in female adults and are located in the left atrium.

ANSWER: A

35. Physiologic effects of the intraaortic balloon pump (IABP) include which of following?

A. Increased cardiac afterload.
B. Increased coronary blood flow.
C. Decreased left ventricular end-diastolic pressure.
D. Decreased left ventricular preload.
E. Increased left ventricular preload.

Ref.: 1, 3

COMMENTS: An electronically synchronized IABP, which inflates during diastole and deflates at the onset of systole, has physiologic effects that both decrease myocardial oxygen consumption and increase coronary blood flow. The IABP decreases systolic blood pressure, decreases time during systole, and improves emptying of the heart (decreased radius). Deflation of the IABP reduces impedance to aortic flow, thereby reducing afterload and improving cardiac output. Left ventricular end-diastolic volume and pressure are reduced, and diastolic coronary blood flow is enhanced, particularly in failing hearts. The pulmonary artery diastolic pressure is decreased, thereby reducing left ventricular preload.

ANSWER: B, C, D

36. Which one or more of the following statements describes the clinical effects of the IABP?

A. IABP in myocardial infarction with cardiogenic shock decreases infarct size.
B. IABP effectively relieves pain in patients with unstable angina.
C. IABP is indicated for support of cardiac failure following cardiopulmonary bypass.
D. IABP is indicated in severe aortic insufficiency to decrease peripheral resistance.

Ref.: 1

COMMENTS: Indications for use of the IABP include the following: cardiac failure after cardiopulmonary bypass, refractory unstable angina, preoperative treatment of septal defects, mitral regurgitation, arrhythmias, ventricular aneurysms, and occasionally cardiogenic shock. The IABP is used to treat cardiogenic shock associated with myocardial infarction; however, only 15–20% of patients can be weaned successfully from this device, and there is no conclusive evidence that the IABP decreases infarct size. The IABP is particularly effective in controlling pain in patients with angina refractory to pharmacologic manipulation. The device has also been successful in the support of patients with cardiac failure following cardiopulmonary bypass; most such patients can be weaned successfully, with excellent long-term survival. Severe aortic insufficiency is a contraindication to use of the IABP because regurgitation and cardiac failure are exacerbated.

ANSWER: B, C

37. Which of the following is/are indications for placement of a permanent cardiac pacemaker?

A. Sick sinus syndrome.
B. Complete atrioventricular (AV) block.
C. Mobitz type I AV block.
D. Mobitz type II AV block.
E. Stokes-Adams attacks.

Ref.: 1

COMMENTS: There is some disagreement regarding the indications for temporary or permanent cardiac pacing. Most agree that indications for permanent pacing include the following: severe or symptomatic sick sinus syndrome; Mobitz type II AV block (because it frequently leads to complete AV block); complete AV block; symptomatic bilateral bundle branch block; and bifascicular or incomplete trifascicular block with intermittent complete AV block following myocardial infarction. Stokes-Adams attacks, which consist of intermittent syncopal episodes and sometimes convulsions, are manifestations of complete heart block. Mobitz type I AV block (Wenckebach's block) rarely necessitates pacing.

ANSWER: A, B, D, E

38. Open chest massage may be indicated in patients with which of the following?

A. Blunt thoracic trauma.
B. Penetrating thoracic trauma.
C. Barrel chest.
D. Spinal deformities.

Ref.: 1, 3

COMMENTS: External cardiac massage transmits pressure and flow energy to the cardiovascular system by direct cardiac compression. The stroke work is generated through forceful displacement of the chest wall, which compresses the ventricles, closes the mitral valve, opens the aortic valve, and produces unidirectional pressure and flow. Intrathoracic pressure, once considered a more plausible explanation for the beneficial effect of closed-chest massage, accounts for less than 25% of cavitary cardiac pressure. Stroke volume is optimized by compressions of high velocity, moderate force, and brief duration. Coronary artery flow occurs during diastole and is optimized at a compression rate of 100–120/min. In hospitalized cardiac arrest victims, successful resuscitation may not be achieved with closed-chest massage; in such cases data suggest that after 15 minutes of unsuccessful closed-chest massage one should convert to open-chest resuscitation. Cardiac output and diastolic aortic profusion are better with open cardiac massage. Open methods are used when arrest occurs after cardiac surgery and in cases of thoracic injury when there is suspected cardiac tamponade, massive intrathoracic hemorrhage, penetrating cardiac injury, or an open pericardium. It may be necessary in patients with a barrel chest, emphysema, or spinal deformities because closed-chest resuscitation is sometimes unsuccessful in such settings. Most patients who arrest in the field following blunt thoracic trauma cannot be successfully resuscitated even by open-chest massage. Those who survive the initial episode may have a dismal outcome.

ANSWER: A, B, C, D

39. With regard to blood conservation during cardiac surgery, which of the following statements is/are true?

A. Transfusion of blood components during or after cardiac surgery is largely unavoidable.
B. The risks associated with transfusions are primarily associated with red blood cells, not plasma.
C. Patients can safely recover and be discharged with a hematocrit as low as 25%.
D. Antifibrinolysins, such as aprotonin, dramatically reduce bleeding and should be routinely used during cardiac surgery.

Ref.: 5

COMMENTS: Strict blood conservation should be practiced. This statement relates largely to meticulous hemostasis during surgery. During routine procedures, transfusions can usually be avoided. The risks associated with the transfusion of blood components such as platelets and plasma are similar to those associated with the transfusion of red blood cells. Hematocrit values as low as 25% can generally be tolerated. Aprotonin, an antifibrinolytic agent, has been shown to reduce postoperative blood loss, but its cost and potential side effects do not justify its use during routine cardiac procedures.

ANSWER: C

40. Which of the following statements regarding adult cardiac transplantation is/are true?

A. Despite improved immunosuppression, the 5-year survival following a cardiac transplant is approximately 50%.
B. The number of cardiac transplants performed annually in the United States is limited by the number of donors rather than suitable recipients.
C. Although rejection and infection are problematic during the early postoperative period, the development of coronary occlusive disease in the transplanted heart affects long-term survival.
D. With improved medical therapy available, the number of patients awaiting a heart transplant has remained relatively constant.

Ref.: 3, 4, 5

COMMENTS: Results following cardiac transplantation have continued to improve owing largely to improved immunosuppression. Currently, the 1-year survival is approximately 80% and the 5-year survival 65–70%. The number of transplants performed annually is limited almost solely by the number of available donors. The development of coronary occlusive disease in the transplanted heart, "graft vasculopathy," remains a major determinant of long-term survival. Many researchers believe that it is a manifestation of a low-intensity, chronic form of rejection. The number of cardiac transplants performed annually has remained relatively constant, whereas the number of patients waiting continues to increase.

ANSWER: B, C

REFERENCES

1. Sabiston DC Jr: *Textbook of Surgery*, 15th ed. WB Saunders, Philadelphia, 1997.
2. Baue AE, Geha AS, Hammond GL, et al: *Glenn's Thoracic and Cardiovascular Surgery*, 7th ed. Appleton & Lange, Norwalk, CT, 1999.
3. Schwartz SI, Shires GT, Spencer FC: *Principles of Surgery*, 7th ed. McGraw-Hill, New York, 1999.
4. Greenfield LJ, Mulholland M, Oldham KT, et al: *Surgery*, 2nd ed. Lippincott-Raven, Philadelphia, 1997.
5. Grillo HC, Austin WG, Wilkins EW Jr, et al: *Current Therapy in Cardiothoracic Surgery*. BC Decker, Philadelphia, 1989.

CHAPTER 43

Urology

1. Which of the following statements is/are true regarding renal vascular anatomy?

   A. Renal arteries are end-arteries.
   B. The right renal artery usually crosses ventral to the vena cava.
   C. The left renal vein usually crosses ventral to the aorta.
   D. The right adrenal and gonadal veins typically empty into the right renal vein.
   E. Multiple renal arteries are seen in approximately 20–30% of patients.

Ref.: 1, 2

COMMENTS: Approximately two-thirds of normal kidneys are supplied by a single renal artery arising from the aorta, near the upper aspect of the second lumbar vertebra. Each renal artery has approximately five segmental branches that are end-arteries; occlusion of the segmental vessels therefore causes infarction. Renal arterial anomalies are more often present in abnormally located kidneys. Venous drainage of the kidney often involves collateral vessels, particularly on the left side via the gonadal, adrenal, and lumbar veins. The renal vein itself is usually singular on the left but is multiple on the right side approximately 10% of the time. Because the aorta in normal individuals lies to the left side of the vena cava, the right renal artery crosses behind the vena cava and the left renal vein crosses ventral to the aorta. This is consistent with the general anatomic principle that major systemic veins pass ventral to their associated arteries. The longer length of the left renal vein is advantageous when the left kidney is used as a donor organ during renal transplantation.

ANSWER: A, C, E

2. Regarding the management of renal trauma, which of the following statements is/are true?

   A. Contusions are treated by observation until the gross hematuria subsides.
   B. Parenchymal lacerations secondary to blunt trauma require routine exploration because of the risk of secondary hemorrhage or infection.
   C. Retroperitoneal flank hematomas encountered during laparotomy should be explored.
   D. On exploring a perinephric hematoma, Gerota's fascia is opened first and vascular control obtained.
   E. Nonvisualization of the kidney on computed tomography (CT) requires immediate operative exploration.

Ref.: 1, 2, 3, 4, 5

COMMENTS: As with any visceral organ, a spectrum of renal injuries may occur following **blunt trauma**. Renal contusions are the most common renal injury and are managed conservatively with bed rest and observation. Parenchymal lacerations confined to the renal cortex may also be treated nonoperatively if the patient is stable. Deeper lacerations extending into the calyceal system may require primary surgical repair. When an expanding retroperitoneal hematoma is encountered, it should be explored. However, when a nonexpanding perinephric hematoma is encountered, high dose intravenous urography should be done if no other imaging study is available to evaluate the potentially injured kidney and to confirm the presence of a contralateral functioning kidney. Preoperative CT provides accurate staging, allowing one to determine the best treatment modality. • The key surgical principle and the approach to the injured kidney is to *obtain control of the vascular pedicle first*. Exposure of the pedicle is via an incision in the small bowel mesentary medial to the inferior mesenteric vein over the aorta. If Gerota's fascia is incised first, the tamponade effect may be released and a significant hemorrhage can result. Initial vascular control allows accurate assessment of the extent of injury and may permit primary repair or partial nephrectomy rather than removal of the entire organ. Also, if a nephrectomy is necessary, the presence of a functioning contralateral kidney is verified. • **Penetrating renal injury** usually requires exploration, but nonoperative management for low-stage injury is advocated by some. • Traditional management of nonvisualization of the kidney is further evaluated with renal angiography. Recently, spiral CT has provided adequate evaluation of the renal vessels. Nonvisualization of the renal artery may be caused by total avulsion of the renal artery and vein, renal artery thrombosis, absence of the kidney, and severe contusion resulting in major vascular spasm. If a kidney fails to visualize on the arteriographic image, exploration and revascularization are indicated if salvage of the kidney is possible.

ANSWER: A

3. Which of the following occurs in most patients with renal cell carcinoma?

   A. Hypertension.
   B. Erythrocytosis.
   C. Hematuria.
   D. Acute varicocele.
   E. Fever.

Ref.: 1, 2, 3

COMMENTS: Among the many symptoms that have been associated with renal cell carcinoma, hematuria, pain, and abdominal mass are the most common. Only 10% of patients present with the classic triad of hematuria, pain, and abdominal mass. Hypertension (25%) may result from renal vascular compression but is more commonly seen with Wilms' tumor. Fever (17%) is thought to result from tumor necrosis. A small percentage of patients exhibit erythrocytosis (1–5%), which has been related to the production of erythropoietin-like substances by the tumor. It is more common, however, for patients with renal cell carcinoma to present with anemia than with erythrocytosis. A small percentage of patients with renal tumors develop renal vein thrombosis and a subsequent acute varicocele (3%). Hematuria occurs in about 60% of patients. • Renal cell carcinomas occur in an approximate 2:1 male/female ratio. Most patients are diagnosed during the sixth and seventh decades of life. Most renal cell carcinomas are now detected incidentally on ultrasonography or CT scans; thus most masses are not palpable on physical examination. • The TNM staging system classifies a T1/T2 tumor as confined to the kidney, with tumors larger than 7.0 cm at a higher stage (T2). T3 tumors involve the renal veins, inferior vena cava, or perinephric tissues that are confined by Gerota's fascia. T4 tumors extend beyond Gerota's fascia. Nodal status is stratified by size, number of nodes, and whether metastatic disease is present or absent. Lesions that involve the inferior vena cava may still be cured with surgical therapy, and such involvement is not considered a contraindication to surgery.

ANSWER: C

4. Transitional cell cancers of the renal pelvis are best treated by which of the following?

A. Nephrectomy.
B. Nephroureterectomy with excision of the ureter to the level of the bladder.
C. Radical nephroureterectomy with excision of the bladder cuff.
D. Nephroureterectomy and total cystectomy.
E. Radiotherapy.

Ref.: 1, 2, 3

COMMENTS: Transitional cell cancers of the renal pelvis and ureter are notable for their multicentricity and their tendency to spread by direct extension to other parts of the uroepithelium. Approximately 30% of patients have a recurrence in the ureteral stump. For this reason, radical nephroureterectomy with excision of a cuff of bladder at the ureteral orifice is the preferred treatment. Simple nephroureterectomy results in significantly diminished survival compared to the more radical procedure. There is no specific role for radiotherapy in the primary treatment of these lesions. Long-term cystoscopic surveillance is necessary postoperatively, as in approximately 25% of patients a subsequent bladder tumor arises. In selected cases (e.g., solitary kidney or chronic renal disease), local resection of low grade noninvasive tumors of the renal pelvis or ureters have produced long-term survival. Meticulous long-term postoperative surveillance including cystoscopy, intravenous urography, urethroscopy, and urine cytologic examination are essential in these circumstances.

ANSWER: C

5. Regarding treatment of renal cell carcinoma, which of the following statements is/are true?

A. Induction chemotherapy followed by nephrectomy yields the best overall results.
B. Radical nephrectomy involves removal of the kidney, adrenal gland, perinephric fat, Gerota's fascia, and regional lymph nodes.
C. Regional lymphadenectomy for lesions extending outside the kidney improves postoperative survival.
D. CT- or ultrasound-guided biopsy of the renal mass should be performed prior to nephrectomy.

Ref.: 3, 4

COMMENTS: The treatment of renal cell carcinoma and the subsequent prognosis is determined by the anatomic extent of the disease. Treatment of the local disease focuses on tumor removal by radical nephrectomy. Solid renal masses are rarely biopsied, and they are diagnosed after pathologic examination of the kidney. Surgery alone offers an excellent prognosis in patients with early lesions confined within the renal cortex. A survival advantage for those having regional lymphadenectomy has not been established. Metastases frequently occur by hematogenous routes as well and may negate any theoretic advantage of even more radical local surgery, although the presence of a limited volume of tumor thrombus in the vena cava with right-sided carcinomas may not adversely affect the long-term outcome if completely removed. In the presence of distant metastases nephrectomy may still be appropriate to control bleeding, pain, or infection; but it has not been shown to result in increased survival. Chemotherapy for renal cell carcinoma has met with poor results. Immunotherapy may result in remission of the cancer in a small percentage of cases. In selected circumstances, patients with isolated metastases have benefited from resection of their metastatic disease.

ANSWER: B

6. During ultrasonic examination of the abdomen to look for gallstones in a 64-year-old woman with symptoms typical of cholelithiasis, an asymptomatic left solid renal mass is incidentally detected. Which of the following should be the next examination?

A. Excretory urography.
B. Renal angiography.
C. CT of the abdomen.
D. Radionuclide scanning of the urinary tract.
E. Renal biopsy.

Ref.: 6

COMMENTS: See Question 7.

7. A precontrast (A) and postcontrast (B) CT examination of the abdomen in this patient is shown. What is the most likely diagnosis?

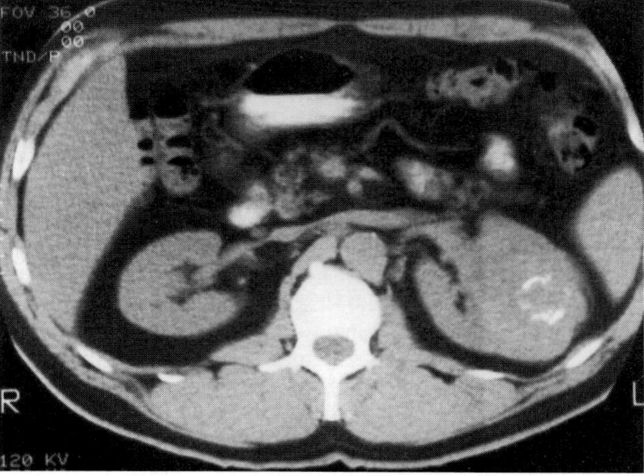

A

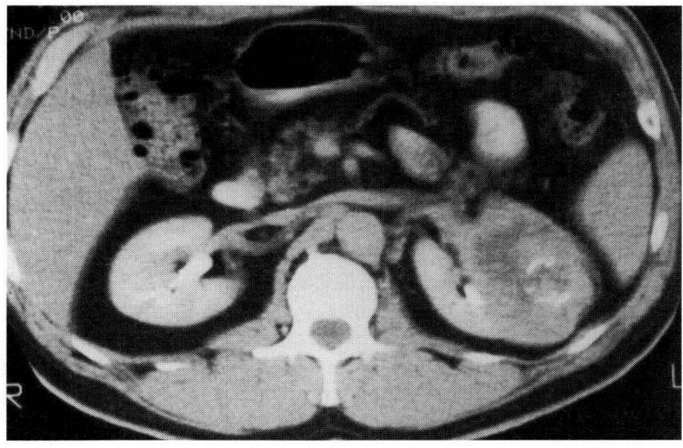

B

A. Calcified simple cyst.
B. Calcified renal artery aneurysm.
C. Calcified renal cell carcinoma.
D. Calcified metastasis to the kidney.

Ref.: 7

COMMENTS: In the above example, the most likely diagnosis is a calcified **renal cell carcinoma**, as there is a solid intrarenal mass with central calcification. CT of the abdomen is the single most useful examination for the workup of patients suspected of having a renal cell carcinoma. In addition to confirming the solid nature of a renal mass, it can demonstrate local extension, venous and caval involvement, and distant metastases to the liver, adrenal, and visualized skeleton. Calcification as seen in this patient is present in 8–18% of renal cell carcinomas, in contrast to about 1% of simple renal cysts. The classic triad of flank pain, gross hematuria, and a palpable renal mass is seen in fewer than 10% of patients at presentation. Small asymptomatic renal cell carcinomas are frequently discovered during abdominal sonography and CT examinations done for other reasons. Renal cell carcinoma, which probably arises from the proximal tubular epithelium, is the most common *primary* renal cancer, accounting for approximately 86% of all primary malignant renal cancers. Of the remainder, 12% are Wilms' tumor and 2% are renal sarcomas. The above comments refer to *primary* renal tumors. The most common *asymptomatic* renal masses are metastatic, with lung as the most frequent primary site. A **calcified renal artery aneurysm** would demonstrate opacification of the lumen on the postinfusion scan. **Calcified metastases** to the kidney are extremely uncommon, having been reported only in patients with primary osteosarcoma elsewhere. A **calcified simple cyst** would demonstrate a radiolucent center with peripheral ring calcification.

ANSWER:
Question 6: C
Question 7: C

8. For which of the following type(s) of renal calculi is growth not affected by manipulation of urinary pH?

A. Cystine.
B. Uric acid.
C. Ammonium magnesium phosphate (struvite).
D. Calcium oxalate.
E. Calcium phosphate.

Ref.: 3, 4

COMMENTS: Renal calculi result from a variety of metabolic conditions. Determination of the stone composition is important for both recognition of the underlying abnormality and institution of appropriate therapy aimed at removing the stone and preventing recurrence. Most urinary calculi (up to 75%) are **calcium oxalate** stones; approximately one-half of these are mixtures of calcium oxalate and phosphate. Calcium phosphate and calcium oxalate stones are not generally altered by variations of urinary pH within the normal range. **Ammonium magnesium phosphate (struvite)** stones are the next in frequency and are usually associated with infection. They form in alkaline urine, and solubility is increased by acidic urine. The problem is that in the presence of infection urea-splitting organisms form ammonias and an alkaline urine; therefore adequate pH manipulation cannot be obtained without control of the infection. **Uric acid** stones are typically radiolucent and solubility is increased by alkalization. The solubility of cystine is increased in alkaline urine; but because **cystine stones** are not crystal in nature, but composed of amino acids, they are not easily pulverized by extracorporeal shock lithotripsy. Stone composition is also related to the ability to visualize stones on plain radiographs. Calcium-containing stones in particular are radiopaque; however, ammonium magnesium phosphate (struvite) and cystine stones may also be visualized.

ANSWER: D, E

9. Which of the following is/are indications for endoscopic, percutaneous, or open surgical removal of renal calculi?

A. Progressive renal damage.
B. Intractable pain.
C. Persistent or progressive obstruction.
D. Intractable urinary tract infection.
E. Detection of any calculi.

Ref.: 1, 2, 3

COMMENTS: The simple presence of a renal or ureteral calculus alone is not an indication for intervention by invasive techniques. Medical management, including analgesics, antibiotics, and appropriate urinary pH adjustments, often result in the spontaneous passage of stones. Smaller stones (<4 mm), in particular, can be expected to pass 90% of the time. There is no evidence that excessive hydration facilitates the passage of renal or ureteral calculi; indeed, it may increase pain. Surgical management is indicated when calculi produce persistent obstruction, intractable pain, or a stone associated with impaired renal function. Techniques for stone removal include ureteroscopic manipulation, percutaneous nephrolithotomy, open nephrolithotomy, and extracorporeal shock wave lithotripsy.

ANSWER: A, B, C, D

10. Extracorporeal shock wave lithotripsy (ESWL) can fragment stones in which of the following urinary tract locations?

A. Renal calyx.
B. Upper two-thirds of ureter.
C. Ureter overlying sacrum and pelvic bones.
D. Lower ureter.
E. Bladder.

Ref.: 3, 4

COMMENTS: Initially, only stones in the kidney were considered appropriate for ESWL. Subsequently, stones located anywhere along the course of the ureter have been successfully treated by this modality. ESWL is accomplished more readily for calculi at the renal level. For this reason, some urologists advocate an initial attempt at manipulating a ureteral stone into the kidney. Ureteral stones located in the bony pelvis can be treated by placing the patient in the prone position so the shock wave enters ventrally and avoids skeletal attenuation. Localization of stones for ESWL is usually accomplished fluoroscopically after a ureteral catheter has been placed for contrast instillation. Some stones can be localized by ultrasonography. Although ESWL has been used to disintegrate bladder stones, most urologists prefer cystoscopic visualization and direct intracorporeal ultrasonic or electrohydraulic lithotripsy. Lower ureteral stones are most commonly treated with ureteroscopic removal.

ANSWER: A, B, C, D, E

11. In a male patient with a pelvic fracture due to blunt trauma, retrograde urethrography demonstrates disruption of the membranous urethra. Which one or more of the following constitute(s) appropriate initial treatment?

A. Passage of a transurethral catheter.
B. Suprapubic cystostomy.
C. Urethrostomy.
D. Retropubic repair.

Ref.: 1, 2, 3,4

COMMENTS: Blunt pelvic trauma is the most common cause of urethral injury. Disruption usually occurs at or above the membranous portion of the urethra, as the anterior prostatic and membranous portions are relatively fixed by the puboprostatic ligaments and the urogenital diaphragm. Urethral injury should be suspected if blood is noted at the meatus or if the patient is unable to void clear urine. Passage of a catheter should *not* be attempted under these circumstances; a retrograde urethrogram should be obtained. In selected cases a urologist may attempt passing a catheter retrograde in patients with minimal disruption. The risk of inserting the catheter is that partial disruption may convert to complete disruption. In most cases, if urethral injury is confirmed, treatment initially should be accomplished with suprapubic cystotomy. A punch cystostomy can be done if the bladder is palpable and no contraindications exist, such as extreme obesity, suprapubic surgical scars, or the presence of an abdominal hernia. Perineal urethrostomy does not divert the urine proximal to the site of injury and is of no value in such a situation. Immediate retropubic surgical realignment has a place in selected clinical situations such as major bladder neck laceration, prostatic fragmentation, or severe dislocation of the prostate with severely displaced bony fragments. In most cases, however, current results suggest that the complications of incontinence, stricture, and impotence are minimized by performance of suprapubic cystostomy and delayed repair. Penetrating urethral injuries, on the other hand, can often be treated by initial repair and urinary diversion.

ANSWER: B

12. Resection of a sigmoid cancer necessitates excision of a segment of the left pelvic ureter with the specimen extending 3 cm distal to the bifurcation of the common iliac artery. Possible options for reconstruction include which of the following?

A. Transureteroureterostomy.
B. Ureteroneocystostomy.
C. Boari's bladder flap.
D. Psoas bladder hitch ligatures.
E. Cutaneous ureterostomy.

Ref.: 3, 4

COMMENTS: In this situation, simple in situ ureteroneocystostomy is not possible. An end-to-side anastomosis of the severed ureter to the opposite ureter (transureteroureterostomy) may be successful but may jeopardize the contralateral ureter. An isolated segment of ileum can be used to bridge the gap between the divided ureter and bladder. The ileum can be tapered distally and implanted into the bladder in the fashion of a ureter so as not to reflux (ileal ureter). A broad U-shaped flap (Boari flap) can be rotated off the bladder, fashioned into the shape of a cylinder, and anastomosed to the severed ureter. Another solution is to mobilize the bladder extensively and hitch it to the psoas muscle as high as possible, at which point a ureteral implantation is performed (psoas hitch). With this technique, the bladder can often be brought as high as the common iliac artery. Mobilization of the kidney may give 2–3 cm of ureteral length distally. If time is of the essence or the abdomen is grossly contaminated, the cut end of the ureter can be brought to the skin as an intubated cutaneous ureterostomy with anticipated later reconstructive repair (rarely performed).

ANSWER: A, C, D, E

13. Which one or more of the following are principles of repair of an intraoperative ureteral injury?

A. Use of nonabsorbable suture materials.
B. Spatulation of transected ends.
C. Extensive ureteral dissection to minimize tension.
D. Drainage.
E. Intraureteral stent.

Ref.: 3, 4

COMMENTS: Ureteral injuries are usually iatrogenic and occur during the course of retroperitoneal dissection of various abdominal and pelvic operations. In cases of transection, repair should be carried out using absorbable suture material and an indwelling intraureteral stent. Nonabsorbable sutures should be avoided because they may serve as a nidus for calculus formation. Extensive ureteral dissection should be avoided to preserve the segmental blood supply. Spatulation reduces the incidence of anastomotic stricture in the severed ureter. Drains should be placed to accommodate any anastomotic leak. When injury involves the lowest ureteral segment, ureteroneocystostomy may be preferable. Percutaneous (or open) nephrostomy serves to divert urine from the repair site, facilitating healing at the anastomotic site.

ANSWER: B, D, E

14. A properly constructed cutaneous ureteroileostomy (ileal conduit) should do which of the following?

A. Provide an adequate reservoir for urine storage.
B. Prevent ureteral reflux.
C. Require catheterization for emptying.
D. Separate the urinary and fecal streams.

Ref.: 1, 2, 3, 4

COMMENTS: The use of an isolated segment of ileum to serve as a conduit between the ureters and the skin has become the most common form of urinary diversion and is the standard against which all other diversions are measured. It is used for patients after cystectomy, as well as those with other indications for supravesical diversion. Large bowel is useful as a conduit because of the ease of creating an antireflux ureterointestinal anastomosis. Continent urinary reservoirs are fashioned from colon or small bowel (or both) and require periodic catheterization. Continent reservoirs offer patients even greater control of urinary function and are well accepted. In selected cases complete neobladders, fashioned from bowel, may be attached directly to the urethral remnant. The purpose of constructing an ileal conduit is to create a route (unidirectionally within the conduit) for transport of urine; it is not a reservoir for storage. Stasis in the bowel segment predisposes to infections, stone formation, and ureteral reflux. Stasis also promotes absorption of electrolytes and may result in hyperchloremic acidosis. Some degree of ureteral reflux can be expected normally with an ileal conduit.

ANSWER: D

15. Regarding bladder cancer, which of the following statements is/are true?

A. Adenocarcinoma is the most common histologic type.
B. Prognosis is related to histologic grade of the tumor.
C. Painless hematuria is the most common presenting symptom.
D. Prognosis is related to the presence or absence of muscular invasion of the bladder wall.

Ref.: 1, 2, 3

COMMENTS: Cancer of the urinary bladder has a peak incidence in the 50- to 70-year-old group of patients and is more common in men than in women. Ninety percent of these tumors are transitional cell in type; squamous cell cancer and adenocarcinoma occur infrequently. Painless hematuria, either gross or microscopic, is the most common initial manifestation. Approximately 30% of patients present with symptoms of bladder irritability (urgency, frequency, dysuria). The prognosis is directly related to both the stage and the histologic grade of the cancer. It is necessary therefore that an attempt be made to obtain adequate tissue during the biopsy to determine the depth of microscopic involvement. Bladder malignancies metastasize via both lymphatic and hematogenous routes to lung, liver, bone, and other sites.

ANSWER: B, C, D

16. Appropriate treatment of superficial low-grade transitional cell bladder tumors may include which one or more of the following?

A. Transurethral resection and electrocoagulation.
B. Systemic chemotherapy.
C. Intravesical chemotherapy.
D. Intravesical bacillus Calmette-Guérin (BCG).

Ref.: 3, 4

COMMENTS: Only about 10% of patients presenting with superficial low-grade cancers have their lesions progress to invasive cancer. Generally, endoscopic ablation of superficial cancers is definitive therapy. Systemic chemotherapy for superficial tumors has not been shown to be of value. Intravesical chemotherapy, however, with agents such as thiotepa, mitomycin and doxorubicin is useful for treatment and prophylaxis of recurrent cancers. Of all the intravesical agents, immunotherapy with BCG seems most effective against both superficial disease and in particular carcinoma in situ.

ANSWER: A, C, D

17. Preferred treatment for muscle invasive bladder cancer involves which of the following?

A. Radical cystectomy.
B. Preoperative irradiation and radical cystectomy.
C. Preoperative chemotherapy and radical cystectomy.
D. Radiation therapy alone.
E. Intravesical chemotherapy.

Ref.: 1, 2, 3, 4

COMMENTS: In the United States, radical cystectomy is the preferred treatment for muscle-invasive bladder cancer. Preoperative radiation therapy has not been shown to increase survival after radical cystectomy. The role of partial cystectomy with muscle invasion is limited secondary to a high local recurrence rate (approximately 50%). Lesions confined to the mucosa can be treated with transurethral resection, fulguration, or intravesical chemotherapeutic agents; then a careful surveillance program must be maintained. The treatment of lesions with submucosal invasion has been controversial as to whether intravesical chemotherapy is appropriate and as to the necessary extent of surgical resection. Certainly, intravesical therapy is of no value for high grade invasive cancer. In Britain and Europe, radiation therapy continues to be a common form of treatment for invasive bladder cancer with salvage cystectomy used for irradiation failure. In the United States, radical cystectomy alone is the preferred treatment. The 5-year survival rate of patients with muscle invasion following cystectomy is only 50%, and the major cause of death is distant metastatic disease. There is interest in the use of adjuvant chemotherapy before of after cystectomy, but a survival benefit is yet to be proved. Because combination chemotherapy (with methotrexate, vinblastine, doxorubicin (Adriamycin), and cisplatinum (MVAC) in patients with advanced disease has yielded response rates of 50–70%, these agents now are being used prior to cystectomy when muscle invasion is present. Complete response rates with MVAC alone have been disappointing (10–15%).

ANSWER: A

18. Regarding bladder trauma, which of the following statements is/are true?

A. Rupture usually is extraperitoneal when associated with pelvic fracture.
B. A single-view retrograde cystogram in the emergency room demonstrates most significant bladder injuries.
C. Primary closure is generally indicated for extraperitoneal ruptures.
D. Intraoperative injury usually requires repair with a suprapubic cystostomy.

Ref.: 1, 2, 3, 4

COMMENTS: Bladder injury may result from blunt or penetrating trauma or may occur during pelvic operations. When associated with pelvic fracture, the site of injury is usually extraperitoneal, having been caused by the shearing force of the pelvic fracture. Extraperitoneal rupture without pelvic fracture is an infrequent occurrence. Isolated extraperitoneal bladder rupture is treated with 7–10 days of Foley catheter drainage. Blunt injury without pelvic fracture is associated with intraperitoneal rupture, particularly if the bladder is full at the time of injury, and results in perforation typically at the dome of the bladder. Bladder injury should be suspected in any patient with lower abdominal trauma if there is any hematuria or if the patient is unable to void. Single-view cystography may miss a significant injury. Anterior, posterior, lateral, and oblique films, and in particular postvoid films, are necessary. The usual treatment of intraperitoneal rupture involves a two-layer watertight closure with absorbable sutures and transurethral or suprapubic bladder drainage. Iatrogenic injury recognized at the time of an operation generally does not require suprapubic cystotomy but does require repair with absorbable sutures and urethral catheter drainage for 5–7 days. It is necessary also to be vigilant that the Foley catheter does not become obstructed, such as with blood, causing the bladder to become distended.

ANSWER: A

19. Which of the following is true regarding management of a patient with benign prostatic hyperplasia (BPH)?

A. All patients with complaints of prostatism should undergo therapy.
B. Patients with BPH have an increased risk of prostate cancer.
C. Initial therapy usually consists of medical therapy with α-blockers (terazosin and doxazosin) or 5α-reductase inhibitors (finasteride).
D. Absolute indications for surgical therapy include recurrent urinary tract infection, recurrent gross hematuria, bladder stones, and renal insufficiency.

Ref.: 1, 2, 3, 4

COMMENTS: The indications for treatment of BPH are based on the patient's symptoms. Most patients are treated initially with medical therapy using 5α-reductase inhibitors or α-blocking agents that act on the prostatic smooth muscle. 5α-Reductase inhibitors inhibit the conversion of testosterone to dihydrotestosterone, which is the active agent responsible for BPH. Indications for surgical management include recurrent urinary tract infection, recurrent gross hematuria, worsening renal function, failure of medical management, or the presence of bladder stones. The presence on rectal examination of a normal-sized prostate does not exclude obstruction by BPH. BPH occurs in most men with an increased incidence with increasing age; it is not a risk factor for the development of prostate cancer. It should be noted, however, that the usual transurethral prostatectomy or open surgery does not remove all the prostate tissue, and prostate cancer can occur following removal of the prostate for benign disease.

ANSWER: C, D

20. Regarding prostate-specific antigen (PSA), which of the following statements is/are true?

A. It is a better serum marker for prostate cancer than acid phosphatase.
B. It is produced by both benign and malignant prostate tissue.
C. As an immunohistochemical marker, PSA has been able to establish whether a metastatic adenocarcinoma is of prostatic origin.
D. Elevation of PSA in a patient with prostatic cancer usually precludes a surgical cure.
E. A normal PSA is less than 10 ng/ml.

Ref.: 3, 4

COMMENTS: PSA is the best marker for prostate cancer and the first organ-specific marker in all of cancer biology. It is produced by both benign and malignant prostate tissue. Although age-specific reference ranges have been proposed, most would consider a normal PSA as less than 4 ng/ml. As an immunohistochemical marker, PSA is much more accurate and specific than prostatic acid phosphatase, which can be elevated in association with nonprostatic cancers, bone disorders, and liver abnormalities. Additionally, acid phosphatase is not generally elevated with early prostate cancer. Elevated PSA does not necessarily imply escape beyond the capsule and surgical incurability, although high values are often associated with bulky lesions. In contradistinction, an elevated acid phosphatase level in an individual with prostate cancer usually signifies extensive local or metastatic disease.

ANSWER: A, B, C

21. One hour after a prolonged transurethral prostatectomy (TURP), a 70-year-old man with mild coronary artery disease experiences bradycardia, hypertension, confusion, nausea, and headache. The most likely cause is:

A. Hyperkalemia.
B. Hypokalemia.
C. Hypernatremia.
D. Hyponatremia.
E. Anemia.

Ref.: 3, 4

COMMENTS: The patient is most likely suffering from transurethral resection (TUR) syndrome, which is caused by excessive absorption of irrigating solution resulting in hyponatremia. The usual irrigation fluid is 1.5% glycine, which has an osmolarity of 200 mOsm/L compared to the normal serum osmolarity of 290 mOsm/L. Excessive systemic absorption of the irrigating solution can result in a dilutional hyponatremia, hypoproteinemia, and ultimately a decreased serum osmotic pressure. Extremely low sodium levels (<110 mEq/L) may result in severe cerebral edema causing seizure. The treatment of TUR syndrome traditionally consists of terminating the procedure as rapidly as possible, administration of furosemide (Lasix) intra- or postoperatively, and use of 0.9% NaCl (and in severe cases 3% NaCl) solution over 3–6 hours.

ANSWER: D

22. Which of the following is true regarding benign prostatic hyperplasia (BPH)?

A. BPH arises in the periphery of the prostate gland.
B. The prevalence of BPH increases with age.
C. All patients with BPH should undergo medical or surgical treatment.
D. Indications for surgical treatment include recurrent urinary tract infections (UTI), bladder stone, renal insufficiency, or persistent hematuria.

E. Most patients after a TURP experience retrograde ejaculation.

Ref.: 1, 2, 3, 4

COMMENTS: Unlike prostate cancer, which arises in the periphery of the gland, BPH arises in the transitional zone of the prostate gland. The incidence of BPH is approximately 50% at age 50 and increases to approximately 80% with men entering their eighth decade of life. Patients are traditionally treated with medical therapy first if symptoms warrant and then undergo surgical therapy in the face of medical failure. Indications for surgical therapy include recurrent UTIs, the presence of bladder stones, worsening renal function, or recurrent hematuria. Although impotence and incontinence are rare following a TURP, most patients after a TURP experience retrograde ejaculation as a result of resection of the bladder neck. Patients should be appraised of this preoperatively.

ANSWER: B, D, E

23. A 60-year-old man in good general health presents with an asymptomatic prostate nodule. PSA is noted to be 9 ng/ml, and biopsy confirms adenocarcinoma (Gleason III+III) on one side. Bone scan does not reveal any evidence of metastatic disease. Which of the following therapies is appropriate?

A. Transurethral prostate resection.
B. Radical prostatectomy.
C. Orchiectomy.
D. Diethylstilbestrol.
E. Local radiation therapy.

Ref.: 1, 2, 3, 4, 6

COMMENTS: When a prostatic nodule is detected, a PSA level should be obtained followed by transrectal ultrasonography and biopsy. If prostate cancer is found, a bone scan may be obtained to rule out evidence of metastatic disease. In addition, a chest radiograph and possibly a serum acid phosphatase level are obtained preoperatively. Treatment of localized prostate cancer is by radical prostatectomy or external beam radiotherapy depending on physician and patient preference. There are many new experimental and investigational modalities utilized for treatment of prostate cancer. Radical prostatectomy consists of removing the entire prostate and seminal vesicles. A staging pelvic lymph node dissection is often performed prior to prostatectomy. If the lymph nodes are grossly enlarged, they are sent for frozen section; and the operation is usually terminated if cancer has spread to the lymph nodes. Tables have been established that predict the likelihood of positive margins and lymph node involvement based on the clinical stage, PSA, and Gleason score.

ANSWER: B, E

24. An asymptomatic 76 year-old man presents with a hard, irregular prostate, elevated acid phosphatase, PSA 53 ng/ml, and multiple osteoblastic lesions in the lumbosacral spine. Biopsy of the prostate reveals a moderately differentiated adenocarcinoma. Which one or more of the following therapies is/are indicated?

A. Transurethral prostate resection.
B. Radical prostatectomy.
C. Hormonal therapy.
D. Radiation therapy.
E. Cytotoxic chemotherapy.

Ref.: 1, 2, 3, 4

COMMENTS: The treatment of locally advanced or metastatic prostate cancer is palliation. The primary method of therapy is by hormonal manipulation, consisting of bilateral orchiectomy or the administration of luteinizing hormone-releasing hormone agonists (e.g., leuprolide) and testosterone-blocking agents (e.g., flutamide). Exogenous estrogens such as diethylstilbestrol are not used often because of their associated increased incidence of thromboembolic disease. Hormonal therapy is the primary means of palliating bone pain, obstructive uropathy, and the general debility of metastatic disease. Use of early versus delayed hormonal therapy is controversial, and a survival benefit for initiating hormonal therapy prior to the onset of symptoms has yet to be proven. When hormonal treatment fails to palliate, transurethral resection of the prostate to relieve obstruction or local radiotherapy to palliate painful or bulky metastasis is employed. Chemotherapy is not particularly useful, although protocols are forthcoming for hormonal refractory prostate cancer. Radical prostatectomy is not indicated in the presence of metastatic disease.

ANSWER: C

25. Regarding prostate cancer, which of the following is/are true?

A. Prostate cancer causes symptoms early in the course of disease.
B. Transrectal ultrasonography alone (without biopsy) can accurately predict prostate cancer.
C. Prostate cancer most commonly spreads to the lung and liver.
D. Most lesions are adenocarcinoma.
E. Bony metastases are usually osteolytic.

Ref.: 1, 2, 3, 4

COMMENTS: Carcinoma of the prostate is the most common nonskin cancer in men over the age of 65 and is the second most common cause of cancer death in the male population. Histologically, most of these lesions are adenocarcinomas; squamous cell carcinoma and sarcomas of the prostate are rare. No definite etiologic factors have been established. Most prostate cancers arise in the periphery of the gland and are asymptomatic until urinary obstruction or symptoms of metastases develop. More than half of the prostate nodules detected on examination are malignant. Prostate-specific antigen (PSA) determination in conjunction with an annual rectal examination has evolved as the optimal means of early detection of prostate cancer. Transrectal ultrasonography and prostate biopsy are indicated in men with an elevated PSA or abnormal rectal examination. After regional lymph nodes, bone metastasis (usually osteoblastic) occur most commonly, but widely metastatic disease can be found at almost any site.

ANSWER: D

26. Regarding radical prostatectomy, which of the following are true?

A. It may be done via both the retropubic and the perineal routes.
B. Following successful surgical treatment, the PSA drops to virtually zero within 24 hours.

C. Urinary incontinence develops in most patients after radical prostatectomy.
D. All patients, regardless of age, with localized prostate cancer should undergo this treatment.

Ref.: 3, 4

COMMENTS: Radical prostatectomy may be done through the retropubic or the perineal route. The advantage of a retropubic approach is that a limited staging pelvic lymphadenectomy can be done at the same time. Fewer than 5% of patients develop total incontinence after radical prostatectomy. A higher percentage, however, do develop some mild stress incontinence. Almost all patients develop erectile dysfunction immediately postoperatively, but the use of a nerve-sparing prostatectomy preserves potency in up to 80% of select patients. The PSA drops to 0 after successful prostatectomy, but the half-life of PSA is approximately 2–3 days, so the PSA does not reach its nadir for approximately 3 weeks postoperatively. Patients considered candidates for surgical therapy should have localized disease and a life expectancy of at least 10 years.

ANSWER: A

27. Match the illustrations with the pathology below.

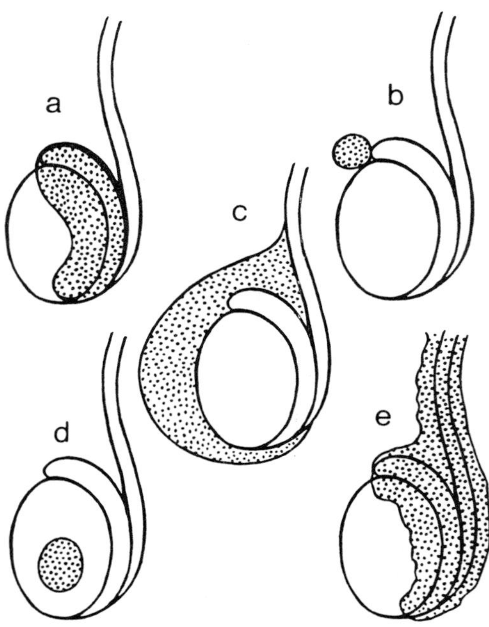

A. Testicular tumor.
B. Spermatocele.
C. Chronic epididymitis.
D. Acute/subacute epididymitis.
E. Hydrocele.

Ref.: 1, 2, 3, 4

COMMENTS: **Hydrocele** can be idiopathic or secondary to a disease process such as epididymitis, trauma, mumps, or tuberculosis. Typically, it is a nontender, translucent mass. It can obscure palpation of the testis; and it is important to be aware of this in young men because as many as 20% of acute hydroceles are secondary to testicular tumors. If a mass with all the characteristics of a hydrocele empties when the patient is in the supine position, likely there is a patent processus vaginalis. Hydroceles in adults require treatment only when symptomatic, but in children they may require treatment if persistent. **Spermatocele** is a simple or multiloculated cyst at the head of the epididymis and usually requires no treatment unless it is symptomatic. It transilluminates and can be palpated as being discrete from the testes. **Epididymitis**, if acute, leaves the patient with an exquisitely tender scrotum whose skin may be red and edematous. There may be a mass, but often this is difficult to appreciate because the patient does not permit a deliberate examination. With **chronic epididymitis**, the mass is nontender and firm and can cause beading of the entire vas deferens. If, in addition, a draining sinus tract is present, the most likely cause is tuberculosis. **Testicular cancer** is the most serious condition present in the scrotum, and a mass therein must be so viewed until proved otherwise. The mass is usually firm, cannot be transilluminated, and is not tender. If it is tender, it may be as a result of a tumor bleeding into the testicle. Ultrasonic examination of the testicle along with tumor markers have greatly facilitated making a diagnosis in such a clinical setting.

ANSWER: A-d; B-b; C-e; D-a; E-c

28. A 14-year-old boy presents to the emergency room with a 4 hour history of acute, severe left scrotal pain. Examination reveals a left high-riding testicle with severe pain upon palpation. Urinalysis does not reveal any evidence of red blood cells or white blood cells. Which one or more of the following is/are the treatment of choice at this point?

A. Heat, scrotal elevation, and antibiotics.
B. Manual attempt at detorsion.
C. Analgesics and reexamination.
D. Doppler examination to assess testicular blood flow.
E. Radioisotope scan to assess testicular blood flow.
F. Surgical exploration.

Ref.: 1, 2, 3, 4

COMMENTS: When examining the acutely painful scrotum, one should attempt to differentiate epididymitis from testicular torsion, but it may not be possible. Doubtful cases should be treated as testicular torsion until proved otherwise. Because irreversible testicular ischemia occurs within 4 hours when there is complete torsion, prompt surgical exploration is indicated even if there is diagnostic uncertainty. Use of a Doppler examination may be helpful for assessing the testicular blood flow. Nuclear medicine scans also are reliable and must be used judiciously. Manual detorsion is not usually successful but can be done when the scrotum is not swollen. It may relieve pain, but exploration is still necessary because residual torsion may still exist. At the time of exploration, the involved testis should be anatomically fixated as well as detorsed. The contralateral testis should undergo a similar procedure prophylactically, as the same anatomic abnormality may be found in both testes.

ANSWER: F

29. The anatomic abnormality found with torsion of the testicle in adolescents most commonly involves which of the following?

A. Intravaginal torsion of the spermatic cord.
B. Extravaginal torsion of the spermatic cord.
C. Torsion of the appendix testis.

D. Torsion of the appendix epididymis.

Ref.: 1, 2, 3, 4

COMMENTS: There are two types of torsion of the testicle. In the neonate, torsion of the spermatic cord occurs before attachment of the gubernaculum, allowing torsion of the entire testicle and tunica vaginalis. This is called **extravaginal torsion**. The second type of torsion usually occurs in adolescents and older men and is called **intravaginal torsion** of the spermatic cord. By this time, the tunica vaginalis is fixed to the dartos fascia and cannot twist. Intravaginal torsion is most commonly associated with a long mesenteric attachment between the cord and the testes and epididymis, which allows the testicle to rotate (producing the "bell clapper" deformity), and torsion can therefore occur within the tunica vaginalis. Since this deformity is often bilateral, fixation of the contralateral testis should be performed at the time the testicular torsion is corrected. Regarding the appendix testis and the appendix epididymis, torsion of these appendages can produce acute pain and swelling similar to torsion of the spermatic cord, but it does not result in testicular infarction. Transillumination may reveal the "blue dot" sign representing the infarcted structure. Exploration is sometimes required to exclude testicular torsion.

ANSWER: A

30. Which of the following is/are true regarding varicocele?

A. Varicoceles occur more commonly on the left side.
B. Varicoceles are associated with infertility.
C. Varicoceles occur in about 40% of men.
D. Varicoceles are often associated with testicular tumors.
E. Varicoceles feel like a "bag of worms" on physical examination.

Ref.: 1, 2, 3, 4

COMMENTS: Varicoceles are found in approximately 15–20% of the adult male population but are seen even more commonly in infertile men. Varicoceles have not been found to be associated with testicular tumors. They have been associated with diminished sperm count, decreased sperm motility, and abnormal sperm morphology. In infertile patients with an abnormal semen analysis, varicocelectomy often improves the semen analysis. Physical examination of the scrotum reveals a large group of veins palpable within the scrotum that has been described as a "bag of worms."

ANSWER: A, B, E

31. A 65-year-old man is unable to void after an abdominoperineal resection. Postvoid residuals have been 600–800 ml. The treatment of choice is which of the following?

A. Chronic Foley catheterization.
B. Transurethal resection of the prostate (TURP).
C. Clean intermittent catheterization.
D. Transurethral sphincterotomy.
E. α-Blockers alone.

Ref.: 1, 2, 3, 4

COMMENTS: Bladder dysfunction has been reported in 10–50% of patients following abdominal perineal resection or other major pelvic surgery. The type of voiding dysfunction that occurs is dependent on the specific nerve involved and the degree of the injury. Patients are best treated by clean intermittent catheterization. Most (>80%) resolve over 3–6 months. The use of a chronic indwelling catheter is a reasonable choice in some patients, but the risk of infection is higher with chronic catheterization than with intermittent catheterization. The use of α-blockers alone or transurethral resection of the prostate (TURP) is unlikely to be successful. Transurethral sphincterotomy does not treat the underlying problem and may result in incontinence.

ANSWER: C

32. Match the following regarding testicular tumors on the left with the appropriate treatment/sign on the right.

A. Seminoma	a. Radiation therapy
B. Nonseminomatous	b. Retroperitoneal lymph node dissection
	c. Elevated α-fetoprotein (AFP)
	d. Elevated human chorionic gonadotropin (hCG)
	e. Chemotherapy for advanced disease

Ref.: 1, 2, 3, 4

COMMENTS: The most common solid tumor in a young male is a seminoma. About 95% of testicular masses are of a germ cell origin. Germ cell tumors are divided into seminoma and nonseminomatous germ cell tumors. Nonseminomatous germ cell tumors include tumors of the following histologic types: embryonal cell carcinoma, yolk sac tumor, choriocarcinoma, teratoma. Clinically stage I seminomas (confined to the testis) are treated with prophylactic radiotherapy to the retroperitoneal lymph nodes to eliminate any chance of failure in the retroperitoneum. Higher stage seminoma (visible adenopathy in the retroperitoneum or lung metastasis) are best treated with chemotherapy. An elevated hCG level is seen in 5–10% of seminomas, but if an elevated AFP level is found, the tumor is considered a nonseminomatous tumor. The treatment of clinical stage I nonseminomatous germ cell tumors is controversial but consists of either retroperitoneal lymph node dissection or surveillance. Elevated AFP and β-hCG levels may be seen in patients with nonseminomatous germ cell tumors. For patients with bulky retroperitoneal disease or visceral metastasis, treatment consists of combination chemotherapy.

ANSWER: A-a,d,e; B-b,c,d,e

33. Appropriate treatment of a painless solid testicular mass in a 28-year-old man includes which of the following?

A. Preoperative determination of tumor markers.
B. Incisional biopsy via a scrotal incision.
C. Incisional biopsy via an inguinal incision.
D. Orchiectomy via a scrotal incision.
E. Orchiectomy via an inguinal incision.

Ref.: 1, 2, 3

COMMENTS: During the workup of a patient with a testicular tumor, serum should be obtained for determination of the α-fetoprotein (AFP) level and the β-subunit of human chorionic gonadotropin (β-hCG), as these tumor markers are elevated in many patients with testicular cancer. The primary diagnostic and therapeutic manuever is orchiectomy, and it should be carried out via an inguinal incision with early clamping of the vessels. If the presence of a testicular mass is confirmed, an orchiectomy should be performed. Rarely, the testicle suspected of being involved with cancer may be affected by a benign condition, yet even here the best treatment is often orchiectomy. A scrotal approach is contraindicated, as it does not permit control of the testicular vessels prior to manipulation of the testicle, which may dislodge tumor cells into the venous drainage. Also, with such an approach cells from the biopsy specimen may spill into the scrotum and subsequently spread tumor via the scrotal lymphatic drainage to the superficial inguinal nodes or they may seed locally.

ANSWER: A, E

34. Which of the following is/are true regarding testicular tumors?

A. Solid masses of the testis are usually malignant.
B. Testicular tumors are the most common solid tumor in men aged 18–35.
C. The overall survival for patients with testicular cancer exceeds 90%.
D. The most common testicular tumor is seminoma.
E. They are associated with cryptorchidism (undescended testis) in their etiology.

COMMENTS: The most common non-skin cell tumor in men ages 18–35 are testicular tumors of germ cell origin. These tumors, unlike extratesticular tumors within the scrotum that are benign, are almost always malignant. The most common solid testicular mass is a seminoma. Today, survival of patients with testicular tumor exceeds 90% owing to the development of aggressive surgical therapy, tumor markers (AFP and hCG) and *cis*-platinum based combination chemotherapy. Thirty percent of premature male neonates have an undescended testis, but spontaneous descent occurs in most of these infants by 1 year of age. The incidence of undescended testes is approximately 0.8% in 1-year-old infants. Undescended testes must be placed in the scrotum (orchiopexy); they often have an associated indirect hernia that should be repaired by ligation of the sac at the time of orchiopexy. Patients who are found to have cryptorchidism of the testes have a higher chance of developing testis cancer in both the affected and contralateral testes.

ANSWER: A, B, C, D, E

35. A 32-year-old man presents in the emergency room with an exquisitely painful and "woody" feeling penile erection of 18 hours' duration. Effective therapy includes which of the following?

A. Aspiration of blood from the corpora cavernosa.
B. Irrigation of the corpora cavernosa with a dilute solution of papaverine.
C. Creation of a communication between the glans penis and a corporal body with a biopsy needle or scalpel blade.
D. Side-to-side anastomosis between the corpus spongiosum and the corpus cavernosum.
E. Exchange transfusions.

Ref.: 3, 4

COMMENTS: Most cases of prolonged pathologic penile erection in the absence of sexual stimulation (priapism) are idiopathic. Some known causes are sickle cell disease, leukemic infiltration of veins draining the penis, and certain medications such as anticoagulants and antidepressants. Often simple aspiration of blood from the corpus cavernosum alone can cause lasting detumescence. If this fails, irrigation of the corpus with a dilute solution of epinephrine or norepinephrine may work. This has the dual effect of decompressing the corpus and the venous obstruction that goes with it, as well as diminishing arterial flow. Papaverine is used to treat impotence; it increases penile blood flow by directly relaxing vascular smooth muscle. The glans penis is an extension of the corpus spongiosum and is usually not affected by priapism. Shunts between it and the corpus cavernosa created with biopsy needles or scalpel blades or removal of a portion of the glandular corporal septum may provide a path of egress for blood trapped in the penis. If all else fails, formal spongiosum-to-cavernosum shunts may be created. There is a high incidence of impotence after priapism of 24 hours or more. When priapism is secondary to sickle cell anemia, exchange transfusions and other medical therapies including oxygenation, hydration, and alkalinization may be indicated.

ANSWER: A, C, D, E

36. Regarding vasectomy, which of the following statements is/are true?

A. It produces prompt sterility.
B. Duplication of the vas deferens is a common cause of failure.
C. It may be performed through a midline scrotal incision.
D. The pregnancy rate after vasovasotomy done to reestablish patency approaches 50%.

Ref.: 1, 2, 3, 4

COMMENTS: Vasectomy for the purpose of sterilization has become a commonplace procedure safely performed in the outpatient setting. Careful attention must be given to appropriate patient screening, preoperative patient education, and informing patients of the risk and alternative methods of birth control. Patients must also be instructed that viable spermatozoa remain in the seminal tract distal to the site of vasectomy for several weeks after the operation. Careful follow-up examination of the semen must be performed at 6–8 weeks to confirm that the patient is in fact sterile. Vasectomy may be done through a midline scrotal incision or two smaller incisions on either side of the scrotum. The procedure should be considered a permanent form of sterilization, although with microsurgical techniques reanastomosis of the vas deferens can be performed in more than 90% of cases with an average success rate (as attested to by subsequent pregnancy) approaching 50%. The presence of high antisperm antibody levels and a prolonged interval between vasectomy and reanastomosis have a negative effect on preganacy rates after vasovasotomy. Duplication of the vas deferens is a rare cause of failure after vasectomy.

ANSWER: C, D

37. Match the following:

A. Dysuria	a. Painful urination
B. Strangury	b. Difficulty or straining with voiding
C. Hesitancy	c. Delayed voiding in response to attempts at voiding
D. Prostatism	d. Symptoms associated with benign prostatic hypertrophy

Ref.: 3, 4

COMMENTS: Dysuria is defined as painful urination, and strangury is defined as difficulty or straining with voiding. Pneumaturia refers to the presence of air in the urine and is associated with recent instrumentation or enterovesical fistula. Prostatism refers to the symptoms of obstruction associated with benign prostatic hyperplasia, and it may be defined as having both obstructive and irritation components. Nocturia, hesitancy, and intermittency are associated with prostatic obstruction. Urgency and daytime frequency are considered urge-related prostatism.

ANSWER: A-a; B-b; C-c; D-d

REFERENCES

1. Sabiston DC Jr: *Textbook of Surgery*, 15th ed. WB Saunders, Philadelphia, 1997.
2. Schwartz SI, Shires GT, Spencer FC: *Principles of Surgery*, 7th ed. McGraw-Hill, New York, 1999.
3. Gillenwater JY, Grayhack JT, Howard SJ, Duckett JW: *Adult and Pediatric Urology*, 3rd ed. Mosby, St. Louis, 1996.
4. Walsh PC, Retik AB, Vaughan ED, Wein AJ: *Campbell's Urology*, 7th ed. WB Saunders, Philadelphia, 1998.
5. Wessels H, McAnich JW, Meyer A, Bruce T: Criteria for nonoperative treatment of significant penetrating renal lacerations. *J Urol* 157:24, 1997.
6. Partin AW, Yoo J, Carter HB, et al: The use of prostate specific antigen, clinical stage and Gleason score to predict pathological stage in men with localized prostate cancer. *J Urol* 150:110, 1993.
7. Pollack HM: *Clinical Urography*. WB Saunders, Philadelphia, 1990.

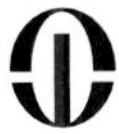

CHAPTER 44

Gynecology

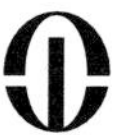

1. Which of the following statements is/are true regarding embryologic development of the female genital tract?

A. The uterus represents fusion of the müllerian ducts.
B. The internal genitalia are partially derived from the ectoderm.
C. The development of the female genitalia occurs independent of androgenic influence.
D. Urologic and gynecologic developmental anomalies rarely coexist.

Ref.: 1, 2

COMMENTS: Urogenital development in the male and female results from the appropriate migration and fusion of the müllerian and wolffian ducts. Prior to the eighth week of development, there is no evident morphologic sexual differentiation. Subsequently, müllerian development and fusion result in formation of the uterus and vagina. Normal müllerian development is inhibited by testicular androgens, as has been proved by studies that demonstrated that castrated male rabbit fetuses uniformly undergo normal müllerian development. As fetal development proceeds, the müllerian structures join with the endodermally derived structures of the urogenital sinus to complete the development of the internal genitalia. The external genitalia are derived from the ectoderm and include the vulva, the major and minor labia, and the clitoris. Embryologically, müllerian and wolffian abnormalities frequently coexist, and thus surgeons must be alert to the possibility of urologic abnormalities in patients with developmental gynecologic abnormalities.

ANSWER: A

2. A 23-year-old woman presents to you after undergoing a diagnostic laparoscopy. After pathologic examination of a specimen, she is diagnosed with endometriosis, which agrees with her history of pelvic pain. She wants to discuss options for treatment. You counsel her that:

A. Endometriosis is a diffuse disease, and often surgical correction by itself is not adequate.
B. Multiple medical options exist for suppressing this disease.
C. Medical treatment is curative for this process.
D. Cauterization of implants cures the disease.

Ref.: 3

COMMENTS: Endometriosis is defined as endometrial tissue found outside the endometrial cavity. To make the diagnosis, two of three findings must be present on the histologic examination: endometrial glands, endometrial stroma, and hemosiderin-laden macrophages. Many theories have been postulated concerning the origin of the endometrial implants, but no one theory explains all findings. When considering treatment for this disease, numerous options exist. We know that surgical treatment is effective in "debulking" the disease, but this treatment affects only the visible or superficial findings and not the deeper implants, which may not be readily visible. Endometrial implants can invade to 10 mm and so may not be readily visible on laparoscopy. Therefore medical therapy is often given in conjunction with surgery. The goal is to induce a pseudopregnancy state so the normal menstrual fluctuation is nonexistent. Pregnancy is one option to suppress the implants if it is so desired. Other options include a continuous dose of oral contraceptive (typically of moderate androgenicity), continuous Depo-Provera (every month to suppress menses), gonadotropin-releasing hormone agonists, or antagonists for 3- to 6-month periods. A shortcoming of medical therapy is that once the therapy stops the implants often reactivate and the pain returns. It is important during counseling that the chronic nature of the disease is stressed to the patient and that continuous reevaluation be performed.

ANSWER: A, B

3. Match the supportive structures of the uterus in the left column with their appropriate description in the right column.

A. Round ligament	a. Contains the ovarian artery, vein, and nerve
B. Broad ligament	b. Contains uterine vessels
C. Infundibulopelvic ligament	c. Provides anteversion or flexion of the uterus
D. Uterosacral–cardinal ligament complex	d. Supports the uterus at the apex of the vagina

Ref.: 3, 4

COMMENTS: A number of ligamentous structures support the uterus. The **round ligament** provides accessory support to maintain anteversion of the uterus, thereby ensuring stability during times of increased intraabdominal pressure. The **broad ligament** provides a route for the entrance and egress of blood vessels and lymphatics. The **infundibulopelvic ligament** contains the ovarian vessels and nerves. It also provides some support for the ovary. The **uterosacral–cardinal ligament**

complex is the most important suspensory apparatus of the uterus. It includes a meshwork of fibers that hold the cervix and upper vagina over the levator plate.

ANSWER: A-c; B-b; C-a; D-d

4. Regarding menopause, which of the following statements is/are true?

A. The primary physiologic event is depletion of the number of ovarian follicles.
B. Menopausal symptoms tend to be gradual in onset, with marked variability in the age of onset.
C. A dry vagina, hot flashes, osteoporosis, and increased cardiovascular risk are sequelae of menopause.
D. Progesterone should not be used to treat the symptoms of menopause because of the risk of inducing uterine bleeding.
E. Menopause may be asymptomatic.

Ref.: 3

COMMENTS: Menopause refers to the gradual cessation of ovarian function and occurs at an average age of 50 years, although this may vary. The initial event is thought to be a decrease in the number of ovarian follicles. As these cells degenerate they fail to respond to gonadotropin, and as a consequence less estrogen is produced. Subsequent manifestations of estrogen depletion include hot flashes, vaginal drying, increasing risk of myocardial infarction, and osteoporosis. Estrogen replacement therapy (ERT) is highly effective in ameliorating these symptoms. Prior to institution of ERT, the patient should have a breast and pelvic examination along with screening mammography and a cervical Papanicolaou smear. Contraindications to ERT include a history of endometrial cancer, active thromboembolic disease, and undiagnosed abnormal vaginal bleeding; a history of breast cancer is a relative contraindication. Note that hypertension is **not** a contraindication for ERT. Estrogen *always* should be prescribed together with some form of progesterone in women who have a uterus, as it prevents the development of endometrial hyperplasia and cancer. Women without a uterus should be given unopposed estrogen. Some women may have ''breakthrough bleeding'' on an estrogen-progesterone regimen, but it does not preclude the regimen's use. If there is any question whatever about the cause of such bleeding, an endometrial biopsy can be used to differentiate hormonally induced bleeding from that due to malignancy.

ANSWER: A, B, C, E

5. Match each clinical problem in the left column with its etiology in the right column.

A. A 76-year-old woman with frequent urine loss since her stroke	a. Urinary fistula
B. A 50-year-old woman with urinary leakage when coughing	b. Urethral syndrome
C. A 25-year-old woman with urinary frequency	c. Stress incontinence
D. A 63-year-old woman with dribbling 2 months after a hysterectomy	d. Urge incontinence
E. A 32-year-old woman with dribbling, dysuria, and dyspareunia	e. Urethral diverticulum

Ref.: 3

COMMENTS: Urinary incontinence is a common problem in the United States; it is estimated that 28–40% of all mature women have some degree of leakage. **Stress incontinence** is the most common type; the patient has urine loss when there is increased intraabdominal pressure, such as with coughing and sneezing. Although the etiology is multifactorial, typically there is an anatomic defect at the bladder neck. **Urge incontinence** or detrusor muscle instability is also a prevalent cause of incontinence. It is the most common form of incontinence among the elderly and in those with neurologic diseases such as stroke, Parkinson's disease, or multiple sclerosis. The symptoms include a strong sensation of urgency and an inability to inhibit urine loss. This can happen during activity or while resting. Sensory disorders include **urethral syndrome** and **interstitial cystitis**, both of which present with irritative voiding symptoms such as frequency, dysuria, and urgency. These diseases usually occur in young women who have negative urine cultures. **Urinary fistula** is another cause of incontinence. This is an important consideration in women with the onset, or worsening, of incontinence after pelvic surgery. The classic triad of dribbling, dyspareunia, and dysuria suggests a **urethral diverticulum**. These women may have a tender suburethral mass. Frequently, they give a history of frequent urinary tract infections. The diagnosis can be confirmed with urethroscopy or a voiding cystourethrogram.

ANSWER: A-d; B-c; C-b; D-a; E-e

6. Which of the following therapeutic approaches to the problem of stress urinary incontinence in the female is/are considered acceptable?

A. Kegel pelvic muscle exercises.
B. Drugs.
C. Transvaginal surgical repair.
D. Transabdominal surgical repair.

Ref.: 3

COMMENTS: Stress urinary incontinence is the result of an anatomic defect at the bladder neck. Both medical and surgical therapy is available for this problem. Kegel **pelvic muscle exercises** are an effective treatment for mild stress incontinence and consist of intermittent contractions of the levator ani muscles. Like any exercises, however, if they are not done properly and on a consistent basis they are not effective. **Drugs** have been used to treat stress urinary incontinence. Imipramine or the sympathomimetic-like phenylpropanolamine can improve stress incontinence by increasing urethral pressure. When the drug is discontinued, however, the symptoms return. Surgery is the only permanent treatment of stress incontinence. One hundred (more or less) operations have been described for the treatment of this condition. The goal of all of them is to support the bladder neck. Operations in current use utilizing transabdominal retropubic urethropexy include the **retropubic** Marshall-Marchetti-Krantz procedure and the Burch procedure. Retropubic approaches utilizing a needle suspension, such as the Stamey and Pereyra procedure, have less associated morbidity but are also less effective than transabdominal approaches. **Transvaginal operations** such as the Kelly-Kennedy plication and anterior colporrhaphy are older, less effective operations. Concomitant hysterectomy should not be performed unless there is a separate indication for it.

ANSWER: A, B, C, D

7. Match each clinical presentation in the left column with the appropriate diagnosis in the right column.

A. First trimester bleeding; os closed; no tissue passed; fetus with heartbeat seen on ultrasonography	a. Incomplete abortion
B. First trimester bleeding; tissue protrudes through os	b. Ectopic pregnancy
C. First trimester bleeding; os closed; ultrasonography shows a sac without a fetal pole; adnexa are clear	c. Septic abortion
D. Abdominal pain, fever, uterine tenderness; urine pregnancy test positive	d. Threatened abortion
E. First trimester with urine pregnancy test result positive; abdominal pain; os closed; ultrasonography shows nothing in uterus	e. Missed abortion

Ref.: 3

COMMENTS: *Any woman* with first trimester bleeding is considered to have an **ectopic pregnancy** until proven otherwise. The most common cause of maternal death in the United States is from complications of ectopic pregnancy. Other diagnoses include abortion, molar pregnancy, genital lacerations, and cervicitis. After clinical examination a patient with suspected ectopic pregnancy should have a quantitative serum human chorionic gonadotropin β (β-hCG) level determined and an ultrasound study done if she is hemodynamically stable. Some important points to keep in mind when ectopic pregnancy is a consideration include the following: (1) A sac with a fetal pole (embryonic structure seen on an ultrasound study prior to visualization of the heartbeat) should be seen on a transabdominal ultrasound scan if the quantitative hCG level is greater than 6000 IU. (2) A woman with a viable, intrauterine pregnancy should have a quantitative hCG level that roughly doubles every 48 hours. (3) Most pregnancies cannot be visualized on abdominal ultrasonography until 6 weeks' gestation. **Abortion** is loss of pregnancy prior to 20 weeks' gestation. An **incomplete abortion** means that there has been passage of some, but not all, fetal and placental tissue; often the cervical os is open. A **threatened abortion** means that the pregnancy is still viable (β-hCG level is doubling appropriately), and the os is closed. A **missed abortion** presents as nonviability on ultrasound examination (sac but no fetal pole) and a declining serum hCG; the os is closed. Finally, a **septic abortion** is any type of abortion accompanied by uterine infection. Infection occurs in about 1–2% of all spontaneous abortions.

ANSWER: A-d; B-a; C-e; D-c; E-b

8. A 19-year-old woman comes to the emergency room complaining of right lower quadrant pain, nausea, and vomiting. Her last menstrual period was 6 weeks ago. Which of the following are true statements?

A. A quantitative β-hCG level and a pelvic ultrasound examination are crucial diagnostic tests.
B. If an unruptured ectopic pregnancy is found at laparoscopy, an attempt should be made to remove the products of conception and spare the fallopian tube.
C. Laparotomy is generally reserved for laparoscopic failures or for patients who are in unstable condition as a result of acute blood loss.
D. It generally is advisable to perform an appendectomy to avoid future diagnostic confusion because of the high incidence of recurrent ectopic pregnancy.

Ref.: 3

COMMENTS: With the availability of ultrasonography and sensitive assays for the β-subunit of hCG, ectopic pregnancy can be diagnosed much earlier than was previously the case. Laparoscopy has become the preferred procedure to diagnose and treat unruptured ectopic pregnancy. An incision is made on the antimesenteric side of the fallopian tube, immediately over the implantation site, and the products of conception are removed using gentle traction. Although it seems that the incidence of repeat ectopic pregnancy should be high, the recurrence rate is not significantly increased. On the other hand, in appropriately selected patients the incidence of subsequent intrauterine pregnancy is substantially increased when conservative procedures are performed.

ANSWER: A, B, C

9. Match each of the following clinical conditions in the left column with the appropriate feature in the right column.

A. *Trichomonas* vaginitis	a. Acid environment, marked pruritus
B. *Candida* vaginitis	b. Estrogen withdrawal
C. Bacterial vaginosis	c. Alkaline environment
D. Atrophic vaginitis	d. Foul, "fishy" odor predominant; positive "whiff" test; vaginal pH >6.0

Ref.: 3

COMMENTS: Vaginitis can be caused by infections, allergic reactions, neoplasms, and foreign bodies. The most common infectious causes are *Candida*, *Trichomonas*, and bacterial vaginosis (formerly nonspecific vaginitis or *Gardnerella* vaginitis). Atrophic vaginitis occurs when estrogens available to the vagina fall below certain physiologic levels. This is common with a natural menopause. It can happen also after surgical or radiation-induced castration or with administration of antiestrogen drugs.

ANSWER: A-c; B-a; C-d; D-b

10. Regarding endometriosis, which of the following statements is/are true?

A. Reflux of endometrial tissue through the fallopian tubes is the only recognized explanation for the occurrence of endometriosis.
B. The severity of pain bears a fairly direct relation to the size of the endometrial implants present.

C. Gastrointestinal bleeding or obstruction may be caused by endometriosis.
D. Inducing a "pseudopregnant" state with hormone manipulation may relieve the symptoms of endometriosis.
E. As many as one-third of patients with endometriosis are asymptomatic.

Ref.: 3

COMMENTS: Endometriosis is caused by the presence and growth of endometrial cells outside the uterine cavity. Several theories are proposed as an attempt to explain the pathogenesis of endometriosis. The most popular theory is that endometriosis results from retrograde menstruation. The presence of endometriosis in the lung and other areas distant from the uterus suggests that endometriosis also may result from activation of embryologic nests of tissues present at birth. Most endometrial implants are found in the pelvis, with the ovaries being the most common site involved. Other common places for implantation include the cul-de-sac and uterosacral ligaments. Endometrial implants are found on the serosa of the large bowel (most often rectosigmoid areas) and the small bowel; when on the small bowel they can cause bowel obstruction and bleeding. The classic symptoms of endometriosis are dysmenorrhea and infertility, thought to be the result of cyclic bleeding within the ectopic tissue. Dyspareunia and abnormal bleeding also are symptoms of endometriosis. Up to one-third of patients with endometriosis, however, are asymptomatic. There does not appear to be any correlation with the extent of the disease and the severity of pain. Medical therapy for endometriosis usually involves hormone manipulation, including establishment of a "pseudopregnancy" state with birth control pills. A "pseudomenopause" can be induced with danazol or gonadotropin-releasing hormone (GnRH) agonists, which inhibit ovarian function. Patients who have completed their childbearing or who are refractory to medical management may be treated surgically with a hysterectomy and bilateral salpingo-oophorectomy.

ANSWER: C, D, E

11. Regarding carcinoma of the cervix, which of the following statements is/are true?

A. It is the most common malignancy of the female genital tract.
B. Most are squamous cell carcinoma.
C. Early childbearing and multiple sexual partners appear to be risk factors.
D. There possibly is a viral etiology.
E. The death rate from this disease has declined in recent years.
F. A Papanicolaou (Pap) smear is 100% sensitive for cervical cancer.

Ref.: 1, 2

COMMENTS: Endometrial cancer is the most common gynecologic malignancy. Cancer of the cervix is the *second most common type*, accounting for approximately 40% of all gynecologic malignancies. Approximately 95% of cervical cancers are squamous in type; and usually they begin at the squamocolumnar junction of the cervix. Early pregnancy and multiparity appear to be risk factors for the development of cervical carcinoma. Further, there is an increased incidence in women with a history of multiple sexual partners, suggesting a possible viral etiology. This has been supported by the association of cervical carcinoma with several viruses (herpes simplex type II, papilloma virus, and cytomegalovirus). Screening Pap smears have assisted early detection and have led to improved cure and survival rates in recent years.

ANSWER: B, C, D, E

12. Regarding the Papanicolaou (Pap) smear, which of the following statements is/are true?

A. It is approximately 95% accurate when screening for cervical carcinoma.
B. A negative smear result effectively rules out the presence of carcinoma.
C. Abnormal-appearing epithelial cells that are not frankly malignant suggest an underlying inflammatory process.
D. A definitive histologic diagnosis cannot be made on the basis of the smear results alone.

Ref.: 1, 2

COMMENTS: Wide use of the Pap smear has made it possible to screen large populations of women for cervical carcinoma. Results of the Pap smear are accurate approximately 95% of the time; however, as with any screening technique, false-negative or false-positive findings may occur. Because it is a cytologic technique, it may indicate the presence of malignant cells but does not give information about the degree of invasiveness. Definitive diagnosis requires colposcopic evaluation and a tissue diagnosis. The Pap smear also aids in the detection of preinvasive, dysplastic lesions.

ANSWER: A, D

13. Regarding carcinoma in situ of the uterine cervix, which of the following statements is/are true?

A. It can be diagnosed definitively by Pap smear.
B. It has a predisposition for developing into invasive carcinoma.
C. Its proper treatment requires hysterectomy.
D. Local radiation therapy is the preferred treatment.

Ref.: 1, 2

COMMENTS: Carcinoma in situ of the cervix usually is asymptomatic and therefore is most often suspected because of abnormal results of a Pap smear. The definitive diagnosis requires a cervical biopsy showing malignant cells confined to the superficial layers of the cervical epithelium without invasion through basement membrane. As with in situ carcinoma at other sites, carcinoma in situ of the cervix is associated with a high incidence of concurrent or future development of invasive carcinoma. For this reason aggressive therapy is indicated, which usually means either hysterectomy or, in women who wish to retain the ability to bear children, conization of the cervix. Other cytodestructive techniques, such as laser therapy, cryosurgery, and electrocoagulation, are not acceptable treatments because they do not provide a specimen whose margins can be examined microscopically for completeness of excision. Radiotherapy has also been employed but offers no benefit over conization and has considerably more significant side effects.

ANSWER: B

14. Match each clinical finding for carcinoma of the cervix in the left column with the appropriate clinical stage in the right column.

A. Bladder mucosal involvement	a. I
B. Involvement of the lower one-third of the vagina	b. II
C. Hydronephrosis	c. III
D. Parametrial involvement	d. IV
E. Attachment to the lateral pelvic wall	

Ref.: 1, 2

COMMENTS: As with other malignancies, clinical staging of carcinoma of the cervix influences treatment and has a strong relation to prognosis. The clinical staging of the primary tumor is accomplished by physical examination, intravenous pyelography, cytoscopy, proctoscopy, or computed tomography (CT). **Stage I** tumors are confined to the cervix. **Stage II** tumors may involve the upper two-thirds of the vagina (IIA) or the parametrial tissues (IIB). **Stage III** tumors extend through the parametrial tissues to the pelvic side wall, extend to the lower one-third of the vagina, or result in ureteral obstruction. **Stage IV** tumors may invade the bladder or rectal mucosa, or they may have spread outside the pelvis.

ANSWER: A-d; B-c; C-c; D-b; E-c

15. Match each characteristic in the left column with the tumor(s) to which there is an association in the right column.

A. Nulliparity	a. Cancer of the cervix
B. Late first pregnancy	b. Cancer of the endometrium
C. Obesity	c. Cancer of the breast
D. Prolonged use of unopposed estrogens	
E. Primarily adenocarcinoma	
F. Positive family history	

Ref.: 1, 2

COMMENTS: Endometrial and breast cancers share a number of epidemiologic characteristics. Nulliparity and late first pregnancy both increase the risk of developing these cancers. This is in contrast to cancer of the cervix, which occurs with greater frequency in patients with early sexual activity or with multiple partners. There is an association between obesity and carcinoma of the endometrium and breast, although the association is much stronger for endometrial cancer. Prolonged, unopposed use of estrogen for management of menopausal symptoms is thought to increase the risk of breast carcinoma slightly; birth control pills have not been shown to increase this risk. Once again, however, this association is much more pronounced with endometrial carcinoma. Although cancer of the cervix, endometrium, and breast can affect more than one member of a family, only with breast cancer is a positive family history considered a significant risk factor.

ANSWER: A-b,c; B-b,c; C-b,c; D-b,c; E-b,c; F-c

16. Which of the following is the most common form of uterine sarcoma?

A. Mixed müllerian tumor.
B. Endolymphatic stromal myosis.
C. Stromal sarcoma.
D. Leiomyosarcoma.

Ref.: 1, 2

COMMENTS: Uterine sarcomas are not common, accounting for fewer than 5% of all uterine malignancies. They tend to occur in the postmenopausal patient and generally carry a poor prognosis. These tumors arise primarily from two tissues: endometrial sarcomas from the endometrial glands and stroma and leiomyosarcomas from the uterine muscle itself. **Leiomyosarcoma** is the most common uterine sarcoma. It rarely arises from a previous leiomyoma; but when it does, the prognosis appears to be more favorable. **Mixed müllerian tumors** contain both adenocarcinomatous and sarcomatous elements. **Endolymphatic stromal myosis** and its more aggressive counterpart, **stromal sarcoma**, represent invasion of the myometrium by stromal cells of the endometrium. All of these tumors, when confined to the uterus, are treated by hysterectomy.

ANSWER: D

17. Match each ovarian tumor in the left column with its appropriate characteristics in the right column.

A. Teratoma	a. Masculinizing
B. Granulosa-theca cell tumor	b. Totipotential cell
C. Sertoli-Leydig cell tumor	c. Thyroid tissue
D. Struma ovarii	d. hCG
E. Choriocarcinoma	e. Elaborate estrogen

Ref.: 1, 2

COMMENTS: Many of the unusual ovarian tumors are characterized by their capacity to elaborate humoral substances or to manifest pluripotentiality in their growth patterns; they have varying malignant potential. A **teratoma** is a germ cell tumor that arises from the totipotential ovarian germ cell and may contain differentiated tissues that are grossly or histologically recognizable (e.g., brain, teeth, hair, muscle, bone). In its benign form (cystic teratoma or dermoid), simple excision suffices. Careful inspection or bivalving of the opposite ovary must be performed because of the incidence (15–20%) of bilaterality. **Granulosa-theca cell tumors** usually elaborate estrogen and have been associated with precocious puberty in young patients and endometrial carcinoma in the older age groups. **Sertoli-Leydig cell tumors** (arrhenoblastomas) are associated with androgen output and masculinization, and they have a malignant potential of 25%. **Struma ovarii** refers to the presence of thyroid tissue and is considered a component element in some dermoid cysts. Occasionally hyperthyroidism results. **Choriocarcinoma** is a rare primary tumor of the ovary that elaborates chorionic gonadotropin, which also occurs in this variation of trophoblastic disease. Treatment for all of these tumors depends on the extent of disease when diagnosed, but in their early stages many are appropriately treated by unilateral oophorectomy.

ANSWER: A-b; B-e; C-a; D-c; E-d

18. A 22-year-old woman with intermittent pelvic pain underwent an ultrasound examination; the image is displayed below. Which of the following is/are true of this lesion?

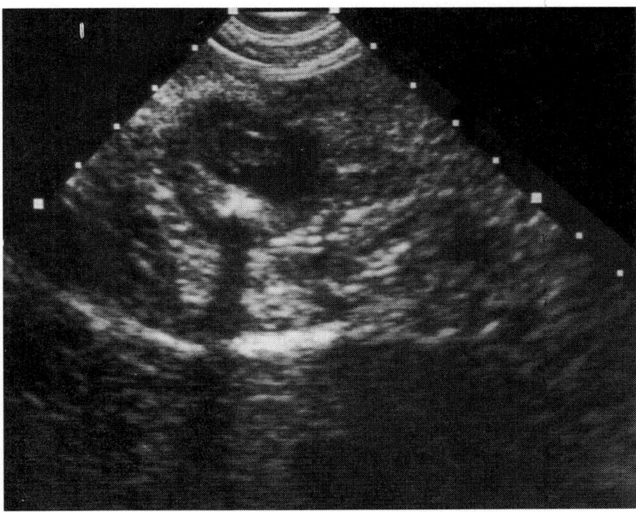

A. Bilateral in 15–20% of cases.
B. Responds to antibiotic therapy.
C. Is often malignant.
D. Pain is aggravated with menstruation.
E. Diagnosis may be made on plain film, CT, or magnetic resonance imaging (MRI).

Ref.: 5

COMMENTS: The *ultrasound* image displays a cystic teratoma, as evidenced by the calcification and fat within it. This is the most common germ cell tumor in the female pelvis and is most frequently seen in patients younger than 20 years of age. Histologically, tissue from all three germ layers are present. The term "dermoid cyst" is used interchangeably; however, a true dermoid tumor has elements derived only from the ectoderm. The tumors are bilateral 15–20% of the time and are almost always benign, having a less than 1% risk of malignant degeneration. They rarely rupture because of the thick capsule that surrounds them, but torsion is fairly common. • The sonographic appearance may be variable; it may be predominantly cystic or complex with internal calcifications. Fat-fluid levels may be identified, or the lesion may be diffusely echogenic. The presence of echogenic material suggests the presence of fat, which is most helpful for establishing the diagnosis. • *Plain films* of the pelvis may reveal fat, bone, or teeth. *CT* may display low attenuation values consistent with fat; calcifications also may be identified. Recently, *MRI* protocols were established specifically to examine for fat.

ANSWER: A, E

19. Match the extent of involvement in the left column with the appropriate stage of ovarian adenocarcinoma in the right column.

A. Unilateral fallopian involvement	a. Stage I
B. Both ovaries involved	b. Stage II
C. Studding of the outer surface of the bladder	c. Stage III
D. Malignant pleural effusion	d. Stage IV
E. Involvement of the undersurface of the diaphragm	

Ref.: 1, 2

COMMENTS: See Question 20.

20. Regarding ovarian adenocarcinoma, which of the following statements is/are true?

A. At laparotomy, peritoneal fluid or washings should be routinely sent for cytologic examination.
B. Total abdominal hysterectomy and bilateral salpingo-oophorectomy should be reserved for patients with bilateral ovarian involvement.
C. "Debulking" ovarian tumors (i.e., removing as much gross tumor as possible plus the abdominal metastases) may contribute to improved survival.
D. Chemotherapy has done little to improve survival.
E. Primary carcinoma of the breast, stomach, and colon are the most common sources of metastases to the ovary.

Ref.: 1, 2

COMMENTS: Primary adenocarcinomas of the ovary may be **serous**, **mucinous**, or **endometrioid**. Most patients present with advanced-stage disease. There is no effective screening test for ovarian carcinoma. They are staged as follows: **stage I**, one or both ovaries; **stage II**, extraovarian involvement but contained within the true pelvis; **stage III**, involvement of the abdomen outside the true pelvis; **stage IV**, spread beyond the abdominal cavity or within the liver. Peritoneal washings must be obtained for cytologic examination when the abdomen is opened for suspected ovarian carcinoma. • With rare exceptions (e.g., a small, unilateral ovarian tumor in a patient who insists on retaining her childbearing capability), the operative therapy of ovarian carcinoma is total abdominal hysterectomy and bilateral salpingo-oophorectomy with debulking of as much gross intraabdominal disease as possible. It includes routine omentectomy, because the omentum is a common site for histologic metastasis not grossly apparent at the time of laparotomy. • Some evidence suggests that cytoreductive ("debulking") surgery improves the response to chemotherapy and consequently improves survival. Adjuvant chemotherapy (usually cisplatin-based) is generally required. Overall 5-year survival is poor. • The ovary also may be the site of metastasis from other epithelial tumors. About 6% of ovarian cancers encountered during exploration for a pelvic mass are metastatic, usually from primary cancers of the gastrointestinal tract, breast, thyroid, or lymphatic tissue.

ANSWER:
Question 19: A-b; B-a; C-b; D-d; E-c
Question 20: A, C, E

21. Which of the following statements is/are true regarding the evaluation of ovarian masses?

A. In infants and young children they are most often malignant germ cell tumors.
B. During the reproductive years, cystic masses smaller than 5 cm may be simply observed.
C. Clinical characteristics usually suffice to distinguish benign from malignant lesions.
D. Laparoscopy provides little practical information because all patients with ovarian masses require laparotomy for management.

Ref.: 1, 2

COMMENTS: Pelvic masses in females may arise from the genital tract, lower urinary tract, gastrointestinal tract, or mesenchymal structures of the pelvis; they may be developmental, inflammatory, or neoplastic. The evaluation of a pelvic mass that is thought to represent ovarian pathology is best accomplished initially with careful bimanual pelvic examination (when appropriate according to age) and ultrasonography. In the absence of extensive disease in the pelvis or fixation of the mass, the clinical diagnosis of ovarian malignancy may be difficult. **Ultrasonography** may demonstrate features suggestive of malignancy, including solid components, irregular borders, and ascites. A firm diagnosis depends on tissue examination. **Laparoscopy** is a safe method for evaluating pelvic masses and may provide sufficient diagnostic information (e.g., case of simple ovarian cyst or endometriosis), precluding the need for laparotomy. In *infants and young children*, one must be alert to nonovarian causes of pelvic masses, including Wilms' tumor, imperforate hymen, and bladder abnormalities. Ovarian tumors in this age group are rarely malignant and most likely are benign teratomas. In *women of reproductive age*, cystic masses smaller than 5 cm usually represent benign follicle cysts and may be followed through one or two menstrual cycles. Treatment with oral contraceptives may hasten resolution of these cysts. Larger masses, those with hard consistency, or those that persist should be further investigated with laparoscopy or laparotomy. In *postmenopausal* women, ovarian masses should be evaluated and operation performed when they are discovered because the probability of malignancy increases sharply after the age of 50 years. A plan of observation and follow-up is not applicable to the infant or young girl. In these patients any enlargement mandates surgical exploration because spontaneous resolution is unlikely.

ANSWER: B

22. Which one or more of the following items accurately characterize(s) Meigs syndrome?

A. Hydrothorax.
B. Ascites.
C. Chylothorax.
D. Malignant ovarian tumor.
E. Curable by excising the ovarian fibroma.

Ref.: 1, 2

COMMENTS: **Meigs syndrome** refers to the coexistence of hydrothorax, ascites, and an underlying benign ovarian tumor, usually a fibroma. The pathophysiology of the ascites and pleural fluid is unclear, but they may result from lymphatic obstruction of the ovary. Excision of the ovarian fibroma is usually accompanied by resolution of the findings. Many ovarian malignancies are also associated with ascites and pleural effusion, which some refer to as "pseudo-Meigs" or "malignant Meigs" syndrome.

ANSWER: A, B, E

23. Match each vaginal cancer in the left column with its appropriate characteristics in the right column.

A. Clear cell carcinoma	a. Most common primary vaginal malignancy
B. Sarcoma botryoides	b. Most common vaginal malignancy
C. Squamous cell carcinoma	c. Diethylstilbestrol exposure in utero
D. Involvement from malignancies of adjacent organs	d. Seen in young children

Ref.: 1, 2

COMMENTS: **Primary cancer** of the vagina is rare; most commonly, cancerous involvement is the result of extension from primary tumors of the adjoining vulva, cervix, or endometrium. **Squamous cell carcinoma** is the most common primary vaginal malignancy. This is not unexpected, because the vagina is lined by squamous epithelium. These tumors most often occur in postmenopausal women, although there are notable exceptions: **Sarcoma botryoides**, a bulky, polypoid sarcoma, occurs in infants and young children; and **clear cell carcinoma** (mesonephroma), an adenocarcinoma, frequently occurs in the adolescent or young adult offspring of mothers who took diethylstilbestrol during pregnancy. Treatment for these tumors may be by operation (frequently requiring partial or total pelvic exenteration), irradiation, or a combination of the two.

ANSWER: A-c; B-d; C-a; D-b

24. Which of the following vulvar abnormalities is/are considered to be risk factor(s) for invasive malignancy?

A. Hypertrophic dystrophy without atypia.
B. Lichen sclerosis.
C. Vulvar intraepithelial neoplasm III.
D. Paget's disease.

Ref.: 3

COMMENTS: Tissue diagnosis is required for these vulvar lesions. **Vulvar dystrophies** are of two types: lichen sclerosis and hyperplastic dystrophy (with or without atypia). **Lichen sclerosis** has no significant relation to vulvar malignancy. It is a patchy, white lesion that produces pruritus and is thought to be related to chronic irritation. **Hyperplastic dystrophy without atypia** is not a premalignant condition. Atypical changes, however, begin the spectrum of intraepithelial neoplasia. **Vulvar intraepithelial neoplasia (VIN I, II, III)** is a preinvasive or in situ squamous carcinoma that requires surgical excision. It is frequently multifocal, and it is premalignant. **Paget's disease** appears as an ulcerative, eczematoid vulvar lesion, with the histologic finding of large, foamy pagetoid cells. As with Paget's disease of the breast, this finding is suggestive of an underlying adenocarcinoma (in approximately 2% of cases). In the vulva it is thought to arise from the apocrine sweat glands. Paget's disease usually requires wide surgical excision and careful follow-up.

ANSWER: C, D

25. Which of the following statements regarding invasive squamous cell carcinoma of the vulva is/are true?

A. The "typical" patient is elderly, nulliparous, and obese.
B. The primary tumor is usually unilateral.
C. The regional lymph nodes most likely involved are those along the ipsilateral common iliac vein.
D. Bilateral regional lymph node metastases are rare.
E. The proper treatment for most cases is radical vulvectomy, with bilateral superficial inguinal lymph node dissections.

Ref.: 1, 2

COMMENTS: Invasive vulvar malignancies account for approximately 4% of all cancers of the female genital tract; and among them, squamous carcinoma accounts for most. Epidemiologically, these tumors occur with greater frequency in elderly, nulliparous, obese women. They may present anywhere on the vulva but are usually unilateral. Nonetheless, the rich lymphatic networks that interdigitate across the midline result in a high incidence of bilateral lymph node metastases, most often in the inguinal region caudal to the inguinal ligament. For this reason, proper curative treatment for this tumor is total radical vulvectomy, with bilateral inguinal lymphadenectomy. The role of prophylactic iliac lymphadenectomy is controversial, but most reserve this procedure for cases in which the superficial inguinal nodes are grossly involved. The overall cure rate for invasive squamous cell carcinoma of the vulva is approximately 50%, but it may be as high as 80–90% in women with negative regional lymph node results at biopsy.

ANSWER: A, B, E

26. Regarding endometrial carcinoma, which of the following statements is/are true?

A. Postmenopausal hormone replacement with progesterone increases the risk of the development of endometrial cancer.
B. Endometrial cancer is the most common malignancy of the female genital tract.
C. Endometrial cancer commonly arises in uterine leiomyomas.
D. Endometrial cancer is staged surgically.
E. Currently, there is no role for radiation therapy in the treatment of endometrial cancer.

Ref.: 3

COMMENTS: Surgery and radiation therapy, alone or in combination, are the principal treatment modalities for endometrial carcinoma. As with carcinoma of the cervix, surgery alone is reserved for the early stages of the disease. Endometrial carcinoma is staged surgically because there is no reliable way to do so preoperatively. The principal value of staging endometrial cancer is to determine appropriate adjuvant therapy, if any, and to estimate the prognosis. Extension of the tumor beyond the corpus (stage II, III, or IV) is most often treated by surgery and irradiation in combination. Once endometrial cancer is diagnosed, estrogens are contraindicated because of their suspected role in the promotion of endometrial carcinoma. Postmenopausal hormone replacement with progesterone, however, does not increase the risk of endometrial cancer. The overall 5-year survival following appropriate therapy of endometrial carcinoma is in the range of 50%, but it can be as high as 80% for patients with stage I disease.

ANSWER: B, D

27. Match each clinical finding in the left column with the appropriate stage for endometrial carcinoma in the right column.

A. Confined to corpus	a. I
B. Rectal mucosal involvement	b. II
C. Cervix involvement	c. III
D. Vaginal involvement	d. IV
E. Ovary involvement	

Ref.: 1, 2

COMMENTS: The staging for endometrial cancer has been completely revised. Corpus cancer is now surgically staged. Fractional dilatation and curettage (D & C), commonly used to differentiate between stages I and II, is no longer necessary. The staging is as follows: **Stage I**, confined to the corpus. The degree of myometrial involvement and histopathologic grading are important considerations for substaging. **Stage II**, extension to the cervix. **Stage III**, involvement of the adnexa, vagina, or positive peritoneal cytology. **Stage IV**, involvement of the bowel or bladder mucosa or the presence of distant metastases.

ANSWER: A-a; B-d; C-b; D-c; E-c

28. Which of the following statements is/are true regarding trophoblastic disease?

A. The risk of malignant, metastatic trophoblastic disease following partial hydatidiform mole is 3–5%.
B. Patients at high risk for metastatic trophoblastic disease include women with twins and women who smoke more than two packs of cigarettes per day.
C. Hysterotomy is preferable to suction curettage when emptying a 16-week gestational size uterus.
D. Patients with nonmetastatic or low risk gestational trophoblastic disease are 100% curable by chemotherapy.
E. Complete hydatidiform moles are of paternal origin and carry a 20% risk of malignant sequelae.

Ref.: 1, 2, 3

COMMENTS: Gestational trophoblastic disease is categorized as **hydatidiform mole** (partial or complete) and **gestational trophoblastic neoplasia** (metastatic and nonmetastatic). About one-half of the cases of gestational trophoblastic neoplasia follow molar pregnancy; one-fourth follow normal pregnancy; and one-fourth follow ectopic pregnancy or abortion. Complete moles are of paternal origin, are diploid, and carry a 20% risk of malignant sequelae. Partial moles are of maternal and paternal origin, are triploid, and rarely are followed by gestational trophoblastic neoplasia. Hydatidiform moles are effectively and safely evacuated using suction curettage. • *Low-risk* gestational trophoblastic neoplasia is one in which the initial serum human chorionic gonadotropin (hCG) titer is less than 40,000 mIU/ml, the disease is present less than 4 months, and there has been no prior chemotherapy. It usually is treated with single-agent chemotherapy. *High-risk* gestational trophoblastic neoplasia has one or more of the following present: an initial serum hCG titer of more than 40,000 mIU/ml, disease present longer than 4 months, brain or liver metastases, and failure of prior chemotherapy. It is treated with multiple-agent chemotherapy.

Prognostic Classification of Gestational Trophoblastic Neoplasia

1. Nonmetastatic GTN
2. Metastatic GTN: Disease outside the uterus
   A. Good prognosis:
      1. Disease present less than 4 months (short duration)
      2. Pretreatment hGC less than 40,000 mIU/ml
      3. No prior chemotherapy
   B. Poor prognosis:
      1. Disease present more than 4 months (long duration), or
      2. Pretreatment hCG greater than 40,000 mIU/ml, or
      3. Presence of brain or liver metastases, or
      4. Failure of prior chemotherapy

From Herbst AL, Mishell DR, Jr, Stenchever MA, Droegemueller W: *Comprehensive Gynecology*, 2nd ed. Mosby-Year Book, St. Louis, 1992, p 934.

ANSWER: A, D, E

29. Complete the following phrase to make one or more true statements: Leiomyomas of the uterus . . .

A. Being mesenchymal rather than epithelial in origin, are not under hormonal influence.
B. Being found within the wall of the uterus rather than within the endometrial cavity itself, are not associated with bleeding.
C. May be the cause of habitual abortion or infertility.
D. If larger than 2 cm, have a significant likelihood of malignant degeneration.
E. Should be treated surgically if there is failure of medical therapy or rapid growth and obstruction of the urinary tract.

Ref.: 1, 2

COMMENTS: Uterine leiomyomas (fibroids) are fairly common, occurring in approximately 50% of women. They present as whorls of interlacing smooth muscle and are characterized according to their location within the uterus: submucosa, intramural, or subserosal layers. Although mesenchymal in origin, they definitely are under hormonal influence and have been seen to grow in response to estrogen administration. The simple presence of leiomyomas is not an indication for treatment, as most are probably asymptomatic. Complications may develop, however, as a result of the size and specific location of the tumor. Fibroids in a submucosal location may bleed significantly, resulting in iron deficiency anemia. They may be pedunculated and undergo a twist of their stalk, with subsequent infarction. They also may be the source of infertility and habitual abortion because of their interference with normal uterine function during pregnancy. Only 1–2% of uterine leiomyomas are thought to undergo malignant transformation, but this point must be considered whenever there is a rapid increase in size of a previously stable tumor. Leiomyomas causing significant problems may be managed by either local excision (myomectomy) or hysterectomy, depending on other clinical circumstances.

ANSWER: C, E

30. Which of the following is/are true concerning the progestin agents found in oral contraceptives?

A. The progestins can be categorized by their androgenic activity and are classified as low, medium, or high androgenic progestins.
B. Norgestimate and desogestrel are examples of medium androgenic progestins.
C. Low androgenic progestins tend to have the lowest side effect profile.
D. When starting a woman on an oral contraceptive, it is best to start her on a medium androgenic formulation.

Ref.: 3

COMMENTS: The first oral contraceptive formulation was introduced in 1960 and contained 9.75 mg of progestin. Since that time, the progestin quantity has been reduced to a level of 0.075 to 2.5 mg depending on the progestin itself. The purpose of the progestin was to inhibit ovulation by suppressing the luteinizing hormone surge. The estrogen component was added to limit breakthrough bleeding. Recently, a new class of progestin, termed the gonanes, was introduced and was found to have a low androgenic effect. Progestins are classified as having high adrogenicity (norgestrel 0.3 mg, norethindrone acetate 1.5–2.5 mg, and levonorgestrel 0.15 mg), medium androgenicity (levonorgestrel triphasic, norethindrone 1.0 triphasic or monophasic, northindrone acetate 1.0 mg, ethynodiol diacetate 1.0 mg, and levonorgestrel 0.1 mg), or low androgenicity (norgestimate, desogestrel, or norethindrone 0.4–0.5 mg monophasic). Typically, it is better to start a patient on the lowest androgenicity, given that the patient then experiences fewer side effects. Exceptions to this rule include specific indications for the oral contraceptive: Women with functional ovarian cysts and endometriosis, those with blood dyscrasias, and those with dysmenorrhea typically do better on a moderate androgenic progestin.

ANSWER: A, C

31. Match each of the following hormones or events with the appropriate letter on the chart of a typical menstrual cycle.

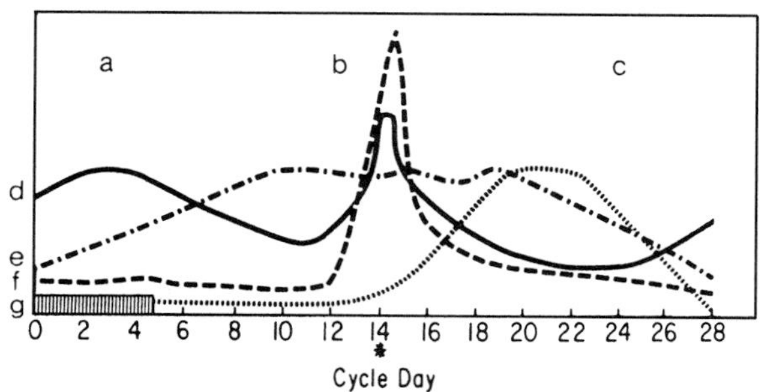

A. Estrogen.
B. Progesterone.
C. Follicle-stimulating hormone (FSH).
D. Luteinizing hormone (LH).
E. Menses.

Ref.: 1, 2

COMMENTS: The typical menstrual cycle occurs as a result of fluctuating levels of gonadotropic and steroid hormones as indicated in the diagram. The physiologic events stimulated by these hormonal fluctuations can be considered in two phases: the proliferative or follicular phase (from the first day of menses to the day of ovulation) and the secretory or luteal phase (from ovulation to the onset of subsequent menses). Estrogen predominates during the proliferative phase, allowing follicular development and endometrial proliferation. Ovulation occurs as a direct result of a midcycle LH surge. The small estrogen surge may also lead to midcycle spotting. If fertilization does not occur, the oocyte begins to break down within 24 hours. The second half of the cycle is a progesterone-dominant time. Finally, in the absence of an implanted ovum, the superficial layers of the endometrium are shed, and FSH again begins rising to stimulate the next cycle of follicular proliferation.

ANSWER: A-e; B-g; C-d; D-f; E-a

32. Which of the following is/are noncontraceptive benefits of oral contraceptives?

A. Decreased incidence of dysmenorrhea.
B. Increased cycle regularity and decreased blood loss.
C. Decreased incidence of ectopic pregnancy and pelvic inflammatory disease.
D. Decreased incidence of benign breast disease.
E. Decreased risk of cervical cancer.
F. Decreased risk of sexually transmitted diseases.

Ref.: 3

COMMENTS: Oral contraceptives provide excellent protection against unwanted pregnancy provided they are taken properly. Often patients are unaware of the numerous noncontraceptive benefits these pills confer: a reduction in dysmenorrhea with increased cycle regularity; increased iron stores for women with heavy menses by decreasing the blood loss with menses; decreased risk of ectopic pregnancy (approximately 400-fold) and decreased incidence of pelvic inflammatory disease (thought to be secondary to thickened cervical mucus); decreased incidence of benign breast conditions including fibromas and fibrocystic changes; decreased risk of endometrial and ovarian cancers depending on how long the pills have been used; and possible decreased incidence of rheumatoid arthritis, increased bone mineral density, and decreased incidence of functional ovarian cysts (mainly with moderate-dose oral contraceptives). Recently, the U.S. Food and Drug Administration (FDA) has approved one formulation for treatment of acne vulgaris, the first FDA-approved noncontraceptive use. Contraceptive pills have little impact on cervical cancer and sexually transmitted diseases.

ANSWER: A, B, C, D

33. Which of the following statements is/are true regarding pain associated with the menstrual cycle?

A. The term "primary dysmenorrhea" refers to painful menses associated with identifiable predisposing gynecologic causes.
B. Dysmenorrhea often is effectively treated by nonsteroidal antiinflammatory drugs, oral contraceptives, or both.
C. The premenstrual syndrome may produce symptoms throughout the entire menstrual cycle.
D. Mittelschmerz is pain occurring between the 10th and 14th days of the cycle from rupture of a graafian follicle; it may be confused with ectopic pregnancy.

Ref.: 2

COMMENTS: A careful history of the time course of pain presumed to be of menstrual cycle origin is useful for determining the cause of it. **Dysmenorrhea** refers to pain occurring during menses and is considered to be either primary (idiopathic) or secondary. Although no exact cause of **primary dysmenorrhea** has been identified, prostaglandins have been implicated. As a result, treatment involving prostaglandin synthetase inhibitors, such as ibuprofen, have been used successfully in many instances. With **secondary dysmenorrhea**, specific abnormalities such as endometriosis, congenital malformations, and uterine myomas have been identified as causes of the pain. The use of oral contraceptives also has been effective in reducing the severity of dysmenorrhea, possibly through the inhibition of endometrial development and prostaglandin synthesis. **Premenstrual syndrome** refers to a constellation of systemic and psychological abnormalities (e.g., anxiety, depression, irritability, edema, acneiform eruptions) that occur within the 10-day period preceding menses. The diagnosis can be excluded if the symptoms occur earlier in the cycle. **Mittelschmerz** (midcycle pain) occurs between the 10th and 14th days of the cycle and is thought to be related to local pelvic peritoneal irritation from a ruptured ovarian follicle. Its characteristic timing and fairly abrupt onset also may mimic the presence of an ectopic pregnancy or gastrointestinal pathology such as appendicitis.

ANSWER: B, D

34. Which of the following conditions may cause hypomenorrhea or amenorrhea?

A. Hyperthyroidism.
B. Cushing syndrome.
C. Excessive aspirin use.
D. Recent death in the family.
E. Sheehan syndrome.
F. Low body weight.
G. Recent weight gain.
H. Training for the marathon.

Ref.: 1, 2

COMMENTS: Amenorrhea or hypomenorrhea may be due to a number of abnormalities of the central nervous system hypothalamic-pituitary-ovarian axis. **Hyperthyroidism** is characteristically associated with hypomenorrhea. Although hypothyroidism classically causes menorrhagia, progressive or persistent hypothyroidism may eventually result in amenorrhea. **Cushing syndrome** can cause amenorrhea, possibly through the inhibitory effect of excessive adrenal androgen production. Primary pituitary problems, such as **Sheehan syndrome** (postpartum pituitary necrosis) or pituitary tumors, also may cause amenorrhea. **Severe stress**, either psychological or metabolic, commonly causes aberrations in the menstrual cycle and may result in temporary amenorrhea. These entities have in common altered pituitary function causing abnormal hormonal interplay. For example, it is not uncommon for women having a major operation to miss a menstrual period. **Significant weight loss** or persistence of marked low body weight also has been commonly associated with amenorrhea. *Female athletes*, especially those involved in endurance sports, also have a significant likelihood of being amenorrheic. Investigation of amenorrhea involves a careful medical and social history, as well as an appropriate endocrinologic assessment.

ANSWER: A, B, D, E, F, H

35. Which of the following statements is/are true concerning pelvic inflammatory disease?

A. Acute pelvic inflammatory disease (PID) usually is a polymicrobial infection of organisms ascending from the vagina and cervix.
B. Approximately one in four women with acute PID experiences other medical sequelae.
C. Oral contraception provides a preventive effect by inhibiting the development of PID.
D. Nausea and vomiting are early symptoms of acute PID.
E. Laparoscopy is the best method to establish accurately the diagnosis of acute PID.
F. Surgery is reserved for patients who fail to improve with antibiotic therapy.

Ref.: 3

COMMENTS: Pelvic inflammatory disease (PID) is a spectrum of inflammatory disorders of the upper genital tract in women. PID may include salpingitis, endometritis, tuboovarian abscess, and pelvic peritonitis. Bacterial organisms cultured from tubal fluid commonly include *Neisseria gonorrhoeae*, *Chlamydia trachomatis*, endogenous aerobic and anaerobic bacteria, and mycoplasma species. *N. gonorrhoeae* and *C. trachomatis* coexist in up to 40% of patients. • The risk factors associated with PID include early age at first intercourse, multiple sexual partners, lack of contraception, and living in an environment in which there is a high prevalence of sexually transmitted disease. • Women who use oral contraception have a lower incidence of PID. This is thought to be due to thicker cervical mucus produced by the progesterone (progestin) component of the pill, which inhibits sperm and bacterial penetration. • Patients with acute PID present with a wide range of clinical symptoms, which commonly include abdominal pain, vaginal discharge, and fever. Nausea and vomiting are late symptoms of acute PID. The diagnosis based on clinical criteria alone has been found to have high false-positive and high false-negative rates. • Diagnostic laparoscopy allows a much more precise diagnosis of this entity. Once thought to be strictly a surgical disease, broad-spectrum antibiotic coverage now is thought to be the initial treatment of choice, with surgery being reserved for those who fail to improve with antibiotic therapy or for patients with recurrent disease who do not care to retain their fertility.

ANSWER: A, B, C, E, F

36. Ultrasonography is based on the reflection of sound in human tissues. Which of the following conditions affect reflectivity?

A. Size of the transducer head.
B. Atomic number of the tissue being scanned.
C. Acoustic impedance.
D. Frequency of the transducer.
E. Angle of the incident sound beam.

COMMENTS: Ultrasonography employs sound waves with a frequency measured in megahertz (millions of cycles per second), compared to audible sound, which is measured in cycles per second (20–20,000 cycles per second). Ultrasound waves require a medium in which to be propagated. The more tightly bound a substance, the faster the sound wave travels. Several principles of wave physics apply to ultrasonography: The strength of the returning echoes is related to the angle at which the beam strikes the acoustic interface. The more perpendicular the beam, the stronger the reflecting echoes. The strength of the returning echoes also depends on differences in acoustic impedance between the various tissues in the body. Acoustic impedance is determined by multiplying the acoustic density of the tissue by the speed of sound in this tissue. The greater the difference in density between the two structures, the stronger the returning echoes. Structures having different acoustic impedance are much easier to distinguish from one another than structures of similar acoustic texture. • Because much of the sound beam is absorbed or scattered as it travels through the body, it undergoes progressive weakening. Transducers are chosen according to the structures being examined. The higher the frequency of the transducer, the less the penetration and the greater the resolution. The frequency of the transducer has nothing to do with the reflection of sound. • The wider the transducer head, the more the beam can be focused; however, as the transducer heads become larger, they are increasingly bulky and cumbersome to use. Small transducer heads can be used to scan between interspaces, or they may be angled into the pelvis. The size of the transducer head has nothing to do with reflectivity. • Atomic number is important for absorption of x-rays in soft tissues but plays no role in the formation of the ultrasound image.

ANSWER: C, E

37. Match each venereal infection listed in the left column with its appropriate characteristics in the right column.

A. Syphilis
B. Gonorrhea
C. Chancroid
D. Granuloma inguinale
E. Lymphogranuloma venereum
F. Condyloma acuminatum
G. Genital herpes

a. Painful ulcer caused by *Haemophilus ducreyi*
b. Associated with cervical dysplasia
c. Purulent discharge; intracellular diplococci
d. Inguinal lymphadenopathy caused by *Chlamydia trachomatis*
e. Painless ulcer; positive darkfield picture
f. Painful vesicles; intranuclear inclusion bodies
g. Nontender ulcers; Donovan bodies

Ref.: 6

COMMENTS: Many of the infections listed above are easily treated if diagnosed early, but they have potentially serious and long-term sequelae if missed or neglected. Primary **syphilis** usually presents as a painless ulcer (chancre). The diagnosis is made by several serologic tests [reactive plasma reagent (RPR), a test for *Treponema*; fluorescent treponemal antibody test (FTA-ABS)]. The preferred treatment is penicillin. **Gonorrhea** can present as a purulent urethritis or cervicitis, although many women who harbor this organism are asymptomatic. The diagnosis is made by identifying vaginal discharge with intracellular gram-negative diplococci or with a positive culture. The treatment favored currently is ceftriaxone and doxycycline. Doxycycline is given because of the concomitant high incidence of *Chlamydia* infections in persons with gonorrhea. Both patient and partner should be treated. Reculture should be done 1–2 months after treatment to detect both treatment failures and reinfection. **Chancroid**, caused by *Haemophilus ducreyi*, presents as a painful genital ulcer; painful inguinal lymphadenopathy is present in about one-half of all chancroid cases. Treatment includes either ceftriaxone or erythromycin. **Granuloma inguinale** is a chronic, ulcerative bacterial infection of the vulva. The diagnosis is established by identifying Donovan bodies in smears or specimens from the ulcers. Tetracycline is effective treatment. **Lymphogranuloma venereum** is caused by *C. trachomatis*. Inguinal lymphadenopathy is the most common clinical manifestation. The diagnosis is made by culturing the pus or aspirate from a tender lymph node. Tetracycline or erythromycin is effective therapy. **Condyloma acuminatum**, or venereal wart, is caused by the human papilloma virus (HPV). There is a strong association between this virus and genital dysplasia and carcinoma. Any woman with condyloma should be screened with a Pap smear. No therapy has been shown to eradicate HPV effectively. Lesions can be removed by a number of methods, including podophyllum application and excision with electrocautery or with laser. Recurrence is fairly common. **Genital herpes** is a viral disease that may be acute, chronic, or recurring. This infection begins as multiple painful vesicles in the genital area, and the initial episode may be associated with systemic symptoms of fever and malaise. There is no known cure for this problem at present. Pap smears of herpes lesions show intranuclear inclusion bodies and multinucleated giant cells. Definitive diagnosis is made by culture or biopsy. Systemic acyclovir treatment accelerates healing but does not eradicate the infection.

ANSWER: A-e; B-c; C-a; D-g; E-d; F-b; G-f

38. Which of the following statements is/are true regarding the course of the ureter?

A. The ureter is retroperitoneal in location in both its abdominal and pelvic portions.
B. The iliopectineal line serves as the marker for the pelvic portion of the ureter.
C. The ureters run downward and laterally along the anterior surface of the psoas major muscle.
D. The right ureter crosses the common iliac artery at its bifurcation, whereas the left ureter crosses 1–2 cm above the bifurcation.
E. The ureter can be found in the lateral leaf of the parietal peritoneum.
F. Upon entering the cardinal ligament, the ureter is 1–2 cm lateral to the uterine cervix.
G. The uterine artery lies on the anterolateral surface of the ureter for 2.5–3.0 cm.

Ref.: 3, 4

COMMENTS: Any pelvic surgeon needs to know the course of the ureter and its associations with other organs in the pelvis. The ureters typically are 28–34 cm in length and are divided into two segments: abdominal and pelvic portions. It is retroperitoneal throughout its entire course. The abdominal ureters run downward and medially along the anterior surface of the psoas major muscle. The iliopectineal line serves as the marker for the pelvic portion of the ureter. The ureters run along the common iliac artery and then cross over the iliac vessels as they enter the pelvis. Often a slight variation exists between the two ureters in their association with the common iliac vessels. The right ureter tends to cross at the bifurcation of the common iliac artery, whereas the left ureter crosses 1–2 cm above the bifurcation. From here, the ureter can be found on the medial leaf of the parietal peritoneum and in close proximity to the ovarian, uterine, obturator, and superior vesical arteries. The uterine artery lies on the anterolateral surface of the ureter for 2.5–3.0 cm. Upon entering the cardinal ligament, the ureter is approximately 1–2 cm lateral to the uterine cervix and is surrounded by a plexus of veins. The ureter then runs upward and medially in the vesical uterine ligaments to pierce the bladder wall obliquely. Prior to entering the bladder, the ureter is in close contact with the anterior vaginal wall.

ANSWER: A, B, D, F, G

39. A 29-year-old woman presents to your office for a second opinion. She has been suffering from chronic pelvic pain for 16 months, and an ultrasound examination and physical examination have been essentially normal. Her prior physician tested her CA 125 and the value returned as 52 U/ml (normal for that laboratory was less than 35 U/ml). She states that he informed her that she probably has cancer and needed to see an oncologist immediately. Which of the following could be an explanation for her elevated CA 125?

A. Pancreatitis.
B. Endometriosis.
C. Pregnancy.
D. Pelvic inflammatory disease.
E. Inflammatory bowel disease.
F. Germ cell tumor of the ovary.

Ref.: 3

COMMENTS: Much has been learned about the CA 125 test over recent years. Originally conceived to detect nonmucinous epithelial ovarian adenocarcinomas, this test has been found to be far more reliable in the postmenopausal patient than it is in the premenopausal patient. In the premenopausal patient, as depicted in the above scenario, any intraabdominal inflammatory process can elevate this marker, including endometriosis, uterine leiomyomas, pregnancy, inflammatory bowel disease, pelvic inflammatory disease, appendicitis, pancreatitis, menstruation, among others. When evaluating chronic pelvic pain in this patient population, the CA 125 assay is not the test to order. It is best utilized when evaluating a postmenopausal patient with an ovarian mass or as a baseline value when epithelial ovarian cancer has been found, to judge how the chemotherapy treatments are progressing. A rising CA 125 level in the face of ongoing chemotherapy often indicates failure of treatment. Germ cell tumors of the ovary, not being included in the epithelial ovarian cancer category, would not produce an elevated CA 125 level.

ANSWER: A, B, C, D, E

40. The following patients present with complaints of abdominal bleeding. Match each clinical scenario in the left column with the likely etiology in the right column:

A. An 18-year-old sexually active woman with spotting 7 weeks after last menses	a. Anovulatory bleeding
B. A 65-year-old woman with bleeding for the first time since menopause 10 years ago	b. Coagulopathy
C. A 37-year-old woman with regular menses becoming significantly heavier	c. Endometrial polyp
D. A 30-year-old woman with highly irregular menses	d. Threatened abortion
E. A 13-year-old girl with extremely heavy first menses	e. Endometrial hyperplasia

Ref.: 3

COMMENTS: Abnormal uterine bleeding is a common gynecologic complaint. It is defined as dysfunctional uterine bleeding if there is no demonstrable organic cause, implying an endocrinologic origin. The age of the patient and the timing of her cycle may provide a clue. In sexually active reproductive-age women with abnormal bleeding, pregnancy must always be ruled out as the first etiology. Regularly timed cycles suggest normal ovulatory function; therefore organic lesions such as submucous fibroids, endometrial polyps, and adenomyosis may produce heavy, regular cycles (menorrhagia). Irregular cycles are frequently due to disruption in normal ovulatory function and may even be due to anovulation. It is important to identify and treat these women, as failure to move into the progesterone dominant luteal phase of the cycle gives them prolonged unopposed estrogen exposure. Postmenopausal women with the onset of vaginal bleeding require thorough endometrial evaluation, as the bleeding may herald malignant or premalignant pathology, such as endometrial hyperplasia. Up to 50% of young women presenting with heavy bleeding at menarche are diagnosed as having a coagulopathy.

ANSWER: A-d; B-e; C-c; D-a; E-b

41. Which of the following surgical procedures are recommended to support the vaginal apex in a patient with post-hysterectomy vaginal prolapse?

A. Abdominal sacrocolpopexy.
B. Paravaginal repair.
C. Sacrospinous ligament suspension.
D. Uterosacral ligament plication.
E. Rectocele repair.

Ref.: 7, 8

COMMENTS: Patients who present with pelvic organ prolapse require pelvic examination with intent to identify all defects that may be altering normal vaginal support. Support may be defective to the anterior vaginal wall (cystocele), the posterior vaginal wall (rectocele), or the vaginal apex (enterocele) in any combination. **Sacrocolpopexy** is an abdominal approach to apical vaginal prolapse designed to bridge the vagina to the sacrum via a medical mesh or donor fascial graft. **Uterosacral ligament plication** relies on the patient's own ligamentous support to achieve the same purpose. It may be performed abdominally or transvaginally as a McCall's culdoplasty. **Sacrospinous ligament suspension** sutures the vaginal apex to the sacrospinous ligament with a transvaginal approach. **Paravaginal repair** is utilized to repair a cystocele secondary to loss of lateral vaginal support; a rectocele implies a defect in posterior vaginal support.

ANSWER: A, C, D

42. Which of the following is an absolute contraindication to hysteroscopy?

A. Uterine bleeding.
B. Submucosal fibroid.
C. Endometrial carcinoma.
D. Acute pelvic infection.
E. Uterine septum.

Ref.: 8, 9

COMMENTS: Hysteroscopy is an excellent method for directly visualizing the uterine cavity. It may be performed in the office or operating room and allows definitive diagnosis and treatment of intrauterine pathology, such as uterine septum, endometrial polyp, and submucosal fibroids, with one procedure. It may be performed in the presence of active uterine bleeding as the continuous-flow system flushes away debris. Potential exists for carcinoma dissemination, however, so it is not typically used to evaluate and stage known endometrial carcinomas. It is routinely utilized for the workup of patients with abnormal or postmenopausal uterine bleeding. Acute pelvic infection is an absolute contraindication due to spread of the infectious process to the upper genital tract through the fallopian tubes and into the peritoneal cavity.

ANSWER: D

43. Risk factors for pelvic organ prolapse include all of the following *except*:

A. Vaginal delivery.
B. Chronic asthma.
C. Prior vaginal hysterectomy with anterior colporrhaphy.
D. Cesarean delivery.

Ref.: 7

COMMENTS: The primary risk factor for the development of pelvic organ prolapse is prior vaginal delivery. Pregnancy itself and even the first stage of labor do not increase the risk as women who undergo elective cesarean section or whose babies are delivered abdominally prior to the second stage of labor are at no increased risk for pelvic organ prolapse. It is not known whether episiotomy at the time of vaginal delivery is protective of the pelvic floor for the development of urinary incontinence or prolapse. Other risk factors for prolapse include chronic increases in abdominal pressure, such as with chronic asthma or cough, constipation, or heavy lifting. Pelvic surgery itself may place a patient at risk for subsequent prolapse if the normal support structures of the vagina are disrupted. Extensive dissection of the vaginal wall, such as with anterior colporrhaphy, may also cause denervation injuries.

ANSWER: D

REFERENCES

1. Sabiston DC Jr: *Textbook of Surgery*, 15th ed. WB Saunders, Philadelphia, 1997.
2. Schwartz SI, Shires GT, Spencer FC: *Principles of Surgery*, 7th ed. McGraw-Hill, New York, 1999.
3. Herbst AL, Mishell DR Jr, Stenchever MA, Droegemueller W: *Comprehensive Gynecology*, 3rd ed. Mosby-Year Book, St. Louis, 1994.
4. Williams PL, Warwick R, Dyson M, Bannister LH: *Gray's Anatomy*, 38th ed. Churchill Livingstone, New York, 1995.
5. Cullen PW: *Ultrasonography in Obstetrics and Gynecology*, 3rd ed. WB Saunders, Philadelphia, 1994.
6. CDC: Sexually transmitted disease surveillance. U.S. Department of Health and Human Services, Public Health Service, Centers for Disease Control, Center for Prevention Services, Division of STD-HIV Prevention, Surveillance and Information Systems Branch, Annual 1989.
7. Nichols DH, Randall CL: *Vaginal Surgery*, 4th ed. Williams & Wilkins, Baltimore, 1998.
8. Nichols DH: *Gynecologic and Obstetric Surgery*, 1st ed. Mosby-Yearbook, St. Louis, 1993.
9. Thompson JD, Rock AR: *Te Linde's Operative Gynecology*, 7th ed. JB Lippincott, Philadelphia, 1992.

CHAPTER 45

Neurosurgery

1. Regarding neuronal function, which of the following statement(s) is/are true?

   A. The resting membrane potential is dependent on sodium and potassium ion concentrations and the sodium/potassium-dependent ATPase pump.
   B. The action potential is dependent on changes in the permeability to ions, specifically sodium and potassium.
   C. Myelin provides the axon with necessary insulation to provide better conduction of the action potential.
   D. Acetylcholine is the major neurotransmitter at the neuromuscular junction.
   E. The sections of myelin along an axon are called nodes of Ranvier.

Ref.: 1

COMMENTS: Neuronal physiology depends on a semipermeable membrane that, along with a membrane-bound ATPase pump, keeps two important ions—sodium and potassium—at markedly different concentrations. An action potential is a self-propagating ionic current that results from opening voltage-gated channels, allowing a drastic change in the permeability of sodium and potassium ions. Myelin is produced by Schwann cells to cover axons on the peripheral nerves and by oligodendrocytes to cover axons of the brain and spinal cord. Myelin offers insulation to decrease the diffusion of ionic current needed to propagate the axon potential and therefore increase the velocity of the action potential. The axon is lined by myelin sheaths, which are interrupted by areas of bare axon called nodes of Ranvier. This arrangement allows a faster, interrupted style of conduction known as saltatory conduction. The neuromuscular junction involves the release of acetylcholine from synaptic vesicles as a result of an action potential and the acetylcholine receptor on the muscle cell. Activation of this receptor causes ionic permeability changes, leading to release of calcium from the sarcoplasmic reticulum with activation of actinomycin and subsequent muscular contraction. The hallmark neurologic disorder involving the neuromuscular junction is myasthenia gravis, which is an autoimmune disorder involving the blocking of an acetylcholine receptor.

ANSWER: A, B, C, D

2. Regarding diagnostic procedures used to evaluate the central nervous system (CNS), which of the following statements is/are true?

   A. Computed tomography (CT) is the best available radiographic test for soft tissue evaluation.
   B. Magnetic resonance imaging (MRI) is the most useful initial test in the evaluation of spinal cord compression.
   C. Magnetic resonance angiography (MRA) eliminates the risk associated with cerebral angiography.
   D. Pneumoencephalography has been replaced by CT scans.
   E. Water-soluble contrast material has decreased the incidence of arachnoiditis following myelography.
   F. MRI produces less bony artifact than does a CT scan.

Ref.: 2, 3, 4

COMMENTS: **Angiography** is the main method of demonstrating vascular lesions and is useful for preoperative evaluation of neoplasms and certain cases of trauma. Its major danger—stroke as a result of vessel manipulation—may be eliminated by the use of MRA, but the images obtained with MRA are of slightly inferior quality. **Pneumoencephalography**, once used to enhance definition of the subarachnoid spaces, has been almost completely replaced by the CT scan; this definition can be enhanced even further if necessary by injection of soluble contrast material prior to performance of the CT scanning. **Myelography** is the radiographic study of the spinal cord and spinal canal after subarachnoid injection of contrast material; the use of water-soluble contrast media has decreased the incidence of postprocedure arachnoiditis. In most institutions myelography has been replaced by the CT scan or MRI, including its use for evaluation of intervertebral disc disease. The **CT scan** is at present the most useful diagnostic tool for identifying acute hemorrhage or fracture. Modern units provide resolution in the range of 1 mm. The major disadvantage of CT scans is the artifact created by the bone coverings of the CNS. **MRI** is superior to CT scan in many cases because it does not expose the patient to radiation, is associated with minimal bone artifact, yields high-grade differentiation of gray-white matter, and can directly scan in multiple planes. MRI is the best diagnostic tool for soft tissue evaluation. Hence MRI is the most useful initial test for cord compression.

ANSWER: B, C, D, E, F

3. Which of the following statements is/are true regarding scalp injuries?

A. The blood supply to the scalp lies between the periosteum and the galea.
B. Most scalp laceration hemorrhages can be controlled by applying direct pressure.
C. Subgaleal hematomas must be drained to avoid abscess formation and extensive scalp elevation.
D. The largest arteries providing blood supply to the scalp are the superficial temporal and occipital arteries originating from the vertebral artery.
E. Galeal lacerations should be closed when possible.
F. If a scalp laceration extends below the zygoma, the ipsilateral facial nerve may be injured.

Ref.: 2, 3

COMMENTS: The scalp consists of five layers: skin, subcutaneous, galea aponeurotica, loose areolar tissue, periosteum. The skin and galea are the layers of surgical importance, with the blood supply lying between the skin above and the galea below. The blood supply to the scalp is rich, and so lacerations can be accompanied by significant blood loss. When the underlying skull is intact, this blood loss can be controlled by simple pressure. If the skull is fractured, direct pressure may be hazardous to the underlying brain; pulling the retracted galea back over the wound edge with forceps often controls such hemorrhage. Contusions causing subgaleal hemorrhage can lead to the formation of large subgaleal hematomas that can elevate extensive portions of the scalp off the skull. For this condition, compression dressings can reduce the extent of hematoma formation. If the overlying scalp is viable and there is no evidence of infection, subgaleal hematomas should be left alone to resolve naturally, a process that may require several weeks. If the hematoma is infected, it is necessary to evacuate it. The occipitalis and frontalis muscles insert on the galea, and their contraction tends to separate areas of galeal disruptions; therefore even small lacerations of the galea should be closed. As for nonoperative treatment of subgaleal hematomas, large lacerations with significant loss of galeal or subgaleal tissue should be treated with compression dressings after appropriate débridement and closure to minimize the chances of postoperative subgaleal hematoma and infection. The largest arteries supplying the scalp, the superficial temporal and occipital arteries, originate from the external carotid arteries.

ANSWER: B, E, F

4. Which of the following statements is/are true regarding hydrocephalus?

A. It represents a primary process in up to two-thirds of patients.
B. It is classified as communicating or noncommunicating.
C. With communicating hydrocephalus, obstruction to cerebrospinal fluid (CSF) flow is outside the ventricular system.
D. With proper shunting, patients with hydrocephalus usually have intelligence equal to that of matched control groups without hydrocephalus.
E. Hydrocephalus ex vacuo is more common in the elderly.

Ref.: 2, 3

COMMENTS: Hydrocephalus is a secondary, not a primary, problem. Causes of hydrocephalus include aqueductal stenosis, dysfunction of arachnoid granulations, subarachnoid scarring, and CSF blockage by clot or tumor. Hydrocephalus is classified as communicating or noncommunicating. With **communicating hydrocephalus**, obstruction to flow is outside the ventricular system. With **noncommunicating hydrocephalus**, there is obstruction to flow of the CSF inside the ventricular system. The clinical features of **infantile hydrocephalus** include diastasis of the cranial sutures, weakness of upward gaze (the setting sun sign), enlarging head circumference, and a bulging anterior fontanelle. Clinical features of hydrocephalus past 1 year of age (when the cranial sutures are closed) include headache, nausea, vomiting, visual loss, and lethargy. In some cases this progresses to coma and death without proper treatment. Most cases of hydrocephalus are treated by pressure-activated shunts, the most common being the ventriculoperitoneal (VP) shunt. Although treated patients usually attain acceptable levels of intelligence (and some, in fact, are very bright), overall patients with shunts do not do as well intellectually as nonhydrocephalic matched control groups. It largely depends on the cause of the hydrocephalus. **Hydrocephalus ex vacuo** refers to enlarged ventricles secondary to cerebral insult or atrophy. Therefore it is more common in the elderly.

ANSWER: B, C, E

5. Regarding intracranial pressure (ICP) monitoring, which of the following is/are true?

A. Normal ICP is 0–15 mm Hg or 0–20 cm H_2O.
B. Risk factors for elevated ICP after head injury include age less than 40, open basal cisterns on CT scan, and systolic blood pressure over 90 mm Hg.
C. In patients with a Glasgow Coma Scale (GCS) score of 3–8 after resuscitation who have an abnormal head CT scan, intracranial pressure monitoring is appropriate.
D. Although ventricular pressure monitoring is the reference standard for ICP, it has a higher risk of causing hemorrhage and infection.
E. The ICP treatment threshold is usually 10 mm Hg.

Ref.: 5, 6

COMMENTS: Because of the approximately 1% risk of hemorrhage and 5% infection risk with ICP monitoring, this procedure is not appropriate for all patients with head injury. ICP monitoring is appropriate in patients with a GCS score of 3–8 with an abnormal head CT scan or for select patients with normal CT and risk factors for elevated ICP such as age over 40 and systolic blood pressure less than 90 mm Hg. Ventricular catheter ICP measurements are accurate but carry a higher risk for complications than intraparenchymal monitors. The normal ICP is 0–15 mm Hg, but the ICP is usually not treated in most centers until it rises to 20 mm Hg.

ANSWER: A, C, D

6. Which of the following statements is/are true regarding traumatic cerebrospinal fluid (CSF) leaks?

A. Most are due to basilar skull fractures.
B. Most close spontaneously.
C. The risk of infection is greater with rhinorrhea than with otorrhea.
D. They require immediate surgical repair to avert infection.
E. They may be observed for up to 14 days if there is no evidence of infection.

F. Intracranial air on CT scan is indirect evidence of a CSF leak.

Ref.: 2, 3, 5

COMMENTS: Most traumatic CSF fistulas close spontaneously. They should be managed in the hospital under close supervision. Placement of a lumbar drain to divert the fistula can be helpful. The risk of persistent drainage and infection is greater with rhinorrhea than with otorrhea. Otorrhea or rhinorrhea that persists for more than 10–14 days despite lumbar drainage is an indication for repair of the torn dura if the site of the CSF leak can be found. The overall incidence of CSF leak with head injury is 0.25–0.50%.

ANSWER: A, B, C, E, F

7. Regarding brain injury, which of the following statements is/are true?

A. The extent of brain injury is a function of the mechanism of injury.
B. Contusions may occur on the side of the brain opposite the side of initial impact.
C. Contusions tend to involve the anterior portions of the frontal and temporal lobes.
D. Diffuse axonal injury is usually an incidental finding.
E. The effects of secondary edema and hematoma enlargement may be delayed for several days.
F. There is no role for surgery for gunshot wounds to the head in patients with a Glascow Coma Scale (GCS) score of less than 8.

Ref.: 2, 3, 5

COMMENTS: Localized force can cause damage to the scalp, skull, and underlying brain in the immediate area of injury. The resulting neurologic deficit relates to the area of the brain directly involved and usually produces brief or no loss of consciousness. Applications of generalized force to the skull, such as that caused by impact of the head against an immovable object, allow diffuse transmission of energy, causing injury to the whole brain. In such a case, the brain insult is generalized, often producing altered consciousness; and its severity relates to the mechanism of injury. For example, the injury may be the result of linear or rotational acceleration/deceleration of the brain against the confining cranium, such as when the head hits an immovable object. When the brain strikes the rigid skull, contusions occur in the area where the force is applied as well as against the opposite inner surface of the skull (contrecoup injury). Rotation of the brain within the skull may cause tearing of axons, resulting in diffuse axonal injury within the white matter, a so-called shearing injury, which is often severe. The undersurface of the frontal lobes, the anterior portions of the temporal lobes, the posterior portions of the occipital lobes, and the upper portion of the midbrain are more likely to suffer contusions because they are relatively more confined by bone or dural shelves. The contusion may be clinically silent initially if the involved area of the brain has no demonstrable clinical function. These injuries often become apparent days after the injury as edema accumulates, creating the effects of an intracranial mass. Occasionally, a hematoma accumulates in the area of contusion 24–72 hours after injury, a situation seen more often in elderly persons. Gunshot brain injuries are often severe because of damage caused by the bullet and the associated shock wave that travels along the path. The primary injury, bleeding, swelling, and infection cause high mortality rates, but surgical débridement can lead to significant improvement, even in some patients with a GCS score of 3–8.

ANSWER: A, B, C, E

8. Regarding the evaluation and care of head-injured patients, which of the following statements is/are true?

A. Hypotension is often the direct result of intracranial trauma.
B. Decerebrate posturing is a common response to diffuse cortical injury.
C. A score of 5 on the Glasgow Coma Scale (GCS) is associated with a poor prognosis.
D. Inappropriate secretion of antidiuretic hormone (ADH) should be suspected when the serum sodium level exceeds 150 mEq/L.
E. Inappropriate secretion of ADH should be treated with administration of exogenous solute.

Ref.: 2, 3

COMMENTS: The initial care of the head-injured patient must focus on maintenance of ventilation, control of hemorrhage, and maintenance of the peripheral circulation. Continued hypotension and tachycardia are rarely the direct result of head trauma and should alert the examiner to the existence of a systemic hemorrhage. In fact, intracranial hemorrhage with elevated intracranial pressure often manifests as hypertension and bradycardia. As soon as possible, there should be a careful neurologic examination and documentation of the level of consciousness; it is a baseline against which the patient's progress is measured. Decerebrate posturing (extension and internal rotation of the extremities, neck extension, and arching of the back) implies compression of, or damage to, the brain stem and often requires immediate therapy. In a patient unconscious for more than 6 hours, the Glasgow Coma Scale is useful for predicting eventual outcome. It measures motor (M), verbal (V), and eye (E) responses on scales of 1–6, 1–5, and 1–4, respectively. It is recorded as a sum of the highest score in each category. Patients with a score lower than 5 have a mortality rate higher than 50%. Patients who have lost the reflex capability to protect their airway should be intubated and their stomachs decompressed by a nasogastric tube. A Foley catheter should be placed and serum and urine electrolytes monitored. Inappropriate secretion of ADH should be suspected when serum osmolality and sodium levels fall in association with an increase in urinary osmolality. Restriction of water intake or the use of solute diuretics may be necessary to control this problem. The body temperature must be closely monitored, because head injuries may be accompanied by the loss of capacity for superficial cutaneous vasodilation and sweating, leading to hyperthermia.

ANSWER: C

9. Which one or more of the following is/are true statements regarding the treatment of cerebral edema?

A. CT scans should be obtained to exclude the diagnosis of intracranial hemorrhage or a mass lesion before starting therapy.
B. Barbiturates are used to capture free radicals.
C. Steroids are useful for treatment of head trauma.
D. Hypercapnia induces cerebral vasoconstriction and is useful for decreasing intracerebral blood volume.

E. Lumbar puncture to drain CSF is contraindicated.

Ref.: 2, 3, 5

COMMENTS: The brain responds to injury by forming edema. The bony confines of the skull impose a narrow tolerance for swelling before the intracranial pressure equals the arterial pressure. When this occurs, perfusion stops and neuronal death follows in 4–5 minutes. The onset of edema usually is slow and reaches a maximal level within 48–72 hours. The progress of cerebral edema is best followed by the use of intracranial pressure-monitoring devices. These devices are commonly used to monitor patients with altered consciousness following head injury or patients with Glasgow Coma Scale scores lower than 8. After a baseline CT scan is obtained to rule out intracranial hemorrhage or a mass lesion, treatment is started as soon as possible to minimize the progress of edema. This can be accomplished by: (1) elevating the head of the bed 15–30 degrees; (2) intermittent drainage of CSF by a pressure-monitoring catheter placed in the frontal horn of the lateral ventricle; (3) hyperventilation to PCO_2 levels of 28–35 mm Hg to induce vasoconstriction; and (4) the use of fluid restriction and solute diuretics to minimize edema. Barbiturates are thought to provide protection for the injured brain by decreasing metabolic demands and by capturing free radicals that have been released through cell destruction. Steroids are thought to decrease inflammation and swelling, but their effectiveness in the treatment of cerebral edema resulting from head trauma has not been established (unless given prior to the injury, as in experimental brain trauma). Lumbar puncture is contraindicated because the nonuniform distribution of elevated pressure between the supratentorial space, infratentorial space, and spinal canal may lead to herniation of the cerebellum through the foramen magnum or temporal lobe herniation with consequent compression of the brain stem.

ANSWER: A, B, E

10. Regarding subarachnoid hemorrhage, which of the following statements is/are true?

A. A normal CT scan of the brain excludes the possibility of a subarachnoid hemorrhage.
B. Aneurysms occur most frequently on the basilar artery.
C. Hydrocephalus develops in 2–4% of patients after subarachnoid hemorrhage.
D. Surgical correction within 48–72 hours is recommended in patients who are neurologically intact and have an uncomplicated aneurysm.
E. The use of hypertension, hypervolemia, and calcium channel blockers is recommended for treatment of vasospasm.
F. Aneurysms with a narrow neck can sometimes be packed with coils via an endovascular approach.

Ref.: 2, 3, 6

COMMENTS: Sudden headache followed by altered consciousness is the usual clinical pattern following subarachnoid hemorrhage (SAH). Focal neurologic deficits may occur, but they are less common than those seen after occlusion of major intracranial arteries. The sequelae vary depending on the size of the hemorrhage and range from headache to death. Although CT scan is the diagnostic method of choice to confirm an SAH, approximately 10% of patients with documented hemorrhages have a normal CT scan within 24 hours of SAH. It is important, therefore, to perform a lumbar puncture when SAH is suspected and the CT scan is negative for SAH. Angiography is required to confirm the presence of an aneurysm. Most intracranial aneurysms arise from the large intracranial arteries of the circle of Willis and at the origin of the vertebrobasilar arteries. The most common sites of SAH, in decreasing order of prevalence, are the internal carotid artery, anterior cerebral artery, middle cerebral artery, and vertebrobasilar system. Multiple aneurysms are present 20% of the time. When multiple, they tend to be symmetric in distribution or arise from the same parent artery. Most aneurysms are congenital and probably are the result of defects in the muscular and elastic layers of the intracerebral arteries. They have a saccular or berry-like shape, hence the name berry aneurysm. The incidence of silent aneurysms is the same in patients with and without hypertension, but rupture is more common in patients with hypertension. The incidence of rupture is highest in patients between the ages of 40 and 60 years. The goal of treatment is to isolate the aneurysm from the force of systolic blood flow. This should be attempted as early as possible because the likelihood of secondary rupture is approximately 20% by 2 weeks after SAH. It is recommended that surgical correction be performed within 48–72 hours in patients who are neurologically intact with an approachable aneurysm. A relative contraindication to early surgical intervention is the presence of a neurologic deficit resulting from spasm of the circle of Willis caused by the irritating effect of blood in the CSF. The rationale for early surgical correction—that the patient then can be treated aggressively for vasospasm—is based on the concept of maximizing cerebral perfusion. A calcium channel-blocking agent (nimodipine), relative hypertension, and hypervolemia are recommended for treatment of vasospasm. Other treatments are advocated, however, and there is no proven effective treatment for symptomatic cerebral vasospasm as a result of subarachnoid hemorrhage. The incidence of hydrocephalus is 15–20% in patients after a subarachnoid hemorrhage, and many of these patients eventually require a shunt for this complication. Some aneurysms with a narrow neck can be coiled under fluoroscopy. Long-term results of this approach are pending.

ANSWER: D, E, F

11. Which one or more of the following statements is/are true regarding subdural hematomas?

A. Acute subdural hematomas are usually unilateral and have a poorer prognosis than chronic subdural hematomas.
B. Adequate treatment of an acute subdural hematoma generally consists of drainage through burr holes.
C. Chronic subdural hematomas frequently recur.
D. The diagnosis of subacute subdural hematomas can be made reliably by CT scan.
E. Chronic subdural hematomas should be suspected in elderly patients with progressive changes in mental status, even without a definite history of trauma.

Ref.: 2, 3, 5

COMMENTS: Subdural hematomas are caused by rupture of veins traversing the subdural space or by arterial bleeding from parenchymal laceration. Their presentation and treatment depend on the rapidity of hematoma formation. All types of subdural hematomas (acute, subacute, chronic) have in common the presence of a decreased level of consciousness out of proportion to the observed focal neurologic deficit. **Acute subdural hematomas** are those that cause progressive neurologic deficit within 48 hours of injury. They usually follow severe head trauma, are unilateral, have both arterial and venous sources of bleeding, and can progress rapidly. The diagnosis should be considered in any patient with a severe head injury who shows deteriorated neurologic status or who is unresponsive with a focal neurologic deficit. The hematomas are solid and easily visualized by CT scan. They also may produce a pineal gland shift visible on skull films. They can be bilateral, and adjacent intracerebral hematomas often are present. Treatment requires formal craniotomy with removal of solid clot and control of bleeding points. **Subacute subdural hematomas** are defined as those more than 48 hours, but less than 2 weeks, old. The patients usually are less severely injured than those with acute subdural hematomas, and marked fluctuation of the level of consciousness or headache should alert surgeons to the diagnosis. With large hematomas, third nerve paresis with pupil dilatation is a warning that midbrain compression due to temporal lobe herniation is occurring. CT scans may not identify the mass because the hematoma becomes isodense 10–12 days after its formation and there may be bilateral hematomas. If the clot is completely liquefied, burr holes are therapeutic as well. If solid clot is found, craniotomy is indicated. **Chronic subdural hematomas** most often occur in infants and elderly people, frequently without a clear history of antecedent trauma. They can occur months to years after the initial injury and should be suspected in patients with a decreasing or fluctuating mental status out of proportion to the focal neurologic deficit. The hematoma is liquid, and drainage via burr holes is usually all that is necessary for treatment. Chronic subdural hematomas frequently recur when they are associated with multiple subdural membranes. In some of these cases, craniotomy to strip the membranes is necessary. Subdural peritoneal shunting may also be necessary.

ANSWER: A, C, E

12. Which of the following statements about surgical treatment of epilepsy is/are true?

A. Surgery for focal epilepsy without an associated lesion is considered only after a significant trial of medical therapy.
B. Surgery for primary generalized epilepsy is rarely indicated.
C. The chance for rendering a patient seizure-free with temporal lobectomy for temporal epilepsy is about 20%.
D. Hemispherectomy, the surgical removal of an entire hemisphere, is an accepted modern procedure in some cases of epilepsy.
E. With modern medicines now available, epilepsy surgery is becoming less common.
F. The cerebellum is often implicated in focal epilepsy.

Ref.: 2, 3, 6, 7

COMMENTS: The surgical treatment of epilepsy is a valuable option for well selected patients. Patients who are medically intractable, who are proven to have a localizable seizure focus, and who can accept the risks and consequences of surgery are candidates for surgery. Most seizure foci in adults are in the temporal lobe where surgical removal is associated with a seizure-free rate of 60–70% in most series. Primary generalized (idiopathic) epilepsy is rarely aided by surgery. Advances in differentiating primary and focal onset seizures and advances in surgery have made epilepsy surgery a progressively more common therapeutic choice. Other surgical treatments are tailor-made for specific problems. **Corpus callosotomy** for drop attacks and **hemispherectomy** for a patient with a dysfunctional epileptogenic hemisphere are rare but useful procedures in carefully selected patients. Most recently, **multiple subpial transection (MSPT)**, a procedure that selectively isolates a seizure focus, has been shown to be useful.

ANSWER: A, B, D

13. Current uses of stereotaxis in neurosurgery include which of the following?

A. Ablations of globus pallidus interna for Parkinson's disease.
B. Treatment of spinal cord injury.
C. Biopsy of brain tumors.
D. Placement of ventricular catheters.
E. Stimulation of the *ventralis intermedius nucleus* thalamus for essential tumor.
F. Radiosurgery for treatment of arteriovenous malformation (AVM).

Ref.: 3, 6

COMMENTS: **Stereotaxis** has been a useful aid in localizing, biopsying, or ablating lesions in the brain. A stereotactic frame is placed on the patient's head, and a CT or MRI scan is obtained. This image shows the lesion or target in relation to posts on the head frame. With these points as a reference, X, Y, and Z coordinates with possible trajectories to the target are chosen. This allows the surgeon to pass a probe through a small hole in the skull to the target with millimeter accuracy. This approach is being used in some patients with Parkinson's disease and patients with essential tremor. The basic idea of stereotaxis with a frame is being used for **stereotactic irradiation** targeted at AVMs and some tumors.

ANSWER: A, C, D, E, F

14. Which of the following statements is/are true regarding subarachnoid hemorrhage?

A. It is one of the most common intracranial hemorrhages following head trauma.
B. It usually produces meningismus (stiff neck and headache).
C. Rapid dilution of the blood by the CSF prevents accumulation of a mass-producing clot.
D. It may produce communicating hydrocephalus as a late complication.

Ref.: 2, 3

COMMENTS: One of the most common intracranial hemorrhages following head injury is subarachnoid hemorrhage. It usually causes signs of meningismus (stiff neck, headache) and changes in the patient's mental status. Because the hemorrhage is small and rapidly diluted by the CSF, no localized mass effect occurs; therefore this type of hemorrhage after trauma has little surgical significance. Rarely, it leads to progressive communicating hydrocephalus requiring shunting.

ANSWER: A, B, C, D

15. Which are true statements about vascular malformations?

A. Arteriovenous malformations (AVMs) are the most common vascular malformations in the brain.
B. Venous angiomas commonly bleed, and surgical removal is usually required.

C. To plan surgical excision of a cavernous angioma properly, angiography should be performed.
D. AVMs are congenital lesions consisting of feeding and draining vessels with a central nidus that bypasses the capillary phase.
E. AVMs are graded for surgical prognosis by size, location, and venous drainage.
F. Ten percent of AVMs have an associated aneurysm.

Ref.: 2, 6

COMMENTS: Vascular malformations in the brain include venous angiomas, cavernous angiomas, capillary telangiectasias, and **arteriovenous malformations**. AVMs get more attention than the other, more common lesions because of their propensity to cause seizure or life-threatening hemorrhage. Most AVMs are symptomatic when found. During the era of MRI, the other lesions are commonly incidental findings. In fact, CT or MRI is necessary to find a **cavernous angioma**, which is not visible on the angiogram. AVMs have irregular vessel walls, and 10% have aneurysms. These irregularities lead to a 2–3% incidence of hemorrhage per year. This risk must be balanced against surgical risks as measured by lesion size, location, and drainage pattern.

ANSWER: D, E, F

16. Which of the following statements is/are true regarding peripheral nerve injuries?

A. Neurapraxia requires surgical resection of the nerve root involved if pain is to be eliminated.
B. Denervation atrophy of muscles becomes irreversible after 12–15 months.
C. Restoration of sensory loss is not possible after the muscle atrophy following denervation is complete.
D. Axonal regeneration progresses at a rate of 1 mm per day after a 10- to 20-day lag period.

Ref.: 2, 3

COMMENTS: There are several classifications of nerve injuries. The Seddon classification uses three terms to classify nerve injuries: neurapraxia, axonotmesis, and neurotmesis. With **neurapraxia**, anatomic continuity of the nerve is preserved, and often there is incomplete motor paralysis with little muscle atrophy and considerable sparing of sensory and autonomic function. Operative repair is not indicated, and the quality of recovery is excellent. **Axonotmesis** is the loss of axonal continuity without interruption of the investing myelin tissue. There is complete motor, sensory, and autonomic paralysis and progressive muscle atrophy. Operative repair is not indicated, and recovery occurs at the rate of about 1 mm per day. **Neurotmesis** is a more severe injury with significant disorganization within the nerve or actual disruption of continuity of the nerve and its investing tissues. Recovery is impossible without operative repair. After disruption, axonal sprouting begins within 10–20 days. If not repaired, scar tissue blocks the entrance of axonal sprouts into the distal nerve; instead, the axons coil into a disorganized neuroma that can be quite painful. After operative repair, distal growth occurs at the rate of 1 mm per day after the initial 10- to 20-day lag described above. The degree of recovery is a function of patient age (younger is better), type of nerve involved (pure motor or sensory nerves recover better than mixed nerves), level of nerve injury (distal is better), and duration of denervation (shorter is better). If more than 12–15 months is required for regenerating axons to reach a denervated muscle, a significant degree of denervation atrophy will have occurred, which is irreversible. In contrast, sensory loss may be recovered after prolonged periods of denervation, and so a nerve repair can provide protective sensory function in the atrophied distal extremity.

ANSWER: B, D

17. Which one or more of the following statements is/are true concerning brain tumors?

A. There is no uniformly accepted system of classification for brain tumors.
B. Brain tumors may be classified according to tissue of origin, location, and malignant potential.
C. Gliomas are the most common type of primary brain tumor.
D. Glioblastoma multiforme is the most common type of glioma in adults.
E. There is no benefit to be gained by operating on tumors metastatic to the brain.
F. The most common brain metastasis in men is from prostate cancer.

Ref.: 2, 3, 6, 7

COMMENTS: No uniformly accepted system of classification for brain tumors has been developed. One system developed by Kernohan and Sayre is based on naming the tumor for the cells present in the adult nervous system, vascular tissue, and developmental defects (e.g., astrocytoma, medulloblastoma, oligodendrocytoma) combined with grading the malignancy (where appropriate) from grade I (least malignant) to grade IV (most malignant). Another method classifies tumors according to location: intraaxial neuroectodermal (gliomas), intraaxial nonneuroectodermal (e.g., metastases, blood vessel tumors), and extraaxial (meningiomas). Most primary brain tumors are **gliomas**, the most common of which, in adults, is the highly malignant glioblastoma multiforme (astrocytoma grades III and IV). The most commonly used grading system for astrocytomas is that of the World Health Organization, which includes low-grade astrocytomas, anaplastic astrocytomas (intermediate malignant potential), and glioblastoma multiforme (malignant). Other gliomas include medulloblastomas, oligodendrogliomas, and ependymomas. **Nonglial tumors** include meningiomas, pituitary tumors, neurilemmomas, blood vessel tumors, and metastatic tumors. Approximately 25% of patients who die of cancer have **brain metastases** on autopsy. The most common brain metastases are from lung, breast, melanoma, and kidney cancers. Half of all patients with brain metastases will have a single metastasis. If these patients do not have widespread disease, they are considered for surgery.

ANSWER: A, B, C, D

18. A 53-year-old banker with a history of lung cancer presents to your office with difficulty ambulating. On examination he has nystagmus, dysmetria, and an ataxic gait. What statements are true concerning this patient?

A. There is likely to be an abnormality in the cerebellum.
B. The most common tumor in the adult posterior fossa is metastatic.
C. Radiation therapy is better than surgical treatment when dealing with solitary metastatic brain lesions.

D. Additional symptoms in this patient that include confusion, nuchal rigidity, and cranial nerve palsies are highly suggestive of meningeal carcinomatosis.

Ref.: 2, 3, 7

COMMENTS: Metastatic brain tumors constitute at least 25% of adult brain tumors. This patient's symptoms are suggestive of cerebellar dysfunction. In the adult population, the most common tumors found in the posterior fossa are metastatic lesions. Another common presentation of metastatic disease to the central nervous system (CNS) is **meningeal carcinomatosis**. Symptoms suggestive of this disease include confusion, nuchal rigidity, pain, and multiple cranial nerve palsies. Diagnosis is usually obtained by performing a lumbar puncture with isolation of malignant cells and cerebrospinal fluid (CSF) cytology. When dealing with patients with a metastatic brain lesion, the first question to address is whether it is a solitary lesion or multiple lesions. If it is a solitary lesion and the patient has at least a 6-month expected longevity from the systemic cancer, and if the lesion is in a surgically accessible region, surgical resection followed by limited brain radiation therapy is strongly recommended. If the lesions are multiple, biopsy may be done (to confirm the diagnosis only) and whole-brain radiation therapy is strongly recommended.

ANSWER: A, B, D

19. With peripheral nerve injury:

A. Recovery is influenced by the etiology of the injury, patient age, type of nerve injured, and severity of injury to nearby vessels and bone.
B. Causalgia refers to the etiology of nerve injury.
C. Electromyography (EMG) is not useful during the first week of peripheral nerve injury.
D. Injuries to peripheral nerves during surgical positioning are usually neurotmesis and have a good prognosis for recovery.
E. Surgical repair with an interposed nerve graft to relieve tension on the repair gives results as good as primary repair.

Ref.: 1, 2, 3, 7

COMMENTS: Traumatic peripheral nerve injury requires surgical repair in cases of neurotmesis, where a nerve and its connective tissues are disrupted. This is common with penetrating trauma and less common with compression injury, such as that seen with surgical positioning. Early repair of the severed nerve has the advantage of clearer anatomy and a longer period allowed to regenerate, but late repair also has advantages. The timing of surgical repair is controversial and depends on many factors, which are weighed in each case. When the repair is done, a primary repair in a pure nerve (pure motor or pure sensory) near the target muscle gives the best results. With peripheral nerve injury the site of injury and nerve activity can be detected by EMG only after 2–3 weeks. A rare late consequence of peripheral nerve injury is **causalgia**. Causalgia is a painful condition causing burning sensations in the distribution of a partially injured mixed peripheral nerve. Treatment is with phenoxybenzamine or sympathectomy in intractable cases.

ANSWER: A, C

20. Which of the following statements is/are true regarding spinal cord tumors?

A. Spinal cord tumors occur as frequently as intracranial tumors.
B. Like intracranial tumors, most spinal cord tumors are malignant.
C. Spinal cord tumors are divided according to location into extradural and intradural tumors.
D. Intradural tumors are divided by location into extramedullary and intramedullary tumors.

Ref.: 2, 3, 7

COMMENTS: Spinal cord tumors are one-sixth as common as intracranial tumors. Although most intracranial adult tumors are malignant, 60% of spinal cord tumors are benign. Many of the malignant spinal cord tumors seem to have a better prognosis than their intracranial counterparts. Metastatic tumors occur as frequently as primary tumors. Spinal metastases and primary spinal neoplasms (malignant and benign) are classified according to their relation to the dura and spinal cord. They are divided into extradural and intradural groups, the intradural group being divided into the extramedullary and intramedullary locations.

ANSWER: C, D

21. Match the nerve root on the left with the dermatome and myotome it innervates on the right.

A. C6
B. T4
C. T10
D. L1
E. L5

a. Dermatome: posterior thigh, large toe; myotome: extensor hallucis longus and anterior tibialis
b. Dermatome: inguinal area; myotome: iliopsoas
c. Dermatome: thumb, index finger; myotome: biceps
d. Dermatome: anterior and posterior chest; myotome: intercostal muscles
e. Dermatome: abdominal level of the umbilicus; myotome: abdominal muscles

Ref.: 6, 7

COMMENTS: There are 31 paired spinal nerves providing afferent and efferent innervation to the body. Compression of a spinal nerve can lead to pain, numbness, or weakness in the distribution of that spinal nerve. This is known as **radiculopathy**. When the radiculopathy presents with pain only, certain ones mimic common medical conditions. A left-sided midthoracic radiculopathy can be mistaken for cardiac disease. A right-sided lower thoracic radiculopathy can mimic gallbladder disease, and an L1 or L2 radiculopathy can be mistaken for hernia symptoms. Disc herniations at these levels are uncommon. Common levels for disc herniation are C5–6, C6–7, L4–5, L5–S1. The disc herniation usually causes a radiculopathy in the nerve root paired with the lower vertebrae (C5–6 causes C6 radiculopathy).

ANSWER: A-c; B-d; C-e; D-b; E-a

22. Which of the following statements is/are true regarding the signs and symptoms of spinal cord tumors?

A. Local signs can result from involvement of the anterior motor horn cells.
B. Local signs occur in a segmental distribution, allowing localization of the tumor in a rostral-caudal orientation.

C. Flaccid paralysis is the result of slow onset of tumor compression.
D. Spastic paralysis is the result of slow onset of tumor compression.
E. Long-tract signs allow localization of the tumor to a point at or cephalad to the highest level of involvement.

Ref.: 2, 3, 7

COMMENTS: Local signs are segmental changes that allow rostral-caudal localization. Local motor signs result from involvement of the anterior motor horn cells or anterior spinal roots and lead to weakness and loss of reflexes, fasciculation, and atrophy in a dermatome and myotome pattern. Local sensory signs are the result of involvement of the dorsal root or dorsal root entry zone, producing localized pain, radicular or radiating pain, and loss of sensation over a dermatome distribution. Local sensory signs may result from involvement of fibers crossing in the anterior commissure caused by a central lesion of the spinal cord. The sensory deficit is loss of pain and temperature sensation with persistence of touch, a condition called "sensory dissociation." Long-tract signs indicate that the lesion is at or cephalad to the highest point of involvement. Motor changes depend on the rapidity of onset, with rapid loss of function leading to flaccid areflexic paralysis and slow progressive loss leading to spastic paralysis at the time of presentation. Other tract signs can include loss of pain and temperature sensation (anterolateral fasciculus involvement), loss of position and vibratory sense (dorsal column involvement), weakness, spasticity, hyperreflexia, and Babinski's sign (resulting from posterolateral fasciculus involvement).

ANSWER: A, B, D, E

23. Which of the following statements is/are true regarding the anatomy of the blood supply to the brain?

A. The cervical portion of the internal carotid artery gives off the internal and external maxillary arteries.
B. The petrous portion of the internal carotid artery gives off branches to the orbit.
C. The circle of Willis is fully developed in only 18% of the population.
D. The vertebral artery has communications with the thyrocervical trunk and posterior branches of the external carotid artery.

Ref.: 2, 3

COMMENTS: The major blood supply to the brain is conveyed by the paired internal carotid and vertebral arteries. The internal carotid artery is divided proximal to distal into the cervical portion (which has no branches) and the petrous, cavernous, and intradural portions. The petrous portion has branches that anastomose with the internal maxillary artery, a branch of the external carotid artery. Branches of the cavernous portion include arteries to the cavernous sinus, semilunar arteries, and meningeal arteries (which anastomose with meningeal branches of the internal maxillary artery). These communications create important extracranial–intracranial anastomoses that become significant with certain occlusive lesions. The intradural branches of the internal carotid artery include the ophthalmic artery (which has anastomoses with terminal branches of the external maxillary artery) and the anterior cerebral, middle cerebral, posterior communicating, and anterior choroidal arteries. The vertebral arteries have anastomotic branches to the thyrocervical trunk of the subclavian artery and to the posterior branches of the external carotid artery. After crossing the dura, the vertebral arteries join to form the basilar artery, which supplies the brain stem. The basilar artery ultimately divides into the posterior cerebral arteries. The circle of Willis, fully developed in 18% of the population, is therefore formed by branches of the internal carotid and vertebral arteries. The anterior cerebral arteries (joined by the anterior communicating artery) and the posterior communicating arteries of the internal carotid artery join the posterior cerebral arteries of the basilar artery to create the circle of Willis.

ANSWER: C, D

24. In regard to spinal cord injury, match the syndrome on the left with its definition on the right.

A. Brown-Sequard
B. Anterior spinal
C. Posterior spinal
D. Cauda equina
E. Central cord

a. Unilateral or bilateral loss of motor and sensory in the distribution of multiple nerve roots
b. Bilateral motor and pain sensation loss in arms more than legs
c. Ipsilateral motor and position sense loss, contralateral pain, and temperature loss
d. Bilateral loss of position and vibration sense with preservation of motor and pain sensation
e. Bilateral loss of motor and pain below the lesion, with position and vibratory sense spared

Ref.: 2, 7, 8

COMMENTS: The syndromes of spinal cord injury are named according to the area of injury and have deficits related to the tracts running in that area of the spinal cord. The anterior two-thirds of the spinal cord holds the corticospinal tracts and the spinothalamic tract. Injury to this area via compression or infarct leads to paralysis and loss of pain and temperature sense below the level of the lesion. The posterior spinal cord holds the dorsal columns, which are involved in position and vibratory sense. Lesions in this area result in loss of these modalities below the level of the lesion. The cervical central spinal cord consists of gray matter, crossing fibers of the spinothalamic tract and motor fibers to the upper extremities. Injury here is often caused by neck hyperextension and leads to weakness and pain loss in arms more than legs, along with loss of bowel and bladder control. A hemisection of the spinal cord leads to the Brown-Sequard syndrome. Deficits associated with this syndrome are ipsilateral motor loss, position and vibratory sense loss, contralateral pain, and temperature loss due to the crossing fibers of the spinothalamic tracts. The nerve roots of the cauda equina arise from the distal spinal cord at L1–L2. Compression of nerve roots of the cauda equina leads to variable loss of all functions in the nerve roots involved.

ANSWER: A-c; B-e; C-d; D-a; E-b

25. Which of the following is/are common early complications of acute cervical spinal cord injury?

A. Ileus.
B. Hydronephrosis.
C. Hypertension.
D. Spasticity.
E. Bradycardia.
F. Deep vein thrombosis.

Ref.: 2, 8

COMMENTS: With cervical spinal cord injury, there is a loss of **sympathetic tone**, as the outflow of the sympathetic fibers is mainly through the thoracic spinal cord. It leads to an imbalance in autonomic control favoring the parasympathetic system. The result is a slowing of gastrointestinal motility, weakening of bladder contracture leading to distension and hydronephrosis, and loss of peripheral vascular tone with secondary venous pooling, hypotension, and thrombosis. Bradycardia results from unopposed vagal tone. Reflexes are usually hypoactive initially with a spinal cord injury, with spasticity a late complication.

ANSWER: A, B, E, F

26. Which of the following statements is/are true regarding brain abscesses?

A. The brain is highly susceptible to infection as a result of its high glucose content.
B. The brain is extremely effective in walling off infections.
C. Brain abscesses are classified as acute, chronic, and subacute.
D. Prompt drainage is indicated for all types of brain abscess.
E. Corticosteroids may inhibit abscess wall formation.

Ref.: 2, 3, 6

COMMENTS: The brain is generally resistant to infection unless previously damaged by trauma, hemorrhage, or anoxia. Once infected, the brain is effective in walling off the infection and is capable of isolating the abscess from the uninvolved brain and systemic circulation, making sterilization by systemic antibiotics difficult. The three major sources of brain abscesses include (1) direct extension from middle ear, mastoid, and nasal sinus infections (commonly affecting the temporal lobe and cerebellar hemispheres); (2) hematogenous spread (as occurs in cyanotic heart defects with right-to-left shunts); and (3) direct trauma. The most common organisms are ***Streptococcus***, ***Pneumococcus***, and ***Staphylococcus***. Brain abscesses are classified as **acute**, following a course similar to and difficult to differentiate from subdural empyema; **chronic**, often presenting with progressive neurologic deficit and an expanding mass with a longer history (2 weeks to 2 months); and **subacute**, presenting with a picture somewhere between acute and chronic. MRI is the most accurate indirect means of making the diagnosis and is helpful before performing surgical drainage. The treatment comprises medical measures (antibiotics) or surgical drainage or excision. Medical therapy requires 6–8 weeks of intravenous antibiotics and the use of corticosteroids if severe edema and mass effect are present. On follow-up films, if an increase in the size occurs, surgical drainage must be considered. Medical therapy is best used in patients with multiple lesions and those with relatively small lesions. Abscesses also can be treated with surgical drainage or excision. Again, antibiotics for 6–8 weeks are required; and as with medical treatment, it may take longer than 10 weeks to have significant resolution of the capsule and its enhancement seen on CT scan. Seizures are common sequelae of brain abscess. Brain abscess recurs in 8–10% of patients who initially present with a brain abscess.

ANSWER: B, C, E

27. Match each clinical description with the appropriate unenhanced CT brain film shown here (a–d).

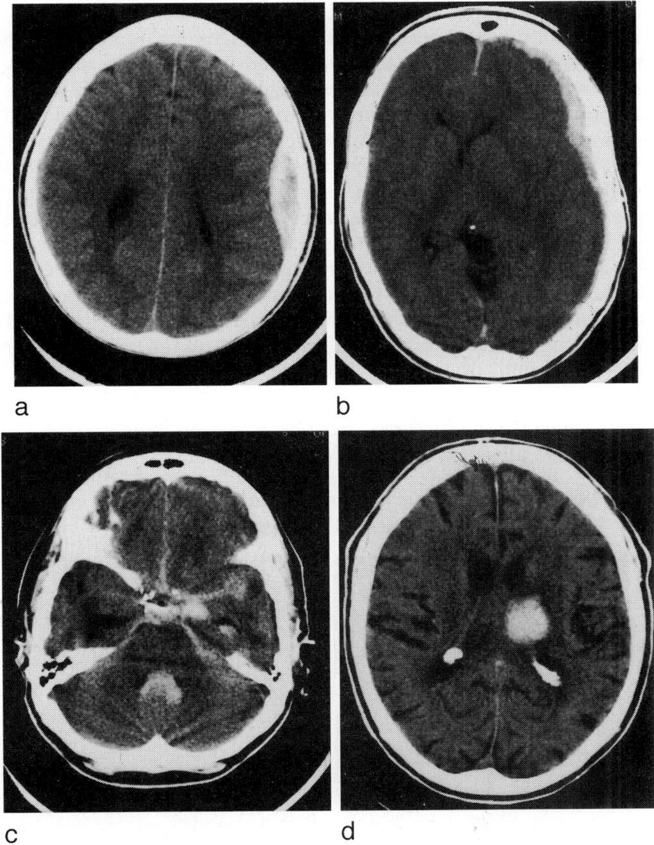

A. A 61-year-old woman fell at home and presented to the emergency room with lethargy and confusion.
B. A 75-year-old man with a long history of hypertension became acutely unresponsive.
C. A 24-year-old man was involved in a motor vehicle accident. Plain skull films in the emergency room revealed a fracture.
D. A 52-year-old woman had an acute onset of severe headache and shortly thereafter became unresponsive.

Ref.: 5, 9

COMMENTS: All of the CT images shown demonstrate intracranial hemorrhage appearing as high-density collections that can be either intraaxial (within the brain parenchyma) or extraaxial (outside the brain parenchyma). Extraaxial hemorrhage is further subdivided into epidural hematoma (EDH), subdural hematoma (SDH), and subarachnoid hemorrhage (SAH). **Epidural hematoma**, which is often associated with skull fracture, occurs following significant head trauma and is usually the result of arterial bleeding between the dura and inner table of the calvarium. The dura does not strip easily from the inner table, even under arterial pressure. As a consequence, an EDH acquires a biconvex configuration, as seen in image *a*. **Subdural hematoma** also occurs following head trauma, but the injury may be mild, particularly in the elderly. Bridging veins between the dura and arachnoid are torn, because the arachnoid strips easily from the dura, and the SDH assumes a crescentic configuration around the hemisphere, as seen in image *b*. **Subarachnoid hemorrhage** (SAH) may be posttraumatic or spontaneous as a result of a ruptured aneurysm. Spontaneous SAH typically presents with acute severe headache. The subarachnoid space—the space between the arachnoid and pia mater—is filled with cerebrospinal fluid. Blood in this compartment can flow relatively freely between the basal cisterns, sylvian fissure, and cortical sulci and may rupture into the ventricular system. In image *c*, which shows a spontaneous SAH secondary to a ruptured aneurysm, blood is noted in the basal cisterns as well as in the fourth ventricle. Posttraumatic SAH tends to remain localized in association with the region of contusion. Individuals with hypertension are predisposed to spontaneous **intraparenchymal hemorrhage** (IPH). Hypertensive hemorrhage occurs most frequently in the basal ganglia, followed in frequency by the brain stem, cerebellum, and occasionally the cortex. In image *d*, a spontaneous thalamic hemorrhage is shown. IPH also may be the result of underlying lesions, including infarction, tumor, and vascular malformation, or it may occur following a trauma (e.g., contusion).

ANSWER: A-b; B-d; C-a; D-c

28. Match each clinical description with the appropriate gadolinium-enhanced MRI images shown here (a–d).

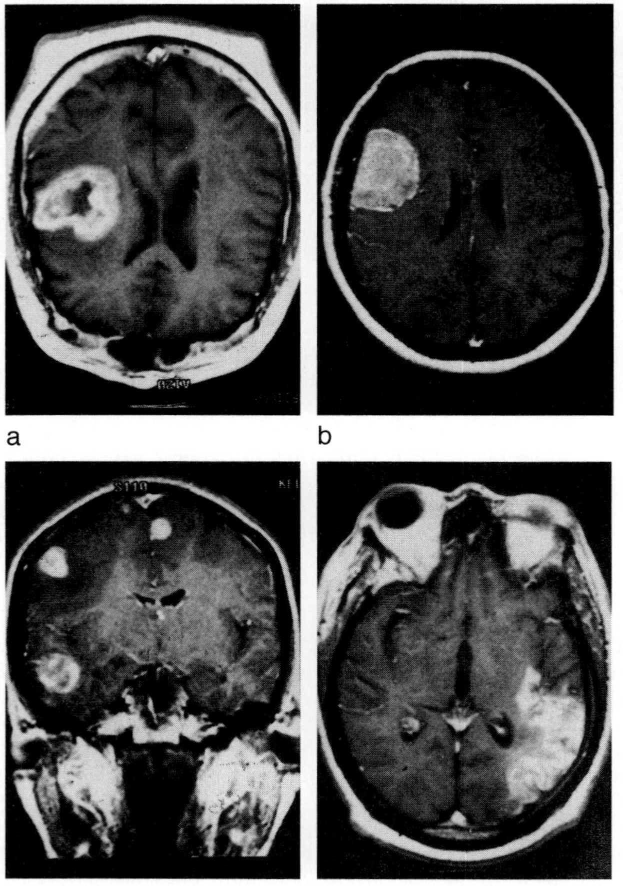

A. A 43-year-old woman with a history of breast carcinoma presented with confusion.
B. A 61-year-old man with no significant past medical history developed seizures and the gradual onset of hemiparesis.
C. A 52-year-old woman had mild head trauma; plain films of the skull demonstrated sclerosis of the calvarium.
D. An 81-year-old man had an acute onset of aphasia 2 weeks prior to the scan.

Ref.: 6, 9

COMMENTS: Gadolinium-DTPA is an MRI contrast medium that increases the intensity ("brightness") of tissues in which it is distributed. Thus it changes the appearance of MRI scans in the same way that radiopaque contrast medium changes the appearance of CT scans. Gadolinium-enhanced MRI is highly sensitive for detecting a wide variety of CNS lesions. Although not always specific, there are features that help distinguish various lesions. Image *a* is that of a **glioblastoma multiforme** (high-grade astrocytoma) and demonstrates a single peripherally enhancing lesion with central necrosis and surrounding edema. The tumor margins are somewhat ill-defined and irregular, and the thickness of the enhancing wall varies. Pathologically, viable tumor cells are almost invariably found outside of the enhancing portion of the tumor. **Meningioma**, demonstrated in image *b*, is a (usually) benign nonglial neoplasm thought to arise from meningothelial cells of arachnoid villi; therefore it typically occurs along dural surfaces. Because of their slow growth, meningiomas may produce few or no symptoms. Radiographically, meningiomas usually are smooth, rounded, sharply defined extraaxial masses that enhance homogeneously following administration of contrast. Hemorrhage and necrosis are uncommon. Often there is sclerosis of the overlying calvarium that can be seen on plain radiographs or CT scan. Most **cerebral metastases**, as seen in image *c*, are multiple, supratentorial, and tend to occur at the junction of gray and white matter. Lung, breast, melanoma, kidney, and colon are the most common sites of origin. Radiographically, metastases typically are enhanced, and hemorrhage and necrosis within them is common. Even small lesions may have significant surrounding edema and mass effect. Not all enhancing intracranial lesions, however, are neoplastic. Image *d* demonstrates gyriform enhancement in a **subacute cortical infarction**. This enhancement occurs approximately 1–3 weeks following the acute event. Cortical enhancement also may be seen in cases of encephalitis. Intracranial abscesses and granulomas may be indistinguishable from primary tumors or metastatic disease, although they tend to have thinner, more uniform walls.

ANSWER: A-c; B-a; C-b; D-d

29. Which of the following is/are true regarding cerebral perfusion pressure (CPP)?

A. CPP is defined as the mean arterial pressure (MAP) minus the intracranial pressure (ICP).
B. CPP should be kept above a minimum of 30 mm Hg.
C. With head trauma, low CPP may aggravate cerebral ischemia caused by mass lesions, vasospasm, and altered vascular autoregulation.
D. ICP increases dramatically with blood pressure changes up to 30 mm Hg in head-injured patients.

Ref.: 5

COMMENTS: Studies have shown that the management of critically ill head-injured patients should take into account the CPP. This was a logical extension of evidence indicating that cerebral ischemia (global and local) was a major factor in the poor outcome of those with severe head injury. Because CPP is a direct factor in cerebral blood flow, increasing the CPP in a patient at risk for cerebral ischemia may improve outcome. Experimental evidence shows that modest increases in MAP increase CPP without significant changes in ICP.

ANSWER: A, C

30. Regarding the anatomy of the peripheral nerve, match each anatomic structure in the left column with the appropriate description or function in the right column.

A. Neuron
B. Endoneurium
C. Perineurium
D. Epineurium
E. Sheath of Schwann

a. Sheet-like structure composed of fine strands of collagen; present along the axons of myelinated and unmyelinated nerve fibers
b. Sheath of connective tissue that surrounds each peripheral nerve fiber and Schwann cell
c. Thin sheet of connective tissue surrounding each fascicle of a nerve trunk
d. Dense collagenous layer of connective tissue that serves as a sheath for all peripheral nerve trunks
e. Cell that serves as the anatomic, trophic, and functional unit of the nervous system

Ref.: 10

COMMENTS: The **neuron** consists of a cell body and one or more axons, which together transmit and receive the messages at the nervous system. The **endoneurium** is a sheath of delicate connective tissue consisting of collagen, ground substance, and an occasional fibroblast that surrounds each peripheral nerve fiber and Schwann cell. The **perineurium** is a thin sheet of connective tissue that surrounds each fascicle of a nerve trunk, protecting it from stretch injury and maintaining a constant intrafascicular pressure. The **epineurium** is a much thicker, fibrous layer of connective tisse that is the outermost layer of a nerve trunk. Peripheral nerves have an additional outer basement membrane known as the **sheath of Schwann**; myelin is formed when the Schwann cell membrane becomes wrapped in a double layer around the peripheral nerve. It serves to insulate the axon, enhancing conduction of the nerve impulse. The microanatomy of the peripheral nerve plays a role in nerve repair. The epineurium readily holds sutures, and epineurial repair is the most commonly used technique of neurorrhapy. Its major drawback is the uncertainty of fascicular alignment. Although the indications for fascicular (perineural) repair are somewhat controversial, there are some situations (such as ulnar nerve transection at the distal forearm) when fascicular repair is preferred, especially in mixed nerves where fascicular alignment is so critical.

ANSWER: A-e; B-b; C-c; D-d; E-a

REFERENCES

1. Kandel ER, Schwartz JH (eds): *Principles of Neural Sciences.* Part II. Edward Arnold, London, 1981.
2. Schwartz SI, Shires GT, Spencer FC: *Principles of Surgery*, 7th ed. McGraw-Hill, New York, 1999.
3. Sabiston DC Jr: *Textbook of Surgery*, 15th ed. WB Saunders, Philadelphia, 1997.
4. Ross JS, Masaryk TJ, Modic MT, et al: Intracranial aneurysms: evaluation of MR angiography. *Am J Radiol* 155:159, 1990.
5. Narayan RK, Rosner MJ, Pitts LH, et al: *Guidelines for the Management of Severe Head Injury.* Brain Trauma Foundation, Chicago, 1995.
6. Schmidek HH, Sweet WH: *Operative Neurosurgical Techniques*, 3rd ed. WB Saunders, Philadelphia, 1995.
7. Way LW: *Current Surgical Diagnosis and Treatment*, 10th ed. Appleton & Lange, Norwalk, CT, 1994.
8. Menezes AH, Sonntag VK, Benzel EC, et al: *Principles of Spinal Surgery*. McGraw-Hill, New York, 1996.
9. Atlas SW: *Magnetic Resonance Imaging of the Brain and Spine.* Raven Press, New York, 1991.
10. Aston S, Seasley R, Thorne C (eds): *Grabb & Smith's Plastic Surgery*, 5th ed. Lippincott-Raven, Philadelphia, 1997.

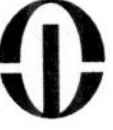

CHAPTER 46

Orthopedics

A. Clinicopathologic Principles

1. With regard to normal articular cartilage, which of the following statements is/are true?

   A. It contains predominantly type I collagen.
   B. It is relatively hypocellular.
   C. It receives its nutrition via capillaries in the subchondral bone.
   D. Its mechanical behavior can be described as viscoelastic.

Ref.: 1

COMMENTS: Articular cartilage is composed of relatively few cells within an extracellular matrix consisting predominantly of type II collagen and proteoglycans. The large, highly negatively charged proteoglycans hold positively charged ions and water in the tissue by electrostatic and osmotic forces. Under compressive loading, these smaller molecules are expressed from the tissue, which results in a greater negative charge density in the tissue. When the load is removed, the positive ions and water are reabsorbed. This is the molecular basis for the viscoelastic property of the tissue, which is vital to its role of smoothly transmitting forces across bony articulations. The cartilage receives its nutrition from the synovial fluid. Movement of nutrients into and out of the tissue is dependent on the cyclic loading of the tissue, which occurs during use of the joint. When musculoskeletal injuries are treated, the advantages of immobilization (e.g., fracture healing) must be weighed against the potential metabolic injury to the cartilage of associated joints.

ANSWER: B, D

2. With regard to bone growth and repair, match each term in the left column with one or more appropriate characteristics in the right column.

A. Endochondral ossification	a. Longitudinal growth
B. Membranous ossification	b. Fracture healing
C. Heterotopic ossification	c. Flat bone growth
	d. Soft tissue injury

Ref.: 1, 2

COMMENTS: Bone growth occurs primarily by endochondral ossification or membranous ossification. The truncal bones and spine are formed principally by **endochondral ossification**. The process consists of formation of a cartilage model and subsequent replacement of the cartilage by bone. This process occurs at the growth plate. The skull, mandible, and clavicles are formed primarily by **membranous ossification**, a process that consists of the development of bone directly from mesenchymal cells of the periosteum. Fracture healing is a complex process in which a composite tissue of bone, cartilage, and fibrous tissue is formed and subsequently is remodeled to form mature bone. The reparative tissue is bone callus. **Heterotopic ossification** is the formation of bone within the soft tissue. It is associated with certain fractures and surgical procedures and may be a significant source of morbidity.

ANSWER: A-a,b; B-b,c; C-d

3. Lateral herniation of the sixth cervical intervertebral disc usually produces which of the following?

   A. Compression of the fifth cervical nerve root.
   B. Compression of the sixth cervical nerve root.
   C. Compression of the seventh cervical nerve root.
   D. Spinal cord compression alone.
   E. Concurrent nerve root and spinal cord compression.

Ref.: 1, 2

COMMENTS: Most patients with cervical disc degeneration have only symptoms of local and referred pain. **Lateral herniation** of a cervical disc may produce nerve root compression with radicular symptoms. **Central (posterior) herniation** occurs less commonly and may result in spinal cord compression. There are eight cervical nerve roots; the first exits from the spinal canal between the occiput and the atlas. Nerve root compression produced by herniation of a cervical disc affects the nerve root immediately below it.

ANSWER: C

4. Which of the following diagnostic studies may be useful in the evaluation of de Quervain's disease?

   A. Adson test.
   B. Chest radiography.
   C. Nerve conduction studies.
   D. Cervical spine radiography.
   E. Finkelstein test.

Ref.: 1, 2

COMMENTS: Pain in the hand or forearm (or both) may result from various musculoskeletal or neurologic disorders. Neurogenic pain may reflect involvement at any level from the spinal cord to peripheral nerves. The cause can be determined from the history, physical examination, and appropriate laboratory tests. Radiologic studies are important for evaluation of cervical vertebral abnormalities and lung tumors. Nerve conduction studies confirm the clinical diagnosis of median nerve compression. The Adson test involves elevation of the first rib (a deep breath), contraction of the scalene muscle (turn head to examined side), and stretching it (extending the neck). The test may be positive with thoracic outlet syndrome (as may other such tests), but it is not diagnostic. The Finkelstein test (patient grasps own thumb within clenched fist and then makes an ulnar deviation of the wrist) produces pain in patients with tenosynovitis of the abductor pollicis longus and extensor pollicis brevis (de Quervain's disease).

ANSWER: E

5. Acute cervical nerve root compression caused by disc herniation may be treated by which of the following?

A. Short-term bed rest, soft cervical collar, and cervical traction.
B. Prompt institution of active resistance exercises.
C. Radiation therapy for progression of any neurologic deficit.
D. Surgical decompression to prevent progression of neurologic deficit.

Ref.: 1, 2

COMMENTS: In most acute cases, recumbency, sedation, and traction immobilization of the neck are indicated. When pain has subsided or the attacks are less severe, exercises may be initiated to improve flexibility. Progression of the neurologic deficit and evidence of spinal cord compression are indications for an operative procedure, usually laminectomy and sometimes spinal fusion or disc removal. Radiation therapy is given for relief of symptoms caused by malignant disease and if there is bone stability; if there is not, bone stability may be obtained by a surgical procedure.

ANSWER: A, D

6. Match each spinal condition in the left column with the appropriate phrase in the right column.

A. Spondylolisthesis	a. Defined as subluxation of a vertebral body
B. Spondylolysis	b. Defined as a bone defect of the neural arch
C. Both spondylolisthesis and spondylolysis	c. Commonly involves L5
D. Neither spondylolisthesis nor spondylolysis	d. Usually results from trauma

Ref.: 1, 2

COMMENTS: **Spondylolisthesis** is anterior subluxation of a vertebral body, most commonly involving the fifth lumbar vertebra. It usually results from a structural defect in the pars interarticularis (**spondylolysis**), which may be inherited. Degenerative joint disease and stress fractures are other causes of spondylolisthesis. Neither of these terms should be confused with **spondylosis**, which is a general term for degenerative vertebral disease.

ANSWER: A-a; B-b; C-c; D-d

7. Which of the following tumors is seen most frequently in the spine?

A. Primary CNS tumor.
B. Primary bone tumor.
C. Metastatic breast cancer.
D. Metastatic colon cancer.

Ref.: 1, 2

COMMENTS: Spinal tumors are classified as intradural or extradural. **Extradural** tumors are usually metastatic cancers or primary bone tumors (the metastatic lesions are more common). Breast, lung, prostate, and kidney are frequent primary sites. Other malignant extradural tumors include myeloma, lymphoma, plasmacytoma, and chordoma osteogenic sarcoma. **Intradural** tumors are usually primary central nervous system (CNS) tumors. They may be benign or malignant.

ANSWER: C

8. With regard to coccydynia, which of the following statements is/are true?

A. It may be of traumatic origin.
B. It is often associated with radicular symptoms.
C. It is best treated by excision of the coccyx.
D. It is often associated with anal sphincter incompetence.

Ref.: 1, 2

COMMENTS: Pain in the coccyx or lower sacrum can be caused by trauma, arthritis, or disc protrusion. The pain must be clinically differentiated from other forms of perineal pain, including proctalgia fugax, intergluteal fold inflammation, low pilonidal cyst infection, and dorsal perirectal abscess. The symptoms of coccydynia may be aggravating and progressive, but there is no radicular component or impairment of sphincter function. Treatment is usually nonoperative, consisting of heat, cushioned seating, and antiinflammatory medications. Only rarely is operative intervention required.

ANSWER: A

9. All of the following are common initial symptoms of lumbar intervertebral disc herniation except:

A. Low backache.
B. Sciatic pain.
C. Simultaneous backache and sciatic pain.
D. Incontinence.

Ref.: 1, 2

COMMENTS: Herniation of an intervertebral disc may proceed vertically or horizontally. **Vertical herniation** into the body of the vertebra (Schmorl's node) has no clinical significance. **Horizontal involvement** can be a bulge in the annulus, herniation of the nucleus, or extrusion of the nucleus. Usually herniation is *posterolateral* and therefore accompanied by unilateral nerve root compression. About half of the patients have presenting symptoms of low back pain, and sciatic pain may develop later. Approximately one third of patients first experience sciatica, however, and in the rest sciatica and back pain occur simultaneously. *Anterolateral* nuclear herniation is often associated with spondylosis (degenerative vertebral disease). Incontinence, which indicates spinal cord or cauda equina compression, is rarely associated with herniated nucleus pulposus, but it may represent progressive neurologic injury requiring immediate surgical decompression.

ANSWER: D

10. Which one or more of the following physical findings would not be consistent with an L5–S1 disc herniation?

A. Positive straight-leg-raising test on the side of the herniation.
B. Positive Lasègue's sign on the side of the herniation.
C. Sensory deficit.
D. Absent knee jerk.
E. Absent ankle jerk.

Ref.: 1, 2

COMMENTS: Examination of a patient with low back pain includes careful observation of movement, spinal curvature, and range of motion. **Straight-leg-raising** with the patient in the supine position produces ipsilateral pain when there is nerve root compression. Aggravation of the pain may be produced by subsequent dorsiflexion of the foot. **Lasègue's sign** is elicited with the patient in the supine position and the hip and knee flexed to 90 degrees. The knee is then extended. Pain in the back and leg with less than 180 degrees of knee extension constitutes a positive result. Neurologic examination may reveal **hypesthesia** and **weakness** according to the nerve root involved. Herniation at the L5–S1 level may be accompanied by a diminished **ankle jerk**. If the **knee jerk** is absent, compression is occurring at a higher level (L3–L4). The **femoral stretch test** (extension of the hip with flexion of the knee) may be positive in this instance.

ANSWER: D

11. With regard to treatment of a herniated intervertebral disc, which of the following statements is/are true?

A. Rest, analgesics, and heat/cold modalities provide relief in most cases.
B. Laminectomy is performed in all cases to prevent paraplegia.
C. Epidural steroids may provide some relief in selected cases.
D. Injection of chymopapain is indicated in patients with extruded disc fragments.

Ref.: 1, 2

COMMENTS: An initial trial of **conservative treatment** is indicated in patients without progressive neurologic deficits. Most patients (>85%) have substantial improvement within 6 weeks. Epidural steroids have been found effective in patients with spinal stenosis and may have some beneficial effect in patients with sciatica. **Operative management** is indicated for substantial or progressive neurologic deficit, in refractory cases, or for those with severe sciatica. Paraplegia rarely occurs with isolated disc injury. **Chymopapain (proteolytic enzyme) injection** into the disc may be beneficial in selected patients with small central disc herniations but not when there is frank extrusion.

ANSWER: A, C

12. With regard to pyogenic osteomyelitis of the vertebral column, which of the following statements is/are true?

A. It is most commonly caused by tuberculosis.
B. It is usually associated with paravertebral abscess.
C. It is most common in the thoracic region.
D. It is most common in the elderly.
E. It is most common in men.

Ref.: 1, 2

COMMENTS: Pyogenic osteomyelitis of the vertebral column is most commonly caused by hematogenous spread of *Staphylococcus aureus* from other sites. These infections most commonly occur in adolescents and young men and most commonly involve the lumbar region. Paravertebral abscess formation, although rare, is seen with increasing frequency in immunocompromised patients. Tuberculous osteomyelitis may occur in patients with active human immunodeficiency virus (HIV) syndrome. Treatment of pyogenic osteomyelitis includes immobilization, antibiotics, and surgical débridement or drainage. An anterior operative approach is usually advised. Bone grafting may be required.

ANSWER: E

13. Principles of tendon transfer include which of the following?

A. The muscle used should retain its full strength after transfer.
B. Joint contractures should be corrected before operation.
C. Synergistic muscles provide better results.
D. The selected muscle must have adequate excursion.

Ref.: 1, 2

COMMENTS: Tendon transfer is used to restore function, muscle balance, and strength to joint motions in patients with various paralytic conditions. There are four main requirements for tendon transfer: (1) A muscle with adequate strength must be available, because one grade of strength is lost after transfer as a result of loss of the direct line of action between the muscle origin and insertion. (2) The muscle must have adequate excursion to allow sufficient range of motion of the joint. (3) The joint must have passive range of motion before transfer. (4) Synergistic muscles generally provide better results, although tendon transfers of nonsynergistic muscles can be successful with proper rehabilitation.

ANSWER: B, C, D

14. With regard to Dupuytren's contracture, which of the following statements is/are true?

A. It results from severe tenosynovitis.
B. It is most common among manual laborers.
C. It may be treated with steroid injection and physical therapy.
D. Successful surgical treatment requires complete excision of the palmar fascia.

Ref.: 1

COMMENTS: Contracture of the palmar aponeurosis is believed to be inherited, although other factors may affect the extent of its expression. It is associated with epilepsy, tuberculosis, and alcoholism. Contrary to common notions, its incidence is not higher in manual laborers. There are several clinical types of involvement that vary in severity. Nonoperative treatment, consisting of exercise, local injections of steroids, and even radiation therapy, has been successful. Partial fasciectomy is useful for limited contractures; more severe cases require radical excision of the palmar fascia.

ANSWER: C

15. Volkmann's ischemic contracture involves which one or more of the following?

A. Ischemic injury to the deep flexor muscles of the forearm.
B. Ischemic injury to the extensor muscles of the forearm.
C. Compromised blood flow in the anterior interosseous artery.
D. Compromised blood flow in the posterior interosseous artery.

Ref.: 1, 2

COMMENTS: Volkmann's contracture is the result of ischemic damage to the muscles of the deep flexor compartment of the forearm (flexor digitorum profundus and flexor pollicis longus) secondary to compromise of flow in the anterior interosseous artery. This contracture can be a complication of supracondylar fracture, forearm fracture, brachial artery puncture, hemophilia, and various forms of trauma. The median nerve, which lies close to the anterior interosseous artery, may be involved in this process; and in severe cases the ulnar nerve can be involved as well. Because the damage occurs within a few hours of the insult, initial treatment must be prompt and definitive.

ANSWER: A, C

16. Which of the following statements is/are true?

A. Osgood's disease and Sever's disease may present in a similar manner.
B. Legg-Calvé-Perthes disease may be confused with septic arthritis of the hip.
C. Slipped capital femoral epiphysis (SCFE) commonly occurs in thin adolescent girls.
D. All of these conditions generally require operative correction.

Ref.: 3

COMMENTS: Traction apophysitis may occur in rapidly growing children as an overuse type of injury. **Osgood's** (tibial tubercle) and **Sever's** (calcaneus) disease are the most common locations. Numerous factors have been implicated, including vascular disturbance, repetitive overuse, and genetic factors. Symptomatic improvement is generally the rule with rest, analgesics, and occasional immobilization. **Legg-Calvé-Perthes** is the pediatric equivalent of avascular necrosis of the proximal femur. It is most common in the 6- to 11-year age group. Symptoms include acute or subacute onset of hip pain, limp, and loss of motion, which may be confused with septic arthritis. Bone scans or magnetic resonance imaging (MRI) may be helpful, although hip aspiration may be necessary to rule out joint infection. **Slipped capital femoral epiphysis** (SCFE) presents with similar symptoms but is usually seen in endomorphic boys between the ages 11 and 15 years. Treatment of SCFE is surgical stabilization with screw fixation or open epiphyseodosis.

ANSWER: A, B

17. With regard to scoliosis, which of the following statements is/are true?

A. Congenital scoliosis is the form most likely associated with paraplegia.
B. The prognosis for both paralytic and idiopathic scoliosis is related to age of onset.
C. Idiopathic scoliosis is progressive.
D. The site of curvature affects the prognosis of idiopathic scoliosis.

Ref.: 1

COMMENTS: The specific treatment of scoliosis depends on several clinical considerations. Because untreated **congenital scoliosis** is the form that most often results in paraplegia, affected patients must be closely observed throughout their growth period. The two most important prognostic factors for **idiopathic scoliosis** are age of onset and site of the curve. This form progresses during growth; and because the onset occurs before the age of 10 years the prognosis is poor and the deformity often severe. With **paralytic scoliosis** the prognosis depends more on age at onset than on the location of the primary curve.

ANSWER: A, B, C, D

18. While obtaining a posterior iliac bone graft, the surgeon encounters major arterial bleeding at the base of the wound. The artery most likely to be damaged is the:

A. Inferior gluteal.
B. Superior gluteal.
C. Lateral femoral circumflex.
D. Iliohypogastric.

Ref.: 4

COMMENTS: The superior gluteal artery exits the pelvis via the sciatic notch just above the piriformis muscle. Lying deep to the gluteus medius muscle, the artery may be lacerated during bone graft harvesting. The lacerated artery may retract back into the pelvis, making hemostasis difficult. Arterial embolization or retroperitoneal exploration may be necessary for control.

ANSWER: B

19. Which of the following is a consistent feature of osteoporosis?

A. Increased serum alkaline phosphatase.
B. Decreased serum phosphorus.
C. Impaired mineralization of osteoid.
D. Increased susceptibility to fracture.
E. Hyperparathyroidism.

Ref.: 5

COMMENTS: Osteoporosis, defined as decreased bone mass, most commonly occurs in postmenopausal women. A relative lifelong calcium deficiency, early menopause, and genetic factors contribute to the etiology. Serum laboratory values are normal and are used to exclude other conditions. Bone density is best measured using radiographic techniques (DEXA scanning) of the spine, radius, or calcaneus. To minimize the increased risk of fracture, treatment strategies included calcium supplementation and hormonal replacement. Some medications (alendronate) may increase bone mass.

ANSWER: D

20. A 33-year-old patient has numbness of the medial side of the leg and foot, no patellar tendon reflex, and weakness of the tibialis anterior muscle. The nerve root involved is:

A. First sacral.
B. Second lumbar.
C. Third lumbar.
D. Fourth lumbar.
E. Fifth lumbar.

Ref.: 5

COMMENTS: See Question 21.

21. The most appropriate diagnostic test for the patient in Question 20 is:

A. Electromyography.
B. Bone scan.
C. Magnetic resonance imaging (MRI).
D. Computed tomography (CT).

Ref.: 5

COMMENTS: The patient presents with complaints typical of sciatica due to a herniated disc between the third and fourth vertebra affecting the L4 nerve root. Electromyography is commonly used in cases of suspected peripheral neuropathy or cervical radiculopathy but rarely for isolated herniated disc of the lumbar spine. Bone scanning or CT imaging may be helpful in suspected cases of spondylolysis or spondylolithesis. MRI provides the best examination of soft tissues including the intervertebral disc and nerve roots.

ANSWER:
Question 20: D
Question 21: C

22. The parents of a 14-month-old child indicate she has been crying and has refused to walk since she fell last night. She had recently begun to walk. Radiographs reveal a displaced spiral midshaft fracture of the femur. In addition to stabilization of the fracture, the physician should order:

A. Serum calcium, phosphorus, and alkaline phosphastase assays.
B. Skeletal survey.
C. MRI of the femur.
D. Bone biopsy.
E. Urine mucopolysaccharide screen.

Ref.: 3

COMMENTS: Spiral fractures are due to a twist or torsional injury and are rare in toddlers or small children. A skeletal survey is indicated to rule out injuries in various stages of healing in cases of suspected child abuse. Fractures due to metabolic bone disease (i.e., nutritional rickets) occur more commonly as transverse metaphyseal fractures and are associated with chronic radiographic changes.

ANSWER: B

REFERENCES

1. Schwartz SI, Shires GT, Spencer FC: *Principles of Surgery*, 7th ed. McGraw-Hill, New York, 1999.
2. Sabiston DC Jr: *Textbook of Surgery*, 15th ed. WB Saunders, Philadelphia, 1997.
3. Morrissey RT, Weinstien SL: *Lovell and Winters Pediatric Orthopaedics*, 4th ed. Lippincott, Philadelphia, 1996.
4. Browner BD, Jupiter JB, Levine AM, Trafton, PG: *Skeletal Trauma*. WB Saunders, Philadelphia, 1992.
5. Deg R: *Principles of Orthopaedic Practice*. McGraw-Hill, New York, 1992.

Orthopedics

B. Trauma

1. Proper care of an open fracture generally includes which of the following?

A. Culture of the wound.
B. Antibiotic prophylaxis.
C. Tetanus prophylaxis.
D. Complete surgical débridement.
E. Immobilization of bony fragments.

Ref.: 1, 2

COMMENTS: With an open fracture the skin or mucosal barrier is broken, introducing the possibility of infection from contamination of the fracture site. Management is aimed at preventing infection and allowing bony union. These goals can best be attained through recognition of potential contamination, antibiotic and tetanus prophylaxis, débridement of devitalized tissues, and immobilization of fractures. Culture specimens should be obtained from all wounds associated with open fractures when patients present and at the time of débridement. Soft-tissue management is based on the same principles as for other types of injury, depending on wound size, degree of contamination, and time interval between injury and treatment. The method of fracture stabilization depends on the fracture configuration, the degree of contamination, and the nature of the associated soft-tissue injury.

ANSWER: A, B, C, D, E

2. Which of the following injuries is/are associated with serious risk of vascular injury?

A. Supracondylar fracture of the humerus.
B. Supracondylar fracture of the femur.
C. Knee dislocation.
D. Trimalleolar fracture.
E. Colles' fracture.

Ref.: 2

COMMENTS: Although arterial injury may accompany any fracture or dislocation, it is more common with certain injuries, such as supracondylar fractures of the humerus or femur and posterior dislocation of the knee. Mechanisms of arterial injury include laceration by bony fragments; traction with resultant spasm, entrapment, and compression by fracture fragments; and compression caused by elevated compartmental pressure. Each of these may occur after manipulative closed reduction or casting. Clinical findings suggestive of vascular compression are known as the **five P's**: pain, pallor, pulselessness, paralysis, and paresthesia. Pain is typically out of proportion to that anticipated and often is not relieved by standard analgesic techniques. The severely injured extremity should be reevaluated frequently even if there is no initial suggestion of vascular compromise. Arteriography should be performed if there is any question of vascular injury. All patients with posterior knee dislocation should undergo arteriography because of the high incidence of arterial trauma associated with this injury. Definitive therapy must be instituted promptly because irreversible muscle injury may occur after 6–8 hours of ischemia. Supracondylar fractures of the humerus associated with brachial artery injury may result in flexion contracture of the forearm (Volkmann's ischemic contracture). Inability to extend the fingers actively or passively without pain is the earliest sign of ischemic contracture.

ANSWER: A, B, C

3. Torus fractures and greenstick fractures have in common which one or more of the following characteristics?

A. At least partial continuity of the cortex.
B. Higher rate of nonunion than with other fractures.
C. Best treated by internal fixation.
D. Caused by repeated stress.
E. Occur only in children.

Ref.: 1, 2

COMMENTS: A **torus** fracture is a wrinkle or buckle of the cortex, usually found in the metaphyseal region of long bones of children. The distal radius is a common site. The fracture results from failure of the cortex under compression. There may be angulation of alignment, but displacement does not occur. **Greenstick** fractures, in contrast, involve disruption of the cortex under tension. Partial continuity of the cortex is present with both fractures. These fractures occur in children and heal readily. They rarely necessitate internal fixation. Whereas repeated stress results in a fatigue or stress fracture, it plays no role in the mechanism of injury for torus or greenstick fractures. Stress fractures commonly occur in young soldiers required to force-march and in athletes.

ANSWER: A, E

4. Which of the following types of peripheral nerve injury associated with extremity trauma is/are usually best treated by delayed surgical repair?

A. Neurapraxia.
B. Axonotmesis.
C. Neurotmesis.
D. Digital nerve injury.

Ref.: 2

COMMENTS: Fractures of the extremities may be associated with peripheral nerve injuries, of which there are three major types. **Neurapraxia** implies a physiologic interruption of nerve conduction caused by the inability of the neurons to reestablish their membrane potentials. With severe stretch injuries, the motor deficit is typically more prominent than the sensory loss. The abnormality usually resolves within 6 weeks after injury. **Axonotmesis** occurs when there is both axonal and myelin loss (wallerian degeneration) even though the Schwann sheath is intact. In this circumstance, there may be complete motor and sensory loss, although axonal regeneration usually ensues in a proximal-to-distal manner. Most fractures cause nerve injuries in continuity (neurapraxia or axonotmesis). These deficits should have follow-up observation and electrodiagnostic studies and be allowed to heal spontaneously. The most severe lesion is **neurotmesis**, or complete division of the nerve. Neurotmesis necessitates precise apposition of the nerve ends. Primary repair is most appropriate in the presence of sharp **lacerations** without adjacent stretch and for digital nerve injuries. Most cases are best treated by delayed repair once the soft tissue injury has resolved.

ANSWER: C

5. Match each fracture or dislocation in the left column with one or more appropriate associated injuries in the right column (each of which may be selected once, more than once, or not at all).

A. Anterior dislocation of shoulder
B. Supracondylar fracture of the humerus
C. Posterior dislocation of the knee
D. Fracture of distal radius
E. Fracture of the neck of the fibula

a. Median nerve
b. Axillary nerve
c. Peroneal nerve
d. Brachial artery
e. Popliteal artery

Ref.: 3

COMMENTS: Blunt trauma can produce a variety of limb-threatening injuries. Anterior dislocation of the shoulder results from axial loading of the externally rotated, extended arm. The humeral head is driven forward out of the glenoid cavity. The axillary nerve is injured in 5–30% of cases. Posterior dislocation typically results from axial loading of the flexed or adducted arm. Axillary nerve injury is rare. Most supracondylar fractures of the humerus are of the extension type; the end of the proximal fragment is driven through the overlying brachialis muscle into the brachial artery and the median nerve. Posterior dislocations of the knee often compromise the popliteal artery. Fractures of the distal radius and the fibular neck can produce compression of the median nerve and common peroneal nerve, respectively.

ANSWER: A-b; B-a,d; C-e; D-a; E-c

6. Nonunion of fractures is more common with or in which of the following?

A. Infection.
B. Children.
C. Extensive soft-tissue injury.
D. Closed reduction.
E. Hypercalcemia.

Ref.: 1, 2

COMMENTS: Nonunion is complete failure of a fracture to unite by bone. There are two types: **Fibrous nonunion** is healing of a fracture by fibrous tissue; there is some potential for bony union, provided the fracture is immobilized and that local deterrents such as infection are eradicated. Once the bone ends have become sclerosed, union should be encouraged by autogenous bone graft. **Pseudoarthrosis** results from continued movement at the fracture site, thereby stimulating the formation of a false joint with a synovial-like capsule. Factors conducive to nonunion include severe disruption of the periosteal sleeve, loss of blood supply, continuation of shearing forces at the fracture site, distraction, interposition of soft tissue, infection, and preexisting bone disorder (i.e., pathologic fracture). In young adults the most common causes of nonunion are excessive soft-tissue destruction and infection. At the time of operative reduction and fixation of the fracture, periosteal stripping and devitalization must be avoided. Rickets and osteomalacia are caused by vitamin D deficiency, a primary effect of which is hypophosphatemia because of decreased renal tubular absorption of phosphate. If operative repair of a bone deformity is attempted before correction of the metabolic abnormality, nonunion is likely to occur.

ANSWER: A, C

7. Pathologic fractures may result from:

A. Primary bone tumors.
B. Metastatic bone tumors.
C. Benign bone cysts.
D. Osteogenesis imperfecta.

Ref.: 1, 2

COMMENTS: Pathologic fractures occur spontaneously or as a result of minor trauma in bones with a preexisting pathologic condition. Although any primary or metastatic malignant process may be responsible, benign conditions frequently are the cause. In adults osteoporosis may result in pathologic fractures; in children developmental and metabolic diseases such as osteogenesis imperfecta, osteopetrosis, and nutritional deficiencies may be responsible. Benign bone cysts and tumors also may be associated with fractures.

ANSWER: A, B, C, D

8. With regard to stress fractures, which of the following statements is/are true?

A. They are associated with an underlying congenital disorder of bone formation.
B. They commonly affect the femoral neck.
C. They are best detected as a result of strong clinical suspicion and a positive bone scan.
D. They usually necessitate internal fixation for adequate union.

Ref.: 1, 2

COMMENTS: Stress or fatigue fractures are the result of repeated forces that cause accelerated osteoclastic activity with a loss of normal structural mass and subsequent new periosteal bone formation. Patients complain of local pain during the early phase. Radiographic findings at this time reveal only subtle osteoporosis; hence a bone scan may be necessary for establishing the diagnosis. Should the repetitive stress continue, a fracture results. The usual locations of such fractures include the femoral neck, the distal second and third metatarsal shafts, the proximal tibia, the distal fibula, and the calcaneus. The treatment of stress fracture is immobilization and cessation of the responsible activity.

ANSWER: B, C

9. Match each Salter and Harris classification with the corresponding physeal injury in children illustrated below.

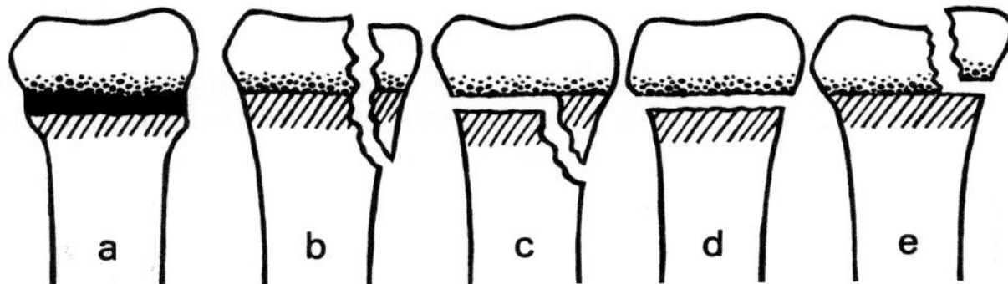

A. Salter I.
B. Salter II.
C. Salter III.
D. Salter IV.
E. Salter V.

Ref.: 2

COMMENTS: The Salter and Harris classification applies to patients in whom the physeal plate has not yet fused. **Salter I** injury is complete separation of the physeal plate from the metaphysis without recognized bony fracture on radiography. The epiphysis may be displaced. **Salter II** injury is partial separation of physeal plate with extension into the metaphysis. This extraarticular fracture commonly occurs at the distal radial or tibial physis. **Salter III** injury is partial separation of physeal plate with extension of the fracture into the epiphysis. It represents an intraarticular fracture. **Salter IV** injury is a fracture that extends from the metaphysis to the bony epiphysis, crossing the physeal plate. The most common injury is fracture of the lateral condyle of the humerus. **Salter V** injury is a crush injury to the physeal plate. It is important to recognize the presence and type of epiphyseal plate injury because the physeal plate is the center of longitudinal bone growth, and injuries may result in abnormalities of length or in angular deformities. **Type I** and **type II** fractures are treated by closed reduction and usually carry an excellent prognosis. Accurate reduction is necessary for **type III** injuries because of an intraarticular component; nevertheless, the prognosis is good if the blood supply to the fractured portion is not impaired. **Type IV** and **type V** injuries are more likely to cause growth disturbances. Whenever an epiphyseal fracture exists, the patient and the parents should be cautioned that growth abnormalities may result.

ANSWER: A-d; B-c; C-e; D-b; E-a

10. Which of the following statements with regard to fractures in children compared to those in adults is/are true?

A. Nonunion is more common.
B. Compound fractures are more common.
C. More angulation and shortening may be acceptable.
D. Long bone shaft fractures more often require open reduction.

Ref.: 2

COMMENTS: Fractures must be approached differently in children and adults. Certain degrees of angulation, displacement, and shortening are acceptable, depending on the fracture site and the age of the child, because some correction occurs during the remaining growth of the bones. Factors that affect the ability of the bone to remodel include (1) the age of the child at the time of injury, (2) the distance of the fracture from the physis, and (3) the plane of deformity in relation to the plane of motion at the nearest joint. Epiphyseal injuries, however, must be properly recognized and treated to minimize the risk of growth disturbance. Compound fractures and nonunion of fractures are much less common in children. In general, shaft fractures in long bones should be treated by closed techniques to avoid the risk of infection or physeal disturbance.

ANSWER: C

11. When pain persists after closed reduction and casting, the immediate concern should be:

A. Inadequate immobilization.
B. Neural injury.
C. Muscle spasm.
D. Pressure point necrosis.
E. Ischemia.

Ref.: 2

COMMENTS: Although several factors may be responsible for limb pain after casting, ischemia is the most serious. After plaster casting, the extremity should be elevated and the digits exposed. Adequate immobilization should substantially relieve pain. Unrelenting pain is always suggestive of ischemia and is an indication for splitting the cast with parallel cuts through the padding on both sides of the extremities. Loss of reduction of the fracture has less serious consequences than prolonged limb ischemia. Other causes of pain include nerve injury, muscle spasm, and pressure-point necrosis; but persistent pain always suggests ischemia. Failure to recognize it may lead to muscle necrosis and serious disability. Localized burning pain may occur as a result of pressure-point necrosis from the cast over a bony prominence and is treated by cutting a cast window.

ANSWER: E

12. Which of the following is/are correct regarding clavicular fractures?

A. Most commonly occur at the junction of the proximal and middle thirds of the clavicle.
B. Treated with figure-of-eight splint in adults.
C. Treated with figure-of-eight splint in children.
D. Closed treatment preferred but nonunion still common.

Ref.: 1, 2

COMMENTS: Clavicular fractures most commonly occur at the junction of the middle and distal thirds of the clavicle, but in older patients fractures of the distal tip are more common. Although accurate reduction is difficult to maintain, both children and adults may be treated with a figure-of-eight or similar splint apparatus; in adults, the arm is also placed in a sling. The splint is left in position for 2 weeks in children and for 2–4 weeks in older individuals. In children, reduction of the fracture is not essential because the bone remodels with time. In adults a cosmetic deformity may result, but it is most often well tolerated and masked by overlying soft tissue. Nonunion is uncommon with closed treatment. Operative treatment of clavicular fractures is indicated only with impending skin necrosis, severe displacement, or multiple associated skeletal injuries. Open reduction of clavicular fractures is associated with a 50% incidence of nonunion and is generally indicated only for unacceptable cosmetic deformity.

ANSWER: B, C

13. With regard to dislocation of the acromioclavicular joint, which of the following statements is/are true?

A. It is most common in elderly patients with lax ligaments.
B. It is best detected with the patient examined in the supine position.
C. Radiologic diagnosis is made with stress views.
D. Operative treatment is usually not necessary.

Ref.: 2

COMMENTS: In young patients a sudden strong, downward force on the shoulder produces acromioclavicular dislocation as a result of disruption of the acromioclavicular and coracoclavicular ligaments; the stability of the distal clavicle is dependent primarily on the coracoclavicular ligaments. In elderly patients, whose bones are more porotic, a similar mechanism of injury results in fracture of the distal clavicle. Patients are best examined in the seated position, as the dislocation may reduce spontaneously in the supine patient; radiologic confirmation may require stress (distraction) views of both acromioclavicular joints. Treatment, which is focused primarily on relieving symptoms, consists of wearing a sling to support the weight of the arm. Operative treatment is seldom indicated, although persistent pain with incomplete dislocations (subluxations) may require excision of the distal end of the clavicle.

ANSWER: C, D

14. With regard to fractures of the proximal humerus, which of the following statements is/are correct?

A. They most commonly involve the anatomic neck.
B. Fractures of the surgical neck risk avascular necrosis.
C. They usually necessitate open reduction and internal fixation because of displacement.
D. Early mobilization is indicated in elderly patients.

Ref.: 1, 2

COMMENTS: The **surgical neck** (below the tuberosities) is the most common site of a proximal humeral fracture. The proximal fragment tends to remain in the neutral position, and the distal fragment (shaft) tends to be pulled medially by the pectoralis major muscle. Closed reduction and immobilization for 1–2 weeks is the main method of treatment. Fractures of the **anatomic neck** (above the tuberosities) are important because of the high incidence of associated avascular necrosis of the head. Proximal humeral fractures in children generally are Salter type II physeal injuries. Fractures of the **greater tuberosity** should be reduced if displaced more than 1 cm, and open reduction and fixation may be necessary. In elderly patients shoulder motion should begin as early as 7–10 days after reduction to prevent shoulder stiffness (adhesive capsulitis). Minimally displaced fractures at any site may be treated with a simple shoulder immobilizer.

ANSWER: D

15. Which of the following are indications for immediate operative treatment of humeral shaft fractures?

A. Radial nerve injury.
B. Median nerve injury.
C. Brachial artery injury.
D. Unsuccessful closed reduction.
E. Fractures in adults.

Ref.: 1, 2

COMMENTS: Neurovascular injuries are not uncommon with humeral shaft fractures, the most common being traction injury to the radial nerve. As with other nerve injuries secondary to fractures, function is usually recovered spontaneously. The median nerve is not in sufficient proximity to be at serious risk. Surgical neurorrhaphy is indicated if nerve function has not recovered in 4–6 months. When repair of the brachial artery is required, open reduction with internal fixation of the humeral shaft is necessary to protect the vascular repair. Although most fractures can be treated by closed reduction through some form of casting or traction, open reduction for closed shaft fractures is necessary if bone apposition cannot be obtained. Age is not a criterion for open versus closed reduction of fractures of the humeral shaft.

ANSWER: C

16. A 7-year-old is brought to the emergency room complaining of pain and deformity in his right elbow. His mother states that he fell from a tree on an extended outstretched arm. The radial pulse is absent, and the neurologic examination is normal. A prompt radiograph demonstrates an extension supracondylar fracture. Appropriate management at this time should consist of which *one* of the following?

A. Immediate arteriography.
B. Closed reduction, reexamination of vascular status, immediate percutaneous pinning.
C. Closed reduction, reexamination of vascular status, immobilization in maximal flexion at the elbow.
D. Immediate open exploration of the brachial artery.

Ref.: 4

COMMENTS: Supracondylar fractures of the humerus in children most often occur from a fall on an extended outstretched arm. Because of the high incidence of neurovascular injury associated with this fracture, accurate assessment of the median, radial, and ulnar nerves and the brachial artery is imperative. Immediate reduction under general anesthesia using fluoroscopy in most cases restores the radial pulse and peripheral circulation. Reduction is achieved by traction on the extended arm followed by pronation and maximal flexion at the elbow to restore alignment. The elbow is reextended to ensure adequacy of the radial pulse, but fractures with significant displacement and brachial artery compression are often unstable, precluding cast immobilization. These fractures are stabilized with percutaneous pinning to maintain bone stability while allowing more extension at the elbow. If arterial circulation is not restored with bone reduction, immediate arteriography, brachial artery exploration, and repair are indicated. Forearm compartment fasciotomy is indicated with any extended ischemia.

ANSWER: B

17. Which one or more of the following humeral fractures in children usually necessitate(s) an operation for correction?

A. Anatomic neck.
B. Surgical neck.
C. Shaft.
D. Supracondylar.
E. Lateral epicondyle.

Ref.: 1, 2

COMMENTS: Humeral fracture of the surgical neck, anatomic neck, and shaft are best treated by closed reduction. Supracondylar fractures are common fractures about the elbow in children and usually are treated satisfactorily by closed reduction and percutaneous pinning. Fractures of the lateral epicondyle in children are Salter type IV injuries and are therefore intraarticular. Malunion or nonunion may result in limb deformity, limitation of motion, or both. Operative correction is therefore indicated. All of the other fractures listed above are best treated by closed reduction.

ANSWER: E

18. Monteggia's fracture is best described as which of the following?

A. Ulnar styloid fracture and radial head subluxation.
B. Proximal ulnar fracture and radial head subluxation.
C. Radial head fracture and ulnar styloid subluxation.
D. Radial neck fracture and ulnar styloid subluxation.

Ref.: 1, 2

COMMENTS: Monteggia's fracture, sustained by a fall on the extended, outstretched arm, is characterized by a fracture of the proximal ulna with subluxation of the radial head. This deformity results from forced pronation or from a direct blow on the ulna, which causes proximal ulnar fracture. The radial head dislocates anteriorly in 60% of cases. Treatment consists of closed reduction for children; adults, however, require rigid internal fixation of the ulna with the forearm placed in supination to maintain reduction of the radial head. If the radial head is anterior, the elbow is maintained in 110 degrees of flexion; when the radial head is posterior, the elbow is placed in 70 degrees of flexion.

ANSWER: B

19. With regard to fractures of the forearm, which of the following statements is/are true?

A. They are more common in adults than in children.
B. Anatomic reduction is necessary in adults even if open operation is required.
C. Pronation usually provides the greatest stability for proximal fractures.
D. Supination usually provides the greatest stability for distal fractures.

Ref.: 1, 2

COMMENTS: Fractures of the forearm occur more often in children than in adults. As a general rule, whenever a fracture or dislocation of one bone of the forearm is present, associated subluxation or fracture of the other bone should be sought. Because of the interrelation necessary for normal function, anatomic reduction is necessary. If this cannot be accomplished by closed technique for single-bone fractures in adults, open reduction is indicated. Fractures of both bones in adults necessitate open reduction. Open reduction is not indicated in children. Fractures that most often necessitate open reduction are displaced fractures of the proximal third of the forearm and oblique fractures of the radius. After reduction, the arm is immobilized with the elbow at 90 degrees and the hand at the position of greatest stability, which varies according to the site of the fracture. In general, 30 degrees of angulation at the fracture site in an infant corrects itself, depending on the patient's age and the proximity of the fracture to the epiphysis. With fractures of the proximal third of the forearm, the proximal radius is in supination; thus the arm is immobilized in supination. With fractures of the distal third, greater stability is achieved by immobilizing the arm in pronation.

ANSWER: B

20. Complications of Colles' fractures include which of the following?

A. Shoulder stiffness.
B. Wrist stiffness.
C. Carpal tunnel syndrome.
D. Avascular necrosis of the ulnar styloid.

Ref.: 1, 2, 4

COMMENTS: Fractures of the distal radius, which may involve the articular surface, are common in adults over the age of 50 years. More common in women than in men, the injury occurs from a fall on the outstretched hand. Examination typically reveals a dorsal deformity of the wrist and hand and occasionally median nerve injury. Serious deformity requires reduction to restore length and proper carpal joint alignment. Unstable fractures not maintained in a cast require use of external fixation or pin fixation. Prolonged cast immobilization or positioning the wrist in excessive palmar flexion can result in joint stiffness and median nerve compression.

ANSWER: A, B, C

21. A 25-year-old skater complains of wrist pain after slipping on the ice and falling on an outstretched hand. There is specific point tenderness over the anatomic snuffbox. There is no deformity. Which of the following is the most likely diagnosis?

A. Colles' fracture.
B. Navicular (scaphoid) fracture.
C. Lunate subluxation.
D. Scaphoid-lunate subluxation.

Ref.: 1, 2

COMMENTS: See Question 23.

22. Which of the following radiographs should be obtained on the patient described in Question 21?

A. Posteroanterior (PA) view of the wrist.
B. Lateral view of the wrist.
C. Oblique view of the wrist.
D. Ulnar deviated view of the wrist.

Ref.: 1, 2

COMMENTS: See Question 23.

23. Radiographs of the patient described in Question 21 reveal no fracture or dislocation. Appropriate treatment at this time should be which of the following?

A. Ice packs, elastic wrap, and rest.
B. Dorsal wrist splint.
C. Plaster cast, including the thumb, up to the elbow.
D. Plaster cast, including the thumb and elbow.

Ref.: 1, 2

COMMENTS: The same mechanism that produces Colles' fracture in older patients results in scaphoid fracture in young adults. It is not uncommon for this fracture to go undetected on initial radiographs. Less commonly, hyperextension injuries of the wrist may cause lunate dislocation or disruption of the normal scaphoid-lunate relation. The ulnar-deviated PA view of the wrist brings the scaphoid into full profile. PA and lateral views demonstrate displacement of the lunate. Oblique radiographs may demonstrate a nondisplaced scaphoid fracture. If the patient has tenderness over the scaphoid, a fracture should be suspected despite negative radiographs. The patient should be treated with plaster cast immobilization, including the thumb and elbow. After 3 weeks, radiographs with the arm out of plaster should be repeated. If the tenderness is gone and the radiographs still are negative, no further cast immobilization is necessary. In the unlikely circumstance that tenderness persists (with negative radiographs), a bone scan can be performed for confirmation of the scaphoid fracture. Adequate treatment is important because of the risk of avascular necrosis of the proximal fragment or of nonunion inasmuch as the arterial supply enters the distal third of the navicular bone consistently. Both complications inherent in this fracture can produce posttraumatic arthritis of the wrist. By immobilizing the elbow pronation or supination, which causes motion at the fracture site, is prevented. Most scaphoid fractures require at least 6 weeks of immobilization, and up to 3 months may be needed.

ANSWER:
Question 21: B
Question 22: A, B, C, D
Question 23: D

24. With regard to fractures of the bones of the hand, which of the following statements is/are true?

A. After reduction of metacarpal neck fractures, moderate rotational deformity is acceptable.
B. An avulsion fracture associated with mallet finger is treated the same as an extensor tendon avulsion without fracture.
C. Crush injury of the distal phalanx can be treated by finger splinting.
D. Bennett's fracture involves an intraarticular fracture of the carpometacarpal joint of the thumb.

Ref.: 1, 2

COMMENTS: Fractures of the bones of the hand are among the most common problems encountered in the emergency room, and they must be treated properly to avoid or minimize any subsequent disability. Correction of **rotational** deformities with metacarpal fractures is important and is determined clinically: When flexed, each finger should point toward the scaphoid. Correction of angulation in the ulnar and radial planes is also important. Intraarticular fractures generally necessitate anatomic reduction. Open fractures (e.g., metacarpal neck fracture with an overlying soft-tissue injury by a tooth) must be recognized because of the potential for serious infection. A **mallet finger** results from avulsion of the extensor tendon, with or without a bone fragment, from its insertion on the distal phalanx. This causes dropping of the finger and loss of the last 20 degrees of active extension. When avulsion occurs with a fragment of bone involving one-third or more of the articular surface, open reduction and wire fixation are required. If the bone chip is small or does not involve the joint, treatment is the same as with pure tendon avulsion, that is, finger splint with the distal phalanx in hyperextension. A **crushed finger** requires meticulous débridement and repair of the soft tissues, including the nail bed. The often associated comminuted fracture of the distal phalanx requires only finger splinting for relief of pain. **Bennett's fracture** involves the carpometacarpal joint of the thumb and usually is sustained by a blow against the tip of the outstretched thumb.

ANSWER: C, D

25. Which of the following describes the preferred primary treatment of a femoral neck fracture?

A. Skeletal traction for nondisplaced fracture in a nonambulatory patient.
B. Internal fixation for nondisplaced fracture in an ambulatory patient.
C. Internal fixation for displaced fracture in elderly patients.
D. Femoral head prosthesis for displaced fracture in young patients.

Ref.: 1, 2

COMMENTS: Femoral neck fractures are intracapsular and most often occur in the elderly. In adults the blood supply to the femoral head is via the metaphyseal vessels (here interrupted by the fracture), the artery of the ligamentum teres, and the ascending cervical (retinacular) vessels. These fractures are classified into four types on the basis of displacement: **Type I** is an impacted or incomplete fracture; **type II** is a nondisplaced complete fracture; **type III** is partially displaced fracture; and **type IV** is a completely displaced fracture. Goals of treatment are relief of pain, early mobilization, and prevention of avascular necrosis of the femoral head. The risk of avascular necrosis is high and increases substantially with the degree of displacement and the length of time this fracture is left unreduced. Type I and type II fractures may be treated nonoperatively in unstable or previously nonambulatory patients. In general, however, the preferred treatment of a nondisplaced femoral neck fracture is internal fixation to prevent further displacement. Because nonunion and avascular necrosis are more likely in instances of displaced fractures, replacement of the femoral head with a prosthesis is preferred in patients physiologically more than 70 years of age. In younger patients, attempts should be made to reduce and internally fix displaced fractures.

ANSWER: A, B

26. Appropriate initial treatment of a femoral shaft fracture includes which one or more of the following?

A. Internal fixation at fracture site.
B. Closed intramedullary nailing in adults.
C. Skeletal traction in children.

D. Application of a cast brace.

Ref.: 1, 2

COMMENTS: Skeletal traction and closed intramedullary nailing are thought to be superior to methods of internal fixation that involve operation at the fracture site because they carry a lower risk of infection. Femoral shaft fractures in children are treated by closed methods with an initial period of skeletal traction because of the risk of damage to the physeal plate and subsequent growth abnormalities. A cast brace may allow earlier mobilization of patients in whom a midshaft or distal femoral fracture was treated initially by skeletal traction.

ANSWER: B, C

27. With regard to the technique of inserting a Steinmann pin for skeletal traction and femoral shaft fractures, which of the following statements is/are true?

A. The pin is inserted lateral to medial at the tibial tubercle.
B. The pin is inserted medial to lateral in the supracondylar femur.
C. The pin should be placed as anterior as possible in the supracondylar position.
D. The pin is placed in the proximal tibia when there is associated knee injury.

Ref.: 2

COMMENTS: Steinmann pins for skeletal traction are easily inserted after administration of a local anesthetic and may be placed proximal to the femoral condyles or across the proximal tibia. The position of the pin can be controlled with greater precision at the point of entry than at its exit; hence the side involving more hazard is penetrated first. In the supracondylar position, the pin is placed as far posterior as possible to avoid the suprapatellar pouch and is advanced medial to lateral to avoid injury to the femoral vessels. At the tibial tubercle, the pin is inserted lateral to medial to avoid injury to the common peroneal nerve. When there is associated knee injury, the pin is inserted above the knee so traction is not applied across the injured joint.

ANSWER: A, B

28. A 19-year-old man jumps over a fence. Upon landing, his knee suddenly gives out. Although he is able to stand and ambulate, he complains his knee is unstable. Examination reveals moderate swelling and tenderness. The Lachman test is positive. Plain radiographs of the knee are normal. Aspiration of the knee reveals hemarthrosis without fat droplets. The likelihood the patient suffered a tear of the anterior cruciate ligament is:

A. 10%.
B. 30%.
C. 50%.
D. 75%.
E. 100%.

Ref.: 4

COMMENTS: Traumatic hemarthrosis of the knee due to **anterior cruciate ligament (ACL) tears** most commonly occurs with twisting, noncontact injuries. The best clinical method for identifying tears of the ACL is the **Lachman test.** It is performed by applying an anterior force on the tibia with the knee held at 30 degrees of flexion. Tears of the ACL are noted with increased anterior movement of the tibia relative to the femur compared to that of the uninjured extremity. Immediate swelling of a joint or extremity is usually due to fracture. Ligament injuries typically produce joint swelling within 2–4 hours after the injury, whereas meniscal injuries typically swell within 12–24 hours. The presence of a **traumatic hemarthrosis** without evidence of fracture may represent tears of the anterior cruciate ligament in as many as 75% of cases. Associated meniscal tears may be present in up to 65% of cases. Although a careful history, physical examination, and plain radiographs allow diagnosis in most cases, magnetic resonance imaging (MRI) remains the ancillary diagnostic test of choice for evaluating soft tissue injuries about the knee. The accuracy of MRI is 85–100%, and MRI has essentially replaced diagnostic arthroscopy in most cases.

ANSWER: D

29. An 18-year-old football player sustains a direct blow to the lateral aspect of the knee. Clinical examination reveals a grade III tear of the medial collateral ligament. He has no other demonstrable injury. The physician should recommend:

A. A hinged knee brace for 8 weeks.
B. A brace locked at 5 degrees of flexion for 6 weeks, then unlocked for 6 weeks.
C. A cylinder cast for 6 weeks.
D. Arthroscopic repair of the deep medial collateral ligament.
E. Open repair of the superficial medial collateral ligament.

Ref.: 4

COMMENTS: The **medial collateral ligament** (MCL) is the primary restraint to valgus loads of the knee and is injured with direct blows to the lateral aspect of the knee. Unlike the cruciate ligaments, the MCL is an extraarticular structure with an excellent ability to heal with functional treatment. Diagnosis of MCL injuries is confirmed by the presence of abnormal valgus laxity of the knee when held at 25 degrees of flexion. Patients with excessive valgus laxity with the knee in full extension have a more complex injury involving the capsule and cruciate ligaments. Patients treated with immediate protected motion obtain a stronger, more rapid healing response than those treated operatively or those immobilized in a cast.

ANSWER: A

30. With regard to meniscal injuries, which of the following statements is/are true?

A. Mechanism involves rotational forces.
B. The lateral meniscus is injured more commonly than the medial meniscus.
C. Diagnosis requires arthroscopy.
D. Operative correction requires meniscectomy.

Ref.: 2

COMMENTS: The tibia rotates slightly as the knee flexes and extends. Forceful rotation causes the cartilage to straighten and become taut; if the force is excessive or continuous, a tear results. The medial meniscus is injured three times more frequently than the lateral mensicus. Diagnostic arthroscopy can improve the accuracy of diagnosis of intraarticular lesions and is employed routinely whenever a meniscectomy is considered, but it is not necessary for diagnosis. Magnetic resonance imaging gives accurate information of ligamentous and meniscal injuries and of associated fractures. When the tear is within the peripheral third of the meniscus and is less than 3 cm in length, meniscal repair is justified. In the presence of an associated tear of the anterior cruciate ligament, the shearing stress on a repaired meniscus drastically decreases its chance of healing successfully.

ANSWER: A

31. With regard to tibial fracture, match each characteristic in the left column to the appropriate location of the fracture in the right column.

A. Associated ligamentous injury
B. Usually necessitates open reduction
C. Open fracture
D. More common in the elderly
E. Prophylactic fasciotomy

a. Shaft
b. Plateau
c. Both
d. Neither

Ref.: 1, 2

COMMENTS: Tibial shaft fractures are usually the result of direct trauma, whereas plateau fractures usually result from indirect forces. **Plateau fractures** are more common among middle-aged and elderly persons. With certain exceptions, treatment is by closed methods. Tibial plateau fractures may necessitate surgical repair if the medial collateral ligament is disrupted or if there is displacement or compression of the tibial plateau. **Tibial shaft fractures** are caused by substantial trauma and are often associated with severe soft-tissue injury; 30% are open fractures. It is important to consider the possibility that compartmental syndromes may develop after tibial shaft fractures; the mechanism involved is swelling within a tight fascial compartment. The arteries may continue to pulsate even as muscle ischemia develops. The clinical diagnosis depends on loss of motor power, paresthesias, tenderness of the compartment to palpation, and pain with passive stretch. Careful observation is mandatory for all tibial shaft fractures, and prompt measurement of compartmental pressures, fasciotomy, or both should be performed whenever signs of the compartmental syndrome are present. Resting compartment pressures typically fall below 10 mm Hg. Pressures higher than 30 mm Hg typically warrant fasciotomy. The anterior and peroneal compartment of the lower leg are the most commonly involved. Prophylactic fasciotomy should be considered for open fractures with severe soft-tissue injury.

ANSWER: A-b; B-d; C-a; D-b; E-a

32. With regard to the assessment of ankle injury, which of the following statements is/are true?

A. Ability to walk immediately after injury excludes fracture.
B. Medial tenderness after abduction injury is suggestive of injury to the deltoid ligament.
C. Lateral tenderness after adduction injury is suggestive of lateral collateral ligament injury.
D. Stress radiographs should be avoided because they are painful and do not help with the diagnosis.

Ref.: 1, 2

COMMENTS: Ligamentous and bony injuries of the ankle frequently result from rotational or abduction/adduction forces. An important goal of treatment is to maintain ankle stability. Initial evaluation should include a history of the mechanism of injury and examination for the site of tenderness, swelling, or deformity. If the patient was able to walk after the injury, the ankle may be stable; but an undisplaced fracture or ligamentous disruption may nevertheless be present. Adequate radiologic evaluation requires standard anteroposterior and lateral views as well as a mortise view obtained in a 15- to 20-degree medial oblique position. The most common ankle injury is **lateral collateral ligament** strain as the result of an adduction force. Tenderness distal to the medial malleolus is suggestive of **deltoid ligament** injury; this injury is seen with abduction and external rotation injuries. Integrity of the lateral collateral ligament and deltoid ligament can be assessed with stress films, which may require the help of local or general anesthesia.

ANSWER: B, C

33. With regard to the treatment of ankle injuries, which of the following is least likely to benefit from operative correction?

A. Tibiofibular ligament disruption.
B. Lateral malleolar fracture.
C. Bimalleolar fracture.
D. Trimalleolar fracture.

Ref.: 1, 2

COMMENTS: The principles of treatment of ankle fractures include anatomic reduction of all fractures, internal fixation, and early motion. Closed reduction and maintenance by casting have been standard treatment. However, instability is inherent in all bimalleolar and trimalleolar fractures, and this fact has led to more aggressive treatment practices, including operative intervention to achieve greater stability, even if anatomic reduction has already been achieved by closed means. The most common isolated malleolar fracture involves the lateral malleolus and is treated with closed reduction and a cast for 6–8 weeks. Bimalleolar fractures usually result from forceful abduction or external rotation of the supinated foot. The posterior malleolus is important for maintaining the anteroposterior (AP) stability of the ankle joint. For trimalleolar fractures with small posterior fragments, the need for surgical intervention is determined primarily by the status of the medial and lateral malleoli. When the posterior fragment involves 30% or more of the articular surface, however, or when there is AP instability, internal fixation of the posterior malleolus and the medial and lateral malleoli is required. The distal tibiofibular joint is important for ankle stability, and disruption generally necessitates operative correction.

ANSWER: B

34. Match each type of hip injury in the left column with the characteristic position of the injured limb in the right column. Each choice may be used more than once or not at all.

A. Anterior hip dislocation
B. Posterior hip dislocation
C. Displaced femoral neck fracture
D. Intertrochanteric femoral fracture

a. External rotation, shortened
b. Internal rotation, shortened
c. Abduction, flexion, and external rotation
d. Adduction, flexion, and internal rotation

Ref.: 2

COMMENTS: Proximal femoral fractures and hip dislocations manifest with the injured limb in characteristic positions. When combined with a history of the mechanism of injury, the position of the limb suggests the diagnosis even before radiologic confirmation. Posterior dislocations occur commonly as the result of an axial force applied to a flexed, adducted hip, as may occur with a dashboard injury. If the hip is in neutral position or slightly abducted, an acetabular fracture may accompany the dislocation. Anterior dislocations are less common.

ANSWER: A-c; B-d; C-a; D-a

35. Complications of hip dislocation include which of the following?

A. Sciatic nerve injury.
B. Avascular necrosis.
C. Degenerative arthritis.
D. Compartmental syndromes.

Ref.: 2

COMMENTS: Avascular necrosis of the femoral head and the later development of degenerative arthritis are the most common complications of hip dislocations. **Avascular necrosis** occurs in about 20% of patients, and the incidence is directly related to delay in reduction. Approximately half of patients who have a hip dislocation later acquire **posttraumatic arthritis**. Chondral and osteochondral fractures of the femoral head are more common with posterior dislocations, increasing the risk for arthritic deterioration. Computed tomography is the most effective diagnostic imaging test used to evaluate bone injury. **Sciatic nerve injury** is a potential complication when the hip dislocates posteriorly. A compartmental syndrome is not a complication of hip dislocation.

ANSWER: A, B, C

36. Match each mechanism of injury in the left column with a fracture of the spine in the right column.

A. Axial load on the head	a. Teardrop fracture
B. Extension	b. Jefferson fracture
C. Hyperflexion	c. Hangman's fracture
D. Flexion-rotation	d. Dislocation
E. Avulsion	e. Clay shoveler's fracture

Ref.: 1, 2

COMMENTS: Although spinal fractures are common, fewer than 10% are associated with neurologic deficit. In patients with a history of trauma who complain of pain or tenderness in the neck, a fracture must be suspected. The neck should be immobilized. A complete neurologic examination, followed by adequate radiographic evaluation with full view of levels C1 to T1, is mandatory. Fracture of the posterior arch of the atlas (**Jefferson fracture**) is caused by an axial load. Fracture through the pedicles of C2 (**hangman's fracture**) is caused by a severe extension injury. Compression fracture of the cervical spine (**teardrop fracture**) is frequently caused by hyperflexion of the neck, as in diving accidents; it is associated with a high incidence of neurologic damage. **Dislocation of the cervical spine** occurs most commonly between C5 and C6. The injury results from a flexion-rotation force with dislocation of the facets and concomitant capsular ligament rupture. Severe muscular contraction can avulse the spinous processes, as in the **clay shoveler's fracture**.

ANSWER: A-b; B-c; C-a; D-d; E-e

37. Indications for operation in patients with acute fractures or dislocations of the cervical spine include all of the following except:

A. Unstable fractures or dislocations.
B. Progressive neurologic deficits.
C. Established neurologic deficit.
D. Persistent bone fragments in the spinal canal.

Ref.: 1, 2

COMMENTS: Patients with unstable fractures or dislocations may be treated by stabilization procedures. Reduction and stabilization are indicated in patients who present with minimal neurologic findings that subsequently progress. In patients with fragments in the spinal canal, operative intervention is mandatory in the presence of a neurologic deficit. The role of surgery for patients with acute fractures and dislocations and established neurologic deficits is controversial.

ANSWER: C

38. Which of the following statements regarding spinal cord trauma is/are true?

A. Immediate intravenous infusion of methylprednisolone (5.4 mg/kg/hr) following spinal cord injury may reduce neurologic sequelae.
B. Progressive neurologic deficit warrants nonoperative observation.
C. Most (85%) cervical spinal injuries are detected on plain lateral radiographs.
D. A soft cervical collar provides adequate stability for most bone cervical injuries.

Ref.: 4

COMMENTS: Multicenter studies have verified the efficacy of intravenous steroid infusion for decreasing spinal cord injury with trauma. The best results occur if treatment begins within the first 8 hours after the accident. Controversy persists as to the timing and method of surgery following spinal cord injury associated with malalignment or canal compromise. However, progressive neurologic deficit requires immediate decompression and stabilization. Plain radiographs of the cervical spine, including open mouth views, are essential for diagnosing the fracture, with lateral radiographs being the most sensitive. Computed tomography remains the standard for evaluating spinal fractures and canal compromise. Soft cervical collars restrict less than 10% of cervical flexion/extension and are ineffective in providing stability. Rigid collars can restrict flexion/extension, but a halo vest is necessary to control rotation and is indicated for unstable cervical spine injuries.

ANSWER: A, C

39. A 42-year-old man feels a sudden sharp pain in the lower calf after jumping for a basketball. Examination reveals weak plantar and dorsiflexion of the ankle with diffuse ecchymosis. Examining the patient prone with his legs over the edge of the examining table shows that he has no palpable defect, but squeezing the calf muscle fails to produce ankle plantar flexion. The diagnosis is:

A. Subfascial hematoma.
B. Torn Achilles tendon.
C. Torn plantaris tendon.
D. Torn gastrocnemius.
E. Torn posterior tibial tendon.

Ref.: 4, 5

COMMENTS: Eccentric contraction of the calf muscles in men typically in their thirties and forties can result in lower leg muscle and tendon injuries. Those with occasional participation in recreational sports are at greatest risk. The Thompson test, performed by squeezing the calf muscles and producing no ankle plantar flexion with the patient in the prone position, is pathognomic for tears of the Achilles tendon. Gastrocnemius muscle tears occur under similar circumstances, but there patients typically have more proximal swelling and a negative Thompson test.

ANSWER: B

40. A 15-year-old boy is seen in the emergency room with a gunshot wound to the thigh. Examination reveals one bullet wound in the posterior lateral aspect of the mid-thigh. There is obvious deformity of the femur and a dense peroneal nerve palsy. Anteroposterior and lateral radiographs of the femur are shown. The physician should recommend:

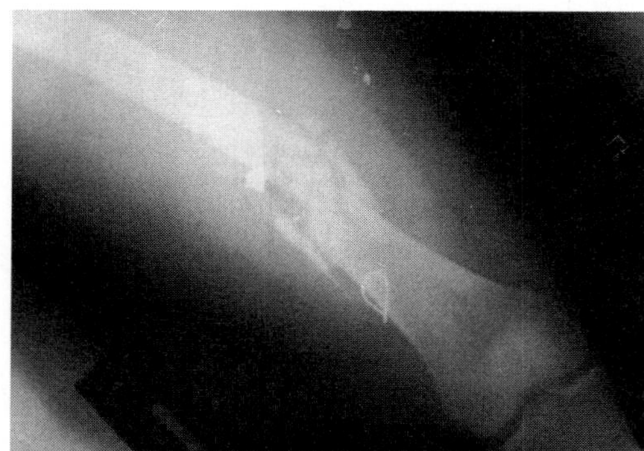

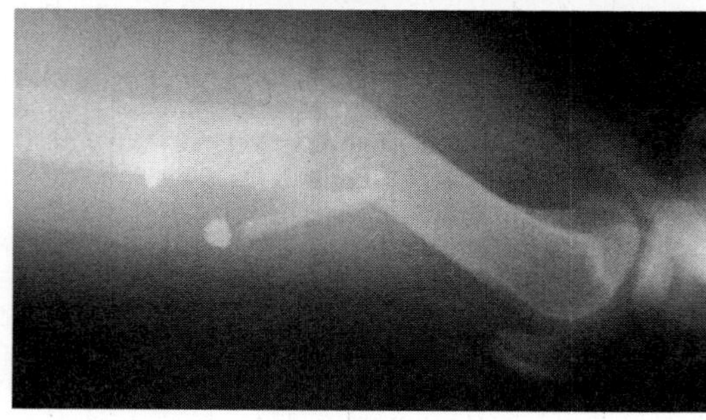

A. Closed intramedullary (IM) nailing of the femur with a locked nail.
B. Skeletal traction followed by long leg casting.
C. Exploration of the peroneal nerve and plating of the femur.
D. Bullet extraction, peroneal nerve exploration, IM nailing of the femur.

Ref.: 4

COMMENTS: Gunshot fractures of the femur are generally treated in the same manner as a closed femoral shaft fracture. With low-velocity gunshot wounds the track is débrided locally at the skin, but a formal extensive débridement is not necessary. Most nerve injuries in this case involve neurapraxia due to the concussive effect of the bullet and do not require exploration. A small percentage of gunshot fractures are due to a close-range shotgun blast or military-style high-velocity bullets. These fractures are similar to type III open fractures and require extensive débridement, delayed fixation, and possibly external fixation.

ANSWER: A

41. A 25-year-old man is seen in the emergency room with a gunshot wound to the shoulder. The radiograph reveals the bullet near the glenoid with a fracture of the inferior glenoid rim. The CT scan reveals that the bullet remains intraarticularly. The physician should recommend:

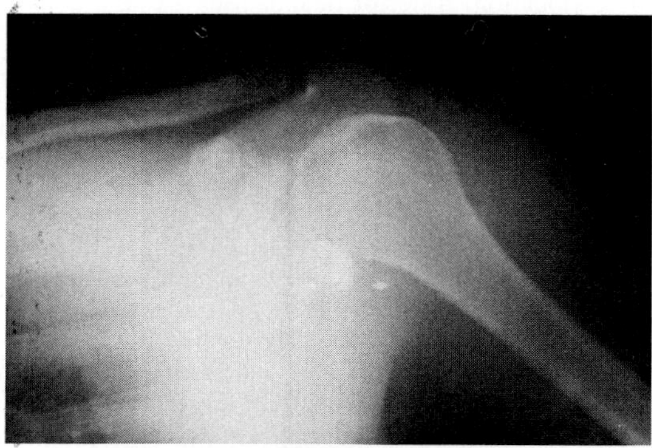

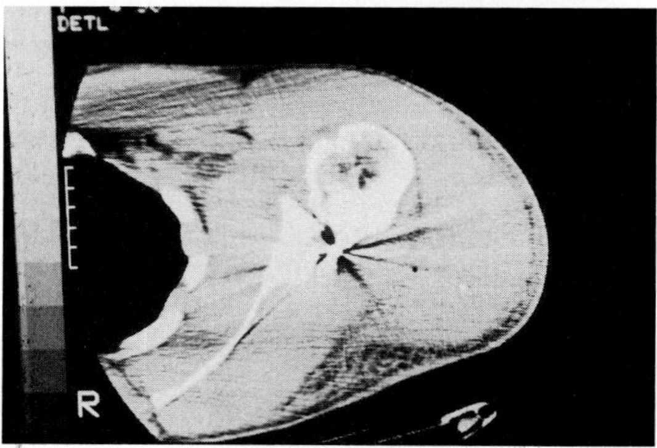

A. Sling immobilization with oral antibiotics.
B. Sling immobilization with intravenous antibiotics.
C. Open or arthroscopic débridement of the bullet fragments, intravenous antibiotics.
D. Delayed exploration if infection develops.

Ref.: 4, 5

COMMENTS: Whereas the bullet in bullet wounds in the soft tissues of extremities rarely require removal, retained intraarticular foreign bodies should be débrided while the joint is inspected and treated for damage to the articular surfaces. Arthroscopic débridement is the method of choice unless fracture care necessitates wide exposure.

ANSWER: C

REFERENCES

1. Sabiston DC Jr: *Textbook of Surgery*, 15th ed. WB Saunders, Philadelphia, 1997.
2. Schwartz SI, Shires GT, Spencer FC: *Principles of Surgery*, 7th ed. McGraw-Hill, New York, 1999.
3. Mattox KL, Moore EE, Feliciano DV: *Patterns of Injury*. Appleton & Lange, Norwalk, CT, 1988.
4. Browner BD, Jupiter JB, Levine AM, Trafton PG: *Skeletal Trauma*, 2nd ed. WB Saunders, Philadelphia, 1998.
5. Deg R: *Principles of Orthopaedic Practice*. McGraw-Hill, New York, 1992.

Orthopedics

C. Acquired Diseases

1. Match each type of joint in the left column with the appropriate example in the right column.

A. Fibrous joint — a. Knee
B. Fibrocartilaginous joint — b. Skull sutures
C. Synovial joint — c. Pubic symphysis

Ref.: 1

COMMENTS: Joints may be categorized according to the tissue type by which they are joined. A **fibrous** joint (synarthrosis) represents two bones joined by fibrous tissue, as exemplified by the suture lines in the skull. **Fibrocartilaginous** joints (symphyses) are those in which the bones are joined by hyaline cartilage or fibrocartilage, examples being the pubic symphysis and the intervertebral discs. **Synovial** (diarthrodial) joints are movable joints in which cartilage-covered bone ends articulate within a synovium-lined capsule, permitting more motion to occur. Most joints of the extremities are synovial joints. The type of motion a synovial joint permits is determined by the contour of the articular surfaces, the anatomy of the supporting connective tissues (capsule and ligaments), and the external forces applied to it.

ANSWER: A-b; B-c; C-a

2. Which of the following organisms are the two most commonly found in pyogenic arthritis?

A. *Escherichia coli.*
B. *Staphylococcus aureus.*
C. *Haemophilus influenzae.*
D. Hemolytic streptococci.

Ref.: 1, 4

COMMENTS: Pyogenic, or septic, arthritis, which is an orthopedic emergency, is a severe joint condition that, if not diagnosed and managed early in the clinical course, will likely result in permanent joint disability. It is most often caused by hematogenous spread of organisms from other infected sites. Direct infection by way of traumatic wounds and extension of adjacent osteomyelitis are also seen. The most common causative organisms are *Staphylococcus aureus* and hemolytic streptococci, although in children *Haemophilus influenzae* is also commonly seen. The clinical manifestation is that of local tenderness, swelling, and extreme pain on motion. The specific diagnosis is made by joint aspiration with immediate Gram stain and culture. Crystal analysis should be performed on the joint fluid to rule out crystal arthropathy, especially gout and pseudogout. Administration of systemic antibiotics should be started promptly and the joint surgically drained on an urgent basis. Drainage can be performed using arthroscopic or open surgical techniques. Adequate débridement of all devitalized tissue is necessary to prevent recurrent abcess formation.

ANSWER: B, D

3. The most common site of skeletal tuberculosis is which of the following?

A. Knee.
B. Hip.
C. Spine.
D. Humerus.

Ref.: 1

COMMENTS: Skeletal tuberculosis remains a significant problem in most of the Asian and African countries. Tuberculosis is now more commonly seen in immunocompromised patients (e.g., human immunodeficiency virus infection, chemotherapy) typically in large urban areas. Although skeletal tuberculosis is rare in the United States (1% of all cases of tuberculosis), its incidence has increased since 1980. The most common site of involvement is the spine. Peripheral joint tuberculosis also occurs and usually involves synovium, bone, and cartilage. Untreated, joint tuberculosis usually results in complete joint destruction, deformity, and pain. In contrast to septic arthritis, the clinical course of skeletal tuberculosis is insidious; symptoms may last weeks to months before the patient seeks medical advice. Worsening of the pain at night is a characteristic feature. The diagnosis requires recovery of organisms from the involved joint or bone. Treatment involves antituberculous drug therapy, rest (bracing), and general supportive and nutritional measures. Surgical management is indicated for patients with advanced lesions, including those with caseation or severe joint destruction.

ANSWER: C

4. Which of the following statements regarding human immunodeficiency virus (HIV) syndrome are true?

A. Musculoskeletal involvement is rare.
B. HIV arthropathy is best treated with methotrexate and azathioprine (AZT).
C. Pyogenic arthritis may occur despite low synovial white blood cell (WBC) counts ($<10{,}000/mm^3$).
D. HIV arthopathy may be confused with psoriatic arthropathy.

Ref.: 3

COMMENTS: Infection with HIV can lead to a variety of musculoskeletal manifestations. The most common is a sterile polyarthritis, which presents in a manner similar to psoriatic arthropathy with atypical skin lesions, joint swelling, and arthralgias. Treatment typically involves nonsteroidal antiinflammatory drugs (NSAIDs), although some patients respond to a combination of AZT and etidronate. Immunosuppressive medications including methrotrexate are not recommended. Pyogenic joint infections, although uncommon, can be difficult to diagnose. HIV patients may be unable to mount the appropriate response, leading to false-negative synovial analysis. Synovial WBC count may remain within normal limits making diagnosis difficult. Treatment however, is similar to that for non-HIV patients: aggressive surgical drainage and intravenous antibiotics.

ANSWER: C, D

5. With regard to the clinical features of gonococcal arthritis, which of the following statements is/are true?

A. It occurs predominantly in females.
B. It usually begins as a migratory polyarthralgia.
C. The hip, knee, and shoulder are the most common sites of infection.
D. Even with proper treatment, mild residual loss of joint motion usually results.

Ref.: 1

COMMENTS: Gonococcal urethritis in males usually is symptomatic and causes the patient to seek early medical treatment. In contrast, gonococcal cervicitis or vaginitis in females frequently is asymptomatic, and the sequelae of septicemia and arthritis are therefore more common among females (4:1). Initial symptoms usually include migratory polyarthralgia with a variable febrile course. The infection usually localizes in the knee, elbow, or wrist. Diagnosis requires recovery of gonococcal organisms from the septic joint. Treatment includes a 2-week course of penicillin and appropriate joint immobilization. With proper treatment, there is usually full recovery of joint function.

ANSWER: A, B

6. Radiographic findings of rheumatoid arthritis include which of the following?

A. Subluxation.
B. Osteoporosis.
C. Bone erosions.
D. Joint deformity.

Ref.: 4

COMMENTS: There are many radiographic abnormalities in patients with rheumatoid arthritis, depending on the stage of the disease process and the specific joints involved. The earliest findings are those related to the destructive effects of the hyperplastic synovium and are best seen on radiographs of the hands. Fusiform swelling, particularly in the area of the proximal interphalangeal or metacarpophalangeal joints, is common. As the disease progresses, periarticular bone erosions produced by osteoclastic resorption occur. This cortical irregularity is made apparent by the development of periosteal new bone formation in response to the synovial inflammation. Osteoporosis occurs as a result of disuse, as well as inflammation in the surrounding tissues. Further progression results in subluxation of the involved joints and joint deformity (particularly ulnar deviation at the metacarpophalangeal joints).

ANSWER: A, B, C, D

7. With regard to joint fluid assessment, which of the following statements is/are correct?

A. Joints should be aspirated with a 22-gauge or smaller needle to prevent hemarthrosis.
B. The mucin clot test helps differentiate inflammatory from degenerative joint abnormalities.
C. The normal gradient of glucose concentration between plasma and joint fluid is approximately 50 mg/dl.
D. Most joint fluid crystals can be adequately assessed with standard microscopic illumination techniques.

Ref.: 1

COMMENTS: Aspiration of a joint to obtain fluid for testing is commonly required for evaluation of joint abnormalities. It should be accomplished through scrupulously sterile technique. In general, the use of an 18-gauge or larger needle is recommended to be able to aspirate the more viscous fluid associated with certain pathologic processes. The fluid obtained should be routinely examined for color, appearance, and viscosity and sent for a Gram stain examination, bacterial culture, mucin clot test, white blood cell count, crystal examination, and measurement of glucose concentration. The mucin clot test is a good qualitative assessment of the character of the protein–polysaccharide complex of synovial fluid. A firm, rope-like clot that does not easily fragment suggests normal polymerization and is seen in normal joints and those with degenerative arthritis. Poor mucin clots suggest the presence of one of the inflammatory arthritides. Similarly, the gradient between joint fluid and plasma glucose concentration may suggest the presence of infection or rheumatoid arthritis. In such conditions, this gradient may be 50 mg/dl or greater; in the normal situation, the gradient is less than 10 mg/dl. Assessment of joint fluid crystals also is important, particularly if gout and pseudogout are possible diagnoses. This requires examination of the joint fluid under polarized light to see the rod-shaped urate crystals, which with gout manifest a strongly negative birefringence.

ANSWER: B

8. With regard to rheumatoid arthritis, which of the following statements is/are true?

A. Its incidence peaks during the sixth and seventh decades of life.
B. It occurs more commonly in women.
C. It is easily distinguished from other autoimmune disorders.
D. A negative rheumatoid factor assay rules out the disease.
E. The clinical manifestations of rheumatoid arthritis are limited to joint disorders.

Ref.: 1

COMMENTS: Rheumatoid arthritis is a systemic disease that may involve the musculoskeletal, cardiovascular, respiratory, and nervous systems. Its incidence peaks during the fourth and fifth decades of life, and it has a marked predominance in females. Because multiple systems may be involved, it is sometimes difficult to differentiate rheumatoid arthritis from other autoimmune disorders. A positive rheumatoid factor is seen in 90% of adult patients and in only 20% of juvenile patients with rheumatoid arthritis. Thus a negative assay does not rule out the disease. From a surgical standpoint, the most significant changes in rheumatoid arthritis are those affecting the synovial joints and the adjacent tendons, tendon sheaths, and bursae. Surgeons treating these disorders must be aware of the cardiopulmonary and other systemic effects of rheumatoid arthritis as well as the side effects of drugs (e.g., steroids, NSAIDs, methotrexate) used to treat this disease.

ANSWER: B

9. With regard to the management of rheumatoid arthritis, which of the following statements is/are true?

A. Medical management is the mainstay of treatment of early rheumatoid arthritis.
B. Appropriate physical therapy reduces the pain of rheumatoid arthritis but does not affect the progressive joint destruction and disability from the underlying disease.
C. Synovectomy of involved joints should be performed along with initial medical therapy in newly diagnosed cases to prevent progression of the disease.
D. Synovectomy is most effective at the knee joint.

Ref.: 1

COMMENTS: Patients with rheumatoid arthritis are best managed in a multidisciplinary way, with input from the rheumatologist, orthopedist, and physical and occupational therapists. Although management of early or less severe cases involves appropriate medical intervention (analgesics and antiinflammatory medications), physical therapy and counseling with regard to physical activities may be of great benefit early in the course of the disease process. Such therapy not only relieves the associated pain but also plays a major role in maintaining strength and joint mobility and delaying joint deformity. Synovectomy has been beneficial in relieving pain and preventing or delaying joint destruction in selected patients. It should be performed, however, only when there is evidence of disease progression despite adequate antiinflammatory treatment and modification of activity. Synovectomy appears to have the greatest benefit in the management of rheumatoid arthritis of the knee and does not appear to modify the disease process when it involves the metacarpophalangeal or metatarsophalangeal joints.

ANSWER: A, D

10. Which of the following statements characterizes osteoarthritis?

A. The earliest recognizable changes occur in the subchondral bone.
B. The articular cartilage is involved late in the disease process.
C. There is a strong correlation between clinical symptoms and radiographic changes.
D. The amount of chondroitin sulfate is increased in the articular cartilage.
E. None of the above.

Ref.: 1

COMMENTS: **Osteoarthritis** is a term that refers to degenerative changes in synovial joints. The earliest changes seen are those in the articular cartilage. On gross examination the cartilage may appear softer and more yellow than usual, and on biochemical examination it is found to have a decrease in the normal amount of chondroitin sulfate. Because cartilage is not normally seen on radiographs these early changes, which may be symptomatic, are not seen radiographically. Thus at times there is poor correlation between the clinical and radiographic findings. This process is more one of degeneration than of inflammation; accordingly, some authors believe that the terms **degenerative joint disease** and **osteoarthrosis** more accurately describe the process.

ANSWER: E

11. The classic clinical manifestation of osteoarthritis includes which of the following?

A. Joint pain occurring on motion and relieved by rest.
B. Frequent involvement of the metacarpophalangeal joints.
C. Normal synovial fluid/blood glucose gradient.
D. Fairly abrupt onset of symptoms.

Ref.: 4

COMMENTS: Osteoarthritis may be considered a primary disease in which there is no antecedent joint disorder or a secondary entity that is related to previous joint trauma, rheumatoid disease, gout, or other forms of inflammatory arthritis. The onset usually is insidious; the primary symptom is joint pain brought on by motion and weight-bearing and relieved by rest. Primary osteoarthritis is a disease of the elderly, usually manifesting in persons 60 years and older. It is most common in the large weight-bearing joints, especially the hips, knees, and spine. Secondary osteoarthritis may be found in any joint that has been previously altered by trauma, rheumatoid arthritis, or other inflammatory conditions. The elbows, wrists, and metacarpophalangeal joints are rarely involved. Laboratory examinations are usually unrevealing; and in the absence of an underlying inflammatory process, the synovial fluid reveals few abnormalities.

ANSWER: A, C

12. With regard to the nonoperative management of osteoarthritis, which of the following statements is/are true?

A. Resting the clinically involved joint is the key to successful nonoperative management.
B. Weight loss in obese patients may significantly alleviate symptoms.
C. Antiinflammatory medications present risks (gastric ulceration and antiplatelet effects) that outweigh the benefit they confer, and they should be avoided for this form of arthritis.
D. Range-of-motion and muscle-strengthening exercises aggravate the osteoarthritic joint and should be avoided.

Ref.: 4

COMMENTS: Most patients with osteoarthritis are successfully treated with conservative management, the basic principle of which is rest and immobilization of the involved joint or joints. A careful search should be made for possible aggravating factors (e.g., occupational trauma, obesity), and modification of such life style-related factors should be made if possible. There is some controversy over the risk versus benefit of intraarticular steroid injections, but most investigators agree that oral NSAIDs are helpful and frequently indicated for treatment. When the acute symptoms have resolved, range-of-motion and muscle-strengthening exercises should be employed to maintain maximal joint function and promote joint stability.

ANSWER: A, B

13. Match each surgical procedure used for osteoarthritis of the hip in the left column with the appropriate descriptive statement in the right column.

A. Arthrodesis
B. Proximal femoral osteotomy
C. Hemiarthroplasty (replacement of the femoral head and neck)
D. Total hip arthroplasty

a. Produces the best short- and medium-term results
b. Joint sepsis is the most frequent indication
c. Is the best procedure for young patients with early osteoarthritis
d. Contraindicated when the acetabulum is severely diseased

Ref.: 1

COMMENTS: A number of operative procedures are available to treat disorders of the hip. **Arthrodesis** (fusion of the hip joint) is most frequently indicated when the presence of pyogenic or tuberculous sepsis precludes prosthetic arthroplasty. It also represents an alternative in young patients with severe degenerative joint changes. **Osteotomy** of the proximal femur involves transection of the femoral shaft and displacement or angulation of the femoral head and neck. It allows articulation of less severely involved cartilage of the femoral head with the acetabulum. It results in excellent pain relief and improved joint motion in carefully selected young patients with early osteoarthritis. **Hemiarthroplasty** (replacement of the femoral head and neck) is used mainly for subcapital fractures of the femur; it requires a normal acetabulum. **Total hip replacement** is indicated when both the femoral head and acetabulum are involved. It has the best short- and medium-term results of all of the procedures available. However, complications from infection or loosening of the prostheses may be severe and debilitating. The tendency to avoid its use in the young population has been based on unanswered questions about the long-term performance of the prostheses, particularly the risk of loosening. Research in the fields of bioengineering and bioprosthetics is extremely active in this regard.

ANSWER: A-b; B-c; C-d; D-a

14. With regard to chondromalacia of the patella, which of the following statements is/are true?

A. The initial changes usually occur on the lateral aspect of the patella.
B. The pain is aggravated by knee flexion, kneeling, and descending stairs.
C. Radiographs show characteristic changes early in the course of the disease process.
D. The progressive nature of the disease warrants early surgical intervention.
E. Patellectomy is the only form of surgical therapy that has proved successful.

Ref.: 1

COMMENTS: Chondromalacia of the patella, as its name implies, is a disease process of the cartilage of the patella. The hallmarks are softening and discoloration of the cartilage. The initial changes are usually seen on the medial aspect of the patella. The characteristic clinical manifestation is an insidious onset of anterior knee or peripatellar pain aggravated by knee flexion, direct pressure (as when kneeling), and descending stairs. As with other forms of cartilage injury, radiographs are frequently negative and not diagnostic, especially during the early stages of the disease. Most patients with this problem are adequately managed by conservative treatment, which involves strengthening the quadriceps muscle and avoiding knee flexion. For advanced cases, surgical intervention may be warranted. The spectrum of surgical management includes local shaving or resection of the involved cartilage (chondroplasty), realignment of the quadriceps mechanism, and total knee replacement (for degeneration involving the trochlea of the femur). Patellectomy is rarely performed.

ANSWER: B

15. With regard to hallux valgus, which of the following statements is/are true?

A. Exostosis removal is usually effective.
B. Most patients are asymptomatic.
C. It is much more common in populations in which shoes are not worn.
D. Silastic arthroplasty is the surgical procedure of choice in most instances.

Ref.: 1

COMMENTS: **Hallux valgus** refers to the lateral division of the great toe and medial deviation of the first metatarsal. It is popularly considered synonymous with **bunion**, which refers more specifically to the large exostosis and overlying soft tissue bursa that frequently occur in association with hallux valgus. This is primarily a disease of the shoe-wearing population (improper shoe fitting). Whereas the anatomic abnormality is fairly common, the associated symptoms of intermittent pain over the involved metatarsophalangeal joint occur relatively infrequently. Conservative treatment with the use of molded insoles and metatarsal arches to redistribute the body weight is usually successful. When symptoms persist despite conservative measures, surgical intervention may be warranted. Surgical management may include simple exostectomy, soft tissue repair, osteotomy of the metatarsal, or fusion, depending on the pathophysiologic mechanism and other factors. Prosthetic arthroplasty generally is not employed for this condition.

ANSWER: B

16. With regard to gout, which of the following statements is/are true?

A. It commonly manifests as a monoarticular arthritis of the metatarsophalangeal joint of the great toe.
B. Diagnosis requires demonstration of urate crystals in synovial fluid.
C. There is a direct correlation between clinical evidence of gout and the serum uric acid level.
D. Because of the inability of medical management to control chronic disease, surgical intervention is usually required at some point in the clinical course.

Ref.: 1

COMMENTS: Gout is a metabolic disease that may manifest in a primary form (inborn error of metabolism) or a secondary form (e.g., myeloproliferative disorders, leukemia, hemolytic anemia). The clinical manifestations of gouty arthritis are caused by the effects of inflammation on the surrounding cartilage, subchondral bone, and periarticular soft tissues as a result of urate crystal deposition in the synovial fluid. Although the likelihood of clinical symptoms increases with higher serum uric acid levels, it is not uncommon for significant hyperuricemia to be present without clinical symptoms and for clinical symptoms to be present without hyperuricemia. The classic clinical manifestation is that of an acute attack of monoarticular arthritis, most often involving the metatarsophalangeal joint of the great toe, most often occurring in men over age 30. Management of the acute attack involves rest and anti-inflammatory medication (e.g., colchicine, NSAIDs). Upon resolution of the acute symptoms, long-term management with allopurinol to reduce serum uric acid levels may be needed. Surgery is rarely indicated for management of acute or chronic gouty arthritis; however, excision of large tophaceous deposits may provide symptomatic relief, and joints that are severely involved may require arthrodesis or arthroplasty.

ANSWER: A, B

17. With regard to slipped capital femoral epiphysis, which of the following statements is/are true?

A. It is more prevalent in males.
B. It is rarely bilateral.
C. It commonly manifests with knee pain.
D. It is often associated with loss of normal internal rotation.
E. It is rarely managed surgically because of the risk of permanent epiphyseal damage.

Ref.: 4

COMMENTS: Slipped capital femoral epiphysis is a relatively rare entity that occurs predominantly in adolescent boys. It represents a separation of the capital femoral epiphysis through the growth plate region above the zone of calcified cartilage. The cause of the physeal disruption is unknown, but the muscular forces across the hip result in the characteristic medial and posterior displacement of the capital epiphysis. The clinical findings include pain in the area of the hip aggravated by motion, pain referred to the knee, and loss of normal internal rotation. The process is bilateral in 25% of cases. Treatment is based on the principles of preventing further slippage and minimizing existing deformity by early fusion of the growth plate. This is achieved most often by surgically pinning the femoral head and neck to engage the epiphysis.

ANSWER: A, C, D

18. Which of the following statements accurately characterize Charcot's joint?

A. It occurs as a consequence of various forms of neurologic disorders.
B. Its onset is usually acute.
C. Characteristic radiographic findings are those of dense sclerosis of the subchondral bone.
D. Treatment may involve arthrodesis.

Ref.: 1

COMMENTS: Charcot's joint, or neuropathic joint, is caused by significant articular and periarticular destruction secondary to repeated trauma to structures rendered insensitive by underlying neurologic disorders (e.g., tabes dorsalis, diabetes). The clinical course usually begins with insidious onset, and the patient is often unaware of the joint disability until it becomes severe with gross instability and significant effusion. Radiographs usually reveal marked bone destruction and abnormality of the joint space, which may contain loose bone fragments. The foot is most commonly involved in diabetics, but the hip and knee are frequently involved. When conservative management with a properly fitted weight-bearing brace fails, arthrodesis is frequently indicated.

ANSWER: A, D

19. Shoulder pain may be caused by which of the following entities?

A. Spinal arthritis.
B. Lung cancer.
C. Umbilical hernia.
D. Diaphragmatic irritation.
E. Angina.

Ref.: 4

COMMENTS: See Question 20.

20. Match each primary shoulder disorder in the left column with the appropriate clinical characteristic in the right column.

A. Subacromial bursitis	a. Pain extending along the proximal humeral groove
B. Bicipital tendinitis	b. Unrelenting pain unimproved by position
C. Supraspinatus tendinitis	c. Limitation of internal rotation and full abduction
D. Rotator cuff tear	d. Surgical repair sometimes required

Ref.: 1

COMMENTS: When evaluating shoulder pain, clinicians must be alert to the numerous clinical entities that, although anatomically unrelated, may cause pain referred to the shoulder. These entities include cervical arthritis with nerve root irritation, Pancoast's tumor, cardiac angina, and abdominal conditions associated with diaphragmatic irritation. Of the primary shoulder disorders that characteristically produce pain, lesions of the rotator cuff, bicipital tendinitis, and subacromial bursitis are the most common. The **rotator cuff** consists of the common tendinous insertion of the supraspinatus, infraspinatus, teres minor, and subscapularis muscles. In positions of full elevation or abduction, the rotator cuff may contact the acromion or coracoacromial ligament and cause irritation of the intervening bursa. Repeated injury may cause degeneration and lead to **subacromial bursitis**. This entity is usually characterized by fairly severe and unrelenting pain that is unimproved by position and may even necessitate the use of narcotics for relief. A **rotator cuff tear** represents a physical disruption of the tendinous structure with varying degrees of associated inflammation. Most rotator cuff tears are partial, and initial conservative management with shoulder immobilization is usually successful. With total rupture, open surgical repair of the tear is often preferred, but conservative management can be successful. With **supraspinatus tendinitis**, the pain is more insidious in onset and of lesser degree. It frequently limits the motions of internal rotation and full abduction, which are painful. **Bicipital tendinitis** produces symptoms similar to those of supraspinatus tendinitis. However, the distribution of pain and tenderness is more distal over the proximal humeral or bicipital groove. With these four inflammatory entities, treatment with rest, analgesics, NSAIDs, and occasionally steroid injection is usually successful.

ANSWER:
Question 19: A, B, D, E
Question 20: A-b; B-a; C-c; D-d

21. Which of the following statements about osteomyelitis in the adult is/are true?

A. Magnetic resonance imaging (MRI) is most effective for evaluating medullary involvement.
B. MRI is most effective for evaluating cortical involvement.
C. Treatment includes appropriate antibiotics, excision of all necrotic tissue augmented by the use of antibiotic-impregnated beads, deadspace management.
D. Chronic osteomyelitis can lead to the development of squamous cell carcinoma.

Ref.: 3

COMMENTS: The diagnosis of osteomyelitis is based on clinical judgment coupled with laboratory studies and imaging techniques. Plain radiographs are helpful but may fail to identify early infection. Indium-labeled leukocyte scintigraphy is more accurate than technetium or gallium scintigraphy for the diagnosis, but MRI is the most effective technique for evaluating medullary involvement. MRI is unable to identify cortical osteomyelitis if there is no cortical disruption or medullary involvement. Appropriate antibiotics and aggressive surgical management are the mainstays of treatment, but late reconstruction of bone loss can be difficult. A complication of longstanding chronic osteomyelitis is the development of squamous cell carcinoma, which occurs in 0.2–1.7% of patients. Treatment in these cases often requires amputation.

ANSWER: A, C, D

REFERENCES

1. Frymoyer JW (ed): *Orthopaedic Knowledge Update 4*, 1st ed. American Academy of Orthopaedic Surgeons, Rosemont, IL, 1993.
2. Crenshaw AH: *Campbell's Operative Orthopedics*, 8th ed. Mosby-Year Book, Chicago, 1992.
3. Schwartz SI, Shires GT, Spencer FC: *Principles of Surgery*, 7th ed. McGraw-Hill, New York, 1999.
4. Kasser JR (ed): *Orthopaedic Knowledge Update 5*, 1st ed. American Academy of Orthopaedic Surgeons, Rosemont, IL, 1996.
5. Simon SR (ed): *Orthopaedic Basic Science*. American Academy of Orthopaedic Surgeons, Rosemont, IL, 1994.

Orthopedics

D. Neoplasms

1. With regard to suspected soft-tissue tumors of the musculoskeletal system, which is the imaging modality of choice?

   A. Plain tomography.
   B. Computed tomography (CT).
   C. Magnetic resonance imaging (MRI).
   D. Thermography.
   E. Ultrasonography.

Ref.: 1

COMMENTS: For the workup of suspected soft-tissue tumors plain films are usually obtained first, but in reality their contrast resolution is not sufficient for differentiating between soft-tissue tumors and adjacent normal tissue. They may, however, demonstrate phleboliths in hemangiomas, bone destruction secondary to adjacent malignant tumors, and dystrophic calcification within tumors; and they are excellent for ruling out bone lesions and detecting myositis ossificans. It is generally agreed that **MRI** is the next step in imaging evaluation. MRI has superb soft-tissue contrast, enabling immediate delineation of tumors and adjacent normal tissue such as fat and muscle. In addition, MRI demonstrates the anatomy with great clarity, enabling anatomic localization of the tumor. **Plain tomography** shows little that was not obvious on plain films. **CT** often does not demonstrate the margins of lesions, particularly intramuscular lesions, as well as does MRI. **Thermography**, basically a map of regions of increased temperature, has no role in the evaluation of soft-tissue masses. **Ultrasonography** is helpful for distinguishing cystic from solid lesions but does not depict the anatomy as well as MRI.

ANSWER: C

2. A 13-year-old girl presents to the emergency room with severe right knee pain that has been present for 3 months and that has become progressively more severe. There is no history of trauma. The pain has been characteristically worse in the evening, keeping the patient from sleeping. Her past medical history is otherwise unremarkable. On physical examination, there is a large, extremely tender soft-tissue mass fixed to the distal femur posteromedially. There is knee flexion contracture measuring 10 degrees and severe pain on range of motion of the knee beyond 90 degrees. Results of all the laboratory examinations are within normal limits except for an alkaline phosphatase level of 340 IU/L. A technetium 99 diphosphonate bone scan reveals a monostotic lesion with intense uptake in the right distal femur. A CT scan of this area shows a destructive lesion of the distal femur with a large posteromedially based soft-tissue mass. A chest radiograph and a CT scan of the chest are normal. The figure shows anteroposterior and lateral radiographs of the right distal femur. An incisional biopsy of this lesion confirms the pathologic diagnosis. Which of the following is the most appropriate treatment for this patient?

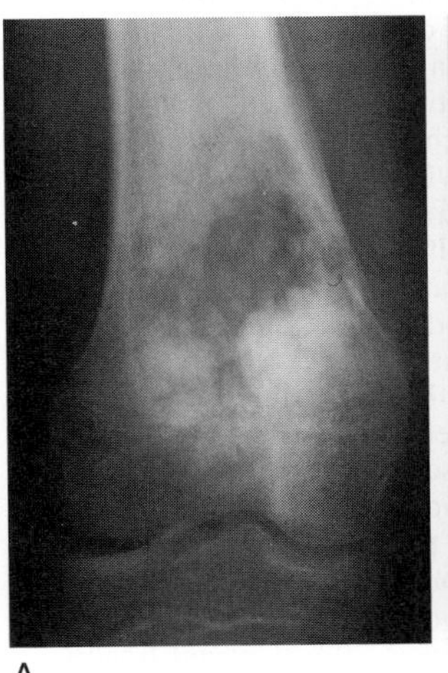

A

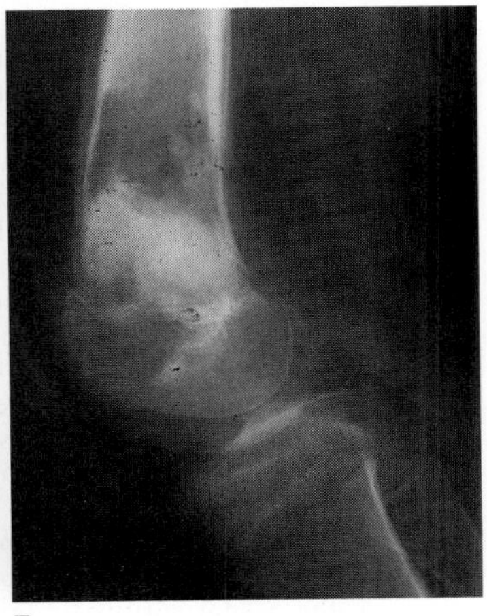

B

   A. Excision of the lesion with autogenous iliac bone graft.
   B. Systemic chemotherapy followed by 6000 rad of radiation.
   C. Neoadjuvant systemic chemotherapy followed by en bloc resection of the distal femur with reconstruction.
   D. Above-knee amputation.

Ref.: 1

COMMENTS: There is a destructive lesion of the metaphysis of the distal femur with matrix ossification within the lesion. In addition, there is evidence of a Codman's triangle and cortical destruction with soft-tissue extension. In a 13-year-old such radiographic findings most likely indicate an osteosarcoma. The current treatment of osteosarcoma consists of neoadjuvant chemotherapy for approximately 3 months; the feasibility of limb salvage is then determined. En bloc resection with reconstruction is a reasonable choice. Excision with autogenous iliac bone graft is totally unreasonable for this sarcoma of the distal femur; it is a procedure reserved exclusively for benign tumors of bone. Chemotherapy plus irradiation would be a reasonable choice for Ewing's sarcoma; Ewing's sarcoma, however, has a different radiographic manifestation and location. Finally, above-knee amputation is a reasonable choice for the treatment of osteosarcoma; however, some form of chemotherapy is usually employed for treatment of osteosarcoma. Amputation alone is not a reasonable choice.

ANSWER: C

3. Features of osteogenic sarcoma include which of the following?

A. The most common site of involvement is the diaphysis of the femur.
B. It occurs in 10% of male patients with Paget's disease.
C. Metastases occur mainly via the lymphatic system.
D. The first symptom usually is pain resulting from a pathologic fracture.
E. Spicules of bone within the tumor produce a typical appearance on radiography.

Ref.: 1, 2, 3

COMMENTS: Osteogenic sarcoma is uncommon, occurring in about 1 in 775,000 population. As a primary tumor, it is seen most commonly during the second decade of life. The most common site of involvement is the metaphysis of the femur, followed by the upper end of the tibia and the humerus; the radius, ulna, ilium, and scapula are less commonly affected. Osteogenic sarcoma in older patients frequently arises from preexisting Paget's disease. Such sarcomatous degeneration occurs in 10% of male patients with Paget's disease; it carries a poorer prognosis than does primary osteogenic sarcoma and may arise simultaneously at multiple sites. When the tumor extends to or originates underneath the periosteum, the periosteum is raised off the bone, producing a soft-tissue swelling. Spicules of bone within the tumor produce a sunburst appearance on the radiograph. Usually, the first symptom is pain unrelieved by rest, secondary to periosteal irritation. This pain often precludes ambulation, and so pathologic fractures are an uncommon occurrence. Metastatic spread is primarily hematogenous and most commonly to the lungs, often producing a clinical picture of bronchitis or pneumonia. In the past, standard treatment was local radiation therapy with delayed amputation; the 5-year survival rate was 20%. Current treatment combines surgery with multiple cytotoxic drugs, including methotrexate, cisplatin, ifosfamide, and doxorubicin (Adriamycin). The 5-year survival rate now is greater than 70%. Considerable success is being reported with limb salvage surgery in combination with pre- and postoperative chemotherapy.

ANSWER: B, E

4. Match each clinical statement in the left column with the appropriate disease in the right column.

A. History of painful swelling with loss of joint function; occurs most commonly in patients 10–30 years old
B. Benign tumor arising from cartilaginous tissue that commonly calcifies
C. Occurs as a primary tumor in the older age groups and as a tumor secondary to osteochondroma and enchondromatosis
D. Occurs during the years of active bone growth and often manifests as a pathologic fracture without previous symptoms
E. Occasionally behaves in a malignant manner despite having a benign histologic appearance

a. Chondroma
b. Benign chondroblastoma
c. Chondrosarcoma
d. Osteoclastoma (giant-cell tumor)
e. Unicameral bone cyst

Ref.: 1, 2, 3

COMMENTS: Chondroma is a benign neoplasm arising from cartilaginous elements of developing bone and often undergoes calcification. It is common in the small bones of the hand or foot. When located in the medullary canal, it is referred to as an **enchondroma**. Multiple enchondromas primarily found on one side of the skeleton characterize Ollier's disease. Multiple enchondromas found with soft-tissue hemangiomas represent Maffucci syndrome. On radiographs, the lesions are densely calcified with a popcorn-ball appearance. Malignant degeneration occurs only within multiple enchondromas. **Benign chondroblastoma** occurs during the first and second decades of life, before closure of the epiphyseal line. There is often a history of painful swelling with loss of joint function. On radiographs it appears as an osteolytic epiphyseal lesion containing calcium deposits. Treatment consists of curettage and grafting with cancellous bone. **Chondrosarcoma** arises from chondroblasts and may be either primary (in older patients) or a secondary malignant change of such preexisting conditions as osteochondroma or enchondromatosis. The pelvis, ribs, sternum, and femur are the bones most commonly involved. Radiographs show destruction of trabecular bone or cortex associated with an expanding soft-tissue mass containing irregular areas of calcified tissue. The degree of cellularity, the amount of matrix formed, and the severity of nuclear irregularities seem to be correlated with survival rate, which ranges from good to poor. **Osteoclastoma**, or giant-cell tumor, contains a highly vascular cellular stroma with many giant cells. They are seen commonly in the ends of long bones in the vicinity of the knee and the lower end of the radius. On radiographs they appear as clear cystic tumors in the metaphyseoepiphyseal area. They may penetrate the articular cartilage but only rarely extend into the joint. These tumors occasionally behave with malignant characteristics despite a benign histologic appearance. Local recurrence is as high as 50% with curettage alone, and adjuvant cauterization is therefore recommended. **Unicameral bone cyst** occurs in the metaphyseal area of long bones, such as the upper end of the humerus and femur. It often manifests during years of active bone growth as a pathologic fracture without previous symptoms. In contrast to the giant-cell tumor, the unicameral bone cyst is relatively avascular. Treatment consists of curettage of the cystic cavity and of bone grafting to restore continuity.

ANSWER: A-b; B-a; C-c; D-e; E-d

5. With regard to Ewing's tumor and lymphoma of bone, which of the following statements is/are true?

A. Both tumors mostly affect patients under 20 years of age.
B. Ewing's tumor is frequently associated with febrile attacks.
C. Ewing's tumor begins in the diaphyseal marrow; and as it extends to the periosteum, new bone formation occurs, creating so-called "onion skinning."
D. Lymphoma of bone responds well to irradiation and chemotherapy, but relapse is common.

Ref.: 1, 2, 3

COMMENTS: Ewing's tumor is a small, round-cell malignancy arising from the diaphyseal marrow of long bones in patients under 20 years of age. The tumor extends from the medulla to the periosteum; and as new bone is formed, "onion skinning" parallel to the shaft is visible on radiographs. A history of trauma is not uncommon, and there are frequently associated febrile attacks and leukocytosis. The tumor is capable of lymphatic and hematogenous spread, and death usually results from pulmonary metastases. The tumors are radiosensitive but tend to recur. Newer treatments involving the use of various chemotherapeutic agents have improved survival; in carefully selected patients the limb can be salvaged. **Lymphoma** of bone (formerly called reticulum cell sarcoma) occurs in patients between ages 20 and 40 and most commonly affects the femur, tibia, ilium, and humerus. Pain, which precedes formation of a visible tumor, is often the first complaint. On radiographs, the lesions appear osteolytic at the end of the diaphysis, later extending throughout the length of the bone. Sometimes there is a pathologic fracture. Radiation therapy combined with surgery and chemotherapy has given the best survival rates.

ANSWER: B, C, D

6. Match each clinical statement in the left column with the corresponding lesion in the right column.

A. Most often located in the jaw	a. Aneurysmal bone cyst
B. Located in the metaphysis; histologically consists of cavernous spaces interspersed with osteoid tissue	b. Adamantinoma
C. Manifests as a single cystic swelling associated with destruction of bone	c. Neurilemoma
D. Most commonly found in the sacrococcygeal region	d. Chordoma
E. A benign vascular tumor more commonly found in the skull and vertebral column than in other bones	e. Hemangioma

Ref.: 3

COMMENTS: Aneurysmal bone cyst is an osteolytic lesion found in the metaphyses of long bones in young people. Histologically, the characteristic findings are cavernous spaces within fibrous tissue, without endothelial lining. Local curettage with or without bone graft usually is adequate treatment. **Adamantinoma** occurs most frequently as an enamel-containing tumor in the jaw. This tumor is treated with wide excision, and often requires bone grafting. A rare histologically similar tumor that occurs in the tibia or other long bones is also designated adamantinoma, although this type does not contain enamel. The treatment of choice for adamantinoma of a long bone is en bloc resection. **Neurilemoma** is a nerve sheath tumor that may grow in bone. In that setting, it manifests on radiographs as cystic swelling with associated destruction of bone. Usually it occurs singly with a benign clinical course; local removal, when possible, provides adequate treatment. Deformity of bone and fracture may occur. **Chordoma** is a rare malignant neoplasm arising from embryonic remnants of the notochord and is found in the sacrococcygeal region. The tumor is radioresistant, the only hope for cure being complete surgical excision. **Hemangioma** is a vascular tumor that rarely affects bone, most commonly doing so in the skull and vertebral column; in the latter location, it can lead to collapse of the vertebral body. Most of these tumors are benign, but excision is advised whenever possible.

ANSWER: A-b; B-a; C-c; D-d; E-e

7. Match each statement in the left column with the corresponding soft-tissue tumor in the right column.

A. Occurs in the deep muscle masses as a painful swelling; is locally invasive but does not metastasize	a. Fibrosarcoma of muscle
B. Malignant small-cell tumor with a high incidence of blood-borne metastases	b. Liposarcoma
C. Arises from sequestered synovioblastic cells	c. Rhabdomyosarcoma
D. Usually manifests as a large painful tumor mass, most commonly in the musculature of the thigh	d. Synovial sarcoma
E. Is one of the more common malignant soft-tissue tumors and occurs primarily in the soft tissues of the extremities	e. Desmoid tumor

Ref.: 1, 2, 3

COMMENTS: Fibrosarcoma of muscle can occur either as a well-differentiated or an anaplastic tumor. Usually it manifests as a large painful tumor mass in the thigh. **Liposarcoma** also occurs either as a differentiated or an anaplastic tumor arising from the soft tissues of the extremities. Liposarcomas most commonly occur in middle-aged patients and equally often in men and women. The thigh-popliteal area and the inguinal and gluteal regions are most commonly involved. These tumors arise de novo and do not represent malignant transformation of a lipoma. Their radiosensitivity is variable; curative treatment is best achieved by wide surgical excision. **Rhabdomyosarcoma** is a small-cell malignancy originating from striated muscle cells. It is a tumor of infants and young adults and has high incidence of hematogenous spread. It is rarely radiosensitive; treatment is multimodal, combining systemic chemotherapy with wide local resection. **Synovial sarcoma** arises from sequestered synovioblastic cells present in subcutaneous tissue and muscle. There is no obvious continuity with joint tissue. It is capable of local infiltration; radical excision should be performed and include the main muscle mass surrounding the tumor. **Desmoid tumor** is a low-grade fibrosarcoma capable of local invasion but not hematogenous metastases. Usually it manifests as a painful tumor in the deep muscles, tends to occur in younger people, and can recur after inadequate resection. Treatment therefore is radical surgical excision.

ANSWER: A-e; B-c; C-d; D-a; E-b

8. A 31-year-old woman has an enlarging and painful mass of the right thigh. Since its first appearance approximately 6 weeks ago, it has progressively enlarged. The patient has otherwise been healthy, and there is no history of trauma. On examination, there is a mass involving the medial aspect of her right thigh; it is extremely tender but mobile, with no fixation to the underlying bone. Results of the neurovascular examination of the right lower extremity are within normal limits. Results of all laboratory studies, including complete blood cell count, serum chemistry studies, and chest radiograph, were within normal limits. The accompanying figure shows a CT scan of the right thigh and T_1- and T_2-weighted MRI studies of the same area of the thigh. Which of the following is the most likely diagnosis for this patient's condition?

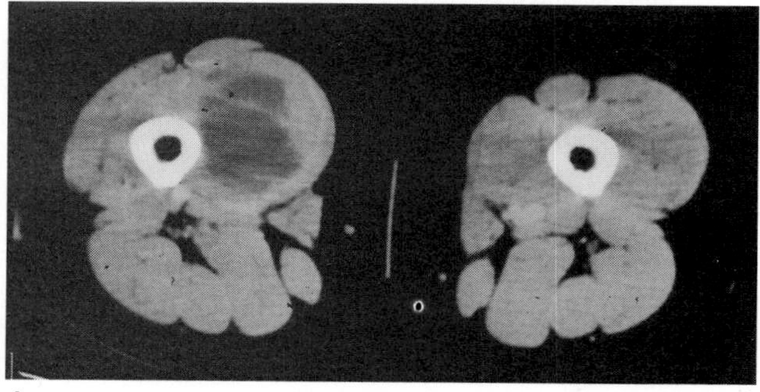

A

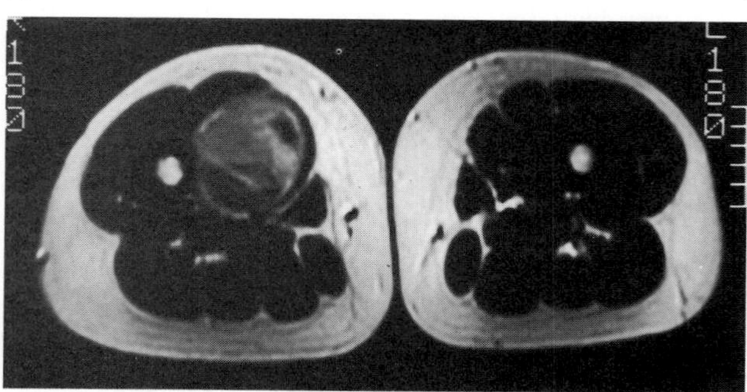

B

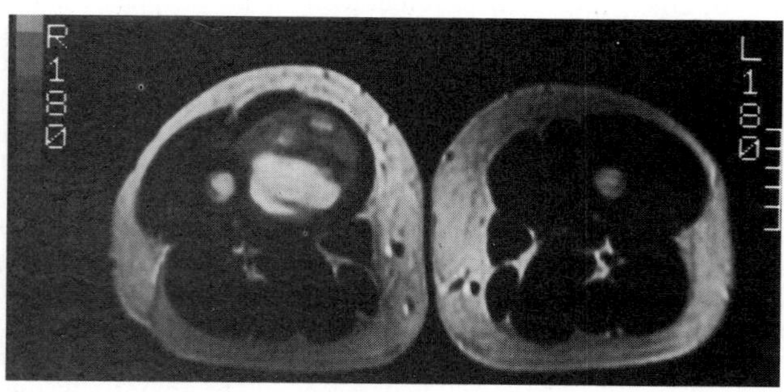

C

A. Aneurysm of the femoral artery.
B. Hematomas.
C. Lipoma.
D. Liposarcoma.

Ref.: 1

COMMENTS: Imaging of the extremity shows a heterogeneous tumor of the medial thigh composed of several tissue densities. This is evident on both the CT scan (Fig. A) and the MRI examinations (Fig. B). The T_2-weighted MRI scan (Fig. C) shows areas of significant tumor enhancement surrounded by areas that are less enhanced, again confirming the heterogeneity of the tumor. This is a rather typical appearance of a soft-tissue **sarcoma** (liposarcoma). The other choices are unreasonable. **Aneurysm of the femoral artery** is unlikely because the artery is well visualized on the CT scan and MRI studies without evidence of abnormality. A **hematoma** also is unlikely because of the lack of history of trauma and the heterogeneity on the imaging studies. **Lipoma** is an unreasonable choice because the tumor shown here is not a fat-density tumor and has a heterogeneous signal on MRI.

ANSWER: D

9. With regard to the treatment of malignant tumors of soft tissue, which of the following statements is/are true?

A. Because they are generally well encapsulated, excisional biopsy around the capsule is the procedure of choice for establishing the diagnosis.
B. Biopsy is generally unnecessary because the diagnosis can be made on the basis of physical examination and radiographic findings.
C. Incisional biopsy, when required, should be performed through an incision that can easily be encompassed at the time of definitive surgical treatment.
D. When soft-tissue sarcomas are diagnosed in the extremity, they are best treated by forequarter or hindquarter amputation.

Ref.: 1, 2, 3

COMMENTS: Rapidly growing soft-tissue tumors compress surrounding normal tissue to form a pseudocapsule. Microscopic nests of cells are often found beyond this pseudocapsule, making simple enucleation unacceptable. Although characteristics consistent with malignancy are often detectable on physical examination and other radiologic studies, a tissue diagnosis is essential before definitive surgical therapy because the natural histories of the various soft-tissue tumors vary widely. Low-grade tumors such as desmoid tumor and low-grade fibrosarcomas and liposarcomas are locally invasive but rarely metastasize. Thus aggressive primary surgical excision is the treatment of choice. In contrast, osteosarcoma, Ewing's tumor, and rhabdomyosarcoma are examples of tumors with high propensities for distant metastases. For these tumors, treatment by operation alone does little to prolong life; multimodal treatment with the use of adjuvant antineoplastic drugs and irradiation is indicated. An incisional biopsy for diagnosis should be performed in a manner that does not preclude wide excision of the tumor through undissected tissue planes. Because many of these tumors are capable of distant metastases, radical amputation does little to prevent death from distant disease. Amputation is indicated when the anatomic location requires it, examples being tumors arising high in the buttock, high in the thigh, or near the shoulder. For tumors that inextricably involve the neurovascular supply to the limb, amputation may be necessary for successful treatment.

ANSWER: C

10. With regard to metastatic tumors of bone, which of the following statements is/are true?

A. Skeletal metastases can arise from virtually all types of malignant tumors but most frequently are from tumors of the breasts, prostate, thyroid, kidneys, and lungs.
B. Metastatic bone tumors are the result of hematogenous spread ending in bony capillary beds.
C. Most patients with bone metastases complain of pain.
D. Bone metastases are a grave prognostic sign; once they appear survival is rarely longer than 3 months.

Ref.: 2

COMMENTS: Although the most common cancers metastasizing to bone are those of the breasts, prostate, thyroid, kidneys, and lungs, nearly all types of malignant tumors can do this. The usual route is via the bloodstream, originating in veins leaving the primary tumor and then passing through the pulmonary circulation and on to the bony capillary beds. The high incidence of metastasis to the axial skeleton probably is attributable to hematogenous dissemination through the vertebral venous plexus (of Batson). Sixty-five percent of patients with radiographic evidence of bone metastases complain of pain; tenderness to palpation is present in fewer than 20%. Many patients with bone metastases live many months or years, particularly those with breast and prostate cancer responsive to hormonal manipulation.

ANSWER: A, B, C

11. Which method of diagnosis is most sensitive for the detection of bone metastases?

A. History and physical examination.
B. Radiography.
C. Technetium bone scan.
D. Measurement of serum alkaline phosphatase.
E. Measurement of serum calcium.

Ref.: 3

COMMENTS: About 65% of patients with bone metastases complain of pain, and about 15% have palpable tenderness. The **alkaline phosphatase** level is normal in up to 40% of patients. **Radiographs** are not adequately reliable because at least 50% of the medulla must be destroyed before a lesion is seen on a bone film. **Tomograms** of the bone are more sensitive. **Technetium bone scan** is by far the most sensitive screening test for bone metastases. **Hypercalcemia** may be the result of bone destruction by metastases; but when the kidneys are functioning, hypercalciuria is usually found, in association with normal serum calcium levels. Hypercalcemia resulting from bronchogenic carcinoma may be caused by a parathormone-like hormone secreted by the tumor. Mammary carcinomas frequently produce hypercalcemia, which may be a result of the excretion of specific osteolytic steroids derived from the mammary carcinoma.

ANSWER: C

12. With regard to treatment of skeletal metastases, which of the following statements is/are true?

A. The pain that arises from skeletal metastases may be diminished if the hypercalcemia is treated.
B. There is an 80% chance of pain relief after hormonal therapy.
C. Radiotherapy to the localized area of pain is indicated when hormonal therapy is ineffective.
D. Large lytic lesions, particularly of the femur, should be treated initially with radiation followed by internal fixation to avoid a pathologic fracture.

Ref.: 3

COMMENTS: In most instances, treatment of skeletal metastases is palliative. Pain occurs in association with hypercalcemia; and once the latter is treated, the pain may be relieved. Patients with hormonally dependent tumors often experience significant relief from pain after hormonal manipulation; however, not all skeletal metastases are hormonally sensitive. If hormonal therapy fails, or for tumors that are not hormonally dependent, radiotherapy to a localized area of pain often produces relief. Large lytic lesions with impending fracture should undergo prompt internal fixation followed by irradiation. Radiotherapy given preoperatively may predispose to pathologic fracture, lessening the effectiveness of the fixation. Vertebral metastases with subsequent compression fracture involving the spinal cord may be treated by decompression laminectomy. Radiotherapy alone in this setting can control pain but does not improve an established paraplegia.

ANSWER: A, C

13. Indications for bone scintigraphy do not include which of the following?

A. Evaluation of the nature and physical limits of a primary bone tumor.
B. Elevation of alkaline phosphatase levels that is not explained by obvious liver disease.
C. Bone pain unexplained by pertinent radiographs.
D. Evaluation of abnormal serum calcium/phosphate levels.
E. Workup of potentially metastasizing tumors.

Ref.: 3

COMMENTS: Although there has been a general decline in the use of bone scintigraphy for preoperative evaluation of potentially metastasizing tumors (for cost-containment reasons), the bone scan remains the most sensitive method for detecting osseous metastases. Bone scintigraphy often provides the most direct answer to whether the skeleton is responsible for aberrations in serum alkaline phosphatase and calcium/phosphate levels, pinpointing offending bones and frequently defining the pathologic process involved. Bone pain, which cannot be adequately explained by radiographs of the offending site, remains one of the more important and frequently employed indications for skeletal scintigraphy. Bone scintigraphy does *not* define the nature or the extent of the primary lesion. CT, plain and tomographic roentgenography, and even MRI, with far better resolution, are more productive in this regard. However, the bone scan remains the most efficient and effective tool for differentiating *monostotic* from *polyostotic disease*.

ANSWER: A

14. A 32-year-old woman has a 3-month history of left knee pain that began after a 2-hour aerobic exercise class. Since that time, the pain has become progressively worse and now is present with activity as well as when at rest. On examination, there is an antalgic component to her gait and marked tenderness over the mediofemoral condyle; range of motion in the knee is normal, and there is no effusion. Results of all laboratory tests are within normal limits, including a complete blood cell count and calcium, phosphorus, and alkaline phosphatase levels. The figures shown here are anteroposterior and lateral radiographs of the left distal femur and knee joint. A technetium 99 diphosphonate bone scan shows intense uptake in the mediofemoral condyle; there are no other osseous lesions. Which of the following is the most likely diagnosis in this patient?

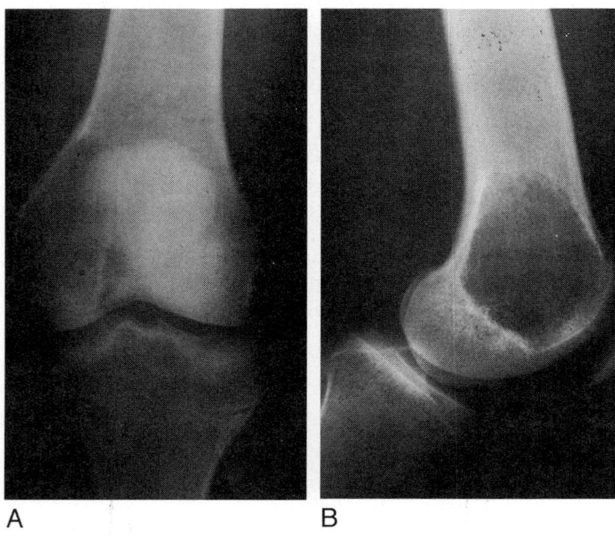

A. Metastatic carcinoma to bone.
B. Hyperparathyroidism.
C. Giant-cell tumor.
D. Osteosarcoma.

Ref.: 1

COMMENTS: **Giant-cell tumor** of bone occurs in skeletally mature individuals. It usually manifests as an eccentric lytic lesion of bone located in the epiphysis and metaphysis. The knee is the most common location. **Metastatic carcinoma** is unlikely because of the age of the patient and because on bone scan it is shown to be a monostotic lesion. Metastatic carcinoma rarely involves the epiphysis and metaphysis of the bone. **Hyperparathyroidism** is the second best choice, and radiographically it can closely resemble a giant-cell tumor. Normal serum calcium, phosphorus, and alkaline phosphatase levels make this diagnosis unlikely. Another possible diagnosis is **osteosarcoma**. This is the most common primary osseous malignancy, usually occurring in the metaphysis around the knee joint. Osteosarcoma is extremely destructive and usually manifests with a significant soft-tissue mass. Radiographic evidence of bone formation is usually present. This tumor also occurs in younger individuals unless it is a secondary osteosarcoma.

ANSWER: C

15. The bone most commonly affected by a simple bone cyst is the:

A. Femur.
B. Tibia.
C. Humerus.
D. Ulna.
E. Carpal bone.

Ref.: 1

COMMENTS: Unicameral bone cysts typically present as solitary fluid-filled cysts in the long bones of children. The humerus is the most common location. The lesion typically abuts the growth plate and may present in association with a pathologic fracture. Treatment consists of immobilization until the fracture heals and then definitive treatment consisting of methylprednisolone acetate injection or open curettage and bone grafting. Incomplete healing is common with most treatment methods, and careful follow-up is essential.

ANSWER: C

REFERENCES

1. Schwartz SI, Shires GT, Spencer FC: *Principles of Surgery*, 7th ed. McGraw-Hill, New York, 1999.
2. Sabiston DC Jr: *Textbook of Surgery*, 15th ed. WB Saunders, Philadelphia, 1997.
3. Schajowicz F: *Tumors and Tumor-Like Lesions of Bone and Joints.* Springer-Verlag, New York, 1981.

CHAPTER 47

Amputations

1. Match the characteristic in the left column with the appropriate amputation in the right column.

A. Tissues are cut circularly and allowed to retract initially; may be closed secondarily or placed with skin traction.
B. Antagonist muscles are sutured across the bone end.
C. Transected muscles are attached to bone by suturing through drill holes placed at the distal bone.
D. Skin, fascia, and muscle are transected based at level of amputation, then closed over the bone.
E. Used when extremity is grossly infected and patient is septic.
F. Usually requires revision.

a. Conventional.
b. Osteomyoplastic.
c. Myodesis.
d. Open "guillotine."

Ref.: 1

COMMENTS: The **conventional** amputation uses curved skin and fascial flaps based at the level of amputation. When care is taken to ensure proper approximation of soft tissue over the bony stump, it lends itself to the potential of good rehabilitation. Fitting for a prosthesis is delayed until healing has occurred. The **osteomyoplastic** amputation (suturing antagonistic muscles across the bone end) and the **myodesis** amputation (attaching muscles directly to the bone) typically are used for special situations (i.e., young patients with trauma). They provide improved function and allow the application of immediate postsurgical prosthetic devices. The **open** or "**guillotine**" amputation is reserved for emergency situations, unstable patients, or the presence of severe sepsis. The wound is left completely open, and the bone usually protrudes after soft tissue contraction occurs, thus requiring revision. This situation can be obviated by employing appropriately elongated skin flaps or even by countering this tendency with postoperative skin traction. The stump usually is not amenable to easy rehabilitation.

ANSWER: A-d; B-b; C-c; D-a; E-d; F-d

2. Principles of postoperative management after amputation include which one or more of the following?

A. Splinting of the stump dressing to avoid shifting in position.
B. Compression dressing over the stump to avoid postoperative edema and hematoma.
C. Exercise and positioning to avoid contracture.
D. Early evaluation and care by a qualified physical therapist and prosthetist.
E. Use of stump stocking to mold the stump for eventual prosthesis fitting.

Ref.: 1, 2

COMMENTS: Conventional postoperative care begins with application of a light compression dressing in the operating room, followed by repeated application of elastic dressings to avoid stump edema. Damage to the skin can result from excessively compressive dressings applied over bony prominences (i.e., the anterior tibial area in a below-knee stump). Stump exercises and stretching prevent contracture after primary wound healing has taken place. Progressive training after suture removal allows the eventual application of a permanent prosthesis. Alternatively, application of a rigid dressing in the operating room allows the immediate use of a prosthetic device; immediate prosthetic fitting, however, need not be employed to use the rigid dressing. Rigid dressings offer the advantage of immediate use of the extremity. Wound healing may be enhanced by maximum control of edema and hematoma and by better tissue immobilization. When treatment is successful, resumption of full activity can be expected to occur within 4–6 weeks. All of the listed choices are important for proper amputation management.

ANSWER: A, B, C, D, E

3. Regarding proper selection of the level of amputation, which of the following statements is/are true?

A. The extent of resection for malignant tumors must not be compromised for functional considerations.
B. The use of skin grafts and flaps to conserve bony length is appropriate in healthy, stable trauma patients.
C. Unless 4 inches or more of tibia can be preserved, the knee joint should be sacrificed.
D. The presence of contracture should not influence the level of amputation.

Ref.: 1, 2

COMMENTS: As a general principle, the longer the amputation stump, the more functional is the limb. However, when performing amputations for malignancy, adequate tumor excision, not preservation of stump length, is the primary concern. The irregular damage to skin caused by trauma can be treated by skin grafts and flaps to preserve bony length. Full-thickness skin should be maintained for weight-bearing surfaces. Amputations in patients with peripheral vascular disease succeed best when performed at levels that have adequate nutritional blood flow to the skin. Below-knee stumps as short as 2 inches can be successfully fitted with prostheses, but function is much better if at least 4 inches of stump is maintained. Preservation of the knee joint allows a bent-knee, end-weight-bearing prosthesis to be used and is usually preferable to a long above-knee stump. Amputations above the knee should remove at least 4 inches of femur to facilitate fitting a prosthetic knee joint. Relative contraindications to below-knee amputation include the presence of hip or knee contracture, which negates its functional advantage.

ANSWER: A, B

4. Useful preoperative methods to evaluate adequacy of blood flow in patients with peripheral vascular disease undergoing amputation include which one or more of the following?

A. Clinical assessment of cutaneous blood flow.
B. Cutaneous PO_2 and PCO_2.
C. Status of peripheral pulses.
D. Doppler systolic blood pressure.

Ref.: 1, 2

COMMENTS: The healing ability of an amputation stump is determined by the adequacy of the nutritional blood flow to the skin. This can be assessed clinically (e.g., skin temperature, capillary refill) or by empiric measurement techniques such as transcutaneous PO_2 and PCO_2 measurements. Palpable popliteal pulses are associated with a higher success rate for below-knee amputations, but their absence is not considered as contraindication. A Doppler systolic blood pressure in the calf of more than 74 mm Hg is associated with a high success rate for below-knee amputations but has a high false-negative rate and should not be used as the single criterion for evaluation. Ankle to brachial pressures may be useful for predicting the outcome of forefoot amputations. Ultimately, the degree of capillary and small vessel bleeding at the incision site may be an indication of the likelihood of achieving primary healing. Among ambulatory patients with impaired circulation and diabetes, recent series report that as many as 80% of patients with successful healing had a below-knee amputation. This is in contrast to studies during 1960–1970 that reported 80% of all successful amputations were above the knee.

ANSWER: A, B, C, D

5. True statements regarding amputations of the toes or feet include which one or more of the following?

A. Transphalangeal amputations may be used so long as the necrosis is distal to the proximal interphalangeal joint.
B. When the entire toe must be removed, disarticulation is preferred over transmetatarsal amputation.
C. Toe amputations should never be attempted in patients who do not have pedal pulses.
D. Rehabilitation after a transmetatarsal amputation requires no special prosthesis.

Ref.: 1, 2

COMMENTS: Transphalangeal amputations may be used if the necrosis is distal to the proximal interphalangeal joint, and whereby relatively healthy skin flaps can be reapproximated without tension. When the entire toe must be amputated, a transmetatarsal level is preferred over disarticulation to avoid problems with the bulky metatarsal head and the poor vascular supply to the articular cartilage. Patients with palpable popliteal and pedal pulses who have transmetatarsal amputations do better than those without, but their absence is not considered an absolute contraindication. Ambulation may be started after the incision is healed; no special shoe is required, but a shoe filler improves gait.

ANSWER: A, D

6. Syme's amputation is best suited for which of the following?

A. Preservation of leg length.
B. Most peripheral vascular disorders involving the feet.
C. A foot destroyed by trauma.
D. Anticipation of lower extremity weight-bearing.

Ref.: 1, 2

COMMENTS: Syme's amputation is created at a bone level just distal to the tibial flare with preservation of the heel pad. It maintains the length of the lower extremity and allows creation of an end-weight-bearing stump. It is usually performed when most of the foot has been destroyed by trauma. Rarely, it is successful in patients with diabetes or peripheral vascular insufficiency. In most cases it requires a complex prosthesis that some patients find cosmetically unacceptable.

ANSWER: A, C, D

7. Knee disarticulation has which of the following advantages?

A. In children it is useful for maintaining the epiphysis for bony growth.
B. In adults it is used to preserve bony length when severe ischemia contraindicates a below-knee amputation.
C. It provides maximal length with good end-weight-bearing characteristics.
D. It is easily fitted with a simple prosthesis.

Ref.: 1, 2

COMMENTS: Knee disarticulation is most often used in children because it allows maintenance of the epiphysis for bony growth. It is rarely used in situations in which there is impaired circulation and is rarely performed in adults. The procedure preserves maximum length, provides a good end-weight-bearing stump, and lends itself to a good fit between stump and socket. However, because the femoral condyles are preserved the stump is bulky, which can make prosthesis fitting difficult. The anterior flap is left longer than the posterior flap, and the patella is preserved if it is not involved by disease.

ANSWER: A, C

8. Indications for an above-knee amputation include which of the following?

A. Absent popliteal pulses.
B. Diabetes mellitus.
C. Gangrene proximal to the malleoli.
D. Calf muscle rigor.
E. Knee or hip contractures.
F. Patient with minimal potential for rehabilitation and ambulation.

Ref.: 1, 2

COMMENTS: Assessment of the vascular status at the level of amputation is important, but the absence of popliteal pulses or the presence of diabetes are not in themselves absolute indications for an above-knee amputation. Rigor of the calf muscles and the presence of gangrene of the skin at the level where the flaps would be constructed for the below-knee amputation are sufficient indications for an above-knee amputation. Because knee and hip contractures make rehabilitation after below-knee amputation unlikely and because the above-knee amputation has the highest healing rate and the lowest reamputation rate in patients with severe peripheral vascular disease, patients so afflicted do best with an above-knee amputation.

ANSWER: C, D, E, F

9. Which of the following statements is/are true regarding hip disarticulation and hemipelvectomy?

A. Prostheses are unavailable for ambulation.
B. The usual indications are bone tumors, soft tissue tumors, and occasionally extensive trauma.
C. Flaps are brought together posteriorly after hip disarticulation.
D. The entire ilium must be removed during hemipelvectomy.

Ref.: 1, 2

COMMENTS: The indications for hip disarticulation are tumors of bone or soft tissue and, in some cases, extensive trauma. Hemipelvectomy is indicated when an upper thigh tumor cannot be excised by disarticulation alone. The posterior flap after hip disarticulation is closed anteriorly so the patient can sit comfortably on the socket of the prosthesis. Whenever possible, a leaf of ilium and the pelvic rami are preserved during the hemipelvectomy to act as support points for the prosthesis. Both amputations can be fitted with a special (Canadian) prosthesis that allows ambulation.

ANSWER: B

10. Of the following statements, which is/are true regarding lower limb prostheses?

A. They require less energy to use than does crutch walking.
B. The shorter the stump, the greater the stump tip pressure.
C. The main pressure point in the below-knee prosthesis is the stump end.
D. A suspension belt is mandatory for all above-knee prostheses.

Ref.: 1, 2

COMMENTS: Prostheses are designed to restore function, mobility, and appearance. Except in cases involving diabetics with above-knee amputations, properly fitted prostheses have lower energy requirements than crutch walking. Socket design has as its goals patient comfort and an even distribution of forces on the stump. The longer the stump, the greater is the surface area over which these forces can be distributed. Above-knee sockets are usually of the quadrilateral total contact design and are suspended by stump suction or pelvic belts. The below-knee prostheses most commonly used are the patellar tendon-bearing type or the patellar tendon supracondylar type.

ANSWER: A, B

11. Regarding amputations distal to the elbow, which of the following statements is/are true?

A. Digital tourniquets should be avoided when possible.
B. Scar placement is of little concern.
C. After suprametacarpal amputation, opposing tendons should be fixed to preserve muscle tone and strength.
D. The precise nature of the operation requires a general anesthetic.

Ref.: 1, 2

COMMENTS: Most patients undergoing lower extremity amputations have peripheral vascular disease, and the use of tourniquets is not necessary. For the upper extremity, however, tourniquets (cuff pressure best tolerated at 280 mm Hg) are frequently used to provide a blood-free field so critical nerve and tendon structures can be identified. Because of the risk of thrombosis, digital tourniquets such as rubber bands should be avoided. Scars should be minimized and placed as far as possible from bone, tendon, nerve, and points of pressure. To best preserve muscle strength, tone, and hence function, opposing tendons should be fixed anatomically. In general, arm amputations are more precise operations than leg amputations. The goal of amputation of the proximal arm is preservation of as much viable tissue as possible; for distal arm amputations, it is preservation of the grasping function of the hand. Adequate anesthesia can often be accomplished by regional block. This is preferred in trauma patients, who may present with a full stomach, because it avoids the risk of vomiting and aspiration.

ANSWER: A, C

12. Which of the following statements is/are true regarding amputations of digits?

A. A shorter volar flap and a longer dorsal flap are desired.
B. The root of the nail should always be preserved.
C. During removal of the distal phalanx, the distal middle phalangeal cartilage should be preserved.
D. Amputation at the metacarpophalangeal joint is preferable to amputation through the proximal phalanx.
E. Even the smallest stump of the thumb is preferable to complete amputation with prosthesis.

Ref.: 1, 2

COMMENTS: A longer volar flap is desired so the scar can be positioned away from pressure-bearing surfaces. However, bone and viable tissue should never be sacrificed to obtain ideal scar placement. Unless more than half of the nail bed can be preserved, the nail root should be removed. If the distal phalanx must be removed, the exposed middle phalangeal cartilage should be resected. Given a choice, resection through the proximal phalanx is preferred over a metacarpophalangeal amputation. As is the case with the thumb, any stump, no matter how short, has function. When a digit must be removed in its entirety, preservation of function of the hand as a unit is the goal and may require a variety of secondary procedures.

ANSWER: E

13. Regarding wrist disarticulation, which of the following statements is/are true?

A. It provides better prosthesis control than does a long forearm amputation.
B. The stump is stronger than that left when the amputation is through the carpal bones.
C. The severed tendons and ligaments of the hand must be fixed to prevent their retraction and atrophy.
D. Preservation of the styloid processes is necessary for prosthetic fitting.

Ref.: 1, 2

COMMENTS: Wrist disarticulation has several advantages over more proximal amputations. It preserves length and provides better control of the prosthesis. Although it is less strong than when the carpal bones remain, it accommodates a less conspicuous prosthesis. The styloid processes are removed to permit a smoother fit. The tendons of the hand are transected with the muscles at rest and fixed to periosteum to prevent retraction and atrophy.

ANSWER: A, C

14. Which of the following statements is/are true regarding forearm amputations?

A. Unless adequate muscle mass and length can be preserved, an above-elbow amputation is preferred to enhance prosthetic function.
B. Skin mobility is preserved by avoiding excessive dissection between skin and fascia.
C. A short stump of the ulna or radius can be lengthened secondarily.
D. Cineplastic operations using biceps or pectoralis muscles can provide function to artificial limbs when the amputation stump is extremely short.

Ref.: 1, 2

COMMENTS: Dissection is kept to a minimum to avoid immobilization of skin by subsequent scar formation. Pronation and supination are preserved by striving for a longer stump. Also, the procedure is conducted as atraumatically as possible to avoid fibrosis. Even an extremely short below-elbow stump is preferable to an above-elbow amputation. Functional control of a prosthesis fitted over a short stump can be provided by a cineplastic operation using the ipsilateral biceps or pectoralis muscle after the initial stump has healed. Other secondary procedures include the use of bone flaps or grafts to lengthen short stumps of the ulna or radius.

ANSWER: B, C, D

15. Relative to infection of the diabetic foot, which of the following statements is/are true?

A. The infection within the foot usually is less severe than it appears on clinical evaluation.
B. The pain expressed by the patient usually is less than one would expect in relation to the degree of infection.
C. The infection rarely has a bony or tendinous element at its base.
D. The factors contributing to the ulceration and infection in the diabetic foot are neuropathy, peripheral arterial occlusive disease, and perhaps impairment of leukocyte phagocytic function.
E. Conservative measures usually fail, necessitating amputation.

Ref.: 1, 2

COMMENTS: The diabetic foot ulcer may be due to pressure on a dysesthetic extremity that may or may not be associated with peripheral-vascular arterial insufficiency. There often is a bony or tendinous element at the base of the ulcer. The infection usually is more extensive in the foot than appears clinically. After adequate débridement, many extremities are salvageable. Aggressive open débridement is essential. Unless the need for amputation is urgent, there first should be an evaluation for arterial reconstruction.

ANSWER: B, D

REFERENCES

1. Frymoyer JW (ed): *Orthopaedic Basic Science*. American Academy of Orthopaedic Surgeons, Rosemont, IL, 1993.
2. Kasser JR (ed): *Orthopaedic Knowledge Update 5*, 1st ed. American Academy of Orthopaedic Surgeons, Rosemont, IL, 1996.

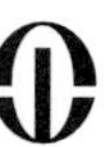

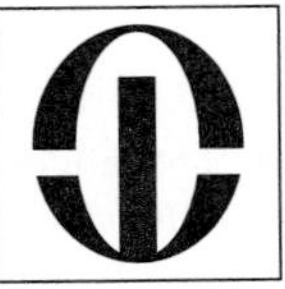

CHAPTER 48

Hand Surgery

1. Match each of the following nerves with the correct labeled structure on the diagram.

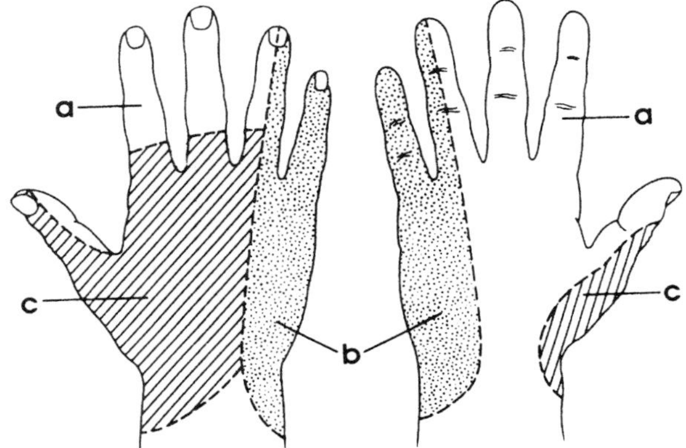

A. Median nerve.
B. Radial nerve.
C. Ulnar nerve.

Ref.: 1, 2, 3, 4

COMMENTS: There is considerable overlap in the sensory innervation of the hand. The usual innervation is as depicted in the illustration. Despite the overlap, there are certain autonomous zones useful for evaluating individual nerve function: the **median** nerve on the flexor aspect of the index finger beyond the distal interphalangeal joint; the **ulnar** nerve on the flexor aspect of the little finger beyond the distal interphalangeal joint; and the **radial** nerve on the dorsal web space of the thumb. Light touch with a piece of cotton and two-point discrimination are the most valuable sensory tests. Light touch is helpful for assessing sensation after acute injury or when examining children. Soaking a digit in water and looking for wrinkling ("pruning") of the skin or checking for sweating or moisture of the skin can also be helpful when examining uncooperative patients.

ANSWER: A-a; B-c; C-b

2. True statements regarding the intrinsic muscles of the hand include which of the following?

A. The intrinsic muscles originate in the forearm and insert on the metacarpals.
B. The palmar interossei pull the fingers to the midline and flex the metacarpophalangeal (MCP) joints of the index, ring, and little fingers.
C. Their innervation is derived from the radial, median, and ulnar nerves.
D. The dorsal interosseous muscles spread the fingers, flex the MCP joints, and extend the proximal and distal interphalangeal joints.
E. The intrinsic muscles of the index, long, and ring fingers consist of the palmar and dorsal interossei and the lumbrical muscles.

Ref.: 1, 2, 3

COMMENTS: The intrinsic muscles have their entire course confined to the hand and include the thenar and hypothenar muscles, the lumbricals, and the interosseous muscles. Together they flex the MCP joints, extend the interphalangeal joints, and spread and close the fingers. When functioning normally, they provide the hand with a transverse and longitudinal arch. The thumb thenar muscles provide radial abduction, palmar abduction, and opposition of the thumb. Their innervation is derived from the median and ulnar nerves, the distribution of which is variable. The classic pattern is **median innervation** of the first two lumbricals and the muscles of the thenar eminence, excluding the ulnar head of the flexor pollicis brevis. The **ulnar nerve** innervates the hypothenar muscles, the interosseous muscles, the ulnar head of the flexor pollicis brevis, and ulnar two lumbricals. The median nerve is tested by palmar abduction of the thumb and opposition. The ulnar innervated intrinsics are responsible for finger abduction and adduction, providing the physiologic basis for the classic test for ulnar nerve motor function, which is abduction and adduction of the long finger. The lumbrical muscles have their origins on the flexor tendons and insert on the extensor hood mechanism, providing additional balance and smooth motion of the digits. They too flex the MCP joint and extend the proximal interphalangeal joints.

ANSWER: B, D, E

3. True statements regarding the techniques of hand surgery include which of the following?

A. Epinephrine should never be used with local anesthesia.
B. Digital blocks are best placed using the ring technique.
C. When providing pain relief to allow assessment of passive digital movement, a radial, ulnar, or median wrist block is employed.
D. A rubber-band tourniquet at the base of the digit is a safe, effective means to provide a bloodless field.
E. Tourniquet ischemia is tolerated for 30 minutes in the unanesthetized arm and for 2 hours in the anesthetized arm.

Ref.: 1, 2, 3, 4

COMMENTS: Because of possible irreversible constriction and vascular complications, epinephrine should never be used in local anesthetics employed during hand surgery. The ring block raises venous pressure and may compromise digital vascularity. Digital blocks therefore are established by injecting the web space on both sides of the involved fingers and across dorsal surfaces. The nerves to the radial side of the index finger and the ulnar side of the little finger are located in the subcutaneous tissue on the volar surface of the corresponding metacarpal head. Wrist blocks anesthetize intrinsic muscles; therefore digital blocks should be used to provide pain relief during assessment of *passive* digital motion. (Active distal motion would be compromised by the anesthetic.) • Despite numerous studies, the absolute limits of tourniquet time have never been firmly established and tend to vary among individuals. The most widely accepted tourniquet time is 2 hours. Pressures should remain between 200 and 250 mm Hg but occasionally may have to be inflated to 350 mm Hg to obtain hemostasis. If reinflation is required, a "breather" period of at least 20 minutes is recommended. Tourniquets are applied as high on the arm as possible over adequate smooth padding, and care must be taken to prevent leakage of iodophor or other solutions underneath this cuff, as they may cause skin blistering and necrosis. Arm exsanguination is accomplished by distal-to-proximal wrapping with an elastic bandage before tourniquet pressure is applied. This method should not be used in the face of infection or if a malignant tumor is present in the extremity. Rubber-band tourniquets at the level of the finger should never be used; they apply high pressure over a narrow area and can cause irreversible neurovascular damage. Specially designed "safe" digital tourniquets are available and should be used instead (e.g., Tourni-cot).

ANSWER: A, E

4. True statements regarding the placement of hand incisions include which of the following?

   A. Palm incisions should parallel the skin creases or cross them obliquely.
   B. It is better to err on the volar aspect than the dorsal aspect when placing incisions on the side of the digit.
   C. Incisions on the volar side of the digit must cross the interphalangeal flexion creases transversely.
   D. Dorsal skin incisions should cross skin creases transversely or obliquely.

Ref.: 1, 2, 3

COMMENTS: There are several principles one must follow when planning hand incisions. Whenever possible these incisions should be designed along lines that undergo no change of length with motion. Those on the palm should run parallel to the skin creases or across them obliquely as the blood supply in this region comes straight up into the skin. Digital incisions should be placed dorsal to the midlateral line on the side of the digit through the midaxial line, which is exactly neutral between flexion and extension. This line is determined by connecting the most dorsal points of the interphalangeal joint creases when the finger is in a flexed position. Oblique incisions connecting these points (Bruner Volar zigzag incisions) are also an excellent approach, giving full exposure to the entire palmar side of the digit. The line marking the change in character between the dorsal and volar skin of the digit is also a useful landmark. Given a choice, it is far better to err when placing an incision dorsally rather than on the volar aspect of the side of the digit because the volar incisions may form a bridging scar. Skin incisions on the dorsum of the hand and digits should cross skin creases transversely, obliquely, or over the mid-dorsum when between joints. In the rheumatoid hand, incisions that cross the skin of the dorsal wrist should be longitudinal or minimally curved to avoid slough of a distal-based flap.

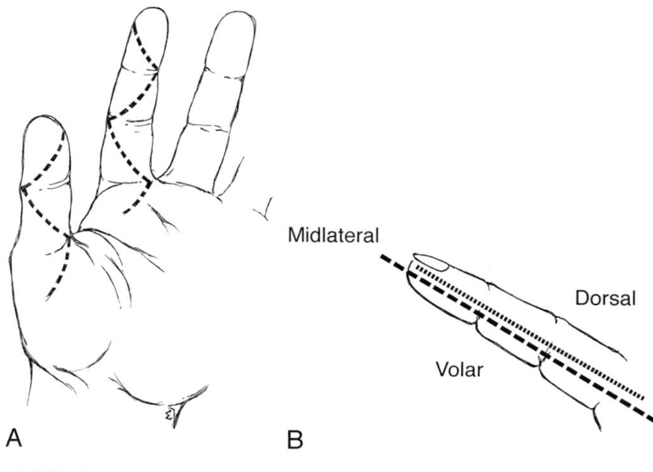

ANSWER: A, D

5. True statements regarding evaluation of the extrinsic flexors and extensors of the hand include which of the following?

   A. The flexor digitorum profundus flexes the proximal interphalangeal joint.
   B. The flexor digitorum profundus flexes the distal interphalangeal joint.
   C. The flexor digitorum superficialis inserts on the proximal end of the distal phalanx.
   D. The flexor pollicis longus flexes the metacarpophalangeal joint.
   E. There are two extensor tendons to the little finger.

Ref.: 1, 2, 3

COMMENTS: The extrinsic muscles of the hand originate in the forearm, and their tendons insert on the phalanges (flexor digitorum profundus, flexor digitorum superficialis, extensor digitorum communis) and thumb (flexor pollicis longus, abductor pollicis longus, extensor pollicis brevis). The flexor digitorum profundus inserts on the base of the distal phalanx and flexes the *distal* and *proximal* interphalangeal joints. The function of the flexor digitorum profundus to the index finger is isolated in 85% of patients. The tendons to the ulnar three digits often act as a single unit and should be tested both simultaneously and individually. Profundus function is evaluated by holding the proximal interphalangeal and metacarpophalangeal joints of the finger being examined in extension. The flexor digitorum superficialis inserts on the volar surface of the middle phalanx and flexes the proximal interphalangeal joint. It is evaluated by holding the adjacent fingers in extension and asking the patient to flex the proximal interphalangeal joint of the involved finger. When examining superficialis injuries to the little finger, simultaneous flexion of both the ring and little fingers at the proximal interphalangeal joint should be tested because their superficialis tendons may share a common muscle belly. The flexor pollicis longus is responsible for flexion of the distal phalanx of the thumb but also flexes the metacarpophalangeal joint. The main extensors of the metacarpophalangeal joints are the extensor digitorum communis passing to each of the four fingers. Additionally, there is the extensor digiti minimi to the little finger and the extensor indicis proprius to the index finger; these are independent extensors and must be taken into account when assessing the extent of injury. Transection of an extensor tendon results in extensor lag of that digit at the metacarpophalangeal joint. The frequent presence of double tendons to the index and little fingers may confuse the diagnosis. The extensor pollicis brevis extends the proximal phalanx of the thumb, and the abductor pollicis longus extends the first metacarpophalangeal joint. Damage to either of these tendons results in loss of their corresponding function.

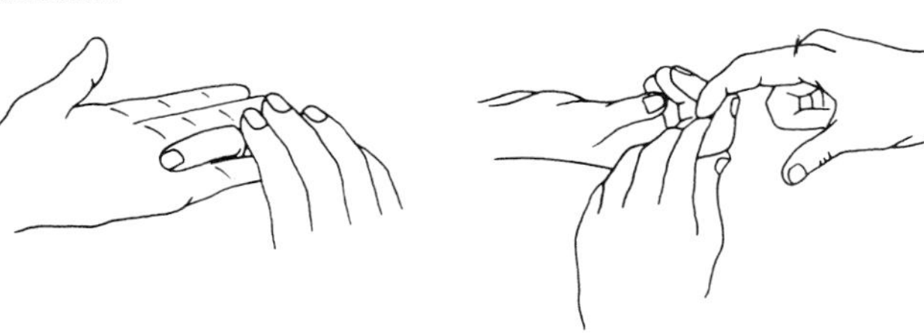

Superficialis testing Profundus testing

ANSWER: A, B, D, E

6. Match the muscle tendon unit in the left column with its appropriate innervation in the right column.

A. Flexor digitorum superficialis
B. Extensor digitorum communis, extensor indicis proprius, extensor digiti minimi, extensor pollicis brevis, abductor pollicis longus
C. Flexor digitorum profundus to index and middle fingers
D. Flexor digitorum profundus to ring and little fingers

a. Median nerve
b. Radial nerve
c. Ulnar nerve

Ref.: 1, 2, 3

COMMENTS: Innervation of the extrinsic muscles is derived from the radial, median, and ulnar nerves. Although variations may occur, the usual pattern of innervation to the extrinsic muscles of the hands are as follows: The innervation of the flexor digitorum superficialis is entirely median, and that of the extensor group is entirely radial. The ulnar nerve innervates the flexor digitorum profundus tendons to the fingers on the ulnar half of the hand, and the median nerve innervates the profundus tendons to the index and middle fingers. Injury to the forearm can potentially lead to abnormalities of digit and thumb flexion and extension due to nerve damage. Flexion and extension of the digits and thumb should always be evaluated in patients presenting with forearm injuries.

ANSWER: A-a; B-b; C-a; D-c

7. You are called to examine a 30-year-old painter who cut the palm of his right hand with a fresh razor blade. On examination you note a 2 cm clean laceration at the base of the long finger. Metacarpophalangeal joint flexion is intact, but he cannot flex either interphalangeal joint in that finger. The injury is 1 hour old. Your diagnosis is which of the following?

A. Lacerated flexor digitorum superficialis tendon.
B. Lacerated flexor digitorum profundus tendon.
C. Combined flexor digitorum superficialis and profundus laceration.
D. Laceration of the intrinsic muscles to the long finger.
E. Median nerve transection.

Ref.: 1, 2, 3

COMMENTS: See Question 8.

8. Your immediate treatment plan for the patient described in Question 7 should include which of the following?

A. Plans for immediate tendon repair (within 6 hours) to avoid the hazards of delayed tendon anastomosis.
B. Wrist block anesthesia, extension of the skin wound along proper incision lines, and exploration to confirm your diagnosis.
C. Careful cleansing and irrigation of the wound, placement of an appropriate dressing or simple sutures, and hand immobilization prior to definitive primary surgical repair some time within the first 2 weeks.
D. Cleansing the wound, primary skin closure, hand immobilization, and outpatient follow-up visits because this injury will require free-tendon graft reconstruction 6 weeks after injury.

Ref.: 1, 2, 3

COMMENTS: Flexion of the metacarpophalangeal joint is a function of the intrinsic muscles and can persist in the face of extrinsic flexor muscle and tendon injury. The goal of flexor tendon repair is restoration of interphalangeal joint flexion. Flexor tendon repair demands meticulous attention to detail and, whenever possible, should be performed by a hand surgeon. The character of the wound, the nature of the injury, the degree of contamination, and the time between injury and definitive treatment determine whether primary or delayed repair is performed. Proper wound cleansing, dressing, immobilization, and prophylactic antibiotics allow delay of primary repair if a hand surgeon is not immediately available. If there is a question about the degree of contamination or if the initial wound treatment has been delayed beyond several hours, making primary closure hazardous, delayed repair after 2–14 days may be performed. This allows the presence or absence of infection to be clearly established. Many experts believe this type of delay does not significantly alter the ultimate outcome of the repair. Tendon injuries with grossly contaminated wounds, those with significant tendon loss of wounds, or wounds with significant associated injuries to the soft tissue, bone, nerve, or blood vessels may be treated by secondary repair in 3–6 weeks, after the wounds have been stabilized, the infection cleared, and edema formation subsides.

ANSWER:
Question 7: C
Question 8: C

9. True statements regarding metacarpal fractures include which of the following?

A. They are commonly known as Bennett's fracture.
B. They are commonly known as the "boxer's fracture."
C. They most often involve the distal metacarpal of the little and ring fingers.
D. Physical examination is the most effective means of assessing the degree of angulation.

Ref.: 1, 2, 3

COMMENTS: Metacarpal fractures commonly result from hitting an object with a clenched fist. They usually involve the distal metacarpal of the fifth and fourth fingers and are known as "boxer's fractures." The metacarpal head is displaced palmward; pain, swelling, and some loss of knuckle prominence are the usual physical findings. Associated lacerations should be treated as human bites until proven otherwise. Swelling usually masks the degree of angulation, and a lateral radiograph is needed for accurate evaluation. Each finger should be individually flexed to the palm to assess the degree of rotational deformity. During flexion the fingers normally point to the scaphoid tubercle. Deviation from this alignment allows estimation of the rotational deformity. The usual treatment is closed reduction followed by immobilization of the involved and adjacent digits, placing the metacarpophalangeal joint in 65–90 degrees of flexion and the interphalangeal joints in full extension. Unstable or multiple metacarpal fractures often require open reduction and internal fixation. Metacarpal shaft fractures require reduction and immobilization; percutaneous k-wires or plate and screws for internal fixation often are required if the fracture is unstable.

ANSWER: B, C

10. True statements regarding injuries of the thumb include which of the following?

A. Bennett's fracture is an intraarticular avulsion fracture of the base of the metacarpal.
B. Abduction force applied to the thumb most often injures the interphalangeal joint.
C. The valgus stress test is used to diagnose disruption of the ulnar collateral ligament system at the first metacarpophalangeal (MCP) joint.
D. The term "gamekeeper's thumb" refers to injuries of the MCP joint of the thumb.
E. The valgus stress test should not be performed when a fracture is suspected or in children suspected of having epiphyseal injury.

Ref.: 1, 2, 3, 4

COMMENTS: **Bennett's fracture** is an intraarticular avulsion fracture at the base of the thumb metacarpal. The ligaments remain attached to the bone fragment, the abductor pollicis longus subluxes the metacarpal laterally, and the fracture is unstable. The usual treatment is traction reduction with percutaneous wire fixation of the metacarpal to the trapezium and adjacent carpus, although open reduction and internal fixation may be required. Abduction force applied to the thumb may result in disruption of the ulnar collateral ligament system at the first MCP joint. It commonly occurs when skiing, ball handling, or supporting a fall with the thumbs. It also may result from repetitive low-grade abduction force, as is encountered when using the thumb to dislocate rabbit's necks—hence the name "gamekeeper's thumb." The diagnosis is based on the finding of valgus instability of the MCP joint. An angle of more than 30 degrees of laxity is usually considered a complete rupture. When the diagnosis is made, open repair of the ligament is indicated because of the ulnar collateral ligament has retracted proximal to the adductor aponeurosis to the thumb. This interposed aponeurosis now prevents the ligament from healing back to its insertion, even with casting and immobilization.

ANSWER: A, C, D, E

11. True statements regarding phalangeal fractures include which of the following?

A. Volar angulation of proximal phalangeal fractures causes a flexion deformity of the proximal interphalangeal joint.
B. Collateral ligament tears of the interphalangeal joints require open repair.
C. Fractures of the base of the middle phalanx tend to have apical dorsal angulation.
D. Fractures of the neck of the middle phalanx tend to have apical volar angulation.
E. In the presence of distal phalangeal fracture, an associated subungual hematoma must not be opened to avoid osteomyelitis.

Ref.: 1, 2, 3

COMMENTS: Closed **distal phalangeal fractures** are often the result of crush injury and involve nail bed damage as well. If the nail bed and plate are intact, subungual hematomas are drained and the nailbed underneath is meticulously repaired after careful antiseptic preparation of the digit. Displaced fractures involving injury to the nail matrix require exploration to ensure that no matrix is interposed in the fracture, and repair of the nailbed tends to better reduce the fragments of bone. The most important aspect of open fractures of the distal phalanx is not the bone but the repair of skin and soft tissue damage. Failure to do so predisposes to chronic osteomyelitis. **Fractures of the middle phalanx** may or may not involve damage to the collateral ligaments at the interphalangeal joints. Tears of these ligaments with or without small chip fractures usually respond to closed realignment, splinting, and appropriate rehabilitative motion. Dorsal and volar dislocations at these joints require precise reduction, and open procedures with internal fixation are frequently necessary. Distal fractures of the middle phalanx usually have apex volar angulation because the proximal segment is flexed by the flexor digitorum superficialis. Fractures at the base of the middle phalanx usually have apical dorsal angulation because of distal segment flexion by the flexor digitorum superficialis and proximal segment extension by the central slip of the extensor mechanism. Most middle phalangeal fractures respond to closed reduction and external immobilization. **Proximal phalangeal fractures** have a relatively long fulcrum, and even minimal displacement or rotational abnormalities exhibit significant rotation and deviation of the digit distally. For that reason meticulous reduction is required, and postreduction examinations should be performed in extension and flexion checking digital orientation in both positions.

ANSWER: A, C, D

12. True statements regarding extensor tendon injuries include which of the following?

A. Extensor tendon lacerations have a good prognosis because of their subcutaneous location.
B. The extensor retinaculum must be closed over extensor tendon repairs to prevent bow-stringing.
C. Avulsion of the extensor tendon at the base of the distal phalanx results in the boutonnière deformity.
D. Disruption of the central extensor tendon at the base of the middle phalanx results in the mallet deformity.

Ref.: 1, 2, 3

COMMENTS: The extensor tendons occupy a subcutaneous position except at the wrist. The overlying skin is nearly as mobile as the excursion of the extensor tendons and, after repair, rarely restricts their function. An exception to this is at the wrist, where the extensor retinaculum overlies the tendons. Injuries at this level are repaired by transposition of the tendons into the subcutaneous tissue with closure of the retinaculum deep to the repair or complete its release if gliding is impeded. The **boutonnière deformity** results from disruption of the central extensor tendon near its insertion into the dorsum of the base of the middle phalanx. Eventually, the lateral bands are displaced toward the palm, lose their extensor function, and become proximal interphalangeal joint flexors. The patient is unable to initiate extension from the flexed position but sometimes can maintain extension if the digit is passively placed in that position. Without treatment the proximal interphalangeal (PIP) joint becomes fixed in flexion, and the distal interphalangeal (DIP) joint assumes a position of hyperextension. Immobilization of the PIP joint at 0 degrees of extension for 6–8 weeks achieves good results. Dynamic extension splinting is now recommended whenever possible. This involves keeping the PIP joint extended at 0 degrees and allowing DIP joint motion, with the theory that it allows tendon gliding and dynamically the lateral bands will "snap back" up into their proper position. Injuries to the extensor insertion into the dorsum of the distal phalanx results in the **mallet deformity**. Often no fracture can be seen. Even if it is associated with a fracture and the fragment is small, dorsal splinting with the joint in 0–10 degrees of hyperextension for 6–8 weeks provides good results. If more than one-third of the articular surface is displaced with the avulsed tendon, and volar subluxation of the distal phalanx occurs, open reduction and internal fixation are advised.

ANSWER: A

13. True statements regarding hand infections include which of the following?

A. The relatively avascular environment of the synovial sheaths makes them resistant to infection.
B. One-third of hand infections have a mixed flora.
C. Treatment of human bite wounds includes aggressive cleansing and antibiotic therapy before suturing.
D. Cellulitis of the hand must be drained before loculation occurs.
E. The organisms most commonly isolated from hand infections are penicillinase-producing staphylococci.

Ref.: 1, 2, 3, 4

COMMENTS: Hand infections are potentially serious because of the superficial location of the hand's bones and joints; the high density of relatively avascular tendons, fat, and synovium; and the ease of spread through the synovial sheaths due to constant flexion and extension. Staphylococci are present in nearly 80% of hand infections and are frequently penicillin-resistant. One-third of hand infections contain mixed flora and frequently include β-hemolytic streptococci, *Escherichia coli*, *Proteus*, and *Pseudomonas*. In human bites anaerobic organisms can also be present in a high percentage, with *Eikenella corrodens* also known to be a significant contributor. Drainage procedures are reserved to decompress loculations of pus; cellulitis without fluctuance is treated with immobilization, elevation, antibiotics, and frequent reexamination. The empiric use of antibiotics is indicated for severe infections, with appropriate changes in therapy being made when culture and sensitivity results are available. All complex infections should be drained in the operating room with proximal tourniquet control. Distal-to-proximal wrapping to obtain a bloodless field, as used during elective hand surgery, is contraindicated. Human bites should be vigorously cleansed, treated with antibiotics (including anaerobic coverage), and left open to close secondarily. Because of the superficial location of the tendons and metacarpophalangeal joints, human bites (usually from a punch) should be vigorously treated. The motion of the skin, tendon, and joints in different planes helps spread infection and cover drainage paths, trapping bacteria. Extension of the wound with formal joint exploration in an operating room is often required.

ANSWER: B, E

14. Which of the following statements is/are true?

A. Paronychia occurs in the digital pulp of the finger.
B. A felon is an infection around the margin of the nail bed.
C. Finger felon or paronychia has the potential to cause tenosynovitis.
D. The deep structures of the hand are protected from subcutaneous abscesses of the palm by the superficial palmar fascia.
E. The versatile "fish-mouth" incision is used for draining both pulp and paronychial infections.

Ref.: 1, 2, 4

COMMENTS: Subcutaneous abscesses of the volar surface of the hand often follow small puncture wounds or infection of superficial blisters. Pain and swelling are confined to the area of inflammation and are not increased with minor tendon motion. Loculations should be drained, as they have the potential of tracking to the dorsum of the hand. A **felon** is an infection of the pulp of the fingertip that can lead to deep ischemic necrosis, osteomyelitis, or both because of the presence of compartmentalizing septa that prevent expansion as pressure increases. Sharp pain and tenderness out of proportion to the amount of swelling are characteristic. The pulp space must be drained by dividing the septa before tissue necrosis occurs. The fish-mouth incision, once popularized, is now extremely discouraged. **Paronychial** infections are around the margins of the nail plate, often caused by hangnails, manicure trauma, or small foreign bodies. *Staphylococcus* is the usual offending organism. Early cases can be treated with warm soaks and antibiotics, but abscesses must be drained, often requiring resection of the overlying proximal nail plate. Unattended superficial infections may spread to deeper compartments such as the tendon sheaths. Likewise, deep compartment infections frequently spread to neighboring bursa and web spaces.

ANSWER: C

15. True statements regarding tenosynovitis include which of the following?

A. Infections of the flexor sheath of the little finger more often extend to the thumb than to the adjacent ring finger.
B. A flexor tendon sheath infection causes the involved finger to assume a position of mild extension at all joints.
C. The involved digit becomes uniformly swollen, and active or passive extension elicits pain.

D. By definition, deep palmar space infections involve the flexor tendons.

Ref.: 1, 2, 3, 4

COMMENTS: Infection of the synovial sheaths of the flexor tendons is a serious problem that requires prompt appropriate treatment. The tendons are relatively avascular and are characterized by poor natural resistance to infection. Although anatomy varies, the sheath of the little finger is often continuous with the ulnar bursa, which in turn is directly adjacent to the radial bursa, which extends to the flexor sheath of the thumb. Kanavel (from Cook County Hospital) described four classic findings of pyogenic tenosynovitis. The infected digit becomes uniformly swollen and assumes a position of mild flexion at all joints. Active or passive extension elicits local pain, and there is exquisite tenderness over the course of the sheath. Surgical drainage is mandatory and is accomplished by a longitudinal incision on the side of the digit along the axis of joint motion. The incision is placed on the ulnar side of the digit if palmar spread is suspected. Placement of irrigating catheters within the sheath and systemic antibiotics are important adjuncts to surgical therapy. The deep palmar space is located between the flexor tendons and the metacarpals in the palm. It is divided into the thenar space and midpalmar space at the level of the third metacarpal, where a vertical septum extends between the metacarpal and sheath of the long finger flexor tendons. Infections here present as localized, tender swellings and must be drained using an appropriate incision.

ANSWER: A, C

16. True statements regarding the forearm compartment syndrome include which of the following?

A. The classic four P's—pain, pallor, paralysis, pulselessness—accurately describe the syndrome.
B. The underlying cause is increased tissue pressure in the deep flexor compartment of the forearm.
C. The deep flexor compartment is fed only by the anterior interosseous artery, which becomes occluded as tissue pressure rises.
D. The median, radial, and ulnar nerves become strangulated by deep flexor compartment fibrosis.
E. The hand loses intrinsic muscle function and becomes numb in the median and ulnar distributions.

Ref.: 1, 2, 3, 4

COMMENTS: The elevation of tissue pressure in the deep flexor compartment of the forearm leads ultimately to occlusion of flow through the anterior interosseous artery. The result of this occlusion is dense, fibrotic degeneration of the muscular contents of the deep flexor compartment. Originally described by Volkmann as the result of tight bandaging at the elbow, it can be caused by a number of insults that have elevation of tissue pressure as their common denominator. The fibrosis that results causes a fixed flexion contracture of the wrist and fingers and a "strangulation neuropathy" of the median and ulnar nerves. The nerve involvement causes loss of intrinsic muscle function and numbness in the respective sensory distributions of the ulnar and median nerves. The radial artery does not pass through the deep flexor compartment and maintains its patency. The early clinical signs of increasing tissue pressure are tenderness over the forearm muscles, pain with passive finger extension, and paresthesias in the distribution of the median and ulnar nerves. Once the diagnosis is made, complete fasciotomy from elbow to wrist is indicated. Treatment of late cases involves major reconstructive surgery.

ANSWER: B, C, E

17. True statements regarding replantation of the hand include which of the following?

A. Single digits (other than the thumb) are uncommonly replanted except in children.
B. The amputated part may tolerate cool ischemia for up to 24 hours if there is no significant avascular muscle mass.
C. Bleeding from the proximal part is ideally treated with pressure rather than clamping.
D. A history of heavy smoking, diabetes mellitus, hypertension, and Raynaud's phenomenon are relative contraindications to replantation.
E. Replantation above the elbow is contraindicated.

Ref.: 1, 2, 3, 4

COMMENTS: Replantation is a highly specialized procedure best performed by a team of replantation surgeons. The procedure is long and requires that the patient be carefully evaluated for associated injuries before committing to a replantation attempt. Distal amputations properly cooled immediately after injury may be viable for up to 24 hours. The part should be wrapped in sterile saline-soaked dressings and placed in a plastic container (a sterile urine cup is one easily available), which is then submerged in ice water. The part should never be frozen, "salted," or come in contact with the surrounding liquid. Single digits are less frequently replanted except in children or if there is a sharp noncrushing cut at the level of the middle phalanx distal to the splitting of the superficialis tendon. The hand and thumb are always considered for replantation unless definite contraindications exist or the extremity was not properly preserved. Amputations above the elbow are considered for replantation (particularly in children), as even a partial success can convert an above-elbow to a below-elbow stump for future rehabilitation. Guillotine amputations are the injuries that present most favorably for replantation.

ANSWER: A, B, C, D

18. False statements regarding digit amputations include which of the following?

A. Any length of thumb that can be saved should be preserved.
B. The middle finger can assume the role of primary pinch if the index finger is lost.
C. Any length of index finger that can be saved should be preserved to maintain its pinching function.
D. Metacarpophalangeal joint amputations of the middle and ring fingers leave a space open in the clenched fist through which objects held in the palm may fall.
E. Traumatic loss of the thumb can be treated by digital transposition or by toe transfer.

Ref.: 1, 2, 3

COMMENTS: Planned or traumatic amputations within the hand must take into consideration a number of factors, including the patient's handedness, age, occupation, and concern for aesthetics. The thumb is the most important digit; as much of its length as possible should be preserved. The index finger amputated proximal to the proximal interphalangeal joint loses its ability to pinch, and the brain naturally switches the pinching to the long finger. All attempts to preserve length distal to the proximal interphalangeal joint should be made, but if the digit is painful or insensate, or "gets in the way," the patient may be best served by transection through the middle metacarpal (ray amputation), as the long finger can assume the role of primary pinch. Loss of little finger length proximal to the proximal interphalangeal joint may also be best treated by ray amputation. Central finger amputations (long and ring fingers) near the metacarpophalangeal joint can cause bothersome spaces in the clenched fist that can be treated by transfer of the adjacent peripheral finger with its metacarpal to fill the space. Using this basic principle, when multiple digits are amputated at once, combinations of digits "on-top plasties" should be considered.

ANSWER: C

19. True statements regarding carpal tunnel syndrome include which of the following?

A. The carpal tunnel syndrome is entrapment of the ulnar nerve in the carpal canal.
B. It is most commonly traumatic in origin.
C. The associated pain and numbness is often nocturnal, with referral of the pain to the shoulder and neck.
D. Injection of steroids into the carpal canal is contraindicated.
E. Electromyography and nerve conduction studies help confirm the diagnosis and exclude more proximal nerve entrapment.

Ref.: 1, 2, 3, 4

COMMENTS: Carpal tunnel syndrome is entrapment of the median nerve in the carpal canal with resultant nerve injury. Most commonly, it is idiopathic in origin, but it can be seen following Colles' and Smith's fractures or lunate and perilunate dislocations or it can be part of the presenting symptoms of rheumatoid arthritis, gout, diabetes mellitus, hypothyroidism, or amyloidosis. Carpal tunnel syndrome may be related to one's occupation, caused by repetitive strain, such as working on an assembly line or on a computer keyboard for prolonged periods. Proximal entrapment due to Pancoast tumors, brachial plexis abnormalities, cervical spine disease, and compression in the forearm (pronator teres syndrome) must be excluded as a diagnosis. Presenting symptoms include pain and numbness along the median nerve distribution, often nocturnal because of peripheral vasodilation that increases venous congestion and pressure on the nerve. Fetal sleeping habits with the wrists flexed, also can increase pressure inside the carpal canal at night. The pain may refer to the shoulder and neck, making the diagnosis more difficult. Physical findings include thenar atrophy, increased symptoms with forced wrist flexion (Phalen's test), and a positive Tinel's sign (tingling felt after percussion over the nerve at the wrist). Initial treatment consists of splinting, nonsteroidal antiinflammatory agents, and possibly a steroid injection into the carpal canal. Thenar atrophy, weakness, and failure to respond to conservative therapy are indications for surgery, which involves release of the portion of the flexor retinaculum that is entrapping the nerve. This release can be performed "open" or in some cases endoscopically with excellent success.

ANSWER: C, E

20. True statements regarding stenosing tenovaginitis include which of the following?

A. One form is also known as "trigger finger."
B. It is also known as the "swan-neck deformity."
C. It can cause locking of the digit in flexion or extension.
D. Surgical correction should be performed with wrist-block anesthesia.
E. When seen at the wrist level it is called Dupuytren's contracture.

Ref.: 1, 2, 3, 4

COMMENTS: Stenosing tenovaginitis of the fingers and thumb is a common cause of hand pain and loss of function. Limitation of free gliding of the tendon within its fibroosseous tunnel is due to a disproportion in size between the flexor tendons and the fibroosseous sheath. It is associated with a "popping or snapping" sensation that, in the extreme situation, can even cause locking of the digit in extension or flexion. Treatment is with nonsteroidal antiinflammatory agents and steroid injections. Failure to respond to medical treatment is an indication for surgical decompression with release of the A-1 pulley. Wrist-block anesthesia is used for operation so free active excursion of the tendon can be demonstrated following release of the constricting area. DeQuervain's syndrome is tenovaginitis of the first dorsal compartment leading to pain and tenderness on the radial dorsal aspect of the wrist. If conservative measures fail, release of this compartment surgically is recommended.

ANSWER: A, C, D

21. True statements regarding Dupuytren's contracture include which of the following?

A. Dupuytren's contracture involves the palmar aponeurosis.
B. Males are affected more often than females, and the contracture is primarily caused by excessive alcohol consumption.
C. It begins as a nodule formation, ultimately leading to contracture at the metacarpophalangeal and proximal interphalangeal joints.
D. Four clinical types have been described.
E. Aggressive nonsurgical treatment can influence the course of the disease.

Ref.: 1, 2, 3, 4

COMMENTS: Dupuytren's contracture occurs 10 times more frequently in males and primarily affects people of northern European origin. It appears to be transmitted as an autosomal gene influenced by multiple exogenous factors, such as injury, liver disease, alcoholism, pulmonary disease, seizure disorders, and chronic bowel disease. It begins as nodule formation within the palmar fascia in line with the pretendinous bands. Gradually, the skin becomes dimpled, and contractures form at the level of the metacarpophalangeal and proximal interphalangeal joints. Four clinical types—senile, middle-aged, young fulminant, and feminine—have been identified. There is no known effective medical therapy. Surgical options include open fasciotomy, radical excision of the palmar fascia, and partial palmar fasciectomy (which is most often performed). Postoperative splinting and hand therapy are critically important to the success of such therapy. Care must be taken to avoid injury to skin flaps and the digital nerves, which can be pushed to the surface and out of anatomic position, especially associated with spiral bands.

ANSWER: A, C, D

22. Which of the following statements is/are true concerning peripheral nerve injury?

A. Nerve repair is progressively less effective if performed 2 months after surgery.
B. Nerve repair is best performed using 4–15× magnification.
C. Nerve repair is best performed in a fashion that minimizes tension across the repair.
D. Regeneration may be followed clinically by observing the distal progression of Tinel's sign.

Ref.: 1, 2, 3

COMMENTS: Nerve injuries result from stretching or compression (neurapraxia) or transection. Neurapractic injuries carry a better prognosis than do transection injuries. Nerve injuries do not need to be repaired at the time of injury, but it is thought that the results are progressively worse if repair is delayed beyond 6 months when the distal nerve tubules have contracted and the new axons can no longer grow distally. Occasionally, repair delayed for up to 2 years is successful, especially in children. Although it is a matter of choice, most surgeons perform a careful epineural repair rather than repair the individual fascicular bundles. Recovery after repair begins with return of function starting proximally. Regenerating axons grow down the distal nerve sheath at an approximate rate of 1 mm per day. Distal progression of Tinel's sign (tingling felt after percussion over the growing nerve) usually follows the start of regeneration.

ANSWER: B, C, D

23. Regarding burns of the hands, which of the following statements is/are true?

A. Full-thickness dorsal burns cause scarring, which prevents flexion contractures.
B. Loss of the extensor tendons is often treated by joint fusion to prevent contractures due to unopposed flexion forces.
C. An important part of treatment includes splinting in the "safe" position.
D. Partial-thickness burns are best treated with whirlpool débridement and splinting.
E. Deep partial-thickness burns require meticulous application of topical antibiotics and débridement after "declaration" of full thickness losses over 2–3 weeks.

Ref.: 1, 2, 3

COMMENTS: Treatment of hand burns must begin as soon as possible. Although the injury to the hand may be complex, certain principles must be followed. Proper dressing should be applied and the hand splinted in a "safe" position whenever possible. Destruction of extensor tendons results in flexion contractures unless the tendons and skin are reconstructed or the joints are fused in the appropriate position. Superficial partial-thickness burns should be débrided of superficial necrotic tissue using whirlpool baths. Deep partial-thickness and full-thickness burns are best treated by early full-thickness or tangential excision and skin grafting. This allows early initiation of occupational hand therapy to prevent stiffness and contractures.

ANSWER: B, C, D

24. Match each item in the left column with the appropriate item in the right column.

A. Median nerve palsy	a. Claw deformity of ring and little fingers
B. Ulnar nerve palsy	b. Loss of wrist extension
C. Radial nerve palsy	c. Loss of thumb palmar abduction and opposition
	d. When injured in the forearm a ring finger superficialis transfer can be used to restore function

Ref.: 1, 2, 3

COMMENTS: **Median nerve** palsy at the wrist results in an inability to perform proper opposition or palmar abduction. Transfer of the flexor digitorum superficialis of the ring finger (median nerve innervation proximal to the wrist) to the insertion of the abductor pollicis brevis is frequently the treatment of choice (superficialis opponens plasty). Median nerve injuries at the elbow result in denervation of the flexor digitorum superficialis, and in this case transfer of the abductor digiti minimi (ulnar innervation) or extensor indicis proprius (radial innervation) is used. **Ulnar nerve** palsy at the wrist results in a claw deformity of the third and fourth fingers. It results from metacarpophalangeal joint hyperextension with secondary flexion of the interphalangeal and distal phalangeal joints. The flexor digitorum superficialis to the little finger can be moved to the base of the proximal phalanx of the ring and little fingers to restore metacarpophalangeal joint flexion. The profundus tendons to the small and ring finger are innervated by the ulnar nerve. **Radial nerve** disruption over the mid or distal humerus causes loss of wrist extension, metacarpophalangeal joint finger extension, and thumb abduction and extension. The common transfer used to repair this deformity is the pronator teres to the extensor carpi radialis brevis, the flexor carpi ulnaris (ulnar innervation) to the extensor digitorum communis, and the palmaris longus (median innervation) to the extensor pollicis longus.

ANSWER: A-c; B-a; C-b

25. Which of the following statements regarding syndactyly is/are true?

A. Syndactyly is often associated with polydactyly.
B. Release should be accomplished by the age of 1 year if digits of differing growth rates are involved.
C. It may be related to an autosomal dominant genetic pattern.
D. Males are more frequently affected than females.

Ref.: 1, 2, 3

COMMENTS: Syndactyly is a common congenital deformity that varies in severity from a thin skin web between normal digits to complete fusion of bony elements with a common nail. It may be inherited in an autosomal dominant pattern and is associated with several syndromes, including the Poland and Apert syndromes. Often both hands and feet are involved, and males are affected more frequently than females. The timing of operation is debatable. Syndactyly involving distal bony structures in digits of differing growth rates is often treated by surgical division of the distal syndactyly before 1 year of age. When there is no concern about the differential growth rate, surgery is delayed 2–3 years. Because of reports of recurrences when performed earlier, complete release of syndactyly before age 1 frequently results in an unacceptable degree of scarring. When more than two digits are involved, the releases are staged with 6 months between operations to avoid compromise of the middle digits' blood supply. Most frequently (unless the syndactyly is small) full-thickness skin grafts are harvested from the groin as needed to close a portion of the surgical defect. Geometric calculations reveal that separating two digits always requires addition of tissue.

ANSWER: B, C, D

26. Match the hand lesions in the left column with the descriptive common features in the right column.

A. Ganglion cyst
B. Giant cell tumor of tendon
C. Inclusion cyst
D. Lipoma
E. Glomus tumor

a. Arises from the short vinculum near the interphalangeal joints
b. When arising from the distal interphalangeal joint, it is called a mucous cyst
c. Fibrous capsule lined with squamous epithelium found on the flexor aspect of the palm and fingers
d. Most commonly found around the thenar eminence and possibly in the carpal canal
e. Painful tumor found underneath the nail

Ref.: 1, 2, 3, 4

COMMENTS: Ganglion cysts are often seen in any of four locations: the dorsum of the hand or wrist; the flexor side of the wrist adjacent to the radial artery; arising from the flexor sheaths (often at the base of the digit); or arising from the distal interphalangeal joints (where they are known as mucous cysts). **Giant cell tumors** of the tendons are benign and arise from the short vinculum near the interphalangeal joints or from the joint synovium itself. Both tendons in the flexor sheath are usually involved by the tumor, which lies deep to the neurovascular bundle. **Inclusion cysts** result from implantation of the epithelium with or without a foreign body and present as a cyst on the flexor aspect of the palm or finger. **Lipomas** often present over the thenar eminence but can even be found within the carpal canal and have been associated with carpal tunnel syndrome. The **glomus tumor** originates from the vasculomusculoneuroglomus of the nailbed that regulates blood flow. Growth of this tissue within the closed space of the fingertip may cause nerve pressure and exquisite pain. Magnetic resonance imaging (MRI) studies are highly successful for confirming the diagnosis, and surgical treatment involves removal of the nail plate with complete excision.

ANSWER: A-b; B-a; C-c; D-d; E-e

27. Match the common anatomic defect in the left column with the associated type of arthritis in the right column.

A. Metacarpophalangeal joint anterior subluxation-dislocation with extensor lag and ulnar drift
B. Can be diagnosed with a blood test
C. Related to repetitive strain at high stress joints
D. Interphalangeal joints of fingers and thumb and the metacarpophalangeal joint of the thumb often affected
E. Heberden's nodes
F. Bouchard's nodes

a. Rheumatoid arthritis
b. Osteoarthritis

Ref.: 1, 2, 3

COMMENTS: Rheumatoid arthritis is a systemic disease that can involve any or all of the tendon systems and joints of the hand. Often there is significant involvement at the wrist and in the metacarpophalangeal and interphalangeal areas. The management of rheumatoid arthritis is complex and involves the hand surgeon, rheumatologist, hand therapist, and social worker. **Osteoarthritis** commonly involves multiple hand joints and most frequently occurs in postmenopausal women. The joints most commonly involved are the interphalangeal joints of the fingers and thumb and the metacarpophalangeal joint of the thumb. Heberden's nodes are osteophytes at the distal interphalangeal joint; Bouchard's nodes are found at the proximal interphalangeal joint. Disabling involvement of the distal interphalangeal joint is often treated with arthrodesis. Severe involvement of the first metacarpophalangeal joint of the thumb often requires autologous or implant arthroplasty or fusion.

ANSWER: A-a; B-a; C-b; D-b; E-b; F-b

28. A 35-year-old mechanic presents 1 hour after a high-pressure oil solvent injection injury to his right index finger sustained while cleaning his spray apparatus. The finger is slightly swollen and erythematous. Sensation is intact. He is able to flex and extend all joints, though with mild discomfort. The most appropriate treatment at this point would be:

A. Ice and elevation; reexamination in the office in 24 hours.
B. Ice, elevation, and oral antibiotics; reexamination in 24 hours.
C. Elevation, intravenous antibiotics; hospital admission for close observation with frequent vital signs, sensibility, and circulation checks.
D. Urgent wide surgical drainage and débridement of the digit and palm to remove all tissue containing the solvent.

Ref.: 1, 2

COMMENTS: High-pressure solvent injection injuries often initially appear deceptively benign. Despite this appearance, urgent wide surgical opening of the digit and hand is required to prevent rapid progression of a severe inflammatory response, compartment syndrome, and digital loss. Similar problems can be seen with paint and grease injected under pressure. Extensive cases have been known to have fluid forced all the way up to the wrist. Ice, elevation, and antibiotics are all important aspects of management to reduce the inflammatory response and prevent digital compartment syndrome and infection; but they are not definitive treatment by themselves. The intense inflammatory response to the solvent will lead to digital compartment syndrome and tissue necrosis unless wide surgical opening of the digit and hand is performed urgently (even before the inflammatory response is obvious). As with tendon sheath infections, the solvent quickly tracks proximally along the flexor tendon sheath into the palm, and aggressive wide opening and débridement into the palm is required. Subcutaneous tissue containing the solvent should be débrided while preserving vital structures whenever possible. Repeated débridement is often required. Stiffness is a common long-term complication, if the digit can be salvaged.

ANSWER: D

29. You are called to the emergency room to evaluate a 42-year-old man who, after 14 hours in subfreezing temperatures, has frostbite of his left index, middle, and ring fingers down to the level of the proximal interphalangeal joint. You should:

A. Plan to amputate the involved areas within the next 6 hours.
B. Begin gradual rewarming of the involved area by immersion in a waterbath (35°–39°C).
C. Splint the hand and administer tetanus immunoglobulin, provide elevation, begin oral antibiotics, and discharge home for follow-up in 48 hours.
D. Begin rapid rewarming of the involved area by immersion in a waterbath at 40°–44°C.

Ref.: 4

COMMENTS: Tissue destruction secondary to frostbite is the result of direct cellular injury through the formation of extracellular ice crystals and through vascular impairment as the result of intense invasive constriction, shunting, stasis, and endothelial damage. The frozen extremity should be rewarmed rapidly in a warm bath carefully maintained at 40°–44°C until flushing of the digital pads is observed (usually about 30 minutes). Gradual warming allows continued tissue injury and is not indicated. Parenteral analgesics may be required during the rewarming period. Loose dressings and topical aloe vera or bacitracin should be applied to intact blebs and Silvadene dressings to the ruptured blebs and to exposed skin. It takes at least 2 weeks for demarcation to occur, so amputation should be delayed until after this acute period. Splinting and elevation do not address the issue of tissue damage. The intense care listed above requires hospitalization, especially for observation during the first 48 hours. The patient should not be discharged home until the wounds are under control, although the patient need not remain in the hospital until demarcation and surgery, if necessary. The tetanus immunization status must always be checked and supplemented as necessary for frostbite and burn injuries.

ANSWER: D

30. A 36-year-old man is involved in a common industrial mishap where he sustains a phenol burn. Which of the following antidotes can most effectively minimize skin destruction?

A. Alcohol.
B. Sodium bicarbonate.
C. Propylethylene glycol.
D. Calcium gluconate.
E. Balanced salt solution.

Ref.: 4, 5

COMMENTS: Propylethylene glycol applied directly to the burn areas is the treatment of choice. If it is not available, glycerol is the best second choice. Phenol burns not only affect the skin locally but, if absorbed systemically, can cause toxic affects. For this reason, using soap and water is not recommended as it would dilute the concentration in the phenol burns and prevent formation of a thick scar, which acts as a barrier preventing further absorption of phenol. Calcium gluconate is used for the immediate treatment of hydrofluoric acid exposure. These patients usually present several hours after exposure (most commonly when etching glass or cleaning aluminum) with pain about the nails and fingertips. Injection of a 10% solution of calcium gluconate is required without delay to prevent further symptoms and tissue destruction.

ANSWER: C

31. A 70-year-old mechanic sustains "pinching" amputation when his dominant long finger is caught between a garage door pulley and the belt. There is loss of the volar two-thirds of the pulp skin with exposed subcutaneous tissue. The most appropriate reconstruction would be:

A. Sterile dressing changes with topical antibiotics and closure by contracture and epithelialization.
B. Full-thickness hypothenar skin graft.
C. Split-thickness skin graft.
D. V-Y Advancement flap.
E. Replantation.

Ref.: 4

COMMENTS: Fingertip amputation is one of the most common hand injuries. The mechanism of injury, age, gender, general condition, and hand dominance of the patient, as well as the orientation and location of the amputation, are integral parts involved in the decision-making and planning of the reconstruction. Reconstructions that require prolonged immobilization in "unsafe" positions, such as a thenar flap or a cross-finger flap, are not recommended in older individuals. The amputated part, if properly cared for and free of crush avulsion injury, can be defatted, meticulously sutured back, and used for a salvage procedure. Microvascular replantations have been successful even as far distal as the midnail but generally are not performed for fingertip injuries except in certain countries where complete digits are of cultural significance. In this particular case, a hypothenar skin graft is best. It provides nonglaborous skin matching the other digits and resists contracture and hypersensitivity. Sensibility, which is an important factor with all of these grafts, is similar to those achieved with the flaps. The V-Y advancement flap would have been a good option, except that the orientation of this amputation does not lend itself to its use. It is best used with straight transverse amputations. A split-thickness skin graft would be too thin and presents with texture- and color-match problems, as well as difficulties with wound breakdown and hypersensibility. Allowing the wound to heal by contracture and epithelialization is a good option when there is only soft tissue loss; but, again, the orientation should be such that the tissues can contract to cover the defect. The broad surface area described here would not be satisfactory for this method of healing.

ANSWER: B

REFERENCES

1. Sabiston DC Jr: *Textbook of Surgery*, 15th ed. WB Saunders, Philadelphia, 1997.
2. Schwartz SI, Shires GT, Spencer FC: *Principles of Surgery*, 7th ed. McGraw-Hill, New York, 1999.
3. Crenshaw AH (ed): *Campbell's Operative Orthopaedics*, 8th ed, vol 1. Mosby-Year Book, St. Louis, 1992.
4. Green DP, Pederson WC: Green's *Operative Hand Surgery*, 5th ed. Churchill Livingstone, Philadelphia, 1998.
5. Bentivegna PE, Deane LM: Chemical burns of the upper extremity. *Hand Clin* 6:253–259, 1990.

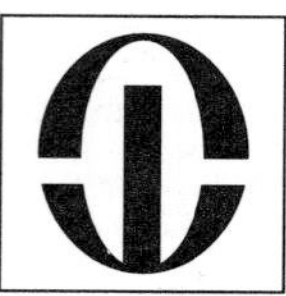

CHAPTER 49

Plastic and Reconstructive Surgery

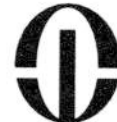

1. Regarding the skin, which of the following statements is/are true?

A. The skin is composed of dermis, epidermis, and an underlying subcutaneous padding; all structures involved are derived from mesoderm.
B. The dermis serves primarily to support the epidermis.
C. The amount of pigmentation of the skin is determined by the absolute number of melanocytes present.
D. Skin thickness varies widely according to anatomic location; this difference is due almost entirely to the varying thickness of the epidermis.

Ref.: 1, 2

COMMENTS: The **dermis** is entirely mesodermal in origin (except for its neural supply). The **epidermis** is composed of four cell types: the keratinocyte (the most common); the melanocyte; Merkel cells, which originate from neural crest cells (all of these are ectodermal in origin); and Langerhans cells, which are mesenchymal. Dermal collagen is 80% type I and 15% type III. The pigmentation of the skin is related to the size and activity of melanosomes, which are organelles synthesized and secreted by melanocytes and absorbed by adjacent keratinocytes. Sunlight and various hormones (melanocyte-stimulating hormone, adrenocorticotropic hormone, estrogen, progesterone) stimulate melanosome production. The thickness of the epidermis varies little; skin thickness variability is almost entirely due to differences in dermal thickness.

ANSWER: B

2. Which of the following statements regarding the orientation of skin incisions is/are correct?

A. Skin incisions should usually be oriented parallel to the long axis of the underlying muscle.
B. Lines of minimal tension parallel skin lines.
C. The long axis of underlying muscles is usually perpendicular to skin lines.
D. In some anatomic locations, the best incision is chosen independent of the orientation of the underlying muscle.

Ref.: 1, 2, 3, 4

COMMENTS: In most anatomic areas, skin lines represent lines of minimal tension (so-called Langer's lines). Incisions in these areas should be made parallel to these lines to result in the narrowest possible scar. These lines of minimal tension generally run perpendicular to the long axis of underlying muscles. In some circumstances, however, the choice of an incision is made independent of the underlying orientation. Examples are vertical incisions in the preauricular area and circumareolar incisions of the breast. Other examples are those incisions made at the rims or borders of the eyelids, lips, nose, and ears.

ANSWER: B, C, D

3. Regarding the blood supply of a skin graft, which of the following statements is/are true?

A. Initially, the graft survives by the active uptake of nutrients and serum by the endothelial cells of graft capillaries.
B. A skin graft does not become ischemic unless the graft bed is poorly vascularized.
C. The process of capillary ingrowth begins approximately 48 hours after grafting, with generalized blood flow established by the fifth or sixth postgraft day.
D. Capillary buds from recipient bed vessels have been shown to form anastomoses with graft vessels and to invade the graft directly.

Ref.: 1, 2, 3, 4

COMMENTS: A skin graft survives initially by plasmatic circulation, a passive imbibition of serum by the graft. This phase lasts 24–48 hours, depending on the degree of proliferation of the grafted wound. In a fresh wound, the serum imbibition phase of a skin graft lasts approximately 48 hours. During this phase the graft is ischemic and undergoes significant weight gain, as the plasmatic circulation is essentially from bed to graft only. At the end of 48 hours, capillary buds grow from the recipient bed, probably in response to a vasoactive agent released by the anaerobic metabolism of the graft. These buds grow across the fibrin meshwork between the graft and recipient bed. Evidence suggests that circulation is ultimately restored by a combination of actions. Anastomoses are formed between invading vessels and graft arteries and veins. Capillary ingrowth may occur directly into the graft, or neovascularization may occur along preexisting degenerated graft vessels. By the end of the first postgraft week, some of the final remodeling of the microvasculature has begun with differentiation into afferent and efferent vessels. It is at this point that true circulation is restored. Return of the venous circulation occurs later in the process, and its delayed return is one of the reasons for the required elevation of the extremity after grafting. This explains the initial pink appearance of the early graft, which changes to blue or purple because of venous insufficiency later.

ANSWER: C, D

4. Which of the following statements regarding the techniques of wound closure is/are correct?

A. Forceps with fine teeth are less traumatic to skin than forceps without teeth.
B. Questionably viable tissue at the wound margin should be preserved because it frequently regains vascularity within 2 days of the injury.
C. Sutures on the face should be kept in approximately 10–14 days to reduce tension on the wound during that time.
D. Even modest undermining of skin edges should be avoided, because it devascularizes the overlying skin and impedes wound healing.

Ref.: 1, 2, 4

COMMENTS: Successful closure of a surgically created or traumatic wound requires proper coaptation of well vascularized tissues without tension. Gentle handling of tissues is always recommended and is facilitated by the use of small "piercing" forceps rather than "crushing" forceps (i.e., those without teeth). Skin hooks may even be used to tug gently on the edges. Devitalized or questionably viable tissue should be removed prior to closure when the tissue is not deemed critical. Tension on a wound impedes healing and leads to widening of the scar. At times tension can be avoided by undermining the wound edges. A rich network of subdermal vessels provide adequate vascular supply to the skin edges, so long as the undermining has not been excessive. For best cosmetic results sutures are removed at variable times, depending on the vascularity and tension of the tissues coapted. On the abdomen sutures can be removed at 5–7 days, with the edges then reinforced with adhesive strips. On the face, sutures are removed sooner. The sutures themselves do not add to the cosmetic appearance but are a "necessary evil" to coapt the tissues properly. Early removal of sutures or staples with the addition of adhesive strips allows support of the wound without leading to the crosshatch marks created by permanent epithelialization of the sutures or staple holes themselves. Cyanoacrylates are now being used as "surgical glue" in an effort to reduce inflammation and provide adhesion at the coapted edges, thereby avoiding the use of sutures with their associated complications.

ANSWER: A

Ref.: 4

5. Which one or more of the following recipient beds is unlikely to support a split-thickness skin graft?

A. Muscle with its overlying fascia intact.
B. Muscle without overlying fascia.
C. Tendon with its paratenon intact.
D. Tendon without its paratenon.
E. Nerve with its perineurium intact.
F. Bone without its periosteum.

Ref.: 1, 2, 3, 4

COMMENTS: Proper "take" of a split-thickness skin graft applied to a recipient bed depends on adequate vascularization of the bed, avoidance of shear forces, avoidance of deadspace or tenting of the graft over the bed, and absence of infection within the wound (defined as more than 10^5 bacteria/gm of tissue). Muscle, with or without its fascia intact, is an excellent recipient site for split-thickness skin grafts. Although less well vascularized, tendon with its paratenon intact, nerve with its perineurium intact, and bone with its periosteum intact can also support a split-thickness skin graft.

ANSWER: D, F

6. Regarding the use of split-thickness and full-thickness skin grafts, which of the following statements is/are true?

A. A split-thickness skin graft undergoes approximately 10% shrinkage of its surface area immediately after harvesting.
B. A full-thickness skin graft undergoes approximately 40% shrinkage of its surface area immediately after harvesting.
C. Secondary contraction is more likely to occur after adequate healing of a full-thickness skin graft than a split-thickness skin graft.
D. Sensation does not return to areas that have undergone skin grafting.
E. Skin grafts may be exposed to moderate amounts of sunlight without changing pigmentation.

Ref.: 1, 2, 3, 4

COMMENTS: Skin grafts are considered to be *full-thickness* when they are harvested at the dermal–subcutaneous junction. *Split-thickness* skin grafts are those that contain epidermis and variable partial thicknesses of underlying dermis. They may be considered as thin, medium, or thick split-thickness skin grafts and usually are in the range of 0.018–0.060 inch in thickness. Cells from epidermal appendages deep to the plane of graft harvest resurface the donor site of a split-thickness skin graft in approximately 1–3 weeks depending on the depth. • When a skin graft is harvested, there is immediate shrinkage of the surface area of the graft. This process is known as primary contraction and is due to recoil of the elastic fibers of the dermis. The thicker the skin graft, the greater this immediate shrinkage, with full-thickness skin grafts shrinking approximately 40% of their initial surface area, and split-thickness skin grafts shrinking approximately 10% of their initial surface area. This must be considered when planning the amount of skin to harvest for coverage of a given size defect. • Contractile myofibroblasts in the bed of a granulating wound interact with collagen fibers to cause a decrease in the wound's surface area, a process known as *secondary contraction*. Secondary contraction is greater in wounds covered with split-thickness grafts than in those wounds covered with full-thickness grafts. The amount of secondary contracture is inversely proportional to the amount of dermis included in the graft, not the absolute thickness of the graft. Dermal elements hasten the displacement of myofibroblasts from the wound bed. • Sensation may return to areas that have been grafted so long as the bed is proper and not significantly scarred. Although not completely normal, it is usually adequate for protection. This process begins at about 10 weeks and is maximal at 2 years. • Skin grafts appear to be more sensitive to melanocyte stimulation during ultraviolet sunlight exposure than is the normal surrounding skin. Early exposure to sunlight after grafting may lead to permanently increased pigmentation of the graft and should be avoided. Dermabrasion or application of hydroquinones may be of benefit for reducing this pigmentation.

ANSWER: A, B

7. Situations in which a full-thickness skin graft is preferred to a split-thickness skin graft include which one or more of the following?

A. Contaminated wounds.
B. Small facial wounds.
C. Wounds in an irradiated field.
D. Burn wounds.
E. In hair-bearing regions.

Ref.: 2, 4

COMMENTS: Thicker grafts have a higher rate of failure in situations where a wound is more likely to be compromised by vascular insufficiency, hematoma, or infection. For this reason, thinner split-thickness skin grafts generally are preferred in instances where the recipient site for a graft is suboptimal. With extensive burn injury, multiple grafts are often required from limited donor sites; therefore the technique of harvesting thin split-thickness grafts—and earlier skin regrowth—may increase the availability of donor tissue. For wounds in which the most normal final appearance and less contraction is desired, as on the face or hands, full-thickness skin grafts are preferred. Full-thickness grafts are used when hair production is required. Accessory skin structures (i.e., hair follicles, sweat glands, sebaceous glands) transplanted with a graft survive but must be included in the graft; partial-thickness or full-thickness grafts are the only ones deep enough to include the pilosebaceous apparatus.

ANSWER: B , E

8. Match the type of flap in the left column with the appropriate nature of its blood supply in the right column.

A. Z-plasty
B. Forehead flap
C. Deltopectoral flap
D. Omental flap
E. Rhomboid flap

a. Random pattern
b. Axial pattern

Ref.: 1, 2, 3, 4

COMMENTS: See Question 9.

9. Match the type of flap in the left column with the appropriate description or example from the right column.

A. Transposition flap
B. Interpolation flap
C. Advancement flap
D. Island flap
E. Myocutaneous flap
F. Free flap

a. V-Y flap
b. Microvascular anastomosis required
c. Rotation about a point to an adjacent defect
d. Rotation about a point to nearby but not adjacent defect
e. Attached pedicle of vessels
f. Transverse rectus abdominis myocutaneous (TRAM) flap

Ref.: 1, 2, 3, 4

COMMENTS: Flaps are defined according to the nature of their blood supply. A **random flap** derives its blood supply from the dermal-subdermal plexus, in contrast to an **axial flap**, which derives its blood supply by a direct, usually named, cutaneous artery. **Random flaps** usually are those used to reorient a wound in a different direction or to close small defects. Examples are a Z-plasty, a simple rotation flap, an advancement flap, and a transposition flap. A *simple rotation flap* usually is semicircular and is "slid" over the recipient site for closure. An *advancement flap* is moved directly forward to cover a defect without rotation around a pivot point. A *V-Y flap*, a commonly employed *advancement flap*, frequently is used to close small defects in the finger or eyelid areas. *Transposition* flaps are those that involve rotation around a pivot point to a defect that is adjacent to the donor site. A rhomboid *flap* is a type of transposition flap in which a rhomboid-shaped flap is transposed to cover an adjacent defect with primary closure of the donor site. An *interpolation flap* is another type of transposition flap that involves rotation around a pivot point but is used to cover a defect that is nearby but not directly adjacent to the donor site. **Axial flaps** generally are used to cover larger defects more distant from the donor site. Although historically the primary determinant for the design of skin flaps has been the length/width ratio, axial flaps can be designed with a much greater length/width ratio than random flaps, demonstrating that the length to which a flap survives is determined principally by its blood supply, not its width. Examples are the midline forehead flap (supratrochlear artery), deltopectoral flap (perforating branches of the internal mammary artery), or omental flap (gastroepiploic arteries). An *island flap* is a type of axial flap in which a segment of tissue is carried on a vascular pedicle that has been skeletonized and is without overlying skin at the base to allow greater flap mobility. A myocutaneous flap provides blood supply through the overlying skin or subcutaneous tissue (or both) via muscular perforators. Examples are the perforators emanating from the rectus muscles about the umbilical region supplying the **TRAM** flap or the latissimus dorsi myocutaneous flap. **Free flaps** involve complete severing of the nutrient vessels with reanastomosis to vessels in the vicinity of the recipient site. This nearly always requires microvascular surgical technique.

ANSWER:
Question 8: A-a; B-b; C-b; D-b; E-a
Question 9: A-c; B-d; C-a; D-e; E-f; F-b

10. Necrosis of a pedicle flap is usually due to which of the following?

A. Arterial thrombosis.
B. Venous thrombosis.
C. Arterial spasm.
D. Venous spasm.
E. Trauma from manipulation of a compromised flap.

Ref.: 2

COMMENTS: All flaps must be observed closely during the immediate postoperative period following transfer because of possible compromise of their circulation. An initial dusky coloration may be due to venous spasm or excess tension on the flap, each resulting in compromised venous return. Development of a sharp line of color demarcation portends venous thrombosis, which is the most common cause of flap necrosis. Arterial insufficiency is not usually responsible for flap failure. Complications such as excessive tension, infection, or hematoma can eventually lead to venous thrombosis. Treatment of a seriously compromised flap requires immediate attention and may involve taking down a dressing; removing tight sutures; changing the position of an extremity or head and neck; returning a flap to its donor site; using heparin, aspirin, or low-molecular-weight dextran; and (experimentally) using hyperbaric oxygen. The patient must also be examined for systemic causes such as hypovolemia, hypotension, or hypoxia.

ANSWER: B

11. Regarding myocutaneous flaps, which one or more of the following statements is/are true?

A. A myocutaneous flap is a free graft of full-thickness skin with a small shaving of underlying muscle.
B. A myocutaneous flap is predicated on the skin receiving its blood supply by perforating vessels from the underlying musculature.
C. A myocutaneous flap fails if it is transferred to a poorly vascularized wound.
D. Only myocutaneous flaps supplied by arteries larger than 0.8 mm in diameter can be transferred as free flaps.
E. Rib, with its overlying pectoralis muscle and skin used for mandibular reconstruction, is an example of an osseomyocutaneous flap.

Ref.: 2, 4

COMMENTS: The development of myocutaneous flaps for reconstruction of soft tissue defects is based on the fact that skin frequently receives blood supply from vessels perforating the underlying somatic musculature. When the blood supply to the underlying muscle is by way of a discrete vessel, the muscle and its overlying skin may be transferred to a distant site on a pedicle containing only the nutrient vessels. It is critical that both the artery and vein within the pedicle remain patent for successful transfer of the flap. In some circumstances, bone closely associated with the muscle and skin may be transferred en bloc, providing an osseomyocutaneous flap (e.g., rib and its overlying pectoralis muscle and skin used for mandible reconstruction or latissimus dorsi muscle with a portion of scapula). Transfer of these flaps to distant sites requires the use of microvascular surgery. The vessels that supply the flap are isolated, transected, and anastomosed to vessels near the recipient site; refinements in technique and in instrumentation allow the routine transfer of flaps on vessels as small as 0.5 mm. Myocutaneous flaps are widely used in head and neck, breast, upper and lower extremities, and other areas of reconstructive surgery where well vascularized soft tissue covering of bone, tendon, nerve, or vascular structures is required. Myocutaneous or muscle flaps can be used to introduce additional blood supply to an area of impaired vascularity. Clinical examples include transfer of a latissimus dorsi myocutaneous flap to the anterior chest wall to correct an area of necrosis after radiation therapy and the transfer of vascularized muscle to the lower extremity after débridement of chronic osteomyelitis. In both of these examples, tissue with an excellent blood supply is imported to bring about the healing of a wound or infection not responding to more conservative measures.

ANSWER: B, E

12. Which of the following statements is/are true?

A. Reduction mammoplasty only rarely relieves the back pain that accompanies macromastia.
B. Gynecomastia in the adolescent should be treated surgically if the condition does not resolve in 6 months.
C. Hypomastia is best corrected by injection of liquid silicone into the breast.
D. Ptosis of the breast is said to exist when the nipple lies below the level of the inframammary fold.

Ref.: 1, 2, 3

COMMENTS: **Macromastia** is an abnormal enlargement of the breast, which may be a result of hormonal imbalance or obesity or may be idiopathic. For some women the breasts become so large they cause chronic back, shoulder, or neck pain. Women may also develop numbness of the ulnar side of the hand due to nerve compression about the chest and shoulder region, as well as skin changes of the shoulders from pressure of brassiere straps and inframammary areas of skin maceration or infection from constant moisture. These conditions usually are markedly improved by reduction mammoplasty, which involves resecting portions of the breast parenchyma and overlying skin and repositioning the nipple and areola. Extremely large breasts may require partial mastectomy with recontouring of the breast and free nipple grafting. **Gynecomastia** is enlargement of the male breast due to an increase in glandular tissue. In the adolescent it is frequently a physiologic response to the hormonal changes of puberty; it may be unilateral or bilateral, and it usually reverses itself. For this reason, surgery should be postponed until gynecomastia has been present for 2 years. In the adult, gynecomastia may result from underlying liver disease; pituitary, testicular, or adrenal tumors; or the use of certain drugs (e.g., digitalis, estrogens, some antihypertensives, and even marijuana). It must be differentiated from male breast carcinoma, especially when it is unilateral in presentation and presents with pain, drainage, or rapid enlargement. Resection of the breast tissue confirms the diagnosis and corrects the cosmetic abnormality. **Hypomastia** refers to insufficient volume of breast tissue and may be corrected, for cosmetic reasons, with the placement of a silicone prosthesis completely below the breast tissue or pectoralis muscle. Direct injection of silicone, fat, or any other substance into the breast tissue, specifically, is not an appropriate method to correct hypomastia. **Ptosis** of the breast exists when the nipple is present at a level below that of the inframammary crease. This may occur in breasts of any size and may lead to chronic skin changes in the inframammary crease. Reduction of the skin envelope (mastopexy) can alleviate the ptosis. This is a common procedure also seen in breast reconstruction after mastectomy to obtain symmetry.

ANSWER: D

13. Select the true statement(s) regarding techniques of breast reconstruction.

A. When a silicone implant is used for a single-stage breast reconstruction, frequent problems include an inadequate skin envelope leading to excess tension with possible skin necrosis or wound dehiscence.
B. Breast reconstruction with a tissue expander involves placement of the expander in a submuscular pocket, closure of the wound, and immediate introduction of sufficient saline solution to match the size of the opposite breast.

C. When the latissimus dorsi myocutaneous flap is used for breast reconstruction, a silicone implant is usually placed underneath the flap.
D. The trapezius myocutaneous flap may be used to reconstruct a breast even if the vascular pedicle to the latissimus dorsi muscle has been interrupted.
E. The transverse rectus abdominis myocutaneous (TRAM) flap survives on vessels that run longitudinally in a plane superficial to the anterior rectus sheath.

Ref.: 1, 2, 3, 4

COMMENTS: Breast reconstruction following mastectomy is an important aspect of breast cancer therapy for obvious cosmetic and psychological reasons. There are two main avenues available for breast reconstruction: (1) the use of tissue expanders and silicone implants and (2) transfer of vascularized tissue by means of a myocutaneous flap. **Tissue expander** breast reconstruction has several advantages: the avoidance of scars other than the mastectomy incision, creation of natural native breast skin that has the best textural and color match, less operative morbidity, and a shorter operative time. The simplest method of breast reconstruction is placement of a **silicone implant** in a submuscular pocket. This method has three potential disadvantages: (1) inability to reach a symmetric volume, (2) poor projection due to an inadequate skin envelope, and (3) the lack of a naturally ptotic breast shape with a well defined inframammary fold. The surgeon may avoid these disadvantages by placing a **tissue expander** (*not* a simple silicone implant) in a subpectoral, subserratus pocket. Saline solution is added to the expander intermittently over a several-month period. It leads to stretching of the overlying muscle and skin and the creation of some additional skin as well due to increased mitosis at the epidermal level. At a second-stage operation, the surgeon replaces the expander with a permanent implant. An alternative is the use of a single-stage expander, which has a removable valve. **Myocutaneous flap** reconstruction is particularly well suited to patients who have an *inadequate amount* of local skin remaining after the mastectomy, a poor quality skin envelope, skin that has been damaged from previous radiation therapy, or loss of the pectoralis major muscle, such as with the defect following radical mastectomy. The **latissimus dorsi** myocutaneous flap pedicled on the thoracodorsal vessels can transfer sufficient skin to the chest wall and is particularly useful to replace the pectoralis major muscle in a radical mastectomy defect. The flap depends on an intact thoracodorsal vascular pedicle. Usually an implant must be placed underneath this flap to achieve adequate volume and projection of the breast mound. The **TRAM** flap obtains its blood supply from the superior epigastric vessels that run *within* the rectus abdominis sheath, with perforating branches supply the overlying skin and fat of the abdominal wall. When there is sufficient volume of skin and fat such that a natural breast mound can be created without the need for an implant. The TRAM flap or a free gluteal flap with their own fatty tissue and skin offer one of the best methods for matching the shape of a broadly based ptotic breast. The short pedicle and improper arc of rotation of the **trapezius** myocutaneous flap precludes its use for breast reconstruction.

ANSWER: A, C

14. Regarding postmastectomy breast reconstruction, which of the following statements is/are true?

A. The presence of positive axillary nodes is a contraindication to reconstruction.
B. Delayed reconstruction (i.e., 3 months or longer after mastectomy) is generally preferred over immediate reconstruction.
C. The status of the skin flaps (vascular supply and degree of tension) is the key consideration when deciding on immediate versus delayed reconstruction.
D. Nipple reconstruction is usually delayed for several months following reconstruction of the breast mound.
E. In most cases, excellent symmetry can be achieved without the need for surgery on the uninvolved breast.

Ref.: 1, 2, 3

COMMENTS: The presence of positive axillary lymph nodes, anticipated adjuvant chemotherapy, and postoperative chest wall irradiation are not in and of themselves absolute contraindications to reconstruction. However, one must weigh the possible increased risk of infection (related to chemotherapy-induced leukopenia) and the possibility of a suboptimal cosmetic result from postreconstruction irradiation against the psychological advantage to the patient of the reconstruction itself. Postmastectomy reconstruction may be carried out immediately or in a delayed fashion (at least 3 months after mastectomy), depending on the desires of the patient, the anticipated need for adjuvant treatment, and most importantly the status of the skin flaps in terms of vascular supply and degree of tension on closure. Excess tension or poor vascular supply to the mastectomy flaps necessitates delayed reconstruction. There does not appear to be any significant difference in the final cosmetic outcome comparing immediate with delayed reconstruction. In either case, **nipple reconstruction** is usually deferred for several months following completion of the breast mound reconstruction to allow the breast to settle into its final position. The prominent papule of the nipple can be created from a flap of skin and subcutaneous tissue on the breast mound. A skin graft can then be used for the surrounding areolar part of the nipple, or it can be done after the flap has healed. Some advocate that the nipple and areola be tattooed to the appropriate color. This approach avoids the need to harvest skin from remote sites and minimizes patient discomfort. The ultimate goal of breast reconstruction is to achieve **symmetry** of the two breasts. In many patients this necessitates a reduction mammoplasty, mastopexy, or submuscular augmentation on the uninvolved side.

ANSWER: C, D

15. Select the true statement(s):

A. Women with breast augmentation implants have a significantly increased risk of developing breast carcinoma than do those with nonaugmented breasts.
B. When breast cancer is diagnosed in a patient with silicone breast augmentation implants, it is more likely to be at an advanced stage than when diagnosed in nonaugmented breasts.
C. Patients with silicone breast implants require a modification of conventional mammographic techniques to obtain optimal visualization of the breast parenchyma.
D. Silicone deposits have been noted in the lymph nodes of patients with silicone breast augmentation implants but not in the lymph nodes of patients with other implanted silicone medical devices.

E. Epidemiologic studies have clearly demonstrated a cause-and-effect relation between breast implants and the development of collagen vascular diseases.

Ref.: 5

COMMENTS: Recent media coverage of the possible hazards of breast implants has produced a great deal of confusion among patients with these medical devices. It is important to base recommendations to patients on scientifically valid data. Well designed studies have demonstrated that patients with breast implants *do not have* an increased risk of developing breast carcinoma. In addition, when breast carcinoma develops in a patient with breast implants, it is not at a more advanced stage than when it develops in a patient without breast implants. It is important to be aware of the need to modify conventional mammographic techniques when performing imaging studies on patients with breast implants. The Eklund modification involves compression of the implant and displacement of the breast parenchyma away from the implant with a modification of the conventional mammographic views. If this modified technique is not employed, significant portions of the breast parenchyma are obscured by the radiopaque silicone. Although occasional reports have surfaced documenting the presence of minute deposits of silicone in the lymph nodes of patients with breast implants, such deposits have also been found in the lymph nodes of patients with other implanted silicone medical devices (joint implants) as well. The significance of this finding is unclear and its association with other disease states unproved. At present, there is no clear-cut documentation of an increased incidence of collagen vascular disease in patients with silicone breast implants, nor is there any proven cause-effect relation between the two.

ANSWER: C

Ref.: 5, 6

16. Regarding pressure sores, which of the following statements is/are true?

A. Preservation of the underlying bony prominence is key to the successful management of pressure sores.
B. After débridement of devitalized tissues, closure of the defect is usually satisfactorily achieved with local skin flaps.
C. Superficial ulcers often heal spontaneously after débridement if subsequent pressure can be avoided.
D. An ischial sore is the most common decubitus ulcer.
E. Pressure of 40–80 mm Hg applied to tissue continuously for 8 hours may result in irreversible microvascular changes and an ischemic ulcer.

Ref.: 1, 4

COMMENTS: Continuous pressure on tissues, if severe enough for a long enough time, results in venous, then capillary, and then arterial compression with subsequent ischemic necrosis of the tissue, leading to a pressure ulcer. A pressure of 40–80 mm Hg applied continuously to tissue over 4 hours results in temporary microvascular changes and edema. If it continues for an 8-hour period, it may lead to permanent microvascular changes and the development of a pressure ulcer. It is a misnomer to describe any ulcer as a decubitus ulcer unless the clinician is sure that it resulted from pressure while the patient was in the decubitus or recumbent position. The astute clinician would best describe any of these pressure-induced injuries as pressure sores or ulcers, thereby matching their clinical appearance with the underlying pathophysiology described above. Superficial ulcers usually heal spontaneously if devitalized tissue is débrided and subsequent pressure is avoided. Deeper ulcers, especially those involving exposed bone in the base of the ulcer, also require débridement, followed by the transfer of well vascularized tissues into the defect. Reduction of the underlying bony prominence is critical to prevent recurrence of the pressure sore. Local skin flaps often fail because of tension and poor vascularity. The most successful closure of deep pressure ulcers involves the placement of myocutaneous flaps into the defect. Partial epithelialization of a long-standing ulcer impedes subsequent healing, and débridement of the ulcer must be carried back to nonepithelialized tissue for a graft to be successfully placed.

ANSWER: C, E

17. Which of the following statements regarding maxillomandibular disproportion is/are true?

A. Retrognathia is defined as an abnormally small mandible positioned abnormally posteriorly.
B. Prognathism is not satisfactorily correctable without the use of synthetic prostheses.
C. Most operative corrections of developmental mandibular problems with wire fixation allow normal use of the mandible within 3 weeks of the surgery.
D. Hypoplasia is the most common developmental deformity of the maxilla.
E. Maxillary osteotomies are used for correction of both hypoplasia and hyperplasia of the maxilla.

Ref.: 1, 2, 3

COMMENTS: Developmental mandibular deformities may result from the mandible being malpositioned or abnormally large or small. With **retrognathia** the mandible is of normal size but is malpositioned posteriorly. Correction involves osteotomies through the mandibular rami. With **micrognathia** the mandible is properly positioned but is abnormally small in its anterior portion; it can be corrected by a horizontal osteotomy, which brings the chin prominence forward. With **prognathism** the mandible is overdeveloped and prominent. Surgical treatment involves osteotomy with posterior repositioning. For all of these surgical corrections, if the bone segments are held in position by wires, intermaxillary fixation of the mandible is required for 10–12 weeks for proper healing of the osteotomies. An increasing number of surgeons make use of rigid fixation techniques involving plates and screws. With rigid immobilization of the fragments, the time in intermaxillary fixation is reduced or even eliminated. Of the maxillary anomalies, **hypoplasia** is the most common and is often seen in association with cleft palate. It may be treated by a maxillary osteotomy with repositioning of the isolated lower maxillary segment. Maxillary **hyperplasia** is evidenced clinically by a long face with exposure of the gingiva when smiling. This may be corrected with maxillary osteotomy and a resection of a vertical segment of maxilla with an upward repositioning of the lower segment of the maxilla.

ANSWER: D, E

18. Match each vascular abnormality in the left column with one or more appropriate descriptive statements in the right column.

A. Capillary hemangioma (port-wine stain)	a. Flat, dark red; does not involute; treated best with tunable dye laser
B. Immature hemangioma (strawberry mark)	b. Associated with gigantism of the affected part
C. Cavernous hemangioma	c. May enlarge during periods of infection; no documented cases of carcinoma developing
D. Cystic hygroma	d. Most spontaneously involute
	e. Microembolization may be required

Ref.: 1, 2, 3, 4

COMMENTS: The surgeon must be aware of the differential characteristics of the above-listed vascular lesions insofar as their natural history, size, and location may affect the appropriateness and difficulty of surgical intervention. The **capillary hemangioma** (port-wine stain) is a form of vascular malformation and presents as a flat, uniformly dark red cutaneous lesion that is present at birth and does not involute. The tunable dye laser, which can select the appropriate wavelength for destroying the lesion, has markedly improved treatment of this lesion. **Immature hemangioma** (strawberry mark) is a form of capillary hemangioma and is raised and brighter red in color than a port-wine stain. Usually, it is not present at birth but may become apparent within several weeks and then grow rapidly during the early months of life. Observation is appropriate, as most of these lesions involute spontaneously by age 7 years. Often anxious parents wishing for prompt erasure of such a blemish need repeated reassurance. Corticosteroids, radiation therapy, and even emergency surgery may be required for large lesions obstructing the rapidly maturing eye, airways, or small lumens. These cases must be treated immediately as must the lesions that bleed or are large enough to consume platelets leading to coagulopathy (Kasabach-Merritt syndrome). The **cavernous hemangioma** (venous malformation, in recent terminology) is situated in deeper subcutaneous tissues and appears as a swollen blue mass; it may be associated with gigantism of the involved part of the body. It is present at birth and seldom involutes. Excision may be hazardous because of the risk of hemorrhage and should be reserved for patients with significant associated functional or cosmetic disability. In certain situations microembolization treatment may be required to thrombose vessels and reduce lesion size. The **cystic hygroma** is a lymphatic malformation that most often presents in the head and lateral neck region. These lesions may enlarge and become tender during periods of upper respiratory infection. Some cystic hygromas involute but not if there is a venous component to the lesion. Complete excision of both venous and lymphatic malformations is frequently impossible because of the diffuse insinuation of these lesions into local tissues without regard to tissue planes.

ANSWER: A-a; B-d; C-b,e; D-c

19. Regarding the embryology and anatomy of the craniofacial region, which of the following statements is/are true?

A. The first embryonic structures that form the face are not evident until late during the first trimester (week 10).
B. The maxillary and mandibular processes differentiate from the first branchial arch.
C. The external ear develops from a single mesenchymal projection, the absence of which causes microtia.
D. Ossification of the craniofacial skeleton occurs by endochondral and intramembranous bone formation.
E. Normal development of the soft tissues of the face depends on normal bone growth, an independent process inherent in the bone itself.

Ref.: 2

COMMENTS: By the *fourth week* of embryonic life, primitive facial structures are evident. Migration of *mesenchyme* forms the frontonasal prominence, the nasal, otic, and optic placodes, and the maxillary and mandibular processes. By the eighth week, rapid morphologic change creates a nearly completely developed face. The external ear develops from six small hillocks surrounding the first and second branchial arches. Bony development is thought to occur in response to soft tissue forces. A distinction of the craniofacial skeleton is that ossification occurs by two separate processes: **endochondral** (replacement of preformed cartilage by bone) at the cranial base and **intramembranous** (mesenchymal differentiation to osteoblasts, which lay down bone without a cartilaginous framework) throughout the rest of the craniofacial skeleton. This has clinical significance with regard to craniofacial bone grafting and the improved results seen with bone grafts using a cranial donor site.

ANSWER: B, D

20. Regarding reconstruction of nose and lip defects, which of the following statements is/are correct?

A. A composite graft of cartilage and skin from the ear should not be employed for reconstruction of the nasal alar rim because of the high risk of graft necrosis.
B. A full-thickness skin graft is an appropriate form of reconstruction for soft tissue loss at the tip of the nose.
C. A forehead rotation flap is useful for reconstruction of major nasal defects.
D. The Abbe flap involves the transfer of lower lip tissue around to the upper lip and commissure.

Ref.: 1

COMMENTS: Nose: Reconstruction of *minor* soft-tissue defects of the nose (e.g., following excision of a superficial basal cell carcinoma) may be achieved by a full-thickness skin graft or rotation of a flap from tissue adjacent to the defect. When there is loss of cartilage, as may occur at the nasal ala, a composite graft of skin and cartilage taken from the ear results in an excellent reconstruction when the defect is less than 1 cm. This helical rim tissue is similar to the alar rim and can be found nowhere else in the body. *Major* nasal losses require a bone graft or cartilage grafts for the framework and provision of internal and external soft-tissue lining. *Total* nasal reconstruction is accomplished by anterior mobilization of the septal cartilage to provide midline support and reconstruction of lateral support with cartilage grafts. Lining is provided from adjacent mucosa; skin coverage is provided with a two-staged midline forehead flap based on the supratrochlear vessels. **Lip:** Defects of the lip usually can be closed primarily unless they involve more than one-third the length of the upper lip or are in close approximation to the commissure. The most important aspect cosmetically of primary closure of a lip defect is *proper apposition* of the vermilion border and multilayered closure. Even a slight "step-off" of vermilion apposition is noticeable. *Large* lip defects or those near the commissure require rotation flaps from the opposite lip (Estlander) or cheeks and advancement of buccal mucosa. The Abbe, or lip-switch, flap uses a full-thickness wedge of up to one-third of either the upper or lower lip. Based on the marginal artery, this flap is rotated to cover the defect, with the pedicle divided 10 days later. This technique is best for reconstruction of the central philtral area of the upper lip. The lower lip is longer, and even up to one-half of this lip can be resected, retaining good function and cosmesis.

ANSWER: B, C

21. Which of the following are indications for repair of orbital blow-out fractures?

A. Cosmetically unacceptable enophthalmos.
B. Disabling diplopia.
C. Associated facial fractures.
D. Accompanied severe degree of permanent visual loss.

Ref.: 4

COMMENTS: The indications for surgery for orbital blow-out fractures are not always clear-cut; a fracture in the absence of significant physical signs or symptoms does not invariably require operative intervention. Significant, cosmetically unacceptable enophthalmos and disabling diplopia are the most obvious indications for exploration. If these indications are not present, the need for surgical repair has not yet been substantiated. Likewise, if a patient has permanent visual loss accompanying an orbital blow-out fracture, repair of the floor fracture is probably not justified unless there is marked enophthalmos. Exploration of the orbital floor is not considered an emergency measure; surgery can safely be delayed for up to 14 days without risking irreversible scarring and fibrosis. Patients who initially have no diplopia or lose the diplopia within 14 days of injury should not undergo surgery at all, unless radiographic films show extensive defects in the orbital floor that could cause delayed, marked enophthalmos if not repaired. Surgery under emergency conditions is not justified unless the patient is undergoing a necessary operation for other simultaneously sustained facial trauma. In summary, the basic indications for repairing an orbital floor fracture are prevention of subsequent subjective diplopia and of cosmetically significant enophthalmos.

ANSWER: A, B

22. Select the correct statement(s) about rhinoplasty.

A. A nose deviated from the midline on external examination frequently is accompanied by deviation of the cartilaginous and bony septum.
B. If nasal airway obstruction is present, a window of cartilage and mucosa is excised from the septum so there is free communication between the right and left nasal airways.
C. Osteotomies along the nasal bones and maxilla allow the surgeon to narrow the width of the upper two-thirds of the nose.
D. The rhinoplasty patient must be willing to trade an improved nasal contour for external scars on the nose.

Ref.: 1, 2

COMMENTS: Rhinoplasty is one of the most frequently performed operations in the field of plastic surgery. When the patient is evaluated for rhinoplasty, it is important to carry out a thorough examination of the internal and external nasal anatomy. If the nose has a twisted appearance with deviation from the midline, usually it is the result of nasal trauma from a lateral impact. Such external deformity is often accompanied by internal deviation of the bony and cartilaginous septum. The patient with such a septal deviation may suffer from nasal airway obstruction and may be a candidate for septoplasty. The overlying mucoperichondrium is carefully dissected free from the septal cartilage, and the deviated portion of septum is removed, taking care to leave enough septal cartilage for nasal support. It is important to *preserve* the mucosal lining of the septum because it prevents communication between the right and left nasal airways (when this occurs it is a septal preformation). Narrowing of the upper portions of the nose is accomplished by osteotomies along the nasal bones and maxilla. The tip is improved by altering the anatomy of the alar cartilages through a combination of scoring, partial resection, internal sutures, and cartilage grafts. Most rhinoplasties can be accomplished without external incisions; the surgeon gains access to the nasal anatomy through incisions placed inside the nasal vestibule.

ANSWER: A, C

23. Select the correct statement(s) regarding cleft lip.

A. Cleft lip is an uncommon abnormality, occurring in approximately 1 of every 50,000 live births.
B. Nasal anatomy is normal in patients with unilateral cleft lip but is severely distorted in patients with bilateral cleft lip.
C. Repair of the cleft lip generally is delayed until the patient is at least 6 months old.
D. Once the lip is repaired, the resultant pressure causes narrowing of any associated alveolar cleft.
E. Patients with nasal deformity associated with cleft lip should not undergo nasal surgery until eruption of the permanent dentition.

Ref.: 1, 2

COMMENTS: Cleft lip is one of the more common anomalies treated by the plastic surgeon, with an incidence of approximately 1 in 1000 live births. Cleft lip may occur as an isolated abnormality or may be associated with clefts of the alveolar ridge, hard palate, and soft palate. Typically the "rule of 10's" determines the timing of lip repair: when the hemoglobin is more than 10 gm, the patient is more than 10 weeks old, and the patient weighs more than 10 pounds. At some centers, clefts of the lip are repaired at even earlier ages. With all but the most minimal unilateral and bilateral cleft lips, there are associated nasal abnormalities. In the unilateral variant, there is flattening of the alar–cheek groove and malrotation of the alar cartilage. In the bilateral variant, the columella is extremely short and the nose has a broad, flattened appearance. In general, the trend is to achieve at least partial correction of the nasal abnormality at the time of lip repair. Most patients require additional revisions to the nose when they are older. One advantage of early repair of the lip is that it places tension on the underlying alveolus and tends to narrow any associated palatal cleft.

ANSWER: D

24. Select the correct statement(s) regarding cleft palate.

A. Structures anterior to the incisive foramen are part of the primary palate.
B. If there is a cleft in the secondary palate, there is always an associated cleft of the primary palate.
C. With a soft palate cleft, the palatal musculature is abnormally inserted onto the posterior margin of the hard palate.
D. Problems associated with a cleft palate include hyponasal speech and otitis externa.
E. Speech development is optimized if the palate is closed before age 12 months.

Ref.: 1, 2, 4

COMMENTS: The primary palate (the lip and hard palate anterior to the incisive foramen) and the secondary palate (the hard palate posterior to the incisive foramen) develop from different embryologic structures, resulting in differing degrees of susceptibility to genetic and environmental influences. Hence it is possible to have isolated clefts of either the primary or secondary palates as well as complete clefts of the entire palate. When the soft palate is cleft, the levator palatini muscle, which normally forms a muscular sling across the palate, is abnormally inserted on the posterior border of the hard palate. Restoration of the normal muscular anatomy is thought to play an important role in normal speech development. Contraction of normal palatal musculature propels the posterior margin of the soft palate against the posterior pharyngeal wall to produce velopharyngeal closure. This closing off of the nasopharynx is critical to the normal production of most sounds in the English language. Patients who lack this closure mechanism have hypernasal speech. Most consonants require the buildup of nasal pressure. Cleft palate patients have velopharyngeal incompetence and are therefore unable to produce sufficient nasal pressure to produce most consonant sounds. This situation results in characteristic speech marked by hypernasality, nasal air emissions, weak pressure consonants or plosives (p/t/d), and compensatory articulation consisting of consonant omissions (“og” for “dog”), substitutions, or distortions. It is well known that patients with cleft palate have an increased incidence of middle ear infections and resultant hearing loss, probably related to abnormal muscular dynamics of the eustachian tubes. The development of normal speech in patients with cleft palate appears to be optimized if the palate is closed before the age of 12 months, before abnormal compensatory habits are formed.

ANSWER: A, C, E

25. Select the correct statement(s) regarding midface trauma.

A. If the nose is swollen, it is best to delay treatment of a nasal fracture until the swelling subsides, so the fragments may be reduced more precisely.
B. If a hematoma of the nasal septum is detected during physical examination, it should not be drained, as it would increase the likelihood of infection.
C. Complex nasoorbital fractures are best approached through a coronal incision.
D. A depressed fracture of the zygomatic arch may cause difficulty opening the jaw by impinging on the motor nerve to the muscles of mastication.

Ref.: 1, 4

COMMENTS: Fractures of the nasal bones are best evaluated by physical examination, as radiographs are notoriously misleading. Frequently, the patient with a nasal injury presents with a marked degree of swelling. Reduction is best delayed for several days for the swelling to subside, so the fragments can be reduced more precisely. Even then, many patients require later surgical revision after the fracture fragments have healed. Examination of the patient with midface trauma should always include inspection of the nasal septum for a hematoma. An undrained septal hematoma can lead to necrosis of the septal cartilage with loss of midline nasal support and resultant saddle nose deformity. Application of craniofacial techniques has improved the treatment of midfacial trauma. Complex midfacial injuries, including nasoorbital fractures, are best approached through a coronal incision. Incisions at the upper gingivobuccal sulcus and lower eyelid complete the exposure for the multiply injured midface. A depressed fracture of the zygomatic arch may interfere with jaw motion by directly impinging on the coronoid process or muscles of mastication.

ANSWER: A, C

26. Match the stage of the pressure sore development in the left column with its appropriate characteristics in the right column.

A. Stage I	a. Requires sharp débridement but usually underlying bone not exposed
B. Stage II	b. Partial skin loss
C. Stage III	c. Erythema and pain; no skin loss
D. Stage IV	d. Complete necrosis of tissue superficial to bony prominence, often with infection of bony cortex

Ref.: 2, 4

COMMENTS: **Stage I** pressure sores appear erythematous with some edema and tenderness. Treatment is removal of pressure from these areas with frequent turning or the use of specially designed beds to distribute pressure evenly (Clinitron). Meticulous skin care to avoid maceration, friction, and shear forces is also necessary. **Stage II** ulcers have areas of partial skin loss with a yellow debris. They can be treated with the conservative means listed above plus topical antibiotics (e.g., Silvadene). Reepithelialization can be achieved. **Stage III** ulcers have areas of full-thickness skin loss and subcutaneous tissue exposure. Sharp débridement of devitalized, infected tissue and conservative treatment may allow closure by secondary contracture and scarring with epithelialization. **Stage IV** pressure sores represent full-thickness loss of skin and underlying soft tissue usually with involvement of the bony cortex of the underlying bony prominence. These sores require débridement, control of the septic cellulitic process, and usually excision of the bony prominence and flap closure. Myocutaneous flaps are generally preferable to random rotational flaps because they provide more durable coverage and a better blood supply to deal with infection.

ANSWER: A-c; B-b; C-a; D-d

27. Which of the following is/are true regarding myocutaneous flap repair of pressure ulcers?

A. Prior to planning a flap closure of a pressure ulcer, devitalized tissue needs to be débrided.
B. A pressure ulcer has to be rendered sterile prior to flap repair.
C. Incisions are planned solely with regard to achieving wound closure.
D. The bursa is excised, but the bony prominence usually does not require removal.
E. Wound-approximating sutures or staples are not removed until 3–5 weeks.

Ref.: 2

COMMENTS: Prior to operative repair of a pressure ulcer with a myocutaneous flap, it is necessary to excise devitalized tissue, assess the extent of the wound, and allow resolution of the cellulitic reaction or infection at the viable margins. The open base of the wound, often with exposed bone, is not sterile, but the cellulitic process must be controlled with débridement, wound care, and frequently antibiotics. The entire ulcer bursa and usually the exposed bony prominence is excised to remove devitalized tissue and provide a more even surface for pressure distribution. The incisions are not placed over potential pressure areas; and previous trauma and surgeries, with their associated incisions or alteration in skin blood supply, must be taken into account. These wounds are large and slow in healing with varied tension forces. It is best to have approximated tissues supported by sutures or staples for 3–5 weeks while the healing proceeds. Inherent in all surgical treatment modalities is proper nutrition and the correction of systemic problems such as hypoxia, anemia, hypovolemia, or hypotension. It is important to choose the appropriate antibiotics for treatment of infection and to prevent direct pressure with turning or alternating pressure. The use of pressure distribution beds or mats are usually required. Beware that although these beds can reduce pressures to a safe level of 30 mm Hg over most bony prominences, the heel must still be protected. Pressure sores along the heels and other unusual areas can develop even on a pressure distribution bed.

ANSWER: A, E

28. With regard to differentiation of keloid from hypertrophic scar, which of the following statements is/are correct?

A. A keloid grows beyond the boundaries of the initial scar or injury.
B. Differentiation between the two is by histologic diagnosis; it cannot be determined clinically.
C. Keloids are most often seen in dark-skinned individuals.
D. If left chronically neglected, a keloid can degenerate into a malignancy.
E. They both have increased lysis of collagen at the cellular level.

Ref.: 7

COMMENTS: The differentiation between hypertrophic scarring and keloid is based mainly on clinical examination. A keloid scar overgrows the boundaries of the initial injury, whereas a hypertrophic scar presents as a raised indurated erythematous scar. There may be wound breakdown or pain or itching with decreased function across joints. Light microscopy alone shows the same basic architecture for both lesions, namely increased collagen production and decreased lysis of the collagen with perivascular sclerosis. Keloid and hypertrophic scars occur more commonly in persons with dark skin, but this in and of itself does not help differentiate between the two, and certainly they are seen in all groups. Malignant degeneration to squamous cell carcinoma (Marjolin's ulcer) is seen with chronic open wounds, burns, or ulcers; it is not seen with keloid formation.

ANSWER: A, C

29. Which of the following wounds would most likely require free-flap reconstruction?

A. Open wound of the knee with an exposed total knee prosthesis.
B. Open wound with exposed sternum following coronary artery bypass surgery.
C. Full-thickness resection of the chest wall for tumor with exposed lung.
D. Fracture of the distal one-third of the tibia with an open wound and exposed bone without hardware in the wound.

Ref.: 8

COMMENTS: Open tibial fractures have a high incidence of infection and nonunion, and they require extended hospital stays. The zone of injury is always larger than what is clinically apparent. Replacement of the tissue deficit is a critical part of the treatment, and myocutaneous flaps have led to a significant decrease in the incidence of infection and nonunion. Local muscle flaps are not dependable in this region, as they are usually involved in the zone of injury and may not even be available that far distally. For this reason, free-flap transfer of muscle or skin (or both) from a distant site is the treatment of choice. The other wounds mentioned above do require muscle coverage but can be treated with a local muscle flap, unless the flap has been previously used and failed. In such instances a free flap can be used as a salvage procedure.

ANSWER: D

30. Match the composite tissue transfer on the left with its predominant blood supply on the right.

A. Rectus abdominis myocutaneous free flap	a. Thoracodorsal artery
B. Latissimus dorsi myocutaneous free flap	b. Superior epigastric artery
C. Fibula osteocutaneous free flap	c. Inferior epigastric artery
D. Dorsalis pedis fasciocutaneous flap	d. Anterior tibular artery
	e. Peroneal artery

Ref.: 4

COMMENTS: The above-mentioned free-flaps are widely used for free tissue transfer to replace a wide variety of soft tissue and bony deficits. The blood supply of the **latissimus dorsi flap** comes from the thoracodorsal artery, which gives one branch to the latissimus dorsi and another to the serratus anterior muscles. The latissimus dorsi can be transferred on the thoracodorsal artery itself, or it can be harvested at the level of the subscapular artery to provide a longer, larger pedicle. The **rectus abdominis free flap** is classically based on the inferior epigastric artery; and when it is used as a pedicle flap (e.g., TRAM flaps for breast reconstruction) it is usually based on the superior epigastric artery. The inferior epigastric artery is a branch of the external iliac artery. The **fibular osteocutaneous flap** is based on the peroneal artery. The **dorsalis pedis flap** (dorsum of the foot) is based on the anterior tibial artery. Documenting the blood flow present in the three leg vessels is critical prior to harvesting these flaps and it is extremely helpful also when the leg is the recipient site as well. Arteriograms are usually necessary to assist in planning and to help to avoid tissue necrosis or loss of the foot.

ANSWER: A-c; B-a; C-e; D-d

31. With regard to microvascular free tissue transfer, which of the following is the most important technical feature?

A. Finding an end-to-end anastomosis.
B. Beveling the donor artery if end-to-side anastomosis is performed.
C. Use of a microscope.
D. Ischemia time.

Ref.: 9, 10

COMMENTS: Studies have shown that the patency of end-to-side and end-to-end anastomosis are similar. When the use of end-to-side anastomosis is necessary, beveling the end of the donor vessel is not critical for success and patency. Although most free tissue transfers are done with the use of microscopy, studies have shown that 5.5× magnifying loops have the same patency rate (in excess of 95%). Ischemia time, however, is crucial for a successful transfer, whether at the time of initial surgery or following thrombotic events postoperatively. For this reason, prompt recognition of postoperative thrombosis is essential with immediate intervention mandatory for a successful outcome.

ANSWER: D

32. A 12-year-old girl is brought to your office because she has hypoplasia of the breasts. On closer examination she also has asymmetry of the chest wall itself. Which of the following is most likely associated with this syndrome?

A. Absence of the nipple and areola.
B. Deformity of the thoracoacromial joint.
C. Absence of the sternum.
D. Absence of the sternal head of the pectoralis muscle.

Ref.: 4, 7, 11

COMMENTS: Poland syndrome is a congenital defect with an incidence of about 1 in every 30,000 births. The chest wall anomaly is a hallmark of the syndrome, which includes partial absence of the sternal head of the pectoralis major muscle with possible complete absence of the pectoralis minor muscle. Other muscles around the chest wall can be affected, including the serratus anterior, supraspinatus, external oblique, and latissimus dorsi muscles. Although the sternum may be normal, the ribs can be hypoplastic or even absent. Absence of the nipple is rare and not associated with this syndrome. The upper extremities and the hand can be affected in the form of hypoplasia and possibly with syndactyly. Reconstruction can be started early with a temporary expandable prosthesis that is inflated periodically to match the growing opposite side. Ultimately, during adulthood the chest wall asymmetry must be addressed by reconstruction to obtain maximum aesthetic results.

ANSWER: D

33. A 65-year-old woman with insulin-dependent diabetes mellitus underwent coronary artery bypass grafting using the left inferior mammary artery (IMA). She developed a sternal wound infection. Which one or more of the following flaps is/are appropriate for repair?

A. Bilateral pectoralis flaps.
B. Omental flap.
C. Bilateral rectus abdominis flaps.
D. Latissimus flap.

Ref.: 3, 7, 11

COMMENTS: Sternal wound infections are a potential complication of heart surgery. When the IMA is used in diabetic patients, there is an increased chance of a sternal wound infection. The use of the IMA interrupts the blood flow into the superior epigastric artery (SEA). The SEA is the blood supply to the pedicled rectus abdominis flap. In this patient the bilateral rectus abdominis flap is a poor choice because the left rectus muscle's superior vascular pedicle (i.e., the SEA) has been interrupted. Bilateral pectoralis muscle flaps are an excellent choice for sternal wound repair. Each pectoralis muscle is fully dissected and advanced to the midline. Each muscle can be dismissed for additional mobility. The thoracoacromial artery supplies the pectoralis muscle. The omental flap is also a viable choice. It may be based on the right or the left gastroepiploic vessels. The latissimus flap, although not ideal, can be mobilized to repair a sternal wound. It is based on the thoracodorsal vessels.

ANSWER: A, B, D

REFERENCES

1. Sabiston DC Jr (ed): *Textbook of Surgery: The Biological Basis of Modern Surgical Practice*, 15th ed. WB Saunders, Philadelphia, 1997.
2. Schwartz ST, Shires GT (eds): *Principles of Surgery*, 7th ed. McGraw-Hill, New York, 1999.
3. Jurkiewicz MJ: *Plastic Surgery: Principles and Practice*. CV Mosby, St. Louis, 1990.
4. Aston S, Seasley R, Thorne C (eds): *Grabb & Smith's Plastic Surgery*, 5th ed. Lippincott-Raven, Philadelphia, 1997.
5. Habal MB (ed): *Advances in Plastic and Reconstructive Surgery*, vol. 15. CV Mosby, St. Louis, 1999, Ch 1.
6. Paton D: Management of ocular injuries. In: Deutsch TA, Feller DB (eds): *Paton and Goldberg's Management of Ocular Injuries*, 2nd ed. WB Saunders, Philadelphia, 1985.
7. McCarthy JG (ed): *Plastic Surgery*. WB Saunders, Philadelphia, 1990.
8. Shaw WW, Hidalgo DA: *Microsurgery in Trauma*. Futura Publishing, Mount Kisco, NY, 1987.
9. Serafin D (ed): *Atlas of Microsurgical Composite Tissue Transplantation*. WB Saunders, Philadelphia, 1996.
10. Strauch B: *Atlas of Microvascular Surgery: Anatomy and Operative Approaches*. Theime, New York, 1993.
11. Cohen M: *Mastery of Plastic and Reconstructive Surgery*. Little, Brown, Boston, 1999, p 1252.

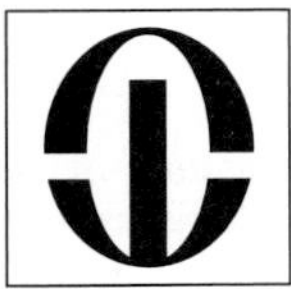

CHAPTER 50

Biostatistics and Data Management

1. Calculate the mean, median, and mode from the following data sample: 1, 2, 3, 4, 5, 5, 10.

A. 4.3, 4, and 5.
B. 4, 4, and 5.
C. 4.3, 5, and 4.
D. 4.3, 5, and 5.

Ref.: 1

COMMENTS: The mean, median, and mode are all measures of central tendency of a data sample. The arithmetic **mean** is the sum of all the observations divided by the number of observations. After ordering the sample from smallest to largest, the **median** is the middle point (for odd sample sizes, half of the remaining observations fall to the left of this value and the other half fall to the right of this value, whereas for even sample sizes the median is the mean of the two middle values). The **mode** is simply the most frequent value in the sample. For a normal distribution, the mean, median, and mode are roughly the same value. The median is often used when reporting biologic data because it is less sensitive to extreme values than the mean.

ANSWER: A

2. Match each statistical measure of spread with its unique characteristic.

A. Variance	a. Sum of the squares of the deviation of each sample point about the mean
B. Standard deviation	b. Variability of sample means drawn from the same population
C. Standard error	c. Individual sample variability about the mean in natural units

Ref.: 1

COMMENTS: The ability to test hypotheses of a sample mean is critically dependent on the degree to which the data points deviate from the mean. The simplest measure of variability is the **variance**: the sum of the squares of the difference between each sample point and the mean. The **standard deviation** is simply the square root of the variance. The standard deviation is a more familiar quantity because it is in the same units as the mean and is not dependent on sample size. The **standard error** of the mean is the standard deviation divided by the square root of the sample size. Unlike the standard deviation, the standard error decreases as the sample size gets larger. The accuracy of a sample estimate of a population mean is dependent on the standard error. If the standard error is large the mean is an unreliable measure, whereas if the standard deviation is small and the sample size is large (small standard error) the sample mean is an accurate estimate of the population mean.

ANSWER: A-a; B-c; C-b

3. The notation P (A or B) is read as "the probability that A or B or both occur." The conditional probability notation P (A/B) is read as "the probability that A occurs given that B occurs." Match the left side of each probability definition equation in the left column with that in the right column.

A. P (A or B)	a. P (A) + P (B)
B. P (A and B)	b. P (A) × P (B)
C. For mutually exclusive events A, B: P (A or B)	c. P (B) × P (A/B)
D. For independent events A, B: P (A and B)	d. P (A) + P (B) − P (A and B)
E. P (A/B)	e. P (A and B)/P (B)

Ref.: 1

COMMENTS: A basic understanding of the probability theory is required for the proper use of statistics. All probabilities fall between zero and one ($0 \leq P(X) \leq 1$). For two events, A, B, that cannot happen at the same time (mutually exclusive events), the probability of A or B occurring is the probability that A occurs plus the probability that B occurs: P (A or B) = P (A) + P (B). However, if both can happen at the same time, the probability that they do would be counted twice and we must therefore subtract the probability that both occur: P (A or B) = P (A) + P (B) − P (A and B). Similarly, the joint probability of two independent events both occurring is the simple product of the probabilities; P (A and B) = P (A) × P (B). However, if the events are not independent (such as the probability of having a high glucose given that one has diabetes), one must multiply one event by the conditional probability of the other event: P (A and B) = P (A) × P (B/A), also P (A and B) = P (B) × P (A/B). Finally, note that the probability of A occurring or A not occurring is always equal to 1 (a specific example of mutually exclusive events).

ANSWER: A-d; B-c; C-a; D-b; E-e

4. With regard to statistical testing, which of the following is/are true?

A. A normal (Gaussian) distribution is required for most statistical tests.
B. When $p > 0.05$ we can accept the null hypothesis.
C. Confidence intervals can be used for hypothesis testing.
D. The p values and confidence intervals can be calculated from data with a binomial distribution.

Ref.: 1

COMMENTS: Data are essentially normally distributed if the probability distribution (histogram) is continuous from positive to negative infinity and has a characteristic, symmetric "bell-shaped" curve. For this data distribution, 95% of the data points fall less than 1.96 standard deviations from the mean. Sample data are usually asymmetric (skewed) or flattened (kurtosis). However, the **central limit theorem** states: Even for nonnormal sample data, as sample size increases, the sample mean approaches normality. This theorem allows us to perform statistical testing on the sample mean of nonnormal data if the sample is large enough. **Hypothesis testing** is the process by which conclusions are drawn in an objective, probabilistic way. Generally, conclusive studies are those in which the probability is less than 5% that the sample data were obtained by chance ($p < 0.05$). In this circumstance we say that the null hypothesis (that our experimental data is not different from the control) is rejected. However, when the probability of a chance finding is greater than 5% ($p > 0.05$), we draw no conclusions (we do not conclude the null hypothesis is true). The **confidence interval (CI)** is a calculated range that encompasses a specified percentage of our sample data. Calculation of the 95% CI is analogous to hypothesis testing. Generally, if the expected value (null hypothesis) does not fall within the 95% CI, the null hypothesis can be rejected. There are mathematic methods for calculating p values and confidence intervals for many types of data in addition to normal data.

ANSWER: C, D

5. Regarding hypothesis testing, which of the following is/are true?

A. A two-sided test is the same as a two-sample test.
B. Type I error is the probability of falsely rejecting the null hypothesis.
C. Type II error is the probability of falsely failing to reject the null hypothesis.
D. Power is equal to one minus the probability of a type II error.
E. The Boneferroni adjustment ensures that significant differences are detected during multiple comparisons.

Ref.: 1

COMMENTS: During hypothesis testing, we usually calculate the difference between the observed and expected results and divide it by the variability of the sample(s). This statistic is then compared to a (normal) distribution; if it falls above or below (two-sided) a set cutoff, we reject that the data came from the same distribution (the null hypothesis). This can be done to compare data to a known value (one sample), to another set of data (two sample) or to multiple sets. **Type I error** (alpha) is the probability of falsely rejecting the null hypothesis. This is usually set to be 5%. When all possible pairs of multiple groups are tested for significance, the type I error increases in proportion to the number of tests. Thus when doing multiple group comparisons, the **Bonferroni adjustment** (or another multiple-comparison procedure) should be used to ensure that alpha is maintained at the fixed level. **Type II error** (beta) is the probability of failing to reject the null hypothesis when it is in fact false. One minus this probability is the **power** of a test. In other words, power is the probability of detecting a significant difference when it exists. Statistical tests are chosen to minimize alpha error and beta error (maximize power). However, any action to minimize one tends to increase the other. In practice, we set the alpha error at a specified level and attempt to maximize power (by choosing the best test and increasing the sample size). "Power calculations" are performed prior to initiating a study to determine the sample size required for a specified power or to determine the power for a set sample size.

ANSWER: B, C, D

6. Match each situation with one statistical test.

A. Compare two means of adequate sample size
B. Compare multiple means of adequate sample size
C. Compare two medians of small sample size
D. Compare multiple medians of adequate sample size

a. Wilcoxon
b. *t*-Test
c. ANOVA
d. Kruskall-Wallis

Ref.: 1

COMMENTS: Data can be divided into three general types: interval, ordinal, and nominal. **Interval data** are on an ordered scale where the distance between values is meaningful. Calculations such as mean and standard deviation can be performed on interval data. **Ordinal data** are ordered (small, medium, large), but the distance between values is arbitrary. Common arithmetic on ordinal data is not meaningful. **Nominal data** are classified into groups without any specific order (surgery, medicine, pediatrics). Specific methods of statistical inference are chosen based on the nature of the data to be compared. In fact, flowcharts have been constructed detailing the decision process for choosing the appropriate statistical test. **Parametric methods** are used for interval data. Parametric methods depend on the assumption that sample data come from a specific, known distribution. Recall that if a sample is large enough, the mean approaches normality (central limit theorem). The independent samples *t*-test (two samples) and the ANOVA (multiple samples) are typical parametric methods used to compare means. **Nonparametric methods** are used when the central limit does not hold and there is no underlying distribution to describe the data. The Wilcoxon rank-sum (two samples) and Kruskall-Wallis (multiple samples) are typical nonparametric methods that require only that the data be ranked (ordered).

ANSWER: A-b; B-c; C-a; D-d

7. Match each situation with one statistical test.

A. Compare two Kaplan-Meier survival analyses
B. Compare multiple Kaplan-Meier survival analyses
D. Test a small sample 2 × 2 table of values for significance
E. Test a large sample multiple row and column table of nominal data for significance

a. Cox proportional hazards
b. Log-rank
c. Fisher's exact test
d. Chi-square

Ref.: 1

COMMENTS: Discrete methods are used for nominal data (see Question 6). Fisher's exact test and chi-square are discrete methods. The **Fisher's exact** test can obtain an exact *p* value for 2 × 2 tables with small numbers of points in each cell (<5) but becomes computationally difficult with larger contingency tables. The **chi-square** easily estimates the *p* value for more complex tables but requires larger numbers (>5 per cell). There is some overlap between nonparametric and discrete methods. For example, the rank-sum or the chi-square for trend test can be used with identical results in some situations. The **Kaplan-Meier** estimator is a nonparametric method to estimate survival probability in a population with varying incidence. The **log-rank** test compares (varying) incidence rates and computes a *p* value. The **proportional hazards model** is a regression model (see Question 8) that can be used to relate survival to many other risk factors.

ANSWER: A-b; B-a; C-c; D-d

8. Regarding regression and correlation, which of the following is/are true?

A. The dependent variable is used to predict the independent variable.
B. In logistic regression, the outcome variable is categorical.
C. Two variables are uncorrelated if they have a negative correlation coefficient.
D. Multiple regression generally refers to more than one outcome variable.

Ref.: 1

COMMENTS: Regression methods are general-purpose models used to predict the value of a dependent variable from one or more independent variables. Multiple regression generally refers to models with more than one independent variable. In **linear regression**, the outcome variable is normally distributed, whereas in **logistic regression** the outcome variable is dichotomous. Often, instead of predicting one variable or another, we wish to determine if there is a relation between two variables. The correlation coefficient quantifies the relation between two variables. A positive **correlation coefficient** means that as one variable increases the other variable increases. A negative correlation means that as one variable increases the other variable decreases. In the unusual circumstance that the correlation coefficient is zero, the variables are uncorrelated.

ANSWER: B

For Questions 9 through 11, please use the table at top of next column. The table represents the results of performing the same diagnostic test for the same diagnosis in two different patient populations.

Diagnostic test	Disease +		Disease −		Total
Population 1					
Test +	(True +) =	90	(False +) =	90	180
Test −	(False −) =	10	(True −) =	810	820
Total		100		900	1000
Population 2					
Test +	(True +) =	9	(False +) =	99	108
Test −	(False −) =	1	(True −) =	891	892
Total		10		990	1000

9. For each population, calculate the prevalence of disease and the relative risk of disease in those who test positive (versus those who test negative).

A. Prevalence of disease in population 1
B. Prevalence of disease in population 2
C. Odds ratio in population 1
D. Odds ratio in population 2

a. 81
b. 1%
c. 89.1
d. 10%

Ref.: 2

COMMENTS: **Prevalence** is the number of patients in a sample who currently have disease divided by the total number of patients sampled. The prevalence is calculated from the column totals only. It is important to distinguish **incidence** from prevalence. Often in epidemiologic studies we wish to determine the number of new cases of a disease occurring during a specified time period (incidence). When we do this, we must be certain not to count all diagnosed cases but only those newly diagnosed during the study period. We can then calculate the relative risk of disease: the incidence in one population divided by the incidence in another population. If incidence cannot be determined, we can still compare risk of disease in two populations using the **odds ratio** (the odds of disease in the exposed divided by the odds of disease in the nonexposed). In the tables above, the incidence of disease cannot be directly calculated, but the relative risk of disease (in those who test positive versus those who test negative) is approximated using the odds ratio TP×TN/FP×FN.

ANSWER: A-d; B-b; C-a; D-a

10. What are the sensitivity and specificity of the test in the table?

A. Sensitivity
B. Specificity

a. 82%
b. 18%
c. 90%
d. 10.8%
e. 89.2%

Ref.: 2

COMMENTS: Sensitivity and specificity are characteristics of tests that are independent of the population tested. **Sensitivity** is defined as the number of patients with disease who also test positive divided by the total number with disease in the sample TP/(TP + FN). **Specificity** is defined as the number of patients without disease who also test negative divided by the total number without disease in the sample TN/(TN + FP). Sensitivity is a measure of the test's ability to detect the disease, whereas specificity is a measure of the test's ability to detect the absence of disease. Recall that the prevalence of disease in these two populations is different, however the sensitivity and specificity of the test does not change across the populations tested. For this test, the sensitivity happens to be equal to the specificity (90%). In general, as one improves either the sensitivity or the specificity of a test, the other is degraded.

ANSWER: A-c; B-c

11. What is the positive predictive value (PPV) and negative predictive value (NPV) of the test for each population?

A. PPV for population 1	a. 99.9%
B. NPV for population 1	b. 50%
C. PPV for population 2	c. 99%
D. NPV for population 2	d. 8%

Ref.: 2

COMMENTS: Positive predictive value (PPV) and negative predictive value (NPV) are characteristics of tests that are dependent on the prevalence of disease in the population tested. **PPV** is defined as the number of patients who test positive who also have the disease divided by the total number who test positive in the sample: TP/(TP + FP). **NPV** is defined as the number of patients who test negative who also do not have the disease divided by the total number who test negative in the sample: TN/(TN + FN). PPV is a measure of the test's ability to predict the presence of disease, whereas NPV is a measure of the test's ability to predict the absence of disease. Note that the PPV and NPV can change dramatically as the prevalence of disease in a population changes. In this example, as the prevalence changes from 10% to 1% the PPV falls from 50% to 8%. Thus, this may be a good screening test for the first population but a poor screening test for the second. In fact, in the second population most positive tests are falsely positive. This is often the case when testing low prevalence populations (even with a highly sensitive and specific test). It is therefore important to use tests selectively for a specific purpose. For example, this test may be extremely useful for the second population to be "certain" that a patient is not a rare individual with the disease (high NPV).

ANSWER: A-b; B-c; C-d; D-a

12. Regarding characteristics of screening tests, which of the following is/are true?

A. The population to be screened should have a high prevalence of preclinical disease.
B. Treatment before the development of clinical disease must reduce cause-specific morbidity and mortality more than treatment after clinical manifestations of disease.
C. Increasing the specificity of the test often increases the positive predictive value.
D. Determining feasibility is as important as efficacy when determining the effectiveness of a screening program.

Ref.: 2

COMMENTS: The PPV of a screening test improves if applied to a population with a high prevalence of disease. In addition, measures taken to improve the specificity in a given population tend to increase the PPV because as the number of negative tests increase a positive test is more likely in a disease-positive patient. The measures taken to improve specificity tend to decrease sensitivity, however, so there is always a trade-off. Obviously, treatment is useful only when it diminishes morbidity and mortality. Furthermore, successful screening requires that early treatment based on screening tests improves morbidity and mortality more than treatment initiated later when disease is clinically detected. Bias in measurement of survival based on earlier detection of disease (lead-time bias) must also be accounted for. Finally, screening tests are of no value if they are not feasible. Considerations of feasibility include acceptability to the population screened, cost-effectiveness, and case yield.

ANSWER: A, B, C, D

13. Match each type of validity with the alternative explanations that could invalidate an association.

A. Internal validity	a. Confounding
B. External validity	b. Chance
	c. Biologically incredible
	d. Bias
	e. Poor generalizability

Ref.: 2

COMMENTS: Epidemiologic studies are generally performed to *demonstrate* a valid statistical association judged to be a cause-and-effect relation. Good **internal validity** is defined by a statistical association that is not due to chance, confounding by other causal factors, or bias introduced in the study design. Generally, it is adequate to demonstrate that an effect is only 5% likely due to **chance** (95% confidence interval shows the effect or $p < 0.05$). A **confounding factor** is defined as an effect that independently causes the outcome and that is unevenly distributed among patients with and without the exposure risk. **Bias** comes into play when there is a methodologic difference in the handling of exposed and unexposed populations. Examples of bias include when participants are enrolled by differing criteria (selection bias), noncomparable information is collected from the different groups (observation bias), or inaccuracies are introduced during data collection (classification bias). Good **external validity** is also required to postulate a cause-and-effect relation. A study is considered to have good external validity if the association demonstrated is a **biologically credible** one (consistent with other observations and theories) and is **generalizable** to clinically relevant populations beyond the narrow group selected for study. Selecting the appropriate population for study can be challenging and often requires balancing internal validity against external validity. Internal validity should prevail, as it is better to demonstrate a conclusive association in a narrow population than to collect generalizable data through questionable methods.

ANSWER: A-a,b,d; B-c,e

14. Match the advantages to each observational study design.

A. Case-control	a. Quick and inexpensive
B. Cohort	b. Valuable when the exposure is rare
	c. Useful when the disease has a long latent period
	d. Optimal for evaluating rare diseases

e. Can demonstrate temporal relations and multiple effects of an exposure
f. Minimizes bias
g. Allows direct measurement of incidence

Ref.: 2

COMMENTS: When conducted properly, observational studies can provide conclusions as compelling as those drawn from intervention studies (randomized controlled trials). In **case-control** studies, patients with the disease of interest are selected from a population and compared with representative non-diseased individuals selected from the same population. Advantages to this design include the following: It is quick and inexpensive; it is useful when there is a long latent period between exposure and disease or the disease is rare; and it can look at multiple etiologies of a single disease. Disadvantages to case-control studies include the following: It is inefficient when the exposure is rare; one cannot directly calculate the incidence of disease or the relative risk (the odds ratio must be used instead); temporal relations can be difficult; and the design is prone to bias. In **cohort studies**, a population is selected and followed for the development of exposures and development of disease over time. Advantages to cohort studies include these factors: It is valuable when exposure is rare; it can examine multiple effects of an exposure; it can demonstrate temporal relations; when performed prospectively bias is minimized; and it can measure incidence and relative risk directly. Disadvantages are that it is generally inefficient for rare diseases; it can be expensive; and complete follow-up and good record-keeping are mandatory.

ANSWER: A-a,c,d; B-b,e,f,g

15. Which of the following is/are true with regard to intervention studies (randomized controlled trials)?

A. Randomization and large sample size generally eliminate confounding.
B. Randomization generally eliminates observation bias.
C. Ethical considerations and issues of feasibility can make intervention studies impractical.
D. The effects of poor compliance with therapy can be eliminated with an "intention to treat" design.

Ref.: 2

COMMENTS: When properly conducted—a difficult proposition—intervention studies can generate a level of validity greater than that of observational studies. The issue of confounding virtually disappears when a study population of adequate size is properly randomized to treatment or control. Proper randomization not only equalizes the prevalence of known confounding factors in each group, it makes the prevalence of unknown factors equal. Blinding both the investigator and the patient successfully (double-blind) as to whether they are in the intervention group or the control group can eliminate observation bias. The "intention to treat" analytic design regards a patient in the treatment group for the duration of study (whether treatment can be completed). This method improves the generalizability of the study. There are, however, unique problems when performing controlled trials. Poor compliance with therapy can bias the results toward the null hypothesis (selection of a known compliant population from the start can help eliminate this effect). Ethical considerations (randomizing therapy) and issues of feasibility (high cost of the study) can make intervention studies impractical. One must achieve uniformly high rates of data collection. Finally, the placebo effect (any therapy tends to improve patients' assessment of well-being) can dramatically alter results.

ANSWER: A, C

REFERENCES

1. Rosner B: *Fundamentals of Biostatistics*, 4th ed. Wadsworth Publishing, Belmont, CA, 1995.
2. Hennekens CH, Buring JE: *Epidemiology in Medicine*. Little, Brown, Boston, 1987.